Pathology of the cerebral blood vessels

Pathology of the
CEREBRAL BLOOD VESSELS

William E. Stehbens

M.D. (Syd.), D.Phil. (Oxon.), F.R.C.Path., F.R.C.P.A., M.R.A.C.P.

Professor of Pathology, Albany Medical College of Union
University, and Director of the Electron Microscopy Unit,
Veterans Administration Hospital, Albany, N. Y.

With 322 illustrations

The C. V. Mosby Company

Saint Louis   1972

PREFACE

The high mortality and frequent disability occasioned by diseases of blood vessels supplying the brain have engendered much disquiet. Notwithstanding the fact that vital statistics indicate cerebrovascular diseases to be of unquestionably greater import than nonvascular diseases of the brain, current textbooks of general pathology and neuropathology deal only superficially with cerebral blood vessels. Although the clinical aspects have not been neglected, pathology has assumed but a minor role. This state of affairs is a reflection of the perfunctory interest in cerebrovascular diseases displayed by neuropathologists and general pathologists, and so it is not surprising that the field has not been investigated intensively. Advances in electron microscopy, histochemistry, physiology, and pathology have made apparent the serious need for a text dealing exclusively with the cerebral blood vessels, which differ structurally, physiologically, and pathologically from those of extracranial sites. This, therefore, is a comprehensive treatise on diseases of the blood vessels supplying the brain and spinal cord. The coverage is not encyclopedic, being restricted of necessity by publication costs. Historical aspects have been for the most part omitted and comparative pathology touched upon lightly. Nevertheless, the mass of information widely dispersed in the literature has been reviewed and appraisals of the conflicting theories so rife in the field are proffered, with emphasis on the etiology and underlying mechanisms in the pathogenesis of disease. The application of new information and concepts in general pathology and physiology, both experimental and observational, adds considerably to the scope of the book. The bibliography is extensive. The book is intended for general pathologists, neuropathologists, neurologists, neurosurgeons, and neuroradiologists and as a reference book for psychiatrists, students, and clinicians in general.

It is my earnest desire that criticisms and provocative speculations will not only focus more attention on cerebrovascular diseases in general, but will stimulate a renewal of interest in scientific research and investigations in this field, which has been so long neglected.

Sincere thanks are due to Dr. George Margolis, Dr. V. J. McGovern, Professor F. R. Magarey, Dr. K. D. Barron, and Dr. V. N. Tompkins for making material available and to the authors acknowledged in the text who have permitted citations of their work or reproductions of their illustrations. The librarians of the Albany

v

Medical College and Albany Veterans Administration Hospital are especially remembered for their patience and invaluable assistance.

My thanks are also due to Miss B. McLean, Mrs. M. Egy, Miss S. Ingvarsson, and Mr. J. E. Walden, who assisted in various ways during the preparation of the manuscript and to the Department of Medical Illustration of the Veterans Administration Hospital for some of the photography. Dr. W. A. Thomas and Dr. K. D. Barron read the manuscript.

The investigations incorporated in the text were supported financially by the National Heart Foundation of Australia, N.I.H. Grants HE 12920 and HE 14177, and Veterans Administration Research Funds.

I am indebted to my mother for providing the opportunity to study medicine and I acknowledge with gratitude the continued encouragement, aid, and interest of my wife, Jean.

William E. Stehbens

CONTENTS

1 / Anatomy of the blood vessels of the brain and spinal cord

The vascular system of the brain and spinal cord exhibits morphological peculiarities not seen in other organs. The reason for the differences appears to be bound up with phenomena responsible for the unique functions of the highly specialized tissues of the central nervous system.

Arterial supply to the brain

The arterial supply to the brain is derived from two carotid and two vertebral arteries, which enter the skull through its base.

Common carotid artery

Anatomy. The right common carotid artery begins at the bifurcation of the innominate (brachiocephalic)[221] artery. The left arises independently from the aortic arch. Each of these arteries terminates by dividing into internal and external carotid arteries at the level of the upper border of the thyroid cartilage in the environs of the fourth cervical vertebra.

Variations. The point of origin of the three great vessels from the arch varies[58] as does the number of vessels arising from it. A "normal" pattern is found in 65% to 70%.[124] The right common carotid artery can arise independently from the aorta and its site of origin is inconstant.[27] The left common carotid artery is even more variable than the right, not infrequently arising from a common stem with the right common carotid and subclavian arteries. This was observed nine times in 130 subjects.[221] In rare instances, the common carotid arteries are absent and then the internal and external carotid arteries arise directly from the aorta.[7]

The termination of the common carotid may be as high as C1 or as low as T2.[124]

Quain,[173] investigating the level of bifurcation in 295 subjects, found the bifurcation at the normal level in 184 individuals (62.4%), at the level of the hyoid bone in 60 subjects (29.4%), above the hyoid bone in 10 subjects (3.4%), at the middle of the thyroid cartilage in 26 subjects (8.8%), and opposite the cricoid cartilage in five subjects (1.6%).

Toole and Patel[223] found the bifurcation at the "normal" level in only 50% of individuals and Lie[124] ascertained it was usually at a higher level in children than in adults. Periodically a common carotid artery will not divide at all, but is continued directly into the internal carotid artery whence branches, generally arising from the external carotid artery, take origin.

Internal carotid artery

Anatomy. The internal carotid artery may conveniently be divided into four segments: cervical, petrosal, cavernous, and terminal or cerebral. The cervical segment lies posterolateral to the commencement of the external carotid. The initial portion and the terminal section of the common carotid form a slight fusiform dilatation, the carotid sinus.

The cervical segment of the internal carotid artery ascends in the neck veering with some tortuosity laterally and dorsally to the base of the skull. The artery then enters the carotid canal in the petrous portion of the temporal bone where it is closely related to the eustachian tube and tympanum.[198] This then, the petrous segment, courses upward and bends abruptly, passing almost horizontally forward and medially to the apex of the petrous temporal bone. It leaves the canal, traversing

1

the upper part of the foramen lacerum, ascends along the side of the body of the sphenoid bone, and enters the middle cranial fossa. It is extradural in position for a short distance and surrounded by areolar tissue before entering the cavernous sinus where angiograms show a circular constriction.[221]

The cavernous segment ascends for a short distance and proceeds horizontally forward until it underlies the anterior clinoid process. It then bends upward, grooving the medial side of the anterior clinoid process to leave the sinus. If both anterior and middle clinoid processes are bridged by bone, it leaves the sinus through the foramen thus formed. The carotid groove is an S-shaped shallow indentation on the side of the sphenoid body, where the artery lies close to the sphenoid sinus.[198] While in the cavernous sinus, the artery is supported by numerous fibrous strands and trabeculae that give the sinus a coarse spongelike appearance yet is excluded from the circulation by the sinus endothelium. On its lateral side, from above down, lie the oculomotor, trochlear, and ophthalmic division of the trigeminal and the abducent nerves. The carotid artery traverses

the dura mater, and its terminal or cerebral segment (somewhat narrowed in angiograms) bends backwards below the optic nerve, from whence it travels upward and laterally, with the optic nerve and chiasm lying medially and the oculomotor nerve laterally. Below the anterior perforated substance it divides terminally into the middle and anterior cerebral arteries. The cerebral segment is supraclinoid in position and the very variable direction is best appreciated angiographically. The carotid siphon is the series of curvatures made by the cavernous and cerebral segments of the internal carotid artery. Angiograms demonstrate the tortuosity well (Fig. 1-1). The internal carotid artery does not branch in the neck.* The small caroticotympanic artery arises from the petrous segment in the carotid canal and enters the tympanum through a small canal in the petrous temporal bone. An inconstant pterygoid branch passes to the pterygoid canal to anastomose with the artery of the canal. Several small branches arise from the cavernous segment

---

*Branches of the external carotid artery occasionally arise from the internal or common carotid artery instead.[151]

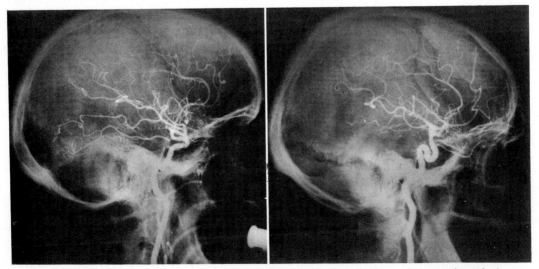

Fig. 1-1. Two carotid angiograms demonstrating different degrees of tortuosity of the siphon. Terminal segments of internal carotid arteries are smaller than the more proximal segments despite absence of branches of significant size.

and disperse to the nerves within the sinus, the walls of the cavernous and petrosal sinuses and the dura mater of the anterior and posterior fossae. Parkinson[162] described the following:

1. A meningohypophyseal trunk (constant in 200 cases) sends branches to the tentorium, the clivus and dorsum sellae, and hypophysis cerebri
2. An artery supplying the walls of the inferior cavernous sinus (present in 80% of the dissections)
3. A capsular artery (an intercarotid anastomosis anterior to the hypophysis)
4. An anterior meningeal branch assisting in the supply of the dura in the anterior cranial fossa[221]

Two additional branches of the cavernous segment, the marginal tentorial artery and the basal tentorial artery, arise at the same level as the primitive trigeminal artery[124] and supply the tentorium cerebelli. The marginal tentorial artery is of importance angiographically when associated with (1) increased intracranial pressure caused by supratentorial lesions and (2) increased vascularity caused by arteriovenous formations, ependymoma, acoustic nerve tumor, and malignant gliomas[204] and meningiomas of the tentorium[124] and falx.[20,67] The superior hypophyseal artery, a perforating branch from the internal carotid near its bifurcation, proceeds to the tuber cinereum, the pituitary stalk, and the neurohypophysis. Blood supply to the adenohypophysis is from a complex portal system extending from the tuber cinereum via the stalk to the adenohypophysis. Collateral vessels may be found between this portal system and neighboring hypothalamic vessels.[105,172]

All major branches of the internal carotid artery arise from the terminal or cerebral segment, that is, the ophthalmic, posterior communicating, anterior choroidal, anterior cerebral, and middle cerebral arteries.

Variations

Level of origin. The level at which the internal carotid commences is variable and the artery appears to undergo disproportionate lengthening during postnatal growth.

Tortuosity, coiling, and kinking of the cervical segment. The cervical segment often exhibits tortuosity, at times bilateral. Such sigmoid tortuosity increases the risk of injury to the carotid artery at tonsillectomy and indeed, on occasions, presents as a pulsating swelling bulging into the pharynx.[108,109]

Cairney[35] dissected the carotid vessels in 36 elderly subjects and found definite tortuosity, bilateral in two instances, in 12 of 76 arteries. The first bend was medially or otherwise laterally directed with variation also in the plane of the tortuosity. In 20 fetuses (5 months' gestation to full term), there was tortuosity in 4 (bilateral in one instance). Parkinson and associates[163] described 40 patients with a pulsatile swelling in the neck caused by a kink in the common carotid artery. They stressed the important role of hypertension, arteriosclerosis, and hemodynamics in the etiology. Severe degrees of tortuosity affect the internal carotid more often than the common carotid artery and angiography reveals the frequent nature of such changes.

Quattlebaum and associates[174] reported three elderly patients with transient hemiparesis. Pronounced elongation with kinking was accentuated in certain positions of the head. In 1000 consecutive angiograms Metz and associates[140] found kinking (angulation of 90% or less) or the formation of a complete loop in 161 cases (16%). They occur in every decade but predominantly between 41 and 70 years with mean age and blood pressure in the more severe degrees of kinking less than in subjects with milder grades of tortuosity. In another series[15] of 71 subjects diagnosed clinically as occlusive cerebrovascular disease, tortuosity or kinking of the carotid arteries was present in 17 individuals (24%) mostly with advanced atherosclerosis.

Weibel and Fields[237] investigating such arterial configurations divided them into three groups:

Table 1-1. Prevalence of carotid tortuosity in angiograms*

Angiography	Age group	Bilateral tortuosity	Unilateral tortuosity	Bilateral coiling	Unilateral coiling	Bilateral kinking	Unilateral kinking
Bilateral	Under 50 years	15%	6%	3%	3%	0.5%	3%
	Over 50 years	25%	12%	4%	3%	2%	4%
Unilateral	Under 50 years		27%		2%		4%
	Over 50 years		59%		4%		3%

*From Weibel, J., and Fields, W. S.: Tortuosity, coiling, and kinking of the internal carotid artery.
1. Etiology and radiographic anatomy, Neurology **15:**7, 1965.

1. *Tortuosity.* Any S- or C-shaped elongation or undulation in the course of the internal carotid artery
2. *Coiling.* Elongation or redundancy of the internal carotid artery resulting in an exaggerated S-shaped curve or in a circular configuration
3. *Kinking.* Angulation of one or more segments of the internal carotid artery associated with stenosis in the affected segment

The need for classification of the degree of tortuosity and redundancy of the artery is obvious but the above classification is not ideal. Weibel and Fields[237] examined 2453 carotid arteries from 1407 subjects. The proximal end of the tortuous segment of the internal carotid artery was seen most frequently at from 2 to 8 cm. above the common carotid bifurcation (peak incidence at about 3 cm.), coiling occurred most often between 4 and 9 cm. (peak incidence around 6 cm.), while kinking occurred mostly between 2 and 5 cm. (peak at about 3 cm.). In each case there was wide variation and bilateral symmetry was frequent. The prevalence of tortuosity, coiling, and kinking is shown in Table 1-1. Tortuosity is more frequent in older patients and kinking is associated with tortuosity more often than with coiling of the internal carotid arteries. Of the group having bilateral angiograms, 29% of those with bilateral tortuosity had neither a stenotic lesion nor an aneurysm as against 37% of those with unilateral tortuosity. This incidence of obviously severe degenerative changes whether primary or second-ary is inordinately high. Those who were submitted to unilateral angiography only, included many young patients. Of this group, 65% with tortuosity had neither stenosis nor aneurysms compared to 76% in the group displaying no tortuosity, coiling, or kinking.

Despite (1) the greatest prevalence of tortuosity in the middle aged and elderly and (2) the greater prevalence of aneurysms and atherosclerotic stenotic lesions in association with tortuosity, Weibel and Fields[237] supported the contention[108,109] that tortuosity is caused by the persistence of a curvature at the junction of the third aortic arch and dorsal aorta (fifth week of embryonic life) from which vessels the internal carotid develops. The main support for this concept appears to be (1) the occurrence of tortuosity among some of the younger patients investigated by them, (2) the finding of tortuosity in some fetuses by Cairney,[35] and (3) the 12.5% incidence of tortuosity or coiling in 70 carotid angiograms of children under 15 years by Lie.[124] However bilateral tortuosity can hardly be regarded as supporting a developmental origin, for the same findings can be used equally well to substantiate a theory of widespread degenerative change in arteries even of the young. Fisher[60] found that pathological examination of histological sections from two specimens revealed comparatively little atherosclerosis, which led him to conclude that the tortuosity was congenital. The result of a study of two cases is far from conclusive and further-more his contention introduces without elucidation the vexed problem: "What is atherosclerosis?" Tortuosity may occur in association with elastic tissue destruction, just as medial and intimal fibrosis may be present in the absence of gross lipid ac-cumulation. In general, tortuosity indicates a loss of elasticity of the vessel wall, and tortuosity could indicate the same thing in the young, particularly in the absence of large-scale, detailed investigations of the histological and physical properties of such arteries. Until results from such a study are forthcoming the hypothesis that even slight carotid tortuosity in the young is a "con-genital abnormality" is only for the cred-ulous and another instance of the invoca-tion of the convenient catch-all. One should remember that gross atherosclerosis and hypertension are not essential for the production of tortuosity. Comparison of the tortuosity with that of the splenic artery would be more meaningful.

The frequent coexistence of aneurysms and tortuosity was a striking feature of the angiographic study made by Weibel and Fields.[237] They gave no criteria for aneu-rysmal dilatation and it is likely that they were in reality viewing evidence of ar-teriectasis.

Though not universally accepted as such,[237] coiling and kinking are associated with and should be regarded merely as variants of tortuosity, the eventual mani-festation probably being dependent on both resilience and function of the peri-vascular connective tissues.

Absence of the internal carotid artery. Total absence of the internal carotid ar-tery is extremely rare and mostly uni-lateral.[5,59,107,124,128] Altmann[5] collected 11 instances to 1947, and Lie found 24 cases of the "aplasia." Absence of the artery was bilateral in four instances.

Lie[124] states that the internal carotid ar-tery can safely be assumed to be absent if no bony carotid canal can be found. Arteriog-raphy reveals only the presence or absence of a functional lumen, not the presence or

absence of the artery. One of the following states[124] may be found:

1. Total absence of one or both internal carotid arteries, or of both internal and external carotid arteries on one side
2. Replacement of the internal carotid by a fibrous cord with or without a small lumen. Histological detail of such cords is not clear. They could be secondary phenomena.
3. Absence of the intracranial segment of the internal carotid
4. Absence of the cervical and petrous seg-ments of the internal carotid
5. Gross narrowing (hypoplasia) affecting the whole internal carotid artery or all of it from a short distance above the bifurcation of the common carotid artery

As a consequence of the absence of an internal carotid artery the corresponding area of supply in the brain is provided with blood from other vessels and second-ary compensatory variations occur in these vessels. The area may be supplied from (1) the basilar artery and the contralateral in-ternal carotid artery,[128,225] (2) branches from the internal maxillary, which enter the cranium through the foramen ovale and foramen rotundum to form a common trunk supplying ophthalmic and cerebral branches,[124] (3) the basilar and vertebral arteries entirely via two enlarged posterior communicating arteries, while the ophthal-mic arteries arise from the posterior com-municating arteries.[59,107]

Lie[124] found incomplete internal carotid arteries on four occasions in the literature. The artery terminated in a large posterior communicating artery in one case[116] and in the other three cases, only the cavernous and cerebral segments were present. The collateral flow was derived from either the contralateral internal carotid, the ophthal-mic,[124] or from the multiple anastomotic channels in the petrous portion of the tem-poral bone together with the ophthalmic artery.[58] In the case reported by Lagarde and colleagues[116] the contralateral internal carotid supplied the area, though their illustration of the topography was unreal-istic and the alleged aneurysm of the ante-rior communicating artery may have been merely a fenestration.

"Hypoplasia" of the internal carotid artery is a term used to describe unusually small internal carotid arteries. Lie[124] reviewed several cases. In a 53-year-old woman, Smith, Nelson, and Dooley[205] reported bilateral "hypoplasia" with a large intracerebral hematoma and small ophthalmic, posterior communicating, middle cerebral, and anterior cerebral arteries. The vertebral, basilar, and posterior cerebral arteries were large, and anastomoses with the meningeal and intracerebral perforating arteries were prominent. The internal carotid arteries abruptly tapered above their origin. Histologically all the great arteries of the neck exhibited intimal fibrosis and atherosclerosis. The history of an unidentified malady at the age of two and the tapering of the arteries are suggestive of an acquired disease of unknown nature.[123] Lie[124] believed the arterial narrowing was caused by involution and that collateral circulation occurs as a compensatory consequence. At this stage it is wisest to be skeptical about aplasia and hypoplasia.

Variation in the size of the cervical segment of the internal carotid artery depends on the area of brain that it ultimately supplies. The presence of a carotid-basilar anastomosis will be reflected in the size of the cervical internal carotid. Such variation was stressed by Lehrer[120] who found differences in the caliber of the vessels on each side to be from 5% to 40% in 25% of 142 patients subjected to bilateral angiography. The caliber of the cervical segment was found to be larger on the side where the anterior cerebral artery was enlarged in association with a small proximal segment of the contralateral anterior cerebral.

Lie[124] recorded a large intercarotid anastomosis and absent cervical and petrous portions of the right internal carotid artery. The large vessel branched from the left carotid siphon, crossed the midline, and continued into the right carotid siphon. It probably represents the enlargement of one of the naturally occurring small intercarotid anastomoses normally found between the two carotid arteries.

Carotid-basilar anastomoses. Carotid-basilar anastomoses are unusual anastomotic channels linking the internal carotid to the basilar artery in the postnatal state in man. They are thought to be universal in horses[51] and caused by the development and perpetuation of vessels that are prominent in the early embryo. They are either absorbed or alternatively persist as small insignificant branches in the adult circulation[154] in which their precise incidence is impossible to determine without careful postmortem angiographic studies in combination with anatomical dissection of the vessels from a large series of cadavers. Gross examples are readily found by angiography despite difficulties inherent in the angiographic recognition of the trigeminal artery.[168] A carotid-basilar anastomosis of small caliber more readily passes unrecognized. It is convenient to divide them into three groups depending on the name of the embryonic vessel from which the anastomosis is derived, that is, primitive trigeminal artery, primitive otic (acoustic) artery, and the primitive hypoglossal artery.

Primitive trigeminal artery. A persistent primitive trigeminal artery is the most common of the three types of carotid-basilar anastomosis.[147,222] Fields, Bruetman, and Weibel[58] found 8 instances while investigating 2000 patients over a 4- to 5-year period.

The primitive trigeminal artery provides blood to the longitudinal neural arteries, which in the 3- to 4-month embryo fuse to form the basilar artery. Its importance is temporary and its function is normally usurped in the 5 to 6 mm. embryo by the posterior communicating arteries from the internal carotid. By the time the embryo is 14 mm. in length, it has disappeared.

The first anatomical report[173] of its persistence was in 1844 and a few isolated cases were published subsequently[23,91,150,215] until Sunderland[217] found three cases in 210 dissecting room cadavers. In 1950, Sutton[219] published the first angiographic description

Table 1-2. Incidence of persistent trigeminal artery

Author	Number of cases	Number of angiograms	Number of dissections	Incidence as percentage
Blackburn (1907)[23]	1	—	220	0.45
Sunderland (1948)[217]	3	—	210	1.43
Harrison & Luttrell (1953)[88]	3	582	—	0.52
Stenvers et al. (1953)[210]	1	750	—	0.13
Gessini & Frugoni (1954)[71]	2	160	—	1.25
Poblete & Asenjo (1955)[171]	2	828	—	0.24
Schaerer (1955)[191]	1	60	—	0.17
Rupprecht & Scherzer (1959)[183]	6	Nearly 3000	—	0.2
Schiefer & Walter (1959)[193]	8	1657	—	0.48
Campbell & Dyken (1961)*[36]	4	1076	—	0.37
Bingham & Hayes (1961)[22]	2	1600	—	0.13
Lamb & Morris (1961)[117]	3	1500	—	0.2
Madonick & Ruskin (1962)[130]	3	3000	—	0.1
Passerini & DeDonato (1962)[164]	9	4000	—	0.23
Gilmartin (1963)[80]	3	2207	—	0.14
Eadie et al. (1964)[52]	17	4500	—	0.38
Fields et al. (1965)[58]	8	2000	—	0.4
Krayenbühl & Yaşargil (1965)[114]	14	7305	—	0.19
Dickmann et al. (1967)[49]	7	2000	—	0.35
Lie (1968)[924]	6	3218	—	0.19
Fields (1968)[57]	9	1600	—	0.6
McCormick (1969)[133]	5	—	2000	0.25

*Campbell and Dyken[36] found trigeminal arteries in 0.1% of angiograms at the Indiana University Medical Center and 3 in 76 angiograms at the New Castle State Hospital.

of the anastomosis. A veritable spate of reports has appeared since. Table 1-2 indicates the frequency of its incidence from the literature. Wollschlaeger and Wollschlaeger[250] in 1964 collected 134 recorded cases. Additional cases to a total of 170 have been reported.[25,50,124,209,245,251]

The primitive trigeminal artery arises from the internal carotid artery at an angle of at least 90 degrees as it enters the cavernous sinus[124] and is proximal to the siphon. It runs posteriorly in the cavernous sinus medial to the trigeminal nerve and either penetrates the sella turcica or perforates the dura mater near the clivus (approximately half of the cases).[110,124] The artery communicates with the basilar artery below the origin of the superior cerebellar and above the anterior inferior cerebellar arteries. Angiographically, the shunt of blood and contrast medium to the basilar circulation in carotid angiography is characteristic,[250] but the shunt varies considerably in size. When large, the trigeminal artery supplies most of the blood to the basilar artery and the inferior half or

two thirds of this artery and the vertebrals are compensatorily small. At autopsy the vessel will be seen emerging from the dura and joining the basilar artery. The discrepancy in size between the upper and lower segments of the basilar should alert one to the possibility of finding an anastomosis. If small, the trigeminal contributes little to the vertebrobasilar circulation, and such cases are very likely to be overlooked at both autopsy and angiography.

In one instance a left primitive trigeminal artery supplied its fellow of the opposite side and then both vessels joined the basilar artery.[29] In the remaining reported cases, the artery was unilateral, the right side predominating slightly.[250]

Controversy exists concerning the significance of the primitive trigeminal artery, which is not generally related to any special pathological entity.[124,241,250] Not all instances of this anastomosis find their way into medical literature, and only emphasis on an association with a particular disease entity or a review is likely to be sanctioned for publication. In association with cere-

Table 1-3. Association of persistent trigeminal artery and intracranial arterial aneurysm

Author	Sex	Age in years	Site, trigeminal artery	Site of aneurysm
Slany (1938)[203]	F	48	Right	1. Left middle cerebral 2. Right internal carotid
Poblete & Asenjo (1955)[171]	F	54	Right	Cavernous segment of right internal carotid
Phillipides et al. (1952)[169]	M	53	—	Basilar
Murtagh et al. (1955)[147]	M	62	Left	Left middle cerebral
Schaerer (1955)[191]	M	40	Right	Left middle cerebral
Davis et al. (1956)[47]	—	—	—	Trigeminal
Mount & Taveras (1956)[146]	M	42	Right	Left internal carotid
Wiedenmann & Hipp (1959)[240]	M	40	Right	Right anterior cerebral
Meyer & Busch (1960)[141]	F	24	Right	1. Basilar 2. Right posterior cerebral 3. Anterior cerebral
Brenner (1960)[30]	F	25	Right	Anterior communicating
Lamb & Morris (1961)[117]	F	62	Left	Right posterior communicating
Bingham & Hayes [1961][22]	M	52	Left	Anterior communicating
Passerini & DeDonato (1962)[164] 1.	F*	71	Left	Cavernous sinus
2.	M	27	Left	Anterior communicating
Bossi & Caffaratti (1963)[25]	M	61	Right	Trigeminal
Wise & Palubinskas (1964)[245] 1.	F	52	Left	Left internal carotid
2.	F	52	Left	Anterior communicating
Eadie et al. (1964)[52]	(No details of five cases available)			
Djindjian et al. (1965)[50] 1.	—	—	—	Anterior communicating
2.	—	—	—	Junction of posterior communicating and internal carotid
3.	—	—	—	Junction of posterior communicating and internal carotid
4.	—	—	—	—
Krayenbühl & Yaşargil (1965)[114]	—	—	Homolateral	Internal carotid and posterior communicating
Wolpert (1966)[251] 1.	F	57	Right	Trigeminal
2.	M	35	Left	1. Left posterior communicating 2. Basilar (junction with anastomosis), basilar bifurcation
Lie (1968)[124]	F	64	Right	Anterior communicating
Bull (1969)[32]	F	43	Right	Trigeminal artery (possible)
Stehbens (1970)[209]	M	70	Right	Anterior communicating
McCormick (1970)[134]	M	47	Left	Left internal carotid at origin of ophthalmic
	F	57	Right	Left middle cerebral

*Also reported by Lombardi et al.[127]

bral aneurysms, 36 cases have now been observed (Table 1-3). The presence of the artery is alleged to indicate that mechanical weaknesses, sufficient to predispose the patient to aneurysm formation,[251] may occur in the encephalic arteries. No such deficiency in the wall has been demonstrated. The fact that the primitive artery existed as an endothelial tube in an embryo of some 4 to 5 mm. has been assumed to be sufficient verification of a developmental weakness of the cavernous segment and of a predisposition to the formation of aneurysms and carotid-cavernous fistulas[251] whether they be of spontaneous or traumatic origin. However the age incidence of the onset of cerebral aneurysms with a persistence of the trigeminal artery hardly suggests a developmental disease, and furthermore the few aneurysms geographically related to the artery appear to be of the "arteriosclerotic" type. Indeed the tri-

Table 1-4. Reported instances of persistent trigeminal artery associated with arteriovenous aneurysms

Author	Age in years	Sex	Side of persistent trigeminal artery	Site of vascular lesion
Saltzman (1959)[186]	69	Female	Left	Left frontal (multiple)
Schiefer & Walter (1959)[193]	51	Male	Left	Left parietal
Campbell & Dyken (1961)*[36]	38	Female	Right	Multiple small angiomas related to middle cerebral artery
Lamb & Morris (1961)[117]	23	Female	Left	Left posterior parietal
Gannon (1962)[68]	46	Female	Right	Right parietal
Eadie, Jamieson, & Lennon (1964)[52] Case 1		Information not available		
Eadie, Jamieson, & Lennon (1964)[52] Case 2		Information not available		
Fields (1968)[57]	25	Female (pregnant)	Left	Right parietooccipital

*Patient had history of traumatic birth with right hemiparesis since infancy.

geminal artery is often ectatic and coexistent hypertension not infrequent.

Sutton[219] and others[36,114,124,193] have recorded a persistent trigeminal artery in association with a cerebral tumor. Passerini and DeDonato[164] in 4000 angiograms found five cases associated with cerebral tumors and, although no causative relationship was put forward, their two cases with cerebral aneurysm were emphasized.

Appearing on a so-called negative angiogram, a primitive trigeminal artery has been held to be the cause of subarachnoid hemorrhage.[112,193] But negative angiograms are not infrequent in subarachnoid hemorrhage and to ascribe the hemorrhage to the anastomosis is but speculation and indicative of observer bias. Saltzman[186] reported a case of an arteriovenous aneurysm in the ipsilateral frontal lobe as did Harrison and Luttrell[88] with the added complication of intracerebral hemorrhage. Eight cases of this association are now known (Table 1-4).

Trigeminal neuralgia, presumably caused by an ectatic anastomotic vessel exerting pressure on the sensory branch of the trigeminal nerve,[100,124] has been recorded as has hyperesthesia. In a few instances the ocular nerves have been involved by this artery.[124,130]

Djindjian and colleagues[50] reported thrombosis of the internal carotid artery where a trigeminal artery originated, and this is not surprising in view of the longevity and severity of atherosclerosis in such cases. Fotopulos[66] recorded thrombosis of the contralateral internal carotid, and a few similar vascular occlusions have been observed.[117,124,164] There is no evidence for contending that the shunt results in a relative deficiency in the region of carotid supply,[165] and hemodynamic studies should establish this as fact. Campbell and Dyken[36] felt that differences could exist in retinal and cerebral arterial pressures on the two sides. The results of ophthalmodynometric measurements in two patients were equivocal.

Primitive otic (acoustic) artery. The primitive otic (acoustic or acousticofacial) artery is usually the first of the three primitive presegmental arteries to disappear. It is quite transitory and of little importance in the blood supply to the posterior cranial fossa.[124]

A few cases supposedly denoting the persistence of this artery have been reported,[5,114,240] but Lie,[124] in reviewing the literature, does not accept them and no indubitable case of the persistence of this anastomosis is extant. All attempts to establish its existence have come to naught. Lie[124] believes that the primitive otic artery should normally arise from the petrous segment of the internal carotid artery and pass with the facial and auditory nerve through the internal auditory meatus turning medially to join the basilar artery between the anterior and posterior inferior cerebellar arteries. If the otic artery is of any size, reduction in dimensions of the vertebral arteries transpires.

Primitive hypoglossal artery. The primitive hypoglossal artery (last occipital or hypoglossal artery[124]), variously held to be single or to consist of 2 or 3 channels, disappears after the otic artery when the embryo is approximately 5 mm long.[124] Regarding the origin of the hypoglossal artery in the adult, Morris and Moffat[145] contend that the primitive lateral basilovertebral anastomoses of Padget are bilateral channels parallel to the longitudinal neural arteries forming, as their name implies, anastomotic vessels between the vertebral and basilar arteries. Morris and Moffat[145] consider that the adult hypoglossal artery is derived from three sources, the first portion being near the carotid artery consists of the primitive hypoglossal artery itself, the second segment is derived from the lateral basilovertebral anastomosis normally communicating with the longitudinal neural arteries (future basilar) by means of transverse anastomosing channels, one of which is thought to constitute the third part. Observations in support of this concept[124] are the following: (1) The postnatal hypoglossal artery is lateral and dorsal to the hypoglossal nerve roots rather than ventromedial as is the embryonic vessel. The anatomical location can be explained only if the lateral basilovertebral anastomosis and a transverse channel to the primitive basilar participate in the eventual development of the hypoglossal artery, (2) The posterior inferior cerebellar artery arises from the lateral anastomotic channel in the embryo and in some instances from the postnatal hypoglossal artery.[145]

Lie[124] found 20 instances of this hypoglossal artery in the adult. Others[58,188] have brought the total to 30; so it is much less common than the trigeminal artery. Gilmartin[80] found two instances in 2207 angiograms, and Wiedenmann and Hipp[240] found two in 7382 angiograms. Most have been demonstrated by angiography,[43,124] and as with the otic artery the authenticity of some reported cases is doubtful.[124] Lie[124] offers four criteria for the diagnosis:

1. The artery should emerge as a robust branch from the cervical segment of the internal carotid artery at the level of the first, second, or third cervical vertebra.
2. After a tortuous course the artery should pass through the anterior condylar foramen (hypoglossal canal) and not the foramen magnum to the posterior cranial fossa.
3. The basilar artery filled just beyond the point of anastomosis with the hypoglossal artery.
4. The posterior communicating arteries should not be visible by angiography.

To compensate, the vertebral arteries are very small. Samra and associates[188] found the hypoglossal arising from the common carotid artery and in Oertel's case[150] it was associated with a persistent trigeminal artery. This anatomical variation is of no great significance[31] and the comment concerning the primitive trigeminal artery is applicable here. Lie[124] considered the variation purely as an accidental finding on arteriograms performed for pathological lesions such as cerebral tumor,[164,196] mental impairment, subarachnoid hemorrhage, and cerebrovascular accidents. Four instances of this carotid-basilar anastomosis in association with a saccular aneurysm have come to light.[118,124,228] Neither histological nor gross examinations of these aneurysms were attempted.

In a mildly hypertensive woman of 57 years dying with multiple cerebellar and occipital lobe infarcts, Gilmartin[80] reported a hypoglossal artery in conjunction with old myocardial infarction. Radiologically there was stenosis of the internal carotid artery with poststenotic dilatation proximal to the origin of the hypoglossal artery. Lie[124] found associated thrombosis of a middle cerebral artery in a 63-year-old woman. Gerlach and associates[70] reported a traumatic carotid cavernous fistula on the same side as the hypoglossal artery.

Carotid-vertebral anastomosis. The proatlantal intersegmental artery embryologically supplies blood from the dorsal aorta to the longitudinal neural artery and thence to the posterior cranial fossa. The counterpart in the adult is an anastomotic vessel arising from the cervical segment of the internal carotid artery and joining the horizontal segment of the vertebral artery in the neck. Lie[124] found three cases in the literature.

Ophthalmic artery

Anatomy. The ophthalmic artery, the first branch of the cerebral segment of the internal carotid artery, arises under cover of the optic nerve at an obtuse angle from the anteromedial aspect of the artery immediately after the internal carotid emerges from the cavernous sinus and passes through the dura mater. Alternatively it may arise from the cavernous segment passing anterolaterally below the optic nerve and through the optic foramen into the orbital cavity where anastomoses with branches of the external carotid artery are frequent.

Variations. Variations of the intracranial segment are extremely rare but replacement by the branch of the middle meningeal artery has been described[27] as has origin from the middle cerebral in the absence of the internal carotid.[128]

Posterior communicating artery

Anatomy. The posterior communicating artery arises from the dorsal convex surface of the cerebral segment of the internal carotid artery. It proceeds posteriorly and medially below the optic tract and above the oculomotor nerve to anastomose with the posterior cerebral artery at a varying distance from the bifurcation of the basilar artery. It gives off a number of small branches to the optic chiasm and tract, the cerebral peduncle, the internal capsule, the medial surface of the thalamus, and the wall of the third ventricle and assists, to a greater or lesser extent than the posterior cerebral, in the supply of the occipital pole and the tentorial aspect of the cerebrum. When the posterior communicating artery is small, it often appears to diminish in caliber as it proceeds backwards indicating that the flow is in that direction. Angiography supports this observation, for the artery fills more frequently in carotid angiograms than in vertebral.

Kaplan and Ford[105] refer to the posterior communicating artery as the proximal portion of the posterior cerebral and to the small arterial segment that is a terminal branch of the basilar (divisional branch of the basilar) as the mesencephalic artery (Fig. 1-2). Haschce[90] named the posterior communicating artery the pars carotica and the divisional branch of the basilar the pars basilaris. Such nomenclature unless universally adopted only adds to the general confusion.

Variations. There are frequent variations in the size of the posterior communicating artery and of the divisional branch of the basilar (proximal segment of the posterior cerebral artery). The role played by each of these two arteries in the supply of the distal segment of the posterior cerebral artery seems to be inversely proportional to that of the other and less often the anterior choroidal artery usurps the role of both.

Fetterman and Moran[56] examined the posterior communicating arteries of 200 brains, derived mostly from old individuals. Those circles of Willis in which the posterior communicating arteries contributed most of the blood to the distal segments of the posterior cerebral arteries were referred to as being of the primitive type.[97,189] The circles in which the basilar contributed most of the blood to the distal segment of the posterior cerebral on both sides were said to be normal or average circles. When the posterior communicating

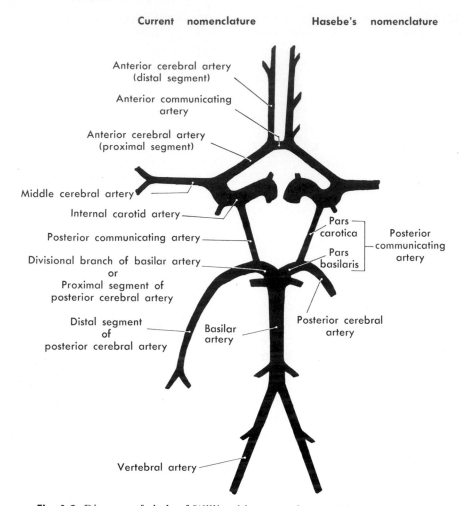

Current   nomenclature   Hasebe's   nomenclature

Anterior cerebral artery
(distal segment)

Anterior communicating
artery

Anterior cerebral artery
(proximal segment)

Middle cerebral artery

Internal carotid artery

Posterior communicating artery

Divisional branch of basilar artery
or
Proximal segment of
posterior cerebral artery

Distal segment
of
posterior cerebral artery

Vertebral artery

Pars
carotica

Pars
basilaris

Posterior
communicating
artery

Basilar
artery

Posterior cerebral
artery

Fig. 1-2. Diagram of circle of Willis with nomenclature of its components.

and the divisional branch of the basilar were approximately equal in caliber on each side, the circle was of the transitional type. Mixed types were frequent and in yet other circles the posterior communicating arteries were either minute or not found. In less than 50% were the circles of Willis the "normal" or standard textbook type. Padget[155] classified the variations of the vessels in the posterior half of the circle into 21 types. Such a classification of vessels of this caliber is virtually pointless and ignores both the individual variability that surely exists[208] as well as postnatal changes. Asymmetry of the posterior communicating arteries is the usual pattern.[77]

Irrespective of the type of variation aris-

ing in this region of the circle of Willis, at least some small anastomosis between the internal carotid and basilar arteries is generally present. Absence of either a posterior communicating artery or the divisional branch of the basilar has been recorded (Table 1-5), but the failure to find small anastomotic vessels in this region can accrue from indifferent dissection and artifacts occasioned during removal of the brain or during fixation.[208]

When the posterior communicating artery is large, the posterior cerebral artery tends to arise from the internal carotid artery rather than the basilar. This configuration, of interest from an embryological viewpoint, is also functional and is said

Table 1-5. Frequency of absence of the posterior communicating artery

| Author | Number of brains examined | Absence of posterior communicating artery cases | |
		Unilateral	Bilateral
Windle (1888)*[244]	200	22	3
Fawcett & Blachford (1905-1906)[54]	700	23	3
Blackburn (1907)[23]	220	1	nil
Stopford (1915)[213]	150	11	nil
Hasebe (1928)[90]	83	3	nil
Godinov (1929)[82]	100	1	nil
Fetterman & Moran (1941)[56]	200	9	1
Von Mitterwallner (1955)[236]	360	1	nil
Vander Eecken (1959)[231]	40	nil	nil
Alpers, Berry, & Paddison (1959)[4]	350	2	nil
Riggs & Rupp (1963)[177]	994	nil	nil
McCormick (1969)† [132]	1000	4	nil

*In most of Windle's cases, some small anastomotic channel was present.
†Not specified whether unilateral or bilateral.

to occur in 15% to 40% of brains.[4,61,101] The caliber of the posterior communicating artery displays considerable variation and so does its length.[82] In this regard the type of skull is naturally relevant.

Anterior choroidal artery

Anatomy. The anterior choroidal artery, a small but fairly constant vessel, arises from the internal carotid artery just distal to the origin of the posterior communicating artery. Directed posteriorly in the interpeduncular cistern, it inclines laterally between the cerebral peduncle and the uncus entering the lower and anterior part of the choroid fissure and terminating in the choroid plexus of the inferior horn of the lateral ventricle. It supplies branches to the optic tract, lateral geniculate body, cerebral peduncle, uncus, posterior part of the internal capsule, lateral part of the thalamus, and the tail of the caudate nucleus as well as to the lentiform and amygdaloid nuclei. Anastomoses with the posterior choroidal and posterior communicating arteries together with the branches in the interpeduncular fossa are frequent.[37,82]

Variations. The anterior choroidal artery is rarely inspected at autopsy. The origin is variable. It can arise from the middle cerebral artery or from the posterior communicating. Beevor[17] contended it arose

from the internal carotid but Carpenter, Noback, and Moss[37] found the origin from that artery in 76.6% of 60 cerebral hemispheres, from the middle cerebral in 11.7%, from the posterior communicating artery in 6.7%, and from the junction of the middle and anterior cerebral arteries in 3.3%. In one hemisphere (1.7%) the anterior choroidal artery was not found. In a larger series (778 hemispheres of 389 brains), Otomo[153] found the origin to be from the internal carotid in 99.2%, from the posterior communicating in 0.4%, from the same site as the posterior communicating in 0.4%, and from the junction of the anterior and middle cerebral arteries in 0.4%. The variations were mostly on the left and the artery was always present. Asymmetry of size was frequent (37.6%) with the artery extremely large in 0.6% usually when in association with a small posterior communicating artery. Von Mitterwallner[236] found the anterior choroidal to be of average or ideal size in 78% of 360 brains. In 2.7% of cases it was absent, in 2.7% double, and in a few it arose either from the middle cerebral or from the internal carotid proximal to the origin of the posterior communicating artery. The limits of the area supplied by the anterior choroidal artery vary widely. No constant clinical picture evolves when this artery is occluded[77] and even when it replaces in part or in whole the origin of the posterior cerebral from the internal carotid or basilar,[236] some anastomosis between the carotid and basilar persists.

Anterior cerebral artery

Anatomy. The anterior cerebral artery, the smaller of the two terminal branches of the internal carotid, arises from the parent stem at the medial end of the Sylvian fissure at an obtuse angle (approximately 135 degrees). The artery can be divided into proximal and distal segments. From its origin the proximal segment passes medially and forward above the optic nerve and chiasm to enter the longitudinal cerebral fissure, whence, just anterior to the lamina terminalis, it approaches and anastomoses in a most variable manner with its fellow of the opposite side. Beyond this anastomosis, called the anterior communicating artery, the anterior cerebral artery or its distal segment changes direction, running forward and upward with its fellow of the opposite side proceeding along the rostrum then around the genu of the corpus callosum. It continues posteriorly on or near the superior surface of the corpus callosum, sometimes under cover of the cingulate gyrus, until finally it anastomoses with a branch of the posterior cerebral artery in the region of the splenium. This recurrent section is referred to as the pericallosal artery.[221]

From the proximal segment of the anterior cerebral artery small slender branches, the anteromedial central arteries[27] enter the anterior perforated substance, the lamina terminalis, and the rostrum of the corpus callosum. They supply the anterior hypothalamus, and to a lesser extent the dorsomedian nuclei of the hypothalamus and possibly branches to the head of the caudate nucleus and the anterior portion of the globus pallidus.[152]

Heubner's artery (the recurrent branch of the anterior cerebral artery[200] or the recurrent lenticulostriate artery[221]) arises from the lateral aspect of the anterior cerebral artery most frequently in the region of the anterior communicating.[2] It courses laterally and backwards along the proximal segment of the anterior cerebral artery to the stem of the middle cerebral artery and penetrates the anterior perforated substance with the medial lenticulostriate arteries. It supplies the anteromedial aspect of the head of the caudate nucleus and adjoining putamen, the anterior limb of the internal capsule, part of the septal nucleus, and cells in the rostrolateral area of the olfactory trigone.[221] It anastomoses with the other lenticulostriate arteries and with cortical branches of the anterior and middle cerebral arteries and may be duplicated totally or in part.[2]

Cortical branches of the anterior cerebral artery are numerous:

1. The orbital branch or branches (one to three in number) are the first branches of the distal segment of the anterior cerebral artery. They extend forward and downward to supply the medial aspect of the frontal lobe below the subrostral sulcus, the gyrus rectus, the olfactory peduncle, and the internal orbital convolutions,[230] reaching to the frontal pole.[44]

2. The frontopolar branch usually arises from the anterior cerebral artery proximally to the maximum bend of the vessel, but may arise from the callosomarginal branch. The frontopolar artery courses forward arborizing to supply the most anterior part of the superior frontal gyrus.[44,230]

3. The callosomarginal artery is the major branch of the anterior cerebral artery. Mostly it arises distally to the origin of the frontopolar artery, and passes backward and upward, terminating in anterior, middle, and posterior internal frontal branches. The anterior internal frontal branch may commence directly from the anterior cerebral near the genu.[221] These branches supply the medial and posterior portion of the superior frontal gyrus and the upper limit of the procentral sulcus.[230]

4. The paracentral branch begins near the middle of the corpus callosum or is from the callosomarginal artery and supplies the paracentral lobulus.[230]

5. The precuneal branch emerges from the recurrent segment of the anterior cerebral (pericallosal artery) and supplies the anterior four fifths of the precuneus.

6. The posterior callosal artery supplies the corpus callosum.

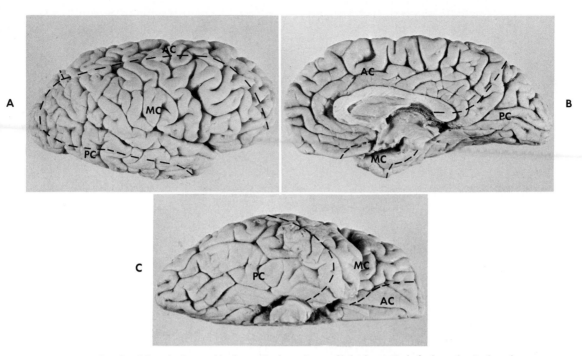

Fig. 1-3. Cerebral hemisphere (**A,** lateral view; **B,** medial view; **C,** inferior view) showing cortical areas of supply. *AC,* Anterior cerebral artery; *MC,* middle cerebral artery; *PC,* posterior cerebral artery.

The classification used here is that of Foix and his colleagues.[65,230] There is need for standardization of nomenclature as various other classifications are in use (Fig. 1-3).

Variations. Variation in the size of the proximal segment of the anterior cerebral artery is frequent. The absence of this segment has been described[23] but must be extremely rare for no instances were reported in a total of 1360 brains.[54,82,236,244] Windle[244] contended it was absent in two brains and then described a threadlike branch in its place. This segment, like the posterior communicating artery, is probably overlooked.

Asymmetry of size is most frequent in the proximal segment of the anterior cerebral artery. Hasebe[90] found inequality of the proximal segment in 3 of 83 brains examined, Windle[244] 3 in 200, Godinov[82] 9 in 100, Riggs and Rupp[177] 119 of 994, Stehbens[208] 22 in 89 (24.7%), and Alpers, Berry, and Paddison[4] 8 in 350 brains.

Seydel[199] found 12 brains with inequality of these vessels in 98 human fetal and newborn brains. The disparity in size of the two vessels whether slight or extreme is usually associated with a shunt of some type through the anterior communicating artery. The anterior communicating artery at times resembles a simple bifurcation with an anastomosis of a small vessel from the contralateral internal carotid artery (Fig. 1-4). Alternatively there may be a shunt either to the contralateral distal segment or to a third or median anterior cerebral artery. Fields, Bruetman, and Weibel[58] assert that at angiography when both distal segments of the anterior cerebral arteries fill from one proximal segment only, it is usually the left anterior cerebral artery that fills rather than the right (in the ratio of 8:1). Anatomical dissections[23,236] do not confirm this theory.

Sedzimir[197] demonstrated angiographically that in 69.3% the anterior and middle cerebral arteries of both sides filled during

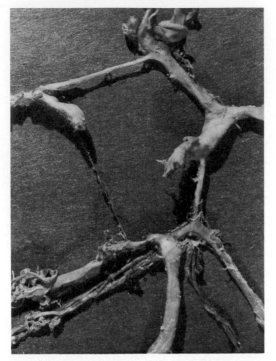

Fig. 1-4. Asymmetrical circle of Willis with a bilocular aneurysm on the anterior communicating artery, which is a bifurcation. Note the inequality of the posterior communicating and of the proximal divisions of the anterior cerebral arteries. (From Stehbens, W. E.: Aneurysms and anatomical variation of cerebral arteries, Arch. Path. **75:**45, 1963.)

contralateral carotid compression; in 23.6% the anterior cerebral artery was the only contralateral vessel displayed during contralateral carotid compression, and in 7.1% no filling whatsoever occurred on the side opposite the angiogram. In a few patients, the collateral circulation thus demonstrated differed when tested on different occasions. The differences were attributed to spasm.

A variation seldom seen is a thin proximal segment of the anterior cerebral artery with the usual anatomical relations. A large vessel arising from the contralateral internal carotid more proximally than the expected site of origin passes anteriorly and medially below the optic nerve to the anterior longitudinal median fissure where, anastomosing with the anterior communi-

cating, it constitutes the main supply of the distal segment of the ipsilateral anterior cerebral artery. McCormick[133] reported a large branch of the proximal supraclinoid portion of the internal carotid artery joining a plexiform anterior communicating artery. The relationship to the optic nerve was not stated. Both proximal segments of the anterior cerebral arteries were small and the distal anterior cerebral arteries were said to fuse. The illustrations however suggested a large median anterior cerebral artery and correspondingly smaller distal anterior cerebral segments. Blackburn[23] referred to cases in which both anterior cerebral arteries arose as separate trunks from the one internal carotid. Duplications occur in the form of fenestrations, island formations, or small branches that course toward and anastomose with the anterior communicating artery.

Moffat[143] reported a variation of academic interest only in a 71-year-old male—the persistence of the primitive olfactory artery. It originated from the left anterior cerebral artery near the anterior communicating, passed forward and downward, and pierced the dura mater on the lesser wing of the sphenoid. Running deep to the dura mater, it reached the cribriform plate, gave off a few dural twigs, a branch to the mucous membrane of the nose, and divided into two branches that pierced the cribriform plate to be distributed to the nasal septum.

Distal segments of the anterior cerebral arteries also exhibit considerable variation in branching, in number, caliber, and location, nor is the correlation between branches and the cortical areas of supply absolutely constant.[9,141] Two or more branches frequently arise from a common stem.[44] Baptista[9] divided variations of the distal segments of the anterior cerebral arteries into the following three major groups:

1. A single unpaired anterior cerebral artery caused by fusion of the two proximal segments near the anterior communicating artery, which supplied the medial aspects of both

hemispheres. Fusion of the anterior cerebral arteries is unusual and may persist for only a short distance. It is considered as an instance of an absent anterior communicating artery but more important is that an anastomosis occurs. It is a finding in 0.5% to 5% of brains.[9]

2. Both anterior cerebral arteries present but one (bihemispheric) vessel supplying one or more branches to the contralateral hemisphere. This type of cross-circulation is well known. Baptista[9] found 45 instances of it in 381 brains—20 from right to left and 25 vice versa.

3. A median anterior cerebral artery (the median artery of the corpus callosum) or azygos anterior cerebral artery[44] is an additional or third vessel of variable length and caliber arising most often from the anterior communicating artery. It supplies one or both hemispheres and occurs more often in the fetus than in the adult,[231] in which Windle[244] found it in 9 of 200 brains. The incidence varies spectacularly—Fawcett and Blachford[54] discovered 23 in 700, Blackburn[22] 2 in 220, Alpers, Berry, and Paddison[4] 28 in 350, and Baptista[9] 50 in 381.

Gradations occurred between the groups and there was little correlation between the anatomical variations and sex, age, or cerebrovascular disease.[9] It is generally held, however erroneously, that beyond the anterior communicating artery no anastomoses will occur between the two anterior cerebral arteries, but they have been encountered.

Anterior communicating artery

Anatomy. The anterior communicating artery is the extremely variable anastomotic communication between the two anterior cerebral arteries when they are in close proximity above and in front of the optic chiasm in the median longitudinal fissure. It would be better labelled the communication or anastomosis of the anterior cerebral arteries.[208] It is more of an anastomotic complex rather than the separate and distinct arterial entity as is currently implied. Its importance lies in (1) the frequency of the anatomical variations particularly when they function as a circulatory shunt and (2) the prevalence of aneurysms at this site.

The median artery of the corpus callosum is sometimes a prominent branch of the anterior communicating artery, accompanying the distal segments of the anterior cerebral vessels. Small branches not infrequently arise from the anterior communicating as Rubinstein[182] emphasized.

Variations. Textbook descriptions of the anterior communicating artery are cursory and misleading. The variability of the topography cannot be sufficiently stressed. Invariably, when dissection is performed carefully, an anastomosis is revealed at this site.

Padget[155] believed that the anterior communicating artery should be half to two-thirds the diameter of the anterior cerebral arteries, and deviations from this arbitrary standard were regarded as anomalous even when the vessel was single and thin. Short communications and slight areas of fusion are frequent, but complete union of the two anterior cerebral arteries is less common. Multiple channels (Fig. 1-5) are particularly common and fairly often overlooked. There are three main types of duplication: (1) When a vessel divides into equal or unequal parts that course for a short distance and then reunite to form a single stem, the entity is termed a duplication. (2) The duplication of the vessel is of a much smaller degree than the first type and is referred to as a fenestration or island-formation on account of the histological appearance of division of the lumen. The external configuration of the wall may widen only imperceptibly. The presence of the island or fenestration may be deduced from the dimpling of the external surface of the vessel. (3) The lumen is traversed by cords or septa consisting of intima including internal elastic lamina and possibly media, but no adventitia. The cords often exhibit considerable elastic tissue degeneration and intimal proliferation. All three types are very common in the environs of the anterior communicating,[61,208] and their true incidence is probably much higher than is deduced from the literature.

Table 1-6 gives the variations of the an-

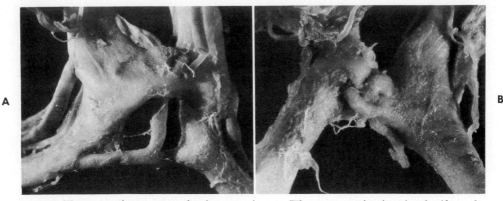

Fig. 1-5. Two anterior communicating arteries. **A,** The communication is plexiform but basically an **H** formation. **B,** Irregular dimpled surface has produced a tangled appearance. Multiple partitioning of the lumen would be observed histologically.

terior communicating artery provided by several authors. Insufficient information was set down in many instances and, though the figures are far from complete, the variability is a gauge of each investigator's punctiliousness. Von Mitterwallner[236] reported that 74.4% of 360 anterior communicating arteries were normal, and obviously he allows some leeway. Fawcett and Blachford[54] found the anterior communicating to be a single vessel in 92.1%, and Windle[244] found it to be normal in 79.5%. Both figures are underestimates largely ignoring variations in branchings, size and caliber, and the vessels associated with a large shunt. Busse[34] found only 173 of 400 anterior communicating arteries conformed to the "normal" pattern, and Riggs and Griffiths[176] found "abnormal" formation of the artery in 47.9% of 566 brains. Fisher[61] concluded from a study of 414 brains that the anterior communicating artery is usually a single vessel of 0.25 to 3 mm. in diameter, and from 0 to 4 mm. in length occasionally reaching 7 mm. He found reduplication of arteries near this anastomosis in 33% of brains and illustrated 63 different patterns.

Middle cerebral artery

Anatomy. The middle cerebral artery, which appears to be the direct continuation of the internal carotid, is the larger of its two terminal branches. It passes horizontally, laterally, and forward into the lateral fissure, often inclining downward slightly as is extends over the insula or island of Reil. It gives off numerous branches with usually a major bifurcation or trifurcation about 2 to 3 cm. from its origin.

Small and numerous central arteries arise from the stem of the middle cerebral artery or from one of the secondary vessels into which the artery divides. These central branches are known as the anterolateral central arteries and are divided into medial and lateral lenticulostriate groups. The medial lenticulostriate arteries enter the brain through the anterior perforated substance to supply the anterior zone of the lentiform nucleus, caudate nucleus, and internal capsule. The larger lateral lenticulostriate arteries penetrate the anterior perforated substance and traverse the lentiform nucleus and the internal capsule with few branches; anterior branches terminate in the caudate nucleus and posterior branches in the thalamus. One of the anterior set of the lateral lenticulostriate arteries, larger than the others, has frequently been considered to be responsible for primary intracerebral hemorrhage, hence its appellation "the artery of cerebral hemorrhage."

The numerous cortical branches of the

Table 1-6. Variations in the anterior communicating artery

Author	Number of brains examined	Absent	Single	Number and type of variation of anterior communicating artery						
				Small area of fusion	Long area of fusion	Double V or Y forms	Treble or plexiform	Large shunt or bifurcation	Median (azygos) anterior cerebral	"Normal"
Windle (1888)[244]	200			8	1	22	3		9	159
Fawcett & Blachford (1905-1906)[54]	700	1	645		4	51	3		23	
Blackburn (1907)[23]	220	2				14		7	2	
Stopford (1915)[212]	150	2				14			7	
Hasebe (1928)[90]	83			} 17		20	29		1	
Godinov (1929)[82]	100		47			29	7			
von Mitterwallner (1955)[236]	360	1		6		74	14	14	25	268
Alpers, Berry, & Paddison (1959)[4]	350			6		} 30		8	28	304
Riggs & Rupp (1963)[177]	802						7	119		
Seydel (1964)[199] (Fetuses & Infants)	98	1		} 38		23	7		9	
Jain (1964)[101]	300					20		19	30	
McCormick (1969)*[132]	1000	1				} 151		42	107	

*Six were described as severely hypoplastic.

middle cerebral artery display considerable variability. They are as follows:

1. The anterior temporal branch and the orbitofrontal originate from the middle cerebral artery proximal to the origin of the more lateral lenticulostriate arteries. The anterior temporal branch with the polar branch[230] supplies the anterior half or two-thirds of the temporal gyri.

2. The orbitofrontal branch supplies approximately the lateral third or half of the orbital surface of the frontal lobe and the middle two-thirds of the inferior and middle frontal gyri.

3. A series of three or more branches from the middle cerebral artery emerge from the lateral sulcus passing upward and backward, (a) the prerolandic to the anterior border of the precentral gyrus, the foot of the middle frontal gyrus, and the opercular part of the inferior frontal gyrus, (b) the rolandic branch to the posterior border of the precentral gyrus and the anterior border of the postcentral gyrus, and (c) the anterior parietal to the posterior border of the postcentral gyrus and the anterior portions of the superior and inferior parietal lobules.[230]

4. The most posterior or terminal branches vary and are often difficult to identify in any particular case and are variously (a) the posterior parietal branch supplying the supramarginal gyrus and the middle portions of the superior and inferior parietal lobules, (b) the angular branch to the angular gyrus, and (c) the posterior temporal branch supplying the posterior half or two-thirds af the superior and middle temporal gyri.

Variations. The size of the stems of the middle cerebral arteries is not constant.[199,236] There is variation in the position of the main division of this artery, the main stem sometimes being some 4 cm. long and sometimes almost nonexistent. Duplicated areas and fenestrations of the main stem are infrequent.

The cortical branches display considerable variation in number, size, and precise location, yet the area supplied by the artery is fairly constant. An accessory middle cerebral artery occasionally arises from the lateral aspect of the proximal segment of the anterior cerebral artery and less often from the internal carotid artery,[101] runs backwards and laterally, and enters the Sylvian fissure to accompany and anastomose with branches of the main middle cerebral artery.

The vertebrobasilar circulatory system
Vertebral artery

Anatomy. The vertebral is the first branch of the subclavian artery, arising from its upper and posterior aspect (Fig. 1-6). Like the internal carotid, it is divisible into four parts. The first segment runs upward and backward from its origin to the foramen in the transverse process of the fourth or less commonly the fifth or seventh cervical vertebra. The second segment ascends vertically to pass through the foramina of the transverse processes of the vertebrae above until it reaches the axis, from whence upon emerging from its foramen transversarium, it proceeds laterally to the corresponding foramen of the atlas likewise more laterally situated at this stage. The third or horizontal segment emerging from the foramen curves backward and medially behind the atlas and lies in the groove on the upper surface of the posterior arch of the atlas. It then proceeds anteriorly to the thickened free edge of the posterior atlanto-occipital membrane to enter the vertebral canal. The fourth or intracranial part, after piercing the dura mater and arachnoid immediately below the skull, veers upward into the cranial cavity through the foramen magnum. It continues upward, passing in front of the roots of the hypoglossal nerve, and inclines to the front of the medulla oblongata, where, at approximately the lower border of the pons,[212] it unites with the contralateral artery to form the basilar artery. The average angle of union is approximately 63 degrees (range, 34 to 118 degrees).[227]

Apart from various muscular branches in the neck,* the vertebral artery (second segment) gives rise to spinal branches that

---

*Muscular branches of the vertebral artery anastomose with branches of the external carotid of each side, the homolateral occipital artery and the subclavian.[148,159,192]

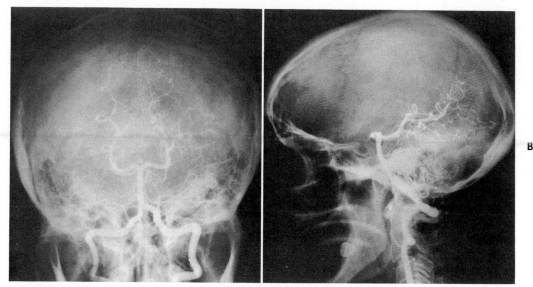

Fig. 1-6. Vertebral angiograms (**A,** anteroposterior; **B,** lateral) showing the curvatures of the vertebral arteries. The long slender terminal branches follow a sinuous course. Compare with Fig. 1-1.

pass through the intervertebral foramina into the vertebral canal, whence they give off small branches along the roots of the spinal nerves to reinforce the anterior and posterior spinal arteries. Small branches supply the vertebrae and intervertebral discs and anastomose with corresponding vessels above and below.

One or two small meningeal branches arise before the vertebral artery pierces the dura mater and are distributed to the posterior fossa, where they anastomose with other meningeal arteries.

The posterior spinal artery arises most frequently from the posterior inferior cerebellar artery,[212] although it can emerge directly from the vertebral after the latter pierces the dura mater. The posterior spinal artery descends over the side of the medulla oblongata giving branches to the fasciculi cuneatus and gracilis[28] and then lies on the dorsal aspect of the spinal cord, medial to the posterior nerve roots. It anastomoses with other segmental spinal branches and the posterior plexiform channels over the posterior aspect of the cord.

The anterior spinal ramus arises from the medial aspect of the vertebral artery a short distance before its termination. It runs obliquely downward and medially in front of the medulla oblongata, uniting with the contralateral vessel to form a common trunk at the level of the decussation of the pyramids. Branches arise from the rami before fusion, subdivide, and form a fine network in the upper portion of the pyramids where several fine filaments terminate. A few filaments as well as branches from the anterior spinal artery (after fusion) enter the anteromedian fissure.[212] Lateral branches, like those of the transverse pontine branches of the basilar, ramify and send penetrating branches to the pyramids and into the anterolateral sulcus. These anterior spinal branches are important to the supply of the midline structures of the medulla and only of secondary consequence in the supply of the spinal cord.

Small bulbar branches from both vertebral arteries and the anterior spinal supply the anterior aspect of the medulla oblongata and central nerve cell masses of the medulla.[105]

The posterior inferior cerebellar artery is the largest and only major branch of the vertebral artery. Sometimes it is entirely absent, but when present, it usually arises from the lateral aspect of the vertebral artery near the lower end of the olive, thence arching upward and laterally on the surface of the medulla between the rootlets of the hypoglossal nerve and then behind the rootlets of the vagus and glossopharyngeal nerves. Below the level of the pons it forms a loop with its convexity towards the pons[212] and proceeds backward and downward to the posterolateral aspect of the medulla oblongata along the inferolateral border of the fourth ventricle. Turning laterally into the vallecula of the cerebellum, it divides into terminal, lateral, and medial branches. The trunk sends many small perforating rami to supply the dorsolateral region of the medulla and sends other branches to the choroid plexus of the fourth ventricle[28] and usually the posterior spinal artery. The medial terminal branch runs posteriorly between the inferior vermis and the hemisphere to supply the vermis and medial part of the base of the hemisphere. It anastomoses with its fellow of the opposite side. The lateral terminal branch supplies the caudal two-thirds of the base and lateral aspect of the cerebellar hemisphere.[105]

Hutchinson and Yates[99] stressed the effect of the second segment of the vertebral artery on its medial aspect to the neurocentral joint within the vertebral canal. The bony osteoarthritic outgrowths at the neurocentral joint displace the artery in a gentle curve or grossly distort it laterally and sometimes anteriorly also. On the other hand ectasia and tortuosity of the vertebral artery, even when not associated with an arteriovenous aneurysm, can cause erosion of the body and pedicle of cervical vertebrae.[253]

Several instances of failure of the vertebral arteries to unite to form the basilar artery have been reported.[21,135,137] A vertebral may terminate in the posterior inferior cerebellar artery whereas the other is continuous with the basilar; an anastomosis across the midline is generally present.

Alternatively two laterally placed basilar arteries may be found with or without transverse anastomoses.

Variations. The left vertebral arteries have been found to arise directly from the aorta in 6% of cadavers.[221] The right vertebral stems from the aorta or the common carotid artery.[27] Origin of a vertebral artery from an intercostal or an inferior thyroid artery has been reported.[27] Flynn[63] demonstrated by angiography a left vertebral artery emerging from the external carotid artery near the third cervical vertebra. It was presumed that it entered the transverse foramen of the second cervical vertebra to pursue an otherwise conventional course. Luccarelli and De Ferrari[129] demonstrated a similiar case angiographically. The external carotid, after giving off the superior thyroid, lingual, and maxillary arteries continued upward as the vertebral artery. An unusual variation, namely, the origin of the vertebral artery from the internal carotid was reported by Ouchi and Ohara.[154] Absence of a vertebral artery is quite rare, but inequality of the two vessels is much more frequent. Stopford,[212] in 150 specimens found the left to be larger than the right in 51%, the right dominant in 41%, and the two vessels of equal size in only 8%. The variation in size so often observed in the intracranial segments is maintained throughout.[99]

A short anastomosis, from which the anterior spinal derives its origin, may unite the two vertebral arteries just below their fusion to form the basilar. Alternatively there may be a degree of duplication of one or both vertebrals, particularly at their upper ends.

Considerable variation exists in the branching patterns of the vertebrobasilar system supplying the brain stem[78] with lateral or transverse arteries numerous and unpredictable. They have been subdivided into short and long lateral or transverse branches and from them small perforating or nutrient vessels arise.

The posterior inferior cerebellar arteries vary in caliber and site of origin, and asymmetry in size of the two sides is usual.[78] Stopford[212] found the artery absent on one or both sides in 24% of brains examined and in 64% to 68% the course was as described above. When one is small, the homolateral anterior inferior cerebellar artery is usually compensatorily enlarged or *vice versa*. Occasionally this vessel is replaced by several small branches from the vertebral or basilar artery. Origin from the anterior inferior cerebellar artery or the lower end of the basilar is infrequent.[212]

Basilar artery

Anatomy. The basilar artery, formed by the union of the two vertebral arteries, ascends along a shallow groove on the ventral surface of the pons. At the upper border of the pons it terminates by bifurcating into the two posterior cerebral arteries. The bifurcation is approximately at the level of the tip of the dorsum sellae but position and course of the basilar vary with the degree of atherosclerosis present. In the infant it is straight.

The basilar artery gives off numerous small pontine branches from its sides (transverse) and from the posterior surface. They supply the pons, the middle cerebellar peduncles, and the roots of trigeminal nerves and do not tend to be arrayed symmetrically.

The internal auditory artery, a slender branch of the basilar, at times originates from the homolateral anterior inferior cerebellar artery. It enters the internal auditory meatus with the facial and auditory nerves supplying the internal ear.

The anterior inferior cerebellar artery is derived from approximately the middle of the basilar and passes laterally over the side of the pons to the anterior aspect of the lower surface of the cerebellar hemispheres. Branches anastomose with the posterior inferior cerebellar arteries.

The superior cerebellar arteries arise from the lateral aspects of the basilar artery immediately proximal to the basilar bifurcation and thus near the upper border of the pons. Each superior cerebellar artery passes laterally, backward, and slightly downward over the upper surface of the pons, immediately below the oculomotor nerve. After winding round the cerebral peduncle, they reach the upper surface of the cerebellum where each divides into medial and lateral branches. The medial branch supplies the upper part of the vermis and the superior medullary velum, while the lateral branch irrigates the upper surface of the cerebellar hemisphere and anastomoses with other cerebellar arteries.

Variations. Variations occasionally occur in the basilar artery, most frequently short segments of duplication or island formations that are not nearly as usual here as in the region of the anterior communicating artery. Riggs and Griffiths[176] found four in 566 subjects. In another brain the vertebral arteries failed to unite, a most unusual phenomenon,[21,135,137] representing the persistence of the longitudinal neural arteries as two distinct vessels. McCullough[135] reported a brain in which the basilar was completely plexiform and von Mitterwallner[236] encountered an instance of duplication for almost the entire length of the pons, with fusion at the upper and lower ends of the artery only.

The anterior inferior cerebellar artery may be replaced by several small branches or, not arising independently from the basilar, it may emerge with the internal auditory or the posterior inferior cerebellar artery by a common stem. It can replace in part or in whole the posterior inferior cerebellar artery and has been known to perforate the abducent nerve.

The superior cerebellar artery, only occasionally double for all or part of its course, is more constant in both size and relationships than the short and long lateral transverse pontine arteries, the concealed perforating branches of which Gillilan[78] stressed.

Altmann[5] mentioned that the basilar artery gave rise to the middle meningeal artery in a 7-month fetus.

Posterior cerebral artery

Anatomy. The posterior cerebral arteries, the largest and terminal branches of the basilar, arise so close to the origin of the superior cerebellar arteries that the basilar appears to divide into four terminal branches. The angle of bifurcation is usually about 100 to 130 degrees, and each artery passes laterally parallel to the superior cerebellar artery though separated from it by the oculomotor and trochlear nerves. Initially there is an upward curve succeeded by a short slight downward inclination as the artery swings around the cerebral peduncle between it and the hippocampal gyrus and uncus. It ascends slightly in its posterior course beneath the splenium of the corpus callosum to the calcarine fissure where it divides into the temporo-occipital and the internal occipital branches.[221] The posterior communicating artery joins the posterior cerebral artery within 1 cm. of the basilar bifurcation. Padget[155] called the segment between the bifurcation and the anastomosis the "divisional" branch of the basilar. Beyond lies the distal segment.

For part of its course the posterior cerebral artery is closely related to the medial edge of the tentorium cerebelli, passing from below upwards and at times establishing contact with the dural margin. Sunderland[218] gives the anatomy of this relationship in detail.

Small posteromedial central arteries arise from the commencement of the posterior cerebral and enter the posterior perforated space medial to the cerebral peduncles to supply the peduncle, the posterior part of the thalamus, the mamillary bodies, and the walls of the third ventricle.

The posterolateral central arteries are small vessels passing round the lateral side of the cerebral peduncle to supply the quadrigeminal and geniculate bodies, the pineal gland, the peduncle, and the posterior part of the thalamus.

Small posterior choroidal branches enter the choroid fissure to ramify in the choroid plexus of the lateral ventricle. Others course over the posterocaudal aspect of the thalamus and penetrate the roof of the third ventricle to ramify in its choroid plexus.

The temporo-occipital branch (posterior cerebral) gives off (1) the anterior cerebral branch, which supplies the inferior part of the inferior temporal gyrus, the anterior part of the hippocampal gyrus, and the fusiform (medial occipitotemporal) gyrus and (2) posterior temporal branches, which supply the inferior two-thirds of the posterior half of the inferior temporal gyrus, the posterior portion of the fusiform (medial occipitotemporal) gyrus, and the lateral part of the lingual gyrus.

The internal occipital branch bifurcates into the parieto-occipital and the calcarine arteries. The parieto-occipital artery supplies the superior part of the cuneus, the posterior edge of the precuneus, and the most inferior portion of the superior parietal lobule.[230] The calcarine branch irrigates the posteromedial aspect of the lingual gyrus, the inferior portion of the uncus, and the occipital pole.

Variations. Phylogenetically, the posterior cerebral artery is a branch from the internal carotid artery.[106] In 30% of brains it remains a major carotid branch on one or both sides,[78] and the divisional branch of the basilar is correspondingly reduced in caliber. Riggs and Griffiths[176] found this variation in 26.7%, whereas in another 35.7% the distal posterior cerebral artery was supplied from both the internal carotid and the basilar. Asymmetry in size is frequent and duplication infrequent.

Intrinsic brain stem arteries

The intrinsic arteries of the brain stem are small vessels, mostly arteriolar supplying gray matter predominantly. The arterial patterns are remarkably constant in the medulla, pons, and midbrain. Gillilan[78] likened them to the supply of the spinal cord and divided them into four groups:

1. The median arteries are the perforating vessels originating singly from medially situ-

ated vessels on the ventral surface of the brain stem and entering the brain stem usually in groups. The longest vessels are generally the largest in caliber and the most central. They supply structures more dorsally situated. The shorter vessels are distributed laterally.

2. The paramedian group constitutes short vessels arising from the short and long transverse arteries, which are branches of the vertebral artery at the medullary level and from the basilar and posterior cerebral at the level of the pons and midbrain. They supply a wedge-shaped zone with the apex directed medially and posteriorly and the base paramedian on the ventral surface.

3. The lateral arterial group consists of penetrating branches mainly from the long transverse arteries (posterior and anterior inferior cerebellar, internal auditory, and superior cerebellar arteries). They supply an area behind and lateral to that of the paramedian arteries and, except in the upper pontine region, reach neither the midline nor the floor of the fourth ventricle. They often enter the brain stem where cranial nerve roots emerge from the medulla.

4. The dorsal group of arteries comprises branches of the longest of the lateral arteries and the posterior cerebral and occasionally the inferior cerebellar artery. They supply the brain stem structures roofing over the ventricular system, including the anterior and posterior medullary vela. Gillilan,[78] Hassler,[93] and Fisher, Karnes, and Kubik[62] provide additional detail.

The circle of Willis

In 1664, in London, Sir Thomas Willis[242] published his classic work including an illustration by Christopher Wren[178] and a description of the polygonal anastomosis that now bears his name.

Anatomy. The circle of Willis is a polygonal anastomotic configuration composed of the anterior communicating artery anteriorly, the proximal segment of each anterior cerebral artery, the two internal carotid and posterior communicating arteries, and posteriorly the basilar bifurcation with its two divisional branches. The structure varies according to the anatomical variability of the constituent parts.

Variations. The so-called normal circle of Willis has been assumed to be symmetrical and its component limbs all constant in size relative to one another[155] as judged by external measurements. Unfortunately such rigid criteria and the narrow philosophical outlook of which they are symptomatic have prevailed.

It is apparent from the anatomy of the circle's individual parts that the polygon is a variable structure. Table 1-7 gives the incidence of a "normal" pattern in the literature, and it is obvious that the classic textbook description of the Willisian circle applies to much less than 50% of human brains.[160] Furthermore, von Mitterwallner[236] and Blackburn[23] admitted to some latitude in their estimates, and Blackburn disregarded slight asymmetry in size.

In the literature there is little agreement

Table 1-7. Frequency of alleged normal pattern of the circle of Willis

Author	Number of brains examined	Number of brains with alleged normal pattern, in percent
Windle (1888)[244]	200	38
Blackburn (1907)[23]	220	29.5
Stopford (1915)[212]	117	39
Hasebe (1928)[90]	83	10*
Riggs & Griffiths (1938)[176]	566	2.8
Fetterman & Moran (1941)[56]	200	Less than 50
von Mitterwallner (1955)[236]	360	27.2
Alpers, Berry, & Paddison, (1959)[4]	350	52.3
Solnitzky (1962)[206]	500	40+
Riggs & Rupp (1963)[177]	994	19.3
Seydel (1964)[199]	98†	21.4
McCormick (1969)[132]	1000	53.8

*Estimated by Padget.[155]
†Fetal and newborn brains.

either with nomenclature of anatomical variations or in the criteria used for determining what constitutes deviation from the alleged normal. A firm means of grading the changes is wanting, for results deviate from investigator to investigator because of varying exactitude and differing criteria of normality employed even by the same author.

Several authors have resorted to mensuration of the vessels of the circle of Willis.[82,160,199] Such procedures, if performed accurately, are quite laborious but in the presence of the extreme variability one ponders on their value and justification.

The term "normal" refers to the average or that which prevails for the most part in nature. It follows that the textbook description so precisely defined by Padget[155] cannot be regarded as normal. Moreover, even Willis' original illustration of the circle (reproduced by Hamby[85]) does not conform to the textbook pattern. A normal circle of Willis is more logically defined as a complete anastomotic polygon that shows considerable variability not only in its components but also in its branches.[208]

When consideration is given to the diameter of the components of the circle of Willis, their length, their mode of branching, and other details of each branch, it should be anticipated that the topography of each cerebral circulation is unique.[208] Furthermore, modifications of arterial topography come with advancing age,[48,155,199,208] the divisional branches of the basilar artery undergoing proportionately greater increase in size than the posterior communicating, probably because of functional need in the area of supply. In postnatal development, the cerebellum increases in weight commensurately more than either the cerebrum or brain stem,[115] and this could well alter the configuration of the circle of Willis. Pathological changes in the vessels, that is, arteriectasis* and com-

pensatory enlargement of collateral vessels modify the topography.[208]

Anatomical variations in the cerebral circulation of animals other than man are prevalent, but studies usually deal with small numbers. However, Stehbens[208] examined 122 circles of Willis of sheep of which 13 (10.7%) were roughly symmetrical, equal on two sides and without visible form of duplication. Plexiform arrangements about the anterior communicating artery occurred in 79 circles (64.8%) and 36.6% exhibited fenestrations elsewhere. In all, there were 97 sheep (79.5%) with some form of duplication. Anatomical variations are thus common in the sheep, and it is highly likely that this holds true for other animals.

Function. Speculation concerning the function of the circle of Willis has been rife and probably more importance has been placed on this anastomotic polygon than on any other anastomotic arcade or circle in the mammalian body. Authors have bestowed upon the circle of Willis more functional significance than is warranted.

An early concept was that the circle was designed to aid mixing of the blood to the primary vessels.[84] Kramer[113] did much to disprove the view. Injection of dye into the carotid and vertebral arteries revealed that the areas of brain stained corresponded in the main to regions supplied by the vessel injected. Little mingling into outside areas occurred, though with carotid injection a small region of the contralateral anterior cerebral artery was usually stained. Vertebral artery injection resulted in staining of the area supplied by the basilar and both posterior cerebral arteries, a finding that is consistent with vertebral angiography in man but conflicts with observations by McDonald and Potter.[136] Rogers,[178] injecting indicators into a rubber and glass model of the circle, saw little cross flow. The pressure and flow variation after occlusion of a carotid inlet resulted in a drop in pressure and flow on the homolateral side such as might be ex-

---

*Atherosclerosis and arteriectasis affect larger vessels more readily than the smaller.

pected if the communicating arteries are anastomoses rather than part of a distributor system. In any case, the diameters of the limbs of the model were not realistic. McDonald and Potter[136] exposed the basilar artery of a rabbit and demonstrated that dye injected into one vertebral artery remained on the ipsilateral side of the basilar and returned by veins on the same side. Furthermore, carotid injection resulted in dye crossing into the contralateral anterior cerebral distribution even though the two anterior cerebral arteries fused for a short distance before dividing again. The applicability of such experiments to the cerebral circulation in man is limited for too much depends on the configuration of the circle. For example, gross disparity in size between the two arteries and between the proximal segments of the anterior cerebral arteries with major shunts through the anterior communicating must be associated with flow across the midline though not necessarily with thorough mixing.

The function of the circle of Willis has been thought to lie in retarding blood flow through its angles, branches, and communicating channels to ensure uninterrupted circulation at regulated pressures.[84] It was thought that the sinuous course of the extradural segments of the internal carotid and vertebral arteries would dampen the systolic peak of pressure and flow to provide a more continuous flow through the cerebral vessels.

A popular theory has it that the circle of Willis is like a distributing station ensuring adequate flow through its many branches. Willis himself intimated as much.[178] There is little in support of the concept on either anatomical or clinical grounds. Flow through the vessels is proportional to the cube of the radius,[160] and consideration of the innumerable anatomical variations and the disparity in size of the components of the circle suggest that equalization of flow could not be achieved in most instances. In practice, the circle often fails to ensure adequate flow to its branches when vessels are either abruptly

occluded by pathological processes or surgical procedures. Consideration of each individual circle of Willis will usually provide some idea of its potential for preservation of flow, aided naturally by the peripheral anastomoses.

Phylogenetically it appears that a transfer of responsibility for supply of the posterior cerebral arteries from the carotid to the vertebrobasilar system is underway. The change is still not finalized for the posterior communicating artery on at least one side is larger than the divisional branch of the basilar in approximately a third of the instances. One would not expect that the posterior communicating arteries would become attenuated[84] (relative separation of the carotid from the vertebrobasilar system) if maintenance of the cerebral circulation by a distributor system were the aim. Brain[26] too thought it unlikely that the circle had evolved as a device to obviate the ill effects of occlusive vascular disease. The circle of Willis probably developed as the result of the proximity of the major vessels of supply to the brain in ontogeny and is caused by hemodynamic factors influenced by the varying need of the developing tissues, about which we have little concrete information.

It is better regarded as an anastomotic circle able to assist in the development of a collateral circulation when and if one of the large arteries supplying the brain is occluded. Its limitations depend on the anatomy of the individual cerebral circulation and the rapidity of the onset of the occlusion. It seems logical not to assume any more specific function for the circle whose prime value is as a potential shunt.

Pathological considerations. It has been often assumed that variations of the circle of Willis are causally related, apart from hemodynamic factors, to the development of saccular aneurysms of the cerebral arteries. But (1) the variations should not be regarded as developmental faults or anomalies, (2) the alleged frequency of aneurysms in association with anatomical variations is based on unscientific evidence, and (3) in other animals the prevalence of arterial variations of the circle of Willis contrasts with the low incidence of cerebral aneurysms. There is little significance in any association of aneurysms and anatomical variations of cerebral arteries.[208]

Several authors have studied the variations of the circle of Willis in the insane,[23,83,189] but as yet there is no conclusive statistical evidence that they are unduly prevalent in the mentally ill. Godinov[82] was interested in the cerebral circulation of individuals of different race, nationality, and skull shape but in these respects, too, no statistics are available.

There has been considerable interest in correlations between anatomical variation of the circle of Willis and cerebrovascular disease, especially encephalomalacia. Saphir[189] believed that cerebral softening and hemorrhage in the absence of definite thrombotic lesions of the cerebral arteries might be explained at times by the occurrence of vascular variations of the circle of Willis. He cited two cases. Griffiths and Riggs[83] analyzed 78 cases of cerebral vascular disease, and of these 81% were attributed to hemodynamic imbalance resulting from variations of the circle of Willis. This high figure appears insignificant when compared to the 97% incidence of variations in a series of brains examined by the same authors.[176] Fetterman and Moran[56] examined 200 brains and found softenings more prevalent in those with variations of the posterior communicating arteries. Much latitude was allowed in judging "normal" size and other anatomical variations were ignored.

Alpers and Berry[3] found "normal" circles in only 33% of 194 brains with softening, some caused by embolism, some thrombosis, and others to causes undetermined. They emphasized the association of thin posterior communicating arteries and encephalomalacia but made no analysis of the size and site of softenings. Furthermore, thin posterior communicating arteries should not be regarded as anomalies if this formation is the ultimate goal of the phylogenetic trend.

Battacharji and associates[14] in a large series discovered more "normal" circles of Willis (52%) in their control brains than in the subjects with cerebral softenings (33%). Two common anatomical variations were small posterior communicating arteries and a carotid origin of the posterior cerebral. There was a statistically significant association between infarction and a unilateral small posterior communicating artery only when in combination with stenosis of one or more neck vessels. An important point that casts doubt on the hypothesis of the anatomical variant contributing to the cause of the infarct is that bilateral small posterior communicating arteries were not very frequently associated with infarcts. The hypothesis has been based on assumptions, both ill-founded, that (1) anatomical variations are anomalies, developmental faults, or abnormalities and hence associated with deficiencies in the circulation or hydraulic imbalance[83] and (2) the circle of Willis serves as an equalizing circuit in respect to the circulation. Severe atherosclerosis[14,189] either augmenting any disparity in size of the posterior communicating arteries and other larger ectatic arteries,[208] or as is more likely, developing in certain vessels under augmented hemodynamic stress because of the presence of some anatomical variations in the circle of Willis, seems to be the essential prerequisite.

Comparative sizes of the components of the circle of Willis can be correlated with volume flow and hence area of supply. Therefore, because the extent of the infarct when a particular vessel is occluded depends on the anatomy of the circle, it is of considerable clinical importance. Infarction of both occipital lobes is likely to occur in basilar artery thrombosis, but not if the posterior cerebral arteries take origin from the internal carotids. Likewise, thrombosis of an internal carotid artery supplying both anterior cerebral arteries via a large homolateral proximal segment will cause, among other changes, infarction of the supply area of the contralateral anterior cerebral and so forth.

Rete mirabile

The rete mirabile, known since Galenic times,[46] is a compact network of intertwining, freely anastomosing small vessels (70 to 230 μ in internal diameter). Their adventitia is relatively thin and is covered by the endothelium of the cavernous sinus or the pterygoid venous plexus in the case of the extracranially situated carotid rete of the cat. The rete displays considerable species variation and has afferents derived to a variable degree from the internal carotid, vertebral, ascending pharyngeal, and occipital arteries. One or more efferent vessels from the rete join the circle of Willis.

The unusual relationship of the rete to a venous sinus or plexus, its proximity to the pituitary gland, and its unusual structure has led to the belief based on inadequate evidence that it performs some metabolic function.[124] Interposed as it is between the heart and the internal carotid artery, the rete has been assumed to discharge a hemodynamic function protecting the circle of Willis and the distal cerebral vessels when a quadruped grazes and the head is low.[124] Yet other animals with similar habits have no rete. No satisfactory explanation of the rete's functional role in animal physiology exists.

The ancients argued about the existence of a rete mirabile caroticum in man. Abortive attempts at rete formation exist on occasions when a compensatory collateral circulation develops between the external and internal carotid arterial systems after occlusion of a major vessel. The sheaf of collateral vessels forms and simulates a rete mirabile, and, to encompass this phenomenon, usage of the term "rete" has unfortunately become common.[238] Lie[124] was able to find three instances of a rete mirabile proper in man,[58,59,142] although a venous lake was not mentioned.

Nishimoto and Takeuchi[149] collected 96 cases of an abnormal cerebrovascular network in Japanese (moyamoya disease[220]). A variety of neurological disorders, often transient, became manifest mostly in young people under 21 years of age. In those under the age of 21, weakness of a limb or limbs was the most frequent sign, often with convulsions, visual disturbances, and nystagmus. In those over 21 years, subarachnoid hemorrhage was the commonest initial manifestation despite its being infrequent in those under 21 years of age. Characteristically both internal carotid arteries exhibited narrowing, usually at the level of the first cervical vertebra but sometimes from the fourth cervical vertebra. Less often it was unilateral and associated with a pathological hemangiomatous dilatation of vessels at the base of the brain and in the pial circulation. The vessels have been interpreted as telangiectasia or even as arteriovenous aneurysm. Controversy is rife as to whether the internal carotid artery is primarily stenosed and the vascular network is a compensatory collateral circulation or whether the entity is basically a congenital vascular malformation.[121,220] Unlike arteriovenous aneurysms the internal carotid artery is narrowed. There appears to be a familial tendency with the behavior of the network appearing to be that of a vascular malformation. Nishimoto and Takeuchi[149] believe it to be peculiar to the Japanese. Comparable cases in non-Japanese have been reported.[33,121] Leeds and Abbott[119] reported two American-born Japanese children with bilateral narrowing of the internal carotid arteries just beyond their origin, with complete occlusion angiographically of the distal segments. Collateral circulation consisted of (1) communications from branches of the external carotid arteries that perforate the dura to anastomose with branches of the internal carotid arteries and (2) enlarged perforating vessels of the anterior choroidal and posterior cerebral arteries. Another instance was interpreted similarly by Weidner and associates[238] as thrombotic occlusion of the anterior and middle cerebral arteries with the development of a compensatory vascular pial network in the form of collaterals, which, Busch[33] believes, take a long time to develop. It is possible that the incidence of subarachnoid hemorrhage is caused by the previously recognized propensity of collateral vessels for rupture. Emphasis should be on the pathological examination of the narrowed or occluded internal carotid vessels and detailed study of the so-called cerebral rete mirabile.

External carotid artery

The external carotid artery is the smaller of the two terminal branches of the common carotid artery, and the reader is referred to standard textbooks of anatomy for detail. The importance in the central nervous system primarily accrues from (1) the abundant anastomoses between its branches and those of its fellow of the opposite side, (2) the actual and potential anastomoses between its extracranial branches and the cerebral arteries, and (3) the fact that it supplies the meningeal arteries.

Anterior meningeal arteries

The anterior meningeal arteries are small branches originating from the ethmoidal arteries medially and those in the lateral part of the anterior cranial fossa are from the anterior branch of the middle meningeal artery.

Middle meningeal arteries

The middle meningeal artery, the largest of the meningeal vessels, is yet a small vessel entering the middle cranial fossa through the foramen spinosum. Entering the skull, it passes forward in a groove on the greater wing of the sphenoid bone and divides into anterior and posterior terminal branches. The anterior terminal branch (larger than the posterior ramus) passes upward along the greater wing of the sphenoid to the anteroinferior angle of the parietal bone where, opposite the pterion, it grooves the bone deeply and is often enclosed in a bony canal. It contin-

ues upward, immediately behind the anterior border of the parietal bone almost to the vertex, and ramifies as it goes. The posterior terminal branch extends backward from the greater wing of the sphenoid to the squamous part of the temporal bone, sending branches upward and posteriorly to the vertex and posteriorly to the occipital region. The middle meningeal artery anastomoses with the contralateral artery, with the accessory meningeal artery, with meningeal branches of the occipital, ascending pharyngeal, ophthalmic, and lacrimal arteries, with the stylohyoid branch of the posterior auricular in the temporal bone, and through the skull wall with the middle and deep temporal arteries.[27]

The accessory meningeal artery arises below the skull either from the middle meningeal or from the maxillary artery and enters the middle cranial fossa through the foramen ovale to supply the trigeminal ganglion and the neighboring dura mater. Meningeal branches are contributed by (1) the internal carotid and the anterior and posterior ethmoidal arteries to the anterior cranial fossa, (2) the internal carotid, ophthalmic, lacrimal, and ascending pharyngeal arteries to the middle cranial fossa, and (3) the vertebral, occipital, and ascending pharyngeal arteries to the posterior fossa.

The meningeal arteries course and ramify in the outer layer of the dura mater, supplying the cranial bones principally, and standing out in relief on the external surface of the dura. Thence they groove the inner table of the skull bones. The thin-walled meningeal veins situated in the dura between the arteries and the bone[27] are difficult to dissect from the arteries, and the intimate relationship of the vessels and cranial bones explains their vulnerability when the skull fractures.[28]

Significance of anatomical variations

Variations of the encephalic arteries of man have been unduly stressed and often classed as congenital abnormalities or anomalies, the criteria for the classification never having been specified. Variations of the superficial cortical vessels, more common than those of the major arteries,[246] have received, in contradistinction, little attention and are not generally regarded as anomalies.

Gillilan[75] divided the arteries into three groups. The basilar, vertebral, and internal carotid arteries belong to group 1, in which few variations occur. The terminal portions of the three pairs of cerebral arteries and the nutrient branches of the vertebrobasilar system, included in group 3, are invariably present. However the origins of the cerebral arteries and of the major branches arising from the vertebrobasilar and internal carotid arteries and of the three associated communicating arteries (group 2) are unpredictable[75] and highly individual.[208] Similarly in the coronary[195] and subclavian arterial trees,[16] patterns are not the same in any two subjects. This probably holds true for the mesenteric circulation and other vascular beds.

Development from angioblasts of a primordial capillary plexus from which all blood vessels of the part are ultimately derived is not peculiar to the head or cranial cavity. Thus, speculations concerning the role of the plexus in the development of hypothetical anatomical variations can be applied correspondingly to the systemic circulation. In the formation of the plexus there is allowance for variability in the subsequent elaboration of supply and drainage channels, which fact indicates a functional adaptation of the net to the demands of the circulation.[53] However, chance, chemical, physical, and hemodynamic factors as well as the vagaries of flow and even minor differences in the angles of bifurcations in such a microcirculation could influence the development of variations in vascular pattern and the dominance or otherwise of major channels.[53] Little is known concerning the regulatory factors governing the entire field of angiogenesis and even less of the genetic factors operative during the de-

velopment of vascular patterns. The anatomical features of the arterial tree predetermined by genetic factors are likewise unknown and cannot be distinguished from those that are fortuitous or secondary to local environmental changes. Painstaking anatomical and angiographic examination of the vascular patterns in the brain and cord of sets of identical twins would be a means of attaining clearer understanding of this aspect. At present, it can at least be stated that identical twins are not identical in every respect, for example, fingerprints are not identical.[243] In three sets of identical twins the superficial veins of the forearm were dissimilar[209] as is said to be the case with the retinal vessels. It appears very likely that the arterial variations of the cerebral circulation under discussion are not genetically determined.

Granted the presence of other anatomical variations, one does not logically presuppose the existence of any structural or functional defect in the vessel wall or a tendency to any specific disease entity. There is thus no basis for making assumptions to the contrary in the case of the cerebral vessels. Yet with no substantiation[208] variations in the circle of Willis have been thought to indicate the presence of congenital deficiencies in the arterial wall sufficient to lead to aneurysm formation and arteriovenous fistulas.

The development of the brain has enabled *Homo sapiens* to master the animal and plant kingdom. At an equal pace with its evolution, modification of the blood vessels has occurred and appears to have been adequate for the purpose primarily because of the remarkable inherent ability of the vessels to proliferate in an organized manner. Streeter[213] has stressed the continual adequacy of the vascular system of the brain at all stages of embryological development, and its adaptability is obviously a characteristic feature. Levenson and Nelson[122] found that injury to the chick embryo's primitive capillary plexus resulted in anatomical variation. The variations compensated for the experimental intervention of the vessels and may therefore be regarded as functional adaptations. It is thus entirely possible that various environmental factors in utero could lead to anatomical variations of vascular pattern by interfering with the primitive capillary beds about the embryonic central nervous system.

Vogel and McClenahan[234,235] studied the cerebral circulation of 15 anencephalic monsters post mortem. Always the cerebral hemispheres were replaced by vascular fibroglial tissue while the midbrain, medulla, cerebellum, spinal cord, eyes, and segments of the cranial nerves were spared or involved to a lesser degree. They concluded that the brain deformity was caused by some disturbance after the optic cups and cranial nerves formed between the third and fifth weeks of embryonic life. In five anencephalics, there was absence or marked "deformity" of the major arteries of the circle of Willis. In an additional eight anencephalic monsters Vogel[233] found many thin-walled endothelial channels with a variable angiomatous appearance. The authors believed that the deformity may have been secondary to curtailment of blood flow or impaired angiogenesis. Such studies however do not prove whether the neural defect is primary or secondary, but it is likely that remodeling of the vascular pattern could still be a secondary manifestation of altered metabolic needs of the developing brain. In the absence of more definite facts concerning the etiology of anencephaly, no conclusion can be reached. An unusual vascular pattern has also been seen in cerebral hemiatrophy,[161] and it is possible that some primary vascular lesion of unknown etiology might have been responsible for the severely shrunken hemisphere, but faulty angiogenesis should not be invoked.

Khodadad and Putscher[111] studied the cerebral vasculature of a stillborn female with cyclopia and numerous other abnormalities. The brain, especially the cerebrum, was grossly deformed, and the arterial supply, as one might expect, was found to be quite bizarre. A stillborn male with arrhinencephalia displayed a similar underdevelopment of the brain and the arterial supply resembled that of the cyclopian. In both brains, one internal carotid was primarily responsible for the supply of the anterior and middle cerebral arteries and the other carotid supplied the posterior cerebral arteries and anastomosed or was continuous with the basilar artery. In the arrhinencephalic the carotid-basilar anastomosis resembled somewhat the trigeminal artery, except that the carotid itself coursed posteriorly from the cavernous sinus to join the basilar. The maldevelopment of the cerebrum was not attributed to vascular factors, and it was thought that neural development dominates vascular development, the arterial variations described being consistent with the principles governing the arterial supply to the brain, namely, functional constancy, economy of distribution, and convenience of source.[1,201]

Collateral circulation

The principal underlying aim of the arterial supply to the brain is the provision of an adequate circulation of the blood to the tissues under physiological and if possible pathological conditions according to the diverse functional needs. It is well known clinically that obstruction or therapeutic ligation of a major artery in the neck will frequently result in no disability whatsoever. The development of ill effects depends variously on the site and the rapidity of onset of an obstruction, and on the anatomical nature of the collateral circulation so often only potential. Gradual arterial occlusion of any vessel is almost invariably accompanied by the progressive development of an adequate compensatory circulation, that is, enlargement of preexisting collateral vessels. Conversely, sudden obstruction of a major artery is frequently associated with disastrous ischemia in the field of supply, the extent of damage also dependent on the efficacy of the peripheral collateral circulation, and always worth remembering is that the topography of the collateral circulation is different for each individual.

Available collaterals. Collateral circulation to the brain is available from a number of sources.

Carotid-basilar anastomoses. Three arterial channels (trigeminal, otic, and hypoglossal arteries), important links between the carotid and vertebrobasilar systems in early embryonic life, generally regress postnatally. When present they are sizable anastomotic channels (described earlier in this chapter).

Circle of Willis. At best, the circle of Willis can be regarded as a potential anastomosis only, and its effectiveness in providing collateral circulation when any artery is occluded is directly dependent on the anatomy and pathological state of the individual circle under consideration. Yet, the futile controversy regarding the functional role of the circle as an anastomotic ring continues. Be that as it may, it is patently fallacious to consider that the collateral circulation in the vicinity of the circle is restricted to the arterial polygon itself, for small anastomoses are also to be found between the branches of these major vessels in the interpeduncular fossa.

Leptomeningeal anastomoses. Anastomoses other than those of the circle of Willis occur over the surfaces of the cerebral hemispheres and cerebellum. Abbie[1] asserted that there was no such thing as a nonanastomotic artery, however small, on the surface of the brain. Anatomists such as Beevor,[18] Fay,[55] and Shellshear[200,201] have enlarged our knowledge of anastomoses, the anatomical features and implications of which have been treated by several other authors more recently.[229,231]

Vander Eecken,[231] using the injection technique to produce a cast from which the brain tissue was removed by maceration, found two types of anastomosis. In the first he included direct end-to-end anastomoses and in the second each artery ramified, the branches being disposed in the form of a candelabrum and anastomosing either terminally or via lateral communications with those of the other artery. Peculiarly enough, though anastomoses occur frequently between branches of different major arteries, they rarely exist between the different branches of a particular artery.[18] Leptomeningeal anastomoses have been explained on the basis of their origin from a primitive capillary network,[230] but this concept does not explain the virtual absence of anastomoses between adjacent branches of each major artery.

Predominantly collateral circulation is found in the anastomoses between the anterior cerebral and middle cerebral, and between the middle cerebral and posterior cerebral. Anastomoses (1 to 3 in number) occur between the anterior cerebral and the posterior cerebral.[231] Anastomoses between the anterior cerebral arteries are seen in the innumerable variations of the anterior communicating artery and also between peripheral cortical vessels.[230,231] Cross circulation from one anterior cerebral artery to the other is facilitated when the anterior cerebral arteries fuse, when there is a large anterior median artery, and in cases in which one anterior cerebral supplies branches to the contralateral hemisphere.

Small anastomoses between perforating branches of both posterior cerebral arteries communicate in the vicinity of the pineal gland and choroid plexus,[104] while the anterior and posterior choroidal arteries habitually anastomose with each other.

In a study by Vander Eecken[231] individual differences occurred in the number, localization, and diameter of the anastomotic vessels, and differences were even found between each of the cerebral hemispheres. There was no distinct difference with age, although from this aspect the number of brains examined was limited.

On the surface of the cerebellum leptomeningeal anastomoses occur between each of the cerebellar arteries and also across the midline to connect with the corresponding arteries of the opposite side. Communications between adjoining branches of the cerebellar arteries are more frequent than in the case of the cerebral arteries.[230,231] Although such communications exist,[104,230] Vander Eecken[230,231] found no anastomoses between the superior cerebellar and the posterior cerebral arteries.

Gillilan[75] demonstrated anastomoses between the pontine branches of the lower basilar and both posterior cerebral arteries. A coloring medium injected into a segment of the lower basilar isolated by ligatures above and below, resulted in a rapid appearance of the colored material in both posterior cerebral arteries and in the upper end of the basilar. The anastomotic vessels were found in the arachnoid tissue between the incisura of the tentorium cerebelli and the posterior aspect of the midbrain.

Fay,[55] in her injection studies of the cerebrum, reported a zone of diminished vascularity situated approximately 2.5 cm. lateral to the superior aspect of the median longitudinal fissure extending anteroposteriorly from the frontal lobe to the parietal lobe. There was a paucity of large arterial branches beneath the cortex in this zone roughly corresponding to the anatomical border between the territories of the anterior and middle cerebral arteries. Such zones of diminished vascularity exist even though functionally such anatomical border zones between territories of supply of adjacent arteries are thought to be susceptible to the hazards of a diminished blood flow.[179] Vander Eecken[231] is the best source for additional detail concerning leptomeningeal anastomoses in man.

Anastomoses between deep perforating arteries and small perforating branches of cortical arteries. Though the cerebral arteries have often been referred to as end arteries, in reality they are not. Numerous precapillary as well as capillary communications exist between neighboring perforating arteries both in the cerebrum and the cerebellum. Vander Eecken[231] stated that anastomoses with a diameter of more than 150 μ are rare between the large perforating arteries entering the brain on the basal surface and almost as exceptional between the perforating branches from the pial arteries. The size of these vessels therefore is such that significant collateral circulation through them is not possible and though the cerebral arteries may not be end arteries, functionally they behave as such.[40,73]

Anastomoses between encephalic and meningeal arteries. Small anastomoses occur (1) between the meningeal branch of the cavernous segment of the internal carotid with the middle meningeal artery, (2) between the ophthalmic artery and orbital branches of the middle meningeal, and (3) between inconstant branches perforating the dura and leptomeningeal arteries on the surface of the brain.[87] Riggs[175] observed two cases in which a branch of the anterior cerebral artery anastomosed with meningeal arteries in the falx cerebri.

Anastomoses between branches of the internal carotid and extracranial arteries. Anastomoses between branches of the external carotid and those of the internal carotid occur at regions where nerves related to the eye, ear, and nose[104] variously exit. Wolff[248] pointed out that phylogenetically the eye and orbit have been the meeting ground of the intracranial and extracranial circulations. In the orbit the anastomoses are small and found between branches of the ophthalmic artery on the one hand and on the other (1) branches to the face and nasal cavity from the internal and external maxillary arteries,[87,104] or (2) frontal branches of the superficial temporal artery, or (3) branches of the middle meningeal artery.[58] As a source of collateral circulation in man, the contribution of these anastomoses to the cerebral circulation is negligible. Gillilan,[76] from an anatomical study of the circulation to the orbit, concluded that one or other of the anastomoses between the internal and external carotid arteries is sufficiently large to ensure an adequate blood supply to the orbit if the ophthalmic is occluded. She made no mention of the maintenance of a sufficient supply to the brain.

Pitts,[170] from an angiographic study of

23 patients with internal carotid artery occlusion, deduced that good evidence of ophthalmic filling was associated with greater disability than occurred in those patients with poor filling and collateral circulation from other sources. More recently Fogelholm and Vuolio[64] reached similar conclusions after investigating a much larger series (90 subjects) and found that the caliber of the ophthalmic artery failed to increase as time elapsed and the disease progressed.

Anastomoses in the auditory region occur between (1) the anterior tympanic branch of the internal maxillary and tympanic branches of the internal carotid[27] and (2) the inconstant artery to the pterygoid canal from the internal carotid to the corresponding branch of the internal maxillary artery. Nevertheless, such communications about the ear normally provide but a minute anastomotic circulation. Kaplan[104] stated that the stapedial artery, if it persisted to adult life, provided a moderate collateral flow in the region of the ear.[104] However, according to Vander Eecken,[231] although this artery has been shown to persist in most individuals, it survives in arteriolar form only.

Anastomoses between branches of the vertebrobasilar system and extracranial arteries. The internal auditory branch of the basilar anastomoses with branches from the stylohyoid artery (external carotid),[27] the communication being insignificant.

Cervical and extracranial anastomoses. Anastomoses between the external carotid and branches (such as the superior thyroid artery) arising from the common carotid artery are generally free, as they are in regard to the corresponding branches of the contralateral external (common) carotid artery, particularly via the facial, lingual, and thyroid arteries.[75] They are prevalent between these vessels and branches of the subclavian artery. Thus the usual consequence of ligation or obstruction of the common carotid artery is that blood reaches the homolateral external carotid artery via this rich collateral circulation, then flows

downward to its origin to enter the internal carotid, and thence proceeds to the brain. When the internal carotid artery is ligated, the collateral circulation comes primarily from the intracranial anastomoses.

The vertebral arteries anastomose extensively via their muscular branches with the deep and ascending cervical arteries and with the occipital.[27,192,232] Anastomoses also occur in the spinal circulation from one side to the other as well as through the anterior and posterior spinal arteries with medullary arteries. Although the anastomoses are considerable in the neck, collateral circulation does not become established with sufficient rapidity to substitute for blocked major conducting arteries to the brain, and as Gillilan[75] pointed out, the nearer the base of the skull that these arteries are interrupted, the fewer are the alternative collateral channels.

Anastomosis of the internal carotid and the vertebral artery via the carotid-vertebral artery before their entry to the skull has been reported on three occasions.[124]

Development of collateral circulation

The foregoing anastomotic pathways are possible sources of collateral circulation when there is acute obstruction of a major arterial vessel, but their enlargement requires time. Considerable enlargement of the collaterals often demonstrated by angiography[180,181] can ordinarily be expected when the occlusion of major vessels is gradual. Extensive collateral circulation also develops in association with arteriovenous shunts. However enhanced circulatory needs often lead to the development of quite an extraordinary degree of large collateral vessels from small preexisting channels, although it is possible that some may be derived from newly formed vessels. To distinguish between newly formed and preexisting collateral vessels is not always possible. Handa and colleagues[86] found that preexisting collateral vessels related to the internal carotid participated to the maximum degree almost immediately in the case of sudden carotid occlusion in the neck of monkeys. However, collateral circulation via the external carotid increased only slowly over ensuing weeks, a state of affairs attributed to the development of new collaterals.

Our knowledge of the mechanisms governing angiogenesis in embryology is very meagre, and likewise the factors reviewed by Liebow[125] initiating and controlling the development of the collateral circulation are uncertain and exceedingly complex. Collateral vessels usually exhibit varying degrees of tortuosity attributable to degenerative changes in the constituents of the wall (the elastica in particular) and associated with the hyperkinetic state.[207] Collateral arterial channels, developing to a remarkable degree in coarctation of the aorta are prone to aneurysm formation. Venous collaterals, as in portal hypertension, often cause serious hemorrhage. Currently explanations of these phenomena are at best speculative; however, some forms of intracerebral hemorrhage have been attributed to bleeding from small intracerebral collaterals formed secondarily to occlusive vascular disease.

Significant anatomical relationships of cerebral vessels

The anatomy of the circulation to the brain is such that the arteries under certain pathological conditions compress cranial nerves, thereby causing secondary nerve lesions. Other pathological states result in gross pressure alterations within the cranial cavity leading to displacement of brain tissue and compression of blood vessels. The effects therefore are of two types—nerve compression and vascular compression.

Nerve compression

Optic nerve and chiasm. The internal carotid artery is applied to the inferolateral and lateral aspects of the optic nerve near the chiasm. Below the optic nerve the ophthalmic artery arises from the internal carotid and runs on the inferolateral aspect of the nerve to the optic foramen. The anterior cerebral artery passes medially above the nerve to reach the median longitudinal fissure. Each of these arteries may compress the optic nerve, and partial optic atrophy can follow in the wake of nerve compression by atherosclerotic arteries.[217] Bergland and Ray[19] suggest that in many instances of optic chiasmal compression seen clinically, the visual loss may be ischemic because of damage to or compression of the small vessels from all the arterial components of the circle of Willis to the optic nerves, chiasm, and tracts.

Slade and Weekley[202] reported that in a patient with an aneurysm of the anterior communicating artery, an unnamed branch of the internal carotid passed through the nerve (diastasis) to reach the frontal pole. Such neurovascular relationships are particularly prone to cause neural disturbances in pathological states of the vessels involved.

Oculomotor nerve. The oculomotor nerve is closely related anatomically to several arteries:

1. The nerve may be wedged in the angle formed by the superior cerebellar and posterior cerebral near their origin from the basilar. If the angle is narrow, some constriction of the nerve may ensue. If the basilar bifurcation is low, the posterior cerebral is more likely than usual to cause angulation of the nerve,[217] and a branch of the posterior cerebral artery may even pass through the nerve (diastasis).[244] If the basilar bifurcation is high, the superior cerebellar artery may cause angulation of the nerve.[218]

2. The posterior communicating artery may groove the oculomotor nerve, compressing it against the dural roof of the cavernous sinus.[217] A large posterior communicating, likely to be atherosclerotic and rigid, has a high chance of causing nerve compression.

3. The internal carotid artery in its cavernous segment endangers the nerve in cases of aneurysmal dilatation. In the intracranial segment, an atherosclerotic or ectatic artery may compress the nerve whereas aneurysms especially at the origin of the posterior communicating artery readily produce oculomotor paresis.

4. Markedly ectatic and tortuous basilar arteries are associated with considerable displacement of the vessel and may elevate and displace the third nerve laterally.[217]

Trigeminal nerve. The three divisions of the trigeminal nerve may be involved in aneurysmal dilatation of the cavernous segment of the internal carotid artery. The nerve may be grooved by either the superior cerebellar or the posterior inferior cerebellar artery. Ectatic S-shaped basilar arteries reach and compress the nerve, producing trigeminal neuralgia.[45] Whether a persistent trigeminal artery can be the cause of trigeminal neuralgia is not known, but coexistence has been reported.[100,124]

Abducent nerve. The abducent nerve, like the trigeminal and the other motor nerves of the eye, may be compressed by enlargement of the cavernous segment of the internal carotid artery. In a study by Sunderland[217] the anterior inferior cerebellar artery on occasions passed through the abducent nerve and not infrequently, when lying ventral to it, deeply grooved the nerve. Though diplopia or convergent squint has been attributed to nerve compression by the anterior inferior cerebellar artery, as with other nerves, grooving may eventuate in the absence of symptoms and signs of disordered function.

A tortuous basilar artery may compress the nerve against the pons and in severe cases elevate it to the level of the upper border of the pons, thereby sharply angulating it. A tortuous and atherosclerotic vertebral artery may compress the nerve at the pontomedullary junction.[217]

Facial and auditory nerves. Sunderland[216] studied the variable anatomical relationship of the anterior inferior cerebellar artery to the facial and auditory nerves. In some cases, the artery reached the internal auditory meatus and in such a confined space, nerve compression is a possibility. The internal auditory artery frequently arises in the meatus from the anterior inferior cerebellar artery and is thus intimately associated with the nerves in the meatus also. The posterior inferior cerebellar artery may loop upward in front of the nerve compressing it against the pons or middle cerebellar peduncle. Tortuous basilar and vertebral arteries, considerably displaced, may compress the nerves, particularly on the left side.[217]

Glossopharyngeal, vagus, accessory, and hypoglossal nerves. The posterior inferior cerebellar artery may deform and stretch these nerves, but displacement or compression is much more likely to occur with an aneurysmal dilatation of a vertebral artery or a tortuous ectatic vertebral artery.

Vascular compression. Veins are more readily compressed than arteries because of their thinner walls and lower intravascular pressure, but the proliferation of venous anastomoses usually ensures adequate drainage in the presence of venous obstruction. Vascular obstruction occurs specifically at several sites, such as the edges of the falx cerebri, tentorium cerebelli, foramen magnum, the interpeduncular fossa, and the rostral portion of the Sylvian fissure. Grossly increased intracranial pressure of course interferes with the general circulation throughout the brain.

Where there is compression of brain tissue against a rigid surface or edge, well-known pressure grooves will be found. Vessels crossing these grooves may be sharply angulated, indented, or compressed. Vital microscopy of living tissues adequately demonstrates just how susceptible small vessels are to pressure, and hemorrhagic necrosis in the depths of these grooves[126] comes as no surprise, for local stasis occurs in the microcirculation. These lesions eventually become glial scars[126] intimating a prior raised intracranial pressure.

Posterior cerebral artery. This artery, because of its important anatomical relations to the dural margin of the tentorium cerebelli[218] may be compressed against the free edge of the tentorium as the vessel courses around the cerebral peduncle. As the herniation of the hippocampal gyrus progresses (supratentorial pressure), the site of compression progressively shifts posteriorly until only that portion of the artery in the calcarine fissure is involved, and accordingly the medial aspect of the occipital lobe is the area most frequently affected. Branches crossing the tentorium may become embroiled and the lesions may be bilateral. The necrosis is usually cortical, hemorrhagic, or ischemic, and if the compression is complete, the white matter likewise becomes necrotic. Lindenberg[126] emphasized the damage to Ammon's horn that follows in the wake of pressure changes. The arterial supply to Ammon's horn from the posterior cerebral artery runs upward perpendicular to the edge of the tentorium and is therefore readily compressed. Necrosis sets in and if the patient survives sufficiently long, sclerosis with cystic changes ensues. Sunderland[218] believes that kinking of the artery where it crosses the oculomotor nerve is conceivably an added factor in the causation of vascular embarrassment in the distribution of the posterior cerebral artery.

The tendency is for branches passing through the interpeduncular fossa to the thalamus, caudal thalamus, and the medial sector of the upper pons and midbrain to be involved. The cerebral peduncles may be elongated and compressed and the mammillary bodies wedged into the interpeduncular fossa in such a way as to compress perforating vessels.[126] In severe cases almost the entire thalamus will be ischemic and usually secondary vascular lesions in the midbrain and pons (dealt with elsewhere) will be apparent.

Anterior choroidal artery. Because of supratentorial pressure, the posterior communicating artery is affected only in very severe cases of herniation. The anterior choroidal artery is more vulnerable and has been found compressed between the herniated hippocampal gyrus medially and the cerebral peduncle laterally. Ischemia caused by the compression involves the amygdaloid nucleus, uncus, hippocampal formation, optic tract, lateral geniculate body, posterior limb of internal capsule carrying the optic radiation, part of the globus pallidus and the cerebral peduncle.[218] Lindenberg[126] found that usually only pallidal branches are compressed and cause necrosis in the medial part of the globus pallidus and that bilateral involvement can simulate carbon monoxide poisoning or hypoxia.

Anterior cerebral artery. This artery may be compressed against the free margin of the falx cerebri, varying branches being affected. The cingulate gyrus usually escapes vascular involvement but can be severely displaced.

Middle cerebral artery. A compression groove in the orbital surface of the frontal lobe caused by the sphenoid ridge may involve cortical branches of the middle cerebral artery. The stem itself usually lies too deep to be affected.

Posterior inferior cerebellar artery. This artery (or branches) may be compressed by the posterior rim of the foramen magnum and the tonsillar necrosis that sometimes occurs is secondary to the vascular compression.

Superior cerebellar artery. Space-occupying lesions in the posterior fossa cause raised subtentorial pressure with herniation of cerebellar tissue through the tentorial notch. Branches of the superior cerebellar arteries on the upper surface of the lateral lobes are likely to be compressed where related to the margins of the tentorium. Collateral circulation generally prevents infarction.[218]

Veins. In supratentorial space-occupying lesions, the basal vein may be compressed between the midbrain and the herniated temporal lobe. With severe herniation the great cerebral vein of Galen may be kinked at the site of entry into the falx to enter the straight sinus. Both of these complications are likely to aggravate intracranial pressure by initiating cerebral edema.

With increased subtentorial pressure the cerebellum is herniated upward through the tentorial notch and can compress the great cerebral vein of Galen against the splenium of the corpus callosum, thereby producing venous obstruction of this vein and the basal veins.

Venous system of the brain

Two sets of veins drain the brain. A superficial or external group and a deep or internal group drain into the dural sinuses and thence into the internal jugular vein.

Superficial cerebral venous system

The superficial cerebral veins, more numerous and of larger caliber than the arteries, lie in the sulci on the surface of the brain. Akin to though not coincidental with the arteriolar plexus, the pial plexus of venules interconnects the large superficial veins in which variations are much more frequent than in the arteries.[246] However, several of the larger veins are sufficiently consistent to be individually named. Anastomoses are abundant between the superficial veins but intercommunication with the deep venous system is negligible.[77] The superficial cerebral veins fall into three main groups—the superior, middle, and inferior cerebral veins.

Superior cerebral veins. Superior cerebral veins drain the cortex and the underlying white matter of the dorsolateral, dorsal, and medial (above the corpus callosum) aspects of the cerebral hemisphere. Their number varies (6 to 16) on the superolateral surface of the hemisphere,[77,246] from which they continue up directly into the superior longitudinal sagittal sinus. They traverse the subdural space for 1 to 2 cm. in a sheath of arachnoid and often two or three units coalesce to form common trunks as they course for 1 to 3 cm. in the dura mater before entering the sinus or the adjacent lateral lacunae. The angle of junction with the superior longitudinal sinus varies. Anteriorly the angle is about 90 degrees, while the angle becomes progressively more acute proceeding posteriorly. The superficial vein or veins on the lateral aspect of the occipital lobe drain upward. No veins join the sinus for a distance of 4 to 5 cm. anteriorly to the torcular.[246]

The number of major veins on the medial aspect of the cerebral hemisphere corresponds more or less to the number on the superolateral surface. They may unite before entering the superior longitudinal sagittal sinus or the sinusoids of the upper part of the falx cerebri. The cingulate gyrus is drained by small veins that proceed into the anterior and posterior cerebral or callosal veins[246] and communicate with the inferior longitudinal sagittal sinus.[167]

Middle cerebral veins. The superficial Sylvian vein is the major vessel in this sector and customarily drains that portion of the brain in the vicinity of the Sylvian fissure (Fig. 1-7). Commencing in the posterior or horizontal limb of the Sylvian fissure, it runs forward and downward along the fissure superficially, courses medially around the temporal pole, and terminates in the cavernous sinus.[105,139] However, Wolf, Huang, and Newman[246] assert that in the region of the pterion the superficial Sylvian vein pierces the dura mater and runs along the lesser wing of the sphenoid as the sphenoparietal sinus and terminates by draining into the cavernous sinus.

The superficial Sylvian vein is quite variable in its course and caliber. Occasionally multiple rather than single, it may be quite a minor vessel, its role being compensatorily taken over by an adjacent

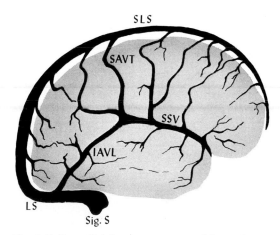

Fig. 1-7. Superficial venous system of lateral surface of the brain. **SLS,** Superior longitudinal (sagittal) sinus. **SSV,** Superficial Sylvian vein. **LS,** Lateral (transverse) sinus. **Sig. S,** Sigmoid sinus. **SAVT,** Greater (superior) anastomotic vein (of Trolard). **IAVL,** Lesser (inferior) anastomotic vein (of Labbé).

vessel.[246] In most brains (91%)[167] an accessory vein courses below and parallel to the superficial Sylvian vein, which at times runs an unusual course proceeding intradurally from the pterion backward along the inner surface of the squamous temporal bone to the tentorium to join the lateral sinus.[246] Alternatively it has been reported to leave the lesser wing and course across the floor of the middle cranial fossa to the superior petrosal sinus or via emissary veins to the pterygoid plexus.[246]

The posterior extremity of the superficial Sylvian vein anastomoses with the superior longitudinal sagittal sinus via the greater (superior) anastomotic vein (of *Trolard*) which may become the primary drainage vessel of the Sylvian area.[77] The Rolandic vein, one of the superior cerebral veins, lies in the central or Rolandic fissure. It drains into the sagittal sinus and usually anastomoses with one of the Sylvian veins.[77] The superficial Sylvian vein anastomoses posteriorly with a superficial temporal vein, the lesser (inferior) anastomotic vein (of Labbé), which drains posteriorly and downward to the lateral (or transverse) sinus. From the adjacent surface of the frontal lobe it receives tributaries, one of which at least is usually quite prominent.[77]

The deep Sylvian veins drain the cortex of the insula and adjacent gyri of the frontal and temporal lobes and continues medially into the inferior cerebral veins. They anastomose with the superficial Sylvian vein or veins.

Inferior cerebral veins. The inferior cerebral veins drain a considerable portion of the lateral aspect of the temporal and occipital lobes as well as most of the basal surface of the frontal, temporal, and occipital lobes.

In the main, veins of the frontal pole and inferior surface of the frontal lobe drain into the superior longitudinal sagittal sinus, but many drain posteriorly into the cavernous and sphenoparietal sinuses and into the basal vein of Rosenthal.[77,167] Laterally at least one large vein drains into

the Sylvian veins.[77] In brains examined by Perese[167] there were no veins along the inferior lateral edge of the frontal lobe bridging the subdural space.

The inferior cerebral veins, including the lesser anastomotic vein of Labbé, drain a considerable portion of the lateral surface of the temporal and occipital lobes mostly entering the transverse sinus. The inferior surface of the temporal lobe is drained into the superior petrosal sinus. lateral sinus, and the basal vein of Rosenthal, while veins of the corresponding surface of the occipital lobe flow into the lateral sinus and the great cerebral vein (vena magna cerebri) of Galen.[167] The lower medial aspect of the occipital lobe including the calcarine area, drains into the internal occipital veins and thence into the great cerebral vein of Galen.[77]

Deep cerebral venous system

The bulk of the cerebral white matter is served by small transcerebral veins arising in the subcortical white matter or centrum ovale. They tend to follow the course of the fibers of the corona radiata toward the lateral aspect of the lateral ventricle where they are joined by venous channels leaving the corpus striatum. Though anastomoses occur between these transcerebral veins and cortical veins draining to the superficial veins,[98,194] the consensus is that such intracerebral communication is limited in extent. Kaplan[103,105] divided these transcerebral veins into three groups. The anterior group joins veins from the anterior part of the basal ganglia to form the septal or anterior subependymal vein, which runs backward along the septum pellucidum.[103,105] The middle group of transcerebral veins drains into the terminal, thalamostriate, or middle subependymal vein, which follows the tail of the caudate nucleus in the roof of the inferior horn of the lateral ventricle into the floor of the body of the ventricle, crossing it obliquely between the caudate nucleus and the dorsal thalamus to the interventricular foramen of Monro.[77]

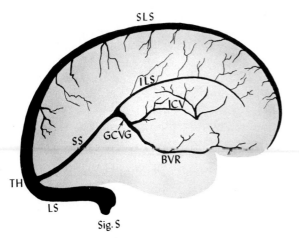

Fig. 1-8. Course of deep cerebral venous system. **SLS,** Superior longitudinal (sagittal) sinus. **ILS,** Inferior longitudinal (sagittal) sinus. **ICV,** Internal cerebral vein (small vein of Galen). **BVR,** Basal vein of Rosenthal. **GCVG,** Great cerebral vein of Galen. **TH,** Torcular Herophili. **LS,** Lateral (transverse) sinus. **Sig. S,** Sigmoid sinus. **SS,** Straight sinus.

The internal cerebral vein (Fig. 1-8), a paired structure, is formed near the interventricular foramen of Monro by the union of the terminal, septal, and anterior caudate veins, veins from the lentiform and caudate nucleus, and a choroidal vein from the plexus of the lateral ventricle. Once formed, this internal cerebral vein (small vein of Galen) bends sharply and posteriorly into the roof of the third ventricle. At the so-called venous angle[77] below the splenium of the corpus callosum, the two internal cerebral veins unite to form the great cerebral vein of Galen. The posterior group of transcerebral veins unite, forming a posterior subependymal vein that courses over the thalamus to join the internal cerebral vein anteroinferiorly to the splenium. The internal cerebral vein also receives venous blood from the corpus callosum, the choroidal plexus of the third ventricle, and the thalamus.[102]

The basal vein (of Rosenthal) commences near the anterior perforated substance formed by the union of (1) the anterior vein of the corpus callosum (collecting blood from the callosum and the anteromedial surface of the cerebral hemisphere), (2) the deep middle cerebral vein (draining the insular and the lenticulostriate veins), and (3) the anterior cerebral vein (draining blood from the orbital surface of the frontal lobe).[77] The basal vein lies deep to the arteries at the base of the brain[105] and runs posteriorly along the optic tract, round the cerebral peduncle under cover of the uncus and hippocampal gyrus to the splenium of the corpus callosum. Here the basal vein joins the homolateral internal cerebral vein or enters the great cerebral vein of Galen. In some brains there is an anastomosis between the basal vein and the petrosal sinuses by means of either the lateral anastomotic mesencephalic vein or the pontine or prepontine plexus. Yet again drainage of the basal vein may take place via a channel in the tentorium cerebelli terminating in the transverse or the straight sinus.[247] Occasionally the vein is altogether absent and its function performed by neighboring vessels.[77] The basal vein receives tributaries from the choroid plexus of the inferior horn of the lateral ventricle (inferior choroidal vein) and from the pons and inferior surface of the adjacent temporal and occipital lobe. A lateral mesencephalic vein running vertically along the posterior aspect of the cerebral peduncle may join the basal vein to serve as the anastomosis between it and the superior petrosal sinus.[77]

The great cerebral vein of Galen is formed by the union of the two internal cerebral veins, and from its origin proceeds posteriorly curving under the splenium of the corpus callosum and thence upward to end together with the inferior longitudinal sagittal sinus in the anterior extremity of the straight sinus. Its tributaries include (1) the internal cerebral veins, (2) the basal veins of Rosenthal, (3) the posterior vein of the corpus callosum from each side draining the posterior part of the gyrus cinguli and the posterior part of the corpus callosum,[77] (4) veins from the pineal and quadrigeminal bodies,[27] (5) the posterior cerebral veins from the inferior surface of the occipital lobes, and (6) veins from the tentorium cerebelli and the superior cerebellar vein from the upper surface of the cerebellum.[27,77] The drainage area of the great cerebral vein is obviously extensive and overlaps with that of the superficial venous systems, especially in the frontal and occipital lobes, and the pons.[194]

Venous drainage of the brain stem and cerebellum

A superficial venous plexus, deep to the arteries is to be found on the surface of the brain stem from the midbrain level and continuing downward.[77] There are two lateral venous channels on the pons, but occasionally a single median pontine vein may be found deep to the basilar artery, anastomosing superiorly with the basal veins on either side. In many brains one or more veins from the upper part of the pontine plexus drain into the cavernous sinus. These vessels bridge the subdural space and are vulnerable to traction in the pons during neurosurgery.[167] The flow of blood from the pontine and upper medullary plexus is in general directed laterally toward the inferior petrosal sinus in the cerebellopontine angle or toward a trigeminal venous plexus in the foramen ovale. Drainage channels from the lower medullary plexus enter the marginal sinus or the vertebral veins,[77] being continuous with the venous channels and networks of the spinal cord.

Deep cerebellar veins emerge from the cerebellum to join the superficial cerebellar veins that form a network over the cerebellar surface and anastomose with venous plexuses over the pons and medulla. Larger venous channels are often arranged at right angles to the folia superficial to the ramifications of the cerebellar arteries.[77] Laterally the superior cerebellar veins drain into the lateral and the superior petrosal sinuses. Other veins drain medially toward the vermis to form a median superior cerebellar vein, which terminates anteriorly in either the great cerebral vein of Galen[27] or a basal vein.[77] Posteriorly there is drainage

from the superior cerebellar venous plexus to the straight sinus.[105] Lateral efferents from the inferior surface of the cerebellum drain into the transverse sinus, the superior[77] and inferior petrosal sinuses,[27] and the occipital sinus.[27,77] A well-formed median inferior cerebellar vein may drain posteriorly to either the straight sinus or one of the lateral sinuses.[27]

Venous sinuses of the dura mater

The cranial venous sinuses are endothelium-lined spaces situated between the two layers af the dura mater. Functioning as venous channels collecting blood from the cerebral, meningeal, and diploic veins of the cranium, they communicate frequently with extracranial veins and end either directly or indirectly in the internal jugular vein.

Superior longitudinal (sagittal) sinus. The superior longitudinal sinus lies superiorly in the midline along the line of attachment of the falx cerebri and the dura mater lining the calvarium. Its lumen is triangular in outline and often traversed by fibrous strands. It grows perceptibly larger after its commencement at the crista galli where it communicates through the foramen cecum with veins of the frontal sinus, with those of the nasal cavity, and rarely with the anterior facial veins.[27] It flows backward along the convex border of the attachment of the falx cerebri, grooves the cranial vault, and usually deviates slightly to the right as it descends along the occipital bone[27] to the internal occipital protuberance, where it usually terminates by becoming the right transverse sinus (in up to 70% of subjects).[72] Communication with the torcular is variable. Occasionally it terminates in the left transverse sinus, and at times it bifurcates and drains blood into both transverse sinuses. The large venous lacunae and the Pacchionian granulations projecting into them, though absent at birth,[77] are present in late childhood and young adult life when there are three or four lacunae on each side. They tend to coalesce subsequently to form one or two more extensive lakes,[77] with perhaps a noticeable thinning of the overlying bone.

This sinus receives the superior cerebral veins and meningeal veins from the dura mater, and as well communicates with the extracranial circulation by means of emissary veins traversing the parietal foramina.

Inferior longitudinal (sagittal) sinus. The inferior longitudinal sinus is a small channel in the posterior half to two-thirds of the inferior or free margin of the falx cerebri. Arising from the confluence of veins in the falx cerebri and running posteriorly to the junction of the falx with the tentorium, it is joined by the great cerebral vein of Galen to form the straight sinus. It receives tributaries from the falx cerebri, from the middle third of the medial surface of the cerebral hemispheres and from the corpus callosum.

Straight sinus. The straight sinus is the direct continuation of the inferior longitudinal sinus after it is joined by the great cerebral vein. It runs posteriorly and downward along the line of union between the falx cerebri and the tentorium cerebelli and receives tributaries from the superior cerebellar veins, the vessels of the falx, and the occipital lobes. It most frequently terminates at the internal occipital protuberance by turning to the left into the left transverse sinus and less frequently bifurcating or turning to the right.

Occipital sinuses. There may be a single or a paired sinus in the attached border of the falx cerebelli. They are continuous with vessels about the posterolateral margins of the foramen magnum, which in turn communicate with the sigmoid sinus on each side and the vertebral veins. Superiorly they may open individually or by a common channel into the right or left transverse sinus with a variable relationship to the torcular. Tributaries are received from the meninges and cerebellum.

Confluens sinuum (torcular herophili). At the internal occipital protuberance the superior longitudinal sinus, the straight sinus and the occipital sinuses communicate to some extent to form the confluens

sinuum (torcular Herophili). Woodhall[252] reviewed the variations of the sinuses in the region of the torcular Herophili, finding five main types.

Common pool type. In this variation (encountered in 9% of 100 brains[252]) the superior longitudinal and the straight sinuses coalesce to form a common pool from which blood passes into both transverse sinuses.

Plexiform type. The longitudinal and straight sinuses may each divide equally or unequally into two branches that are distributed to the two transverse sinuses, but there is usually asymmetry, though intercommunications between the transverse sinuses are frequent. This type occurred in 56% of Woodall's series in which subgroups are numerous.

Ipsilateral type. In this variety (found in 31% of subjects) the superior longitudinal sinus drains to one side, usually the right, and the straight sinus to the contralateral side with intercommunicating channels between the transverse sinuses.

Unilateral type. In 4% of subjects both the superior longitudinal and the straight sinuses empty into one transverse sinus. The contralateral transverse sinus may be minute or absent.

Occipital type. This variation concerns the occipital sinus or sinuses when large enough to carry a significant quantity of blood. The common variation is merely a large single or paired occipital sinus draining blood from the confluens sinuum. The second rare variation is that in which either the superior longitudinal or the straight sinus or both, in a common pool formation, empty directly into a large occipital sinus at the expense of a lateral sinus.[252]

Transverse (lateral) and sigmoid sinuses. The transverse sinuses commence at the internal occipital protuberance. They are unequal in size in approximately 24% of subjects.[252] The right sinus is more often the continuation of the superior longitudinal sinus than the left, which is most frequently the continuation of the straight sinus. At their commencement, some communication is generally present between the sinuses of each side. Each sinus passes laterally along the attachment border of the tentorium cerebelli in a groove in the occipital bone to reach the posteroinferior angle of the parietal bone. The sinus then leaves the tentorium cerebelli and turns downward on the intracranial surface of the mastoid portion of the temporal bone as the sigmoid sinus; it passes thence into the upper surface of the jugular process of the occipital bone and there turns forward and then downward into the jugular foramen to unite with the internal jugular vein.[27] The internal jugular vein usually exhibits a distinct bulbous enlargement, the jugular bulb, at its junction with the sigmoid sinus.[77]

Tributaries that enter the transverse sinus are some of the inferior cerebral and superior and inferior cerebellar veins, a posterior parietal diploic vein and the superior petrosal sinuses. The inferior petrosal sinus enters the terminal portion of the sigmoid sinus. Small veins from the bone and mucosa of the mastoid air cells drain into this sinus and jugular bulb,[77] while connections with extracranial veins occur by means of emissary veins through the mastoid foramen and the posterior condylar canal.[27]

Cavernous sinuses. The cavernous sinuses are situated on either side of the body of the sphenoid bone. They extend from the medial end of the superior orbital fissure where they receive the ophthalmic veins, to the apex of the petrous portion of the temporal bone. The lumen of each sinus is crossed by innumerable fibrous strands imparting a cavernous appearance. The internal carotid artery, surrounded by the sympathetic nerve plexus, traverses the sinus and the oculomotor, trochlear, ophthalmic, and maxillary divisions of the trigeminal. The abducent nerves lie along its lateral wall. Each cavernous sinus communicates with its fellow of the opposite side by the intercavernous sinuses passing in front of and behind the pituitary gland.

Tributaries of the cavernous sinus are the ophthalmic veins (from the eye and orbit), the sphenoparietal sinus, superficial middle cerebral and inferior cerebral veins, and those about the hypophysis cerebri. Additional communications with other sinuses and veins allow multiple avenues for the drainage of blood: (1) the superior petrosal sinus to the transverse sinus, (2) the inferior petrosal sinus to the lowest segment of the sigmoid sinus, (3) emissary veins through the foramen ovale or the sphenoidal emissary foramen to the pterygoid plexus,[27] and (4) basilar sinus to the superior petrosal sinus and the anterior longitudinal vertebral sinuses.

Important anastomoses with extracranial veins are to the pterygoid plexus, to the vertebral veins, and to the facial veins (in the ophthalmic veins). The cavernous sinus is said to be particularly prone to infection from the upper three-fourths of the face and underlying tissues as the result of a spreading thrombophlebitis. The event has become extremely rare in this era of antibiotics.

Superior petrosal sinus. Each superior petrosal sinus is small and begins at the open end of the petrous portion of the temporal bone in the posterior end of the cavernous sinus. It runs backward and laterally along the petrous ridge in the attached margin of the tentorium cerebelli and joins the transverse sinus where the sinus turns downward to become the sigmoid sinus. It receives inferior cerebral, superior cerebellar, and small tympanic veins from the middle ear as tributaries. Occasionally however this sinus is absent.

Inferior petrosal sinus. The inferior petrosal sinus extends from the posteroinferior aspect of the cavernous sinus to terminate in the sigmoid sinus as it passes into the jugular foramen. The tributaries include inferior cerebellar veins, small veins from the inner ear as well as the internal auditory vein,[27] and veins from the pons and upper medulla.

Sphenoparietal sinus. Each sphenoparietal sinus runs medially in the dura mater along the under surface of the lesser wing of the sphenoid bone to terminate in the anterior part of the cavernous sinus. Superficial veins from the middle and inferior cerebral veins drain into the sinus as do veins from the dura mater. It communicates with the superior longitudinal sinus through the meningeal veins, accompanying the middle meningeal artery.

Basilar sinus. The network of the basilar venous sinus is located in the dura on the clivus of the skull and communicates with the cavernous sinuses, the inferior petrosal, occipital, and marginal sinuses, and the anterior longitudinal vertebral veins.[27]

Emissary veins. Emissary veins are channels of varying caliber anastomosing intracranial venous sinuses with the extracranial venous circulation, hence with tributaries of the external jugular vein or of the vertebral venous system. They may be single or plexiform channels in which flow is reversible. There are eight major emissary veins:

1. Parietal, from the superior longitudinal sagittal sinus to scalp veins (posterior occipital veins and diploic veins)
2. Occipital, from the confluens sinuum to the occipital veins and the vertebral venous plexus
3. Mastoid, from the transverse sinus to the posterior or occipital veins
4. Condyloid, from the sigmoid sinus via the posterior condylar canal to the vertebral venous system
5. Hypoglossal, from the sigmoid sinus to the vertebral venous system
6. Pharyngeal, from the cavernous and petrosal sinuses to the pterygoid plexuses via foramina in the floor of the middle cranial fossa
7. Ophthalmic, from the inferior ophthalmic vein to the pterygoid plexus[223]
8. Ethmoidal, from the superior longitudinal sinus via the foramen cecum to the nasal veins

Emissary veins like venous channels within the skull have no valves and consequently provide an accessory route for venous drainage from the brain, though they are secondary in importance to the vertebral venous systems as collaterals.

Meningeal veins. The veins of the dura mater or meningeal veins accompany the corresponding branches of the meningeal arteries. There are two veins that lie on either side of or external to the respective arteries.[27,77] They collect blood from the dura and the diploic veins of the cranium and terminate in the dural venous sinuses.

Vertebral veins. The vertebral veins consist of an internal vertebral (epidural) venous plexus and an external vertebral plexus. The internal vertebral or epidural plexus is situated externally to the dura mater overlying the spinal cord and extending the entire length of the vertebral canal. Two or more anterior and posterior longitudinal channels or sinuses may be in the plexus,[27,105] the anterior channels usually being the larger.[105] The anterior veins are applied to the posterior aspect of the vertebral bodies and intervertebral discs and contain one or more transverse channels on each vertebra resembling the rungs of a ladder. Usually by means of one large vein, these horizontal veins communicate with several converging veins, which emerge from the vertebral body.

The internal vertebral (epidural) venous plexus receives branches from the spinal veins and communicates with the external vertebral venous plexus. This vertebral plexus is drained by a series of intervertebral veins that in the cervical region communicate with the vertebral veins, in the thoracic region with intercostal veins, in the lumbar region with the lumbar veins, and in the sacral region with the lateral sacral veins. Above, the plexus communicates with the network of basilar sinuses, the terminal portions of the sigmoid sinuses, with the plexus of veins accompanying each hypoglossal nerve through the anterior condylar canal and via a plexus surrounding the foramen magnum with the occipital sinuses and the vertebral veins.[27]

The external vertebral venous plexus is a large plexiform arrangement of veins on the external surface of the vertebrae, an anterior plexus lying on the anterior surface of the vertebral bodies, and a posterior plexus lying on the posterolateral surfaces of the vertebrae, in the vertebral grooves, around the spines, and around the articular and the transverse processes of the vertebrae.[27] These venous plexuses communicate with the vessels within the vertebral bodies and with the internal vertebral venous plexus and then drain into the intervertebral veins.

Batson[13] considered these vertebral veins as constituting one venous system—the vertebral, akin to the portal, pulmonary, and caval venous systems. He divided the vertebral system into three intercommunicating divisions, first, the internal vertebral or epidural venous network, second or intermediate, the veins within the bones of the vertebral column itself, and the third or outer division, the external vertebral venous plexus.

Significance. Batson,[11,12] by injecting radiopaque material into the dorsal vein of the penis of a cadaver, was able to outline the prostatic plexus of veins, the lateral sacral veins, the iliac veins, and inferior vena cava. Using a less viscous medium, he demonstrated by postmortem angiography that the opaque material outlined the veins in and about the sacrum, ilium, and spine and several intercostal and intracranial veins. In animal experiments, the abdomen was compressed to simulate coughing or straining and angiography outlined the vertebral system of veins, dye entering even the thoracic spine and intercostal veins. When small mammary veins in a female cadaver were injected, the dye entered the clavicles, intercostal veins, head of the humerus, cervical vertebrae, transverse cranial venous sinus, the superior longitudinal sinus, skull, azygous vein, and superior vena cava. The experimental results led Batson to suggest that the spread of tumor or infection was possible by means of the vertebral system of veins, the absence of valves allowing reversal of flow under certain physiological conditions such as straining, coughing, and the Valsalva maneuver. In this way the venae cavae and lungs could be bypassed, permitting what

appears to be paradoxical embolism, for spread could occur from the pelvis to the spine, skull, brain, etc., without traversing the lung and heart.

Batson[11-13] pointed out also that the vertebral venous system not only possesses rich communications with the spinal cord and spinal column but also with the segmental veins of the thoracoabdominal wall (including breast), with the azygos veins, and hence with the posterior bronchial vein and parietal pleural veins. There were occasional communications with the renal vein and rich anastomoses with the pelvic viscera. Batson extended the thesis and demonstrated that postmortem angiography could outline continuously the vertebral venous system from the pelvic veins to the cranium in which with this technique extensive injection of intracranial veins was possible.

Batson's observations caused controversy even though his basic contention is certainly plausible, and there has been cogent support of the thesis.[6,95] The vertebral venous system is thought to be an extensive venous reservoir of blood, the total capacity of which has yet to be determined. It is relatively stagnant yet appears to have tidal variations with quiet respiration.[13] It is a low pressure system, devoid of valves but with extensive communications,[11,13,95] leading ultimately to all viscera except the heart, ovaries, and testes.[95] It is par excellence a collateral circulation for the obstruction of even such large veins as the superior or inferior vena cava. More pertinent to the present problem however is obstruction or ligation of the internal jugular veins, for the vertebral veins then become the major drainage rout for intracranial blood. Herlihy[95] noted that undue emphasis had been placed on the emissary veins of the skull, which decrease in size with age. No doubt they assist in a collateral venous circulation but their importance is secondary.

Herlihy[95] emphasized the important role of the vertebral veins in the maintenance of cerebrospinal fluid pressure. An increase in cerebrospinal fluid pressure occurs in the Valsalva maneuver and after pressure on the internal jugular vein (Queckenstedt test). Collapse of the veins after death probably accounts for the drop in cerebrospinal fluid pressure at that time. With the possibility of such rapid changes in the volume of blood within the vertebral system and in view of its vast anastomotic communications, the vertebral venous system conceivably acts as a buffer against rises in cerebrospinal fluid merely by affecting the egress of blood from the internal vertebral plexus.

Batson[11-13] discussed at some length the significance of the vertebral venous system in the hematogenous spread of tumors, particularly from the breast, lung, and pelvis to the brain, skull, and vertebral column. The rarity of spinal cord metastases was thought not to substantiate Batson's theory of tumor spread, but Anderson[6] in a personal series found that the incidence of metastases in the cord when compared with those in the brain was roughly proportional to the bulk of the respective organs. However, Gillilan[79] attributed the infrequency of metastatic tumors in the cord to the presence of valves in the medullary veins at their junction with the vertebral venous system. Coman and DeLong[42] injected tumor suspensions into the femoral veins of rabbits and rats. In support of Batson's theory, tumor metastases were more frequent in the vertebral venous system in those animals injected during abdominal compression than in those injected without compression.

Anson and associates[8] emphasized the close relationship of the pararenal venous system to the vertebral veins, and Batson[13] incriminated vascular communications between perirenal vessels and the vertebral system in the production of cerebral air embolism after perirenal injection of air for diagnostic purposes. Collis[41] elaborated on the hematogenous spread of infections via this venous system, whereas Gius and Grier[81] asserted that bilateral removal of the internal jugular veins might augment metastatic spread via vertebral (Rachidian) veins in conditions of uncontrolled disease.

Blood supply of the spinal cord
Arteries of the spinal cord

The spinal cord in man derives its blood supply from a number of sources, and as is consistent with their size, the spinal blood vessels exhibit considerable variation in pattern as well as numerous anastomoses. Strangely enough the anastomotic network about the spinal cord has been likened to the circle of Willis.[224]

Anterior spinal branch of the vertebral artery. The anterior spinal branch of each vertebral artery commences a short distance below the vertebrobasilar junction. Each branch runs downward and medially on the front of the medulla oblongata to unite with its fellow of the opposite side to form the anterior spinal artery. These rami from the vertebral arteries are small, being rarely more than 1 mm. in diameter.[105] They supply primarily the midline structures of the medulla oblongata. The combined anterior spinal artery continues down the spinal cord, supplemented by tributaries from segmental vessels and is responsible for the supply only as far as the third cervical segment.[39]

Variations of the two branches are considerable. In a comprehensive study of 150 brains, Stopford[212] found one or other branch absent in 12% of cases, and in another 3% one branch arose from the angle of fusion of the two vertebral arteries. Of those cases in which the anterior spinal artery had a double origin, there was equality in size of the two rami in only 11% and sometimes one of the rami was duplicated. The level of origin of the two branches varied from the extreme upper end of the vertebral (51% on the right, 59% on the left) to the level of the inferior extremity of the olive or below it (20% on the right, 13% on the left) with many at the midolivary region (29% on the right, 28% on the left). In 6% of subjects the two rami remained separate, in

47% fusion occurred, and in the remaining 47%, one or more transverse branches anastomosed the nonfused rami. Levels of fusion also varied and mostly did not conform to the standard textbook pattern. Seven cases were regarded by Stopford[212] as anomalous because of triple origin or plexiform arrangements.

Radicular arteries. Paired segmental arteries arise from the second portion of the vertebral artery and the deep cervical, ascending cervical, and superior intercostal arteries proceeding to the cervical and upper thoracic segments. In the thoracic, lumbar, and sacral segments are segmental branches from the thoracic and lumbar aorta and from the lateral sacral arteries (branches from the internal iliac arteries) or less frequently from the median sacral. They supply paravertebral muscles, vertebrae, meninges, and nerve roots. Branches from them proceed with the respective segmental nerves through the vertebral foramina where they divide into anterior and posterior radicular arteries.[223] Each radicular artery supplies its nerve roots and ganglia but contributes little to the spinal cord. Occasionally, however, the posterior radicular artery extends to the spinal cord to join the posterior pial plexus.[74] In the sacral region the radicular arteries follow the long nerve roots of the cauda equina upward but none contributes to the spinal arteries. For the most part, each nerve root of the cauda equina is accompanied by at least one small artery.[92] Variations occur, and two or more segmental arteries may arise from a common stem.

Medullary arteries. Special unpaired and unbranched arteries, called the anterior and posterior medullary arteries,[74] arise sporadically from the segmental arteries along the spinal column. Many authors, however, still regard these vessels as radicular arteries and not as distinct and separate vessels.[214,224] The number of unpaired tributaries from the segmental arteries varies (Tureen[224] said 2 to 17, Suh and Alexander[214] 6 to 8, Henson and Parsons[94] 3 to 6, and Gillilan[74] 7 to 10). They anastomose and reinforce the anterior spinal artery. Usually two occur in the cervical region, the larger mostly at the fifth or sixth cervical segment, rarely at the fourth or seventh, and the eighth only infrequently has a medullary artery. One or a few small arteries at times contribute similarly.[74] Two to four small segmental medullary arteries are found in the thoracic zone, two or three of them in the upper thoracic region. An additional vessel is located generally between the fifth and sevenths segments.[74]

The largest anterior medullary artery (of Adamkiewicz) joins the anterior spinal artery most often on the left side at the second lumbar region. Its position varies from the eighth thoracic to the fourth lumbar.[77,214] The artery courses upward along the nerve root to the cord, where at the anterior median fissure it turns caudally at an acute angle as it joins the tapering anterior spinal artery from above. Gillilan[77] believes that the flow is directed downward, but it may divide into ascending and descending limbs that reinforce the anterior spinal artery both above and below. An additional small lumbar medullary artery may join the anterior spinal artery a few segments below. However, quite apart from this contribution, the great anterior medullary artery is responsible for the anterior two-thirds of the spinal cord caudal to its junction with the anterior spinal artery.

Posterior medullary arteries, noticeably smaller than the anterior medullary arteries, number 6 to 8 on each side.[74] On the other hand, Garland and associates[69] state that there are 11 to 23 posterior vessels. Some of these vessels are very small but usually two posterior medullary arteries in the lumbar region are more prominent than the others, and the last large vessel, much less significant than its anterior counterpart,[74] has been called the great posterior medullary artery.

Anterior (median) spinal artery. The anterior spinal artery is a longitudinal channel extending, if somewhat sinuously,

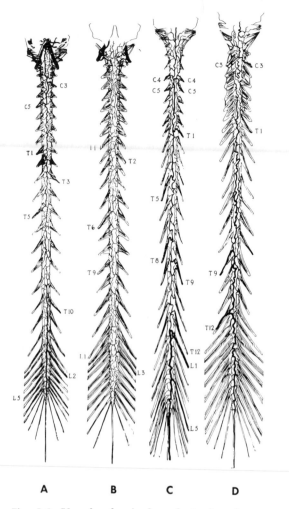

A   B   C   D

Fig. 1-9. Vessels of spinal cord. **A,** Arteries on ventral surface. **B,** Arteries on dorsal surface. Spinal veins are shown on ventral, **C,** and dorsal, **D,** surfaces. Spinal roots are labeled when accompanied by major medullary arteries or veins. (Courtesy Suh, T. H., and Alexander, L.: Vascular system of the human spinal cord, Arch. Neurol. Psychiat. 41:659, 1939.)

the full length of the spinal cord and lying in close relationship to the entrance of the anterior median fissure (Fig. 1-9). It originates superiorly with the union of the two anterior spinal branches of the vertebral artery, though fusion can be delayed and take place in the spinal canal. Regions of duplication are not uncommon especially in the cervical region.[224] The caliber of the anterior spinal artery is not uniform, being narrowest in the thoracic region where it

tapers from above downward, thus indicating the direction of blood flow. In this region it may dwindle to such an extent that it can be difficult to differentiate between it and other pial arteries on the anterior surface of the cord.[74] The artery has its greatest dimension at and just below the junction with the great anterior medullary artery, and then it again tapers from above downward over the lower cord and on to the filum terminale.

Posterior spinal artery. Stopford[212] considered that, though frequently stated to be a branch of the vertebral artery, more often this artery was a branch of the posterior inferior cerebellar artery, from which it arose on both sides in 73% of subjects. It took origin from the vertebral artery on the right side in 18% and on the left in 20%. It had a double origin on the right side in 9% and on the left in 7%. After giving off an ascending branch that runs upward on the posterior columns to the calamus scriptorius, each posterior spinal artery proceeds downward on the posterolateral aspect of the cord, medial to the posterior rootlets and reinforced by segmental vessels. However, the posterior spinal branches from the cranium contribute to a longer length of cervical cord than do the anterior spinal branches of the vertebral.[24]

In the spinal course, the two posterior spinal arteries are not single distinct vessels but rather plexiform channels located on the posterolateral aspect of the cord along the entrance of the posterior nerve rootlets. The posterior medullary arteries are not symmetrically arranged either with their fellows of the opposite side or with the anterior group. Anastomoses occur sporadically between the two posterior spinal plexiform channels, which extend inferiorly to the conus medullaris where they anastomose with the anterior spinal artery.

Pial circulation of the spinal cord

The anterior spinal arteries give off lateral branches, which ramify in the subarachnoid space over the anterior aspect of the cord and anastomose to a limited extent with each other and with similar branches from the posterior spinal arteries. These ramifications and anastomoses however are arteriolar in size, and together with those on the posterior aspect of the cord constitute the spinal pial plexus, which, on account of its size, has been referred to as the vasocorona. The anterior three-fourths of the pial plexus is supplied by the anterior spinal artery and the remainder by the posterior spinal arteries.[69] Tortuosity of these vessels is not uncommon, particularly in the aged.[226] Gillilan[74] points out that at times additional longitudinal channels have been described. However other than the three described (one anterior and two posterior spinal arteries), no distinct channels can be recognized for more than a few segments. The pial network constitutes a potential if variable and limited collateral circulation.

Intrinsic spinal arteries

The anterior spinal artery gives rise to 240 to 300 central sulcal arteries.[69,74] These arteries arise singly at right angles and enter the anterior median fissure, where in the depths of the sulcus they alternate irregularly[226] to the left and to the right. Branched vessels have been reported, Hassler[92] asserting that the bifurcations always occurred in the sagittal plane with the branches passing to each half of the cord. The number of central arteries supplying the cord varies with the segment, being most numerous and of larger caliber in the lumbosacral enlargement and least numerous and smallest in the thoracic region.[74,92,96] The central arteries penetrate the anterior white commissure and arch laterally toward the anterior horn where they immediately break up into a dense capillary network about the anterior horn cells. In corrosion material, Gillilan[74] described the perineuronal capillary network as having a tangled skein appearance. The network anastomoses with that of central arteries above and below and the flow through them is centrifugal. These central arteries supply the anterior two-thirds of the central gray matter, and the anterior spinal artery as a whole supplies roughly the anterior two-thirds of the entire cord. The pial network supplies about one-third to a half of the peripheral spinal white matter, the branches pentrating to a variable extent from segment to segment.[92] These vessels constitute the centripetal system. Vessel density is less in the white matter than in the gray, and a few of the centripetal vessels penetrate more deeply to anastomose with the capillary bed of the anterior gray columns.[74] The rectangular capillary meshes in the white matter are longitudinally orientated in the direction of the nerve bundles, whereas those of the gray matter are arranged transversely, parallel to the crossing axis cylinders.[74]

The posterior third of the cord is supplied by the penetrating branches of the posterior spinal arteries, many entering the cord with the posterior rootlets at the tip of the posterior horn. These vessels, on reaching the posterior gray substance, divide into two branches, which then subdivide immediately into precapillary and capillary vessels.[74] The posterior columns are supplied by other penetrating branches from the posterior pial network and a few anastomoses with the capillary bed of the posterior horn.

During life, the penetrating vessels behave functionally as if they are end arteries,[74] and the variation and small caliber of the anterior spinal artery exclude its being an efficient collateral circulation. The small size of the anterior spinal artery in the thoracic region[74,92] suggests that this region of the cord may be more susceptible to the deprivation of blood, though there is no reason to suppose that the intrinsic blood supply is inadequate.[74] Obviously certain portions of the cord will be more susceptible to anoxia than others, and in this regard collateral circulation and the variable anatomy of the blood supply are of importance.

Veins of the spinal cord

The spinal veins that drain the cord have a pattern similar to that of the arteries, though they are not true *venae comitantes.* The anterior central (sulcal) veins drain blood from both sides of the cord and are less numerous though larger than the central arteries.[96,226] The other intraspinal veins drain toward the surface often in connective tissue septa and join the extensive subarachnoid venous plexus.

Six longitudinal venous channels have been described in the pia mater of the spinal cord—one in the midline anteriorly, one in the midline posteriorly, a pair behind the posterior roots, and yet another pair behind the anterior roots.[28] Gillilan[77] however includes but three major channels. The anterior median vein or anterior spinal vein is the best defined of the venous channels. It is a single or paired vessel, sometimes plexiform, lying near or in the anterior median fissure and draining much of the spinal cord parenchyma by means of anterior sulcal veins. The paired posterior venous channels are plexiform and exhibit pronounced variability. Paired posterior channels are more prominent at the cervical and lumbosacral enlargements. In the cervical region the spinal veins are continuous with intracranial veins of the medulla.

The anterior median or spinal vein is drained by anterior medullary[77] or radicular veins,[214,224] and descriptions differ considerably. Gillilan[79] described 8 to 14 asymmetrical anterior medullary veins, among which a very large vein between the eleventh thoracic to the third lumbar segments, usually on the left side, can be identified as the great anterior medullary vein. The posterior medullary veins are more numerous than the anterior, especially in the cervical enlargement. They accompany the nerve roots peripherally to join the segmental veins, which usually form venous plexuses about the spinal nerves in the vicinity of the intervertebral foramina.[77]

Suh and Alexander[214] have described monocuspid valves at the junctions of spinal veins. They were portrayed as flaplike prolongations that could fold in such a manner as to occlude both tributaries and protruded from the apical region of junctions extending an inordinately long distance proximally into the proximal trunk. The existence of these unusual valvelike structures and their function have yet to be confirmed.

Nerves to the intracranial blood vessels

The vasomotor supply of the meningeal and cerebral arteries consists of both sympathetic and parasympathetic fibers. Parasympathetic vasodilator fibers leave the brain via the facial nerve and at the geniculate ganglion enter the greater superficial petrosal nerve, which gives off a few fibers to the sympathetic plexus on the internal carotid artery.[239] Preganglionic sympathetic fibers (vasoconstriction and vasodilatation) from the upper two thoracic segments reach the stellate and superior cervical sympathetic ganglia from which postganglionic fibers enter the skull by two routes. A plexus from the stellate ganglion extends up the vertebral and basilar arteries and a larger plexus from the superior cervical sympathetic ganglion passes up the external and internal carotid arteries to reach, respectively, the middle meningeal arteries and the circle of Willis.[239]

The sensory innervation of intracranial structures is derived from several sources:

1. Sensory fibers of the trigeminal nerve are believed to innervate pain-sensitive structures within the supratentorial portion of the cranium. Fibers extend along the meningeal arteries. However, the dural sinuses are also innervated. It is furthermore believed that afferent sensory fibers to the internal carotid, together with the anterior, middle, and posterior cerebral arteries, are supplied by the trigeminal nerve.[249]
2. The sensory supply to the subtentorial region of the cranial cavity is even more complex and unresolved. Experimentally induced histamine headaches indicate that the ninth and tenth cranial nerves and upper cervical

nerves are the principal source of afferent fibers for headache in the subtentorial region. It has been deduced that the sigmoid, the occipital, and the inferior aspects of the straight sinus, transverse or lateral sinus, and torcular are supplied by the ninth and tenth cranial nerves. The upper cervical nerves are said to be responsible for the sensory supply of the posterior meningeal, vertebral, and posterior inferior cerebellar arteries.[249]

It appears to be quite possible that there are sympathetic afferent nerve fibers in the internal and external carotid plexuses.[239] The nerve plexuses about the internal carotid arteries lie in or on the adventitia and extend onto the anterior and middle cerebral arteries while another branch extends along the posterior communicating to the posterior cerebral. The posterior cerebral artery, irrespective of its main source of blood, receives its nerve plexus from the internal carotid as is consistent with its phylogenetic origin from the carotid circulation.[241] The vertebral plexuses extend to the basilar and cerebellar vessels and the divisional branch of the basilar artery. These plexuses send branches along their ramifications to the small pial vessels and continue onto the larger intracerebral vessels.[166] Stöhr[211] found the nerves to be virtually absent from the media and never present in the intima. The pial vessels are believed to have both sympathetic and parasympathetic components in conjunction with the afferent or sensory innervation.

Penfield[166] demonstrated that the perivascular nerves within the brain are continuous with the nerve fibers upon the pial blood vessels. Vascular nerves have the same appearance within the cerebrum, cerebellum, medulla oblongata, and spinal cord. They form either a loose plexus or consist of longitudinal fibers on or in the adventitia. The intracerebral vascular nerves are for the most part nonmyelinated and continuous with both myelinated and nonmyelinated fibers on the pial vessel. The endings of the intracerebral nerves are small, grapelike clusters (5 μ or less in diameter) found in proximity to the media.[166] These nerves extend to intracerebral arterioles[138] and are restricted at least in the rat to vessels possessing a perivascular space.[187]

Both myelinated and nonmyelinated fibers have been traced to the choroid plexuses of the ventricles. Ganglion cells have been described in the tela choroidea, but Clark[38] was not able to confirm this observation. Some of the fibers arise from the cervical sympathetic chains while others are derived from the vagus and glossopharyngeal nerves. Some sensory nerves terminate in the epithelium or in the connective tissue, but sensory and vasomotor fibers end in or on the blood vessels.[38,77]

The pial blood vessels of the spinal cord possess both myelinated and nonmyelinated fibers[39] and thus they are similar basically to those of the brain. Little information is available concerning the origin of these nerves.

In electron microscopic studies of the cerebral arteries of the rat, myelinated and nonmyelinated fibers are to be found in the adventitia of the internal carotid artery, the proximal portion of the basilar,[190] and the middle cerebral artery.[187] Elsewhere, the nerves are nonmyelinated[187] and terminate close to the medial muscle fibers.

Embryology of the cerebrospinal blood vessels

Streeter[213] subdivided the development of the cerebral circulatory apparatus into five stages. During the first of these five stages, the primitive capillary plexus evolves, becoming the germinal bed from which all arteries, veins, and capillaries ultimately emerge. The second stage witnesses the development of a primary circulation in which the capillary bed, closely applied to the embryonic brain, is supplied by arterial channels from the aortic arch system and drained by a venous trunk extending to the venous end of the heart. In the third stage, stratification of the tissues of the head occurs, and vessels immediately surrounding the brain separate from those belonging to the membranous skull and its coverings. The fourth stage overlaps the third and encompasses, as the brain develops, a series of major developmental alterations and adjustments culminating in the completed circle of Willis. The fifth stage, includes the histological differentiation of the vessel walls intrinsic to arteries, veins, sinuses, and capillaries.

The proliferation of the primitive capillary plexus is a complex phenomenon. In embryos of higher vertebrates the vascular anlagen are first recognized as localized thickenings of the extraembryonic, undifferentiated mesenchyme and as such have been accepted as being mesodermal in origin, though ectodermal elements may make a contribution to at least some pial vessels.[89] The vasoformative cells or angioblasts, which differentiate from the mesenchyme, proliferate to form dense syncytial masses linked by delicate cytoplasmic processes with similar neighboring syncytia. The angioblastic masses increase in size by division and further differentiation of new angioblasts from the mesenchyme.[184,185] Vacuolation commences within these syncytial masses, and by confluence and extension of the vacuoles a lumen is formed. These spaces, lined by angioblasts or endothelial cells, contain a plasmalike fluid resolved from the disintegration of the cytoplasm and nuclei of the cells. Some angioblasts separate and enter the lumen to form blood cells. The isolated vesicles formed in neighboring syncytial masses subsequently link up to form plexuses of primitive blood vessels. The differentiation of angioblasts from mesenchyme becomes progressively less frequent; eventually it ceases altogether.[53,185] Thereafter all new vessels arise from growth or proliferation of older angioblasts or from budding of the walls of preexisting channels.

Vasculogenesis first commences in the body stalk and wall of the yolk sac, though some differentiation of primordial blood vessels probably occurs locally about the neural tube.[185] At the sixth somite stage an angioblastic plexus along the hindbrain is connected to the first aortic arches by chains of angioblasts. At the stage of 12 somites, a vascular plexus is related to the forebrain, midbrain, and hindbrain and connects with the aorta.[185] These primordial vessels spread over the surface of the brain, particularly the forebrain and midbrain, to form an irregular endothelial vascular meshwork in which initially no differentiation of major channels has occurred.[213] This then is the primordial plexus. The differentiation of this plexus into the adult pattern is achieved by the end of the first trimester. Other authors have dealt with the entity in detail.[53,131,155-158,213]

References

1. Abbie, A. A.: The morphology of the forebrain arteries, with especial reference to the evolution of the basal ganglia, J. Anat. **68:**433, 1934.
2. Ahmed, D. S., and Ahmed, R. H.: The recurrent branch of the anterior cerebral artery, Anat. Rec. **157:**699, 1967.
3. Alpers, B. J., and Berry, R. G.: Circle of Willis in cerebral vascular disorders, Arch. Neurol. **8:**398, 1963.
4. Alpers, B. J., Berry, R. G., and Paddison, R. M.: Anatomical studies of the circle of Willis in normal brain, Arch. Neurol. Psychiat. **81:**409, 1959.
5. Altmann, F.: Anomalies of the internal carotid artery and its branches; their embryological and comparative anatomical significance, Laryngoscope **57:**313, 1947.
6. Anderson, R. K.: Diodrast studies of the vertebral and cranial venous systems to show their probable role in cerebral metastases, J. Neurosurg. **8:**411, 1951.
7. Andrews, E. T., and Howard, J. M.: Congenital anomalies of the carotid artery: a case report, J. Amer. Geriat. Soc. **11:**642, 1963.
8. Anson, B. J., Cauldwell, E. W., Pick, J. W., and Beaton, L. E.: The blood supply of the kidney, suprarenal gland, and associated structures, Surg. Gynec. Obstet. **84:**313, 1947.
9. Baptista, A. G.: Studies on the arteries of the brain. II. The anterior cerebral artery: some anatomic features and their clinical implications, Neurology **13:**825, 1963.
10. Baptista, A. G.: Studies on the arteries of the brain. IV. Circle of Willis: functional significance, Acta Neurol. Scand. **42:**161, 1966.
11. Batson, O. V.: The function of the vertebral veins and their role in the spread of metastases, Ann. Surg. **112:**138, 1940.
12. Batson, O. V.: The role of the vertebral veins in metastatic processes, Ann. Intern. Med. **16:**38, 1942.

13. Batson, O. V.: The vertebral vein system, Amer. J. Roentgen. **78:**195, 1957.

14. Battacharji, S. K., Hutchinson, E. C., and McCall, A. J.: The circle of Willis—the incidence of developmental abnormalities in normal and infarcted brains, Brain **90:**747, 1967.

15. Bauer, R., Sheehan, S., and Meyer, J. S.: Arteriographic study of cerebrovascular disease. II. Cerebral symptoms due to kinking, tortuosity, and compression of carotid and vertebral arteries in the neck, Arch. Neurol. **4:**119, 1961.

16. Bean, R. B.: A composite study of the subclavian artery in man, Amer. J. Anat. **4:**303, 1905.

17. Beevor, C. E.: The cerebral arterial supply, Brain **30:**403, 1908.

18. Beevor, C. E.: On the distribution of the different arteries supplying the human brain, Phil. Trans. Roy. Soc. Series B, **200:**1, 1909.

19. Bergland, R., and Ray, B. S.: The arterial supply of the human optic chiasm, J. Neurosurg. **31:**327, 1969.

20. Bernasconi, V., and Cassinari, V.: Un segna carotidografica tipico di meningioma del tentorio, Chirurgia **11:**586, 1956. Cited by Smith et al.[204]

21. Berry, R. J. A., and Anderson, J. H.: A case of nonunion of the vertebrals with consequent abnormal origin of the basilaris, Anat. Anz. **35:**54, 1909-1910.

22. Bingham, W. G., and Hayes, G. J.: Persistent carotid-basilar anastomosis, J. Neurosurg. **18:**398, 1961.

23. Blackburn, I. W.: Anomalies of the encephalic arteries among the insane, J. Comp. Neurol. **17:**493, 1907.

24. Bolton, B.: The blood supply of the human spinal cord, J. Neurol. Neurosurg. Psychiat. **2:**137, 1939.

25. Bossi, L., and Caffaratti, E.: Su di un caso di aneurisma dell'arteria trigeminale primitiva, Minerva Med. **54:**754, 1963.

26. Brain, R.: Order and disorder in the cerebral circulation, Lancet **2:**857, 1957.

27. Brash, J. C.: Blood-vascular and lymphatic systems. In Brash, J. C., and Jamieson, E. B., editors: Cunningham's Textbook of anatomy, ed. 8, London, 1943, Oxford University Press, p. 1177.

28. Brash, J. C., and Jamieson, E. B.: Cunningham's Manual of practical anatomy, ed. 10, London, 1940, Oxford University Press, vol. 3.

29. Brea, G. B.: Sulla persistenza della anastomosi carotido basilare, Sist. Nerv. **8:**17, 1956. Cited by Lie.[124]

30. Brenner, H.: Ein Fall von kombinierter intrakranieller Gafässmissbildung, Zbl. Neurochir. **20:**244, 1960.

31. Bruetman, M. E., and Fields, W. S.: Persistent hypoglossal artery, Arch. Neurol. **8:**369, 1963.

32. Bull, J.: Massive aneurysms at the base of the brain, Brain **92:**535, 1969.

33. Busch, H. F. M.: Unusual collateral circulation in a child with cerebral arterial occlusion, Psychiat. Neurol. Neurochir. **72:**23, 1969.

34. Busse, O.: Aneurysmen und Bildungsfehler der Arteria communicans anterior, Virch. Arch. **229:**178, 1920.

35. Cairney, J.: Tortuosity of the cervical segment of the internal carotid artery, J. Anat. **59:**87, 1924.

36. Campbell, R. L., and Dyken, M. L.: Four cases of carotid-basilar anastomosis associated with central nervous system dysfunction, J. Neurol. Neurosurg. Psychiat. **24:**250, 1961.

37. Carpenter, M. B., Noback, C. R., and Moss, M. L.: The anterior choroidal artery: its origins, course, distribution, and variations, Arch. Neurol. Psychiat. **71:**714, 1954.

38. Clark, S. L.: Nerve endings in the chorioid plexus of the fourth ventricle, J. Comp. Neurol. **47:**1, 1928.

39. Clark, S. L.: Innervation of the blood vessels of the medulla and spinal cord, J. Comp. Neurol. **48:**247, 1929.

40. Cobb, S.: The cerebral circulation. XIII. The question of "end-arteries" of the brain and the mechanism of infarction, Arch. Neurol. Psychiat. **25:**273, 1931.

41. Collis, J. L.: The etiology of cerebral abscess as a complication of thoracic disease, J. Thorac. Surg. **13:**445, 1944.

42. Coman, D. R., and DeLong, R. P.: The role of the vertebral venous system in the metastasis of cancer to the spinal column, Cancer **4:**610, 1951.

43. Constans, J. P., Dilenge, D., and Jolivet, B.: Un cas de persistance d'une artère hypoglosse embryonnaire, Neurochirurgie **10:**297, 1964.

44. Critchley, M.: The anterior cerebral artery, and its syndromes, Brain **53:**120, 1930.

45. Dandy, W. E.: Lesions of the cranial nerves, J. Int. Coll. Surg. **2:**5, 1939.

46. Daniel, P. M.: Dawes, J. D. K., and Prichard, M. L.: Studies of the carotid rete and its associated arteries, Phil. Trans. Roy. Soc. Series B, **237:**173, 1953.

47. Davis, R. A., Wetzel, N., and Davis, L.: An analysis of the results of treatment of intracranial vascular lesions by carotid artery ligation, Ann. Surg. **143:**641, 1956.

48. DeVriese, B.: Sur la signification morphologique des artères cérébrales, Arch. Biol. **21:**357, 1905.

49. Dickmann, G. H., Pardal, C., Amezúa, L., and Zamboni, O.: Persistencia de la arteria trigeminal, Acta Neurochir. **17:**205, 1967.

50. Djindjian, R., Hurth, M., Bories, J., and Brunet, P.: L'artère trigéminale primitive (aspects artériographiques et signification à propos de 12 cas), Presse Med. **73:**2905, 1965.

51. Du Boulay, G. H.: Some observations on the natural history of intra-cranial aneurysms, Brit. J. Radiol. **38:**721, 1965.

52. Eadie, M. J., Jamieson, K. G., and Lennon, E. A.: Persisting carotid-basilar anastomosis, J. Neurol. Sci. **1:**501, 1964.

53. Evans, H. M.: The development of the vascular system. In Keibel, F., and Mall, F. P.: Manual of human embryology, Philadelphia, 1912, J. B. Lippincott Co., vol. 2, p. 570.

54. Fawcett, E., and Blachford, J. V.: The circle of Willis: an examination of 700 specimens, J. Anat. Physiol. **40:**63, 1905-1906.
55. Fay, T.: The cerebral vasculature, J.A.M.A. **84:**1727, 1925.
56. Fetterman, G. H., and Moran, T. J.: Anomalies of the circle of Willis in relation to cerebral softening, Arch. Path. **32:**251, 1941.
57. Fields, W. S.: The significance of persistent trigeminal artery, Radiology **91:**1095, 1968.
58. Fields, W. S., Bruetman, M. E., and Weibel, J.: Collateral circulation of the brain, Monogr. Surg. Sci. **2:**183, 1965.
59. Fisher, A. G. T.: A case of complete absence of both internal carotid arteries, with a preliminary note on the developmental history of the stapedial artery, J. Anat. **48:**37, 1914.
60. Fisher, A. G. T.: Sigmoid tortuosity of the internal carotid artery and its relation to tonsil and pharynx, Lancet **2:**128, 1915.
61. Fisher, C. M.: The circle of Willis: Anatomical variations, Vasc. Dis. **2:**99, 1965.
62. Fisher, C. M., Karnes, W. E., and Kubik, C. S.: Lateral medullary infarction—the pattern of vascular occlusion, J. Neuropath. Exp. Neurol. **20:**323, 1961.
63. Flynn, R. E.: External carotid origin of the dominant vertebral artery, J. Neurosurg. **29:**300, 1968.
64. Fogelholm, R., and Vuolio, M.: The collateral circulation via the ophthalmic artery in internal carotid artery thrombosis, Acta Neurol. Scand. **45:**78, 1969.
65. Foix, C., and Hillemand, P.: Les syndromes de l'artère cérébrale antérieure, Encéphale **20:**209, 1925.
66. Fotopulos, D.: Die Rolle der Arteria primitiva trigeminal persistans bei Karotisthrombose, Radiol. Diag. **4:**563, 1963.
67. Frugoni, P., Nori, A., Galligioni, F., and Giammusso, V.: Further considerations on the Bernasconi and Cassinari's artery and other meningeal rami of the internal carotid artery, Neurochirurgia **7:**18, 1964.
68. Gannon, W. E.: Malformation of the brain, Arch. Neurol. **6:**89, 1962.
69. Garland, H., Greenberg, J., and Harriman, D. G. F.: Infarction of the spinal cord, Brain **89:**645, 1966.
70. Gerlach, J., Jensen, H.-P., Spuler, H., and Viehweger, G.: Traumatic carotico-cavernous fistula combined with persisting primitive hypoglossal artery, J. Neurosurg. **20:**885, 1963.
71. Gessini, L., and Frugoni, P.: Considerazioni sulla persistenza dell'anastomosi carotidobasilare, Riv. Neurol. **24:**338, 1954. Cited by McCormick.[132]
72. Gibbs, E. L., and Gibbs, F. A.: The cross section areas of the vessels that form the torcular and the manner in which flow is distributed to the right and to the left lateral sinus, Anat. Rec. **59:**419, 1934.
73. Gillilan, L. A.: Observations on the anatomy of the cerebral blood vessels which may influence cerebral circulation, with clinical interpretations, Arch. Neurol. Psychiat. **72:**116, 1954.
74. Gillilan, L. A.: The arterial blood supply of the human spinal cord, J. Comp. Neurol. **110:**75, 1958.
75. Gillilan, L. A.: Significant superficial anastomoses in the arterial blood supply to the human brain, J. Comp. Neurol. **112:**55, 1959.
76. Gillilan, L. A.: The collateral circulation of the human orbit, Arch. Ophthal. **65:**684, 1961.
77. Gillilan, L. A.: Blood vessels, meninges, cerebrospinal fluid. In Crosby, E. C., Humphrey, T., and Lauer, E. W.: Correlative anatomy of the nervous system, New York, 1962, The Macmillan Co., p. 550.
78. Gillilan, L. A.: The correlation of the blood supply to the human brain stem with clinical brain stem lesions, J. Neuropath. Exp. Neurol. **23:**78, 1964.
79. Gillilan, L. A.: Veins of the spinal cord, Neurology **20:**860, 1970.
80. Gilmartin, D.: Hypoglossal artery associated with internal carotid stenosis, Brit. J. Radiol. **36:**849, 1963.
81. Gius, J. A., and Grier, D. H.: Venous adaptation following bilateral radical neck dissection with excision of the jugular veins, Surgery **28:**305, 1950.
82. Godinov, V. M.: The arterial system of the brain, Amer. J. Phys. Anthrop. **13:**359, 1929.
83. Griffiths, J. O., and Riggs, H. E.: Role of anomalies of the circle of Willis in production of cerebral vascular lesions: preliminary report, Arch. Neurol. Psychiat. **39:**1354, 1938.
84. Hale, A. R.: Circle of Willis. Functional concepts, old and new, Amer. Heart J. **60:**491, 1960.
85. Hamby, W. B.: Intracranial aneurysms, Springfield, Ill., 1952, Charles C Thomas, Publisher.
86. Handa, J., Meyer, J. S., Huber, P., and Yoshida, K.: Time course of development of cerebral collateral circulation, Vasc. Dis. **2:**271, 1965.
87. Harrison, C. R., and Hearn, J. B.: A new aspect of collateral circulation in occlusion of internal carotid artery, J. Neurosurg. **18:**542, 1961.
88. Harrison, C. R., and Luttrell, C.: Persistent carotid-basilar anastomosis, J. Neurosurg. **10:**205, 1953.
89. Harvey, S. C., and Burr, H. S.: The development of the meninges, Arch. Neurol. Psychiat. **15:**545, 1926.
90. Hasebe, K.: Arterien der Hirnbasis. In Adachi, B.: Das Arteriensystem der Japaner Kyoto, 1928, Maruzen Co., vol. 1, p. 111.
91. Hasenjäger, T.: Ein Beitrag zu den Abnormitäten des Circulus arteriosus Willisii, Zbl. Neurochir. **2:**34, 1937.
92. Hassler, O.: Blood supply to human spinal cord, Arch. Neurol. **15:**302, 1966.
93. Hassler, O.: Arterial pattern of human brainstem, Neurology **17:**368, 1967.
94. Henson, R. A., and Parsons, M.: Ischaemic lesions of the spinal cord: an illustrated review, Quart. J. Med. **36:**205, 1967.
95. Herlihy, W. F.: Revision of the venous sys-

tem: the role of the vertebral veins, Med. J. Aust. **1**:661, 1947.

96. Herren, R. Y., and Alexander, L.: Sulcal and intrinsic blood vessels of human spinal cord, Arch. Neurol. Psychiat. **41**:678, 1939.

97. Hindze, B., and Fedotowa, A.: Ein Fall von stark ausgeprägter Asymmetrie des Circulus arteriosus Willisii beim Menschen, Z. Morph. Anthrop. **29**:153, 1931.

98. Huang, Y. P., and Wolf, B. S.: Veins of the white matter of the cerebral hemispheres (the medullary veins), Amer. J. Roentgen. **92**:739, 1964.

99. Hutchinson, E. C., and Yates, P. O.: The cervical portion of the vertebral artery: a clinico-pathological study, Brain **79**:319, 1956.

100. Jackson, I. J., and Garza-Mercado, R.: Persistent carotid-basilar artery anastomosis: occasionally a possible cause of tic douloureux, Angiology **11**:103, 1960.

101. Jain, K. K.: Some observations on the anatomy of the middle cerebral artery, Canad. J. Surg. **7**:134, 1964.

102. Johanson, C.: The central veins and deep dural sinuses of the brain, Acta Radiol. Suppl. 107, 1954.

103. Kaplan, H. A.: The transcerebral venous system, Arch. Neurol. **1**:148, 1959.

104. Kaplan, H. A.: Collateral circulation of the brain, Neurology **11** (part 2): 9, 1961.

105. Kaplan, H. A., and Ford, D. H.: The brain vascular system, Amsterdam, 1966, Elsevier Publishing Co.

106. Kaplan, H. A., Rabiner, A. M., and Browder, J.: Anatomical study of the blood vessels of the brain. II. The perforating arteries of the base of the forebrain, Trans. Amer. Neurol. Ass. **79**:38, 1954.

107. Keen, J. A.: Absence of both internal carotid arteries, Clin. Proc. **4**:588, 1946.

108. Kelly, A. B.: Tortuosity of the internal carotid in relation to the pharynx, Proc. Roy. Soc. Med. **17**:1, 1924.

109. Kelly, A. B.: Tortuosity of the internal carotid in relation to the pharynx, J. Laryng. **40**:15, 1925.

110. Kepes, J., and Kernohan, J. W.: Persistent carotid-basilar anastomosis, J. Neuropath. Exp. Neurol. **17**:631, 1958.

111. Khodadad, G., and Putschar, W. G. J.: The cerebral arteries in cyclopia and arrhinencephaly, Acta Anat. **72**:12, 1969.

112. Kloss, K.: Persistierende Carotis-Basilaris-Anastomose als Ursache einer Subarachnoidalblutung, Zbl. Neurochir. **13**:166, 1953.

113. Kramer, S. P.: On the function of the circle of Willis, J. Exp. Med. **15**:348, 1912.

114. Krayenbühl, H., and Yaşargil, M. G.: Die zerebrale Angiographie, ed. 2, Stuttgart, 1965, Georg Thieme Verlag.

115. Krogman, W. M.: Growth of man, Tabulae Biologicae **20**:1, 1941.

116. Lagarde, C., Vigouroux, R., and Perrouty, P.: Agénésie terminale de la carotide interne anévrysme de la communicante antérieure, J. Radiol. Electr. **38**:939, 1957.

117. Lamb, J., and Morris, L.: The carotid-basilar artery: a report and discussion of five cases, Clin. Radiol. **12**:179, 1961.

118. Lecuire, J., Buffard, P., Goutelle, A., Dechaume, J. P., Michel, D., Rambaud, G., Gentil, J. P., and Verger, D.: Considérations anatomiques, cliniques et radiologiques à propos d'une artère hypoglosse, J. Radiol. Electr. **45**:217, 1965.

119. Leeds, N. E., and Abbott, K. H.: Collateral circulation in cerebrovascular disease in childhood via rete mirabile and perforating branches of anterior choroidal and posterior cerebral arteries, Radiology **85**:628, 1965.

120. Lehrer, H. Z.: Relative calibre of the cervical internal carotid artery: normal variation with the circle of Willis, Brain **91**:339, 1968.

121. Lepoire, J., Tridon, P., Montaut, J., Hepner, H., Renard, M., and Picard, L.: Malformations angiomateuses artério-artérilles du système carotidien, Neurochirurgie **15**:5, 1969.

122. Levenson, G. E., and Nelsen, O. E.: Experimentally induced variations in vitelline artery development and circulatory pattern in the early chick embryo, J. Morph. **123**:313, 1967.

123. Lhermitte, F., Gautier, J.-C., Poirier, J., and Tyrer, J. H.: Hypoplasia of the internal carotid artery, Neurology **18**:439, 1968.

124. Lie, T. A.: Congenital anomalies of the carotid arteries, Amsterdam, 1968, Excerpta Medica Foundation.

125. Liebow, A. A.: Situations which lead to changes in vascular patterns. In Hamilton, W. F., and Dow, P.: Handbook of physiology, Section 2, Circulation, Vol. 1, Baltimore, 1963, The Williams & Wilkins Co., p. 1251.

126. Lindenberg, R.: Compression of brain arteries as pathogenetic factor for tissue necroses and their areas of predilection, J. Neuropath. Exp. Neurol. **14**:223, 1955.

127. Lombardi, G., Passerini, A., and Migliavacca, F.: Intracavernous aneurysms of the internal carotid artery, Amer. J. Roentgen. **89**:361, 1963.

128. Lowrey, L. G.: Anomaly in the circle of Willis, due to absence of the right internal carotid artery, Anat. Rec. **10**:221, 1916.

129. Luccarelli, S., and De Ferrari, U.: Studio clinico-radiologico di un caso di origine anomala (della carotide esterna) dell'arteria vertebrale sinistra, Radiol. Med. **46**:963, 1960.

130. Madonick, M. J., and Ruskin, A. P.: Recurrent oculomotor paresis, Arch. Neurol. **6**:353, 1962.

131. Mall, F. P.: On the development of the blood-vessels of the brain in the human embryo, Amer. J. Anat. **4**:1, 1904-1905.

132. McCormick, W. F.: Vascular disorders of nervous tissue: anomalies, malformations, and aneurysms. In Bourne, G. H.: The structure and function of nervous tissue New York, 1969, Academic Press Inc., vol. 3, p. 537.

133. McCormick, W. F.: A unique anomaly of the intracranial arteries of man, Neurology **19**:77, 1969.

134. McCormick, W. F.: Personal communication, 1970.

135. McCullough, A. W.: Some anomalies of the cerebral arterial circle (of Willis) and related vessels, Anat. Rec. **142**:537, 1962.
136. McDonald, D. A., and Potter, J. M.: The distribution of blood to the brain, J. Physiol. **114**:356, 1951.
137. McMinn, R. M. H.: A case of non-union of the vertebral arteries, Anat. Rec. **116**:283, 1953.
138. McNaughton, F. L.: The innervation of the intracranial blood vessels and dural sinuses. In: The circulation of the brain and spinal cord, Ass. Res. Nerv. Ment. Dis. **18**:178, 1938.
139. Mettler, F. A.: Neuroanatomy, St. Louis, 1942, The C. V. Mosby Co.
140. Metz, H., Murray-Leslie, R. M., Bannister, R. G., Bull, J. W. D., and Marshall, J.: Kinking of the internal carotid artery in relation to cerebrovascular disease, Lancet **1**:424, 1961.
141. Meyer, H.-St., and Busch, G.: Karotido-basiläre Anastomose in Kombination mit multiplen Aneurysmen und weiteren Anomalien, Fortschr. Gebiete Roentgenstrahlen Nuklearmed. **92**:690, 1960.
142. Minagi, H., and Newton, T. H.: Carotid rete mirabile in man, Radiology **86**:100, 1966.
143. Moffat, D. B.: A case of persistence of the primitive olfactory artery, Anat. Anz. **121**:477, 1967.
144. Morris, A. A., and Peck, C. M.: Roentgenographic study of the variations in the normal anterior cerebral artery, Amer. J. Roentgen. **74**:818, 1955.
145. Morris, E. D., and Moffat, D. B.: Abnormal origin of the basilar artery from the cervical part of the internal carotid and its embryological significance, Anat. Rec. **125**:701, 1956.
146. Mount, L. A., and Taveras, J. M.: The results of surgical treatment of intracranial aneurysms as demonstrated by progress arteriography, J. Neurosurg. **13**:618, 1956.
147. Murtagh, F., Stauffer, H. M., and Harley, R. D.: A case of persistent carotid-basilar anastomosis associated with aneurysm of the homolateral middle cerebral artery manifested by oculomotor palsy, J. Neurosurg. **12**:46, 1955.
148. Nierling, D. A., Wollschlaeger, P. B., and Wollschlaeger, G.: Ascending pharyngeal-vertebral anastomoses, Amer. J. Roentgen. **98**:599, 1966.
149. Nishimoto, A., and Takeuchi, S.: Abnormal cerebrovascular network related to the internal carotid arteries, J. Neurosurg. **29**:255, 1968.
150. Oertel, O.: Über die Persistenz embryonaler Verbindungen zwischen der A. carotis interna und der A. vertebralis cerebralis, Anat. Anz. **55**:281, 1922.
151. Orr, A. E.: A rare anomaly of the carotid arteries (internal and external, J. Anat. Physiol. **41**:51, 1906.
152. Ostrowski, A. Z., Webster, J. E., and Gurdjian, E. S.: The proximal anterior cerebral artery: an anatomical study, Arch. Neurol. **3**:661, 1960.
153. Otomo, E.: The anterior choroidal artery, Arch. Neurol. **13**:656, 1965.
154. Ouchi, H., and Ohara, I.: Extracranial abnormalities of the vertebral artery detected by selective arteriography, J. Cardiovasc. Surg. **9**:250, 1968.
155. Padget, D. H.: The circle of Willis, its embryology and anatomy. In Dandy, W. E.: Intracranial arterial aneurysms, New York, 1944, Comstock Publishing Co., Inc., p. 67.
156. Padget, D. H.: The development of the cranial arteries in the human embryo, Contrib. Embryol. Carneg. Inst. **32**:205, 1948.
157. Padget, D. H.: The cranial venous system in man in reference to development, adult configuration, and relation to the arteries, Amer. J. Anat. **98**:307, 1956.
158. Padget, D. H.: The development of the cranial venous system in man, from the viewpoint of comparative anatomy, Contrib. Embryol. Carneg. Inst. **36**:79, 1957.
159. Pakula, H., and Szapiro, J.: Anatomical studies of the collateral blood supply to the brain and upper extremity, J. Neurosurg. **32**:171, 1970.
160. Pallie, W., and Samarasinghe, D. D.: A study in the quantification of the circle of Willis, Brain **85**:569, 1962.
161. Parker, J. C., and Gaede, J. T.: Occurrence of vascular anomalies in unilateral cerebral hypoplasia, Arch. Path. **90**:265, 1970.
162. Parkinson, D.: A surgical approach to the cavernous portion of the carotid artery: anatomical studies and case report, J. Neurosurg. **23**:474, 1965.
163. Parkinson, J., Bedford, D. E., and Almond, S.: The kinked carotid artery that simulates aneurysm, Brit. Heart J. **1**:345, 1939.
164. Passerini, A., and DeDonato, E.: Le anastomosi carotido-basilari, Radiol. Med. **48**:939, 1962.
165. Paul, H. A., Prill, A., Pilz, H., and Müller, D.: Cerebrale Funktionsstörungen bei persistierender A. primitiva trigemina, Deutsch. Z. Nervenheilk. **195**:283, 1969.
166. Penfield, W.: Intracerebral vascular nerves, Arch. Neurol. Psychiat. **27**:30, 1932.
167. Perese, D. M.: Superficial veins of the brain from a surgical point of view, J. Neurosurg. **17**:402, 1960.
168. Perryman, C. R., Gray, G. H., Brust, R. W., and Conlon, P. C.: Interesting aspects of cerebral angiography with emphasis on some unusual congenital variations, Amer. J. Roentgen. **89**:372, 1963.
169. Philippides, D., Montrieul, G., de Haynin, G., and Herrenschmidt, M.: Anévrysme de l'artère basilaire identifié par l'artériographie, Presse Med. **60**:1227, 1952.
170. Pitts, F. W.: Variations of collateral circulation in internal carotid occlusion, Neurology **12**:467, 1962.
171. Poblete, R., and Asenjo, A.: Anastomosis carotido-basilar por persistencia de la arteria trigeminal primitiva, Neurocirugia **11**:1, 1955.
172. Popa, G., and Fielding, U.: The vascular link

between the pituitary and the hypothalamus, Lancet **2**:238, 1930.

173. Quain, R.: Anatomy of the arteries, London, 1844, Taylor, and Walton, vol. 2, Cited by Lie.[124]

174. Quattlebaum, J. K., Upson, E. T., and Neville, R. L.: Stroke associated with elongation and kinking of the internal carotid artery: report of three cases treated by segmental resection of the carotid artery, Ann. Surg. **150**:824, 1959.

175. Riggs, H.: Discussion, Arch. Neurol. Psychiat. **72**:117, 1954.

176. Riggs, H. E., and Griffiths, J. O.: Anomalies of the circle of Willis in persons with nervous and mental disorders, Arch. Neurol. Psychiat. **39**:1353, 1938.

177. Riggs, H. E., and Rupp, C.: Variation in form of circle of Willis, Arch. Neurol. **8**:8, 1963.

178. Rogers, L.: The function of the circulus arteriosus of Willis, Brain **70**:171, 1947.

179. Romanul, F. C. A., and Abramowicz, A.: Changes in brain and pial vessels in arterial border zones, Arch. Neurol. **11**:40, 1964.

180. Rosegay, H., and Welch, K.: Peripheral collateral circulation between cerebral arteries, J. Neurosurg. **11**:363, 1954.

181. Rovira, M., and Barluenga, S.: Clinical and angiographic correlations in collateral brain circulation, Angiology **19**:110, 1968.

182. Rubinstein, H. S.: The anterior communicating artery in man, J. Neuropath. Exp. Neurol. **3**:196, 1944.

183. Rupprecht, A., and Scherzer, E.: Über die persistente Karotis-Basilaris-Verbindung, Fortschr. Gebiete Roentgenstrahlen Nuklearmed. **91**:196, 1959.

184. Sabin, F. R.: Preliminary note on the differentiation of angioblasts and the method by which they produce blood vessels, blood-plasma and red blood-cells as seen in the living chick, Anat. Rec. **13**:199, 1917.

185. Sabin, F. R.: Origin and development of the primitive vessels of the chick and of the pig, Contrib. Embryol. Carneg. Inst. **6**:61, 1917.

186. Saltzman, G.-F.: Patent primitive trigeminal artery studied by cerebral angiography, Acta. Radiol. **51**:329, 1959.

187. Samarasinghe, D. D.: The innervation of the cerebral arteries in the rat: an electron microscope study, J. Anat. **99**:815, 1965.

188. Samra, K., Scoville, W. B., and Yaghmai, M.: Anastomosis of carotid and basilar arteries. Persistent primitive trigeminal artery and hypoglossal artery: report of two cases, J. Neurosurg. **30**:622, 1969.

189. Saphir, O.: Anomalies of the circle of Willis with resulting encephalomalacia and cerebral hemorrhage, Amer. J. Path. **11**:775, 1935.

190. Sato, S.: An electron microscopic study on the innervation of the intracranial artery of the rat, Amer. J. Anat. **118**:873, 1966.

191. Schaerer, J. P.: Case of carotid-basilar anastomosis with multiple associated cerebrovascular anomalies, J. Neurosurg. **12**:62, 1955.

192. Schechter, M. M.: The occipital-vertebral anastomosis, J. Neurosurg. **21**:758, 1964.

193. Schiefer, W., and Walter, W.: Die Persistenz embryonaler Gefässe als Ursache von Blutungen des Hirns und seiner Häute, Acta Neurochir. **7**:53, 1959.

194. Schlesinger, B.: The venous drainage of the brain, with special reference to the Galenic system, Brain **62**:274, 1939.

195. Schlesinger, M. J.: Relation of anatomic pattern to pathologic conditions of the coronary arteries, Arch. Path. **30**:403, 1940.

196. Scott, H. S.: Carotid-basilar anastomosis—persistent hypoglossal artery, Brit. J. Radiol. **36**:847, 1963.

197. Sedzimir, C. B.: An angiographic test of collateral circulation through the anterior segment of the circle of Willis, J. Neurol. Neurosurg. Psychiat. **22**:64, 1959.

198. Seftel, D. M., Kolson, H., and Gordon, B. S.: Ruptured intracranial carotid artery aneurysm with fatal epistaxis, Arch. Otolaryng. **70**:52, 1959.

199. Seydel, H. G.: The diameters of the cerebral arteries of the human fetus, Anat. Rec. **150**:79, 1964.

200. Shellshear, J. L.: The basal arteries of the forebrain and their functional significance, J. Anat. **55**:27, 1920.

201. Shellshear, J. L.: The arterial supply of the cerebral cortex in the chimpanzee *(Anthropopithecus troglodytes)*, J. Anat. **65**:45, 1930.

202. Slade, H. W., and Weekley, R. D.: Diastasis of the optic nerve, J. Neurosurg. **14**:571, 1957.

203. Slany, A.: Anomalien des Circulus arteriosus Willisi in ihrer Beziehung zur Aneurysmenbildung an der Hirnbasis, Virch. Arch. **301**:62, 1938.

204. Smith, D. R., Ferry, D. J., and Kempe, L. G.: The tentorial artery: Its diagnostic significance, Acta Neurochir. **21**:57, 1969.

205. Smith, K. R., Nelson, J. S., and Dooley, J. M.: Bilateral "hypoplasia" of the internal carotid arteries, Neurology **18**:1149, 1968.

206. Solnitzky, O.: Abnormalities of the circle of Willis in relation to collateral cerebral circulation, Anat. Rec. **142**:281, 1962.

207. Stehbens, W. E.: Cerebral aneurysm and congenital abnormalities, Aust. Ann. Med. **11**:102, 1962.

208. Stehbens, W. E.: Aneurysms and anatomical variation of cerebral arteries, Arch. Path. **75**:45, 1963.

209. Stehbens, W. E.: Unpublished observations.

210. Stenvers, H. W., Bannenburg, P. M., and Lenshoek, C. H.: Anastomose carotido-basilaire persistante (artériographie et autopsie), Rev. Neurol. **89**:575, 1953.

211. Stöhr, P.: Nerves of the blood vessels, heart, meninges, digestive tract, and urinary bladder. In Penfield, W.: Cytology of cellular pathology of nervous system, New York, 1932, Paul C. Hoeber Inc., vol. 2, p. 381.

212. Stopford, J. S. B.: The arteries of the pons and medulla oblongata, J. Anat. Physiol. **50**:131, 1915.

213. Streeter, G. L.: The developmental alterations in the vascular system of the brain of the

human embryo, Contrib. Embryol. Carneg. Inst. **8**:5, 1918.

214. Suh, T. H., and Alexander, L.: Vascular system of the human spinal cord, Arch. Neurol. Psychiat. **41**:659, 1939.

215. Sunderland, S.: An anomalous anastomosis between the internal carotid and basilar arteries, Aust. New Zeal. J. Surg. **11**:140, 1941.

216. Sunderland, S.: The arterial relations of the internal auditory meatus, Brain **68**:23, 1945.

217. Sunderland, S.: Neurovascular relations and anomalies at the base of the brain, J. Neurol. Psychiat. **11**:243, 1948.

218. Sunderland, S.: The tentorial notch and complications produced by herniations of the brain through that aperture, Brit. J. Surg. **45**:422, 1957-8.

219. Sutton, D.: Anomalous carotid-basilar anastomosis, Brit. J. Radiol. **23**:617, 1950.

220. Suzuki, J., and Takaku, A.: Cerebrovascular "moyamoya" disease, Arch. Neurol. **20**:288, 1969.

221. Taveras, J. M., and Wood, E. H.: Diagnostic neuroradiology, Baltimore, 1964, The Williams & Wilkins Co.

222. Thomas, R. G.: Persistent primitive trigeminal artery (carotid-basilar anastomosis), Brit. J. Radiol. **34**:672, 1961.

223. Toole, J. F., and Patel, A. N.: Cerebrovascular disorders, New York, 1967, McGraw-Hill Book Co.

224. Tureen, L. L.: Circulation of the spinal cord and the effect of vascular occlusion. In: The circulation of the brain and spinal cord, Ass. Res. Nerv. Ment. Dis. **18**:394, 1938.

225. Turnbull, I.: Agenesis of the internal carotid artery, Neurology **12**:588, 1962.

226. Turnbull, I. M., Brieg, A., and Hassler, O.: Blood supply of cervical spinal cord in man. A microangiographic study, J. Neurosurg. **24**:951, 1966.

227. Turner, R. S.: A comparison of theoretical with observed angles between the vertebral arteries at their junction to form the basilar, Anat. Rec. **129**:243, 1957.

228. Udvarhelyi, G. B., and Lai, M.: Subarachnoid haemorrhage due to rupture of an aneurysm on a persistent left hypoglossal artery, Brit. J. Radiol. **36**:843, 1963.

229. Vander Eecken, H. M., Fisher, M., and Adams, R. D.: The arterial anastomoses of the human brain and their importance in the delimitation of human brain infarction, J. Neuropath. Exp. Neurol. **11**:91, 1952.

230. Vander Eecken, H. M., and Adams, R. D.: The anatomy and functional significance of the meningeal arterial anastomoses of the human brain, J. Neuropath. Exp. Neurol. **12**:132, 1953.

231. Vander Eecken, H. M.: The anastomoses between the leptomeningeal arteries of the brain, Springfield, Ill., 1959, Charles C Thomas, Publisher.

232. Vander Eecken, H.: Discussion of "Collateral circulation of the brain", Neurology **11** (part 2):16, 1961.

233. Vogel, F. S.: The association of vascular anomalies with anencephaly, Amer. J. Path. **34**:169, 1958.

234. Vogel, F. S., and McClenahan, J. L.: Anomalies of major cerebral arteries associated with congenital malformations of the brain, Trans. Amer. Neurol. Ass. **77**:132, 1952.

235. Vogel, F. S., and McClenahan, J. L.: Anomalies of major cerebral arteries associated with congenital malformations of the brain, Amer. J. Path. **28**:701, 1952.

236. von Mitterwallner, F.: Variationsstatische Untersuchungen an den basalen Hirngefässe, Acta Anat. **24**:51, 1955.

237. Weibel, J., and Fields, W. S.: Tortuosity, coiling, and kinking of the internal carotid artery. 1. Etiology and radiographic anatomy, Neurology **15**:7, 1965.

238. Weidner, W., Hanafee, W., and **Markham**, C. H.: Intracranial collateral circulation via leptomeningeal and rete mirabile anastomoses, Neurology **15**:39, 1965.

239. White, J. C., Smithwick, R. H., and Simeone, F. A.: The autonomic nervous system, New York, 1952, The Macmillan Co.

240. Wiedenmann, O., and Hipp, E.: Abnorme Kommunikationen zwischen dem Versorgungsgebiet der Arteria carotis interna und der Arteria basilaris (karotido-basilare Anastomosen), Fortschr. Roentgenstr. **91**:350, 1959.

241. Williams, D. J.: The origin of the posterior cerebral artery, Brain **59**:175, 1936.

242. Willis, T.: Cerebri anatome cui accessit nervorum descriptio, London, 1664.

243. Wilson, S. A. K., and Wolfsohn. J. M.: Organic nervous disease in identical twins, Arch. Neurol. Psychiat. **21**:477, 1929.

244. Windle, B. C. A.: On the arteries forming the circle of Willis, J. Anat. Physiol. **22**:289, 1888.

245. Wise, B. L., and Palubinskas, A. J.: Persistent trigeminal artery (carotid-basilar anastomosis), J. Neurosurg. **21**:199, 1964.

246. Wolf, B. S., Huang, Y. P., and Newman, C. M.: The superficial Sylvian venous drainage system, Amer. J. Roentgen. **89**:398, 1963.

247. Wolf, B. S., Huang, Y. P., and Newman, C. M.: The lateral anastomotic mesencephalic vein and other variations in drainage of the basal cerebral vein, Amer. J. Roentgen. **89**:411, 1963.

248. Wolff, H. G.: The cerebral blood vessels—anatomical principles. In: The circulation of the brain and spinal cord, Ass. Res. Nerv. Ment. Dis. **18**:29, 1938.

249. Wolff, H. G.: Headache and other head pain, New York, 1963, Oxford University Press.

250. Wollschlaeger, G., and Wollschlaeger, P. B.: The primitive trigeminal artery as seen angiographically and at postmortem examination, Amer. J. Roentgen. **92**:761, 1964.

251. Wolpert, S. M.: The trigeminal artery and associated aneurysms, Neurology **16**:610, 1966.

252. Woodhall, B.: Variations of the cranial venous sinuses in the region of the torcular Herophili, Arch. Surg. **33**:297, 1936.

253. Zimmerman, H. B., and Farrell, W. J.: Cervical vertebral erosion caused by vertebral artery tortuosity, Amer. J. Roentgen. **108**:767, 1970.

2 / Structure and pathophysiology

Structure of the cerebral blood vessels

Unique macroscopic and microscopic features distinguish cerebral blood vessels from extracranial vessels of comparable size.

Macroscopic features

The lumen of the internal carotid artery mostly in the cavernous and intracranial segments tapers despite the absence of significant branchings prior to its termination. In normal brains of young adults, the cerebral arteries are easily dissected for display and they differ from those of the viscera (spleen, kidney, liver, and lungs), in which the artery enters at the hilum and ramifies, fanning out in arboreal fashion to supply the organ. The cerebral arteries, once attaining the base of the brain, spread out over its surface to run a sinuous course in the sulci and fissures. The arteries tend to be long, thin, and sinuous (Fig. 1-1), diameters diminishing little over long distances. Small vessels penetrate the brain tissue. Large vessels are confined to the cerebrospinal fluid of the subarachnoid space and cisterns.

The arteries of the young possess remarkably thin walls, much more transparent than those of extracranial vessels. Consequently, degenerative changes are readily perceived. Atherosclerotic arteries of older individuals are less transparent. Unlike extracranial and meningeal vessels, the cerebral arteries are devoid of venae comitantes, although intracerebral arteries may have one or two small veins in the same Virchow-Robin space. Drainage of blood is via thin superficial veins emptying primarily into the dural venous sinuses. The deeper portions of the cerebrum drain via the deep transcerebral veins to subependymal collecting veins, the largest vessels within the brain parenchyma and thence to the great cerebral vein of Galen.

The spinal vasculature is basically similar, with arteries and veins coursing in the subarachnoid space and anterior median fissure. Small vessels only enter the cord parenchyma.

Microscopic structure of the arteries

Cerebral arteries are of the muscular variety. Their walls consist of the (tunica) intima, (tunica) media, and the (tunica) adventitia. At birth, the intima is thin and consists of a layer of endothelial cells and a well-developed internal elastic lamina. The endothelium, the same morphologically as elsewhere, consists of a layer of flattened spindle-shaped cells, mostly orientated in the same axis as the artery. The internal elastic lamina seems to be thicker than in extracranial arteries of comparable size.[239] It is fenestrated, the fenestrae being recognizable only in oblique or tangential sections of the lamina. The round or oval fenestrae are relatively evenly distributed holes mostly 2 to 3 μ in diameter (range, 1 to 8 μ).[208] Not infrequently, two are close together or a fenestra is partitioned by cross fibers. The membrane, apart from the fenestrae, is fairly homogeneous, although in some small vessels the lamina appears to have a basic network of more heavily stained fibers. Small cerebral arteries may retain this type of intima into advanced adulthood despite severe atherosclerotic change elsewhere. Intimal thickenings occur at bifurcations, branchings, and sites of union (see Chapter 3).

The width of the media from the cervical to the intracranial segment of the internal carotid gradually reduces slightly. The media of cerebral arteries consists of up to 20 circular muscle layers and its over-all thickness is less than that of extracerebral arteries. [9,220] The muscle fibers pursue a slightly spiral course with a small angle of helix varying from vessel to vessel.[220] This spiral arrangement, of obscure significance, is said to continue uninterrupted into the large branches. The structure at bifurcations was not discussed. Some longitudinally arranged muscle fibers occur in the outer media. Reticulin fibers ensheath individual muscle fibers,[129] and shallow indentations of adventitial collagen (mainly in longitudinal rather than transverse section) extend into the outer part of the media at irregular intervals, dividing it, and imparting a scalloped appearance to its outer edge.

There is much less elastica in the media than in other arteries of comparable size, and fibrils are delicate. The width of the adventitia is less than in comparable systemic arteries (Fig. 2-1). It is composed of collagen in which both reticulin and elastic tissue fibers may be demonstrated. The collagen is less dense in the outermost part of the adventitia, and there is no perivascular supporting tissue and very little elastica. In the adventitia of extracranial ar-teries, the elastic tissue is prominent, concentrated mostly in the inner portion, consists of fibrils and laminae, and is referred to as the external elastic lamina. Cerebral arteries have no external elastic lamina and only a few small fine elastic fibers branching and circularly disposed in the thin adventitia. Meningeal arteries in the dura mater possess more elastic tissue in their adventitia than cerebral arteries.

In the arterial walls of babies, children, and many adults,[208] no vasa vasorum will be found, except for small branches that, as serial sections disclose neither ramify or course in the wall, pass through to supply a perivascular nerve. In man, cerebral arteries do not ordinarily possess vasa vasorum until the development of thickened or atherosclerotic walls. They are then often visible to the naked eye. Winternitz and associates[238] were unable to demonstrate vasa vasorum by their injection technique in undiseased vessels of young humans. They only presumed them to be present for they were demonstrated traversing unaffected segments of sclerotic arteries to reach adjacent diseased foci.

Nerve bundles are really perivascular and course the outermost surface of the ad-

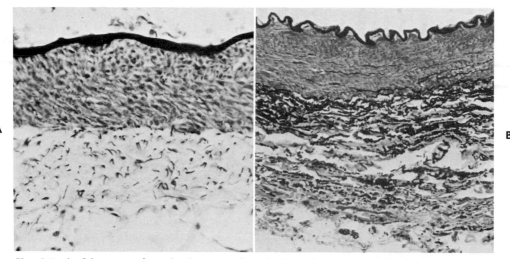

Fig. 2-1. Architecture of cerebral artery of an infant, **A,** contrasts with that of a mesenteric artery of comparable size, **B.** Note scanty thin black elastic fibrils in the adventitia of **A** and abundant elastica in thick adventitia of **B.** There are also a few elastic fibrils visible in media of **B.** (Verhoeff's stain; **A,** ×300; **B,** ×150.)

ventitia of arteries. Some small branches enter the adventitia but cannot be followed further by ordinary light microscopy without special stains.

The structural differences between cerebral arteries and extracranial vessels lie essentially in the distribution of elastic tissue, the thin adventitia, and a somewhat thinner media and less support from perivascular tissues. Triepel[231] thought transition from extracranial to intracranial architecture took place in the posterior fossa near the level of the union of the vertebral arteries to form the basilar, but age and atherosclerotic changes being poorly understood confused him. In infants, no transition zones can be demonstrated at the vertebrobasilar junction. In structure, the intracranial segments of the vertebral and cerebellar arteries are similar to the basilar and other cerebral arteries. When the common carotid and internal carotid arteries are dissected out entirely, cut into segments, and sectioned longitudinally, there is no abrupt transition. Near the bifurcation of the common carotid artery is a gradual or patchy diminution of the elastica in the media and a gradual change from an elastic to a more muscular type of artery. On ascending, there is less elastica in the media and a greater concentration in the adventitia. Traversing the temporal bone, the adventitia is thick with little elastica in this external coat. The media becomes somewhat thinner and the internal elastic lamina more prominent. In the cavernous segment, the slightly thicker adventitia contains a little more elastica than the cerebral segment beyond. A similar gradual transition takes place in the vertebral arteries. Extracranial segments have a thick adventitia with more elastica than is usual in intracranial arteries. The lowest portion of the intracranial segment of the vertebral artery has a slightly larger amount of adventitial elastica. Maximow and Bloom[129] suggested that the structural differences arise because intracranial vessels are not subjected to external pressures or tension. Hassler[83] found that medial

thickening occurred in rabbits when part of the cranial vault was removed. Other structural features were apparently unaltered. The unique structure possibly subserves a special function or requirement exacted only in the skull where the arterial circulation seems to be designed (anatomically and structurally) to obviate the effect of systolic pulsations on the brain or its functions. Wolff[239] concluded that the elastic tissue, being concentrated in the internal elastic lamina, adds rigidity to the cerebral arteries. The media and the adventitia are relatively free of elastic tissue and would not be rigid. This arrangement would greatly dampen systolic pulsations, whereas extracranial arteries with the elastica interspersed throughout the wall possess little shock-absorbing quality. However, the relative thickness of the internal elastic lamina of cerebral arteries has been exaggerated and the functional significance of the specialized architecture remains unresolved.

Medial discontinuities or gaps (defects). Forbus[66] drew attention to discontinuities or gaps in the muscle coat at arterial bifurcations naming them quite inappropriately "medial defects." This misleading term has been partly responsible for the perpetuation of the inadequately substantiated "congenital" or "developmental" hypothesis of the etiology of cerebral aneurysms. The terms "medial gap" or "discontinuity" are more apt as neither infers a specific function or etiology. The term "medial defect" implies a mechanical or structural weakness of the wall, which Forbus[66] believed he proved by finding a medial gap in a stillborn infant. Most authors have accepted his unscientific conclusion. Medial gaps have been assumed to be *loci minoris resistentiae* where arterial aneurysms are liable to occur.

In the infant, medial gaps are wedge-shaped adventitial invaginations into the media, with the apex coming briefly into contact with the internal elastic lamina (Fig. 2-2). They may be seen in only a few serial sections of a fork. Muscle at the edge

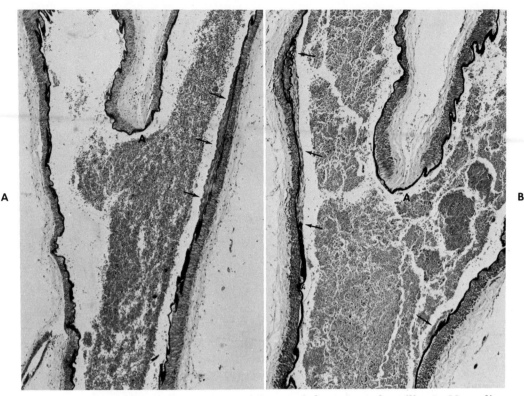

Fig. 2-2. Middle cerebral arterial forks of human infant, **A,** and gorilla, **B.** Note discontinuities of media at *A* and the lateral angle pads (arrows). Virtually no intimal thickening is present at the apices. Note the structural similarity between **A** and **B.** (Verhoeff's stain, ×38.)

of the gap is usually sharply delimited and may taper. The collagen within the medial gap runs longitudinally along the distal sides of the branches and the elastic fibrils are cut transversely. No vasa vasorum or nervi vasorum enter the medial gap. The amount of adventitia and the density of the

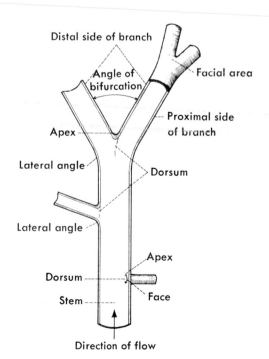

Fig. 2-3. Nomenclature for anatomical sites about the forks of vessels. Apex is the carina where axial stream of blood impinges on the vessel wall at the bifurcation. Apical angle is that subtended by distal sides of daughter branches, and lateral angles are those between proximal side of branches and parent stem. The face is that area on uppermost part of the stem near fork and between entrances to branches. Dorsum is the corresponding area on reverse side of fork. (From Stehbens, W. E.: The renal artery in normal and cholesterol-fed rabbits, Amer. J. Path. 43:969, 1963.)

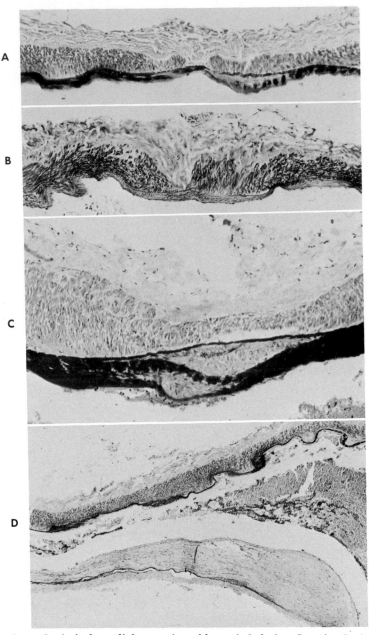

Fig. 2-4. A to **C,** Apical medial gaps in wide-angled forks. Gap in **C** (male aged 30 years) is partial only and adventitia is torn (artifact). In the anterior cerebral artery at its origin, **D,** the lateral angle pad is large and extends distally along proximal side, whereas intima is not thickened on distal (upper) side of vessel. A large lateral angle defect extends almost the full length of this lateral pad, except for small remnants of muscle external to the internal elastic lamina. Note elastic tissue degeneration in **A** and **C.** (Verhoeff's satin, **A, C,** and Mallory's phosphotungstic acid–hematoxylin, **C, D; A** to **C,** ×120; **D,** ×60.)

collagen in the apices of bifurcations vary. In older individuals, the medial gap is generally wider and easily found. It is more distinct and involves the apex (Fig. 2-3) to a greater depth than in the infant. Collagen also is more dense and the media at the edge or in the thinned segment of a partial medial gap exhibits fibrosis. In small arteries, the lateral angle gaps are similar to those at the apex. In larger arteries, lateral angle gaps are more extensive (Fig. 2-4) than apical gaps and appear to develop by a process of thinning of the media with simultaneous replacement by adventitial tissue. Often fibrosis and tapering of the media are prominent and the overlying lateral angle pad is deep. A transverse section from this area may, with the eccentrically thickened or frankly atherosclerotic intima, give the appearance of pressure atrophy of the media. Medial fibrosis, so prevalent as age advances and apparent first in the subintimal zone, often complicates the partial medial gaps. Lipophages, evidence of atherosclerosis, can affect both the media and adventitia of the cerebral arteries but do not extend into medial discontinuities.

Forbus[66] found medial gaps at forks and lateral branchings in 25 of 33 cases studied by random sections. They were found in the coronary arteries of 2 of 9 patients and the frequency was similar in mesenteric arteries. No difference was found between adults and children. Medial gaps have been reported in isolated patients with cerebral aneurysms where their very presence was considered adequate confirmation of a developmental origin of the aneurysm. Tuthill[233] put forward the largely ignored theory that medial gaps were embedding artefacts caused by twisting of the vessels.

Glynn[72] made the first significant attempt to evaluate the role of the medial defect in the pathogenesis of cerebral aneurysms. He examined, by random sectioning, arterial forks from circles of Willis both with and without aneurysms. Combining his results with those of Forbus,[66] he concluded that medial gaps were present in 79% of cases, that they were more frequent in older individuals than in the young, and that factors responsible for their appearance must be sought in postnatal influences.

Carmichael's[26] study of arterial forks depended on macroscopic staining to demonstrate areas of apical thinning that are acquired preaneurysmal lesions.[211] He mistook these preaneurysmal lesions for the medial gaps of Forbus, clearly differentiated from each other since.[211] Later Hassler[83] relying solely on the stereoscopic examination of stained arterial forks studied medial gaps. He believed them to be more prevalent in patients with cerebral aneurysms or polycystic kidneys, but conclusions drawn from inexact techniques need confirmation by the histological study of forks by serial sections, a much more satisfactory method.

In the most comprehensive study of medial gaps, Stehbens[203,204,211] utilized the serial section technique. Medial gaps at the apex were much more frequent in the middle cerebral than in the internal carotid artery, and those at the lateral angle (for nomenclature see Fig. 2-3) were much more frequent in the internal carotid than in the middle cerebral artery (Table 2-1). Lateral angles often exhibited a medial gap when none was present at the apex. Medial gaps were more frequent in acute angles than in obtuse angles, which explains their higher frequency in the middle cerebral bifurcation than in the internal carotid. In the internal carotid artery, lateral gaps when present were found predominantly in the acute angle subtended by the internal carotid and the anterior cerebral rather than in the wider obtuse angle formed with the middle cerebral.[204]

Medial gaps also occur at the basilar bifurcation and at other forks of cerebral, cerebellar, and spinal arteries. In arterial fenestrations or short lengths of duplication, they are found at both ends of the luminal septum. They are common both at the origin of small vessels where the adventitia forms a collarlike sheath around the

Table 2-1. Frequency of medial gaps* in the internal carotid and middle cerebral arteries in man†

Artery	Age group	Number of forks examined	Number of forks with:			
			Complete apical gaps	Partial apical gaps	No apical gaps present	Complete lateral angle gaps
Internal carotid	Under 1 year	35	12 (34.3%)	12	11	1 (2.9%)
	Over 6 years	89	69 (77.7%)	12	8	75 (84.3%)
	All ages	124	81 (65.3%)	24	19	76 (61%)
Middle cerebral	Under 1 year	54	47 (87.0%)	5	2	0
	Over 6 years	83	82 (98.2%)	1	0	18 (21.7%)
	All ages	137	129 (94.2%)	6	2	18 (3.1%)

*A medial gap is complete when the media is completely replaced at one point by the inward extention of the adventitia to the intima. It is partial when the media is incompletely replaced, usually only thinned by the adventitial invagination.[204]
†Adapted from Stehbens, W. E.: Medial defects of the cerebral arteries of man, J. Path. Bact. **78:**179, 1959.

vessel as it traverses the media of the parent trunk and at forks of small peripheral vessels.[204] Medial gaps at the apex of forks increase in number with age quite apart from any qualitative differences, whereas the lateral angle gaps, which Forbus[66] thought the most rare, are not only very common but are usually acquired after birth (Table 2-1). Not one was found in a fetus or infant under 6 months of age.[204]

Smith and Windsor[199] sectioned semiserially 509 bifurcations of cerebral arteries of all sizes from 17 newborn or stillborn infants and found medial gaps in only 32.3% of the forks. The frequency increased with the size of the vessels, but in arteries more than 0.5 mm. in diameter, medial gaps were found in 38.5%. Whether all of the 17 stillborn or newborn infants had medial gaps was not stated nor was the presence of medial gaps related to the common sites for aneurysms. Medial gaps were allegedly found unrelated to bifurcations or branchings. However, in more extensive studies of human and animal arterial forks by the serial section technique, medial gaps of Forbus were always found in association with bifurcations or branchings.[203,204,211] Crompton[35] made a study of medial defects in human cerebral arteries by examining sections at five different levels in each fork and, even with this unsatisfactory tech-

nique, found little resemblance between the distribution of medial gaps and aneurysms on the various arteries.

Medial gaps have been demonstrated with relative ease despite the use of nonserial sections. The most significant finding is that in 48 subjects in which at least four arterial forks were examined by using serial sections, medial gaps at the apex were found in every instance; so these muscle gaps in the media seem to be rarely if ever absent in human cerebral arteries.[204]

In noncerebral arteries, their presence has been confirmed in coronary, mesenteric, renal, and splenic arteries.[66,85,204] Hassler[65,66] found them frequently in these and meningeal arteries but did not find medial gaps in elastic arteries.

Medial gaps have been demonstrated in the cerebral arteries of the dog, horse, sheep,[203] pig,[101] rabbit, cow,[83] chimpanzee, and gorilla[210] (Fig. 2-2). Du Boulay[46] found complete medial gaps in nine of 20 mammals and in four of 48 birds and also saw partial medial gaps. Crompton[36] examined 23 different captive mammalian species (25 animals in all). He found that the media was thicker than in man with no lateral medial gaps whatsoever, but apical medial gaps were demonstrated in all but one animal. His failure to locate intimal pads and elastic tissue degeneration in many of the animals indicates that serial sections were not used.

Large numbers of cerebral arterial forks from a limited number of animals were examined for medial gaps, and as in man, when serial sections of at least four cerebral arterial forks from any mammal were taken, medial gaps were always found.[210] In 115 forks from six dogs, medial gaps were found in 85 (73.9%). In a horse, they were present in all but one of 30 forks.[203] Lower frequencies in other reports appear to depend on the technique used. In extracranial arteries of other animals only one study of medial gaps has been reported.[213] In 36 rabbits, 58 major renal arterial forks were examined by serial section, and 31 (86%) had a complete medial gap on one or both sides. In the remaining five animals, four had a partial gap on one or both sides.[213] Medial gaps were found in random sections of lung, kidney, and heart in several rabbits and in the coronary and mesenteric arteries of a gorilla.[210] It must be concluded that medial gaps are probably universal in the mammal and certainly in man. Morphologically, medial gaps in other animals are identical to those in man. Those in extracranial arteries have considerably more elastica in the adventitial wedge as is consistent with the structure of such vessels. Their functional significance remains uncertain despite a surfeit of theories.

When Forbus[66] introduced the term "medial defect," he assumed there was a deficiency inherent in the medial gap. He pointed out that in aortic development the mesenchyme condenses to form the media about the primitive endothelial tube but stops abruptly at the origin of the aortic segmental branches. Undifferentiated mesenchymal cells later develop as a sheath about the branches independently of the then mature aortic muscle coat. He thought medial gaps or defects resulted from failure of the muscle coats of the aorta and its branches to fuse. However, this sequence of events has never been shown to occur either in the aorta where

medial gaps have not been demonstrated or in cerebral arteries. It is incontrovertible that medial gaps at the apices are often acquired and probably all those at the lateral angles develop postnatally. Such fact detracts considerably from Forbus's hypothesis of a congenital origin. Glynn[72] demonstrated post mortem that medial gaps and areas of the arterial wall from which much of the media had been removed, were capable of withstanding pressures up to 500 mm. Hg. The experiment is unphysiological and a time factor must be considered, but no shred of evidence suggests that medial gaps in themselves are areas of undue weakness in the arterial wall. Moreover, the histological appearance of tissues whether of collagen or elastica gives no accurate indication of their tensile strength. Neither is the apex a proved site of structural weakness caused by the configuration of the bifurcation. Blair[14] found the inherent weakness of branched steel pipes lay in the region of the face and dorsum rather than the apex. Blair's findings need not be applicable to arterial bifurcations, but it can be stated with certainty that no reason exists for belief in the existence of an "inherent" weakness. Hassler's[84] suggestion that medial gaps might rupture and account for unexplained extradural, subdural, and subarachnoid hemorrhage is completely unfounded.

Bremer[17] believed that the adjacent distal walls of the two branches provided mutual support at the apex and that the adventitial wedge was a reinforcement similar to the sharp bow of a boat. As medial gaps are more frequent at acute angles than at forks with wide angles, it seems likely that mechanical factors are responsible at least in part for their occurrence.[204] Hassler[86] reported an increase in their size and aneurysmal evaginations occurring after unilateral carotid ligation in rabbits. His findings are at variance with the experience in man in whom widespread use of carotid ligation has not been complicated by aneurysm formation. Du Boulay[46,47] considered that medial gaps maintained flow through branches when the parent vessel contracted, with their function being of physiological importance. The absence of a distinct nerve supply argues against a sensory function. The increase in the frequency and size of medial gaps after birth suggests they may be degenerative lesions,[204] but we know little of such pathological changes in plain muscle. The explanations provided by Bremer[17] and Du Boulay[47] seem to be plausible.

The role of medial gaps in the pathogenesis of arterial aneurysms is discussed in Chapter 9. That their involvement by aneurysms is only fortuitous is strongly supported by differences in anatomical distribution[210,212] and by the histological study of early aneurysmal formation.[211]

Hassler compared medial gaps of short-term hypertensive rabbits with those in control rabbits and animals subjected to hypertension and then relieved of the hyperpiesis. He concluded that the area of the medial gaps of the hypertensive animals, larger in extent than in control animals, was not reversed by relieving the hypertension. He failed to specify how three-dimensional measurements were made from serial sections nor did he take into account the angle of bifurcation, a feature long known to be of importance in the size of medial discontinuities.[204]

Ultrastructure of cerebral arteries. Ultrastructural studies of blood vessels have been primarily restricted to extracranial vessels, no doubt because of the relative inaccessibility of the brain and spinal cord and the necessity for rapid fixation. Studies have been limited in number and scope, and for the most part quality and high resolution have been lacking, but recent improvements in electron microscopic techniques should ensure interesting results in any subsequent studies of the cerebral circulation.

The encephalic arteries are lined by a layer of flattened spindle-shaped endothelial cells somewhat thicker than that of capillary endothelium. Intercellular gaps or fenestrations are not seen. The nuclei are centrally situated and the cytoplasm contains the usual complement of cytoplasmic organelles. Endoplasmic reticulum is not abundant. Some may be dilated and contain amorphous material of medium density. The micropinocytotic vesicles of Palade[149] are not numerous and only occasional coated micropinocytotic vesicles are present.[214] Mitochondria and membrane-bound electron-dense lysomal structures are seldom met.[38] Tight junctions are presumed to be present between adjoining endothelial cells, which may show some overlapping or interdigitation. Cytoplasmic fibrils, often in bundles, lie mostly in the basal portion of the cytoplasm and could be related to half desmosomes, which have not as yet been studied in cerebral arteries. Microtubular bodies[215] occur sporadically.[97]

Beneath the endothelium, fine granular or fibrillary material of moderate density with the appearance of ground substance and unusually thick multilaminated basement membrane material has been described.[38,59] No high-resolution ultrastructural studies have been made of the extracellular material in the intima of cerebral arteries to correlate it with the light microscopic appearance. Nor have the intimal pads at arterial forks been studied. Smooth muscle cells, collagen, and elastic fibrils occur with an occasional fibroblast.[59] The internal elastic lamina is thick and has a fairly smooth external but very irregular inner surface. Fenestrae, readily recognizable[38] as interruptions in the elastic lamina, may contain connective tissue or cell profiles. In the young, the intima, except at bifurcations, is quite thin.

The media contains a fairly uniformly packed mass of muscle cells each surrounded by basement membrane and intervening collagen. Little elastic tissue is present and there are no nerve fibers. Muscle fibers similar to those elsewhere are surrounded by a basement membrane to which microfibrils and collagen fibers appear to be attached and which may be common to more than one muscle cell.[38] Their fine structure has often been described[38,155] although the function of the cytoplasmic densities, caveolae, and pinocytotic vesicles is unknown. An occasional lipid droplet occurs in the smooth muscle cells even in the young.[38]

The tunica adventitia primarily consists of collagen fibers interspersed with thin elongated fibrocytes and cells like the interstitial cells of Cajal.[38] There are nerve fibers in or on the adventitia of the large encephalic arteries.[39] Myelinated and nonmyelinated fibers are associated with both cerebral and cerebellar arteries.[38,39] Efferent or adrenergic nerve endings containing vesicles with an electron-dense core have been recognized, but there is doubt concerning afferent endings.[39] As yet nerves have not been found about human intracerebral vessels. The outer boundary of the adventitia is of mesothelial-like cells not yet investigated in man. Presuming it to be a fibroblast, Dahl and associates[38] illustrated such a cell with a continuous basement membrane. Though studies are limited in detail,[97,155] the fine structure of the cerebral arteries in other animals is remarkably similar to that of human vessels. Fat cells, though never observed by light microscopy nor in other species, have been reported in the adventitia of the cerebral arteries of pigs.[97]

Both myelinated and nonmyelinated nerve fibers have been found in or on the adventitia of the large cerebral arteries of the rat.[183] No nerves accompany the pial arterioles or intracerebral vessels. Sato[184] contended myelinated nerve fibers were restricted to the internal carotid artery and the proximal portion of the basilar. He found unmyelinated fibers accompanying a few perforating vessels of the internal carotid and middle cerebral arteries even after they had penetrated the brain parenchyma. Nelson and Rennels[143] found nerves in the adventitia of intracranial arteries of the cat, some of the nerves making neuromuscular contacts with the outermost layer of muscle fibers of the media, the minimum distance of separation being 800 Å. The nerve endings contained granular and agranular vesicles of 500 Å in diameter and a few mitochondria.

Intracerebral vessels and capillaries

The finer vessels of the central nervous system can be demonstrated by a variety of techniques, including corrosion specimens, thick cleared specimens, and microangiography. The patterns, which in infants and adults are similar except for the caliber of the vessels,[70] have been studied under physiological conditions mostly,[29,32] but pathological disturbance of this angioarchitecture can occur. Penetrating or nutrient arteries less than 100 μ, except for the lenticulostriate arteries, branch from both the large superficial arteries in the subarachnoid space and the fine intercommunicating network of pial arteries.[70] Alexander and Putman[1] classified the penetrating vessels which were mostly about 34 μ in diameter (range, 16 to 51 μ) as the fourth order of cerebral and cerebellar arteries. Gillilan[70] pointed out that the innumerable small penetrating vessels branching directly from the large arteries had been disregarded. The largest intracerebral vessels, usually 1 mm. or so in diameter, are the subependymal collecting veins. The average diameter of the capillaries in sections of the central nervous system in man ranges from 4.5 to 12 μ,[33] with higher dimensions when fixed by perfusion.

The gray matter of the human brain is much more richly endowed with capillaries than the white matter, the gray matter with the poorest supply being almost twice as richly supplied as the most vascular areas of the white matter.[33] Within the gray matter, there is variation in vascularity that depends more on the number of synaptic junctions than on neuronal mass.[239] The cerebral cortex of the mature brain is much more vascular than at birth because of the greater functional activity in the adult,[29] yet it is less vascular than the liver, kidney, and skeletal or cardiac muscle[239] despite the high oxygen consumption.

Perivascular extensions of the subarachnoid space (Virchow-Robin spaces) encircle only large intracerebral vessels and do not extend to the capillary bed.

Ultrastructure. The Virchow-Robin space has been found to exist only about large parenchymal vessels and does not extend to the capillary bed. The larger parenchymal vessels have not been thoroughly investigated by electron microscopy. The small vessels are lined by a thin layer

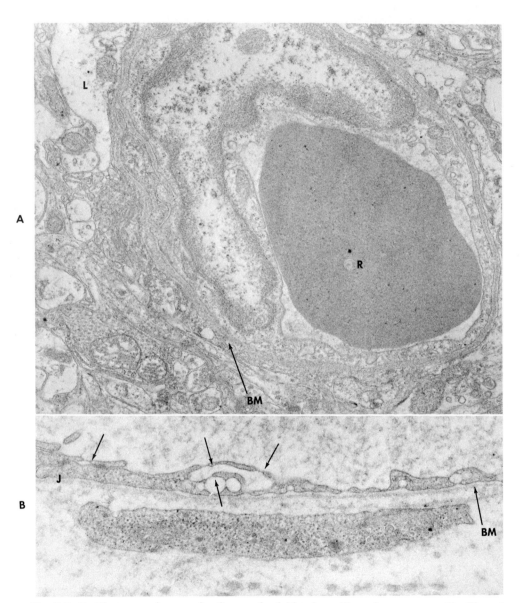

Fig. 2-5. A, Electron micrograph of a cerebral blood capillary from mouse. Capillary is surrounded by a continuous basement membrane, *BM,* and many glial processes but no perivascular connective tissue. Endothelium contains a nucleus and only a few cell organelles. Pinocytotic vesicles are scanty. A low-density glial cell process is at *L* and a red cell at *R.* **B,** Fenestrated endothelium from wall of a vessel in the human choroid plexus. Lumen is at top. Note the basement membrane, *BM,* the junction at *J,* and the unusual location of fenestrae *(arrows)* in walls of large vesicular profiles and overlapping flaps at cell junction. (**A,** ×20,000; **B,** ×30,000.)

of flattened endothelium approximately 0.2 μ thick. The endothelium is devoid of fenestrae and intercellular gaps, although Farquhar and Hartman[51] reported perforations, probably intercellular gaps or stomas, which generally occur in pathological states. The endothelial cells contain the usual cytoplasmic constituents of endothelium but few micropinocytotic vesicles and caveolae (Fig. 2-5). Coated micropinocytotic vesicles and half desmosomes, not yet identified, are probably present.

Surrounding the capillary endothelium is a continuous layer of basement membrane that exhibits occasional zones of duplication.[51] The basement membrane splits to enclose closely applied periendothelial cells or pericytes, which cover less than 50% of the capillary circumference[228] and have denser nuclei than endothelial cells.[51] External to these basement membranes glial cell processes are closely applied, there being a paucity of extracellular space in the brain. Some processes thought to belong to oligodendroglia[120] are wide, containing extremely electron-dense, pale cytoplasm with few organelles. Other authors classify these as astrocytes. Luse[121] suggested the low-density cell processes may constitute a cellular pathway for fluid transport. No doubt these low-density cell processes were responsible for the erroneous belief that a pericapillary space communicated with the subarachnoid space.

Fenestrated endothelium similar to that in the kidney, alimentary tract, and endocrine glands is a feature of the small vessels of the choroid plexus in man (Fig. 2-5) and other animals.[152] It has been observed in the human infundibulum,[12] neurophypophysis, and area postrema,[63,171] which has occasional intercellular gaps.[171]

In other mammals, the ultrastructure of the capillary bed is essentially the same, with no pericapillary space. In immature rats, the capillary basement membrane of the cerebral cortex varies in width and density, thickening with maturity[45] until it is 300 to 500 Å wide in the adult.[130] Arterioles are similar to extracranial ar-

terioles and venules may be quite large and devoid of muscle.[130]

Cerebral veins and dural sinuses

Cerebral veins have extremely thin walls composed primarily of collagen with little muscle. Muscle fibers even in large cerebral veins are scanty and easily overlooked.[239] Maximow and Bloom[129] list the veins of the spinal pia mater, sinuses of the dura mater, and the majority of cerebral veins among those devoid of smooth muscle and consequently of a tunica media.

The thick slightly wavy collagenous sheath about many pial and subependymal veins could be an age change (Fig. 2-6). Elastic tissue is minimal. The dural veins lie between the fibrous layers of the dura mater and are therefore relatively well protected. The thin walls of cerebral veins have been similarly ascribed to the protection from external and environmental pressures afforded by the cranial box, but their structure suggests their state of vasodilatation is a passive response to flow.

Ultrastructural investigations have been made of the arachnoid villi and granulations, though the cerebral venous system has been neglected. In the monkey (macaque), they are covered by a layer of non-fenestrated endothelial cells separated by tight junctions.[191] No distinct basement membrane is demonstrable. In the dog and cat, Andres[4] found fenestrations in the sinus endothelium overlying the villi.

Cerebral microcirculation

The cerebral microcirculation can be examined through a trephine hole or a cranial window, but resolution is considerably limited because epi-illumination rather than transmitted light must be used. The larger pial arteries, on changing direction, throb with each systole, bending and straightening out slightly and exerting gentle traction on the arachnoid.[64] Anastomotic arterial circles can be seen on the cortex. Less frequently, they are venous.[60] Sphincterlike annular constrictions occur at the origin of some arteries that are al-

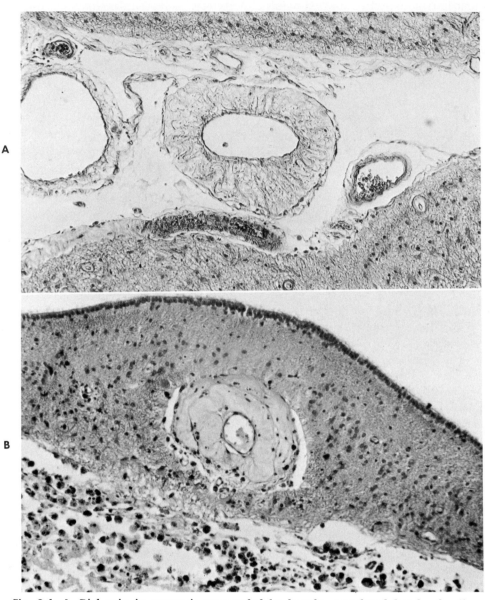

Fig. 2-6. A, Pial vein in center is surrounded by loosely convoluted bands of collagen forming a fairly compact sheath. Vein on left has a thin wall with much less adventitia. **B,** Small subependymal vein surrounded by a bizarre compact sheath of convoluted hyaline fibrous tissue. An old hemorrhagic focus undergoing organization is below and contains many siderophages. A few siderophages are present at periphery of vein. Note survival of a narrow strip of subependymal parenchyma. Venous changes such as these in **A** and **B** are more frequent in the aged. (Hematoxylin and eosin, ×105.)

ways superficial to the veins. Smaller vessels exhibit little or no movement, and according to the oxygen saturation the color of arteries and veins so differs. A clear plasma zone often separates two streams of blood derived from venous tributaries and large drainage channels may exhibit several streamlines because little effective mixing occurs.

Florey[60] found that the cerebral arteries

and arterioles react to mechanical, thermal, electrical, and chemical stimuli by contraction and dilatation. Small thrombi ("white bodies") form in the vessels, but the resolution is low, for individual cells cannot be recognized although their behavior is likely to be similar to that observed in extracranial sites.[195]

Penfield[156] observed the cessation of arterial pulsation (local and general) during a seizure after which hyperemia was seen. Well-oxygenated blood is present in some veins, indicating the arteriovenous shunts noted previously.[157] Flushing and blanching of one or more convolutions may succeed the convulsion and irregular arterial constrictions (postconvulsive spasm) eventuate.

Capillary permeability

Physiologists of yore believed that the balance of forces determined the fluid exchange across the capillary wall, which, it was contended, acted as an inert semipermeable membrane.[202] This mechanical theory was substantiated subsequently by Landis[113] and the "pore" theory of Pappenheimer.[153] The passage of water and lipid-soluble substances was considered to be restricted to pores whose total cross-sectional area was estimated to be less than 0.2% of the histological surface of the capillary endothelium. The estimate correlated well with the contention of Chambers and Zweifach[27] that interendothelial cement substance, the surface area of which was also a small fraction of the histological surface of the capillary wall, was a major factor in controlling capillary permeability. However, the in vivo observations, the basis of the cement theory of Chambers and Zweifach,[27] were shown to be ill-founded,[206,218] and the argyrophilic staining of the so-called cement substance was no more than the peripheral edge of the cell rather than an intercellular adhesive material.[62,206]

Electron microscopy demonstrated greater morphological detail of the endothelium[149] and preexisting views on capillary permeability were modified. There is greater variation in the structure of vertebrate blood capillaries[11] than was hitherto believed. Pores comparable in size to those of Pappenheimer were not seen. The controversy continues despite the existence of various hypotheses explaining the selective permeability of the capillary endothelium. As was natural, the micropinocytotic vesicles first described by Palade[149] were considered as a possible mechanism. From the use of various markers, it seemed that the pinocytotic vesicles transported materials across the vessel wall,[150] but the uptake of tracer particles is slow and there is a lack of variation in the number and morphology of the vesicles despite the noxious influences of metabolic poisons.[61,100,118] Fawcett,[52] describing the formation of large vesicles in the endothelium of capillaries, thought the macropinocytotic vesicles were engaged in gross fluid transport. Coated vesicles, previously found to be associated with the uptake of protein,[178] were then discovered in endothelium.[214] The unconvincing role of pinocytosis as a mechanism of endothelial transport may hinge upon the selectivity of the different types of vesicle and the physicochemical nature of tracer particles.[215]

Luft[119] suggested that capillary permeability was a passive process, with the primary selectivity dependent on the external leaflet of the unit membrane stretched across a fenestra or in the zone of fusion of the outer leaflets of the tight junctions between endothelial cells.

In cerebral vessels, peroxidase even at high dosage is not transported across the endothelial cell. This was attributed to the presence of tight junctions,[106,168] but even the vesicles, though some filled, did not convey the marker to the subendothelial space. Karnovsky,[105,106] examining the transendothelial passage of horseradish peroxidase, concluded that endothelial junctions were the most probable sites of Pappenheimer's[153] small pore system. He believed the endothelial junctions were not closed by tight junctions but by maculae occludentes having gaps about 40 Å wide.

Bruns and Palade[22,23] reaffirmed the presence of tight junctions between endothelial cells. They considered the frequency of open junctions to be very low and vesicular transport to be structurally equivalent to the large pore system of Pappenheimer[153] whereas the site of the small pore system remained uncertain.

The basement membrane has been considered to be a filtration barrier.[150] However, normally, the blood-tissue barrier does not seem to be due to the basement membrane, for the blood-brain barrier appears to be situated internally to it.[168] Like extracerebral capillaries, those within the brain manifest a selective permeability. The mechanism is as yet unknown.

Blood-brain barrier

The concept of the blood-brain barrier stems from the fact that most of the tissues of the body including the meninges stain when dyes (trypan blue, acid aniline dyes, sodium ferrocyanide) are injected intravenously. The brain and cord, however, except for the choroid plexus, neurohypophysis, pineal gland, area postrema, intercolumnar tubercle, subcommissural organ, and to some extent the hypothalamus[122] remain unstained. The conclusion was that in the cerebral vessels a blood-brain barrier provided this apparent selective permeability and excluded the dyes. Ignored was the fact that after repeated intravascular injections, some dye was deposited elsewhere within the brain parenchyma, suggesting that some dye traversed the blood-brain barrier[111] via an alternate route. On the other hand, when much smaller quantities of dye are injected into the cerebrospinal fluid there is parenchymal staining of the brain and severe neurological symptoms ensue.[111] Those regions of the brain which, it was thought, do not possess the blood-brain barrier are surrounded by an interstitial space bounded on each side by a basement membrane. This can be demonstrated experimentally by inducing argyria.[43] The barrier is believed to be incompletely devel-

oped in fetuses and young animals, and a breakdown of the barrier is known to follow cerebral injuries of various types,[126,181] including pathological lesions (infarction, anoxia, edema, epileptic seizures, and X-irradiation)[28] where there is likely to be a change in permeability of the vessel wall and in the injured or necrotic cells.

Bile pigments normally do not stain the brain parenchyma in states of jaundice, and this phenomenon has been attributed to the blood-brain barrier, for other tissues including the meninges can be heavily pigmented. In kernicterus, in which biliary pigmentation occurs in the basal ganglia, thalamus, ependymal lining of the ventricles, dentate nucleus, posterior vermis, cranial nerve nuclei, substantia nigra, corpora quadrigemina, and the gray matter of the spinal cord,[162] or in cerebral softenings in the adult, the blood-brain barrier is considered to be breached.

The higher resolving power of electron microscopy revealed that cerebral capillaries differed little from capillaries elsewhere. The negligible extracellular space in the brain consisting only of an intercellular space no thicker than that between endothelial cells (approximately 200 Å) has been the most striking observation. Little is known of the contents of the intercellular spaces that are narrowed only by zones of attachment. It was thus suggested that the blood-brain barrier might be illusionary rather than an entity because of the relative lack of extracellular space in which dyes could accumulate as is the case in extracerebral tissues.[130] Pathological states such as kernicterus, experimental injury, or softenings[182] are associated with destruction of brain parenchyma, the development of extracellular space, and accumulation of fluid. In such cases, dyes or bile pigments can accumulate and permit parenchymal staining. The dyes as indicators of a physiological barrier are no longer of significance now that the absence of parenchymal staining is dependent on the absence of a substantial amount of extracellular space and fluid. Regions of the brain, such as the area postrema, are characterized by an interstitial space in which dyes may accumulate. The fact that endothelium of the area postrema and of most regions lacking the blood-brain barrier, is fenestrated complicates the issue.[16,63] Furthermore, fluorescein dyes, administered intravenously in the cat, stain the area postrema, and extend into surrounding tissues normally devoid of an extracellular space.[94] The interpretation of this experiment is that an ultrastructural or potential space does not per se act as a barrier.[68]

Other substances cross the capillary wall of extracellular tissues but proceed more slowly across the blood-brain interface.[68] The reduced permeability of cerebral vessels for a wide range of solutes has been attributed to the capillary endothelium of the perivascular astrocytic foot processes. Permeability studies of the cerebral blood capillaries have shown that horseradish peroxidase, when given intravenously as a marker, appeared in micropinocytotic vesicles on the luminal side of the endothelial cells but was not transported across the endothelium.[168] This was attributed to the presence of tight interendothelial cell junctions in cerebral capillaries. It was thought they did not occur in extracellular vessels where transfer of the exogenous peroxidase is easily accomplished.[106] Structural differences between cerebral and extracerebral vessels of the mammal have been challenged by Bruns and Palade,[22,23] who deny the presence of open junctions between endothelial cells of extracerebral vessels such as heart muscle. However, in lower species, peroxidase fails to cross the cerebral capillary endothelium,[16] but under pathological conditions exogenous peroxidase readily crosses the endothelium,[90,91] with the marker not only in the intercellular junctions but even in pinocytotic vesicles and caveolae on both sides of the endothelium and diffusely distributed in the endothelial cytoplasm. At present, there is uncertainty regarding the prime route for the transfer of the peroxidase, though it seems that the barrier for this substance is inherent in the endothleium. Other substances are another matter. It may be that the selectivity displayed by the endothelial cell is unaccompanied by any specific morphological peculiarity.

Cerebral edema

Edema of the brain and cord occurs in a wide variety of pathological conditions, including trauma, ischemic necrosis, infections, and other inflammatory conditions and about hematomas and tumors. It is readily produced experimentally by triethyl tin,[63] stannous chloride, or the intravenous infusion of distilled water.[122] Despite the absence of cerebral lymphatics, cerebral edema can be produced by obstruction of the cervical lymphatics.[63] Extensive edema affects the white matter more markedly than the gray matter. Areas such as subcortical arcuate fibers, the internal capsule, corpus callosum, and the optic radiations in particular tend to be spared.[13] If extensive, the local or general features of a raised intracranial pressure are manifest, the margin of the edematous area, except in ischemic necrosis, is usually not sharp. The affected part appears to be unduly moist, swollen, and with diminished consistency. Microscopically, secondary changes such as demyelination, destruction of axons and gliosis may complicate the edema, though the accompanying disturbances of blood flow and ischemia could be responsible.

Torack[229] observed swollen endothelial cells with a cytoplasm of reduced density in the edematous zone about cerebral tumors. Others have considered the capillary changes inconsistent despite an occasional thick endothelium and increased vacuolization.[117] In rats, Hirano and colleagues[92] observed thinning and unduly folded endothelium in experimental edema. Hills[89] observed the prevalence of macropinocytotic vesicles or vacuoles mostly with clear contents or a small amount of granular material in ischemic lesions.[89] Asssociated with the latter was an increase in the number of cytoplasmic projections extending into the lumen possibly in the formation of the macropinocytotic vesicles described by Fawcett[52] for the transfer of large quantities of fluid. The vacuoles became even more prominent after dehydration of an edematous brain,[121] and it was thought that a reverse shift of fluid was underway.

Severe edema can occur apparently in the absence of striking changes in the endothelium. Statistical evaluation of the number and type of cytoplasmic vesicles in the endothelial cells, no mean feat, is required before the possibility of a change in vesicle population is conceded. The numerous macropinocytotic vesicles observed by Hills[89] may depend on the type of lesion or its severity. It is curious that intercellular gaps and stomas have not been observed in the cerebral circulation, for under similar circumstances endothelial stomas would be fairly readily observed in extracranial tissues. Moreover, it is not known whether the permeability is increased in proliferating cerebral blood vessels, a phenomenon readily demonstrable in extracranial tissues.

The parenchymal edema is itself quite unusual in that much of the fluid accumulation is intracellular, involving the astrocytic foot processes and, according to Luse,[121,122] the oligodendroglia. Glial cell processes enlarge enormously, eventually breaking down to form large extracellular pools sometimes surrounding capillaries.[92,117,121]

The cerebral circulation

The brain and spinal cord are contained within relatively rigid walls and cannot change appreciably in volume. According to the Monro-Kellie doctrine,[187] an increase in the volume of one of the cranial contents will be at the expense of the others and as the volume of the blood and cerebral spinal fluid is more labile, they will be displaced with any increase in parenchymal volume. The cerebral blood pool is said to be fairly constant at about 77 ml. or approximately 2% of the total body

weight.[144,177] The central nervous system is remarkably susceptible to anoxia, and severe ischemia occurs after deprivation of blood flow for more than 2 minutes.

Cerebral blood flow

In healthy young adults, the cerebral blood flow is approximately 50 to 55 ml. per 100 gm. of brain tissue per minute or about 750 ml. per minute for a brain of average weight.[109,114] Higher values are sometimes advanced.[138] The brain, though weighing approximately one-thirtieth of the total body weight,[226] nevertheless receives some 12% to 15% of the total cardiac output.[114,144] In infancy and childhood, it receives a greater percentage of the cardiac output than in the adult, for the flow is twice that of the adult.[108] Studies of the cerebral blood flow determinations of middle-aged hospital patients indicate a progressive fall from the fourth and fifth decades onward.[108] However, many aging but healthy adults have a cerebral blood flow that does not differ significantly from that of healthy young men. Cerebral blood flow is increased by anxiety, hyperthermia, and sleep, even though slightly, and reduced by hypothermia.

Toole and Patel[226] estimate that about 900 ml. of blood flows through the brain per minute and that 300 to 400 ml. from each internal carotid artery supply the ipsilateral orbit and cerebral hemisphere, with most destined for the middle cerebral artery. The vertebral arteries supply approximately 200 ml. of blood to the cervical musculature, the brain stem, cerebellum, occipital lobes, and portion of the temporal lobes. The values determined by investigators vary within moderately wide limits.[74,223] After acute compression of the common carotid artery, flow in the contralateral internal carotid increased by 13% to 38%, and in half of the cases flow in the internal carotid was reversed with 13% to 32% of the collateral flow derived from the superior thyroid artery.[80] In five subjects, flow in the right vertebral artery of the neck was 25 to 87 ml. per minute. In the left vertebral artery of four additional patients, flow varied from 10 to 74 ml. per minute, the mean flow in eight patients was 45 ml. per minute. Compression of either one of the common carotid arteries induced a variable elevation of vertebral flow. Clamping of the subclavian artery proximal to the origin of the vertebral artery caused reversal of flow in the latter and increased flow in the ipsilateral internal carotid.[81]

Rotation of the head to one side can result in carotid compression on the opposite side by the lateral mass of the atlas or in pinching of the vertebral artery between the atlas and the axis, with a corresponding reduction in flow, the effect in general being more pronounced on the vertebrobasilar circulation than on the carotid.[10,226] Toole and Tucker[227] showed that variation in head posture affects carotid and vertebral artery flow of perfused fluid at 100 mm. of mercury in cadavers. In the neutral position, carotid flow is usually equal, but this does not apply in the vertebrals. Turning the head 30 to 45 degrees to either side usually causes abrupt cessation of flow through one vertebral artery and further rotation of 5 to 10 degrees with slight tilting often stops flow through the ipsilateral carotid. Normally, an increase in flow on the side to which the head is rotated tends to compensate for any decrease in flow in the contralateral side.[226] When a normal subject is raised to the erect posture, the resultant 20% drop of cerebral blood flow is offset by the increased arteriovenous oxygen difference.[186]

Exercise of the upper limb has no effect on cerebral blood flow, but if the cardiac output is relatively fixed or if a "steal" phenomenon is present, exercise of the right arm may bring about alterations of flow and pressure gradients sufficient to induce cerebrovascular insufficiency.[225]

Numerous factors are involved in the control of the cerebral blood flow. They operate primarily by means of change in either the pressure head or cerebral vascular resistance,[108] and an adequate cardiac output is a prerequisite. The Valsalva maneuver can reduce the cardiac output and thence the cerebral blood flow below a critical level with giddiness, or even syncope, as the result.[226] Moreover, in cardiac disease associated with a chronically poor cardiac output, the cerebral blood flow may be only 60% of normal, the increased oxygen extraction accounting for only a moderate (13%) drop in oxygen consumption.[185] In the Stokes-Adams syndrome, the cardiac output is so low that no compensatory mechanism can overcome the low cerebral blood flow, and syncope is the outcome.

Autoregulatory mechanisms control cerebral blood flow, but much of the regulation is abolished by extensive surgery, circulatory arrest, severe hypercapnia, hypoxia, and deep anesthesia.[6] Factors known to be involved in these autoregulatory mechanisms are briefly as follows:

Arterial pressure head. Cerebral blood vessels were once thought to possess little or no capacity for intrinsic autoregulation, and cerebral flow was said to passively follow alterations in systemic blood pressure. Venous pressure is normally so low that its role is minor in determining total pressure gradient. The arterial pressure, maintained by numerous homostatic mechanisms (carotid sinus reflex, central control of peripheral vascular tone),[108] is thus of prime importance. Reduction of arterial pressure is accompanied by cerebral vasodilatation, and if it falls to 60 or 70 mm. Hg, syncope secondary to diminished cerebral blood flow is likely. The critical level is higher among hypertensives, and a slow rate of reduction in pressure is tolerated better than a rapid one.[226] Elevation of systemic pressure is accompanied by constriction of cerebral arterioles, but undue increases as occur in hypertensive crises bring in their wake pathological changes in the vessels and parenchyma.

Cerebral vascular resistance. Cerebrovascular resistance is measured in units of pressure head necessary to cause a unit of flow of blood through the brain, the average normal being 1.6 mm. Hg per ml. of blood per minute.[107] Under normal conditions of blood pressure, the cerebral blood flow is maintained by alterations in the cerebrovascular resistance, which depends on blood viscosity and the vasomotor control of the vascular bed.[108,114,201] The viscosity of the blood is largely the concern of the erythrocytes. Two factors significantly affecting the resistance to flow are a reduction in viscosity occurring in anemia and an increase in polycythemia. The flow may be reduced as much as 50% or more in polycythemia.[107] Considerable resistance to flow occurs with erythrocytic aggregation or "sludging" of blood,[195,216] and a greater appreciation of its detrimental effect on the cerebral circulation should accrue from vital microscopy of the retinal or conjunctival vascular beds in disease processes.

The principal element influencing cerebral blood flow is the vasomotor control of the cerebral vessels, especially of the arterioles,[108] and factors affecting the vascular bed are neurogenic, humoral, and organic.

Neurogenic control. Unmyelinated nerves on the cerebral blood vessels are believed to mediate the neurogenic control over the cerebrovascular bed, myelinated fibers being sensory afferents. The sympathetic innervation of the cerebral vessels is characterized as being weak, inconsistent, and without tonic effect,[65,114] whereas the parasympathetic vasodilatation pathway is unknown in man. The role of the vagus, aortic and sinus nerves, and the stellate ganglion in man are yet to be determined.

Humoral control. The normal brain consumes oxygen at the rate of 3.5 cc. per 100 gm. per minute, equivalent to approximately 20% of the total oxygen consumption of the whole body.[114,201] The brain, which is particularly susceptible to oxygen deprivation, utilizes, according to estimations, approximately 25 times as much as an equivalent unit of skeletal muscle even though muscle is more vascular.[142] In children, oxygen consumption is 5 cc. per 100 gm. per minute, which is equivalent to

50% of the total body oxygen consumption. Variations in oxygen usage are associated with intellectual effort, physical, exercise, anxiety, sleep, and temperature. A high oxygen tension exerts a constrictor effect and low tensions a vasodilator effect. Variations in the carbon dioxide tensions have an effect the reverse of that of oxygen, and it would appear that the two gases exert an important regulatory control on the cerebral circulation.[108,140] Destructive lesions in the midbrain, pons, and upper medulla diminish or abolish the responsiveness of the cerebral circulation to alterations in the arterial carbon dioxide tension, suggesting that mediation of the effect of carbon dioxide is via a central pathway.[192] In general, increased activity of the brain results in an augmented cerebral blood flow. Local metabolic effects profoundly influence local cerebral blood flow, and this seems to be an important factor in autoregulation of cerebral vascular tone.

Other authors have dealt with pharmacological agents (hormones and drugs) that bring about changes in cerebral flow by their vasomotor effects.[108,114,140,187]

Organic disease

INTRACRANIAL PRESSURE. The thin-walled encephalic vessels are susceptible to external pressure so that mounting intracranial pressure progressively increases the cerebrovascular resistance. Below a critical level of 450 mm. of water the cerebral blood flow is maintained by a concomitant increase in mean arterial blood pressure. Above this critical level, flow may diminish seriously until eventually the intracranial pressure is such that there is no effective flow in the cranium,[88,110] the vascular tree is not demonstrable angiographically, regional cerebral blood flow studies reveal a small amount of intracranial activity of the radioactive tracer and the virtual absence of isotope clearance is indicative of cerebral death.[20] Quite possibly, however, before the intracranial pressure is grossly elevated, local pressure effects will impair blood flow through the brain parenchyma surrounding the space-occupying lesion.

ATHEROSCLEROSIS AND ARTERIOSCLEROSIS. Chronic brain disease and senile dementia are frequent in older age groups. There is a significant reduction in cerebral blood flow and oxygen consumption.[108,114,185] Progressive narrowing of the cerebral arteries with the involvement of small vessels is held responsible, although Loeb and Meyer[116] consider that cerebral vascular reactivity and the ability to maintain homeostatic equilibrium diminish with advancing years. Cerebrovascular resistance may be twice the normal value. Differentiation of senile changes from those of vascular disease is difficult, and a reduction in cerebral blood flow is not an invariable accompaniment of old age.[200] Both oxygen uptake and cerebral blood flow are reduced in patients with chronic brain syndrome after an acute cerebrovascular accident as would be expected if a considerable area of brain is infarcted.

ORGANIC DEMENTIA OF UNKNOWN ETIOLOGY. Oxygen utilization and cerebral flow are reduced in dementia or amentia whatever the cause. Oxygen uptake is usually inversely proportional to the intellectual impairment.[69]

SEMICOMA AND COMA. In all cases of semicoma and coma, regardless of causation, the oxygen consumption is reduced roughly in proportion to the fall in the level of consciousness. Cerebral blood flow is generally adequate.[107,114]

CEREBRAL TUMOR. Cerebral blood flow is often reduced in subjects with cerebral tumor, particularly when the intracranial pressure is increased. It is believed to be caused by local effects rather than intracranial pressure, moderate elevation of which has no effect on blood flow.[114]

ARTERIOVENOUS ANEURYSMS AND FISTULAS. Arteriovenous aneurysms and fistulas cause an increase in total cerebral blood flow and have been discussed in Chapter 10.

HYPERTENSION. With heightened arterial pressure, it is believed, come increases in cerebral vascular tone and resistance, with the result that cerebral blood flow is within normal limits.[108,114,127] A mean reduction in blood pressure from 60 to 70 mm. Hg is regarded as the critical pressure below which a serious decrease in blood flow and syncope eventuate.[189]

MISCELLANEOUS. In diseases like schizophrenia and disseminated sclerosis, reduction in blood flow is not significant,[108] although there is a decrease with meningovascular syphilis.[107] In idiopathic epilepsy, when no seizures are occurring, flow and oxygen utilization are normal, but they increase during experimentally induced convulsions to at least twice normal values.[159] In man, induced convulsions reduce flow and oxygen consumption, but chronic effects of this therapy are not known as yet.

In migraine, there is evidence that the cranial vessels exhibit more vasomotor reactivity than in normal subjects and for a few days prior to the headache, extracranial arteries appear to be dilated.[232] However, the effect of migraine on the cerebral circulation is inconsistent. O'Brien[145] noted an increased cortex-perfusion rate in seven volunteers with migraine. In another study,[198] one subject had a reduction of cerebral blood flow of up to 67% of the resting flow, another had a high cerebral blood flow, and a third exhibited changes indicative of very fast and very slow perfusion compartments.

Kak and Taylor[103] determined that an increase in cerebral circulation time in patients with subarachnoid hemorrhage was related to the angiographically demonstrable spasm in the cerebral arterial tree.

Regional cerebral blood flow. The regional blood flow is calculated from the rate of clearance of an inert diffusible radioactive tracer rapidly injected into the internal carotid artery and is determined through the intact skull at several regions over the brain simultaneously. Localization of lesions is determined by variation in flow.[93,115,138] Resolution of the clearance curves into a fast and a slow component can be demonstrated and represent the gray matter and the white matter respectively.[237] In normal individuals, there is a wide range of values for the regional cortical flow, with high values generally in the precentral region and low values in the temporal region. High values for flow in the white matter were found in the internal capsule.[237] The technique is said to be of value in determining the consequences of carotid ligation when a value in the frontoparietal region of 25% less than normal indicates the probability of incipient hemiparesis.[99]

In organic dementia, especially in Alzheimer's disease, the average regional cerebral blood flow is significantly reduced and focal flow reduction is found particularly in the temporal region. Consequently, it was suggested that regional blood flow measurements could be used to quantitate to some extent the cerebral effects of organic dementia.[98] Unusually slow circulation times have been found in the frontal and temporal regions of the cerebral hemispheres in patients with dementia caused by cerebrovascular disease.[196]

In one patient with migraine, regional cerebral blood flow during the prodromal stage was found to be reduced to a critical level in the entire internal carotid system, particularly in the parietal lobe and in the upper part of the temporal lobe. During the headache phase of another patient with migraine, flow values were significantly raised in the entire internal carotid system.[197]

In a series of patients with cerebral tumors, the pattern of regional cerebral blood flow was extremely variable and its regulation deranged. The steep initial component in some tumors was indicative of arteriovenous shunting, but the flow patterns were not diagnostic in themselves. There was no correlation between a regional blood flow and hot spots in the brain scans.[151]

As more information becomes available on flow rates, the use of the above technique will increase. The effect of chronically abnormal regional flow rates not only on the parenchyma but also on the arteries and arterioles should be assessed. A labile cerebral circulatory system may exist, and its repercussions on the vascular system would also be of interest.

Cerebral venous flow. The cerebral veins and dural sinuses have virtually no muscle within their media and reduction in volume is compensatory to increased pressure or a space-occupying lesion in accordance with the Monro-Kellie doctrine.[187] In the recumbent position, the venous pressure within the cranial cavity is about 3 or 5 mm. Hg. In the erect posture, the pressure within the cortical veins is zero and in dural sinuses and jugular veins, it is negative.[225]

Blood samples from the internal jugular veins are predominantly of cerebral blood (97.2%).[193] Shenkin and associates[193] estimated that about 66% of the blood from one internal carotid artery appeared in the homolateral internal jugular vein and 34% in the contralateral vessel. However, approximately 22% of the flow in the external jugular vein was found to be cerebral in origin.[142,193]

Blood pressure. Arterial pressure in the cerebral circulation is believed to be similar to that in the neck, with little reduction until in the neighborhood of the very small arteries or arterioles. In selected patients, the mean pressure in the internal carotid artery of the neck has varied from 74 to 137 mm. Hg.[223] Pressure recordings from intracranial vessels have been mainly limited to the internal carotid arterial system, though there is no evidence that the carotid blood pressure differs from the vertebrobasilar.[225] Direct arterial pressure readings indicate that some reduction occurs from the neck to the cerebral arteries,[8,15,240] but in several instances there could have been slight systolic accentuation.

Circulation time. The turnover of the blood in the brain is 11.2 times per minute or twice that of the thorax, which has a value of only 6.1.[144] Rapid serial angiography has revealed that the "normal" cerebral circulation time varies considerably. The carotid circulation time is 7 seconds and that of the vertebrobasilar 8 to 9 seconds.[226] Flow over the cerebellum is much slower than over the occipital lobe,[196] so that under normal circumstances in the adult, cerebrovascular resistance may be higher in the brain stem and cerebellum than in the cerebral hemispheres. The internal carotid circulation is faster in the child than in the adult and faster than in the external carotid artery. In the adult, some reduction occurs with age, no doubt because of tortuosity and arterial disease.[112]

Increased circulation time is a feature of raised intracranial pressure, space-occupying lesions such as a tumor or abscess,[222] cerebrovascular disease,[71] and arteriosclerotic dementia.[116] A decreased circulation time is associated with tumors accompanied by an arteriovenous shunt and with arteriovenous aneurysms.[222]

Little is known of the actual blood velocity in the cerebral circulation. In the basilar artery of the rabbit, a peak velocity of 40 mm. per second has been determined without evidence of retrograde flow.[165] In the cortical arterioles of the mouse brain, a velocity of 3.5 mm. per second was found and in venules an average value of 1.9 mm. per second.[176]

Less is known of the blood flow in the spinal cord, other than that it is slower than in the brain though the regulation is similar.

Laminar and turbulent flow. Disturbances of flow (turbulence, vortices, eddy currents) are said to be involved in the development of vascular lesions whether they are intimal thickenings,[207-209] atherosclerosis, or cerebral ischemic lesions.[96] However, it has been contended that under normal conditions, turbulence of flow could not occur in the vascular system except possibly at the root of the aorta.[102,166] Reynolds[170] expressed numerically the border line between laminar and turbulent flow. The Reynolds number (Re) is a nondimensional constant calculated from the

equation

$$Re = \frac{\rho VD}{\mu}$$

where V is the velocity, D is the diameter of the tube, ρ is the density of the liquid, and μ is the absolute viscosity of the liquid. With steady flow in a simple tube, flow is said to be laminar when the Re is below the critical value of 2000; above 2000 it is turbulent. On this concept the belief that turbulence would not occur in the human vascular system is based. Coulter and Pappenheimer[31] found by experiment that the critical Re for bovine blood flowing in a straight tube was about 2000.* When the Re was calculated, using the mean velocity of blood flow in the arterial segments, values rarely exceeded 2000. But such extrapolation to the vascular system is invalid[205,207] because changes in direction and velocity are liable to induce flow disturbances. Arterial flow is pulsatile, and investigators have estimated that the peak velocity of forward flow in dogs is 15 times that of the mean flow rate.[132] The Re in the human aorta if the diameter is 2.5 cm. is 11,150[205] at the peak velocity of 120 cm. per second at rest, a value considerably higher than that based on mean velocity. There is evidence that turbulence can be induced by a momentary stimulus[190] so that intermittent turbulence in the circulation is a possibility. Flow in glass models simulating arterial bifurcations of 90-degree unions and the carotid siphon was such that turbulence occurred at Reynolds values considerably lower than the accepted critical value of 2000.[205,207] There was also a vigorous flickering motion of the dye filament as it broke off into curling vortices at a bifurcation of 180 degrees. Habib[78] found that the critical Re in pul-

---

*Green[73] gave the value of the kinematic viscosity $\frac{\rho}{\mu}$ for blood as 0.0169 sq. cm. per second for the lower limit of viscosity and 0.0269 sq. cm. per second for the higher. Therefore, $Re = \frac{VD}{0.0169}$ for the lower viscosity and $Re = \frac{VD}{0.0269}$ for the higher viscosity.

satile flow in a straight tube dropped from 1800 to 1100 as the frequency of the pulsations increased from 0 to 150 per minute. Yellin[241] considered that neither the mean nor the instantaneous Re adequately determine the transition of laminar to turbulent flow in a pulsatile system. The previously accepted criterion of a Reynolds number of 2000 is probably not applicable to the cardiovascular system because it disregards bifurcations, curvatures, and pulsatile flow. In fact, the critical Re, which can vary greatly under differing test conditions, is confusing and assuredly obsolete. On theoretical grounds, turbulence might well be expected in the arterial system of man but in actual fact there is uncertainty. McDonald[131,134] injected dye into the rabbit aorta and observed it by high-speed cinematography. Dye was distributed across the lumen in random threads until the end of systole when the filaments reformed, suggesting that vortices and not true turbulence were observed. However, at the aortic bifurcation eddying occurred all the time there was forward flow, being maximal during the phase of rapid systolic ejection. It is likely therefore that a comparable disturbance of flow will occur at other bifurcations of similar or larger size including those of the cerebral arterial tree.[205]

At times in cerebral arteriograms, patterns formed by the injected radiopaque material suggest laminar flow.[222] Direct observation of the basilar artery in the rabbit allegedly revealed that dye injected into one vertebral artery remained strictly on the homolateral side of the basilar with no evidence of eddying or mixing at the union of the streams.[135] These conclusions should be accepted cautiously as high-speed cinematography was not used.

The location of intimal pads or cushions at cerebral arterial forks strongly suggests a relationship to the appearance of eddies in stagnation areas,[208,209] but the detailed examination of flow patterns at forks such as those at the base of the brain is beyond present-day technology. Even in the ab-sence of frank turbulence, conceivably there could be significant flow disturbances at arterial forks. Coulter and Pappenheimer[31] postulated that the axial or red cell column might remain laminar whereas the peripheral or plasma sleeve adjacent to the vessel wall could be turbulent. In the microcirculation, variations in the marginal plasma zone appear at forks, bifurcations, and curvatures in areas corresponding to the site of intimal pads in larger vessels (the face and dorsum cannot be adequately visualized[206,217]).

Rodbard[175] introduced flow chambers of various designs, each being lined by deformable silicone. There were areas of pitting and excavation and mounds or cushions at other sites. Similar flow chambers[83] have been used but with unrealistic diameters of branches and a lack of detail concerning flow conditions. These experimental models have provided useful information concerning stresses on the wall, but though the stresses may be similar, any deductions must be cautiously drawn, for the remodeling of the inert material lining the tubes is not necessarily analogous to the biological responses of human and animal blood vessels. Areas of separation have been demonstrated at sites corresponding to the position of lateral angles in two-dimensional flow models of curves and branchings,[67] and also in a branching tube in which inverse relationships were found between the threshold mean flow rate at which separation occurs and the angle of branching.[76] In both instances, the limbs of the branched models each had the same diameter, and hence the forks are quite unphysiological. Disturbances of flow were found[77] in a similar experimental system using blood. At the lateral angle of the aortic bifurcation of dogs, the use of hot wire anemometry has shown that flow disturbances are severe at low Reynolds numbers. Noticeable are (1) prominent instantaneous change in velocity from moment to moment especially during reversed flow, (2) periodic turbulence, and (3) extremely unstable flow, which could not be classified. These observations accord with those of McDonald[131,134] in smaller arteries.

Pathological lesions can induce turbulence at low Reynolds numbers. The onset has been demonstrated in the poststenotic dilatation in experimental models.[139,173,174] Turbulent flow may be seen in experimental aneurysms and arteriovenous fistulas, and recently it was demonstrated in an experimental model of a berry aneurysm at low flow rates.[54]

Arteriovenous shunts. Pfeifer[157] described leptomeningeal arteriovenous anastomoses and Penfield[156] observed a persistent reddening of veins draining an epileptogenic area of the cortex after a convulsion. Perfusion experiments led Rowbotham and Little[179] to believe that arteriovenous shunts were not unusual on the surface of the brain. They subsequently demonstrated by microdissection the presence of leptomeningeal shunts (varying in diameter from 20 to 160 μ that were under the control of local influences by means of sphincters at the origin of the arteries.[60] The shunts, they considered, explained the imperfect filling of the cortex during injection experiments, the variation in circulation times, the presence of "red cortical veins" after epileptic fits and surgical trauma, the combination of rich surface vascularization in the presence of underlying ischemia, and the anomalous results in cerebral blood flow studies. Hasegawa and associates[82] discovered small arteriovenous shunts both in the cortex and in the subcortical white matter.

Though arteriovenous shunts are prominent features of some pathological lesions, their purpose is not known. The shunting, indicated by "red veins," is readily seen about a few cerebral tumors (Chapter 11) and has been observed in association with trauma, acute infarction,[93,235] epileptogenic foci, cortical scars, and chronic ischemia. It has been referred to as the luxury perfusion syndrome and is essentially a maladaptation of the cerebral circulation in which autoregulation is lost. Feindel

and associates[53] consider this term inappropriate because the presence of the shunt with red veins, a high flow rate, and a diminished arteriovenous oxygen difference is at the expense of the cerebral tissue, which is being deprived of an adequate blood flow. They regard the phenomenon as a relative ischemia or "cerebral steal." Such shunts may also be important in the etiology of arteriovenous aneurysms[179] of which they can be considered a lesser variant. Physiologically, the purpose of the shunts is unknown and pathologically, they appear to be detrimental more often than not.

Cerebral vasospasm. Like vessels of comparable size, the cerebral arteries are capable of active vasoconstriction and a prolonged localized zone of vasospasm may be observed at craniotomy and by angiography in man[101,164] and in experimental animals. It is readily induced by mechanical stimulation of the arteries[146] and topical application of substances such as serotonin and angiotensin may cause vasoconstriction, but the response is most intense with barium chloride.[60,75] Several pharmacological agents including epinephrine cause vasodilatation. The vasospasm at craniotomy is readily relieved by the local application of papaverine and to a lesser extent cocaine is helpful, all of which suggests that a neurogenic factor is involved in the underlying mechanism.[161] It is also pertinent that rhythmic variation in arterial caliber has been observed.[75] There appears to be a gradient of irritability of the cerebral arteries to mechanical stimulation. The response is most prominent in large vessels at the base of the brain and least in peripheral pial vessels. Moreover, there appears to be a species difference in the rapidity of onset.[75] The spasm may be quite localized to a relatively small arterial segment or more diffuse with occasional beading.

In man, vasospasm is most often observed in cases of subarachnoid hemorrhage of aneurysmal origin (in as many as 50% of cases)[2,164] and usually about the distal segment of the internal carotid or the proximal segments of the middle and anterior cerebral arteries. Echlin[49] alleged that the direct application of blood to the cerebral arteries induced spasm, but he did not elaborate upon the nerve endings involved. This observation has not generally been accepted for, in aneurysmal bleeding, angiographic evidence of vasospasm is rarely observed before the fourth day.[75] Its duration is variable, but it persists for a few days and has disappeared 2 weeks after the hemorrhage. The mechanism is obscure. Breakdown products of blood,[164] serum factors in clotted blood, or platelet products[104] possibly serotonin[167] have each been held responsible. Nevertheless, it is usually seen in patients under 50 years of age[188] and is not often observed in patients with severe atherosclerosis.[222] In subarachnoid bleeding, it is associated with a high mortality and frequent neurological deficits.

Vasospasm has been observed in patients with meningitis and head injuries,[75] subdural empyema, and even cerebral arteriovenous aneurysm,[221] but much less frequently than with rupture of an aneurysm. Armstrong and Hayes[7] demonstrated segmental vasospasm of cerebral arteries in a patient with pheochromocytoma and attributed the vasoconstriction to the presence of circulating catecholamines.

The concept that vasospasm is responsible for transient or even more permanent cerebral dysfunction is long standing and has caused much debate.[49,164] Pickering[158] believed that this concept had been accepted uncritically and that organic vascular narrowing could mimic spasm. This may well often be the case, but in aneurysmal subarachnoid hemorrhage it is of poor prognostic significance and, if not the cause of cerebral ischemia and infarction, is believed to be an important contributing factor (see Chapter 9). A reduced circulation time accompanies the vasospasm, but as yet there is no evidence of complete closure of the lumen. Ischemia in association with experimental vasospasm mechan-

ically induced may be caused by a combination of vasoconstriction and embolism from thrombus formed at the site of injury.

Effect of stenoses on flow. Brice and associates[18,19] found that experimental constrictions of the common carotid artery were of little consequence on the pressure gradient or the blood flow until the lumen was reduced to an average of 5 sq. mm. from an average of 35.8 sq. mm. (varying from 17 to 60 sq. mm.). The percentage of reduction was less significant than the absolute cross-sectional area to which the lumen was reduced. A lumen of 2 to 4 sq. mm. represented a reduction of 90% to 80%, and the authors doubt whether lesser degrees of stenosis seen at autopsy were hemodynamically significant even though multiple. The critical degree of stenosis is likely to be less in the presence of occlusion of other major arteries in the neck.[50]

It is well recognized that stenosis of an arterial segment can produce a poststenotic dilatation varying in length but appearing to be dependent on the strength of the thrill and bruit. The presence of stenosis, however, is not invariably followed by such a dilatation, which would not preclude the possibility of structural damage to the wall of the vessel in the poststenotic area. Aneurysmal dilatation and even rupture of the poststenotic area may occur in aortic coarctation, and similar lesions might occur in the large carotid arteries of the neck, though probably not in the smaller intracranial arteries.

The carotid sinus is a slight fusiform dilatation and although frank aneurysmal dilatation is rare at that site, the presumed flow disturbance could conceivably be related to the pathological lesions so frequent at that location.

Cerebral causes of cardiac disturbances. Alterations in the cardiac rate and rhythm have been induced in nine of 22 patients by surgical manipulation of the component arteries of the circle of Willis.[160] These effects appear to be accentuated by hypothermia, and the most profound alterations

Table 2-2. One hundred cases of neurogenic ulceration in cerebrovascular disease*

Type of cerebrovascular lesion	Type of ulceration		Total
	Acute	Chronic	
Acute subarachnoid hemorrhage	13†	0	13†
Acute cerebral hemorrhage‡	30	9	39
Acute thromboembolic infarction	7	2	9
Cerebral infarct without gross hemorrhage or thrombosis	17	22	39
Total number of cases	67	33	100

*Adapted from Dalgaard, J. B.: Cerebral vascular lesions and peptic ulceration, Arch. Path. **69:**359, 1960.
†Nine of these hemorrhages were caused by ruptured aneurysms.
‡Including bleeding hemangioma and secondary intracerebral hemorrhages.

(arrhythmias) can be induced by manipulation or dissection of intracranial arterial aneurysms. A case of fatal ventricular fibrillation has resulted from such a procedure under hypothermia.[160] Actual damage of the myocardial fibers complicates acute cerebrovascular disorders (Chapter 7).

Neurogenic ulceration. Neurogenic ulceration of the upper part of the gastrointestinal tract is a well-established entity complicating severe stress and is notably the result of extensive burns, corticosteroid therapy and a wide variety of lesions of the central nervous system. What is not widely known, despite reports dating back to the nineteenth century, is that similar ulceration can follow cerebrovascular disease. Cushing,[37] in an extensive review of neurogenic ulceration, included an instance of extreme esophageal and gastric malacia postoperatively in a patient who had a craniotomy for a large aneurysm of the basilar artery. Strassman[219] found 26 cases of acute hemorrhagic ulceration and 30 cases of softening or perforation of the esophagus, duodenum, or stomach. All except two cases were associated with intracranial disease and 14 were acute vascular lesions. Dalgaard[41] analyzed 4317 autopsies and found 208 acute and 177 cases of chronic peptic ulceration. Exactly 100 autopsies (2.3%) of the total series revealed both cerebrovascular lesions in association with esophageal, gastric, and duodenal ulceration (Table 2-2). Of the 208 cases of acute peptic ulceration, 32% had cerebrovascular lesions and 18.6% of the 177 cases of chronic ulceration had cerebrovascular pathology. As the chronic ulceration did not appear to be the result of the cerebrovascular accidents, the relationship has little established significance. Acute ulceration was thought to occur a few days after the cerebrovascular incident, though it had appeared as early as 12 hours after the ictus. Dalgaard concluded that cerebrovascular lesions are the most common single cause of acute peptic ulceration encountered at autopsy.[41]

Production of murmurs. An intracranial bruit was first reported early in the nineteenth century by Travers[230] who diagnosed an intracranial arteriovenous fistula. The subject felt a sudden snap on the left side of her forehead and thereafter was aware of a constant noise in the head resembling the blowing of a pair of bellows. It could be arrested by carotid compression and the intensity varied with posture.

Mechanism. The exact mechanism of murmur production in the circulatory system has not been resolved, but several theories have been advanced.

TURBULENCE. Laminar flow is silent, and though turbulent flow is thought to be accompanied by some generation of sound, it is rarely detectable on the exterior surface of the tube in which the flow disturbance is being effected.[133] Bruns[21] estimated that blood must attain a velocity of 2000 cm. per second before any appreciable noise can be generated, and as such a velocity of flow is never reached, turbulence as a cause of murmur was dismissed. However, turbulence cannot be measured quantitatively. Only indirect methods such as distorted dye patterns, high Reynolds numbers and nonlinear pressure-flow curves[172] can be implemented to detect its presence. Though more information about flow in arteries and at forks is called for, the field is at best most difficult to investigate. At the present time, many authors consider that some relationship between turbulence and murmurs exists.[172]

CAVITATION. When water flows through a tube with a constriction, bubbles will form at the neck and will generate sound, if the velocity of flow is sufficiently high. Cavitation, the formation and collapse of these bubbles in the circulation, is a possible source of sound, probably of high frequency.[133] It is yet uncertain whether cavitation exists in vivo and if so to what extent. It has not been seen in vivo, but the bubbles, if they occur, could be transitory. Hugh and Fox[95] argue strongly that cavitation accounts for sound as well as damage to the vessel walls. The present consensus is that cavitation is an unlikely cause of cardiovascular sound, but further investigation is necessary to conclusively exclude the possibility.[134]

PERIODIC WAKE FLUCTUATIONS. Bruns[21] postulated that the bulk of the acoustical energy in murmurs is caused by nearly periodic fluctuations downstream in the wake of an obstacle, such as a stenosis, and that the characteristics of this type of flow are basically similar to those associated with aeolian tones or orifice flow. This concept has much in common with vortex shedding. Rushmer and Morgan[180] consider vortex shedding and periodic wake fluctuations more likely to produce tones with fundamental frequencies and harmonics rather than effecting random frequencies of noise. On these grounds, they consider Bruns' hypothesis to be untenable.

FLITTER. Coarse but rapid oscillation of the vessel wall caused by larger falls in intravascular pressure could cause sound, but this is not currently believed to be the cause of murmurs associated with stenoses and fistulas.

NOISE FROM JETS. Rushmer and Morgan[180] assert that the most common types of heart murmurs develop in the vicinity of turbulent jets produced by flow at high velocities through narrow orifices. The noise is thought to be generated by fluctuations in pressure associated with eddy currents striking the walls of the vessels downstream from the orifice or stenosis without dominant frequencies. The vibrations of the vascular wall might then be transmitted through the tissues to the body surface, and it seems certain that to produce sound sufficiently intense to be heard outside the animal's body, the vessel walls must be vibrated.[133]

In the many pathological states in man, a bruit is associated with flow through a narrow orifice, and so the presence of the murmur, and often a palpable thrill as well, is readily understood. There has been concentration on such lesions, namely, arterial stenoses, coarctation of the aorta, and arteriovenous fistulas. No explanation has been provided for the generation of sound in other states, for example, uterine and mammary souffles and the bruit over the thyroid gland in thyrotoxicosis when flow is considerably augmented. This variety also occurs within the cranium and may be regarded as hyperkinetic in type.

Wadia and Monckton[234] believed that variations and asymmetry in the circle of Willis could be responsible for the production of bruits. The size of such vessels militates against this concept. Although the carotid siphon, wide-angled branches, and the junction of two streams display a tendency to turbulence,[205] there is no evidence as yet that such configurations can produce sound in man.

Significance of murmurs. Assessment of the significance of a bruit of the head and neck is complex, for many murmurs are of no clinical import. Venous hums in the neck may be loud in cases of intra-

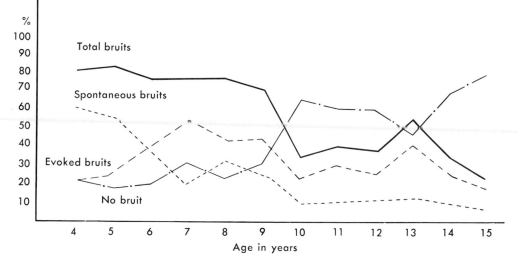

Fig. 2-7. Prevalence of intracranial bruits (spontaneous and evoked) in 513 children according to age. (From Wadia, N. H., and Monckton, G.: Intracranial bruits in health and disease, Brain **80**:492, 1957.)

cranial arteriovenous aneurysm. Physiological murmurs may be heard frequently in the neck and propagation of a cardiac murmur into the neck is not unusual. Murmurs are often present over the head in infants and children, or they may occur in other physiological states but in the adult atherosclerosis is the most common cause of murmurs over the carotid and vertebral arteries.[223]

IN CHILDREN. After the historical observations of Travers (1809-1811), Fisher[57,58] noted sounds with certain physiological functions on auscultation of the head, but related them to such states as chronic hydrocephalus, acute inflammation of the brain, and cerebral abscess. Dodge[44] reviewed the subsequent argument about the significance of murmurs in children and although earlier authors[57,58,236] contended that they were pathological, later authors felt that this was not necessarily so.[42,148] Wadia and Monckton[234] examined 513 children from the age of 4 to 15½ years. Spontaneous bruits occurred in up to 60% of 4 to 5 year olds, diminishing to 20% in those 7 years of age, and then to 10% at 10 years. Thereafter, the fall was slow to 4% at 15½ years of age (Fig. 2-7). The

bruits were mostly unilateral (Table 2-3). The intensity of spontaneous bruits could be augmented by contralateral carotid compression, and their incidence is depicted in Fig. 2-7. The number of subjects in whom bruits (whether spontaneous or evoked) cannot be heard rises steeply at about age 9 or 10 (over 60%) reaching 78% at 15 years of age.

IN ADULTS. Wadia and Monckton[234] examined 228 adults aged 20 to 69 years and found that in only three was a spontaneous bruit audible. One was attributed to arterial disease, and another was associated with migraine. The incidence of bruits evoked by unilateral carotid compression on the other hand was greater but declined slowly after the age of 30 years (Table 2-4). Most bruits evoked were bilateral and in only nine instances was the murmur unilateral. Hammond and Eisinger[79] examined 1000 subjects without neurological disease and found that cervical bruits were present in 87% of those over 60 years. Bilateral bruits were observed in 63% of persons with audible murmurs. Rennie and associates[169] found a high incidence of murmurs (40%) in 70 young medical students of a mean age of 23 years. This

Table 2-3. Incidence of bruits in 513 healthy children (4 to 15½ years of age)*

Bruit	Right	Bilateral	Left	Total
Spontaneous bruits	31	44	21	96†
Bruits evoked by unilateral carotid compression	47	91	31	169

*Adapted from Wadia, N. H., and Monckton, G.: Intracranial bruits in health and disease, Brain **80**:492, 1957.
†This total in the reference source was originally printed incorrectly as 98.

Table 2-4. Incidence of bruits in healthy subjects*

Age of subjects in years	Number of subjects examined	Total number of subjects with bruits	Number with spontaneous bruits	Number with evoked bruits
4-15½	513	267	98	169
20-29	43	21	1	20
30-39	38	9	0	9
40-49	50	10	0	10
50-59	54	10	2	8
60-69	43	2	0	2
Adults only	228	52	3	49

*Adapted from Wadia, N. H., and Monckton, G.: Intracranial bruits in health and disease, Brain **80**:492, 1957.

incidence is in direct contrast with the low figures of other observers (see Table 2-4), and so the problem is raised not only of detection but of interpretation of murmurs. There seems to be considerable argument over the validity of including as murmurs some of the sounds heard in the neck.[136,141] With all subjective assessment, the margin of error can be inordinate, and a serious need is evident for more objective means of differentiating between significant and physiological murmurs. The physical characteristics of the murmurs have not been sufficiently analyzed to enable valid deductions to be made regarding volume, pitch, quality, and transmission, all of which are dependent on the diameter of the vessel, the velocity and viscosity of the blood, the irregularities of the intimal surface including stenoses, the presence of poststenotic dilatations, and the configuration and course of the vessels. Bifurcations with wide angles and the carotid siphon may produce turbulence,[205] but there is no evidence that they cause murmurs, as severe kinks in the carotid

well might. Future technological advances should enable the clinician to accurately localize the site and cause of sound production. It is also possible that pathological effects on the vessel wall may result from the hemodynamic disturbances associated with such sound production.

MURMURS IN PATHOLOGICAL STATES. The presence of spontaneous bruits in adults over 20 years of age is generally of pathological significance.[234] If care is taken to exclude functional or insignificant murmurs, a significant relationship between murmurs of the head and neck and cerebrovascular disease becomes apparent (Table 2-5). The bruits are thought to indicate a degree of stenosis of the lumen or a fistula. The carotid sinus, itself a fusiform dilatation, does not provide disparity in caliber sufficient to cause a murmur. Hyperkinetic conditions of flow particularly in the distal internal carotid artery also cause murmurs, and bruits may occur in association with a prosthetic shunt[123] related to its configuration and the disparity in the size of the lumen. Murmurs need

Table 2-5. Frequency of spontaneously occurring bruits of the head and neck in various states

State of subjects examined	Number of patients	Number of patients with murmurs	Incidence of murmurs as a percentage
Healthy adults (Wadia & Monckton, 1957)[234]	228	3	1.3
Unselected adults without cerebrovascular disease (Siekert, 1966)[194]	200	7	3.5
Unselected adult patients (Dale, 1966)[40]	101	3	3
100 hospitalized patients with a mean age of 52 years* (Crevasse & Logue, 1958)[34]	100	9	9
100 patients with a mean age of 75.7 years (Crevasse & Logue, 1958)[34]	100	8†	8
Adult patients with cerebrovascular disease (Burton, 1966)[24]	75	14	18
Symptoms and signs suggestive of atherosclerotic cerebral vascular lesions (Toole, 1966)[224]	144	55	39
Intermittent claudication of legs without cerebral symptoms (Toole, 1966)[224]	95	19	20
Proved carotid artery stenosis (Peart & Rob, 1960)[154]	103	59	57.3

*Only two of these patients had neurological symptoms.
†Six of the eight had neurological symptoms.

not be audible in the presence of demonstrable arterial stenosis. Moreover, anemia appears to increase the tendency for the commencement of an audible bruit, which may disappear completely on compensation of the anemia.[30,56]

1. *Atherosclerosis.* Murmurs may be audible in the neck or over the head in patients with severe atherosclerosis of the major arteries supplying the brain in either the intracranial or extracranial portions of their course. A systolic murmur (with or without a thrill) may be audible over a partially occluded carotid sinus (the most common site of atherosclerotic involvement). The bruit may be the earliest sign of carotid artery insufficiency.[34] It may be transmitted up the carotid to the cranium, but it is usually inaudible a few centimeters below the carotid sinus. A narrowing in the carotid siphon may also cause a murmur, detected best over the nearest eye.[30,34] In general, murmurs from intracranial sources are heard to advantage over foramina such as the orbit, ear, or a trephine hole. Murmurs over the subclavian and vertebral arteries are much less common

than those produced by carotid occlusions. Toole[224] found bruits over the subclavian or vertebral arteries in five of 144 patients with symptomatic cerebrovascular disease. All could be altered by varying the position of the head or arm.

A disappearance of the murmurs can signify more severe or complete occlusion of the vessel. In any event, a change in intensity and perhaps locale in the middle aged or elderly probably indicates changes in the atherosclerotic disease and changes in the flow patterns in cerebral vessels.[136] The intensity of the murmur has been observed to diminish as signs of arterial insufficiency developed.[123] Compression of the contralateral carotid and exercise may accentuate the bruit. An intracranial systolic bruit may be detected over the eye and perhaps in the temporal region in patients with occlusion of the contralateral internal carotid artery.[48,56] Such a bruit is hyperkinetic in type, probably being caused by increased velocity of flow through the ipsilateral carotid artery by way of compensation.

2. *Arteriovenous aneurysms.* A bruit in the head is heard more often with arteriovenous fistulas or aneurysms than any other patho-

logical state. The presence of a bruit is a well-known diagnostic feature of these lesions, but is a variable sign and occurs only at some time during the natural history of the lesion. Mackenzie[125] stated that it is a distinctive, not necessarily an essential, feature. Potter[163] estimated that a bruit is present in about 20% to 50% of the lesions shown by angiography to be arteriovenous aneurysms. The bruit may be caused by the accelerated and augmented flow through dilated afferent arteries feeding the malformation to the flow of arterial blood into the dilated venous varicosities or to a combination of these factors. In the carotid-cavernous fistula, whether because of trauma or rupture of an aneurysm of that segment of the internal carotid artery, the bruit is derived from the blood flowing through the laceration or tear into the expanded volume of the cavernous sinus, which, with its tributaries, will progressively expand and accentuate the disparity in diameters. Proximal compression of a vessel from which the sound is emanating, usually obliterates the murmur, but in the carotid-cavernous fistula or an arteriovenous aneurysm the bruits may be diminished in intensity only because of a reflex flow of blood to the fistula from collateral or distal vessels. The bruit is usually continuous with systolic accentuation.

The incidence of bruits observed in arteriovenous aneurysms varies considerably in the literature (Table 2-6). Mackenzie[125] observed that in a consecutive series of 50 cases, bruits were detected in 48%. In those patients in whom hemorrhage occurred (either subarachnoid or intracerebral), bruits were rare, but the incidence rose to 65% in those presenting with epilepsy, periodic headache, or hemiparesis.

Table 2-6. Incidence of bruits in intracranial arteriovenous aneurysms

Author	Number of lesions	Number with bruits	Incidence
Dalsgaard-Nielson (1939)[42]	20	5	25%
Olivecrona & Riives (1948)[147]	43	8	18.6%
Mackenzie (1955)[125]	50	24	48%
Wadia & Monckton (1957)[234]	22	18	81.8%
Total	135	55	40.7%

3. *Intracranial arterial aneurysm.* Intracranial arterial aneurysms are at times accompanied by a bruit. First observed by Whitney[236] in an aneurysm of the basilar artery, the phenomenon has been reported repeatedly[54,125] if in only a small proportion of the cases. Once it was thought to be pathognomonic.[125] Less frequently a bruit may be accompanied by a palapable thrill over part of the aneurysmal sac.[25] The bruit can be abolished by compression of the ipsilateral carotid artery but may be momentarily louder after release.[125] There has been no correlation of bruits with the size of the sac or of the entrance. It could well be that bruits occur in large patent sacs. Dalsgaard-Nielsen[42] believed that saccular aneurysms of the vertebral and basilar arteries are more likely to produce bruits than those on the carotid system.

4. *Tumors.* The arteriovenous shunt known to be associated with cerebral tumors may, with increased flow in afferent vessels, cause a bruit. Several authors have noted bruits in association with meningiomas.[125,234] Dalsgaard-Nielsen[42] observed bruits in three of 11 tumors of the fourth ventricle, four of nine patients with Lindau's tumor (hemangioblastoma), nine of 73 gliomas and four of 12 acoustic neurinomas. Wadia and Monckton[234] reported a bruit in a patient with an ependymoma and considerable enlargement of the vessels supplying or draining intracranial tumors is known and has been observed in the case of tumors associated with bruits.[234] Tumors of the glomus jugulare can be extremely vascular and accompanied by a bruit.

5. *Miscellaneous.* Wadia and Monckton[234] found bruits common in thyrotoxicosis and moderately severe anemia, the sound being attributed to the augmented flow and analogous to the murmurs in children. Though anemia has been incriminated as a cause, Fisher[56] did not confirm this in several cases of severe anemia and inferred that the anemia was merely a contributory factor in murmurs arising from pathological vessels.

Paget's disease of the skull may cause a bruit.[234] The affected bones are extremely vascular and associated with an arteriovenous shunt and increased cardiac output. No compression of the internal carotid arteries was observed.

Murmurs have also been reported during attacks of migraine and in increased intracranial pressure, and bruits have been reported in the first few days after cerebral infarction.[3]

McGregor and Medalie[137] discovered a

bruit in an 8-year-old boy with coarctation of the aorta. The common carotid arteries were dilated and tortuous, and at autopsy all the cerebral arteries exhibited gross dilatation and atherosclerosis. No aneurysms and no arteriovenous malformations were detected. The murmur could have been associated with the widespread arteriectasis.

Other reported causes of murmur include fever, exercise, and nervous tension.[5] Mace, Peters, and Mathies[124] recently demonstrated that the incidence of bruits in children (3 months to 5 years of age) was considerably higher in purulent meningitis (82%) than in either a series of febrile (22%) or afebrile (16%) control patients. The bruits were usually transitory lasting 1

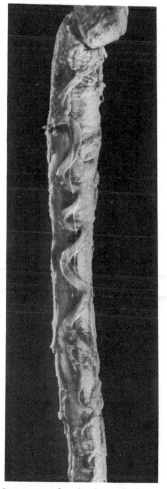

Fig. 2-8. Segment of spinal cord demonstrating grossly enlarged and tortuous anterior spinal artery functioning as a collateral in a patient with coarctation of aorta.

to 4 days after initiation of therapy and could be abolished by lumbar puncture with the removal of some cerebrospinal fluid. Intracranial pressure was thought to be the prime mediator. After their disappearance, the bruits returned on the fifth to the seventh days coincidental with the development of a subdural effusion.

SPINAL BRUITS. The clinical value of cervical and cranial bruits in cerebral vascular abnormalities is appreciated, but spinal bruits have been comparatively neglected. For the most part, the blood vessels supplying the spinal cord are too small to generate sound although under certain circumstances the vessels enlarge. In coarctation of the aorta, the spinal arteries participate in the collateral circulation (Fig. 2-8) and an audible bruit is usually present over the back, but perhaps this is transmitted from the site of stenosis. Arteriovenous malformations of the spinal cord, like those within the skull, are capable of emitting sounds, and bruits have been heard in several instances.[55,128] Palpable thrills have not been noted in association with spinal bruits, almost certainly because of the dampening effect of the intervening tissues.

References

1. Alexander, L., and Putman, T. J.: Pathological alterations of cerebral vascular patterns. In: The circulation of the brain and spinal cord, Ass. Res. Nerv. Ment. Dis. **18:**471, 1938.
2. Allcock, J. M.: Arterial spasm in subarachnoid haemorrhage, Acta Radiol. **5:**73, 1966.
3. Allen, N., and Mustian, V.: Origin and significance of vascular murmurs of the head and neck, Medicine **41:**227, 1962.
4. Andres, K. H.: Zur Feinstruktur der Arachnoidalzotten bei Mammalia, Z. Zellforsch. **82:** 92, 1967.
5. Annotation: The meaning of a murmur, Lancet **1:**710, 1963.
6. Annotation: Cerebral blood-flow and cerebrospinal fluid, Lancet **2:**206, 1968.
7. Armstrong, F. S., and Hayes, G. J.: Segmental cerebral arterial constriction associated with pheochromocytoma, J. Neurosurg. **18:**841, 1961.
8. Bakay, L., and Sweet, W. H.: Cervical and intracranial intra-arterial pressures with and without vascular occlusion, Surg. Gynec. Obstet. **95:**67, 1952.
9. Baker, A. B.: Structure of the small cerebral arteries and their changes with age, Amer. J. Path. **13:**453, 1937.
10. Bauer, R., Sheehan, S., and Meyer, J. S.: Ar-

teriographic study of cerebrovascular disease. II. Cerebral symptoms due to kinking, tortuosity, and compression of carotid and vertebral arteries on the neck, Arch. Neurol. **4:**119, 1961.

11. Bennett, H. S., Luft, J. H., and Hampton, J. C.: Morphological classification of vertebrate blood capillaries, Amer. J. Physiol. **196:**381, 1959.

12. Bergland, R. M., and Torack, R. M.: An electron microscopic study of the human infundibulum, Z. Zellforsch. **99:**1, 1969.

13. Blackwood, W.: Vascular disease of the central nervous system. In Blackwood, W., McMenemey, W. H., Meyer, A., Norman, R. M., and Russell, D. S.: Greenfield's neuropathology, ed. 2, Baltimore, 1963, The Williams & Wilkins Co., p. 71.

14. Blair, J. S.: Reinforcement of branch pieces, Engineering (London) **162:**1, 217, 508, 529, 553, 577, 605; 1946.

15. Bloor, B. M., Odom, G. L., and Woodhall, B.: Direct measurement of intravascular pressure in components of the circle of Willis, Arch. Surg. **63:**821, 1951.

16. Bodenheimer, T. S., and Brightman, M. W.: A blood-brain barrier to peroxidase in capillaries surrounded by perivascular spaces, Amer. J. Anat. **122:**249, 1968.

17. Bremer, J. L.: Congenital aneurysms of the cerebral arteries, Arch. Path. **35:**819, 1943.

18. Brice, J. G., Dowsett, D. J., and Lowe, R. D.: Haemodynamic effects of carotid artery stenosis Brit. Med. J. **2:**1363, 1964.

19. Brice, J. G., Dowsett, D. J., and Lowe, R. D.: The effect of constriction on carotid blood-flow and pressure gradient, Lancet **1:**84, 1964.

20. Brock, M., Schürmann, K., and Hadjidimos, A.: Cerebral blood flow and cerebral death, Acta Neurochirurg. **20:**195, 1969.

21. Bruns, D. L.: A general theory of the causes of murmurs in the cardiovascular system, Amer. J. Med. **27:**360, 1959.

22. Bruns, R. R., and Palade, G. E.: Studies on blood capillaries, I. General organization of blood capillaries in muscle, J. Cell Biol. **37:**244, 1968.

23. Bruns, R. R., and Palade, G. E.: Studies on blood capillaries. II. Transport of ferritin molecules across the wall of muscle capillaries, J. Cell Biol. **37:**277, 1968.

24. Burton, R. C.: Discussion. In Millikan, C. H., Siekert, R. G., and Whisnant, J. P.: Cerebral vascular diseases, Fifth Princeton Conference, New York, 1966, Grune & Stratton, Inc., p. 128.

25. Campbell, E., Perese, D., and Bigelow, N. H.: Excision of multisaccular supratentorial aneurysm of infratentorial origin, J. Neurosurg. **11:**422, 1954.

26. Carmichael, R.: Gross defects in the muscular and elastic coats of the larger cerebral arteries, J. Path. Bact. **57:**345, 1945.

27. Chambers, R., and Zweifach, B. W.: Intracellular cement and capillary permeability, Physiol. Rev. **27:**436, 1947.

28. Clemente, C. D., and Holst, E. A.: Pathological changes in neurons, neuroglia, and blood-brain barrier induced by X-irradiation of heads of monkeys, Arch. Neurol. Psychiat. **71:**66, 1954.

29. Cobb, S.: The cerebrospinal blood vessels. In Penfield, W.: Cytology and cellular pathology of the central nervous system, New York, 1932, Paul B. Hoeber, Inc., vol. 2, p. 577.

30. Cohen, J. H., and Miller, S.: Eyeball bruits, New Eng. J. Med. **255:**459, 1956.

31. Coulter, N. A., and Pappenheimer. J. R.: Development of turbulence in flowing blood, Amer. J. Physiol. **159:**401, 1949.

32. Craigie, E. H.: Postnatal changes in vascularity in the cerebral cortex of the male albino rat, J. Comp. Neurol. **39:**301, 1925.

33. Craigie, E. H.: The comparative anatomy and embryology of the capillary bed of the central nervous system. In: The circulation of the brain and spinal cord, Ass. Res. Nerv. Ment. Dis. **18:**3, 1938.

34. Crevasse, L. E., and Logue, R. B.: Carotid artery murmurs: continuous murmur over carotid bulb—new sign of carotid artery insufficiency, J.A.M.A. **167:**2177, 1958.

35. Crompton, M. R.: The pathogenesis of cerebral aneurysms, Brain **89:**797, 1966.

36. Crompton, M. R.: The comparative pathology of cerebral aneurysms, Brain **89:**789, 1966.

37. Cushing, H.: Peptic ulcers and the interbrain, Surg. Gynec. Obstet. **55:**1, 1932.

38. Dahl, E., Flora, G., and Nelson, E.: Electron microscopic observations on normal human intracranial arteries, Neurology **15:**132, 1965.

39. Dahl, E., and Nelson, E.: Electron microscopic observations on human intracranial arteries. II. Innervation, Arch. Neurol. **10:**158, 1964.

40. Dale, A. J. D.: Unpublished data, cited by Burton.[24]

41. Dalgaard, J. B.: Cerebral vascular lesions and peptic ulceration, Arch. Path. **69:**359, 1960.

42. Dalsgaard-Nielsen, T.: Studies in intracranial vascular sounds, Acta Psychiat. Neurol. Scand. **14:**69, 1939.

43. Dempsey, E. W., and Wislocki, G. B.: An electron microscopic study of the blood-brain barrier in the rat, employing silver nitrate as a vital stain, J. Biophys. Biochem. Cytol. **1:**245, 1955.

44. Dodge, H. W.: Cephalic bruits in children, J. Neurosurg. **13:**527, 1956.

45. Donahue, S., and Pappas, G. D.: The fine structure of capillaries in the cerebral cortex of the rat at various stages of development, Amer. J. Anat. **108:**331, 1961.

46. Du Boulay, G. H.: Some observations on the natural history of intracranial aneurysms, Brit. J. Radiol. **38:**721, 1965.

47. Du Boulay, G. H.: The natural history of intracranial aneurysms, Amer. Heart J. **73:**723, 1967.

48. Dunning, H. S.: Detection of occlusion of the internal carotid artery by pharyngeal palpation, J.A.M.A. **152:**321, 1953.

49. Echlin, F. A.: Vasospasm and focal cerebral ischemia, Arch. Neurol. Psychiat. **47**:77, 1942.

50. Eklöf, B., and Schwartz, S. I.: Critical stenosis of the carotid artery in the dog, Scand. J. Clin. Lab. Invest. **25**:349, 1970.

51. Farquhar, M. G., and Hartman, J. F.: Electron microscopy of cerebral capillaries, Anat. Rec. **124**:288, 1956.

52. Fawcett, D. W.: Comparative observations on the fine structure of blood capillaries. In Orbison, J. L., and Smith, D. E.: The peripheral blood vessels, Baltimore, 1963, The Williams & Wilkins Co., p. 16.

53. Feindel, W. Yamamoto, Y. L., and Hodge, P.: Preferential shunting and multi-compartmental blood flow in the human brain. In Bain, W. H., and Harper, A. M.: Blood flow through organs and tissues, Edinburgh, 1968, E. and S. Livingstone Ltd., p. 232.

54. Ferguson, G. G.: Turbulence in human intracranial saccular aneurysms, J. Neurosurg. **33**: 485, 1970.

55. Fine, R. D.: Angioma racemosum venosum of spinal cord with segmentally related angiomatous lesions of skin and forearm, J. Neurosurg. **18**:546, 1961.

56. Fisher, C. M.: Cranial bruit associated with occlusion of the internal carotid artery, Neurology **7**:299, 1957.

57. Fisher, J. D.: Observations on a cephalic bellows-sound, Med. Mag. Boston **2**:144, 1834.

58. Fisher, J. D.: Observations on cerebral auscultation, Amer. J. Med. Sci. **22**:277, 1838.

59. Flora, G., Dahl, E., and Nelson, E.: Electron microscopic observations on human intracranial arteries, Arch. Neurol. **17**:162, 1967.

60. Florey, H.: Microscopical observations on the circulation of the blood in the cerebral cortex, Brain **48**:43, 1925.

61. Florey, H. W.: The transport of materials across the capillary wall, Quart. J. Exp. Physiol. **49**:117, 1964.

62. Florey, H. W., Poole, J. C. F., and Meek, G. A.: Endothelial cells and "cement" lines, J. Path. Bact. **77**:625, 1959.

63. Földi, M., Csillik, B., and Zoltán, Ö. T.: Lymphatic drainage of the brain, Experientia **24**:1283, 1968.

64. Forbes, H. S.: The cerebral circulation. 1. Observation and measurement of pial vessels, Arch. Neurol. Psychiat. **19**:751, 1928.

65. Forbes, H. S., and Wolff, H. G.: Cerebral circulation. III. The vasomotor control of cerebral vessels, Arch. Neurol. Psychiat. **19**: 1057, 1928.

66. Forbus, W. D.: On the origin of miliary aneurysms of the superficial cerebral arteries, Bull. Johns Hopkins Hosp. **47**:239, 1930.

67. Fox, J. A., and Hugh, A. E.: Localization of atheroma: a theory based on boundary layer separation, Brit. Heart J. **28**:388, 1966.

68. Fox, J. L.: Development of recent thoughts on intracranial pressure and the blood-brain barrier, J. Neurosurg. **21**:909, 1964.

69. Freyhan, F. A., Woodford, R. B., and Kety, S. S.: Cerebral blood flow and metabolism in psychoses of senility, J. Nerv. Ment. Dis. **113**:449, 1951.

70. Gillilan, L. A.: General principles of the arterial blood vessel patterns to the brain, Trans. Amer. Neurol. Ass. **82**:65, 1957.

71. Gilroy, J., Bauer, R. B., Krabbenhoft, K. L., and Meyer, J. S.: Cerebral circulation time in cerebral vascular disease measured by serial angiography, Amer. J. Roentgen. **90**:490, 1963.

72. Glynn, L. E.: Medial defects in the circle of Willis and their relation to aneurysm formation, J. Path. Bact. **51**:213, 1940.

73. Green, H. G.: Circulatory system: physical principles. In Glasser, O.: New Medical physics, Chicago, 1950, Year Book Publishers, Inc., vol. 2, p. 228.

74. Greenfield, J. C., and Tindall, G. T.: Effect of norepinephrine, epinephrine, and angiotensin on blood flow in the internal carotid artery of man, J. Clin. Invest. **47**:1672, 1968.

75. Gurdjian, E. S., and Thomas, L. M.: Cerebral vasospasm, Surg. Gynec. Obstet. **129**: 931, 1969.

76. Gutstein, W. H., and Schneck, D. J.: In vitro boundary layer studies of blood flow in branched tubes, J. Atheroscler. Res. **7**:295, 1967.

77. Gutstein, W. H., Schneck, D. J., and Marks, J. O.: In vitro studies of local blood flow disturbance in a region of separation, J. Atheroscler. Res. **8**:381, 1968.

78. Habib, R. P.: Graduation thesis, Dept. Aeronautical Engineering, University of Sydney, 1959.

79. Hammond, J. H., and Eisinger, R. P.: Carotid bruits in 1,000 normal subjects, Arch. Intern. Med. **109**:563, 1962.

80. Hardesty, W. H., Roberts, B., Toole, J. F., and Royster, H. P.: Studies of carotid-artery blood flow in man, New Eng. J. Med. **263**: 944, 1960.

81. Hardesty, W. H., Whitacre, W. B., Toole, J. F., Randall, P., and Royster, H. P.: Studies on vertebral artery blood flow in man, Surg. Gynec. Obstet. **116**:662, 1963.

82. Hasegawa, T., Ravens, J. R., and Toole, J. F.: Precapillary arteriovenous anastomoses: "thoroughfare channels" in the brain, Arch. Neurol. **16**:217, 1967.

83. Hassler, O.: Morphological studies on the large cerebral arteries with reference to the aetiology of subarachnoid haemorrhage, Acta Psychiat. Neurol. Scand. **36**: (suppl. 154):1, 1961.

84. Hassler, O.: Medial defects in the meningeal arteries, J. Neurosurg. **19**:337, 1962.

85. Hassler, O.: Media defects in human arteries, Angiology **14**:368, 1963.

86. Hassler, O.: Experimental carotid ligation followed by aneurysmal formation and other morphological changes in the circle of Willis, J. Neurosurg. **20**:1, 1963.

87. Hassler, O.: Effect of experimental hypertension on media defects in rabbit arteries, Angiologica **5**:364, 1968.

88. Hedges, T. R., and Weinstein, J. D.: Cerebrovascular responses to increased intracranial pressure, J. Neurosurg. 21:292, 1964.

89. Hills, C. P.: Ultrastructural changes in the capillary bed of the rat cerebral cortex in anoxic-ischemic brain lesions, Amer. J. Path. 44:531, 1964.

90. Hirano, A., Becker, N. H., and Zimmerman, H. M.: Pathological alterations in the cerebral endothelial cell barrier to peroxidase, Arch. Neurol. 20:300, 1969.

91. Hirano, A., Dembitzer, H. M., Becker, N. H., Levine, S., and Zimmerman, H. M.: Fine structural alterations of the blood-brain barrier in experimental allergic encephalomyelitis, J. Neuropath. Exp. Neurol. 29:432, 1970.

92. Hirano, A., Zimmerman, H. M., and Levine, S.: The fine structure of cerebral fluid accumulation, Amer. J. Path. 47:537, 1965.

93. Høedt-Rasmussen, K., Skinhøj, E., Paulson, O., Ewald, J., Bjerrum, J. K., Fahrenkrug, A., and Lassen, N. A.: Regional cerebral blood flow in acute apoplexy, Arch. Neurol. 17:271, 1967.

94. Hoffman, H. J., and Olszewski, J.: Spread of sodium fluorescein in normal brain tissue, Neurology 11:1081, 1961.

95. Hugh, A. E., and Fox, J. A.: Circulatory cavitation "bubbles in the blood," Lancet 2:717, 1963.

96. Hughes, W., Dodgson, M. C. H., and MacLennan, D. C.: Chronic cerebral hypertensive disease, Lancet 2:770, 1954.

97. Imai, H., and Thomas, W. A.: Cerebral atherosclerosis in swine: role of necrosis in progression of diet-induced lesions from proliferative to atheromatous stage, Exp. Molec. Path. 8:330, 1968.

98. Ingvar, D. H., and Gustafson, L.: Regional cerebral blood flow in organic dementia with early onset, Acta Neurol. Scand. 46: suppl. 43:42+, 1970.

99. Jennett, W. B.: Experimental studies on the cerebral circulation: clinical aspects, Proc. Roy. Soc. Med. 61:606, 1968.

100. Jennings, M. A., and Florey, (Lord) H. W.: An investigation of some properties of endothelium related to capillary permeability, Proc. Roy. Soc., Series B, 167:39, 1967.

101. Jennings, M. A., Florey, H. W., Stehbens, W. E., and French, J. E.: Intimal changes in the arteries of a pig, J. Path. Bact. 81:49, 1961.

102. Jerrard, W., and Burton, A. C.: Demonstration of hemodynamic principles in particular of turbulent and stream-line flow, J. Appl. Physiol. 4:620, 1954.

103. Kak, V. K., and Taylor, A. R.: Cerebral blood-flow in subarachnoid haemorrhage, Lancet 1:875, 1967.

104. Kapp, J., Mahaley, M. S., and Odom, G. L.: Cerebral arterial spasm. Part 3: Partial purification and characterization of a spasmogenic substance in feline platelets. J. Neurosurg. 29:350, 1968.

105. Karnovsky, M. J.: The ultrastructural basis of capillary permeability studied with peroxidase as a tracer, J. Cell Biol. 35:213, 1967.

106. Karnovsky, M. J.: The ultrastructural basis of transcapillary exchanges, J. Gen Physiol. 52:64, 1968.

107. Kety, S. S.: Circulation and metabolism of the human brain in health and disease, Amer. J. Med. 8:205, 1950.

108. Kety, S. S.: The cerebral circulation. In Field, J., Magoun, H. W., and Hall, V. E.: Handbook of physiology, Vol. 3, Sect. 1, Neurophysiology, Baltimore, 1960, The Williams & Wilkins Co., p. 1751.

109. Kety, S. S., and Schmidt, C. F.: The nitrous oxide method for the quantitative determination of cerebral blood flow in man: theory, procedure, and normal values, J. Clin. Invest. 27:476, 1948.

110. Kety, S. S., Shenkin, H. A., and Schmidt, C. F.: The effects of increased intracranial pressure on cerebral circulatory functions in man, J. Clin. Invest. 27:493, 1948.

111. King, L. S.: The hematoencephalic barrier, Arch. Neurol. Psychiat. 41:51, 1939.

112. Kuhn, R. A.: The speed of cerebral circulation, New Eng. J. Med. 267:689, 1962.

113. Landis, E. M.: Capillary pressure and capillary permeability, Physiol. Rev. 14:404, 1934.

114. Lassen, N. A.: Cerebral blood flow and oxygen consumption in man, Physiol. Rev. 39:183, 1959.

115. Lassen, N. A., and Ingvar, D. H.: Regional cerebral blood flow measurement in man, Arch. Neurol. 9:615, 1963.

116. Loeb, C., and Meyer, J. S.: Strokes due to vertebro-basilar insufficiency, Springfield, Ill., 1965, Charles C Thomas, Publisher.

117. Long, D. M., Hartman, J. F., and French, L. A.: The ultrastructure of human cerebral edema, J. Neuropath. Exp. Neurol. 25:373, 1966.

118. Luft, J. H.: Fine structure of the vascular wall. In Jones, R. J.: Evolution of the atherosclerotic plaque, Chicago, 1963, University of Chicago Press, p. 3.

119. Luft, J. H.: The ultrastructural basis of capillary permeability. In Zweifach, B. W., Grant, L., and McCluskey, R. T.: The inflammatory process, New York, 1965, Academic Press Inc., p. 121.

120. Luse, S.: Electron microscopic observations of the central nervous system, J. Biophys. Biochem. Cytol. 2:531, 1956.

121. Luse, S. A.: Histochemical implications of electron microscopy of the central nervous system, J. Histochem. Cytochem. 8:398, 1960.

122. Luse, S. A.: Ultrastructure of the brain and its relation to transport of metabolites. In: Ultrastructure and metabolism of the nervous system, Ass. Res. Nerv. Ment. Dis. 40:1, 1962.

123. Lyons, C., and Galbraith, G.: Surgical treatment of atherosclerotic occlusion of the internal carotid artery, Ann. Surg. 146:487, 1957.

124. Mace, J. W., Peters, E. R., and Mathies, A. W.: Cranial bruits in purulent meningitis

in childhood, New Eng. J. Med. **278:**1420, 1968.

125. Mackenzie, I.: The intracranial bruit, Brain **78:**350, 1955.

126. Macklin, C. C., and Macklin, M. T.: A study of brain repair in the rat by the use of trypan blue with special reference to the vital staining of the macrophages. Arch. Neurol. Psychiat. **3:**353, 1920.

127. Mallett, B. L., and Veall, N.: Investigation of cerebral blood-flow in hypertension, using radioactive-xenon inhalation and extracranial recording, Lancet **1:**1081, 1963.

128. Mathews, W. B.: The spinal bruit, Lancet **2:**1117, 1959.

129. Maximow, A. A., and Bloom, W.: A textbook of histology, ed. 4, Philadelphia, 1944, W. B. Saunders Co.

130. Maynard, E. A., Schultz, R. L., and Pease, D. C.: Electron microscopy of the vascular bed of rat cerebral cortex, Amer. J. Anat. **100:**409, 1957.

131. McDonald, D. A.: The occurrence of turbulent flow in the rabbit aorta, J. Physiol. **118:** 340, 1952.

132. McDonald, D. A.: The relation of pulsatile pressure to flow in arteries, J. Physiol. **127:** 533, 1955.

133. McDonald, D. A.: Murmurs in relation to turbulence and eddy formation in the circulation, Circulation **16:**278, 1957.

134. McDonald, D. A.: Blood flow in arteries, London, 1960, Edward Arnold (Publishers) Ltd.

135. McDonald, D. A., and Potter, J. M.: The distribution of blood to the brain, J. Physiol. **114:**356, 1951.

136. McDowell, F., Rennie, L., and Ejrup, B.: Bruits: arterial bruit in cerebrovascular disease. In Millikan, C. H., Siekert, R. G., and Whisnant, J. P.: Cerebral vascular diseases, Fifth Princeton Conference, New York, 1966, Grune & Stratton, Inc., p. 124.

137. McGregor, M., and Medalie, M.: Coarctation of aorta, Brit. Heart J. **14:**531, 1952.

138. McHenry, L. C.: Cerebral blood flow, New Eng. J. Med. **274:**82, 1966.

139. Meisner, J. E., and Rushmer, R. F.: Eddy formation and turbulence in flowing liquids, Circulation Res. **12:**455, 1963.

140. Meyer, J. S.: Interaction of cerebral hemodynamics and metabolism, Neurology **11** (part 2):46, 1961.

141. Meyer, J. S.: Discussion in Millikan, C. H., Siekert, R. G., and Whisnant, J. P.: Cerebral vascular diseases, Fifth Princeton Conference, New York, 1966, Grune & Stratton, Inc., p. 130.

142. Murphy, J. P.: Cerebrovascular disease, Chicago, 1954, Year Book Publishers, Inc.

143. Nelson, E., and Rennels, M.: Innervation of intracranial arteries, Brain **93:**475, 1970.

144. Nylin, G., Blömer, H., Jones, H., Hedlund, S., and Rylander, C.-G.: Further studies on the cerebral blood flow estimated with tho-

rium-B-labelled erythrocytes, Brit. Heart J. **18:**385, 1956.

145. O'Brien, M. D.: Cerebral-cortex-perfusion rates in migraine, Lancet **1:**1036, 1967.

146. Ohta, T., and Baldwin, M.: Experimental mechanical arterial stimulation at the circle of Willis, J. Neurosurg. **28:**405, 1968.

147. Olivecrona, H., and Riives, J.: Arteriovenous aneurysms of the brain, Arch. Neurol. Psychiat. **59:**567, 1948.

148. Osler, W.: On the systolic brain murmur of children, Boston Med. Surg. J. **103:**29, 1880.

149. Palade, G. E.: Fine structure of blood capillaries, J. Appl. Physiol. **24:**1424, 1953.

150. Palade, G. E.: Blood capillaries of the heart and other organs, Circulation **24:**368, 1961.

151. Pálvölgyi, R.: Regional cerebral blood flow in patients with intracranial tumors, J. Neurosurg. **31:**149, 1969.

152. Pappas, G. D., and Tennyson, V. M.: An electron microscopic study of the passage of colloidal particles from the blood vessels of the ciliary processes and choroid plexus of the rabbit, J. Cell Biol. **15:**227, 1962.

153. Pappenheimer, J. R.: Passage of molecules through capillary walls, Physiol. Rev. **33:**387, 1953.

154. Peart, W. S., and Rob, C.: Arterial auscultation, Lancet **2:**219, 1960.

155. Pease, D. C., and Molinari, S.: Electron microscopy of muscular arteries; pial vessels of the cat and monkey, J. Ultrastruct. Res. **3:**447, 1960.

156. Penfield, W.: The circulation of the epileptic brain. In: The circulation of the brain and spinal cord, Ass. Res. Nerv. Ment. Dis. **18:**605, 1938.

157. Pfeifer, R. A.: Die Angioarchitektonik der Grosshirnrinde, Berlin, 1928, Julius Springer. Cited by Wolff.239

158. Pickering, G. W.: Vascular spasm, Lancet **2:** 845, 1951.

159. Plum, F., Posner, J. B., and Troy, B.: Cerebral metabolic and circulatory responses to induced convulsions in animals, Arch. Neurol. **18:**1, 1968.

160. Pool, J. L.: Vasocardiac effect of the circle of Willis, Arch. Neurol. Psychiat. **78:**355, 1957.

161. Pool, J. L.: Cerebral vasospasm, New Eng. J. Med. **259:**1259, 1958.

162. Potter, E. L.: Pathology of the fetus and infant, ed. 2, Chicago, 1961, Year Book Medical Publishers, Inc.

163. Potter, J. M.: Angiomatous malformations of the brain: their nature and prognosis, Ann. Roy. Coll. Surg. Engl. **16:**227, 1955.

164. Potter, J. M.: Cerebral arterial spasm, World Neurol. **2:**576, 1961.

165. Potter, J. M., and McDonald, D. A.: Cinematographic recording of the velocity of arterial blood-flow, Nature **166:**596, 1950.

166. Potter, J. M., and McDonald, D. A.: Cerebral haemodynamics, Lancet **2:**919, 1954.

167. Raynor, R. B., McMurty, J. G., and Pool, J. L.: Cerebrovascular effects of topically ap-

plied serotonin in the cat, Neurology 11:190, 1961.

168. Reese, T. S., and Karnovsky, M. J.: Fine structural localization of a blood-brain barrier to exogenous peroxidase, J. Cell Biol. 34:207, 1967.

169. Rennie, L., Ejrup, B., and McDowell, F.: Arterial bruits in cerebrovascular disease, Neurology 14:751, 1964.

170. Reynolds, O.: An experimental investigation of the circumstances which determine whether the motion shall be direct or sinuous and of the law of resistance in parallel channels, Phil. Trans. 174:935, 1883.

171. Rivera-Pomar, J. M.: Die Ultrastruktur der Kapillaren in der Area postrema der Katze, Z. Zellforsch. 75:542, 1966.

172. Roach, M. R.: An experimental study of the production and time course of poststenotic dilatation in the femoral and carotid arteries of adult dogs. Circulation Res. 13:537, 1963.

173. Robbins, S. L., and Bentov, I.: The kinetics of viscous flow in a model vessel. Effect of stenoses of varying size, shape and length, Lab. Invest. 16:864, 1967.

174. Robicsek, F., Sanger, P. W., Taylor, F. H., Magistro, R., and Foti, E.: Pathogenesis and significance of post-stenotic dilatation in great vessels, Ann. Surg. 147:835, 1958.

175. Rodbard, S.: Vascular modifications induced by flow, Amer. Heart J. 51:926, 1956.

176. Rosenblum, W. I.: Erythrocyte velocity and a velocity pulse in minute blood vessels on the surface of the mouse brain, Circulation Res. 24:887, 1969.

177. Rosomoff, H. I.: Effect of hypothermia and hypertonic urea on distribution of intracranial contents, J. Neurosurg. 18:753, 1961.

178. Roth, T. F., and Porter, K. R.: Yolk protein uptake in the oocyte of the mosquito *Aedes aegypti* L., J. Cell Biol. 20:313, 1964.

179. Rowbotham, G. F., and Little, E.: A new concept of the circulation and the circulations of the brain, Brit. J. Surg. 52:539, 1965.

180. Rushmer, R. F., and Morgan, C.: Meaning of murmurs, Amer. J. Cardiol. 21:722, 1968.

181. Russell, D. S.: Intravital staining of microglia with trypan blue, Amer. J. Path. 5:451, 1929.

182. Rutledge, E. K., and Neubuerger, K. T.: Icterus of the adult brain, Amer. J. Path. 18:153, 1942.

183. Samarasinghe, D. D.: The innervation of the cerebral arteries in the rat: an electron microscope study, J. Anat. 99:815, 1965.

184. Sato, S.: An electron microscopic study on the innervation of the intracranial artery of the rat, Amer. J. Anat. 118:873, 1966.

185. Scheinberg, P.: Cerebral blood flow in vascular disease of the brain, Amer. J. Med. 8:139, 1950.

186. Scheinberg, P., and Stead, E. A.: The cerebral blood flow in male subjects as measured by the nitrous oxide technique. Normal values for blood flow, oxygen utilization, glucose utilization, and peripheral resistance, with observations on the effect of tilting and anxiety, J. Clin. Invest. 28:1163, 1949.

187. Schmidt, C. F.: The cerebral circulation in health and disease, Springfield, Ill., 1950, Charles C Thomas, Publisher.

188. Schneck, S. A., and Kricheff, I. I.: Intracranial aneurysm rupture, vasospasm, and infarction, Arch. Neurol. 11:668, 1964.

189. Schneider, M.: Critical blood pressure in the cerebral circulation. In Schadé, J. P., and McMenemey, W. H.: Selective vulnerability of the brain in hypoxaemia, Philadelphia, 1963, F. A. Davis Co., p. 7.

190. Schubauer, G. B., and Klebanoff, P. S.: Contributions on the mechanics of boundary layer transition, Symposium on boundary layer effects in aerodynamics, National Advisory Committee for Aeronautics, 1955, Paper No. 4.

191. Shabo, A. L., and Maxwell, D. S.: The morphology of the arachnoid villi: a light and electron microscopic study in the monkey, J. Neurosurg. 29:451, 1968.

192. Shalit, M. N., Reinmuth, O. M., Shimojyo, S., and Scheinberg, P.: Carbon dioxide and cerebral circulatory control. III. The effects of brain stem lesions, Arch. Neurol. 17:342, 1967.

193. Shenkin, H. A., Harmel, M. H., and Kety, S. S.: Dynamic anatomy of the cerebral circulation, Arch. Neurol. 60:240, 1948.

194. Siekert, R. G.: Unpublished data, cited by Burton.[24]

195. Silver, M. D., and Stehbens, W. E.: The behaviour of platelets in vivo, Quart. J. Exp. Physiol. 50:241, 1965.

196. Skinhøj, E., Lassen, N. A., and Høedt-Rasmussen, K.: Cerebellar blood flow in man, Arch. Neurol. 10:464, 1964.

197. Skinhøj, E., and Paulson, O. B.: Regional blood flow in internal carotid distribution during migraine attack, Brit. Med. J. 3:569, 1969.

198. Skinhøj, E., and Paulson, O.: Changes in focal cerebral blood flow within the internal carotid system during migraine attack, Acta Neurol. Scand. 46:254, 1970.

199. Smith, D. E., and Windsor, R. B.: Embryologic and pathogenic aspects of the development of cerebral saccular aneurysms. In Fields, W. S.: Pathogenesis and treatment of cerebrovascular disease, Springfield, Ill., 1961, Charles C Thomas, Publisher, p. 367.

200. Sokoloff, L.: Circulation and metabolism of brain in relation to the process of aging. In Birren, J. E., Imus, H. A., and Windle, W. F.: The process of aging in the nervous system, Oxford, 1959, Blackwell Scientific Publications, p. 113.

201. Sokoloff, L.: Aspects of cerebral circulatory physiology of relevance to cerebrovascular disease, Neurology 11 (part 2):34, 1961.

202. Starling, E. H.: The fluids of the body, London, 1909, Archibald Constable and Co., Ltd.

203. Stehbens, W. E.: Medial defects of the cerebral arteries of some mammals, Nature 179:327, 1957.

204. Stehbens, W. E.: Medial defects of the cerebral arteries of man, J. Path. Bact. 78:179, 1959.

205. Stehbens, W. E.: Turbulence of blood flow, Quart. J. Exp. Physiol. 44:110, 1959.
206. Stehbens, W. E.: Properties of endothelium, D. Phil. Thesis, University of Oxford, 1960.
207. Stehbens, W. E.: Turbulence of blood flow in the vascular system of man. In Copley, A. L., and Stainsby, G.: Flow properties of blood, Oxford, 1960, Pergamon Press, p. 137.
208. Stehbens, W. E.: Focal intimal proliferation in the cerebral arteries, Amer. J. Path. 36:289, 1960.
209. Stehbens, W. E.: Discussion on vascular flow and turbulence, Neurology 11 (part 2):66, 1961.
210. Stehbens, W. E.: Cerebral aneurysms of animals other than man, J. Path. Bact. 86:161, 1963.
211. Stehbens, W. E.: Histopathology of cerebral aneurysms, Arch. Neurol. 8:272, 1963.
212. Stehbens, W. E.: Aneurysms and anatomical variation of cerebral arteries, Arch. Path. 75: 45, 1963.
213. Stehbens, W. E.: The renal artery in normal and cholesterol-fed rabbits, Amer. J. Path. 43:969, 1963.
214. Stehbens, W. E.: Endothelial vesicles and protein transport, Nature, 207:197, 1965.
215. Stehbens, W. E.: Ultrastructure of vascular endothelium in the frog, Quart. J. Exp. Physiol. 50:375, 1965.
216. Stehbens, W. E.: Microcirculatory changes in rabbit ear chambers following the infusion of fat emulsions, Metabolism 16:473, 1967.
217. Stehbens, W. E.: Observations on the microcirculation in the rabbit ear chamber, Quart. J. Exp. Physiol. 52:150, 1967.
218. Stehbens, W. E., and Florey, H. W.: The behaviour of intravenously injected particles observed in chambers in rabbits' ears, Quart. J. Exp. Physiol. 45:252, 1960.
219. Strassman, G. S.: Relation of acute hemorrhages and ulcers of gastrointestinal tract to intracranial lesions, Arch. Neurol. Psychiat. 57:145, 1947.
220. Strong, K. C.: A study of the structure of the media of the distributing arteries by the method of microdissection, Anat. Rec. 72:151, 1938.
221. Taveras, J. M., Pool, J. L., and Fletcher, T. M.: The incidence and significance of cerebral vasospasm in 100 consecutive angiograms of intracranial aneurysms, Trans. Amer. Neurol. Ass., 83:100, 1958.
222. Taveras, J. M., and Wood, E. H.: Diagnostic neuroradiology, Baltimore, 1964, The Williams & Wilkins Co.
223. Tindall, G. T., Odom, G. L., Cupp, H. B., and Dillon, M. L.: Studies on carotid artery flow and pressure. Observations in 18 patients during graded occlusion of proximal carotid artery, J. Neurosurg. 19:917, 1962.
224. Toole, J. F.: Bruits, ophthalmodynamometry, carotid compression tests and other diagnostic procedures. In: Cerebrovascular disease, Ass. Res. Nerv. Ment. Dis. 41:267, 1966.
225. Toole, J. F.: Effects of change of head, limb and body position on cephalic circulation, New Eng. J. Med. 279:307, 1968.
226. Toole, J. F., and Patel, A. N.: Cerebrovascular disorders, New York, 1967, McGraw-Hill Book Co.
227. Toole, J. F., and Tucker, S. H.: The influence of head position upon flow through the vertebral and internal carotid arteries: a postmortem study, Arch. Neurol. 3:337, 1960.
228. Torack, R. M.: Ultrastructure of capillary reaction to brain tumors, Arch. Neurol. 5: 416, 1961.
229. Torack, R. M., Terry, R. D., and Zimmerman, H. M.: The fine structure of cerebral fluid accumulation II. Swelling produced by triethyl tin poisoning and its comparison with that in the human brain, Amer. J. Path. 36: 273, 1960.
230. Travers, B.: A case of aneurism by anastomosis in the orbit, cured by the ligature of the common carotid artery. Med.-Chir. Trans. 2:1,1809-1811.
231. Triepel, H.: Das elastische Gewebe in der Wand der Arterien der Schädelhöhle, Anat. Hefte 7:189, 1897. Cited by Wolff.[239]
232. Tunis, M. M., and Wolff, H. G.: Studies on headache, Arch. Neurol. Psychiat. 70:551, 1953.
233. Tuthill, C. R.: Cerebral aneurysms, Arch. Path. 16:630, 1933.
234. Wadia, N. H., and Monckton, G.: Intracranial bruits in health and disease, Brain 80:492, 1957.
235. Waltz, A. G., and Sundt, T. M.: The microvasculature and microcirculation of the cerebral cortex and arterial occlusion, Brain 90: 681, 1967.
236. Whitney, S. S.: Observations on cerebral auscultation, Amer. J. Med. Sci. 6:281, 1843.
237. Wilkinson, I. M. S., Bull, J. W. D., Du Boulay, G. H., Marshall, J., Russell, R. W. R., and Symon L.: Regional blood flow in the normal cerebral hemisphere, J. Neurol. Neurosurg. Psychiat. 32:367, 1969.
238. Winternitz, M. C., Thomas, R. M., and Le Compte, P. M.: The biology of arteriosclerosis, Springfield, Ill., 1938, Charles C Thomas, Publisher.
239. Wolff, H. G.: The cerebral blood vessels—anatomical principles. In: The circulation of the brain and spinal cord, Ass. Res. Nerv. Ment. Dis. 18:29, 1938.
240. Woodhall, B., Odom, G. L., Bloor, B. M., and Golden, J.: Direct measurement of intravascular pressure in components of the circle of Willis, Ann. Surg. 135:911, 1952.
241. Yellin, E. L.: Laminar-turbulent transition process in pulsatile flow, Circulation Res. 19:791, 1966.

3/Atherosclerosis

Atheroma, derived from the Greek for "mush," designates the pultaceous material of high lipid content in advanced intimal plaques. The disease is now termed "atherosclerosis," thus emphasizing the fibrous tissue component of the lesion. Atheroma is but a late stage of atherosclerosis. Arteriosclerosis, used generically, includes atherosclerosis, diffuse hyperplastic sclerosis of small vessels, and Mönckeberg's sclerosis. It is synonymous with atherosclerosis, diffuse hyperplastic sclerosis of small arteries, and also signifies in the arterial wall a generalized increase in fibrous connective tissue accentuated by hypertension. Strong, often conflicting opinion abounds in the field and the terminology should be revised for overlap is considerable and distinction difficult.

This brief survey of cerebral atherosclerosis indicates areas where our knowledge of the pathology remains incomplete and confusing, and emphasizes certain facts that could well provide clues to the etiology.

Pathology of cerebral atherosclerosis

Atherosclerosis is a universal disease occurring to a variable extent in every human. Some have alleged that 31% of patients in the sixth decade exhibit no cerebral atherosclerosis and that even in the ninth decade, 5% remain unaffected,[9,10] but such claims are derived from macroscopic examinations alone. It has never been demonstrated that any adult escapes atherosclerosis if the vessels are examined thoroughly by microscopy. To distinguish between the so-called age changes in human cerebral arteries and atherosclerosis is virtually impossible at present.*

*Barr[11] differentiates senile arteriosclerosis (loss of elastica, ectasia, and gradual infiltration by calcium, lipid, and protein) from atherosclerosis but admits distinction is difficult.

With individual variation, the cerebral arteries undergo progressive increase in caliber with age (ectasia). There is a concomitant variable degree of tortuosity (Fig. 3-1). The earliest macroscopic change is the development of white or opaque areas caused by thickening of the walls, which is frequently related to sites of branching in the facial or dorsal regions and can be diffuse and readily appreciated at the upper end of the basilar. In severely affected brains small distinctly atherosclerotic areas are visible, especially at forks, at the lower end of the basilar, and in the curved terminal segment of the internal carotid ar-

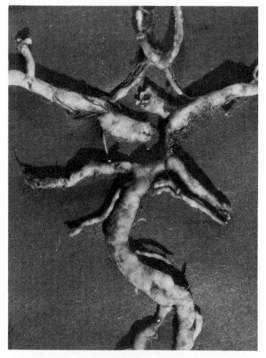

Fig. 3-1. Circle of Willis exhibiting severe atherosclerosis and tortuosity of basilar artery, which forms an S-shaped curvature with one vertebral artery. Note irregularity of surface and external caliber of the arteries.

tery. Early macroscopic lesions, demonstrable in the third decade by gross staining, consist of fatty streaking in the internal carotid and vertebral arteries[114] just after their constriction by the dura mater.

With more severe disease, the arteries appear mottled because of white or yellowish atheromatous plaques contrasting with less affected segments through the walls of which blood or air is often visible. In the occasional patient the atherosclerotic plaques, for reasons unknown, are distinctly orange. When these vessels are sectioned, the lumen is often narrowed and the thickening of the wall eccentric. Yellowish plaques are circumferentially arranged on the basilar artery. A distinctly yellow atherosclerotic nodule is sometimes found at the commencement of small vessels (Fig. 3-2) unaffected in the remainder of their course. Large basal arteries in particular are affected. With increase in severity, the atherosclerosis becomes confluent

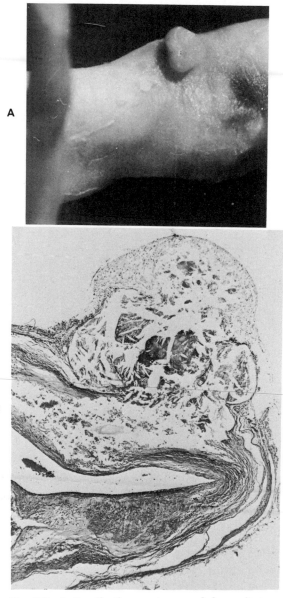

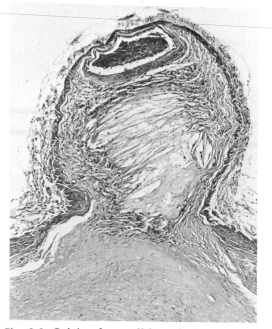

Fig. 3-2. Origin of a small branch (*upper part*) from a large atherosclerotic cerebral artery (*lower part*). Note nodular atherosclerotic involvement of the commencement of the branch. (Hematoxylin and eosin, ×60.)

Fig. 3-3. A, Small atheromatous nodule projecting from surface of middle cerebral artery and simulating a small saccular aneurysm unrelated to a branch. **B,** Section through atheromatous nodule in **A.** Atheromatous material from intima has ruptured externally into adventitia, and periphery of nodule contains many lipophages. (**A,** From Stehbens, W. E.: Aneurysms and anatomical variation of cerebral arteries, Arch. Path. **75:**45, 1963. **B,** Hematoxylin and eosin, ×32.)

in the large arteries, and small flecks and plaques appear in peripheral arteries over the cerebral and cerebellar hemispheres. Atherosclerotic arteries become more rigid and split or even fracture when transected. In external caliber they are larger than unaffected vessels and are displaced from their usual anatomical course by their variable tortuosity. Their uneven knobbled surface (Fig. 3-1), white or yellowish because of the underlying atherosclerosis, often has prominent vasa vasorum and areas of siderotic pigmentation. Small nodules, either firm or pultaceous (Fig. 3-3), can appear on the surface of the arteries, most often the basilar, vertebral, and internal carotid arteries. The vessels may be firm and brittle, though calcification rarely reaches the degree of severity attained by coronary arteries. If the arteries are opened longitudinally, the intimal surface is often of irregular contour. Areas most intensely involved are the upper and lower ends of the basilar, the terminal segment of the internal carotid artery, the first part of the middle cerebral, and the first portion of the posterior cerebral artery.[9] Lesions in the middle and posterior cerebral arteries are allegedly unrelated to bifurcations, but lateral angle pads and their distal extensions lie totally within the daughter branch[162,166] and consequently an atheromatous plaque often extends distally on the appropriate side of the middle cerebral artery from the internal carotid bifurcation. Such lesions may not appear to be related to the arterial fork, but this view would be a misinterpretation. Moreover, macroscopic analysis of the sites of lipid deposition can be fallacious because secondary flow disturbances could complicate the picture. For determination of the earliest sites of lipid deposition reliably, serial frozen sectioning of vessels and forks from children and young adults is essential. Baker and Iannone[8,9] asserted that the earliest manifestations of cerebral atherosclerosis were small zones of intimal thickening. However, from random sections it cannot be appreciated that in the young

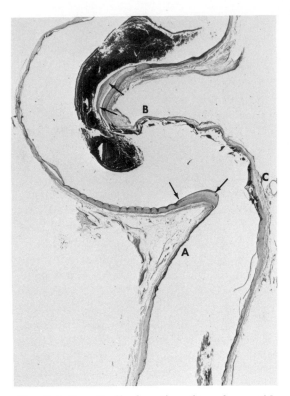

Fig. 3-4. Longitudinal section through carotid siphon showing intimal thickening or pads (*arrows*) downstream in segments protected from impact of flowing blood. Note variation in thickness of vessel wall, which is thinned at **A,** and between **B** and **C.** Calcification is also present between **B** and **C.** Flow is from below upwards. (Verhoeff's stain.)

these pads or cushions are associated with sites of branching.[162,163] Similar intimal pads appear in the carotid siphon (Fig. 3-4) and at other curvatures, but in regard to these sites no systematic studies have been conducted.

Atherosclerosis of the carotid and vertebral arteries in the neck

With increased interest in extracranial arterial occlusion as a cause of cerebral ischemia, atherosclerosis of the extracranial arteries supplying the brain has been investigated. In the carotid arteries the most severe atherosclerosis is usually in the carotid sinus of the common carotid bifurcation[35,55,148] and frequently it is calci-

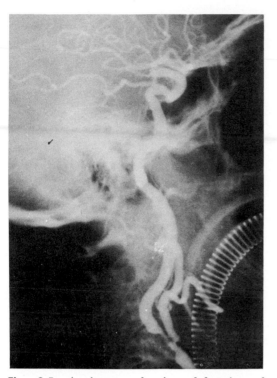

Fig. 3-5. Angiogram showing deformity of lumen of common and internal carotid arteries. Encroachment on lumen is attributed to an atheromatous plaque. Note sinuous course of internal carotid artery in neck. See Fig. 3-6. (Courtesy Dr. J. E. Mincy, Albany, N. Y.)

fied and ulcerated. Dilatation of the sinus, especially in the proximal segment of the internal carotid artery,[126] comes with advancing age. Angiograms demonstrate atherosclerotic plaques as filling defects and confirm the frequency of atherosclerotic involvement of the carotid sinus (Fig. 3-5). A peculiar local vulnerability is suggested, possibly associated with the hemodynamic disturbances induced by the fusiform dilatation constituting the sinus. Mural thrombosis and ulceration are generally not demonstrable in angiograms, but Javid and associates[87] demonstrated by angiography the rapid progression of lesions at this site despite their relative absence from adjacent segments of the carotid arterial tree (both

proximally and distally). The origin of the common carotid artery can be fairly severely affected. The stem, the remainder of the cervical segment, and the petrous segment of the internal carotid artery are less involved, though the cavernous segment tends to be severely diseased. Meyer and Beck[109] removed the petrous and cavernous segments of the internal carotid arteries at 101 autopsies. They found a progressive increase in diameter and length with secondary changes in tortuosity and curvatures. Calcification and intimal thickenings (on the inner curvatures) in association with arteriosclerotic changes were prominent. Samuel[145] observed atherosclerotic intimal thickening on the curvatures of the internal carotid artery and occlusion of the lumen only in the petrous segment. Other authors[53,134] have remarked upon the frequency of calcification in the cavernous segment and its presence in each of the coats of the arterial wall. Calcific deposits appear in the elastic lamina first, in atherosclerotic intimal lesions next, and to a lesser extent in the other coats. Severity increases with age and hypertension (most severely in elderly women). Calcification may limit the development of atherosclerosis[53] but also possible is that each may be a response to different stresses.

The vertebral artery in its extracranial course escapes severe atherosclerosis except at its origin where calcification, stenosis, and ulceration may arise. Fisher and associates[54] contend that vertebral and encephalic arteries exhibit atherosclerosis to a similar degree. Meyer[108] found that atherosclerosis affected the vertebral artery in its ascending cervical course in a segmental manner, with the atherosclerotic patches tending to involve the slightly wider or ectatic segments between the foramina of the transverse processes. Moosy[114] felt the segmental involvement was related to osteoarthritis, but more probably it is associated with ectasia and concomitant degenerative changes.

Moosy[114] found intramural hemorrhage and ulceration more frequently in extracra-

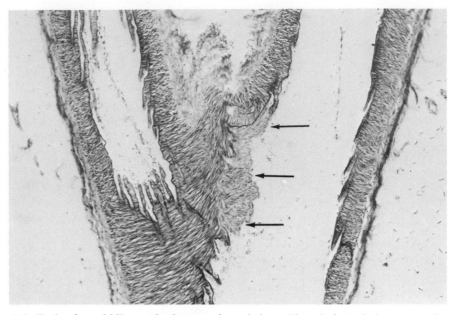

Fig. 3-6. Fork of a middle cerebral artery from infant. Flow is from below upwards. Facial pad *(arrows)* stains less intensely than media suggesting that intermuscular connecnective tissue of the pad is slightly more abundant. (Mallory's phosphotungstic acid—hematoxylin, ×75.)

nial than in intracranial arteries. In the internal carotid artery, the carotid sinus was most affected, and in descending order the cavernous segment, the petrous segment, and the cervical segment. The vertebral arteries were affected at their origin.[114] Solberg and associates[157] in an international survey found that complicated lesions and calicification were uncommon except in the carotid arteries.

Histological changes in the cerebral arteries with age

The histological appearance of advanced atherosclerosis of the cerebral arteries is basically similar to that of extracranial distributing arteries. There is no agreement upon what constitutes the earliest demonstrable lesion:[29,30,113,114] it is said to be a small, raised, yellow intimal "streak" or nodule histologically consisting of a thickened intima containing fat mostly within lipophages. Attention has been focussed on the advanced stages though a stage in the pathogenesis recognizable only by light or electron microscopy should

exist. Observations based on the progressive histological changes of human cerebral arteries seen in the serial sections of over 197 arterial forks (from the fetus to advanced age) will be described.

The intima of the cerebral arteries of all sizes in the infant and fetus consists mainly of an endothelial layer and an internal elastic lamina, with no intermediate layer—a view of a healthy intima that accords with the findings of the Commission for the Study of Cerebrovascular Disease.[25] However, as in the aorta[123,133,191] and other distributing arteries,[34,100,147] cerebral arteries have intimal thickening at sites of branching.[70,163] Serial sections* have revealed that the intimal thickening at cerebral arterial forks is not a diffuse proliferation but occurs as separate pads which later coalesce (such as facial, dorsal, lat-

---

*The need for serial sections in localizing intimal pads is incontrovertible for if they are not used, pads (facial and dorsal) can be overlooked or inaccurately localized, cases in point being the studies of Hassler[75] and Crompton.[31]

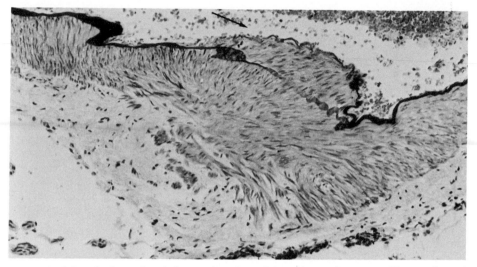

Fig. 3-7. Facial pad of another infant. Direction of flow shown by arrow. Note pale staining of internal elastic lamina deep to the pad and new elastic tissue beneath endothelium. (Verhoeff's elastic stain, ×110.)

eral, and apical pads).[161,163] The facial and dorsal pads (Figs. 3-6 and 3-7) are the earliest to appear (26 weeks in utero). Lateral pads (Fig. 2-2) appear next, and only after facial, dorsal, and lateral pads have enlarged and are coalescing, is the apex involved. Degenerative changes in the internal elastic lamina precede and accompany the pads.[163,164] Lateral pads occur immediately beyond the site where the lateral wall curves into the proximal side of the daughter branch (Fig. 3-8), and in the case of small side branches only one lateral pad will be seen on the side from which the smaller branch took origin.[163] Pads in the fetus consist predominantly of muscle and fine elastic fibrils,[161,163] the muscle for the most part being longitudinally arranged. Accessory incomplete elastic laminae are often present, especially beneath the endothelium in the infant (Fig. 3-7), and very little collagen is demonstrable. The apical pad appears to extend from the facial and dorsal pads and characteristically exhibits less intimal thickening than other pads.[163] By age 7, intimal thickenings about forks and orifices of vessels having coalesced and thickened are not discrete pads. Nevertheless, the greatest thickening still occurs at the sites of the facial, dorsal, and lateral pads even in youth.[144] At the apex, the intima is relatively thin. In the intimal thickenings, the elastica seems to have increased and the elastic laminae are thicker and sometimes numerous. Laminae can be fibrillary, pale, and lacelike or coarse and granular. In tangential section, the elastica is frequently not homogeneous, but fibrillary or granular with the fenestrae absent. In contrast to the internal elastic lamina elsewhere, that beneath the intimal pads, apart from being thin and staining poorly, is often straight rather than wavy in outline. The thickened intima about the forks now contains relatively less muscle and more collagen. Metachromatic ground substance in the intima has increased, but no lipophages are present in the arterial wall. Away from the forks, in the stem and branches, the elastic lamina is thickened and beading is noticeable (Fig. 3-9, *A*). The changes are prominent on the proximal side of the daughter branches, indicating that lateral pads extend peripherally along the proximal surface of the branches (**Fig. 3-10**).

In older individuals the confluent facial, dorsal, and lateral pads are often divided

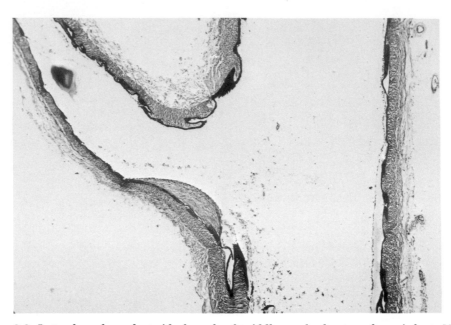

Fig. 3-8. Lateral angle pad at side branch of middle cerebral artery from infant. Note pale-staining elastic lamina deep to the pad and apical medial gap. (Verhoeff's elastic stain, ×37. From Stehbens, W. E.: Focal intimal proliferation in the cerebral arteries, Amer. J. Path. **36:**289, 1960.)

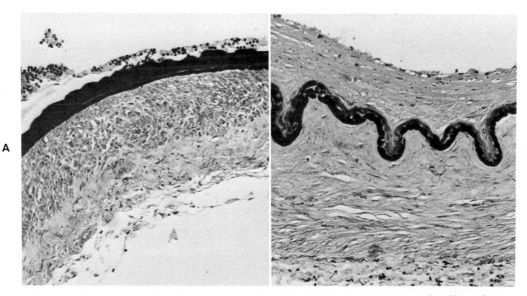

Fig. 3-9. Cerebral arteries displaying considerable thickening with some beading of the internal elastic lamina in **A** (longitudinal section) and beading with fragmentation beneath the intimal thickenings in **B** (transverse section). The functional competence of such elastic tissue changes is uncertain, but the overall thickness of the elastica in such arteries is probably the main reason for the belief that the internal elastic lamina in cerebral arteries is thicker than in extracranial arteries. (Verhoeff's elastic stain, ×110.)

into strata by the new elastic laminae, but the cellularity is reduced. Most commonly, the elastic laminae are fibrillary, granular, or fragmented (Fig. 3-9, *B*). In places, the deepest elastic lamina is heavily stained

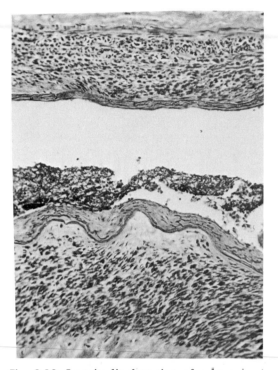

Fig. 3-10. Longitudinal section of a branch of middle cerebral artery. Intima is thicker on proximal side of branch (*below*) than on distal (*above*). There is also subintimal fibrosis of media below. (Mallory's phosphotungstic acid–hematoxylin, ×125.)

and homogeneous apart from fenestrae. The many laminae present simulate the so-called elastic hyperplasia of hypertension seen in smaller arteries. However, the amount of elastic tissue is variable, and as seen in the fixed undistended specimen, the lateral pads in particular often deform the lumen. In general, the intima at the apex is comparatively thin (Fig. 3-11), though the histological features are essentially similar. The intima other than at the forks is diffusely thickened and a layer of material staining gray with Verhoeff's stain lies between the lamina and the endothelium. Small elastic fibrils or definite areas of duplication can appear with the internal elastic lamina thin or fragmented. Occasional muscle fibers are present, becoming more numerous when the intima is thick. Later a number of irregular elastic laminae can be seen and fibrosis, as at the forks, becomes a prominent feature. Like earlier diffuse changes in the internal elastic lamina, this thickening lies mostly along the proximal side of the daughter branches, particularly if the lateral angle is acute. The elastica tends to degenerate less with often only fragments of laminae or hazy fibrillary masses in the intima. Fibrosis and hyalinization are associated with decreased cellularity and lipophages occur in variable numbers. Muscle fibers are less prevalent and may be arranged in strata. Many atypical muscle fibers are commonly stel-

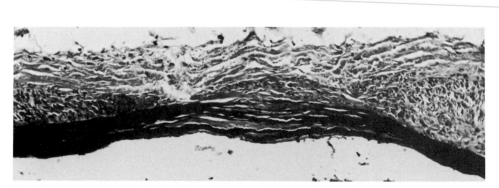

Fig. 3-11. Multiple elastic laminae at apex of internal carotid artery, giving the internal elastic lamina a frayed appearance. Note coarse, dense elastic tissue at edges (Verhoeff's elastic stain, ×155.)

late in shape with large, often irregularly shaped nuclei.

In middle age, the amount of elastica decreases; loose, pale-staining, foamy or hyaline areas usually appear in the deeper portion of the intima (Fig. 3-12), and macrophages accumulate, often in large numbers. Giant cells, calcium stippling, and secondary vascularization are prevalent, the whole typifying atherosclerosis. There is much metachromatic ground substance and fibrinlike material in pools is frequent in the necrotic areas deep in the intima (Fig. 3-13). Thrombosis does not seem to play a part in the development of these plaques because organization of thrombi in the lumen was found in only six of 197 arterial forks examined.

Intimal thickening with lipophages and cholesterol clefts may cover the entire intimal surface of the large arteries (Fig. 3-13, C) though usually the most severe changes appear about the fork at the face, back, and lateral angles. However, progressive degeneration does not always follow the same sequence as the development of the intimal pads, but there is always comparatively less intimal thickening at the apex despite the presence of moderate or severe atherosclerotic thickening at the face, dorsum, and lateral angles. Indeed a general thinning of the media and attenuation of the whole wall has been observed. Intimal thickening is also common at the apex of junctions of vessels (that is, the vertebrobasilar junction and that of the anterior communicating artery with the proximal segment of the anterior cerebral) and tends to be thicker than at the apex of bifurcations (Fig. 3-14). Intravascular cords or bridges crossing the lumen of the artery or septa dividing the lumen are frequent especially near the anterior communicating artery. Elastic tissue degeneration is prominent about these structures and intimal proliferation is thicker on the distal or trailing surface than on the proximal.[166] On occasions the cord, incorporated into the intimal proliferation of the nearby vessel wall, presents a bizarre appearance to the uninitiated.

Calcification of the cerebral arteries is infrequent microscopically and less often macroscopically. Ossification is quite exceptional (Fig. 3-15).

Very small peripheral arteries often escape such changes and only at sites of branchings is there intimal thickening. In others are slight intimal thickenings of little consequence, with gradations up to atheromatous plaques in instances of extremely severe atherosclerosis of the basal arteries (Fig. 3-16).

The media frequently exhibits gross thinning and fibrosis deep to areas of intimal thickening and generalized medial fibrosis is not uncommon when intimal changes are well advanced. Elastic fibrils

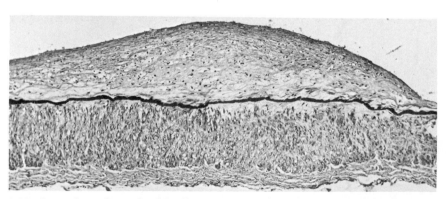

Fig. 3-12. Lateral angle pad with disappearance of much elastic tissue from intima. Loose pale-staining, foamy, or hyaline zones are present deep in intima and innermost portion of media. (Verhoeff's elastic stain, ×80.)

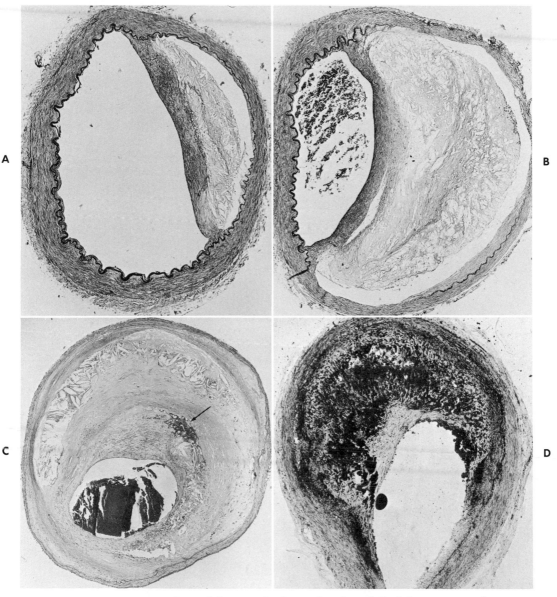

Fig. 3-13. Transverse sections of four cerebral arteries. **A** and **B,** Atheromatous plaque, the base of which is necrotic and of high lipid content, is situated on one side whereas the adjoining intima is virtually unaffected and suggests the existence of a tissue factor governing susceptibility of the wall to atherosclerosis. A more advanced stage, **C,** involves the full circumference of the vessel, the lumen is narrowed, and there is a small hemorrhage (*arrow*) in the intima. Note the extensive destruction of elastica and the medial thinning in **A** to **C.** A fat stain of an atheromatous artery is depicted in **D.** (Verhoeff's elastic stain, **A** to **C;** hematoxylin and fett rot, **D.**)

disappear, metachromasia is moderately prominent, and muscle fibers nearest the intima are replaced by hyaline connective tissue similar to that of the intima (Fig. 3-17). Lipid is frequent in the media beneath a thickened intima containing lipid and foam cells, and cholesterol clefts ultimately appear in such areas. In this way, the media is progressively replaced from within outwards, and the diseased media becomes continuous with and indistinguishable from the atherosclerotic intima

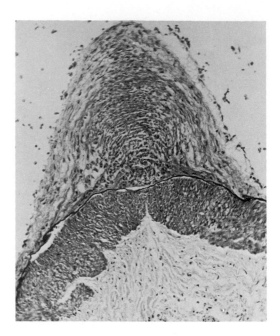

Fig. 3-14. Apical pad at vertebrobasilar junction in infant. Intimal proliferation is considerably thicker than that at the apex of other infants' arterial forks. Internal elastic lamina is thin. (Verhoeff's elastic stain, ×150.)

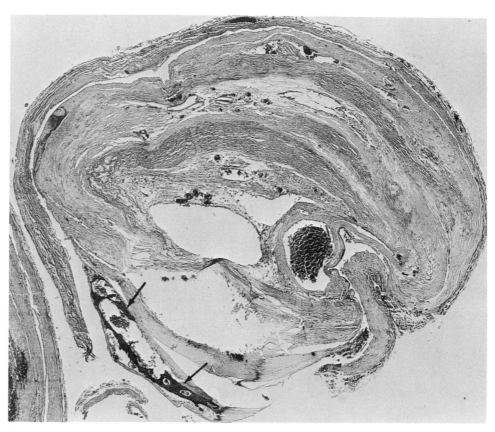

Fig. 3-15. Old recanalized thrombosed cerebral artery with a focus of ossification (*arrows*). Note the absence of large atheromatous areas of necrotic debris.

where the elastic lamina is interrupted. Large blood-filled capillaries penetrate the media to vascularize the wall. There are no atheromatous deposits in the medial gaps.

The innermost part of the adventitia frequently undergoes hyalinization with loss of the elastic fibrils. Metachromasia is faint, if present at all. Foam cells are sometimes seen (Fig. 3-18) and where atheroma is advanced, round cells, and sinusoidal capillaries. Macroscopic nodules projecting from the adventitial surface consist of collections of foam cells round the necrotic center being, in all probability, the result of the herniation of semiliquid contents

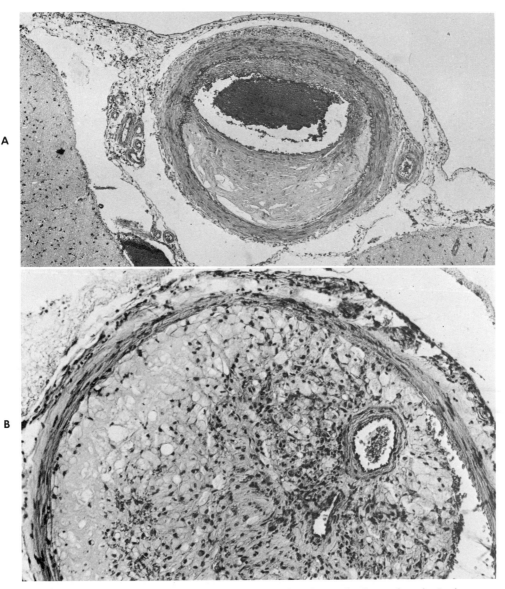

Fig. 3-16. A, Small pial artery displaying moderately advanced atherosclerosis. Intima contains few foam cells in contrast to small pial artery in **B** in which a xanthomatous infiltration of the intima is present in parts (unusual). (**A,** Verhoeff's elastic stain, ×45; **B,** hematoxylin and eosin, ×110.)

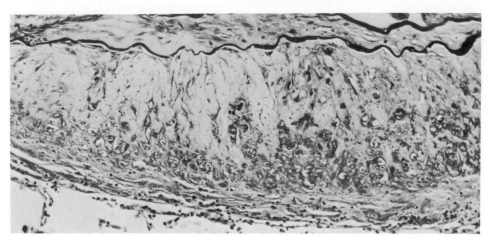

Fig. 3-17. Muscle from inner two-thirds of media has been replaced by pale hyaline tissue. Lipid content of this area would be moderate. Outer media shows vacuolation of muscle. (Verhoeff's elastic stain, ×150.)

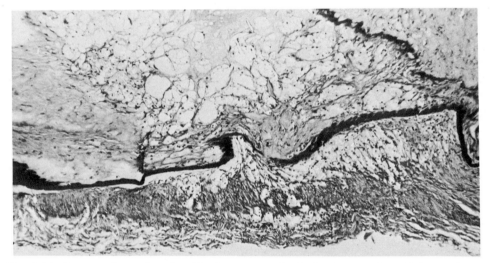

Fig. 3-18. Severe atherosclerosis with degenerate elastic laminae and acellular and hyaline areas in the intima. Foam cells are present in intima, media, and adventitia. (Verhoeff's elastic stain, ×75.)

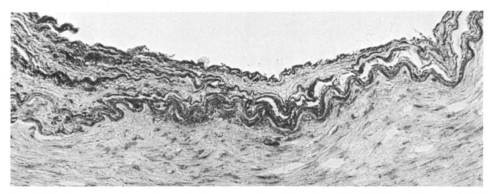

Fig. 3-19. Frozen section of cerebral artery stained for fat. The lipid outlines multiple elastic laminae. (Hematoxylin and oil red O, ×110.)

from the atheromatous intima and media into the adventitia, with subsequent encapsulation by lipophages (Fig. 3-3, *B*). The adventitia tends to be the least affected of all the coats and the intima the most affected. Adventitial changes occur mainly in the elderly and in the presence of severe changes in the intima.

No line of demarcation is evident between the intimal proliferation of infants and the advanced atherosclerosis of adults. In studies of the age changes of the aorta and coronary arteries, similar conclusions were reached,[51,132,191] and French,[62] though conceding it difficult, offered no criteria for clearly distinguishing between the early intimal pads or cushions and pathological changes. Histological manifestations of obvious atherosclerosis (lipophages and/or cholesterol clefts) are usually first seen where the intima is thickest, that is, at the site of the original facial, dorsal, and lateral pads.

Most authors assume that the advent of lipid in the intima is the initial stage of atherosclerosis and that lipid always occurs in a thickened intima often in relation to the elastic laminae (Fig. 3-19). With fat stains, lipid may be demonstrated prior to the appearance of lipophages in paraffin sections or even in quite a thin intima, but there has been no attempt to determine the age at which lipid first makes its appearance microscopically in cerebral arteries. It has been demonstrated in the aorta of the fetus[200] and Duff[41] suggests it may be present in intimal pads at birth. Thus it would seem that the nature of the intimal proliferation in the aorta and distributing arteries in fetuses and infants is of singular import.

Significance of intimal pads (cushions)

Although the significance of intimal pads at arterial forks remains controversial, intimal proliferation is generally taken to be a physiological structure accompanying the increase in blood pressure and vessel size occurring from birth to physical maturity.[59,75,123] The pads, it has been assumed, are concerned with ensuring economy of blood flow throughout the body.[144] This function virtually presupposes neurogenic control but as nerves have never been found in intimal pads, to ascribe to them a sensory function is unwarranted. Furthermore, neither their position nor the arrangement of muscle fibers at arterial forks suggests that they function as sphincters. In small arteries,[59,111] they are believed to be concerned with plasma skimming.

Shanklin and Azzam[151,152] described valves in the cerebral arteries of the rat, mouse, and hamster but could not find them in guinea pigs. Similar structures[143] have been encountered even in extracranial vessels.[107] Facial and dorsal pads can be mistaken for these valves in some planes of section but others appear to be authentic. They have not been found in man.

The elastic tissue changes are indicative of degenerative change,[155,163] and the pads have an intimate relationship to atherosclerosis.[132,163,191] Rotter and associates[144] considered them elective sites for the development of arteriosclerosis in man.* Intimal pads in the cerebral arteries of sheep are sites of predilection (Fig. 3-20) for spontaneous lipid deposition,[170,172] and in the hypercholesterolemic rabbit, intimal pads in the renal artery are also elective sites for lipid deposition.[167] There has not been a detailed study (using serial sections) of the localization of early lipid deposition in human cerebral arteries, but it would seem that intimal pads are either important precursors or an integral stage in the pathogenesis of atherosclerosis.[172]

Anitschkow[6] maintained that lipid deposition in hypercholesterolemic rabbits was determined by local tissue factors. Duff[39,40] believed it followed previous injury only. Duguid and Robertson[47] contended that cholesterol is merely an experimental

---

*Intimal pads have been found in other animals both intracranially and extracranially, and in morphology and localization are similar to those in the human infant.

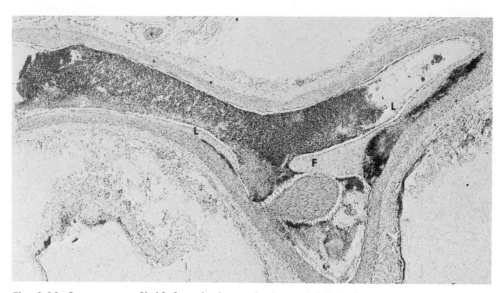

Fig. 3-20. Spontaneous lipid deposits in cerebral arterial fork from a sheep. Dark zones in lateral pads, **L**, represent lipid. Both lateral pads have peripheral extensions and one is confluent with facial pad **F**. Flow is from below upwards. (Hematoxylin and fett rot, ×32. From Stehbens, W. E.: Intimal proliferation and spontaneous lipid deposition in the cerebral arteries of sheep and steers, J. Atheroscler. Res. 5:556, 1965.)

marker of otherwise obscure structural damage. The various views are substantiated by experimental evidence, for in hypercholesterolemic rabbits lipid is deposited in areas previously subjected to trauma.[93,159,193] There is also localization of methyl cellulose at sites of trauma[189] and in the intimal pads of the rabbit renal artery.[175] Trauma may be the local tissue factor referred to by Anitschkow[6] and it is a distinct possibility that intimal pads at forks are the result of stress or damage predisposing them to lipid accumulation. According to Waters[188] acute episodes of hypertension cause damage primarily at sites of branching, and intimal lesions, the result of trauma, are similar histologically to intimal thickenings at arterial forks. Moreover, they are elective sites for lipid deposition.

Rodbard[139,140] and Texon[184] contend that a "suction effect" due to local decrease in static pressure causes intimal thickening at forks. Little is known of stresses at arterial forks, but it seems unlikely that such a mechanism could account for

facial, apical, and dorsal pads. The experiments using tubes lined with silicone rubber[75,139,140] could provide useful information concerning stresses at bifurcations. However, the remodeling of inert material lining these tubes need not be analogous to the biological response of human and animal blood vessels to similar stresses.

Eddy currents at arterial forks have been thought to be a factor influencing the localization of atherosclerosis. The presence of eddy currents has been thought to favor platelet sticking to endothelium and thus initiate thrombosis.[36,117,118] The topography of platelet deposits seen in plastic flow chambers inserted in extracorporeal shunts has been likened to the distribution of atherosclerosis and is said to be the result of hydraulic factors.[36,66,117] It could be postulated that such thrombi at arterial forks organize and result in intimal pads and eventually progress to atherosclerosis. The concept's drawback is a complete absence of supporting evidence from the serial sections of large numbers of cerebral arterial forks from fetuses, infants, and other animals.[161,163] Moreover, in the small vessels of rabbit ear chambers, eddy currents do not favor platelet aggregation or thrombus formation[173] although the latter, in larger vessels, may be influenced by other conditions.

Rindfleisch[137] considered there were grounds for believing that "mechanical irritation" of the vascular wall is a cause of morbid vascular changes. Other authors[47,112] state that the section of the fork exposed to the full stress and impact of the blood is a site of particular involvement. Yet, in actual fact, this region (the apex) is less affected by intimal thickening than are other sites about the fork.[163,167] Indeed, it is a region of thinning or atrophy rather than of thickening.[166]

Both the localization of the pads and the attendant elastic tissue degeneration suggest that they are etiologically related to hemodynamic factors. Moreover, the intimal changes seen early in life seem to be modified by the angle of branching and the size of the vessel. Vibrations associated with frank turbulence do not appear to be responsible for intimal pads though vortices or eddy currents, by producing vibrational injury, could be factors in their genesis.[161,174]

Hassler[75,76] suggested that the intimal pads at arterial forks might so disturb flow as to cause aneurysms. He was aware of only apical and lateral pads, and apparently did not observe facial and dorsal thickenings, and furthermore, little evidence exists to suggest that the pads cause a water-hammer effect or pulse-wave reflexion as he suggested.[76] Intimal pads are better acknowledged as compensatory thickenings in response to stress, which causes the elastic tissue degeneration that precedes and accompanies intimal proliferation at arterial forks.[163,172] There has been little investigation of the effect of hemodynamic processes on the vessel wall though recently their disruptive role has been emphasized,[174] and the relationship of hemodynamic stresses to intimal pads, the important precursors of atherosclerosis,

is of considerable moment in the pathogenesis of atherosclerosis[161] and cerebral aneurysms.[166]

Comparative severity of cerebral atherosclerosis

At birth, cerebral arteries exhibit intimal thickening only at sites of branching, whereas in coronary arteries there is intimal thickening at arterial forks and diffuse changes in the large arteries. In general, gross atherosclerosis of the coronary arteries eventuates at an earlier age and is more severe than that of cerebral arteries and tends to affect young males more severely than young females. Dock[34] claimed that intimal thickening in the coronaries of male infants was more prominent than that in females. The conclusion is questionable as only random sections through the arteries were used, rather than serial sections.

Macroscopic grading of atherosclerosis, employed in the absence of a more satisfactory technique, is imprecise and can produce quite fallacious results.[69] This fact has important implications in epidemiological studies because grading is so often performed by different groups and reproducibility of the results is often a debatable proposition.[28]

The cerebral arteries are one of the sites more severely affected by atherosclerosis. That of the aorta and coronary arteries is usually more severe than is cerebral atherosclerosis,[79,196] but in general the severity of atherosclerosis at one site parallels that at other sites.[196] Nevertheless, individual exceptions occur and it has been noted that cerebrovascular disease is more frequent[15] and more extensive[157] in the black than in the white person. The reverse applies in the case of coronary atherosclerosis.

Fatty streaks of uncertain significance in the aorta and coronary arteries are almost universal in young humans.[104] The coronary fatty streaks, behaving differently from those in the aorta, appear to be more closely related to the development of severe atherosclerosis later in life. Holman and Moosy[80] noted relatively few fatty streaks with early conversion to fibrous plaques in human cerebral arteries, and while differences in size and architecture of the vessels may be responsible for the apparent diversity, histological comparisons would be preferable, for authors believe that there is less fibrosis and much less calcification in cerebral atherosclerosis than in aortic or coronary atherosclerosis.[1]

In young and old males, the thickness of the atherosclerotic intima at different stages of development has been found to be greater in the coronary than in the cerebral arteries.[149] The differences in severity were unexplained but were thought to be responsible for differences in chemical composition.

Böttcher and associates,[16] comparing the lipid content of the aorta and coronary and cerebral arteries in several atherosclerotic patients, found that the triglyceride content was particularly high in the coronary arteries whereas aortic and cerebral arteries remained roughly the same. There was a comparatively high content of cholesterol esters with a low level of free cholesterol (7.6%). As is consistent with macroscopic and microscopic differences in calcification, the chemical analysis of cerebral arteries of 71 subjects revealed that the calcium content is considerably lower than in coronary arteries.[125] Nakamura and Yabuta[120] found that the cerebral arteries contained less acid mucopolysaccharides (particularly chondroitin sulfates) and heparitin sulfate than the carotid sinus, common carotid artery, and aorta, perhaps because of the lesser degree of intimal proliferation in cerebral vessels in comparison with extracranial vessels.

Cerebral atherosclerosis of other animals

Spontaneous. The severe spontaneous atherosclerosis of man is uncommon in other animals,[60] though raised atheromatous and fibrous plaques occur, particularly in birds. Medial calcification, poly-

arteritis nodosa, nonspecific arteritis, or intimal fibrosis have occurred in animals but should be differentiated from true atherosclerosis. Cerebral arteries are even less frequently affected than the aorta and coronary vessels.

In animals in which cerebral arterial forks have been examined by serial sections (sheep, dog, horse, gorilla, steer, pig, chimpanzee) intimal pads similar to those occurring in the human infant have been found,[88,169,172] but they have also been observed in rabbits[75] and several varieties of birds.[38] In some older animals such as the dog and horse, the intimal thickening is more diffuse, having extended beyond the sites of branching. Although intimal changes are believed to have an intimate relationship to atherosclerosis, obvious lipid accumulation is generally believed to be the essence of this disease.[178] In the normal sheep, these intimal thickenings are sites of predilection for lipid deposition,[170,172] but few detailed studies have been made of cerebral arteries.

Spontaneous atherosclerosis of the cerebral arteries of pigs has been observed by several authors[52,67,101] with narrowing of the lumen particularly in the anterior and middle cerebral arteries. Vessels posteriorly were less severely affected[101] and infarction in the distribution of the middle cerebral artery has been observed. The severity has been found to be greater than that in the coronaries in pigs over 8 years of age,[52] but complicated lesions did not occur. Obstructive intimal changes were seen in the spinal arteries of one animal, but in domestic animals, cerebrovascular disease is rarely the cause of death.[72] In an old dog[52] with generalized atherosclerosis, the cerebral vessels were involved though the histological appearance of the lesion was atypical.

Although spontaneous atherosclerosis is quite prevalent in the aorta and even the brachiocephalic artery of many species of birds[60] including pigeons,[131] the cerebral vessels escape. The small size of the vessels and failure to use serial sections may be

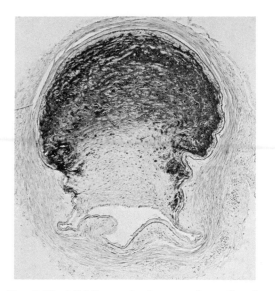

Fig. 3-21. Middle cerebral artery from female chimpanzee (8 years old) that died from a ruptured cerebral aneurysm. Dark-stained area in the thickened intima is lipid. (Hematoxylin and oil red O, ×38. From Stehbens, W. E.: Cerebral aneurysms of animals other than man, J. Path. Bact. **86**:161, 1963.)

responsible for the apparent absence of cerebral involvement.

In rodents, cerebral atherosclerosis is rare, though lipid was found in the media of a few advanced lesions in rats.[190]

Cerebral atherosclerosis is not prevalent in primates. It has not been found in baboons,[105,177,179] and of 80 varied subhuman primates examined macroscopically, it was present in only two chimpanzees. Very severe atherosclerosis, such as in man, and multiple cerebral aneurysms[169] were observed in another chimpanzee (Fig. 3-21). It appears that the chimpanzee might well be a highly suitable animal for experimental studies in cerebrovascular disease.[5,160]

Experimentally induced. After the induction of hypercholesterolemia, large extracranial arteries of experimental animals develop atherosclerotic lesions according to individual and species susceptibility. The cerebral arteries have proved to be more refractory but no adequate reason has yet been proffered.[3,89,124] Pollak[124] observed that ligation of the common ca-

rotid artery in cholesterol-fed rabbits resulted in frequent and severe lipid deposition in that artery, but the cerebral arteries remained free of lipid despite simultaneous epinephrine administration. He noted subsequently that lesions could be produced in the rabbit if the cholesterol were first heated.[125] Bullock and associates[22] could not induce lesions in the cerebral arteries of the cebus and squirrel monkey with an atherogenic diet although with the baboon and chimpanzee the method has been successful. Recently Nyström[122] induced cholesterol atherosclerosis in cockerels. Fat was observed in the intima of the pial arterioles and venules. Imai and Thomas[86] induced lesions in the cerebral arteries of pigs. Others induced lesions in dogs by dietary means.[13,182] Small cerebral infarcts have been thought to be caused by atheromatous emboli though there has been no mention of the ulceration of any lesions. They are probably the result of narrowing of the lumen by the xanthomatous intimal lesions.

Electron microscopy

Ultrastructural investigations of human cerebral atherosclerosis have been extremely limited.[56,103] Martinez[103] concentrated on pial arteries, and Flora and associates[56] examined post mortem the posterior inferior cerebellar artery only. No study of the intimal pads of infants has been made with the elucidation of the progressive development of overt atherosclerosis in mind.

Martinez[103] described the endothelial cells with lipid inclusions as obviously hypertrophied, but arterial endothelium is often thick with prominent and at times dilated endoplasmic reticulum and besides no control material was examined. One prominent feature is the thick multilaminar zone of basement membrane material.[56,103] In thicker intimas, it overlies a variable number of layers of widely separated smooth muscle fibers. The interstitium contains collagen, elastic fibrils, an occasional accessory elastic lamina, and connective tissue microfibrils. Ghost bodies and sporadic cells, either poorly differentiated muscle fibers or fibroblasts[56] with little or no enveloping basement membrane, are occasionally seen.

Early medial changes consist of patchy increases in interstitial connective tissue in which fragments of cell profiles and dense unidentified bodies are found. Lipid in extracranial arteries has been found in smooth muscle cells,[65] believed to ultimately transform to foam cells. Unidentified cells also contain lipid.[56] The relationship of lipid to the extracellular tissues including the internal elastic lamina as occurs in atherosclerosis has not been studied. Calcification commences in the center of elastic fibers. Morphological changes demonstrable by light microscopy in the elastic tissue of cerebral arteries have not been investigated and with basement membrane changes await elucidation.

Nyström,[122] inducing cholesterol atherosclerosis in the cerebral arteries of cockerels, found large vacuoles in the endothelium and lipid-laden macrophages in the intima. Parenchymal vessels also exhibited extensive endothelial vacuolation.

Imai and Thomas[86] fed miniature pigs an atherogenic (high cholesterol) diet. The animals developed atherosclerotic lesions of the cerebral arteries. An electron microscopic study of the middle cerebral arteries was made, but neither macroscopic nor light microscopic studies were reported. The endothelium was thick, was more cellular, and contained more numerous organelles. The intima was thickened due to an increase in smooth muscle cells and in related basement membranes, collagen, and ground substance. There was lipid (vacuoles and phospholipid whorls) within the muscle cells and foam cells and cholesterol clefts within cells and extracellular spaces. In addition, necrotic muscle cells and cell debris were prominent in advanced atheromatous lesions sometimes enveloped or phagocytosed by viable smooth muscle cells or surrounded by as many as three muscle

fibers. Evidence of dietary-induced necrosis was found in the intima and the innermost part of the media.

Complications

Cerebral ischemia. Cerebral ischemia can accrue from severe cerebral atherosclerosis by various means. Progressive enlargement of the atherosclerotic plaque can gradually reduce the size of the lumen. Attention has been focussed on such extracranial stenoses recently, but a significant reduction in flow is likely only if the stenosis reduces the lumen by 80% to 90%.[18,19] Encroachment on the lumen to this extent has been attributed to the organization of a mural thrombus or the incorporation of mural thrombi into the vessel wall. Either will impart to the plaque an eccentric and laminated appearance in accordance with the Duguid hypothesis.[44-46] To what extent mural thrombi contribute to the size of advanced atherosclerotic plaques is difficult to estimate, but strata separated by elastic laminae can occur in intimal pads from an early age and, according to the plane of section, this holds true for lateral pads. Their extensions appear eccentric in cross section. The degree to which small branches of severely atherosclerotic basal arteries are narrowed by intimal disease of the parent artery has not been investigated, but their partial occlusion could contribute to cerebral ischemia.

The role of intimal hemorrhage in arterial occlusion[124] in the presence or absence of a superadded thrombus in the lumen is questionable. Intramural hemorrhages, possibly the result of shearing stresses and dissection without intimal rupture, are seen, but it is unlikely that they ever occlude the lumen.

The formation of an occlusive thrombus, usually complicating severe atherosclerosis, is dealt with separately on p. 117. It can result in severe ischemia. Emboli from these thrombi or atheromatous ulcers between the heart and the cranium are all capable of obstructing small vessels. Additional

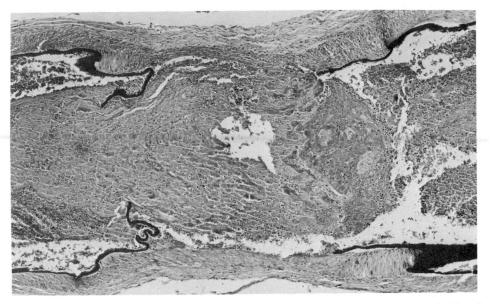

Fig. 3-22. Cerebral artery occluded by a thrombus, which appears to have been initiated by an extensive tear of the internal elastic lamina. The elastic lamina is reflected and embedded in thrombus. There is no atherosclerosis. A less extensive tear with superadded mural thrombus was found in another cerebral vessel of this subject. A more extensive separation of elastic lamina would have constituted a dissecting aneurysm. (Verhoeff's elastic stain, ×45. From Stehbens, W. E.: Contentious features of coronary occlusion and atherosclerosis, Bull. Post-Grad. Comm. Med. Univ. Sydney 19:216, 1963.)

factors such as disease of small perforating arteries, widespread atherosclerosis with multiple narrowings and episodes of hypotension may participate in jeopardizing the critical cerebral blood flow. Some contend that the resultant chronic ischemia is responsible for the widespread nerve cell and tract degeneration that accompany the mental deterioration and dementia of old age.[11]

Thrombosis. Thrombosis in the cerebral arteries is held to be a complication of atherosclerosis in the absence of inflammatory diseases or coagulation defects. Most instances of thrombosis in situ, whether of the carotid sinus or intracranially, are associated with severe grades of atherosclerosis. There are exceptions and Fig. 3-22 depicts a cerebral artery (examined by serial section) containing a thrombus into which is reflected the torn internal elastic lamina.[168]

In the pathogenesis of coronary occlusion, Drury[37] stated that the thrombus usually results from necrosis or rupture of the endothelium overlying an atheromatous plaque. Others drew attention to the tearing of the overlying intima.[14,24,81] Leary[98] believed that necrotic contents of atheromatous abscesses or cavities ruptured into the lumen.

The importance of intimal hemorrhage has been emphasized,[81,124] but it is difficult to imagine how, in the absence of dissection, capillary hemorrhage can form an intramural hematoma sufficient to occlude the arterial lumen.[37]

Tearing, desquamation, or sloughing of the intimal surface overlying an atheromatous plaque, as in the aorta, have been said to result in an atheromatous ulcer, a variable degree of dissection, and superadded thrombosis.[168] The pultaceous, necrotic material within the atheromatous ulcer could place the overlying intima at a mechanical disadvantage[168,174] with tearing or rupture the unavoidable consequence. Dissection and extravasation of blood into the wall, the washing out of necrotic atheromatous debris of high lipid content into the lumen, and thrombosis at the site of intimal damage can all follow concomitantly. Random histological sections of such a lesion can mislead for according to the plane of section the dissection may simulate intramural hemorrhage, or the incorporation of extruded necrotic atheromatous material into a thrombus could well be taken for a fatty degeneration of a thrombus. Serial sections of coronary and cerebral thromboses are essential to determine the pathogenesis and preferably also an improved embedding medium to avoid the histological artefacts.[168] More recently increased emphasis has been placed on the tearing of the intima overlying the atheromatous abscess both in coronary[23,26,64] and cerebral arteries.[27]

The pathogenesis of these tears that initiate thrombosis is unknown but the following explanation is advanced.[174] In lathyrism, the fragility of connective tissues is much increased and arterial tears, dissecting aneurysms, and saccular aneurysms[96] develop. Likewise, fragility of the tissues probably accounts for the dilatation and tearing in the poststenotic dilatations, arteriovenous aneurysms,[174] and saccular aneurysm (Chapter 9). At routine autopsies, pressures much greater than physiological aortic blood pressures are required to produce experimental aortic dissection, and this indicates the virtual impossibility of producing a dissecting aneurysm during life by the access of blood through an intimal defect into a media of normal strength.[138] The loss of tensile strength or mechanical fragility[168,174] apparently precedes and results in the ulcers and tears complicated by thrombosis and dissection in the atherosclerotic intima.

Arteriectasis and tortuosity. Very severely atherosclerotic arteries are not only elongated, wider in external diameter, rigid, and of irregular contour, but also frequently tortuous and deviating as a result from their usual anatomical course,

produce pressure effects on the neighboring brain; compare the S-shaped tortuosity formed by the basilar and a vertebral artery—usually the dominant vertebral artery and generally found in those over 60 years of age with long-standing severe hypertension. Arteriectasis may be associated with either a fusiform or saccular aneurysm. Pressure grooves may be seen on the pons and the pyramid. Cranial nerves, particularly the trigeminal and acoustic nerves, are not infrequently compressed. Trigeminal neuralgia is frequent[32] and glossopharyngeal neuralgia has been reported.[20] The tenth, eleventh, and twelfth cranial nerves may also be compressed, and demyelination may be demonstrable.

The upper end of the ectatic basilar artery may project well into the third ventricle, as demonstrable by angiography and ventriculography.[49,73] Breig and associates[17] encountered three cases of dementia with hydrocephalus caused by pressure of an elongated basilar artery on the third ventricle. Displacement of the tortuous basilar artery can result in indentation of the floor of the third ventricle by the posterior cerebral artery itself displaced upward and toward the midline.

The internal carotid arteries may be even more ectatic than the basilar and compression of the optic nerve pathways can ensue.

Aneurysms. Fusiform and saccular aneurysms of the major cerebral arteries especially of the vertebral and basilar arteries are well known (see Chapter 9). Berry aneurysms are usually not regarded as atherosclerotic despite an unduly high prevalence of atherosclerosis in such patients.[38] The intimal changes about arterial forks that appear to be concerned with aneurysm formation are not usually regarded as atherosclerotic but might at least be an early stage of atherosclerosis.

Senile dementia. Severe cerebral atherosclerosis can be associated with a diminished cerebral blood flow. However, the sporadic involvement of small vessels together with patchy gliosis and ischemic changes accounts for varying grades of mental deterioration.

Epidemiology of cerebral atherosclerosis

Most of the epidemiological studies have centered around coronary artery disease and myocardial infarction. Significant differences both in mortality and morbidity have been demonstrated in different geographic and ethnic groups.[186] Epidemiological studies of cerebrovascular diseases have grouped diseases of varying etiology together and consequently less attention has been paid to cerebral atherosclerosis despite several apparent differences from coronary atherosclerosis.

Deaths from cerebrovascular disease are highest in Japan,[71] the low Japanese mortality for coronary heart disease notwithstanding. Cerebral hemorrhage was said to be more frequent than cerebral infarction, but subsequent surveys have revealed that cerebral infarction occurs more often than cerebral hemorrhage[91,127] and Japanese figures for occlusive vascular disease as a cause of stroke are not appreciably different from those pertaining to the incidence in the United States of America. Occlusive vascular disease of the brain is considered to be dependent on the severity of cerebral atherosclerosis, yet Steiner[176] found cerebral atherosclerosis to be less severe in Orientals than in Caucasians. Recent studies based on macroscopic grading of the cerebral arteries indicate that cerebral atherosclerosis appears macroscopically in the Japanese at an earlier age than it does in Americans in Minnesota. With every decade, the difference in severity increases.[136] Nakamura[119] believes that the distribution of atherosclerosis in the cerebral arteries is basically the same in the Japanese as in Americans, but Resch and associates[136] alleged that in the Japanese early lesions occurred in the small vessels in contrast to large vessel involvement in Americans. No explanation for the differing susceptibility of the coronary and cerebral arteries has been forthcoming, and

comparative studies of such factors as blood pressure and blood flow rates in the cerebral circulation are deemed necessary if the epidemiological findings are valid.

The African is professed to have significantly less atherosclerosis than the North American white or black,[33] but Laurie and Wood[97] contend that cerebral hemorrhage, thrombosis, and severe atherosclerosis are in fact common in Africans. Cerebral atherosclerosis, however, is reportedly less severe in Nigerians than in whites in Minnesota or blacks in Alabama.[192] In the International Atherosclerosis Project,[104] it was concluded that environmental factors are of more importance in determining the severity of atherosclerosis than is racial origin.

Epidemiological studies of environmental factors related to atherosclerosis have concentrated primarily on dietary fats in relation to deaths from coronary heart disease. Kannel[90] concluded from 12 years of the Framingham study that risk factors for ischemic cerebrovascular disease were comparable with those for coronary heart disease.

Cerebral atherosclerosis increases in severity with age when judged by the intimal area involved, the thickness of the plaque, and the frequency of complications.[54,157] This does not preclude individual variation in the same group, for other etiological factors are involved and indeed atherosclerosis to a significant degree occurs in young subjects, as shown by autopsies of young soldiers[50,01] and in aortic coarctation.[165]

Comparisons of the severity of cerebral atherosclerosis in the sexes have provided diverse and conflicting results[8,79,148] with the majority of authors finding no significant difference. Premature severe atherosclerosis with coronary occlusion in childhood accompanies progeria, but little information is available about the cerebral arteries except that they were sclerotic in one instance.[7] In general, it is held that obesity adversely influences the severity of atherosclerosis, but poor correlation between obesity and cerebral atherosclerosis has been found.[10,135] Factors like smoking, hardness of the water supply, endocrine disturbances, exercise, body build, and the like have not been specifically studied in respect to cerebral atherosclerosis.

Etiology of atherosclerosis

A vast and unmanageable quantity of literature is concerned with the etiology of atherosclerosis. For the student commencing readings in this field, several salient features of the nature of atherosclerosis will be documented and followed by a brief résumé of the etiological hypotheses.

Salient features of atherosclerosis

Early stages of atherosclerosis. There is no agreement upon what constitutes the earliest demonstrable lesion whence investigations of the etiology should commence. The primary changes should be ultrastructural. Lipid accumulation in the deepest part of the intima, frequently in relation to the internal elastic lamina, has been emphasized, with lipid regarded as the sine qua non of atherosclerosis.[42,178] Its appearance histologically is thought by many to be the earliest demonstrable stage. However, lipid accumulation in the wall is only one manifestation of atherosclerosis and no constituent of the wall is immune. The intimal proliferation that precedes lipid accumulation is in all probability an earlier stage of atherosclerosis and elucidation of its pathogenesis should provide information pertinent to the etiology of atherosclerosis.

Distribution in the arterial tree. Atherosclerosis is a disease of the major distributing arteries such as the aorta, coronary, cerebral, and mesenteric arteries and those of the lower limb. Yet, small arcuate or interlobular arteries of the kidney and small intracerebral or perforating arteries exhibit changes referred to as arteriorsclerosis or diffuse hyperplastic sclerosis. In the thickened intima proliferative and degenerative changes of the elastica may be demonstrated. Medial fibrosis and hyalinization are frequent. However, if the criterion for atherosclerosis is demonstrable lipid, then changes in these vessels, which contain intimal lipid, often related to the elastic lamina, should also be considered as atherosclerotic—hence the overlap between atherosclerosis and arteriosclerosis (diffuse hyperplastic sclerosis), the difference being perhaps one of severity and size of the vessel involved. Lipid is demonstrable in arteriolosclerosis and the so-called endarteritis obliterans about chronic peptic ulceration.[171] There are similarities between the calcification of Mönckeberg's sclerosis and atherosclerosis. Thus the current concepts of these diseases require revision. They are not the distinct entities that textbooks and authors often suggest.[168]

Salient morphological features. From morphological studies of cerebral arteries and experimental vascular lesions, certain salient features have emerged from the present state of confusion regarding atherosclerosis.

1. In man, the disease appears to be universal and progressive if of slow evolution.
2. The disease progressively increases throughout life, with variation from person to person and vascular bed to vascular bed. Age is but a time factor.
3. The disease is more severe in the systemic circulation than in the pulmonary vasculature and in veins to an extent even less.
4. The larger the artery, the more severe is the atherosclerosis.
5. The disease progressively affects the vessel wall from within outwards; a predilection for sites of branching, unions, and curvatures is evidenced.
6. Hypertension aggravates the disease.
7. The disease involves changes in all constituents of the vessel wall and not lipid alone. Moreover, it is merely an assumption that lipid accumulation is the earliest manifestation of the disease.
8. It appears that lipid accumulation in the vessel wall both in man and the experimental animal must be preceded by some change in the vessel wall, possibly an injury. This local tissue factor, for so long neglected, should receive more attention.
9. The disease affects animals other than man.
10. Great caution must be exercised in the

interpretation of statistical and epidemiological studies of atherosclerosis. Their value depends on the validity of the data collected and the correctness of the interpretation.

Aging or senescence theory

In this theory, it is envisaged that atherosclerosis is a consequence of the progressive and inevitable wear and tear evinced by the advance of age. Katz and Stamler[92] consider that the hypothesis has inhibited progress by fostering an attitude of hopelessness, and it is true that atherosclerosis relentlessly increases in severity with age. For each individual, age is but a time factor indicating the period during which the vessel walls have been subjected to stresses and diverse atherogenic factors. Other elements such as individual variation, tissue susceptibility, and hypertension participate. The concept does not preclude individual variation in severity within the one age group. Moderately severe atherosclerosis was found in young soldiers,[50,61,128] but no similar studies for cerebral atherosclerosis have been performed, though severe cerebral atherosclerosis has been observed in a 23-year-old male with aortic coarctation.[165]

Thrombogenic theory

Rokitansky's theory[46,141] states that mural thrombi in the vessels are endothelialized and incorporated into the vessel wall. The organization and degeneration of the thrombus are said to produce subsequently the familiar atheromatous appearance of the arterial wall. Repeated episodes of thrombosis narrow the lumen, and the arterial intima adopts a laminated appearance. Thrombosis frequently complicates the atherosclerosis in the late stages of the disease, but no evidence exists for a supposed role in its early development. Duguid[44,46] championed the theory but offered little concrete data. Horn and Finkelstein[81] concluded some years ago that it was generally impossible to deduce whether severe arteriosclerotic thickenings of the arterial wall had originated from a thrombus. Once again, random histological sec-

tions, which are so easily misconstrued, could incorrectly be considered to support the hypothesis. Reviews of this hypothesis[1,82,148,180] expose its many inconsistencies. Necrotic grumous material might be expected in venous thrombi, healed valves of mitral stenosis, and bacterial endocarditis and in the laminated thrombi of aneurysms, but it does not appear. In organized or recanalized thrombosed arteries, it is most uncommon (unlike intimal plaques), but blood pigment is usually well in evidence. The distribution of atherosclerosis is quite inconsistent with the thrombogenic theory, for if it were tenable, atherosclerosis would be more prevalent in veins and the pulmonary circulation.

Fibrin in the intima of atherosclerotic arteries,[77,99,195] a phenomenon readily demonstrated in advanced atherosclerosis in man and chimpanzee by light microscopy, has been regarded as strong substantiation of the thrombogenic theory. However, the origin of the fibrin has not yet been determined. Recently it was suggested that fibrin is derived from the insudation of fibrinogen into the wall from either the arterial lumen or vasa vasorum rather than from a thrombus.[180] Then again, platelet thrombi on the vessel wall might become incorporated into the vessel wall and cause increased endothelial permeability to plasma proteins and lipids.[116]

A variation of the theme is that intramural hemorrhage rather than a mural thrombus is the source of the fatty material.[194] Similar objections apply to this hypothesis. In neither hypothesis do the protagonists account for the cause of the thrombus or the hemorrhage, the contribution stems rather from the stimuli provided for research on thrombogenesis.

Lipid theory

Early investigators failed to produce atherosclerosis by mechanical trauma, toxic agents, and repeated injections of epinephrine. Ignatowski[84] fed animal protein (meat, milk, and eggs) to rabbits, which subsequently developed aortic lesions resembling atherosclerosis. It was later realized that the fat content of the diet rather than the animal protein produced the arterial changes. Anitschkow,[6] by cholesterol feeding, initiated the cholesterol era of atherosclerosis research. Many accept cholesterol atherosclerosis of the rabbit as the counterpart of the human disease, but criticisms can be leveled against this experimental model. The well-formed cholesterol lesion often stands up from the surrounding normal intima and is unduly thick in the absence of more diffuse changes. This is reflected in the rapid increase in the mitotic activity in the induced lesions in rabbits[106] and pigs[85] and at the aortic trifurcation in pigs after 3 days of cholesterol feeding.[57] Histologically, the rabbit arterial lesions exhibit circulating lipophages in the blood.[154] Foam cells abound, suggesting a xanthomatous reactions, and there is less fibrosis and hyalinization with the elastic lamina rarely outlined as in spontaneous lipid deposits.[6,168,172] Mesothelial cells in the rabbit also contain lipid.[168] Moreover, the topography of the lesions in the vascular bed differs from that of the human. The accompanying lipid storage in the viscera and subcutaneous tissues[133] and the hemolytic anemia[153] all intimate that the rabbit disease is distinct from human atherosclerosis though akin to hereditary hypercholesterolemic xanthomatosis or hyperlipidemia in man,[102] despite the fact that vascular lesions in hyperlipidemia have not been thoroughly examined.* Others attribute these peculiarities of the experimental model to a species difference and to the accelerated development of the disease in the rabbit. There have been no attempts to explain the crucial and controversial differences by comparing spontaneous lesions in primates, birds, sheep, and pigs with diet-induced lesions in these animals. In the cholesterol-fed rabbit, preliminary injury to the vascular wall precedes and predisposes the wall to lipid deposition.[39,40] Injurious properties of cholesterol feeding or hypercholesterolemic serum have been emphasized.[86,185] Hueper[83] considers that arterial lesions in the hypercholesterolemic rabbit and lesions associated with the administration of methyl cellulose and other macromolecular compounds manifest similarities. Dissimilarities and the unphysiological nature of the experimental atherosclerosis of rabbits and other animals have been stressed; nevertheless, the resemblance to human atherosclerosis is heightened with intermittent or a low daily consumption of cholesterol[12] and when intimal fibrosis develops after the cessation of cholesterol feeding.[1] Regardless of the various merits and demerits, the rabbit remains a useful experimental model to demonstrate local tissue susceptibility.

Epidemiological studies implicate dietary intake of fat in the variation in severity of atherosclerosis and in the mortality of ischemic heart disease. Prevalence in the Western world is accepted as being much greater than in underdeveloped countries, disparities being explained in the main by differences in nutrition, in particular of fat intake. Yudkin[197,198] stressed that apparent relationships of many phenomena demonstrated by epidemiological means could be coincidental without necessarily establishing a cause-and-effect relationship. Standards of living, various indices of community spending power, dietary patterns, the status and state of nutrition, and "way of life," particularly as regards physical activity, can all singly and collectively differ. To select one parameter alone as the responsible element is to run the risk of misconstruing fact. Evidence indicates that the mortality from coronary heart disease among migrants approximates that of native-born inhabitants.[95,142]

Lipid has been recognized as the major, essential component of the atherosclerotic lesion. A large body of evidence relates the severity of atherosclerosis and the mortality from coronary heart disease to dietary fat intake, obesity, and blood cholesterol lev-

---

*Some types of hyperlipidemia are associated with severe and premature atherosclerosis, particularly of the coronary vessels. Cerebral vascular insufficiency may occur, the symptoms allegedly being relieved by an ileal bypass.[21]

els,[68,95,104] and this quite apart from their role in the causation of hypercoagulability and diminished fibrinolytic activity of the blood. A fatty meal, especially of saturated fats, causes hyperlipemia, elevation of serum cholesterol, phospholipid, and lipoproteins more so in the range of 0 to 12 Svedberg flotation units. A reduction in the values follows a dietary regime of low fat content.[95] Clinical studies show that the severity of atherosclerosis is related to serum cholesterol levels, a relationship substantiated by the hereditary hyperlipidemias. However, many individuals with normal blood cholesterol levels suffer from severe atherosclerosis. The low-density lipoprotein blood concentration has likewise been related to the severity of atherosclerosis, but because of the overlap into the normal range, the estimations are of little clinical value in the assessment of the disease in any individual case.

Numerous theories purport to explain the advent of lipid in the vessel wall. The imbibition theory postulates that a loosening of the connective tissue ground substance deep in the intima is associated with increased imbibition of blood plasma and eventual lipid accumulation. An increased permeability of the endothelium of the artery or vasa vasorum has been suggested, and there is the possibility that lipid may originate from thrombus or an intramural hematoma. Evidence certainly denotes that much of the lipid is derived from the circulating lipoproteins, but some is a consequence of the disturbed metabolism in the vessel wall.[68,156]

Polyunsaturated fats have a cholesterol-lowering action, but in the recent international survey it was found that in most populations the sources of fat and carbohydrate are not primary factors in determining the severity of the atherosclerosis.[150] Yudkin[199] asserts that the evidence incriminating sugar is more convincing than that incriminating dietary fat, and in rabbits, atherosclerosis can be induced by a diet rich in meat.[121]

Chronic hypothalamic stimulation intensifies the development of cholesterol-induced aortic atherosclerosis in rabbits.[74] In hypercholesterolemic rabbits, experimental lesions in the thalamus, cerebral cortex, and amygdala have been associated with more extensive aortic calcification and higher serum cholesterol levels.[158] Within 8 to 9 months, chronic ischemic cerebral hypoxia in rabbits results in increased serum lipids including cholesterol and atherosclerotic lesions in the aorta.[187] Such experiments suggest that hypercholesterolemia can be of central origin, that is, endogenous rather than dietary.

Evidence in support of the lipid hypothesis is said to be overwhelming, but the lines of causality are considerably more complex than is frequently supposed.[48,78] Furthermore, glaring incongruities and implications require further elucidation. (1) In experimental animals, the blood lipid cholesterol levels do not correlate well with the severity of atherosclerosis. (2) lipid accumulation can occur in the arteries of some animals (such as sheep) with exceedingly low blood cholesterol levels and a low fat intake.[170,172] Indeed in other animals with high blood cholesterol levels frequently many times the normal values for man, the arteries are free of atherosclerotic changes.[4,58,115] (3) Duff[39] considered that as cholesterol feeding fails to produce arterial lesions in several animal species, dietary cholesterol is not the all-important factor in the pathogenesis of human atherosclerosis. (4) The cerebral arteries in general are peculiarly resistant to cholesterol-induced atherosclerosis but are far from immune in the human disease.

A recent review concludes that the incidence of coronary heart disease and the severity of the underlying atherosclerosis are related to the serum concentrations of certain lipids (notably cholesterol and triglycerides), but no proof exists that the relationship is causal.[181]

Mechanical factors

Eddy currents,[2] "wear and tear,"[2] mechanical irritation,[137] fixation of the aorta by its segmental branches, tugging by branches,[43] shearing strains, and turbulence have all been suggested as possible mechanical factors with a causal relationship to the pathogenesis of atherosclerosis. The bases of these theories derive from vague attempts to explain the peculiar localization of atherosclerosis (see significance of intimal pads). Local tissue factors or hemodynamic trauma have been offered in explanation of the curious localization in the human circulation. The nonuniform distribution of atherosclerosis in the peripheral arterial circulation, its lesser severity in the pulmonary circulation and veins, its localization and severity at sites of branching, unions and curvatures, its dependence on the diameter of the vessel, and even at times the presence of unaffected intima adjoining spontaneous (Fig. 3-13) and induced lesions, as well as the failure of some animals and the cerebral and spinal vessels to respond to an atherogenic diet all indicate the existence of a tissue factor, long neglected, that governs the accumulation of lipid. It would appear that the tissue has to be susceptible to the circulating blood with its lipids, and when it is not susceptible, atherosclerosis does not develop, irrespective of the lipid levels.

Hemodynamic factors can influence the tissue factor by increasing the susceptibility as in hypertension, be it peripheral or pulmonary, or, for that matter, increased venous pressure. It may possibly be affected by hypotension, which usually forecasts longevity. Variation in severity and the distribution of atherosclerosis in the aorta is brought about by coarctation. Not infrequently, atherosclerosis visible in the cerebral arteries is limited to the wall of an aneurysmal sac, and it appears that the hemodynamics within the sac have accelerated the development of the atherosclerosis.

The intimal pads at arterial forks are sites of predilection for spontaneous lipid deposition in the sheep, and for induced lipid deposition in hypercholesterolemic rabbits. Consequently, the pads seem to possess the necessary tissue factor or factors. Their morphology suggests they are compensatory in nature because of a loss of tensile strength consequent upon the degeneration of the internal elastic lamina. The progressive nature of the changes in human intimal pads suggests that the damaging factor,[163] which could be hemodynamic injury as discussed above, persists. The deposition of lipid in arterial walls can be induced by trauma of many varieties, and it is distinctly possible that trauma may be the local tissue factor to which Anitschkow[6] referred. Moreover, intimal lesions resulting from trauma have a similar histology to intimal thickenings at forks.[166] Segments of vessels traumatized mechanically exhibit one important difference; that is, after a period of healing, the scar loses its susceptibility to lipid accumulation.[183] Likewise thrombus-induced plaques accumulate lipid in the hypercholesterolemic rabbit, but if the lesion undergoes complete resolution prior to the commencement of the diet,[63] they do not. Thus, either the intimal pads are not sites of trauma or they are continuously subjected to some form of damage.[163] The latter possibility seems the more correct because in an experimentally induced arteriovenous fistula, the vein becomes dilated and exhibits intimal tears, dissection, and mural hematomas, besides being more susceptible to lipid accumulation than an injured artery would be. Therefore, it seems that the hemodynamic or vibrational injury is what renders the vein susceptible. The arterial fork is subjected to stress associated with the pulse pressure, shear, and hypothetical pressure fluctuations associated with eddy currents. In each instance, the stress is alternating, and there is a possibility that the stresses lead to elastic tissue fatigue (as in the arteriovenous fistula[174]) and consequently render the arterial wall susceptible to lipid accumulation. The possibility that hemodynamic injury of this nature can induce atherosclerosis and lipid accumulation has been tested in arteriovenous fistulas produced in sheep. Disturbances of blood flow associated with the fistula, much more profound than normally present, have not resulted in atheromatous deposits even after 3 years. The lipid observed was the result of organization of a mural thrombus.[174] Moreover, lipid deposits are rarely found in the vessels of a cerebral arteriovenous aneurysm. The chronic vascular changes in these lesions can be regarded as a nonlipid-containing arteriosclerosis. To carry this hypothesis a stage further, we can postulate that the lipid component of human atherosclerosis may be a secondary phenomenon influenced by diet and other factors but that the prime lesion is the progressive intimal thickening occurring throughout life with its attendant elastic tissue degeneration, hyalinization, calcification, and arteriectasis—a combination of reparation and degeneration. The theory goes a long way to resolve many of the difficulties and inconsistencies of current hypotheses of atherogenesis, the influence of hemodynamic factors is more readily explained, and the complications are the result basically of loss of tensile strength. Reversibility, amelioration, or reduction of complications could thus be effected not only by dietary means as suggested by the epidemiological studies[146] but possibly by inducing hypotension. This line of argument being granted, the inescapable conclusion is that alleviation or eradication of the hemodynamic element should preclude lipid deposition, which would then be considered a secondary rather than a primary manifestation of atherosclerosis.

References

1. Adams, C. W. M.: Vascular histochemistry, Chicago, 1967, Year Book Medical Publishers, Inc.
2. Allbutt, T. C.: Arteriosclerosis, London, 1925, Macmillan and Co., Ltd.
3. Altschul, R.: Experimental arteriosclerosis in the nervous system, J. Neuropath. Exp. Neurol. 5:333, 1946.
4. Altschul, R., and Federoff, M. E.: Hypercholesteremia in the prairie gopher (ground squirrel), Arch. Path. 69:689, 1960.
5. Andrus, S. B., Portman, O. W., and Riopelle, A. J.: Comparative studies of spontaneous and experimental atherosclerosis in primates. II. Lesions in chimpanzees including myocardial infarction and cerebral aneurysms, Progr. Biochem. Pharmacol. 4:393, 1968.
6. Anitschkow, N.: Experimental arteriosclerosis in animals. In Cowdry, E. V.: Arteriosclerosis, New York, 1933, The Macmillan Co., p. 271.
7. Atkins, L.: Progeria. Report of a case with post-mortem findings, New Eng. J. Med. 250: 1065, 1954.
8. Baker, A. B., and Iannone, A.: Cerebrovascular disease. I. The large arteries of the circle of Willis, Neurology 9:321, 1959.
9. Baker, A. B., and Iannone, A.: Cerebrovascular disease. VII. A study of etiological mechanisms, Neurology 11 (part 2):23, 1901.
10. Baker, A. B., Iannone, A., and Kinnard, J.: Cerebrovascular disease. VI. Relationship to disease of the heart and the aorta, Neurology 11:63, 1961.
11. Barr, D. P.: Atherosclerosis and its effect on the cerebral circulation. In Wright, I. S., and Luckey, E. H.: Cerebral vascular diseases, New York, 1955, Grune & Stratton, Inc., p. 71.
12. Beckel, F.: Atherogenesis in rabbits fed simulated diet, Arch. Path. 77:563, 1964.
13. Belza, J., Rubinstein, L. J., Maier, N., and Haimovici, H.: Experimental cerebral atherosclerosis in dogs, Ann. N.Y. Acad. Sci. 149: 895, 1968.
14. Benson, R. L.: The present status of coronary arterial disease, Arch. Path. 2:876, 1926.
15. Berkson, D. M., and Stamler, J.: Epidemiological findings on cerebrovascular diseases and their implications, J. Atheroscler. Res. 5:189, 1965.
16. Böttcher, C. J. F., Woodford, F. P., Ter Haar Romeny, C. C., Boelsma, E., and van Gent, C. M.: Composition of lipids isolated from the aorta, coronary arteries and circulus Willisi of atherosclerotic individuals, Nature 183:47, 1959.
17. Breig, A., Ekbom, K., Greitz, T., and Kugelberg, E.: Hydrocephalus due to elongated basilar artery, Lancet 1:874, 1967.
18. Brice, J. G., Dowsett, D. J., and Lowe, R. D.: The effect of constriction on carotid blood-flow and pressure gradient, Lancet 1:84, 1964.
19. Brice, J. G., Dowsett, D. J., and Lowe, R. D.: Haemodynamic effects of carotid artery stenosis, Brit. Med. J. 2:1363, 1964.
20. Brihaye, J., Périer, O., Smulders, J., and Franken, L.: Glossopharyngeal neuralgia, J. Neurosurg. 13:299, 1956.
21. Buchwald, H.: The lipid clinic concept, Hosp. Practice 5 (no. 11):119, 1970.
22. Bullock, B. C., Clarkson, T. B., Lehner, N. D. M., Lofland, H. B., and St. Clair, R. W.: Atherosclerosis in Cebus albifrons monkeys, Exp. Molec. Path. 10:39, 1969.
23. Chapman, I.: Morphogenesis of occluding coronary artery thrombosis, Arch. Path. 80: 256, 1965.
24. Clark, E., Graef, I., and Chasis, H.: Thrombosis of the aorta and coronary arteries with special reference to the "fibrinoid" lesions, Arch. Path. 22:183, 1936.
25. Commission for the Study of Cerebrovascular Disease: Collaborative study of epidemiologi-

cal factors in cerebrovascular disease, Antwerp, 1959, World Federation of Neurology and the National Institute of Neurological Diseases and Blindness (U.S.P.H.S.).

26. Constantinides, P.: Plaque fissures in human coronary thrombosis, J. Atheroscler. Res. **6:**1, 1966.

27. Constantinides, P.: Pathogenesis of cerebral artery thrombosis in man, Arch. Path. **83:**422, 1967.

28. Cranston, W. I., Mitchell, J. R. A., Russell, R. W. R., and Schwartz, C. J.: The assessment of aortic disease, J. Atheroscler. Res. **4:**29, 1964.

29. Crawford, T.: Aetiology and pathology of cerebral atherosclerosis. In Williams, D.: Modern trends in neurology, 2nd series, New York, 1957, Paul B. Hoeber, Inc., p. 82.

30. Crawford, T.: The pathogenesis of atherosclerosis—the trends of recent work. Proc. Roy. Soc. Med. **52:**537, 1959.

31. Crompton, M. R.: The pathogenesis of cerebral aneurysms, Brain **89:**797, 1966.

32. Dandy, W. E.: Intracranial arterial aneurysms, Ithaca, 1944, Comstock Publishing Co., Inc.

33. Davies, J. N. P.: Pathology of central African natives. Mulago Hospital post-mortem studies IX, E. Afr. Med. J. **25:**454, 1948.

34. Dock, W.: The predilection of atherosclerosis for the coronary arteries, J.A.M.A. **131:**875, 1946.

35. Dow, D. R.: The incidence of arterio-sclerosis in the arteries of the body, Brit. Med. J. **2:**163, 1925.

36. Downie, H. G., Mustard, J. F., and Rowsell, H. C.: Swine atherosclerosis: the relationship of lipids and blood coagulation to its development, Ann. N.Y. Acad. Sci. **104:**539, 1963.

37. Drury, R. A. B.: The role of intimal haemorrhage in coronary occlusion, J. Path. Bact. **67:**207, 1954.

38. Du Boulay, G. H.: Some observations on the natural history of intracranial aneurysms, Brit. J. Radiol. **38:**721, 1965.

39. Duff, G. L.: Experimental cholesterol arteriosclerosis and its relationship to human arteriosclerosis, Arch. Path. **20:**81, 259, 1935.

40. Duff, G. L.: The nature of experimental cholesterol arteriosclerosis in the rabbit, Arch. Path. **22:**161, 1936.

41. Duff, G. L.: Functional anatomy of the blood vessel wall; adaptive changes. In: Symposium on atherosclerosis, Washington, 1954, National Research Council Publ. No. 338, p. 33.

42. Duff, G. L., and McMillan, G. C.: Pathology of atherosclerosis, Amer. J. Med. **11:**92, 1951.

43. Duguid, J. B.: Atheroma of the aorta, J. Path. Bact. **29:**371, 1926.

44. Duguid, J. B.: Thrombosis as a factor in the pathogenesis of coronary atherosclerosis, J. Path. Bact. **58:**207, 1946.

45. Duguid, J. B.: Thrombosis as a factor in the pathogenesis of aortic atherosclerosis, J. Path. Bact. **60:**57, 1948.

46. Duguid, J. B.: Pathogenesis of atherosclerosis, Lancet **2:**925, 1949.

47. Duguid, J. B., and Robertson, W. B.: Mechanical factors in atherosclerosis, Lancet **1:**1205, 1957.

48. Editorial: Ambition and disease: the chicken or the egg? Lancet **2:**1291, 1970.

49. Ekbom, K., Greitz, T., Kalmér, M., López, J., and Ottosson, S.: Cerebrospinal fluid pulsations in occult hydrocephalus due to ectasia of basilar artery, Acta Neurochir. **20:**1, 1969.

50. Enos, W. E., Holmes, R. H., and Beyer, J.: Coronary disease among United States soldiers killed in action in Korea, J.A.M.A. **152:**1090, 1953.

51. Fangman, R. J., and Hellwig, C. A.: Histology of coronary arteries in newborn infants, Amer. J. Path. **23:**901, 1947.

52. Fankhauser, R., Luginbühl, H., and McGrath, J. T.: Cerebrovascular disease in various animal species, Ann. N.Y. Acad. Sci. **127:**817, 1965.

53. Fisher, C. M., Gore, I., Okabe, N., and White, P. D.: Calcification of the carotid siphon, Circulation **32:**538, 1965.

54. Fisher, C. M., Gore, I., Okabe, N., and White, P. D.: Atherosclerosis of the carotid and vertebral arteries—extracranial and intracranial, J. Neuropath. Exp. Neurol. **24:**455, 1965.

55. Fisher, C. M., Pritchard, J. E., and Mathews, W. H.: Atherosclerosis of the carotid arteries, Circulation **6:**457, 1952.

56. Flora, G., Dahl, E., and Nelson, E.: Electron microscopic observations on human intracranial arteries, Arch. Neurol. **17:**162, 1967.

57. Florentin, R. A., Nam, S. C., Lee, K. T., Lee, K. J., and Thomas, W. A.: Increased mitotic activity in aortas of swine, Arch. Path. **88:**463, 1969.

58. Florey, H.: Question, Brit. Med. J. **2:**1562, 1961.

59. Fourman, J., and Moffat, D. B.: The effect of intra-arterial cushions on plasma skimming in small arteries, J. Physiol. **158:**374, 1961.

60. Fox, H.: Arteriosclerosis in lower mammals and birds: its relation to the disease in man. In Cowdry, E. V.: Arteriosclerosis, New York, 1933, The Macmillan Co., p. 153.

61. French, A. J., and Dock, W.: Fatal coronary arteriosclerosis in young soldiers, J.A.M.A. **124:**1233, 1944.

62. French, J. E.: Atherosclerosis. In Florey, H. W.: General pathology, ed. 2, London, 1958, Lloyd-Luke (Medical Books) Ltd., p. 351.

63. Friedman, M., and Byers, S. O.: Immunity of the mature thromboatherosclerotic plaque to hypercholesterolaemia, Brit. J. Exp. Path. **46:**539, 1965.

64. Friedman, M., and van den Bovenkamp, G. J.: The pathogenesis of a coronary thrombus, Amer. J. Path. **48:**19, 1966.

65. Geer, J. C., McGill, H. C., and Strong, J. P.: The fine structure of human atherosclerotic lesions, Amer. J. Path. **38:**263, 1961.

66. Geissinger, H. D., Mustard, J. F., and Rowsell, H. C.: The occurrence of microthrombi on the aortic endothelium of swine, Canad. Med. Ass. J. **87:**405, 1962.

67. Getty, R.: The gross and microscopic occurrence and distribution of spontaneous atherosclerosis in the arteries of swine. In Roberts, J. C., and Straus, R., editors: Comparative atherosclerosis, New York, 1965, Harper & Row Publishers, p. 11.

68. Getz, G. S., Vesselinovitch, D., and Wissler, R. W.: A dynamic pathology of atherosclerosis, Amer. J. Med. 46:657, 1969.

69. Giertsen, J. C.: The reliability of macroscopical grading of atherosclerosis, Acta Path. Microbiol. Scand. 50:355, 1960.

70. Glynn, L. E.: Medial defects in the circle of Willis and their relation to aneurysm formation, J. Path. Bact. 51:213, 1940.

71. Goldberg, I. D., and Kurland, L. T.: Mortality in 33 countries from diseases of the nervous system, World Neurology 3:444, 1962.

72. Goldberg, S. A.: Arteriosclerosis in domestic animals, J. Amer. Vet. Med. Ass. 69:31, 1926.

73. Greitz, T., and Löfstedt, S.: The relationship between the third ventricle and the basilar artery, Acta Radiol. 42:85, 1954.

74. Gunn, C. G., Friedman, M., and Byers, S. O.: Effect of chronic hypothalamic stimulation upon cholesterol-induced atherosclerosis in the rabbit, J. Clin. Invest. 39:1963, 1960.

75. Hassler, O.: Morphological studies on the large cerebral arteries with reference to the aetiology of subarachnoid haemorrhage, Acta Psychiat. Neurol. Scand. 36 (suppl. 154):1, 1961.

76. Hassler, O.: Physiological intima cushions in the large cerebral arteries of young individuals, Acta Path. Microbiol. Scand. 55:19, 1962.

77. Haust, M. D., Wyllie, J. C., and More, R. H.: Atherogenesis and plasma constituents 1. Demonstration of fibrin in the white plaque by the fluorescent antibody technique, Amer. J. Path. 44:255, 1964.

78. Hilditch, T. P., and Jasperson, H.: Lipids in relation to arterial disease. A summary of current biochemical evidence, Liverpool, 1959, J. Bibby and Sons Ltd.

79. Hirst, A. E., Gore, I., Hadley, G. G., and Gault, E. W.: Gross estimation of atherosclerosis in aorta, coronary, and cerebral arteries, Arch. Path. 69:578, 1960.

80. Holman, R. L., and Moosy, J.: The natural history of aortic, coronary and cerebral atherosclerosis. In Fields, W. S.: Pathogenesis and treatment of cerebrovascular disease, Springfield, Ill., 1961, Charles C Thomas, Publisher, p. 39.

81. Horn, H., and Finkelstein, L. F.: Arteriosclerosis of the coronary arteries and the mechanism of their occlusion, Amer. Heart J. 19:655, 1940.

82. Hudson, R. E. B.: Cardiovascular pathology, Baltimore, 1965, The Williams & Wilkins Co., vol. 1.

83. Hueper, W. C.: Arteriosclerosis, Arch Path. 39:117, 187, 1945.

84. Ignatowski, A.: Wirkung der tierischen Nahrung auf den Kaninchen-Organismus. Ber. Mil. Mediz. Akad., Petersburg 16:174, 1908. Cited by Anitschkow.[6]

85. Imai, H., Lee, K. J., Lee, S. Y., Lee, K. T., O'Neal, R. M., and Thomas, W. A.: Ultrastructural features of aortic cells in mitosis in control and cholesterol-fed swine, Lab. Invest. 23:401, 1970.

86. Imai, H., and Thomas, W. A.: Cerebral atherosclerosis in swine: role of necrosis in progression of diet-induced lesions from proliferative to atheromatous stage, Exp. Molec. Path. 8:330, 1968.

87. Javid, H., Ostermiller, W. E., Hengesh, J. W., Dye, W. S., Hunter, J. A., Najafi, H., and Julian, O. C.: Natural history of carotid bifurcation atheroma, Surgery 67:80, 1970.

88. Jennings, M. A., Florey, H. W., Stehbens, W. E., and French, J. E.: Intimal changes in the arteries of a pig, J. Path. Bact. 81:49, 1961.

89. Kahn, S. G., and Siller, W. G.: Absence of atherosclerosis in the cerebral arteries of chickens fed an atherogenic diet, Nature 213:720, 1967.

90. Kannel, W. B.: An epidemiologic study of cerebrovascular disease. In Millikan, C. H., Siekert, R. G., and Whisnant, J. P.: Cerebral vascular diseases, New York, 1966, Grune & Stratton, Inc., p. 53.

91. Katsuki, S., and Hirota, Y.: Current concept of the frequency of cerebral hemorrhage and cerebral infarction in Japan. In Millikan, C. H., Siekert, R. G., and Whisnant, J. P.: Cerebral vascular diseases, New York, 1966, Grune & Stratton, Inc., p. 99.

92. Katz, L. N., and Stamler, J.: Experimental atherosclerosis, Springfield, Ill., 1953, Charles C Thomas, Publisher.

93. Kelly, F. B., Taylor, C. B., and Hass, G. M.: Experimental atherosclerosis. Localization of lipids in experimental arterial lesions of rabbits with hypercholesteremia, Arch. Path. 53:419, 1952.

94. Keys, A., Anderson, J. T., and Grande, F.: Prediction of serum-cholesterol responses of man to changes in fats in the diet, Lancet 2:959, 1957.

95. Keys, A., and Grande, F.: Role of dietary fat in human nutrition, III. Diet and the epidemiology of coronary heart disease, Amer. J. Pub. Health 47:1520, 1957.

96. Lalich, J. L.: Factors contributing to the formation of saccular aneurysms in experimental lathyrism, Amer. J. Path. 50:5a, 1967.

97. Laurie, W., and Wood, J. D.: Atherosclerosis and its cerebral complications in the South African Bantu, Lancet 1:231, 1958.

98. Leary, T.: Coronary spasm as a possible factor in producing sudden death, Amer. Heart J. 10:338, 1935.

99. Levene, C. I.: The electron-microscopy of atheroma, Lancet 2:1216, 1955.

100. Levene, C. I.: The early lesions of atheroma in the coronary arteries, J. Path. Bact. 72:79, 1956.

101. Luginbühl, H., and Jones, J. E. T.: The morphology of spontaneous atherosclerotic lesions in aged swine, In Roberts, J. C., and

Straus, R., editors Comparative atherosclerosis, New York, 1965, Harper & Row, Publishers, p. 3.

102. Maher, J. A., Epstein, F. H., and Hand, E. A.: Xanthomatosis and coronary heart disease, Arch. Intern. Med. 102:437, 1958.
103. Martinez, A.: Electron microscopy of human atherosclerotic cerebral vessels. In Jacob, H.: International Congress of Neuropathology, Stuttgart, 1962, Georg Thieme Verlag, vol. 2, p. 164.
104. McGill, H. C., Arias-Stella, J., Carbonell, L. M., Correa, P., et. al.: General findings of the international atherosclerosis project, Lab. Invest. 18:498, 1968.
105. McGill, H. C., Strong, J. P., Holman, R. L., and Werthessen, N. T.: Arterial lesions in the Kenya baboon, Circulation Res. 8:670, 1960.
106. McMillan, G. C., and Duff, G. L.: Mitotic activity in the aortic lesions of experimental atherosclerosis of rabbits, Arch. Path. 46:179, 1948.
107. Menschik, Z., and Dovi, S. F.: Normally occurring intraluminal projections in the arterial system of the mouse, Anat. Rec. 153:265, 1965.
108. Meyer, W. W.: Über die rhythmische Lokalisation der atherosklerotischen Herde im cervicalen Abschnitt der Vertebralarterie, Beitr. Path. Anat. 130:24, 1964.
109. Meyer, W. W., and Beck, H.: Das röntgenanatomische und feingewebliche Bild der Arteriosklerose im intrakraniellen Abschitt der A. carotis interna, Virch. Arch. 326:700, 1955.
110. Mitchell, J. R. A., and Schwartz, C. J.: Arterial disease, Philadelphia, 1965, F. A. Davis Co.
111. Moffat, D. B.: An intra-arterial regulating mechanism in the uterine artery of the rat, Anat. Rec. 134:107, 1959.
112. Moon, V. H.: Atheromatous degeneration of the arterial wall, Arch. Path. 3:404, 1927.
113. Moosy, J.: Development of cerebral atherosclerosis in various age groups, Neurology 9:569, 1959.
114. Moosy, J.: Morphology, sites and epidemiology of cerebral atherosclerosis. In: Cerebrovascular disease, Ass. Res. Nerv. Ment. Dis. 41:1, 1966.
115. Morris, B.: The proteins and lipids of the plasma of some species of Australian fresh and salt water fish, J. Cell Comp. Physiol. 54:221, 1959.
116. Murphy, E. A., Rowsell, H. C., Downie, H. G., Robinson, G. A., and Mustard, J. F.: Encrustation and atherosclerosis: the analogy between early in vivo lesions and deposits which occur in extracorporeal circulations, Canad. Med. Ass. J. 87:259, 1962.
117. Mustard, J. F., Murphy, E. A., Rowsell, H. C., and Downie, H. G.: Platelets and atherosclerosis, J. Atheroscler. Res. 4:1, 1964.
118. Mustard, J. F., Rowsell, H. C., Murphy, E. A., and Downie, H. G.: Intimal thrombosis in atherosclerosis. In Jones, R. J.: Evolution of the atherosclerotic plaque, Chicago, 1963, University of Chicago Press, p. 183.
119. Nakamura, M.: Atherosclerosis of cerebral arteries in Japanese, Jap. Heart J. 8:553, 1967.
120. Nakamura, M., and Yabuta, N.: Difference in acid mucopolysaccharides contents among aortas, carotid and cerebral arteries, J. Atheroscler. Res. 7:83, 1967.
121. Newburgh, L. H., and Clarkson, S.: The production of atherosclerosis in rabbits by feeding diets rich in meat, Arch. Intern. Med. 31:653, 1923.
122. Nyström, S. H. M.: Electron microscopic studies on cholesterol-induced cerebral atherosclerosis in cockerels, Acta Neuropath. 3:48, 1963.
123. Ophüls, W.: The pathogenesis of arteriosclerosis. In Cowdry, E. V.: Arteriosclerosis, New York, 1933, The Macmillan Co., p. 249.
124. Paterson, J. C.: Vascularization and hemorrhage of the intima of arteriosclerotic coronary arteries, Arch. Path. 22:313, 1936.
125. Paterson, J. C., and Cornish, B. R.: Calcium concentrations in sclerotic cerebral arteries, Arch. Path. 62:177, 1956.
126. Peterson, R. E., Livingston, K. E., and Escobar, A.: Development and distribution of gross atherosclerotic lesions at cervical carotid bifurcation, Neurology 10:955, 1960.
127. Phair, J. P., Nefzger, M. D., Namiki, H., and Freedman, R.: Epidemiology of cerebrovascular disease in Hiroshima and Nagasaki, Japan, Circulation Suppl. 3 to Vol. 33 and 34:III-187, 1966.
128. Poe, W. D.: Fatal coronary disease in young men, Amer. Heart J. 33:76, 1947.
129. Pollak, O. J.: Attempts to produce cerebral atherosclerosis, Arch. Path. 39:16, 1945.
130. Pollak, O. J.: Experimental arteriopathies in the rabbit (The devil's advocate). In Roberts, J. C., and Straus, R., editors: Comparative pathology, New York, 1965, Harper & Row, Publishers, p. 291.
131. Prichard, R. W.: Spontaneous atherosclerosis in pigeons, In Roberts, J. C., and Straus, R., editors: Comparative atherosclerosis, New York, 1965, Harper & Row, Publishers, p. 45.
132. Prior, J. T., and Jones, D. B.: Structural alterations within the aortic intima in infancy and childhood, Amer. J. Path. 28:937, 1952.
133. Prior, J. T., Kurtz, D. M., and Ziegler, D. D.: The hypercholesteremic rabbit, Arch. Path. 71:672, 1961.
134. Ratinov, G.: Extradural intracranial portion of carotid artery, Arch. Neurol. 10:66, 1964.
135. Resch, J. A., and Baker, A. B.: Cerebral atherosclerosis, J. Indian Med. Prof. 11:5098, 1964.
136. Resch, J. A., Okabe, N., Loewenson, R., Kimoto, K., Katsuki, S., and Baker, A. B.: A comparative study of cerebral atherosclerosis in a Japanese and Minnesota population J. Atheroscler. Res. 7:687, 1967.
137. Rindfleisch, E.: A manual of pathological histology (translated by Baxter, E. B.: London, 1872, New Sydenham Society, vol. 1, p. 250.
138. Robertson, J. S., and Smith, K. V.: An analysis of certain factors associated with the production of experimental dissection of the aortic

media, in relation to the pathogenesis of dissecting aneurysm, J. Path. Bact. **60**:43, 1948.

139. Rodbard, S.: Vascular modifications induced by flow, Amer. Heart J. **51**:926, 1956.

140. Rodbard, S.: Physical forces and the vascular lining, Ann. Intern. Med. **50**:1339, 1959.

141. Rokitansky, C.: A manual of pathological anatomy (translated by G. E. Day), London, 1852, Sydenham Society, vol. 4, p. 262.

142. Rose, G.: Changing incidence of disease. In Jones, R. J.: Atherosclerosis, New York, 1970, Springer-Verlag, p. 310.

143. Rosen, W. C.: The morphology of valves in cerebral arteries of the rat, Anat. Rec. **157**: 481, 1967.

144. Rotter, W., Wellmer, H. K., Hinrichs, G., and Müller, W.: Zur Orthologie und Pathologie der Polsterarterien (sog. Verzweigungs- und Spornpolster) des Gehirns, Beitr. Path. Anat. **115**:253, 1955.

145. Samuel, K. C.: Atherosclerosis and occlusion of the internal carotid artery, J. Path. Bact. **71**:391, 1956.

146. Schornagel, H. E.: The connection between nutrition and mortality from coronary sclerosis during and after World War II, Document. Med. Geogr. Trop. **5**:173, 1953.

147. Schornagel, H. E.: Intimal thickening in the coronary arteries in infants, Arch. Path. **62**: 427, 1956.

148. Schwartz, C. J., and Mitchell, J. R. A.: Atheroma of the carotid and vertebral arterial systems, Brit. Med. J. **2**:1057, 1961.

149. Scott, R. F., Daoud, A. S., Wortman, B., Morrison, E. S., and Jarmolych, J.: Proliferation and necrosis in coronary and cerebral arteries, J. Atheroscler. Res. **6**:499, 1966.

150. Scrimshaw, N. S., and Guzmán, M. A.: Diet and atherosclerosis, Lab. Invest. **18**:623, 1968.

151. Shanklin, W. M., and Azzam, N. A.: On the presence of valves in the rat cerebral arteries, Anat. Rec. **146**:145, 1963.

152. Shanklin, W. M., and Azzam, N. A.: A study of valves in the arteries of the rodent brain, Anat. Rec. **147**:407, 1963.

153. Silver, M. M., McMillan, G. C., and Silver, M. D.: Haemolytic anaemia in cholesterol-fed rabbits, Brit. J. Haematol. **10**:271, 1964.

154. Simon, R. C., Still, W. J. S., and O'Neal, R. M.: The circulating lipophage and experimental atherosclerosis, J. Atheroscler. Res. **1**: 395, 1961.

155. Smith, D. E., and Windsor, R. B.: Embryologic and pathogenic aspects of the development of cerebral saccular aneurysms. In Fields, W. S.: Pathogenesis and treatment of cerebrovascular disease. Springfield, Ill., 1961, Charles C Thomas, Publisher, p. 367.

156. Smith, E. B., Slater, R. S., and Chu, P. K.: The lipids in raised fatty and fibrous lesions in human aorta, J. Atheroscler. Res. **8**:399, 1968.

157. Solberg, L. A., McGarry, P. A., Moosy, J., Tejada, C., Løken, A. C., Robertson, W. B., and Donoso, S.: Distribution of cerebral atherosclerosis by geographic location, race, and sex, Lab. Invest. **18**:604, 1968.

158. Somozoa, C.: Serum cholesterol levels and aortic medial calcification in rabbits with lesions in the brain, Amer. J. Path. **47**:271, 1965.

159. Ssolowjew, A.: Experimentelle Untersuchungen über die Bedeutung von lokaler Schädigung für die Lipoidablagerung in der Arterienwand, Z. Ges. Exp. Med. **69**:94, 1929-1930.

160. Stare, F. J., Andrus, S. B., and Portman, O, W.: Primates in medical research with special reference to New World monkeys. In Pickering, D. E.: Conference on research with primates, Beaverton, Ore., 1963, Tektronix Foundation, p. 59.

161. Stehbens, W. E.: Intracranial arterial aneurysms and atherosclerosis, Thesis, University of Sydney, 1958.

162. Stehbens, W. E.: Turbulence of blood flow in the vascular system of man. In Copley, A. L., and Stainsby, G.: Flow properties of blood, Oxford, 1960, Pergamon Press, p. 137.

163. Stehbens, W. E.: Focal intimal proliferation in the cerebral arteries, Amer. J. Path. **36**:289, 1960.

164. Stehbens, W. E.: Discussion on vascular flow and turbulence, Neurology **11** (part 2):66, 1961.

165. Stehbens, W. E.: Cerebral aneurysms and congenital abnormalities, Aust. Ann. Med. **11**:102, 1962.

166. Stehbens, W. E.: Histopathology of cerebral aneurysms, Arch. Neurol. **8**:272, 1963.

167. Stehbens, W. E.: The renal artery in normal and cholesterol-fed rabbits, Amer. J. Path. **43**: 969, 1963.

168. Stehbens, W. E.: Contentious features of coronary occlusion and atherosclerosis, Bull. Post-Grad. Comm. Med. Univ. Sydney **19**:216, 1963.

169. Stehbens, W. E.: Cerebral aneurysms of animals other than man, J. Path. Bact. **86**:161, 1963.

170. Stehbens, W. E.: Localization of spontaneous lipid deposition in the cerebral arteries of sheep, Nature **203**:1294, 1964.

171. Stehbens, W. E.: Vascular changes in chronic peptic ulcer, Arch. Path. **78**:584, 1964.

172. Stehbens, W. E.: Intimal proliferation and spontaneous lipid deposition in the cerebral arteries of sheep and steers, J. Atheroscler. Res. **5**:556, 1965.

173. Stehbens, W. E.: Observations on the microcirculation in the rabbit ear chamber, Quart. J. Exp. Physiol. **52**:150, 1967.

174. Stehbens, W. E.: Blood vessel changes in chronic experimental arteriovenous fistulas, Surg. Gynec. Obstet. **127**:327, 1968.

175. Stehbens, W. E., and Silver, M. D.: Arterial lesions induced by methyl cellulose, Amer. J. Path. **48**:483, 1966.

176. Steiner, P. E.: Necropsies on Okinawans, Arch. Path. **42**:359, 1946.

177. Stout, C., and Lemmon, W. B.: Predominant coronary and cerebral atherosclerosis in cap-

tive nonhuman primates, Exp. Molec. Path. **10**:312, 1969.

178. Straus, R., and Roberts, J. C.: Summary of conference. Discussions and editorial comment. In Roberts, J. C., and Straus, R., editors: Comparative pathology, New York, 1965, Harper & Row, Publishers, p. 365.

179. Strong, J. P.: Arterial lesions in primates. In Roberts, J. C., and Straus, R., editors: Comparative pathology, New York, 1965, Harper & Row, Publishers, p. 244.

180. Studer, A.: Thrombosis and atherogenesis. In Jones, R. J.: Atherosclerosis, New York, 1970, Springer-Verlag, p. 20.

181. Sub-Committee, National Heart Foundation of Australia: Dietary fat and coronary heart disease: a review, Med. J. Aust. **1**:309, 1967.

182. Suzuki, M.: Experimental atherosclerosis of the cerebral arteries in dogs: I. A morphologic study, Amer. J. Path. **59**:72a, 1970.

183. Taylor, C. B., Trueheart, R. E., and Cox, G. E.: Atherosclerosis in rhesus monkeys. III. The role of increased thickness of arterial walls in atherogenesis, Arch. Path. **76**:14, 1963.

184. Texon, M.: The hemodynamic concept of atherosclerosis, Amer. J. Cardiol. **5**:291, 1960.

185. Thomas, W. A., Florentin, R. A., Nam, S. C., Daoud, A. S., Lee, K. T., and Tiamson, E.: Plasma lipids and experimental atherosclerosis. In Jones, R. J.: Atherosclerosis, New York, 1970, Springer-Verlag, p. 414.

186. Thomas, W. A., Lee, K. T., and Daoud, A. S.: Geographic aspects of atherosclerosis, Ann. Rev. Med. **15**:255, 1964.

187. Tomus, L., Caluşeriu, I., Ioanes, S., Cordos, Rusu, M., and Iancu, P.: Rôle de l'hypoxie ischémique cérébrale du système nerveux central dans l'athérosclérose du lapin, Atherosclerosis **11**:207, 1970.

188. Waters, L. L.: Dietary fat and arteriosclerosis

—evidence from experimental pathology, Conn. Med. **23**:344, 1959.

189. Waters, L. L., and Duff, R. S.: The role of arterial injury in the localization of methyl cellulose, Amer. J. Path. **28**:527, 1952.

190. Wexler, B. C., and True, C. W.: Carotid and cerebral arteriosclerosis in the rat, Circulation Res. **12**:659, 1963.

191. Wilens, S. L.: The nature of diffuse intimal thickening of arteries, Amer. J. Path. **27**:825, 1951.

192. Williams, A. O., Resch, J. A., and Loewenson, R. B.: Cerebral atherosclerosis—a comparative autopsy study between Nigerian Negroes and American Negro and Caucasians, Neurology **19**:205, 1969.

193. Williams, A. W.: Relation of atheroma to local trauma, J. Path. Bact. **81**:419, 1961.

194. Winternitz, M. C., Thomas, R. M., and LeCompte, P. M.: The biology of arteriosclerosis, Springfield, Ill., 1938, Charles C Thomas, Publisher.

195. Woolf, N., and Crawford, T.: Fatty streaks in the aortic intima studied by an immunohistochemical technique, J. Path. Bact. **80**:405, 1960.

196. Young, W., Gofman, J. W., Malamud, N., Simon, A., and Waters, E. S. G.: The interrelationship between cerebral and coronary atherosclerosis, Geriatrics **11**:413, 1956.

197. Yudkin, J.: Diet and coronary thrombosis. Hypothesis and fact, Lancet **2**:155, 1957.

198. Yudkin, J.: The epidemiology of coronary disease, Progr. Cardiovasc. Dis. **1**:116, 1958.

199. Yudkin, J.: Sugar and coronary thrombosis, Postgrad. Med. **44**:542, 1967.

200. Zugibe, F. T., and Brown, K. D.: Histochemical studies in atherogenesis: human aortas, Circulation Res. **8**:287, 1960.

4/Thrombosis, embolism, infarction, and vascular insufficiency

Basically, stroke indicates an abrupt onset of a neurological deficit irrespective of cause. It has been used synonymously with cerebrovascular disease and to signify cerebral hemorrhage, thrombosis, and embolism but no other vascular lesions of the brain. Mostly, it refers to the sudden onset of symptoms and signs typifying vascular insufficiency or infarction of variable etiology. The neurological disturbance, when associated with severe, perhaps permanent symptoms and signs, is often referred to as a "major stroke." When short lived and manifested by only slight derangement of speech, vision, voluntary motion, cerebration, or somatic sensation, it is usually termed a "little stroke."[14,186] As a medical or scientific term, it lacks precision and, being unacceptable, should be avoided.

Vascular insufficiency, varying from mild transient symptoms of local anoxia to frank massive encephalomalacia, has many causes, all with one feature in common—an inadequate supply of oxygenated blood to the area of the brain affected. Changes in that state and embolism can initiate cerebral ischemia, which is more often the result of pathological changes in the vessel wall causing stenosis or thrombotic occlusion of the lumen.

Cerebrovascular insufficiency
Transient ischemic attacks

In the elderly, bouts of faintness, weakness, loss of consciousness, or other brief neurological episodes are common. The abrupt onset and the total or almost complete recovery suggest a vascular disturbance. Not infrequently, these are the premonitory transient manifestations presaging a major ischemic episode, which may be fatal or permanently disabling.[130] However, such symptoms do not precede all major infarcts and the similarity between these transient attacks and those of hypertensive encephalopathy is more than coincidental.

Alajouanine and associates[10] found that 23 of 40 patients who had experienced a single or several transient ischemic attacks exhibited angiographic evidence of internal carotid or middle cerebral artery occlusion. In 98 patients with signs of cerebral softening and more or less severe aftereffects, 33 (33.6%) had sustained one or more transitory ischemic attacks, which, in the great majority, evinced a distribution corresponding to that of the subsequent infarct. In seven, the attacks subsided completely. They are more frequently associated with an occlusion of the internal carotid than of the middle cerebral artery. Hollenhorst[176] estimates that about 50% of patients with intermittent cerebrovascular insufficiency develop a severe infarct after a lapse of time averaging three years, 25% continue to have the attacks, and 25% recover without further ado. In a more recent study of patients with transient ischemia, almost two-thirds had a permanent stroke within 4 years.[106]

Marshall[243] analyzed 158 cases of cerebrovascular disease with transient cerebral ischemic attacks, mostly between the ages of 45 and 74 years (peak incidence between 55 and 64). The majority of patients, who subsequently had a major cerebral occlusion, had only one or two transient ischemic attacks beforehand. Others, who did not proceed to a major attack, often had several per week for more than a year of observation. Some of the mild attacks cease spontaneously, and do not recur but the eventual outcome is unpredictable. Occasionally, a transient attack is the forerunner of a cerebral hemorrhage or is associated with a neoplasm. Hemiparesis in a transient attack localized in the vertebrobasilar system, is more likely to lead to a major cerebral catastrophe than in attacks with milder symptoms only. The interval between the onset of the minor and of the major ischemic episode is longer than it is with those in the carotid territory which proceed to a major episode. The sex ratio of males to females is about 2:1.

Denny-Brown[92] emphasized that cerebrovascular insufficiency cannot be demonstrated at autopsy. Nevertheless, occasionally residua from the long, drawn-out, and numerous transient ischemic attacks persist, and though demonstration of lesions would prove difficult, it is likely that some permanent neuronal damage is sustained.[14] Indeed focal areas of disturbed regional blood flow have been found many days after the remission of symptoms.[287]

Pathogenesis

Vasospasm. The fleeting nature of many of the seizures suggests a functional disturbance rather than an organic vascular lesion.[10] Vasospasm, traditionally held responsible, is not now regarded as the cause,[91] though on occasions it cannot be completely excluded as a possibility.

Hemodynamic crises. A sudden reduction of systemic blood pressure and flow may interfere with the delicate balance in a precarious cerebral circulation in patients with occlusive or stenotic lesions of the arterial supply to the brain. Episodes of hypotension whatever their cause can contribute to the production of transient neurological symptoms. In experimental occlusion of the internal carotid or middle cerebral artery, animals apparently recovering from the operation, can become hemiplegic after induced hypotension.[92] Gilroy and Meyer[148] provided evidence that symptoms of vertebrobasilar insufficiency (often related to posture) may occur with hypotension associated with anterior pituitary failure and secondary adrenocortical insuffi-

ciency. Hydrocortisone abolishes the hypotension and relieves the symptoms. Another causative factor is the steal phenomenon, in which vascular insufficiency results from the shunting of blood to extravascular tissues at the expense of the cerebral circulation. The attack can be caused by organic obstruction with rapid compensation from the collateral circulation and with subsequent attacks initiated by increased functional demand, vascular steal, or other general circulatory disturbances.[10]

Microembolism. Observations on the retinal circulation during episodic visual disturbances indicate strongly that transient ischemic attacks can often result from microemboli to the brain sloughed off from an ulcerated atheromatous plaque possibly in the carotid sinus or even from an aneurysm. Many patients, who had one or more transient attacks of monocular blindness, subsequently developed thrombosis of the homolateral internal carotid artery (at the level of the sinus) and hence contralateral hemiplegia.[131] It appears that the ocular symptoms herald the subsequent disaster. In a patient subject to frequent, brief ischemic attacks associated with stenosis of the carotid sinus, Fisher[122] observed white emboli passing through the retinal vessels during transient monocular blindness. Finding several similar reports in the literature, he conjectured that transient cerebral ischemic episodes are likewise the result of microembolism. Russell[298] observing a similar case, provided evidence indicating that the white bodies of emboli were platelet aggregates. In 27 of 235 patients (11%) with occlusive disease within the carotid arterial system, and in four of 93 patients (4%) with occlusive disease of the vertebrobasilar system, retinal arterioles were found to contain bright orange, yellow, or copper plaques believed to be atheromatous emboli.[175] This was confirmed subsequently at autopsy.[82] Later studies have established that the emboli, the white plugs, and the small refractile plaques, migrate through the retinal circulation and are often replaced by further emboli.[299,300] Russell[300] referred to a third type, the white embolus that produces segmental blockage of retinal vessels and permanent retinal damage. It is associated with chronic cardiac disease, often vascular, though the embolus does not migrate, no doubt because of its irreversible nature in contradistinction to the other varieties, which break up and gradually pass through the retinal circulation with restoration of flow. Some of these emboli are symptomless.[318]

Such observations suggest that the central nervous system is subject to similar episodes of embolism, many of which do not seem to resolve completely. Furthermore, not all transient ischemic attacks should be regarded as embolic, and Toole and Patel[357] emphasized the conjectural nature of this theory because of the infrequency with which emboli are found at autopsy, but if emboli enter the ophthalmic artery, they are even more likely to enter the cerebral circulation proper. These emboli are derived not only from thrombi complicating atherosclerosis but also from the heart and valves. Transient ischemic episodes, probably embolic in origin, complicate bacterial endocarditis and chronic rheumatic heart disease.

Neck movements. Rotation or extension of the head, when in association with severe atherosclerosis, tortuosity, kinking, or even fibromuscular hyperplasia[283] of the cervical arteries or osteoarthritis of the cervical spine, can cause temporary reduction in blood flow in the presence of inadequate collateral flow.

Miscellaneous. It is also possible that an increased blood viscosity associated with red cell aggregation may render worse the cerebrovascular insufficiency. A low fat diet has been regarded as beneficial in the treatment of transient ischemic attacks.[338] Meyer and Portnoy[256] subjected animals to occlusion of the middle cerebral artery. After recovery, the hemiparesis could be induced to recur by hypoglycemia and relieved by intravenous glucose. Diabetics in whom a transient hemiparesis or localized neuro-

logical disturbance was associated with mild hypoglycemia have been reported.[256,278] Endarterectomy to correct the stenosis of the corresponding internal carotid artery eradicated the tendency to the hypoglycemia-induced transient ischemic attacks in one of the diabetics.[278] Other metabolic disturbances can have a similar effect in precipitating vascular insufficiency.[278]

Subclavian steal syndrome

Under certain pathological conditions, the normal pressure gradients maintaining the flow of blood to the brain may be disturbed and cause diversion of blood from the brain for the supply of the upper limb—the subclavian steal syndrome,[104] or brachial-basilar insufficiency.[267] Found during the last century,[115] its importance has been recognized only within the last 10 years.

Occlusion or severe stenosis of the subclavian artery proximal to the origin of the vertebral artery (Fig. 4-1) can be associated with cerebral ischemia depending on the anatomy of the circle of Willis and the respective sizes of the two vertebral arteries. In patients who have survived the development of this obstructive lesion, the collateral circulation augmenting the flow to the homolateral upper limb is derived from numerous sources, namely, anastomoses of the superior and inferior thyroid arteries, anastomoses between spinal and muscular branches of the vertebral arteries of each side, the anastomosis of the internal mammary with the inferior epigastric, aortic intercostals and the opposite internal mammary artery, the anastomosis of the costocervical with intercostal arteries, the deep cervical anastomosing with the descending branch of the occipital, the scapular branch of the thyrocervical trunk anastomosing with the branches of the axillary artery, and the thoracic branches of the axillary anastomosing with the aortic intercostals, anastomoses between muscular branches of occipital and vertebral arteries, and anastomoses between the external ca-

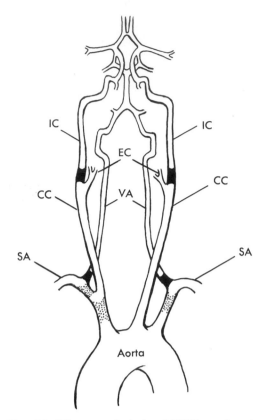

Fig. 4-1. Diagram of circle of Willis and major arteries of neck. Black arterial segments are extracranial sites where stenosis and occlusion are most likely to occur (that is, the carotid sinus and the commencement of the vertebral arteries). Stippled segments are sites of infrequent occlusion causing the common variety of subclavian steal syndrome, with the circle of Willis providing the compensatory collateral flow. **CC**, Common carotid artery. **EC**, External carotid. **IC**, Internal carotid. **SA**, Subclavian artery. **VA**, Vertebral artery.

rotid artery on the one hand and the thyrocervical and costocervical arteries on the other. Mostly these anastomoses are relatively small, though they may contribute blood to the reversed vertebral artery flow.[193] However, if the two vertebral arteries are fairly large, their junction to form the basilar artery is a convenient anastomosis through which blood can be siphoned from the brain to the limb with a consequent reversal of flow through the enlarged homolateral vertebral artery. Such a siphon-

ing effect can compromise the basilar blood flow.[290,291,355] The size of the posterior communicating arteries is of obvious importance in the steal syndrome, and it would be of interest if it could be demonstrated that certain patterns of the circle of Willis showed a proclivity for association with basilar insufficiency. Reivich and associates[290] reported two cases in which the steal phenomenon had been caused by a stenosis. They felt that the carotid circulation assisted in the posterior cerebral circulation when the posterior communicating arteries were sufficiently large. In the same year, Rob[291] ligated the vertebral artery near its origin to relieve symptoms of such a steal. In 207 collected cases, 45% had cerebral symptoms only, 40% complained of cerebral and upper limb symptoms, 10% of symptoms pertaining only to the arm, and 6% had no symptoms.[169] The neurological manifestations can arise from ischemia or actual infarction of the structures supplied by the vertebrobasilar system (upper spinal cord, the brain stem, cerebellum, thalamus, and occipital lobes[356]). In many instances, cerebral insufficiency is either induced or aggravated by exercise of the homolateral arm[169,267] and by rotation of the head in a few instances.[356] Experimentally, systemic vasopressors also increase the reversed vertebral artery flow.[302]

Subclavian steal syndrome has been used to encompass cases in which the innominate artery is significantly narrowed or occluded,[42] but in such cases the shunt is via the homolateral carotid and vertebral arteries. If, however, the homolateral carotid artery is also stenosed or the collateral circulation is poor, the steal occurs via the vertebral artery alone. The homolateral vertebral artery with retrograde flow may supply both the subclavian and the common carotid arteries.[42]

Other variations of the steal are fairly common, blood at times being shunted through the circle of Willis[196,272] as in the case of a woman in whom the reversed vertebral flow resulted from a homolateral carotid angiogram.[272] Such cases usually depend on the presence of multiple stenotic or occlusive lesions and on the topography of the circle of Willis. When the phenomenon is bilateral, the shunt takes place via either the circle of Willis or through collaterals from the external carotid. Other lesions, such as obstruction of the first part of the vertebral artery and a vertebral arteriovenous aneurysm, may also cause reverse flow in part of the vertebral artery and on occasions reversal of vertebral flow seems to occur for no apparent reason.[271]

In a survey of 207 reported cases, the syndrome was two to three times more frequent in males than females (mean age 52.3 years in males and 49 in females).[169] An idea of the frequency of the subclavian occlusion may be gleaned from the study of 1500 patients with cerebrovascular disease.[267] Atherosclerotic obstruction in the subclavian artery proximal to the vertebral artery origin was found in 59 patients, on the left in 33, on the right in 13, and bilateral in 13. Heidrich and Bayer[169] gave the frequency of bilateral subclavian steal as about 1% to 2%. The left subclavian was the cause in 62%, the right subclavian in 28%, and the innominate in 10%. Complete occlusion was more frequently the cause of the syndrome than stenosis[169] in the ratio of 3:1.

The most common cause of this syndrome is unquestionably atherosclerosis, and therefore, in many cases, stenotic or occlusive vascular disease is likely to be observed elsewhere. In one series of 20 patients,[192] 15 had intermittent claudication, 5 had a history of myocardial infarction, and 18 exhibited additional interference with cerebral flow at one or other site in the neck.

The syndrome has been found in several patients with the Blalock-Taussig procedure (anastomosis of subclavian artery to pulmonary artery) for pulmonary atresia[137] and stenosis. Less frequent causes include congenital atresia of the subclavian artery,[16,146] kinking of the subclavian artery in pseudocoarctation,[232] embolism of the sub-clavian or innominate arteries,[80] tumor embolus,[8] the aortic arch syndrome, and aortic aneurysm whereas the origin of the left subclavian artery can be stenosed in aortic coarctation.

The importance of the subclavian steal syndrome lies in its amenability to surgical correction and relief of the symptoms although a recurrence of the stenosis can occur.[67] In some patients, remission of symptoms follows the development of other collateral circulation.

Other forms of steal

Different forms of steal result from arterial occlusions in different locations and the volume and direction of abnormal flow depend on the anatomy of arteries of the neck and cranium, the location of the occlusive arterial lesion, and the balance between demands of the limb or extracranial tissues and the cerebral vascular bed for blood.[357]

Stenosis of the innominate artery and the left subclavian artery results in bilateral reversal of vertebral arterial flow, blood being siphoned from the carotid circulation through both vertebral arteries. Occlusion of the common carotid artery with reversal of flow in the internal carotid and conventional flow in the external carotid has been referred to as the internal-external carotid steal[196] or the external carotid artery steal.[27] The face, scalp, and neck are then supplied at the expense of the cerebral circulation. However, with adequate anastomoses in the distribution of the external carotid, it is possible that the direction of blood flow could be the reverse of that above. Furthermore, therapeutic ligation of the common carotid artery can be succeeded by vertebrobasilar insufficiency after the diversion of blood from the vertebrobasilar system to the carotid tree.[352]

In some instances of occlusion of the external carotid artery, the territory supplied by this vessel is dependent on the vertebral artery for blood, and in other cases it is from the internal carotid artery via the anastomoses between the intracranial and external carotid arteries. Occlusion of the external or common carotid arteries can be the result of surgical procedures. However, in this form of vascular steal, the occlusion is more commonly spontaneous because of atherosclerosis and is, therefore, less likely to occur as an isolated lesion. Rather it is in association with severe occlusive disease of the other major arteries to the brain. In this respect, it differs from the foregoing subclavian steal. Less frequently, a combination of subclavian and external carotid artery steal may exist.[27]

Fisher[127] described five cases in which there was a proximal occlusion of the vertebral artery and collaterals from the external carotid provided blood to the vertebrobasilar system beyond the occlusion.

Aortic arch syndrome

Diseases that diminish or obliterate pulses in arteries arising from the arch of the aorta have been assembled under the term "aortic arch syndrome." In mature cases, no pulses are palpable in the head, neck, or upper limbs. The collateral circulation is well developed, but trophic changes including alopecia and ulceration of the nasal septum, mouth, or skin may follow. The patient suffers frequent transient attacks of syncope, fatigue, vertigo, and renal disturbance. Permanent cerebral damage, sufficient to produce hemiplegia, is a hazard. The carotid sinus is often unduly sensitive and systemic hypertension ("reversed coarctation") can be expected.[296] The causes include (1) Takayasu's arteritis, (2) syphilitic aortitis with or without an associated aneurysm, (3) giant cell arteritis,[184] (4) atherosclerosis and chronic dissection of the aorta, (5) miscellaneous causes, possibly trauma, thrombosis or embolism, and others of unknown etiology.[296] Takayasu's arteritis is probably the most frequent cause of this syndrome. Outside Japan, superadded premature atherosclerosis is not uncommon.[304]

Infarction or encephalomalacia

A cerebral infarct (softening) is a localized area of ischemic necrosis ranging in size from a microscopic focus to massive areas of encephalomalacia involving at times an entire cerebral hemisphere. Less severe degrees of ischemia may elicit severe but reversible neurological dysfunction. Thromboembolic disorders of the central nervous system account for 62% of deaths from cerebrovascular disease (Table 7-1) and as such constitute the commonest organic brain disease. They are precipitated in the main by occlusion of the ar-

Table 4-1. Age distribution of nonembolic cerebral infarction

Authors	0-9	10-19	20-29	30-39	40-49	50-59	60-69	70-79	80 and over	Total
Aring & Merritt (1935)[17]				1	7	25	37	26	8	104
Courville (1937)[72]				9	26	96	151	149	41	472
Pincock (1957)[275]			1	5	5	26	44	30	5	116*
Moosy (1966)[259]				3	12	27	40	41	19	142
Battacharji et al. (1967)[29]					1	2	16	23	15	57
Blackwood et al. (1969)[40]			1	3	13	14	20	6		57
Louis & McDowell (1970)[236]				3	12	45	117	93	30	300
Total			2	24	76	235	425	368	118	1248

*Males only, mean age 63.5 years.

terial supply, less often by obstruction of the venous drainage, and otherwise by circulatory insufficiency.

Nonembolic arterial occlusion

Age and sex distribution. In clinical practice, infarcts of nonembolic origin contribute the bulk of "strokes" and the age-specific incidence figures are similar to the mortality curves for cerebrovascular disease. They are negligible under 35 years of age but climb steeply at 55 years and thereafter. Many patients dying under some other primary classification have had cerebral infarcts of varying severity prior to their demise. Thus, national mortality figures do not reflect the true prevalence. These patients constitute a heterogeneous group, but nonembolic occlusion of the extracranial and intracranial arteries supplying the brain is most often caused by moderate or severe atherosclerosis and its complications. Therefore, most cases are over the age of 50 years (Table 4-1), and the greatest frequency is in the seventh and eighth decades with few examples under the age of 30 years. There is no significant age difference between the lesions of the carotid and those of the vertebrobasilar system.[219] Aronson and Rabiner[19] found that 16% of all autopsies on patients under 15 years had cerebral infarcts. No doubt, most were embolic. Of those over 75 years, 59% exhibited infarcts.

Between 1932 and 1959 at the New York Hospital—Cornell Medical Center,[378] only 77 patients (40 males) under 50 years had a clinical diagnosis of cerebral thrombosis. The age ranged from 6½ to 49 years, with 22 under 40 years of age. Thirty-two were hypertensive. Louis and McDowell[236] found that 56 (6% of the total) of 966 patients with cerebral thrombosis were 50 years or younger, 43 were in the fifth decade, and the youngest was 34 years old. Only four patients had no evidence of hypertension, diabetes, hypercholesterolemia or other diseases to which thrombosis could be attributed.

The abrupt onset of hemiplegia in infancy suggests arterial occlusion, but as most cases do not come to autopsy in the acute phase of the illness, the precise etiology is controversial. Shillito[310] suggested that arteritis could be responsible for many cases of cerebral arterial occlusion in infancy and childhood, including those associated with cardiac disease. Wisoff and Rothballer[382] in 1961 found thrombotic occlusion of the cerebral arteries reported in only 29 children (infancy to 16 years). A few more reports have appeared since.[83,99] Thrombosis secondary to atherosclerosis is less common in the younger individuals. Embolism is generally regarded as the commonest cause of cerebral arterial occlusion in childhood. The sex distribution of cerebral infarction in most studies exhibits a varying male preponderance (Table 4-2). The ratio of males to females[236] is 1.9 in the fifth decade, falling to unity in the ninth.

Pathology of infarction

Macroscopic. Infarcts of the central nervous system are classified as pale or hemorrhagic (red) and recent or old depending on their duration and the stage of resolution.

A pale infarct (ischemic necrosis or anemic infarct) of recent origin, such as in the cerebrum, is usually difficult to recognize macroscopically within the first 24 hours, after which time degenerative and reparative processes are sufficient to make

Table 4-2. Sex distribution in nonembolic cerebral infarction

Authors	Male	Female	Total
Aring & Merritt (1935)[17]	68	38	106
Courville (1937)[72]	323	174	497
Carter (1959)[54]	104	115	219
Fisher (1961)[123]	90	28	118
Eisenberg et al. (1964)[108]	40	51	91
Aronson & Aronson (1966)[18]	130	126	256
Moosy (1966)[259]	76	66	142
Blackwood et al. (1969)[40]	36	21	57
Louis & McDowell (1970)[236]	186	114	300
Total	1053	733	1786

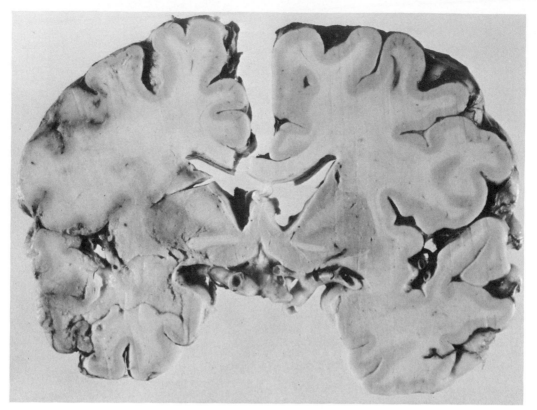

Fig. 4-2. Coronal section through cerebrum with extensive recent softening on left side in the distribution of middle cerebral artery. Note (1) loss of differentiation of gray and white matter in cortex and the lenticular nucleus and (2) fragmentation of softened area. There are a few petechial hemorrhages and some congestion in the softened area.

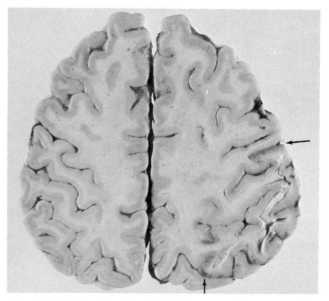

Fig. 4-3. Area of cortical softening (parietal) between the arrows. Note that softened cortex is thicker there, contains a few petechiae, and is poorly demarcated from the white matter in some areas but mostly is separated by an artifactual cleft caused by edema and softening in the subcortical white matter.

its recognition possible. The early infarct is more readily washed away under running water than noninfarcted tissue, though this procedure interferes with the histology. To the naked eye, the earliest demonstrable change is a slight swelling of the infarcted cortex and white matter, and differentiation between the two becomes indistinct (Fig. 4-2). When palpated, the infarcted area is soft. This feature is accentuated by fixation, for the normal brain progressively hardens and the infarct does not. The

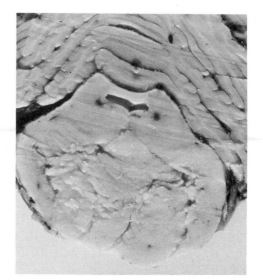

Fig. 4-4. Reasonably well demarcated but extensive softening of the pons caused by basilar artery thrombosis. Note granular and friable nature of softened zone.

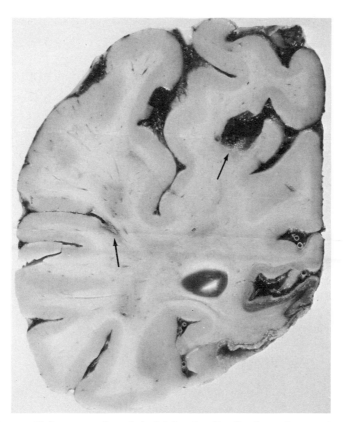

Fig. 4-5. Inferomedial aspect of occipital lobe in distribution of posterior cerebral artery exhibits a small cortical infarct. Readily overlooked, the cortex is much narrowed and granular with a cleft and some pigmentation. There are two areas of softening (*arrows*) indicated by a defect in the cortex; the larger softening also involves the underlying white matter.

swelling may be considerable, with enlargement and flattening of the gyri, narrowing and obliteration of sulci, and a shift of the midline structure to the opposite side with a variable degree of herniation of the brain tissue under the falx cerebri or through the tentorial opening. The cortex is distinctly thicker than the neighboring healthy cortex and the line of demarcation can be abrupt. The subcortical tissue tends to become soft and edematous while a line of separation develops along which a split will readily appear even when the brain (Fig. 4-3) is gently manipulated. This occurs in infarcts involving the cortex alone

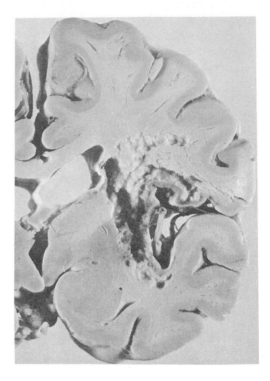

Fig. 4-6. Old softening about insula and lateral fissure of Sylvius. Remnants of cortex persist over irregular cavitation extending to lateral ventricle, but a small zone of subependymal tissue persists. Note the moth-eaten appearance of the margins of the softening.

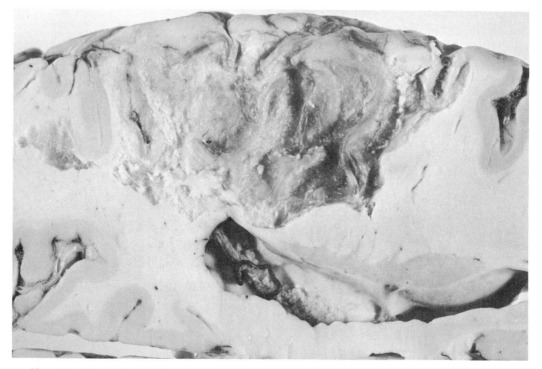

Fig. 4-7. Old cerebral softening with complete destruction of much of the cortex. Meninges and vessels in the lateral fissure are visible. Note spongy and moth-eaten margins and preservation of subependymal tissue.

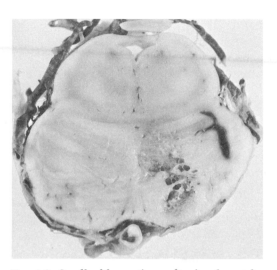

Fig. 4-8. Small old pontine softening by occlusion of perforating arteries. Basilar artery is atherosclerotic and cavity is crossed by trabeculae of irregular dimensions. Unusually large intrapontine vein is seen on right of softening.

and in larger infarcts with concomitant softening of the underlying white matter. A similar phenomenon may arise about the lenticular nucleus with splits separating it from the internal and external capsules. After 1 week, the swelling subsides and the infarcted area is well demarcated, and within 2 weeks, the softened tissue, disintegrating and crumbling, rather resembles cottage cheese (Fig. 4-4). The process of disintegration and resorption of the friable and semifluid infarct continues until resorption, which may take several months, is complete.

In old infarcts, the overlying meninges may be slightly thickened and opaque, wrinkled and depressed to a variable degree. There may be merely a large depression in the brain, but more frequently patches of cortex persist and the gyri appear unusually small and possibly pigmented (yellowish-brown). In sections through the infarcted area the cortex, when visible, is noticeably narrower than normal and yellowish-brown (Fig. 4-5). Small cor-

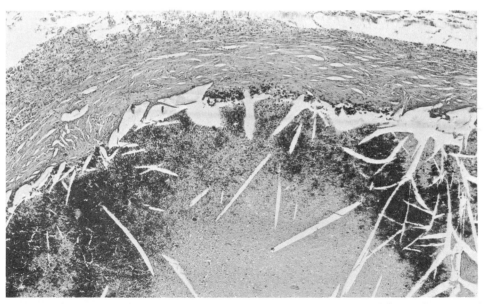

Fig. 4-9. Old infarct exhibiting coagulation necrosis. Cholesterol clefts and zones of calcification are present in the necrotic tissue, which is surrounded by a broad fibrous tissue capsule. Such areas may occur in only part of large infarcts. (Hematoxylin and eosin, ×27.)

tical infarcts, easily missed, are best detected by looking for diminution in thickness or a break in the continuity of the cortex. If the infarct has involved deeper structures beneath it, there is a cystic space (Figs. 4-6 and 4-7) of reduced dimensions because of the collapse of the cortex and a possible localized ex vacuo enlargement of the ventricle. Small cobweblike threads often traverse the cystic space (Fig. 4-8), which communicating through cortical defects with neighboring sulci, may expose pial vessels. The borders of the space are irregular, well demarcated, or have a moth-eaten or spongy appearance (Fig. 4-7). The space may communicate with the lateral ventricle, but more frequently a thin rim of subependymal parenchyma (Fig. 4-6), sometimes less than 1 mm. thick, persists. Occasionally in large infarcts, unabsorbed debris becomes encapsulated and proceeds to calcification (Fig. 4-9).

In the pale infarct or softening, there may be small petechiae (Fig. 4-2) in the gray matter or a slight extravasation of blood into the subarachnoid space. A few cortical petechiae are frequently found mi-croscopically, but in red or hemorrhagic softenings, multiple small hemorrhages of variable size are prevalent, imparting a roseate punctate appearance to the cortex. Their restriction to the cortex is characteristic. If the hemorrhages coalesce, the cortex is diffusely red and hemorrhagic (Fig. 4-10). Involvement of the subcortical white matter may occur when hemorrhages are severe, but as a rule the concomitant softening of the white matter is anemic. On the pial surface, the involved gyri are dark red or brown and usually somewhat mottled with a variable amount of blood in the subarachnoid space. In a hemorrhagic softening, only a portion of the infarct tends to be hemorrhagic and the extent to which it is affected and the severity vary. The hemorrhagic zones sometimes affect the periphery of the infarct and are usually found in the sides or the depths of a sulcus rather than on the summit of the gyri. Hemorrhagic softening never approaches in severity the necrosis and degenerative changes typical of non-hemorrhagic softening,[112] but when it is extensive, the volume of the infarcted area

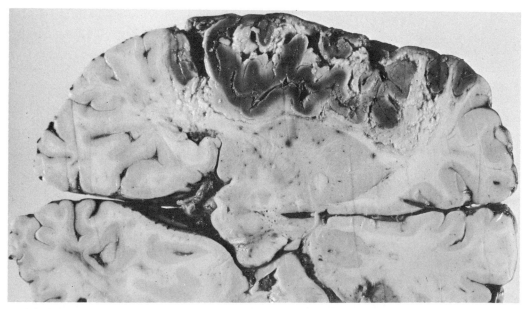

Fig. 4-10. Hemorrhagic softening in distribution of middle cerebral artery above. Cortex is dark and hemorrhagic, underlying white matter is anemic, and a few small hemorrhages are seen in the lenticular nucleus. Slight shift of midline and asymmetrical section through the brain are caused by swelling of the recent infarct.

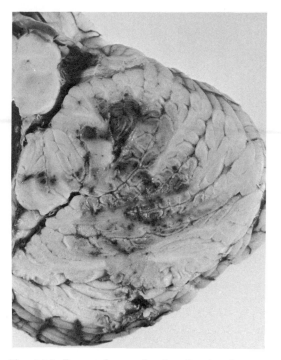

Fig. 4-11. Recent hemorrhagic softening in cerebellum. Molecular layer is predominantly pale. Hemorrhages are most prominent between the molecular and the granular layers, and in the latter, some are in the white matter. Compare with Fig. 4-12.

is much enlarged. In massive infarcts of the middle cerebral artery, there is hemorrhagic infarction in the basal ganglia, particularly the putamen. It is less likely and less severe in the caudate nucleus.[112] Fazio[112] found that in thick benzidine-stained sections, zones of stasis with ecchymoses alternate irregularly with ischemic areas or zones of normal vascularity with hemorrhage preceding necrosis of the parenchyma and vessels.

Softenings in the brain stem are pale, though a few small hemorrhages unpredictable in size and shape may arise. Sometimes they are quite massive (Fig. 4-4). Alternatively, only multiple small infarcts may result. Because of the good collateral circlation via the cerebellar arterial anastomoses,[147] cerebellar infarcts do not tend to be grossly destructive and cystic lesions are not so common as in the cerebrum. Most infarcts involve the white and gray matter of the folia and rarely involve the deep white matter. Generally they are pale, but some exhibit hemorrhagic mottling (Figs. 4-11 and 4-12). In chronic cerebellar infarcts, the architecture of the folia usu-

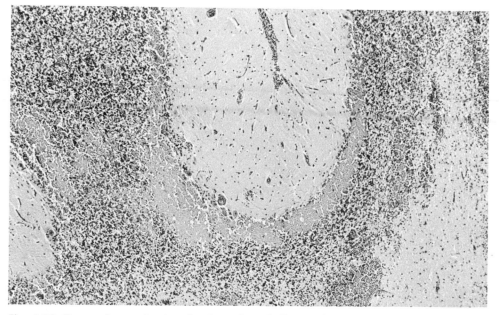

Fig. 4-12. Recent hemorrhagic softening of cerebellum. There is blood in subarachnoid space and hemorrhages in granular layer and to a lesser extent in molecular layer and white matter. It is most severe along the Purkinje zone. Few Purkinje cells are seen. (Hematoxylin and eosin, ×45.)

ally persists even if in a grossly shrunken and withered form.

Infarcts of the brain in the border zones between territories of supply of the major cerebral arteries are believed to occur in cerebral arterial insufficiency. They can be precipitated by hemodynamic crises such as hypotension or a fall in cardiac output The distribution of such infarcts is said to be related to the anatomy of the arterial supply and atherosclerosis.[294] Severe atherosclerosis with multiple stenoses or occlusion in cervical arteries is often present. Romanul and Abramowicz,[294] describing platelet thrombi and recanalization in small vessels related to border zone infarcts, postulated that stasis in these vessels would result in endothelial anoxia and damage, which in turn would induce mural platelet deposition. If flow returns, the platelet deposition ceases and organization results; if the flow remains sluggish, complete occlusion followed by organization and then recanalization is a possibility. Thus, they concluded that the infarcts and vascular

changes are the result of periodic acute circulatory insufficiency in the border zones. It is unlikely, however, that endothelium is as susceptible to anoxia as these authors affirm. More plausible is that microemboli from ulcerated atherosclerotic plaques are less likely to be flushed through such areas of stagnation than through other areas; hence they remain and become organized.

Microscopic. It may be that no pathological change is demonstrable histologically in a cerebral infarct if death swiftly follows the onset of the ischemia. The earliest demonstrable change in the cortex of an anemic infarct is said to be brick-red cytoplasm and slight shrinkage of the nerve cells.[62] Within 6 to 8 hours, polymorphonuclear cells are prominent in the cortical blood vessels, some are in the process of emigration; others may be free in the perivascular space or nearby parenchyma. There is an occasional perivascular ecchymosis. By the end of the first 24 hours, the cortex exhibits evidence of edema, neurones may appear to be undergoing karyo-

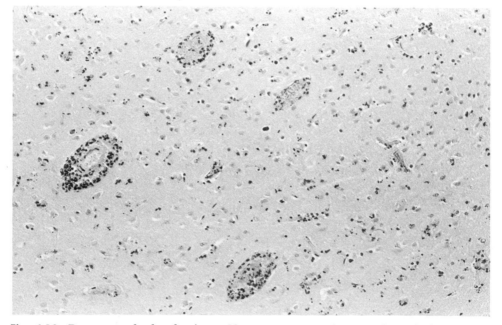

Fig. 4-13. Recent cerebral softeninng. Neurones are mostly necrotic and their nuclei pale or unstained. Polymorphs about vessels are mostly necrotic. Some have infiltrated the tissue. (Hematoxylin and eosin, ×110.)

lysis, polymorphonuclear cells are more prominent (Fig. 4-13), and the sections, due to softening and loss of cohesion of the tissue, exhibit splitting and fragmentation. Otherwise, the appearance is of coagulation necrosis. Leukocytic infiltration increases to a maximum at 2 or 3 days, many leukocytes are necrotic, and the numbers diminish thereafter. Few polymorphs are present after a week.

Several transformed microglia, each with a small dark-staining, round or oval nucleus and dark eosinophilic homogeneous cytoplasm (Fig. 4-14), make their appearance at about 24 hours.[68] They increase in number and become phagocytic, their cytoplasm then being pale pink and foamy (Fig. 4-15), and the nucleus slightly more vesicular. They lie interspersed in the necrotic debris; they are prevalent at the end of 3 days; and they constitute the predominant reactive cell at 7 days, at which stage they vary in size due to the diverse amounts of foamy cytoplasm (Fig. 4-16) and occasionally have two or even three nuclei.

Their numbers increase progressively, replacing the necrotic tissue so that the necrotic zone eventually contains a few vessels, some glial or collagen fibers, and a population of lipophages (gitter cells, foam cells, or compound granular corpuscles). They infiltrate the surrounding brain tissue as well, often aggregating about blood vessels filling the perivascular space, perhaps accompanied by a variable number of lymphocytes (Fig. 4-17). With cell debris completely removed, they diminish in numbers and eventually disappear. In sizable infarcts, they remain for at least 3 months and perhaps in minimal degree for a few years in the case of large infarcts.

The neurones are particularly susceptible. They develop a distinctly smudgy appearance and lose their staining characteristics, while the nucleus undergoes karyolysis (Fig. 4-13). The axones swell concomitantly with degeneration of the myelin sheaths after 24 hours.

In the infarcted cortex, the blood vessels may be necrotic but do not contain much

Text continued on p. 150.

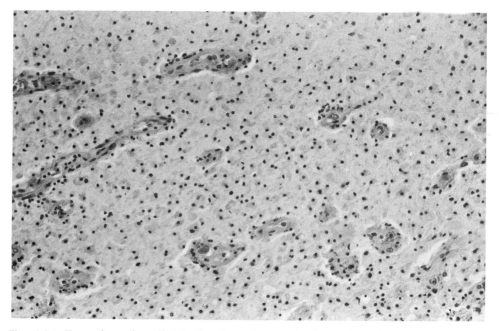

Fig. 4-14. Extensive microglial infiltration of necrotic tissue. Cytoplasm of microglia is not foamy. Note thickening of vessel walls. (Hematoxylin and eosin, ×110.)

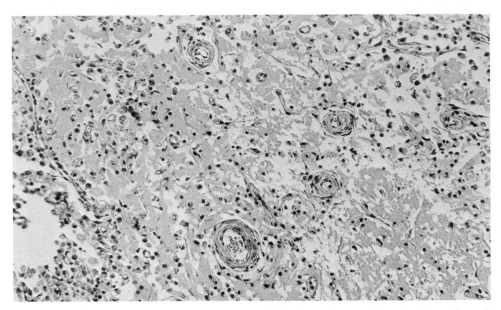

Fig. 4-15. Cerebral softening with extensive infiltration of necrotic parenchyma by microglial cells, which are actively phagocytic and have a foamy cytoplasm. There has been vascular proliferation and the small arteries are concentrically thickened. (Hematoxylin and eosin, ×110.)

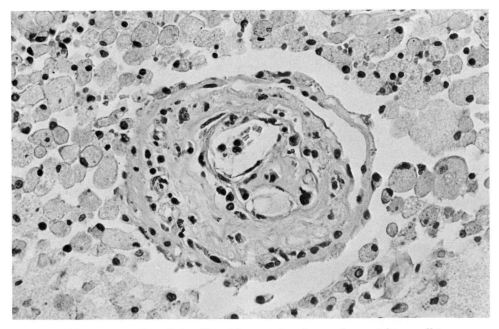

Fig. 4-16. Numerous microglial cells with vacuolated cytoplasm (gitter cells) or compound granular corpuscles. The unusual vessel has a very collagenous wall and may have undergone recanalization or proliferative changes reminiscent of those sometimes seen in cerebral tumors. (Hematoxylin and eosin, ×275.)

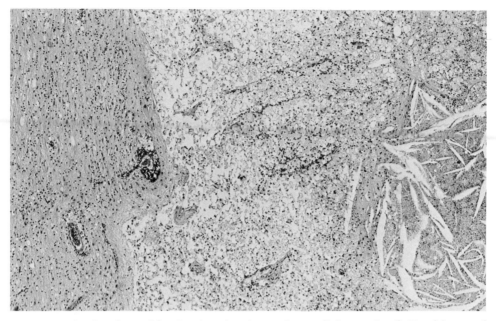

Fig. 4-17. Margin of an old softening showing a dense glial capsule (*left*) with round cells and lipophages about the vessels, then a central zone of microglial activity in which there are some vessels, round cells, and many lipophages, sometimes packed tightly like xanthoma cells, and then an unorganized necrotic area (*right*) in which there are numerous cholesterol clefts but no calcification. (Hematoxylin and eosin, ×45.)

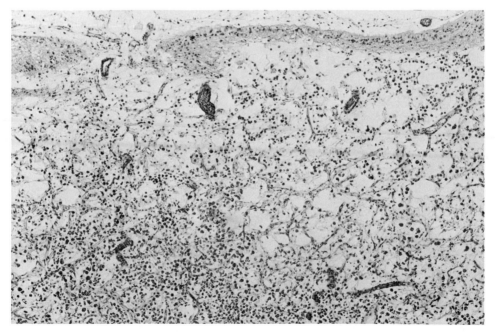

Fig. 4-18. Stage of resolution of infarcted cerebral cortex with interrupted thin superficial lamina of gliosed cortex above. There are numerous blood vessels in the infarcted zone, but lipophages are not numerous. A stage of devascularization will lead to a diminution in the degree of vascularity. Compare with Fig. 4-19. (Hematoxylin and eosin, ×45.)

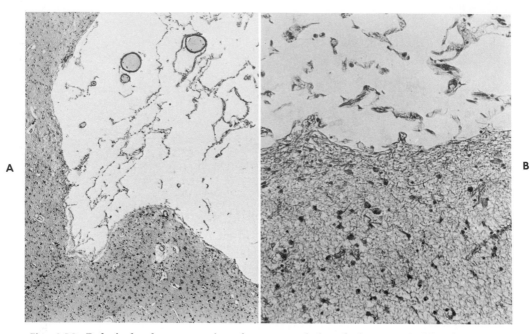

Fig. 4-19. Relatively abrupt margins of two encephalomalacic cysts. **A,** Margin appears to have a membrane. **B,** Marginal fibers are more dense than in the surrounding gliosed brain. A variable number of small glial fibers and at times collagenous trabeculae traverse the cavity, together with a few thin-walled vessels. Compare vascularity with that of Fig. 4-18. (Hematoxylin and eosin; **A,** ×45; **B,** ×110.)

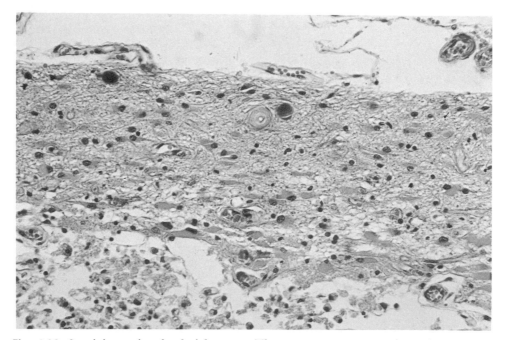

Fig. 4-20. Surviving strip of subpial cortex. There are numerous gemistocytic astrocytes in the cortex bordering the softening, two dark corpora amylacea, and an arteriolosclerotic subpial arteriole. (Hematoxylin and eosin, ×175.)

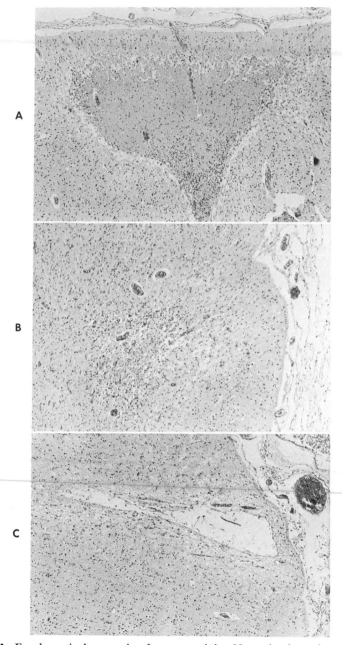

Fig. 4-21. A, Focal cortical necrosis of recent origin. Necrotic tissue in center is undergoing coagulation necrosis. Periphery is edematous and softening has commenced. **B,** Small cortical infarct associated with vascular proliferation and shrinkage with indentation of pial surface. Multiple foci of this nature contribute to cortical granularity. **C,** Resolution of small focus of cortical softening with resultant microcavity. (Hematoxylin and eosin, ×45.)

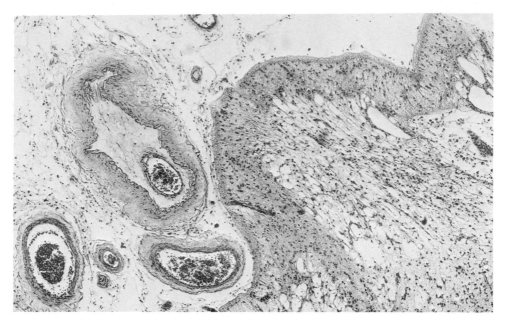

Fig. 4-22. Old cortical softening of insufficient severity to cause complete destruction. Surviving gliosed strip of cortex overlies honeycombed tissue containing vessels, spaces of irregular size and shape, and astrocytes. The lumen of a pial artery is considerably narrowed by acellular collagen, the result of recanalization of a thrombus. (Hematoxylin and eosin, ×45.)

blood. At the periphery, the capillary walls become thickened and more cellular (Fig. 4-14). Ultrastructural studies could identify the cell type responsible, and it is unlikely that the alteration is one of endothelial hyperplasia as has been suggested. The vessels proliferate, and new vessels recognizable by the second week are at times extremely numerous. As resolution proceeds, lipophages become less numerous (Fig. 4-18) and devascularization is the outcome (Fig. 4-19). In healed or resolved infarcts, a few vessels traverse cystic cavities (Fig. 4-19) and arterioles neighboring large infarcts occasionally exhibit pronounced arteriosclerosis, which is possibly coincidental with or caused by the hemodynamic overload during healing (Fig. 4-15). It is less likely to be caused by endarteritis obliterans. Other pial vessels may exhibit degenerative changes, intraluminal thrombi or emboli, or varying stages of organization and recanalization.

A few swollen or gemistocytic astrocytes

may appear in the surrounding brain tissue as early as the fourth day.[62] They are swollen with abundant eosinophilic cytoplasm and have an eccentrically placed nucleus (Fig. 4-20). Occasionally, binucleate forms occur. At the periphery of the ischemic area, gliosis develops and a dense glial scar surrounds the cystic cavity. In the surviving cortex (laminae 1 and possibly 2), gemistocytic astrocytes are often particularly large and numerous. Gliosis is much less prominent about infarcts in the infant than in the adult.

A strip of cortex (most often laminae 3 and 4) may be infarcted over shorter or longer lengths (Fig. 4-21). Ischemia, sufficient to cause partial necrosis, or multiple small cysts, may be the end result of a more severe laminar cortical necrosis imparting a honeycomb appearance (Fig. 4-22), and such being the case, the neighboring parenchyma is often severely gliotic.

The white matter undergoes coagulation necrosis and early demyelination is detect-

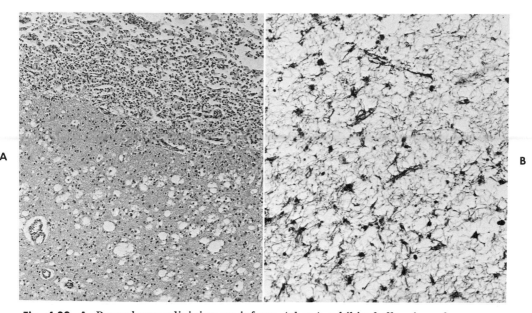

Fig. 4-23. A, Parenchyma adjoining an infarct (*above*) exhibits ballooning of some myelin sheaths (*below*), and, **B,** loose spongy glial network is the end result of severe ischemia of white matter neighboring an infarct. (**A,** Hematoxylin and eosin; **B,** phosphotungstic acid–hematoxylin, ×110.)

able at 24 hours. Vessels contain little blood and the nuclei of the astrocytes and oligodendroglia undergo karyolysis. At the periphery, there is ballooning of the myelin sheaths with some axonal swelling. The infarct becomes clearly demarcated, as it is pale compared to the deeper eosinophilia of the neighboring parenchyma. Organization progresses in much the same manner as in the cortex. In some areas bordering the infarct, there may not be complete, rapid necrosis, and the tissue is replaced by a loose, spongy glial network harboring a few vessels (Fig. 4-23), numerous astrocytes, and at times some residual lipophages. Mostly, however, gliosis is denser and surrounds a cystic cavity, the end result of colliquative resorption. Brain stem infarcts are of this general pattern.

The subarachnoid space itself often reflects the cellular response of the underlying cortex, with polymorphs and perhaps red cells initially and later macrophages and fibroblasts. Occasionally, in very large destructive lesions, this mild meningeal fibrosis may be continuous with similar

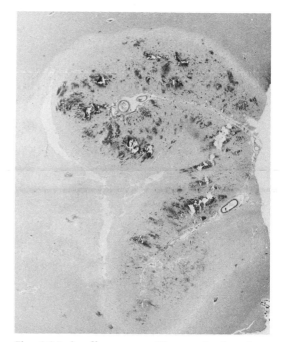

Fig. 4-24. Small segment of hemorrhagic softening. Hemorrhages are confined to the cortex and there is a subcortical zone of demarcation exhibiting pale staining and splitting of the tissue as if it were a plane of cleavage. (Hematoxylin and eosin.)

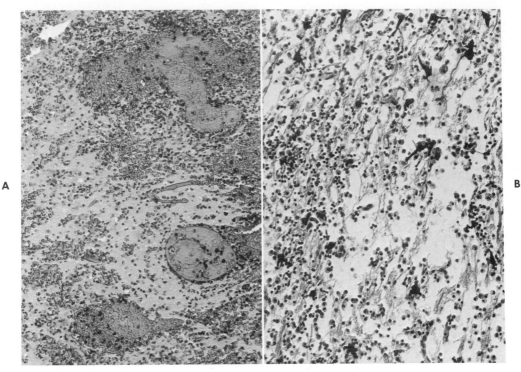

Fig. 4-25. A, Extensive hemorrhage in cortex from a red softening. Note that vessels contain closely packed red cell masses. **B,** Resolution of a hemorrhagic softening. Ferruginated nerve cells. (Hematoxylin and eosin, ×110.)

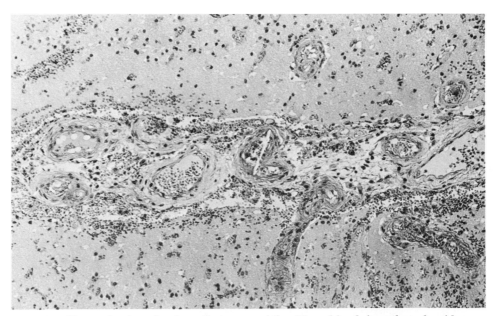

Fig. 4-26. Hemorrhagic softening of recent origin. Note blood in subarachnoid space of sulcus and acicular cholesterol cleft in lumen of small pial artery indicating atheromatous embolism. (Hematoxylin and eosin, ×110.)

fibrosis and gliosis bordering the infarct. Such fibrous tissue reaction is especially likely about areas in which the necrotic brain has not undergone complete colliquative necrosis and resorption, but has persisted partially encapsulated by fibrous tissue. Calcium deposition occurs in the necrotic debris, which contains much lipid and many cholesterol clefts (Fig. 4-9).

In hemorrhagic infarcts (Fig. 4-24), the cortical vessels are usually prominent and contain blood. In some instances, the red cells in the lumen are very closely packed, forming red hyaline masses presumably of agglutinated red cells (Fig. 4-25). Extravasated blood is found in the perivascular spaces and surrounding softened brain (Fig. 4-26). The ecchymoses may coalesce and usually red cells appear in the overlying subarachnoid space. In the tissue reaction, hematoidin and hemosiderin can be found, mostly within macrophages, with much discrepancy surrounding the time these pigments are alleged to appear. Hemosiderin first appears in 2 to 10 days,[12,62,159,352] and hematoidin by the end of the second[352] or third week.[62] Gemistocytic astrocytes in the surviving superficial rim of cortex occasionally contain hemosiderin granules in the periphery of their cytoplasm and a few iron-stained (ferruginated) shrunken nerve cells may be found in the neighborhood (Fig. 4-25). Otherwise, the process of organization and resorption corresponds to that of a pale infarct.

In cerebellar infarction, the degree of damage is usually less. The Purkinje cells, being very susceptible, die early. Their nuclei undergo karyolysis, but an occasional calcified cell body remains. Necrosis of the granular layer occurs and few cells remain. The molecular layer suffers coagulation necrosis (Fig. 4-27) and may exhibit increased eosinophilia. It becomes friable and fragments readily. Macrophages are initially most prevalent in the white matter of the folia, but there is progressive resorption. Arborescent foliation is mostly retained, though a few folia may be completely de-

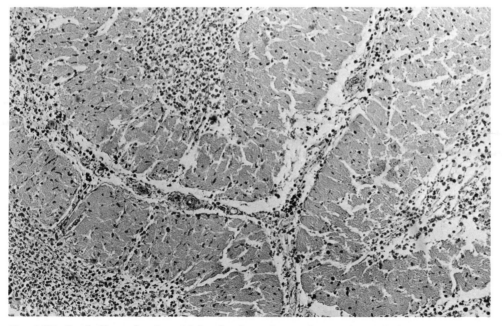

Fig. 4-27. Cerebellar softening. Molecular layer has undergone coagulation necrosis and is fragmented and infiltrated with a few siderophages. Purkinje cells are absent. The granular layer is replaced by macrophages containing lipid and hemosiderin. The sulci also contain siderophages. (Hematoxylin and eosin, ×45.)

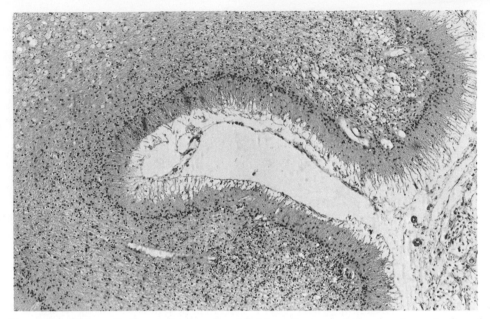

Fig. 4-28. Old cerebellar softening. Superficial surface of molecular layer is frayed. Purkinje cells are absent and the granular layer has mostly disappeared. The white matter contains scattered lipophages and ballooned myelin sheaths, producing a spongy appearance. (Hematoxylin and eosin, ×45.)

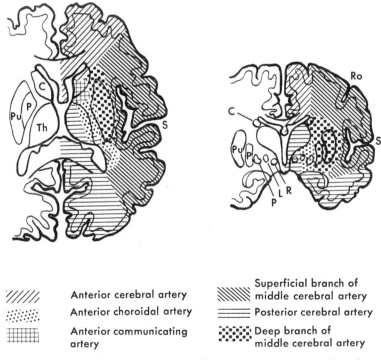

///// Anterior cerebral artery	\\\\\ Superficial branch of middle cerebral artery
:::::: Anterior choroidal artery	≡≡≡ Posterior cerebral artery
▦ Anterior communicating artery	▨ Deep branch of middle cerebral artery

Fig. 4-29. Arterial territories of supply are illustrated on horizontal and coronal section. **C,** Caudate nucleus. **L,** Luys' body or subthalamic nucleus. **P,** Globus pallidus. **Pu,** Putamen. **R,** Red nucleus. **Ro,** Rolandic or central sulcus. **S,** Lateral fissure of Sylvius. **Th,** Thalamus. (Redrawn and modified from Foix, C., and Schiff-Wertheimer (Mme.): Sémiologie des hémianopsies au cours du ramollissement cérébral, Rev. d'oto-neuro-ocul. 4:561, 1926, and Weil, A: Textbook of Neuropathology, New York, 1945, Grune & Stratton, Inc.)

stroyed and the others are reduced in size. The molecular layer is narrower than normal and the superficial half is cystic (Fig. 4-28). After the disappearance of the Purkinje layer and most of the cells of the granular layer, the gray matter is very thin. The white matter may be converted into a loose spongy or multicystic structure with a variable amount of gliosis. Lipophages may be scattered throughout for some time, but they eventually disappear.

In hemorrhagic infarction of the cerebellum, small hemorrhages occur in the molecular and granular layers and a few extravasations appear in the white matter of the folia and subarachnoid space, but blood often tends to form a blood lake in a plane of cleavage between the Purkinje and granular layers. Resorption follows the general pattern already described.

The histochemistry of acute infarction has been reviewed mostly in respect to the neuronal changes.[2,96]

Distribution of infarcts. Cerebral infarcts at autopsy are common[18] and often multiple with three or more separate areas of infarction in a brain. The territory of the middle cerebral artery is that most frequently infarcted and the size of the infarct varies considerably on an individual basis even for the same artery. The distribution of softenings at autopsy is given in Table 4-3 and the territories of supply on the cut surface are depicted in Fig. 4-29.

Infarction caused by occlusion of the internal carotid artery always involves some part of the territory of the middle cerebral artery, but is restricted to that territory in only 36%. In the remaining cases, infarction involves the region of the anterior cerebral also and sometimes the anterior choroidal artery.[58] On occasions, the territory of the posterior cerebral artery is affected, and thus virtually the entire hemisphere is infarcted.

The middle cerebral artery in man is very susceptible to occlusion, and infarcts there account for more than 50% of all the cerebral infarcts. Emboli in the internal carotid artery may extend peripherally and involve the stem of the middle cerebral artery. The major bifurcation or trifurcation of this artery is a common site of embolic impaction. Thrombosis in situ generally involves the main trunk, but occlusion of the peripheral branches is also frequent.[221] With occlusion of the middle cerebral artery, the areas most likely to be damaged are the central and precentral regions, the white matter underlying the affected cortex, the putamen, the outer portion of the globus pallidus, the anterior limb of the internal capsule, the head of the caudate nucleus, claustrum, external capsule, the insula, and part of the frontal lobe. During the stage of swelling, the hemispherical displacement varies from 3 to 14 mm. Of a series of 59 cases, 16 patients died, 15 made a complete recovery, 16 improved slightly, and 12 displayed no improvement during a follow-up period varying from 3 months to 15 years.[221]

Complete occlusion of the anterior cerebral artery is rare; most often the territory of one or several of its branches is affected.

The vertebral artery is usually occluded between the arch of the atlas and the union of the two vertebrals. Occlusions in the intracranial segment may be symptomless. Of 150 cases subjected to vertebral angiography, 37 (24%) had an occlusion of one vertebral artery at the level of the foramen magnum.[348] The occlusion was symptom-

Table 4-3. Distribution of cerebral infarcts at autopsy*

Site	Number
Supratentorial	
Frontal lobe	507
Temporal lobe	320
Parietal lobe	364
Occipital lobe	236
Basal ganglia	611
Subtentorial	
Midbrain	45
Pons	244
Medulla	16
Cerebellum	275

*After Aronson, S. M., and Aronson, B. E.: Ischemic cerebral vascular disease, N. Y. State Med. J. **66**:954, 1966.

less in 29 patients (19%), and associated with brain stem syndromes in 5 (3%). Three patients (2%) had bilateral vertebral or basilar artery occlusions associated with progressive bulbar palsies.

Occlusion of the posterior inferior cerebellar artery, known as Wallenberg's syndrome,[369] or preferably as the lateral medullary syndrome, is occasionally caused by an obstruction of this artery, but more commonly it is the result of vertebral artery occlusion.[87,127]

Thrombosis of the basilar artery has been found once in 300 to 450 autopsies.[217,312] It has also been estimated that it occurs in males more often than females (ratio 2:1) aged from 46 to 84 years (average 63 years).[312] Approximately, two-thirds of the cases are hypertensive.[312] Atherosclerosis of the vertebrobasilar system is usually very advanced, and it is not unexpected that these patients often have been found to have transitory neurological symptoms for months or years before the onset of the final illness.[312] The occlusion may occur at any level in the artery and extend into the posterior cerebral or vertebral arteries.[37,217] The infarcted area of the pons may be large (Fig. 4-4), but since much depends on the size and location of the thrombus, it is remarkably small on occasions. One area of the infarct may be older than another because of propagation of the thrombus and the symptomatology varies accordingly. At times, the softening may be entirely unilateral, possibly because the thrombus commences on one side of the basilar artery and occludes the corresponding branches before the occlusion is complete. Occlusion of the bifurcation alone and the divisional branches of the basilar may cause midbrain infarction. Concomitant involvement of the occipital lobes depends on the origin of the posterior cerebral arteries (carotid or basilar), the adequacy of the collateral circulation (leptomeningeal and posterior communicating arteries), and whether the thrombus extends beyond the divisional branch of the basilar artery. Involvement of the cerebel-

lum, when it occurs, is usually minimal because of the presence of adequate collaterals. The patients not infrequently live for 1 to 2 weeks although on clinical grounds a much more prolonged period of survival is possible.[217,348] The basilar artery can be occluded by incarceration in a skull fracture[313] or even a tumor embolus.[217]

Occlusion of the posterior cerebral arteries occurs in an estimated 10% to 15% of all cases of cerebral infarction.[263] Transtentorial herniation accompanied by compression of the posterior cerebral artery against the tentorium as a rule causes hemorrhagic infarction.

Clinical texts have dealt with syndromes resulting from the occlusion of the encephalic arteries and their branches.[56,123,233,263] Watershed infarcts are situated at the border zones of the major cerebral arteries. They are usually patchy and are distributed along a narrow strip extending almost from the frontal pole to the occipital pole, lateral to the superomedial margin of the cerebral hemisphere.

The infarcts associated with cerebral aneurysms have been dealt with in Chapter 9.

Infarcts associated with venous occlusion tend to correspond to the drainage area of the occluded vein, although venous anastomoses are such that a venous thrombosis may be silent clinically. If, however, the thrombosis has caused infarction, swollen firm veins or distended sinuses are apparent. The infarct is hemorrhagic, but the underlying white matter is more inclined to exhibit petechial or larger hemorrhages, and the subarachnoid hemorrhage is more extensive than the red infarcts of arterial embolism. In extensive thrombosis of the superior longitudinal sinus and tributaries, cerebral swelling, edema, and congestion may raise the intracranial pressure to fatal limits prior to the induction of hemorrhages.[39]

Associated findings

CEREBRAL SWELLING. Like acute infarcts in the viscera, cerebral softenings (both gray and white matter) also swell because of edema and the imbibition of fluid. Consequently, signs of raised intracranial pressure are common during the first week after the ictus. Infarcts in the territory of the middle cerebral artery increase in volume within the first day, and the swelling, as determined by the shift of the midline, reaches a maximum between the second and the sixth days, regressing to normal by the end of the second week.[308] The swelling may shift the pineal gland and compress and deflect the lateral and third ventricles much as any space-occupying lesion. Tentorial herniation can cause secondary pontine hemorrhage, which can be fatal as in 6 of 21 cases (28.6%) studied by Berry and Alpers.[34] In a series of 45 autopsied subjects with supratentorial cerebral infarction and swelling, 78% died within 7 days of the acute infarction. Death was attributed to the effects of brain swelling with transtentorial herniation,[266] and secondary hemorrhage in the brain stem was found in 60%. Compression of the brain stem has also been observed in a number of instances of cerebellar infarction.[226] Compression and distortion of the aqueduct may result in acute obstructive hydrocephalus necessitating ventricular drainage.[384] Ischemic changes can occur in the brain stem although hemorrhage is more likely because of the rapidity of the onset of the swelling.

SECONDARY DEGENERATIONS. In large infarcts involving the motor cortex or its fibers, secondary degeneration of corticospinal fibers will occur with a consequent reduction in size (with asymmetry) of the cerebral peduncle, pons, and corticospinal tracts.

CARDIOVASCULAR DISEASE. The coexistence of severe atherosclerosis not only of the cerebral arteries but also extracranially is very likely in nonembolic infarction. Cardiac disease is fairly frequent and left ventricular hypertrophy or coronary artery disease may well be manifested in the heart.

Electrocardiographic changes simulating myocardial infarction, ischemia, and gross changes in the heart occur in association with subarachnoid hemorrhage (Chapter 7). Similar electrocardiographic findings in patients without significant coronary or cardiac disease[163,223] have been reported in 15% of patients with transient ischemic attacks and 30% of those with major cerebral infarction.[1] The cardiac changes may be coincidental or possibly they are the result of the cerebrovascular disease or vice versa. In any case, the cerebral symptoms and signs can mask those of the heart.

NEUROGENIC ULCERATION. Neurogenic ulceration in cerebrovascular disease is a little recognized entity, but both acute and chronic gastric ulceration can complicate cerebral infarction (Table 2-2).

HYALINE GLOBULES OF THE ADRENAL MEDULLA. Round eosinophilic hyaline globules (3 to 30 μ in diameter), which are usually extracellular and less often in the cytoplasm of both polygonal and chromaffin cells of the adrenal medulla, have been observed in a variety of diseases, particularly bacterial infections.[164] However, their prevalence in chronic neurological disorders is disproportionately high, approximating 15% of cerebral infarcts.

Laboratory studies. The cerebrospinal fluid is generally clear macroscopically, although slight blood staining or xanthochromia may be observed in hemorrhagic infarcts. Pressure is usually below 200 mm. of water, although in an occasional specimen it will reach 400 mm.[253] In 90% of samples, the leukocyte count is normal; in the minority there are counts of up to 200 cells per cu. mm. Polymorphonuclear leukocytes tend to be at their peak at 3 days, but a few macrophages may be present. The protein is either normal (50% of cases) or elevated, but does not exceed 100 mg. per 100 ml. (45%) except in an isolated case.

In experimental cerebral infarction in dogs, the glutamic oxaloacetic transaminase activity in the softened tissue decreases simultaneously with increased activity in the cerebrospinal fluid. This reaches a peak within 4 to 5 days and thereafter decreases roughly in proportion to the extent and severity of the infarct. Serum glutamic oxaloacetic transaminase activity is also increased, though not in proportion to the severity and extent of the infarct.[368] The possibility of using the transaminase level in the cerebrospinal fluid in differentiating cerebral infarction from other diseases of the brain has been disappointing because of the nonspecificity of the test, for increased values occur with cerebral hemorrhage and tumor. The test has been used prognostically as the transaminase level is directly proportional to the size of the infarct.[56] A similar increase in serum creatine phosphokinase follows cerebral infarction, but its specificity in all likelihood resembles that of transaminase.

The blood leukocyte count in cerebral infarction may be at a high normal level or slightly elevated reaching as high as 20,000 per cu. mm. with a massive infarction.[263]

Meyer[254] reported a surprisingly high frequency of hypothyroidism (38%), diabetes mellitus (31%), hypercholesterolemia (44.7%), and gout or hyperuricemia (33%) in subjects with cerebral infarction. Specific figures and normal laboratory values were not provided.

Prognosis. In an analysis of patients with cerebral thrombosis, Robinson and associates[292] determined that 21% died during the initial attack, and of the survivors, 50% died within 4.1 years. The 5-year mortality of 59% was in contrast to an expected mortality of 23%. The mortality in those under 50 years of age tends to be less.[378]

In a study of 100 consecutive patients with cerebral thrombosis, 10 patients died in the acute stages, 15% died within 1 year, 8% in the second year, and thus 33% were dead within 2 years. Of the survivors, only 10% were able to resume their former occupation, 35% managed part-time work only, 28% self-care only, and 17% were bedridden.[81,334]

Pincock[275] noted that 10% of 117 patients with acute cerebral thrombosis died from the initial ictus, and of the survivors, more than 50% were dead within 5 years.

Only 24 (20.5%) were functioning adequately after 8 years. There are recurrences in more than 10% of the survivors for whom the prognosis correspondingly worsens.[81,275]

The prognosis varies with the size of the infarct and the mortality tends to be higher in basilar thrombosis (60%) than in carotid thrombosis.[257] Higher mortality occurs in hypertensives and in those with evidence of cardiac disease.[81] The causes of death include further fatal cerebrovascular accidents, respiratory disease (mostly bronchopneumonia), and quite often coronary thrombosis or congestive cardiac failure.

Angiographic evidence indicates that occlusive vascular disease is unduly prevalent in patients with "chronic brain syndrome,"[207] for serious mental deterioration and dementia are often precipitated by cerebral infarction.[131] In the very young, infarction of the brain during the fetal or neonatal period has also been linked with severe mental retardation.[359]

Pathogenesis of infarction. Experimentally, occlusion of the internal carotid artery or middle cerebral artery causes no stasis, though some vasomotor changes occur in small arterioles on vital microscopy of the cortex.[92] Within 30 seconds of experimental occlusion of the middle cerebral artery, there is dilatation of the collateral vessels of all sizes from large arteries to small arterial anastomoses 50 to 250 μ in diameter. Meyer and Denny-Brown[255] considered that the reduction in pressure caused the dilatation. The oxygen tension falls temporarily but no symptoms develop. When the pressure fell below a critical level of 50 mm. Hg in the monkey, the collateral circulation was inadequate and infarction ensued. The initial dilatation of arterioles is followed by constriction and slow flow. At multiple sites the flow in venules slows, with segmentation and clumping of red cells, and stasis is widespread as the cortex becomes pale and swollen. In the monkey the critical period for the development of infarction was 2 to 5 minutes. Within 5 to 15 minutes venous stasis was reversible, and thereafter, it was persistent and infarction developed with multiple cortical ecchymoses.

The size of the infarct is increased by hypotension.[285] Denny-Brown and Meyer[255] concluded that the development of infarction resulted primarily from damage to the vascular endothelium with resulting edema, hemoconcentration, erythrocytic aggregation (sludging), and stasis. A similar train of events occurred after anoxic anoxia and embolism. Sundt and associates[335] emphasize that the infarct results from a progressive failure of the collateral vessels, possibly because of a locally produced toxic factor, and that restoration of flow a few hours after ligation still reduced the size of the infarct.

A recent, significant observation is that after brief periods of cerebral ischemia, some regions are not perfused after restoration of flow because of vascular obstruction. Ultrastructural studies have revealed that swelling of perivascular glial cells at times reduces small vessels to mere slits. Other vessels are obstructed by small cytoplasmic blebs either projecting from the endothelium locally or impacted because of embolism.[63] It was considered that such vascular changes constitute an early change that perhaps contributes to the irreversibility of the ischemia.

Ligation of the middle cerebral artery may be followed by reddening of the blood in some veins over the ischemic zone associated with either augmented or diminished blood flow.[370] This high oxygen saturation is attributed, not to arteriovenous shunting, but to focal reactive hyperemia with reduced oxygen uptake by the tissue ("luxury perfusion") or partial blockage of vessels by sludging.

During the development of the infarct, white cell sticking and erythrocytic aggregation have been observed, the aggregation of the cellular elements interfering with collateral flow.[93] Red cells escape by diapedesis from stagnant vessels, and these perivascular hemorrhages are augmented by a pressure elevation to normal levels or

above. Fibrinoid necrosis of vessels has been observed in experimental red infarction.[158]

In 373 brains with vascular occlusion (123 with embolism, 89 with thrombosis, and 161 of indeterminate cause), Fisher and Adams[133] found 66 hemorrhagic infarcts. Of the latter, all except three were attributed to embolism. They concluded that apart from venous thrombosis, most hemorrhagic infarcts were caused by arterial embolism. In anemic infarcts, the occlusion was usually proximal to the infarct, but when hemorrhagic, it was often distal to the apex of the anemic section of the infarct. It was considered that in embolism, the infarcted zone or part thereof became hemorrhagic when the embolus moved peripherally, allowing collaterals to expose the necrotic tissue and vessels to a vigorous blood flow. Fisher and Adams[133] asserted that arterial thrombosis had to be proximal to the circle of Willis to cause a red infarct. However, infarcts associated with a dissecting aneurysm of the aorta that occludes branches of the aortic arch may be red, pale, or mixed.[60] Embolic lesions may arise with associated hypotension leading to or contributing to anemic infarction of the brain.

Fazio[112] believed that pale softening is the result of complete blockage sufficiently prolonged to cause infarction that remains uniformly ischemic and in which the onset of necrosis progresses rapidly. Partial occlusion with defective return of the circulation and patchy functional circulatory disturbances in the area preceding the onset of necrosis of the parenchyma and vessels elicit red softening in the pathogenesis of which the collateral circulation is of paramount importance. Simple ligation of the middle cerebral artery distal to the origin of the perforating branches produces pale infarction because blood flow is allegedly inadequate, but with more proximal occlusion, the infarct is in part hemorrhagic.[158] An increase in blood pressure after ligation of the middle cerebral artery causes a hemorrhagic infarct[111] as does ligation in a hypertensive animal, but when the collaterals are occluded by ligation of the anterior and posterior cerebral arteries, the infarct is pale.[111] Low molecular weight dextran, which ordinarily reduces sludging (massive erythrocytic aggregation), protects against such hemorrhagic tendencies.[162]

Experimental cerebral embolism of moderately large emboli produces infarcts that tend to be hemorrhagic.[213] A small steel ball (0.8 mm. in diameter) introduced into the internal carotid artery of 11 dogs lodged in the anterior cerebral artery in three animals and in the middle cerebral in the other eight. However, no macroscopic lesion resulted in six animals. Two major infarcts and three minor infarcts were found in the remainder, cortical infarcts being red and subcortical infarcts pale or anemic.[273]

Thus, hemorrhagic infarcts seem to be dependent ultimately on a collateral flow, the blood pressure only augmenting flow through such vessels into the ischemic zone. The adequacy of the collateral flow is intermediate between that which is sufficient to prevent infarction and that which is insufficient to prevent complete anemic softenings. In transtentorial herniation with compression of the posterior cerebral artery, the red infarction may be attributed to intermittent obstruction whereas in embolism, as Fisher and Adams[133] suggest, collaterals become available as the result of progressive peripheral migration of the embolus. In the case of the steel balls,[273] movement was possibly effected by secondary vasodilatation. However, the embolus must be of sufficient size to obstruct major vessels, for embolic occlusion of minor vessels results in pale infarction.[341] Anticoagulants, of course, may produce hemorrhagic infarcts.

Experimentally, infarction associated with edema and swelling can be fatal[335] and is maximal about the third day.[166] Experimental anoxic-ischemic encephalopathy[228] in rats is associated with edema appearing after 4 hours and attaining a maximum at 19 to 25 hours.[322] The edema fluid is low in protein.

Contributory factors in cerebral infarction

INADEQUATE COLLATERAL CIRCULATION. Infarction will not follow upon arterial occlusion if the collateral circulation (discussed in Chapter 1) is adequate. The degree of arterial stenosis that elicits growth of the collateral circulation is not known. Yates and Hutchinson[387] emphasized that there are alternative arterial routes for all major areas of the brain, except the basal ganglia and the brain stem. The existence of intracerebral anastomoses has given rise to argument. They are small and their significance as collaterals is limited.

Fazio[113] discussing the hemodynamic aspects of infarction indicated that collateral flow is a variety of intracerebral steal and the resultant regional hypotension could contribute to the production of infarcts.

ATHEROSCLEROSIS. Atherosclerosis is the major cause of significant arterial occlusions affecting the cerebral circulation, and collateral vessels may well be severely affected similarly. However, its affect on the collateral circulation aside, atherosclerotic narrowing of more proximal trunks can prevent or limit compensatory augmentation of flow through collaterals.

BLOOD. Anemia may be sufficiently severe to induce parenchymal infarction. Patients with significant narrowing of the cervical arteries to the brain are particularly susceptible to the effects of carbon monoxide,[387] so that frank cerebral infarcts in these patients can be precipitated by relatively small doses of the gas. In patients with chronic lung disease (such as emphysema) or congestive cardiac failure, anoxemia can contribute to the development of cerebral ischemic lesions. So too perhaps with polycythemia in which blood flow may well be retarded.

HYPOTENSION. A fall of blood pressure below the individual's customary level in the presence of other impairments of the cerebral circulation may lead to immediate cerebral ischemia (particularly in the case of hypertensives).[387] Stokes-Adams attacks, surgical or pathological shock, or induced hypotension can induce cerebral ischemia.

Coronary occlusion is not uncommon in these patients, and although cerebral embolism may follow myocardial infarction, encephalomalacia may also be precipitated during the initial phase of shock. The latter is more likely to be pale in contrast to the hemorrhagic infarct associated with the former. Postoperative hemiplegia is not common, and little pathological material is available. It has usually been attributed to a period of hypotension with thrombosis or to vascular insufficiency in an already jeopardized cerebral circulation.

HYPERTENSION. Hypertension augments the severity of atherosclerosis and consequently is more frequent in patients with nonembolic infarction than in control subjects, the prevalence[25,30,281] varying from 47% to 75%. The association is said to be more frequent than hypertension in myocardial infarction[237] and the frequency in lacunar softening is at least 95%. Moreover, hypotensive therapy has reduced the frequency of cerebral infarction in hypertension.[281]

The blood pressure usually rises with the onset of a cerebrovascular accident such as an infarction, and gradually falls to normal values within the early weeks of convalescence. This is thought to be of neurogenic origin.

There is also the possibility, unproved as yet, that ischemia of vasomotor-inhibiting centers of the medulla results in hypertension of central origin.

CARDIAC DISEASE. Cerebral infarction as a complication of cardiac disease is a common autopsy finding in general hospitals where it is usually attributed to embolism complicating mural thrombosis in myocardial infarction, cardiac aneurysm, auricular fibrillation, and acute chronic valvular disease. Vost and associates[365] found that approximately 53.8% of 340 patients with heart disease had a cerebral infarct, yet only 24 arterial occlusions were found between the heart and the brain. The method of determining occlusion of the cervical vessels (by perfusion) was inadequate and would not have revealed severe stenoses. The prevalence of infarction was excep-

tionally high in bacterial endocarditis, but in other types of cardiac disease such as atrial fibrillation, mural thrombus on the left side of the heart, or congestive cardiac failure, the difference was negligible. The authors attributed most of the infarcts to embolism, though the site of obstruction was rarely found. Robinson and associates[292] found that the presence of congestive cardiac failure worsened the prognosis of patients with cerebral thrombosis. Embolism is a hazard of cardiac surgery also.

In 135 cases of congenital cyanotic heart disease, Berthrong and Sabiston[35] found recent or old infarcts in 25 patients (18.3%), a quite significant frequency in view of the age group. In five, thrombi were present in cortical veins or various sinuses. Congestive cardiac failure and embolism were other causative factors, but polycythemia was not implicated, though theoretically it could be expected to play a role.

Etiology of cerebral infarction. Vascular occlusion of a major artery of supply to the brain is often fallaciously regarded as synonymous with cerebral infarction. Whether vascular obstruction will result in a decrease in blood flow sufficient to cause parenchymal ischemia depends on the balance of the various effects of the site of the occlusion and rapidity of its onset, as well as the physiology, pathology, and anatomy of the collateral circulation, the oxygen-carrying capacity of the blood, and the status of the systemic circulation. These factors are sufficiently numerous, variable, and complex to make the clinical and pathological consequences of vascular obstruction so different in the individual response that the issue is difficult to predict.

Though Yates and Hutchinson[387] state that there is no single cause of cerebral infarction, occlusion of the blood supply because of thrombosis or embolism is most commonly the precipitating etiological factor.

The percentage frequency distribution[219] of types in the Cooperative Stroke Study in seven centers in the United States[123] revealed that 57.4% of the 380 patients studied were considered to have a thrombosis (completed or in evolution), 26% thrombosis or embolism, 7.4% embolism, and 8.4% transient ischemic attacks. The carotid arterial system was involved in 74.7%, the vertebrobasilar in 22.1%, and in 3.2%, the localization was uncertain. Kurtzke[219] reviewed other studies and whether based on autopsies, hospital patients, or population surveys, the prevalence of embolism was generally less than that of thrombosis. The ratio of embolism to thrombosis varied from 0.07 to 0.46, and to all ischemic cerebrovascular disease from 0.04 to 0.24.

THROMBOSIS AND STENOSIS. Arterial thrombosis is a frequent precipitating factor in cerebral infarction and is generally caused by the tearing or ulceration of an atheromatous plaque (Fig. 4-30). Careful examination of serial sections is needed for adequate interpretation of the relationship of the thrombus to the intima. Moreover, distinction between a thrombus and a postmortem clot is frequently difficult. Thrombi at autopsy tend to be dry and with a dull surface similar to the underlying intimal surface of the vessel wall, in contrast to the normal shiny surface of the endothelium. Thrombi are usually adherent to the vessel wall though only loosely if of recent formation. Unless severely atherosclerotic and therefore rigid and opaque, the vessels are distended rather than collapsed or retracted, the distended state and dark red-black color of the exposed cerebral vessel suggesting the antemortem nature of the coagulum. This is not the case with nonocclusive mural thrombi and infected thrombi, which tend to be softer, more friable, and even purulent. Macroscopically, most thrombi have a white head largely of platelets and a red tail mainly of rapidly coagulated blood. The plug in the vessel must be carefully examined for pale mottling or gray-white striae, which may be caused by either laminae of fibrin or to the platelet-rich lines of Zahn. Histologically, these are confirmatory evidence for the diagnosis of antemortem thrombus (Fig. 4-31) as are the signs of organization. Usually, but not in-

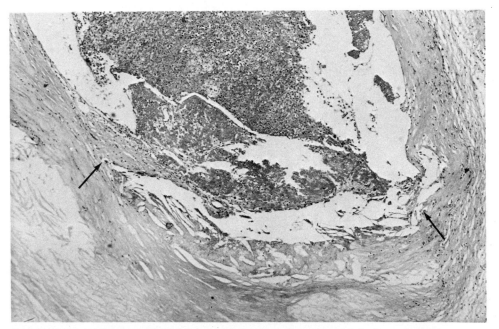

Fig. 4-30. Thrombosis initiated by a tear in the atheromatous intima of basilar artery. Margins of ulcer indicated by arrows. (Hematoxylin and eosin, ×45.)

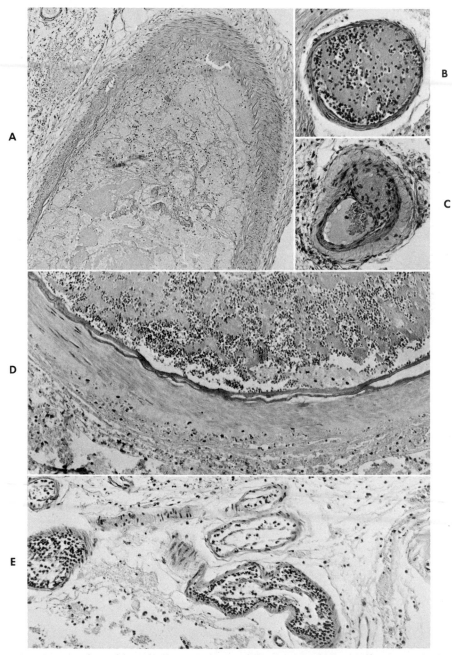

Fig. 4-31. Recent thrombi occluding, **A,** large pial artery and, **B,** small artery. **C,** Small platelet thrombus partially occluding a small artery is being endothelialized and incorporated into the wall. **D,** Large cortical artery is occluded by a recent thrombus and the media is mostly necrotic. **E,** Small vessels in a recent infarct contain many polymorphonuclear leukocytes beneath a raised endothelium, the subendothelial infiltration being attributed to temporary ischemia with subsequent restoration of flow through collaterals. (Hematoxylin and eosin; **A,** ×45; **B** to **E,** ×110.)

variably, a thrombus propagates to the next major branching, but factors covering the propagation have not been clarified. It is more frequent in the cerebral arterial tree than in the coronary arteries, the propagated thrombus being usually dark red. In suspected thrombi, macroscopic and microscopic examination at several different levels will disclose the nature of the plug.[380]

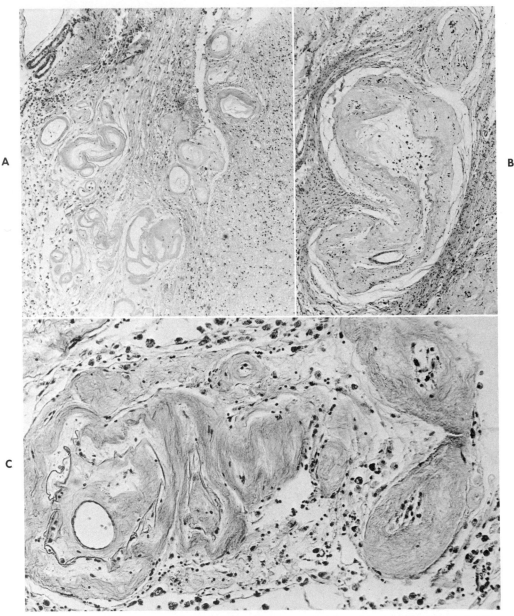

Fig. 4-32. A, Small vessels (resembling ghosts) at margin of an infarct have hyaline walls and lumens occluded by pale acellular material. **B** and **C,** Long-standing occluded vessels. Media is replaced by hyalinized connective tissue, and their lumens are occluded by pale or dense hyaline connective tissue containing an occasional sinusoid and a few siderophages. Such vessels often appear collapsed and their elastic laminae persist for many years. (Hematoxylin and eosin; **A** and **B,** ×45; **C,** ×110.)

Organization of the thrombus has few unusual features. The artery eventually is thin, contracted, and white perhaps with slight brownish coloring of the cut surface. The size of the new vessels in the recanalized thrombus varies as do their mural constituents, but generally they are small and often contracted, and the blood conveyed is probably insignificant in quantity. In the occluded vessels, the internal elastic lamina persists for years (Figs. 4-32 and 4-33), often despite the total absence of residual medial muscle. Small pial vessels not infrequently have the original lumen obliterated by extremely loose pale-staining connective tissue in which a few sinusoidal vessels and an occasional siderophage can be seen. Iron incrustation of the connective tissue in the lumen of recanalized arteries may occasionally be observed. In recanalized cervical segments of the in-

ternal carotid artery, a giant cell reaction to the persistent internal elastic lamina has been observed twice, but the significance is obscure, there being no other evidence of giant cell arteritis.

Narrowing of the arterial lumen is a characteristic feature of atherosclerosis occurring at sites severely affected by the atherosclerosis. The plaques may become ulcerated (Fig. 4-30), providing a source of emboli, but occlusive thrombosis may supervene. It has been estimated that when thrombosis complicates atherosclerosis of the internal carotid artery, it is associated with a preexistent stenosis that reduces the lumen by at least 50% and usually by more than 75%.[58]

Intramural hemorrhage into a plaque is said to play a role in cerebral infarction[259] and in transient ischemic episodes,[388] but this is the case only very sel-

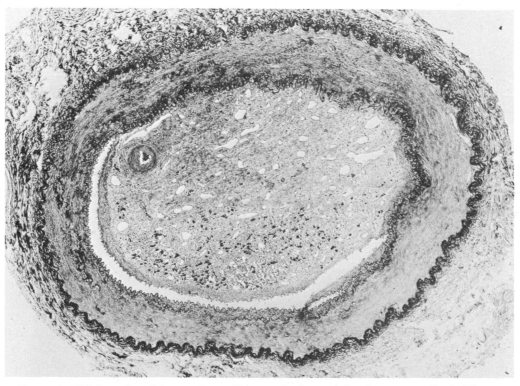

Fig. 4-33. Old thrombosed internal carotid artery in the neck has been recanalized. There are many siderophages in the tissue of organization but no evidence of atheroma. Cleft near internal elastic lamina is an artifact caused by tissue shrinkage. (Verhoeff's elastic stain.)

dom unless there is a considerable degree of dissection. Most instances of "hemorrhage" in an atheromatous plaque are not associated with encroachment on the lumen or constitute a feature of thrombosis on an ulcerated or torn intima as serial sections reveal.[71,325]

In the etiology of cerebral infarction, emphasis has been on local causes. Failure to find the site of the occlusion upon examination of the cerebral vessels led to assumptions that other causal factors including vasospasm and episodes of hypotension were implicated. Causes of cerebral infarction are numerous, but the common, moderate-to-massive cerebral infarct is now known to be often caused by occlusion of extracranial arteries. As long ago as 1855, Gull[155] recorded a cerebral softening in association with occlusion of the left common carotid and innominate arteries. Chiari,[64] in 400 consecutive autopsies, deduced that in six cases emboli from a nonocclusive thrombus on an atherosclerotic plaque in the cavernous segment of the internal carotid artery caused a stroke. Hunt[185] found carotid pulsations in the neck absent in four of 20 cases of hemiplegia and like Chiari emphasized that the entire carotid circulation and not merely the intracranial segment should be investigated. Moniz and associates[258] first demonstrated angiographically thrombotic occlusion of the cervical segment of the internal carotid artery. Hultquist[182] published a monograph on the subject, reporting thromboembolism of the carotid artery in approximately 3% of 1400 routine autopsies. He found ischemic lesions in the brain in only one-third of the cases in which the occlusion was below the origin of the ophthalmic artery. Fisher's subsequent investigations[130,132] stimulated interest in the role of occlusion of the cervical arteries in the causation of cerebral infarcts. He found that spontaneous occlusion of the cervical segment of the internal carotid artery (except when complicating hypotension) is likely to be followed by hemiplegia of severe degree, but frequently

with premonitory and transient symptoms such as paresthesias, paralysis, monocular blindness, aphasia, and headache. One patient had approximately 100 transient ischemic attacks prior to the occlusion of the internal carotid artery in its extracranial course. Atherosclerosis was the primary cause in most cases, although a few were embolic in origin. In 432 consecutive routine autopsies in which the brain was examined, Fisher found complete occlusion of one or both carotid arteries in 28 cases (6.5%). In another 13, the lumen was severely narrowed.[132] In all, there were 45 instances of complete occlusion of the cervical carotid denoting a significance comparable with cerebral hemorrhage and embolism. Not all cases were associated with symptoms, although hemiplegia was almost invariably present. In some cases, neurological symptoms occurred after shock or anoxia only. In six patients, the occlusion was bilateral. In several patients, there was dementia, but it could have been fortuitous.

Numerous pathological and angiographic studies of cervical arteries supplying the brain eventuated. Most estimations of the degree of arterial stenosis appear to be imprecise and subjective, as no indications have been given as to whether the reduction is in the cross-sectional area or in the diameter as shown by angiographic silhouettes, which are known to vary with the view of the angiogram. Estimates are further complicated by the frequent presence of arteriectasis, and in postmortem studies the need for fixation under pressure is obvious.

Of 80 autopsies in which the arteries in the neck were studied angiographically post mortem,[65] in 23 cases (29%) there were no filling defects or only borderline lesions, 31 cases (39%) had mild abnormalities (less than 50% reduction of the lumen), 17 cases (21%) exhibited filling defects in which the lumen was reduced by more than 50%, and the nine remaining cases (11%) had complete or virtually complete ("hairline" narrowing) obstruction of at least one artery. Severe obstruction was more in evidence in the carotid circulation than in the vertebral, and overall the incidence of occlusive or severely stenosing lesions was 11%. Clinical studies have confirmed the prevalence not only of moderate stenosis but also of complete occlusion of the large cervical arteries in aging patients, particularly in those with cerebrovascular disease.[156,246,381]

Of 93 patients autopsied (over 35 years of age), Schwartz and Mitchell[306] found that 90% of the males and 85% of the females had at least one stenosis in the main cervical arteries supplying the brain, with severe narrowing (that is, a reduction of more than 50% in diameter) in 43% of the men and in 35% of the women. In males over 35 years at autopsy one in four had severe stenosis of the carotid sinus. Severe stenosis of the subclavian, innominate and common carotid arteries is less common, but more frequent in males than females. Ulcerated atheromatous lesions in the major cervical arteries occurred in 14% of the 93 patients over 35 years and in five patients thrombi were found. It appeared that if a subject had one stenotic lesion, the presence of a second was likely.

Stenotic and even occlusive lesions are prevalent in these major cervical arteries, but the degree of stenosis is inexact and blood flow is likely to be significantly reduced only when the cross-sectional area is less than 2 sq. mm. Between 2 and 5 sq. mm. a reduction is probable but does not occur when the cross-sectional area is greater than 5 sq. mm.[46] This indicates that the reduction must be 80% to 90% and that the many lesser degrees of stenosis in the literature are insignificant. A pressure drop can eventuate beyond a stenosis, but flow remains the most important criterion for vascular insufficiency. Nevertheless, mild-to-moderate stenotic lesions exhibit progressive changes angiographically, and ulceration, initiating occlusive thrombosis, may occur at any time. Correlations between such stenotic and occlusive lesions with ischemic lesions in the brain have

been attempted, and it has been held that occlusive lesions in these cervical arteries account for between 25% to 42% of the cases of occlusive cerebrovascular disease.[89]

Of 416 brains in which at least one intracranial artery was narrowed to 50% or more of its diameter, Baker and associates found only 36% (149 cases) associated with cerebral infarction, and conversely a similar atherosclerotic narrowing of the relevant artery was found in 50% of 290 brains exhibiting infarcts.[24]

Castaigne and associates[58] studied occlusions of the internal carotid artery in 50 patients at autopsy. They were bilateral in six cases and unilateral in the remainder. Atherosclerosis was the cause of the thrombosis in 60.6% and embolism in 21.3%. Once the initial site of thrombosis in the atherosclerotic group had been determined, it was found that thrombosis had commenced in the sinus in 77.8%, the siphon in 22.2%, and in approximately one-third, the thrombus propagated beyond the bifurcation of the internal carotid. In most of the remainder, it propagated as far as the cavernous segment. Retrograde thrombus occurred in three of the six cases of thrombosis in the siphon but was absent in cases of embolic occlusion of the siphon. Recent and old emboli were frequent in the carotid system in cases of thrombotic occlusion of the carotid.

Hutchinson and Yates[187] found many stenoses and occlusions in the first inch of the vertebral artery, sometimes associated with cerebellar infarcts. They felt that vertebral artery occlusion or stenosis could jeopardize an impoverished carotid arterial flow. Of 83 autopsies of patients with cerebrovascular disease, 40 were found with significant stenosis or occlusion of one or more major cervical arteries. In 22 cases, there were 47 infarcts (29 cerebral, 15 cerebellar, 3 brain stem) and in 16, no occlusion of the related intracranial artery. In only one of the 15 cerebellar infarcts was a cerebellar artery occluded. The frequent association of combined vertebral and carotid occlusive lesions and the apparent interdependence of these arteries in regard to the collateral circulation led Hutchinson and Yates[187] to coin the term caroticovertebral stenosis. In one of their cases, the vertebral arteries maintained a precarious cerebral flow for a time in the presence of chronic occlusion of both internal carotid arteries. In these cases, progression of the vertebral arterial disease could precipitate ischemic lesions in the carotid territory of the cerebrum.

The classic infarcts arising from vertebral arterial occlusion in the neck were considered to be (1) in the territory of the superior cerebellar artery near the junction with the territory of the posterior inferior cerebellar artery and (2) in peripheral areas of the occipital lobes. In carotid artery occlusion in the neck, the infarcts were said to be in the peripheral territory of the middle cerebral artery, the infarcts being incomplete and patchy in distribution, which indicates an inadequacy in the terminal stages of the collateral blood supply.[187] These cerebellar infarcts are often bilateral, symmetrical, and more frequent than the occipital lobe infarcts. The brain stem usually escapes damage when occlusions are in the neck.

Subsequently, Yates and Hutchinson[387] examined the vessels of 100 brains in which the clinical picture indicated cerebral ischemia. At autopsy, cerebral hemorrhage was found in 28 and infarcts in only 35. The clinical differentiation of causes of stroke is thus only of limited reliability. In 35 brains, there were 74 separate major areas of softening, six in the area of the anterior cerebral artery, 34 in that of the middle cerebral, 10 in that of the posterior cerebral, 11 in the basal ganglia, 17 in the cerebellum, and six in the brain stem. Several infarcts involved more than one arterial territory. In 14 cases, thrombi completely occluded an intracranial artery, and in an additional seven cases significant stenosis of an intracranial artery was present. Therefore, at best, in no more than 19 of the 35 cases of cerebral infarction (54%) was an occlusion or significant steno-

sis of an intracranial artery demonstrated. Moreover in all except two of the 14 cases of occluded intracranial artery, a demonstrable infarct was found and even in the exceptions incipient infarcts of 2 hours' duration seemed to be present. The converse did not apply, for occlusions were demonstrable in only 12 of the 35 cases of cerebral infarction and accounted for 15 of the total of 74 infarcted areas.[387]

In the extracranial arteries of the 100 patients,[387] 58 had a significant narrowing or occlusion of one or more of the cervical arteries. There was a slight predominance in males, with most patients being 55 years or more. In 18, the carotid arteries alone were affected, in seven the vertebral arteries alone, and in 33 both vertebral and carotid arteries. Complete occlusion or stenosis of the lumen to 1 mm. in diameter or less was found in the right internal carotid on eight occasions, in the left internal carotid

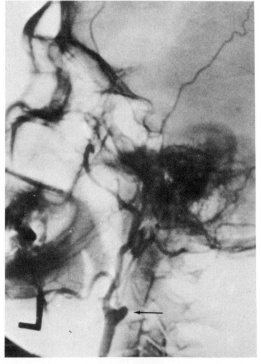

Fig. 4-34. Angiogram demonstrating complete occlusion of internal carotid artery just beyond bifurcation (*arrow*). (Courtesy Dr. M. Tsapogas, Albany, N. Y.)

in 13, in the right vertebral in 10 and left vertebral in six. In five patients, both internal carotid arteries were occluded and in another five, one vertebral and one internal carotid. Occlusion or severe stenosis was most frequent in the carotid sinus (Fig. 4-34) and less so at other sites, but in several, the thrombus had propagated as far as the circle of Willis, which contrasted with the absence of propagation in vertebral artery thrombosis. In vertebral arteries, severe stenosis or occlusion occurred in the first segment in 36, the second part in 17, the third part in eight, and in the intracranial segment in four. There were 19 cases in all in which one or more of the four major extracranial arteries were thrombosed (16 carotid and six vertebral), mostly on an atherosclerotic plaque, though one followed traumatic contusion of the artery.

In a joint study of extracranial occlusion of 4748 patients with symptoms and signs of ischemic cerebrovascular disease, the mean age was 60 years, approximately two thirds were in the preretirement group (under 65 years), men predominated in the ratio of 2:1, and in the age group below 55 years, there were more nonwhites than whites.[117] Four-vessel angiography was successfully performed in 80% (3788 patients), and of these, 25.5% had either no lesions (19.4%) or only inaccessible lesions (6.1%).[167] A total of 74.5% had accessible lesions only (41.2%) or both accessible and inaccessible lesions (33.3%). Multiple lesions were present in 67.3% of patients. Lesions were divided into occlusive and stenotic (Table 4-4), but there was no indication of the severity of the stenosis. The site most frequently involved by stenosis was the carotid bifurcation, especially in or adjacent to the origin of the internal carotid artery (33.8% on the right and

Table 4-4. Frequency of stenotic and occlusive lesions (expressed as percentage of 4748 patients)*

Site of arterial lesion	Stenotic lesion			Occlusion		
	Unpaired	Right	Left	Unpaired	Right	Left
Stem of innominate artery	4.2			0.6		
Innominate bifurcation and adjacent arteries	8.3			0.8		
Left subclavian proximal to vertebral	12.4			2.5		
Common carotid		3.2	4.8		1	2.2
First segment of vertebral		18.4	22.3		4	5.7
Bifurcation of common carotid and adjacent internal carotid		33.8	34.1		8.5	8.5
Cervical segment of internal carotid above carotid sinus		8	9.1		8.6	8.7
Petrous and cavernous segments of internal carotid		6.7	6.6		9	9.2
Second and third segments of vertebral		5.4	5.6		3.2	4.4
Intracranial segment of vertebral		4.9	3.8		2.8	3.2
Internal carotid between ophthalmic and bifurcation		8.3	9.3		2.7	3.1
Internal carotid bifurcation and stem of middle cerebral		3.5	4.1		2.2	2.1
Anterior cerebral		3.2	3.2		1.5	1.7
Basilar	7.7			0.8		
Posterior cerebral		2.6	2.6		0.7	1

*Adapted from Hass, W. K., Fields, W. S., North, R. R., Kricheff, I. I., Chase, N. E., and Bauer, R. B.: Joint study of extracranial arterial occlusion. II. Arteriography, techniques, sites and complications, J.A.M.A. **203**:961, 1968.

34.1% on the left). The next most frequent site was the vertebral arteries (Fig. 4-1) after their origin from the subclavian arteries (18.4% on the right and 22.3% on the left). Complete occlusion of the commencement of the internal carotid artery was found to be as frequent as that of the ascending straight cervical segment and neither area was involved as frequently as the petrous and cavernous segments. These results are at variance with the comparative severity of atherosclerosis at those sites, but no explanation was offered for this discrepancy. The frequency of extracranial and intracranial (large vessels only) occlusion was compared, and, as is apparent from Table 4-4, occlusions proximal to the cranial cavity were more common. Occlusions of the intracranial stem of the internal carotid or the middle cerebral arteries were present in only 10.1% of cases, and occlusions at each of these sites were less frequent than in the vertebral arteries. Arteriographic follow-up studies showed that untreated stenotic lesions progressed and new lesions appeared. The disadvantage of this clinical study is that no pathological correlation was attempted.* The association of the stenotic and occlusive lesions with the symptoms of ischemia was assumed and the frequency of negative arteriograms was not estimated.

In 1951, Johnson and Walker[200] reviewed 107 cases of occlusion of the common or internal carotid artery. Hemiparesis or hemiplegia occurred in 80%, speech disturbances in 60%, paresthesias in 20%, mental disturbances in 15%, and eye signs in 39.3%. Clinically, the entity was manifested by (1) a sudden catastrophic onset (35%) of loss of consciousness, headache, hemiplegia, and perhaps aphasia, (2) a slowly progressive course (25%), or (3) transient attacks (40%) of cerebral ischemia not infrequently terminating in a sudden hemiplegia with aphasia. Males were predominant (ratio 87:20) with a predilection for the 30 to 60 years of age group. The left side was affected in 65% of cases.

Occlusion of an internal carotid or vertebral artery in the neck can be entirely without symptoms. In one series of 143 cases of complete occlusion of the internal carotid artery in the neck, no weakness or paralysis on the opposite side was in evidence at any time in 19 cases.[156] Even bilateral occlusion of the carotid sinuses in the neck is compatible with an adequate cerebral blood flow without clinical evidence of impaired cerebral function. An instance of bilateral carotid and basilar occlusions has been reported with only mild neurological deficit.[98] This is due to the adequate collateral circulation. The circulatory arrangements are more vulnerable to occlusive lesions in other vessels, to increased functional demand, and to decreased collateral flow. Moreover, degrees of neurological disturbance, even when lesions are similar, vary greatly.

The renewed interest in occlusion of extracranial arteries to the brain has obscured the role of intracranial arterial occlusion. In 100 brains with recent large infarcts, Hicks and Warren[171] found only 40 associated with thrombotic occlusion of an intracranial artery with several probably of embolic origin. In the remaining 60 cases, contributory factors such as arterial spasm, hypertension, arteriosclerosis, congestive cardiac failure, and hypotension were invoked in the etiology of the infarct. Adams and Fisher[6] asserted that in large recent softenings caused by atherosclerosis and thrombosis, an occluded vessel can be found in 90% to 95% of cases when cervical and intracranial arteries are examined.

Berry[33] found occluded vessels in 129 of 171 cases (75%) of a single and large cerebral infarct not believed to be embolic. Vessels involved were the middle cerebral (33 cases), internal or *common* carotid (27), basilar and vertebral (24), posterior cerebral (6), cerebellar (5), and small parenchymal and meningeal arteries (9). In

---

*Pathological studies of the large cervical arteries at autopsy are hindered in the United States by the customary embalming of the deceased.

105 cases, there were multiple small infarcts and Berry[33] considered that to find the site of obstruction serial sections were needed.

In 2650 complete brain dissections, Moosy[259] found 58 brains (2.2%) with recent primary infarction exclusive of venous thrombosis and embolism, 84 with both recent and old encephalomalacia (3.2%), and 385 (14.4%) with old infarcts only. In 78 instances (55%) of the 142 brains with recent infarction, an antemortem thrombus was found in an appropriate artery. No dissection of the extracranial vessels was undertaken. In three instances, thrombi were found in intracranial arteries in the absence of a demonstrable infarct. It was said that the collateral circulation compensated adequately, but it is also possible that the patients died too soon for encephalomalacia to develop. Moosy[259] did not dissect the distal segments of the cerebral arteries in his series. The middle cerebral arteries were by far the most frequent site for recent thrombi. In another study of 204 cadavers in which intracranial and extracranial arteries to the brain were dissected, Moosy[260] found 11 patients with recent cerebral infarcts. Thrombi were more frequent in intracranial than in extracranial arteries.[260]

Small areas of encephalomalacia are frequent at autopsy, and probably only microscopic examination of the vessels or even serial sections will demonstrate related occlusions. Possibly many of these cases, especially with multiple softenings, are embolic and secondary to ulcerated atherosclerosis or thrombi in the heart or valve cusps. Failure in many instances to find the thrombus or occlusion responsible can be due variously to an inadequate search, failure to examine the cervical arteries, difficulty in locating small thrombi or emboli related to small infarcts, and finally possible fibrinolysis or breaking up of the clot.

Controversy persists as to whether occlusion of the cervical or its intracranial arteries plays the dominant role in precipitating cerebral infarction. The various studies are not entirely comparable, which obviates a collective analysis. Yates and Hutchinson[387] (pp. 168 and 169) have taken a sound approach and most credence should be given to their results despite the smallness of their series. They emphasize that there is no single cause of cerebral infarction, but that it is caused rather by the failure of the cardiovascular system as a whole to provide an adequate and well-oxygenated supply of blood for cerebral function.

MECHANICAL AND TRAUMATIC OBSTRUCTION. The factors predisposing to vertebral artery occlusion are neck injuries, head traction, and cervical spondylosis and even moderate-to-severe atherosclerosis.[347] In those under 40 years, trauma is the most common cause.[183] The vertebral artery in its extracranial course is often displaced laterally and sometimes severely distorted by osteoarthritic bony outgrowths in the region of the neurocentral joint.[187] Compression of the vertebral artery by osteophytes in cervical spondylosis can be demonstrated by angiography especially on rotation of the head. The most common sites of vertebral artery displacement lie between the fifth and sixth and the fourth and fifth cervical vertebrae, and less often at a higher level.[161,309] Lateral displacement and partial obstruction of the vertebral arteries[177] by herniated cervical intervertebral discs has been demonstrated angiographically, but significant obstruction is unlikely. It has been said that in basilar invagination or impression many of the symptoms and signs might be the result of vertebrobasilar insufficiency.[350] The vertebral arteries seem to be compressed as they cross the arch of the atlas, a theory supported by the aggravation of symptoms and obstruction of the vertebral artery when the head is rotated.[194]

Undue tortuosity of the vertebral artery in the first part of its course or after the artery leaves the transverse foramen of the atlas to pass over the posterior aspect of the atlas is not uncommon. Near the atlas, the artery may become so tortuous and elongated that acute flexion or kinking and obstruction may ensue during extension or rotation of the head.[309] These symptoms accruing from the compression appear ostensibly when severe atherosclerosis affects other major vessels to the brain.[309] Hardin and Poser[162] emphasized the obstruction of the vertebral artery by fascial bands (deep cervical fascia) during rotation of the head.

Chiropractic manipulation of the neck by a rotary motion at times has a fatal outcome, apparently because of a compression injury to the vertebral artery with thrombosis and perhaps embolism peripherally in the vessels of the vertebrobasilar system.[139,347] Ford[138] encountered a boy with excessive mobility of the axis which led to transient obstruction of the vertebral arteries with syncope, vertigo, nystagmus, diplopia, and unsteadiness, symptoms that could be induced by forcing the head backwards. Trauma to the neck admits of a similar dénouement.[52] In one instance, traumatic hyperextension of the neck caused medial dissection and vertebral artery thrombosis.[317] Yates[386] found adventitial hemorrhage in one or both vertebral arteries in 24 fetuses (40% of those examined). The hemorrhage at times stemmed from torn branches of the vertebral artery and in one case, the vertebral artery was thrombosed. External compression of the artery or thrombosis were proposed as principal causes of permanent cerebral ischemic damage in this age group. Incarceration of a vertebral[231] or the basilar artery[313] in fractures of the skull is rare.

Kinking of the internal carotid artery will usually be associated with elongation, tortuosity, and significant degrees of atherosclerosis and may be accentuated by aortic elevation. The anatomical features are discussed in Chapter 1. Most carotid kinks occur 2 to 12 cm. above the bifurcation in the sixth decade or later and are more common in females than males (ratio 2:1). There is an association between kinking and symptoms of insufficiency of cerebral blood flow[297,373] which has led to surgical correction of the course of the vessel or even its resection.[282] Rotation or certain positions of the head may cause the onset of symptoms.[94,297] Extreme kinking of a tube can obstruct or completely occlude it, but no clear evidence shows that the degree of kinking of the carotid as seen in man is sufficient to occlude blood flow. In one patient, arterial insufficiency and internal carotid kinking were associated with a murmur and a palpable thrill derived from the kinking. Moreover, pressure gradients of 20 to 30 mm. Hg have been found across such deformities.[94] It has not yet been demonstrated that thrombosis secondary to the flow disturbances so created results from the kinking. Atherosclerotic stenosis appears to be of importance in such cases.[373] Resection of the kinking has been found to relieve symptoms and reduce the pressure gradient.[94,282] The internal carotid has been obstructed in a case of cervical rib.[301]

Flow through both vertebral and internal carotid arteries is influenced by head position.[358] Boldrey and associates[43] thought that the abrupt turning of the head may lead to damage of the internal carotid artery because of compression and perhaps stretching by the lateral process of the atlas to which the vessel is frequently adherent.

Trauma to the internal carotid artery in the neck, whether with perforating and lacerating wounds of the neck or closed injuries, can result in thrombosis of the artery.[66,173,181] The close relationship of such arterial injuries to dissecting aneurysm has been discussed in Chapter 9. Hughes and Brownell[181] attributed cerebral infarction in two instances to embolism from the site of traumatic medial dissection and thrombotic occlusion of the internal carotid artery in the neck.

Intracranial arteries are rarely compressed though obviously expanding tumors of the base of the skull or pituitary or even massive aneurysms can lead to moderately slow arterial compression which should not progress to infarction.

Head injuries can be complicated by thrombosis of the intracranial segment of the internal carotid artery. The trauma is usually severe, frontal, and associated with a fracture through the floor of the anterior cranial fossa.[307] The internal carotid artery can be damaged where it leaves the dural covering of the cavernous segment[195,307] and a severe injury can also damage the artery more proximally in the cavernous sinus sufficient to cause rupture and false aneurysms and presumably also lead to thrombosis.

MISCELLANEOUS CAUSES OF OBSTRUCTION. Uncommon causes of arterial occlusion whether in the neck or within the cranium include the arteritides, such as giant cell arteritis,[5] syphilis, nonspecific arteritis, and Takayasu's arteritis. Acute cervical lymphadenitis has been said to be a cause of arteritis with thrombosis.[36,143] Thrombo-angiitis obliterans, incriminated in occlusions of the major arteries of the neck, may not be a true entity. Instances have been associated with lupus erythematosus.[5,316] Occlusion of the cavernous segment can complicate cavernous sinusitis. Mucormycosis can obstruct a large artery such as the internal carotid or smaller intracranial vessels, similarly with tuberculous meningitis.

A considerable degree of stenosis can arise when fibromuscular hyperplasia of the internal carotid[283] and superadded thrombosis occlude the lumen.[69] Dissecting aneurysms also produce cerebral infarction (Chapter 9).

Thrombosis of the cervical and intracranial arteries is effected by polycythemia rubra vera,[143] whereas in the puerperium thromboses occur for no known reason.[5] Likewise, thrombosis can complicate the prolonged prophylactic administration of estrogens (oral contraceptives).

Vasospasm is believed to evoke cerebral infarction only when in association with a ruptured cerebral aneurysm (see Chapter 9).

Postoperative complications after endarterectomy. Although a better life expectancy results from surgical correction of occlusive lesions of cervical arteries, some complications occur postoperatively. Postoperative complications consist of the usual infections and hematomas, but dissection of the intimal flap after endarterectomy can cause partial obstruction[265] or thrombotic occlusion of the artery. Occasional false aneurysms appear[284,353] and a thin coating of thrombus forms on the denuded area. Small emboli continue to arise until the surface is completely endothelialized. The time taken for endothelialization to occur is dependent on the extent of the surface area stripped, but if studies of the rabbit aorta[277] are any indication, it can be a lengthy procedure. Thompson and associates[353] have evaluated the surgical procedures. Postoperative thrombosis of an arterial graft with recurrence of the cerebral insufficiency has been reported[265] and retinal emboli have followed endarterectomy.[248]

An unusual complication is chylothorax because of injury of the thoracic duct.[284]

Wade and associates[366] reported the development of hypertension in 29% of 90 patients after unilateral carotid endarterectomy and 38% of 104 subjects after the bilateral procedure. In another study 15 of 27 patients (56%) became hypertensive after unilateral endarterectomy with neurological deterioration in seven. Hypertension developed most frequently in subjects treated for their first ischemic episode and was least common in those with a history of major or minor ischemic attacks.[227] The underlying mechanism of the hyperpiesis is unknown.

In the course of evaluating surgical therapy for internal carotid artery occlusion or stenosis in 900 patients, it was discovered that six patients had subsequently suffered a cerebral hemorrhage.[47] The hemorrhage seemed to arise from an area of previous infarction after the increase of blood pressure in vessels through which normal flow was reestablished or bleeding may stem from the collaterals. The prevalence of this complication in such an age group is not significant.

Embolic arterial obstruction

Large vessel embolism. Embolism is a major cause of cerebral infarction and accounts for anything from 5% to over 40% of cerebral infarcts.[7,203] The age distribution is somewhat lower (peak in the sixth decade) than in nonembolic infarction (peak in the seventh decade, Table 4-1), but the embolic group is so heterogeneous that it is preferable to consider the ages at which major causes of cerebral embolism arise. Thus most patients with bacterial endocarditis are under 40 years, and 70% of those with nonbacterial thrombotic endocarditis are over 40 years of age.[11] Patients with chronic rheumatic heart disease are, in general, younger than those with either hypertensive cardiovascular disease with auricular fibrillation or atheromatous embolism. Those with myocardial infarction fall between these limits.[70] The preponderance of females involved is related to the high incidence of these particular cardiac disorders in women.[206]

Thrombotic emboli in the cerebral arteries cannot always be distinguished from thrombi formed in situ, but the criteria employed are (1) an embolus is an antemortem thrombus, occurring especially at junctions, possibly folded upon itself and not adherent to the wall; (2) there is a likely source of emboli, especially in the presence of multiple emboli throughout the body; (3) the presence of a hemorrhagic infarction usually denotes an embolic cause; and (4) the presence within the embolus of material foreign to the cerebral arteries and obviously derived from a distant site indicates embolism. Cerebral emboli tend to fragment and disappear, which adds to the difficulty.

Large embolic cerebral infarcts are most often the result of cardiac disease. Garvin[145] found cardiac mural thrombi in 4.2% of 6285 consecutive autopsies and in 34.4% of 771 patients with heart disease. The cardiac diseases consist of the following:

1. In chronic rheumatic heart disease with or without auricular fibrillation, thrombi may originate from valves or the auricular appendage.

2. Auricular fibrillation, particularly in association with mitral stenosis, hypertensive cardiovascular disease, or occasionally, thyrotoxicosis, is commonly complicated by cerebral embolism, which is frequently precipitated when rhythm reverts to normal.

3. Myocardial infarction associated with mural thrombosis is a source of embolism in the early stages and during and after healing. In 133 cases of myocardial infarction, Garvin[145] found mural thrombi on the left side of the heart in 60.9%, and in a series[70] of patients with myocardial infarction manifesting embolism, 50% of the patients had cerebral embolism.

4. Bacterial endocarditis is frequently complicated by cerebral embolism, the emboli being either sterile or infected. In the latter case, arteritis can be followed by rupture with or without arterial dilatation. Nonbacterial thrombotic endocarditis causes cerebral embolism.[9,11,359] In 33 cases of nonbacterial endocarditis mostly associated with malignant tumors, Barron and associates[28] found 10 patients (30.3%) with cerebral embolism. Moreover, they found nonbacterial endocarditis to account for a peculiarly high frequency (10.9%) of cases of cerebral embolism at autopsy.[28]

5. Miscellaneous causes encompass cardiac surgery, endocardial fibrosis, foreign bodies,[274] and neoplastic emboli,[87] including those from cardiac myxomas and sarcomas.[204] Neoplastic involvement of pulmonary veins can initiate cerebral embolism, especially during pneumonectomy. Large vessel embolism may occur after traumatic arterial lesions,[181] dissecting aneurysm, ulcerated atheroma, localized arteritis in the neck,[36] or even pulmonary thrombophlebitis in inflammatory lung diseases. Paradoxical embolism is extremely rare.

Emboli most often lodge in the middle cerebral artery, probably because in man the middle cerebral artery is in reality the continuation of the internal carotid and the blood flow through the internal carotid artery is greater than through the external carotid and vertebral arteries. Successive emboli tend to pass along a similar path. Very few, for example, enter the anterior cerebral artery.[239] Similarly, few emboli affect the brain stem, and those in the vertebrobasilar system are inclined to lodge in the posterior cerebral arteries. Solid emboli introduced into the cerebral circulation do not cause vasoconstriction, but a degree of vasodilatation permits them to pass along the arterial tree until they become impacted.

It has been noted that the frequency with which an occlusion of a major cerebral artery is demonstrable by angiography is higher when the interval between the onset of symptoms and the angiographic study[118] is short. In 86 patients with a major cerebral infarct, 49 (57%) had an arterial occlusion; 16 in the cervical segment of the internal carotid, six in the cavernous or intracranial segments, 25 in the middle cerebral, and two in the anterior cerebral artery. The remaining 37 patients exhibited severe atherosclerosis only. In later studies, the occlusions were no longer demonstrable by angiography or necropsy in eight middle cerebral arteries and in two of the distal internal carotid arteries.[118] Experimental pulmonary and cerebral emboli frequently disappear[172] and it is probable that the emboli progressively disintegrate with assistance no doubt from the fibrinolytic activity of the blood. Angiography has demonstrated progressive clearing, confirmed by autopsy at a later date,[76,78,79] but this phenomenon does not apparently occur in cerebral thrombosis.

Bladin,[41] in a series of 54 cases of cerebral embolism, revealed angiographically (1) embolism of the internal carotid artery in 17 cases, two of which had additional emboli (internal carotid and middle cerebral), (2) embolism of the middle cerebral artery in 20 patients, eight in the trunk and 12 in its branches, and (3) no abnormality in 17 cases, presumably because the angiography was delayed for 2 to 3 weeks.[41] Emboli in the internal carotid were usually confined to the upper reaches of the artery, the supraclinoid portion often. Migration into the trunk of the middle cerebral artery and thence to its branches soon followed, seemingly within a matter of hours. In eight cases of embolism of the middle cerebral artery, successive angiograms demonstrated disappearance of the embolus. Actual migration of the embolus from the trunk through the branches with complete clearing of the arterial tree was found in two patients. The salient conclusions were that in the classic embolism of the trunk of the middle cerebral artery at its main bifurcation, the site at which the embolus can be demonstrated is dependent on the time lapse between onset and angiography or autopsy. After 2 to 3 weeks nothing may be found. Migration from the internal carotid artery was said to be more rapid and complete than from the middle cerebral artery. However, clearance and migration are too slow and protracted to prevent ischemic changes and are believed to induce hemorrhage within the infarct.

The emboli may cause gross or microscopic softenings, and multiple emboli may occur in up to 30%[377] or more. Evidence of splanchnic and peripheral embolism is almost the rule. The cerebrospinal fluid may be tinged with blood but is often clear,[377] although red cells may be present microscopically. The pressure is elevated only occasionally and the protein is above normal in approximately 50%. Bacterial endocarditis is particularly prone to produce abnormal findings in the cerebrospinal fluid. A mild leukocytosis is generally present. Wells[377] found that 25% of patients died as the result of the cerebral embolism within 2 hours to 2 months. Several died within 1 hour of the onset. In 35%, a serious neurological deficit persisted. In 40%, there was no neurological deficit or it was only minimal. After the age of 50, the prognosis is considerably worse, and recovery is frequently incomplete or poor. Carter[55] estimated that approximately two-thirds of the patients died within 3 years, with the prognosis depending ultimately on the number and size of the infarcts. The commonest cause of death is cerebral and then cardiac or pulmonary infarctions or cardiac failure.[57] Recurrent emboli may occur in protracted cardiac disease, and the effects on the brain are cumulative and cause chronic neurological and mental deterioration. Towbin[359] found that 4.6% of patients with chronic organic brain disease at autopsy had infarcts caused by recurrent embolism.

Small vessel embolism. Embolism of small vessels is said to be infrequent,[18] but many transient ischemic attacks are caused by embolism of small vessels. Moreover, small cortical infarcts are common at autopsy, and these too may be derived from small emboli discharged from the heart, great vessels, or large cerebral arteries. Many, it has been observed, pass through the retinal circulation and almost certainly many more reach the cerebral circulation. Some cause symptoms and a few can be demonstrated angiographically.[84] Serial sections are probably necessary to demonstrate occlusions in the peripheral pial arteries.

Embolism of atheromatous material from ulcerated atherosclerotic arteries is a well-recognized phenomenon. Arterial ulceration is most frequent in the descending aorta, but other major arteries, including those of the neck, being affected, will also be a source of atheromatous emboli. Vessels of smaller caliber are more likely to undergo occlusive thrombosis with ulceration and so are less likely sources. Consequently, atheromatous emboli have mostly been reported in splanchnic vessels.[135] Renal involvement at autopsy has been estimated at 4.7% in males and 2.7% in females.[150] The lower limbs, frequently severely affected, are rarely examined for such lesions. Similarly, vessels to the spinal cord are probably involved often and are rarely examined post mortem but the lesions have been seen even in vertebral bone marrow.[160] Emboli can originate from ulcerated plaques in the proximal aorta, common carotid, the carotid sinus, or vertebral arteries, and they have been observed in both the cerebrum and cerebellum[321]

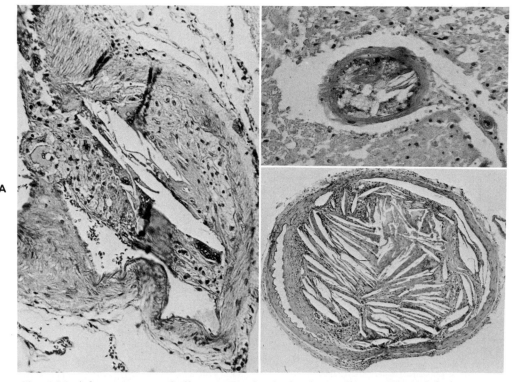

Fig. 4-35. Atheromatous embolism. **A,** Foreign-body giant cells are aggregated about cholesterol clefts, and occluded tissue also contains foam cells. **B,** Small artery is occluded by amorphous debris containing cholesterol clefts. **C,** Larger pial artery is completely occluded. (Hematoxylin and eosin; **A** and **B,** ×110; **C,** ×30.)

where they may be sufficiently severe and widespread to be the direct cause of death.[149]

In extracranial vessels, only small arteries 55 to 900 μ in diameter are affected. In the cerebral circulation, the mean internal diameter of vessels occluded in 16 cases was 116 μ.[321]

Atheromatous emboli produce fairly specific lesions in the vessels. In the early stages, cholesterol clefts may be visible in the blood within the arterial lumen (Fig. 4-26) or incorporated within a thrombus. More often with a variable number of cholesterol clefts in an occluded lumen and a few giant cells about the cholesterol, the end result is recognizable (Fig. 4-35). Eosinophils may be prominent in the early cellular response to the embolus.[109] Lipid is not uncommon in arteriosclerosis of arteries of this caliber, but cholesterol crystals are rarely if ever present, only lipophages and diffuse droplet infiltration. The presence of numerous acicular crystals with a foreign-body giant cell reaction is a characteristic feature. Lipophages are rare and fibrous tissue, a siderophage or two, and a newly formed capillary or sinusoid comprise the remainder of the occluding tissue. Calcific material is also rare. The organized embolus, which need not completely occlude the vessel, may be related to a branch. The architecture of the wall varies from slightly disturbed to completely destroyed. It is believed that the emboli pass through the retinal circulation at least, but no lesions at all similar have been encountered in the lungs. The experimental injection of atheromatous debris[135] or cholesterol crystals (commercial)[320] reproduces the human disease.

Extracranial emboli are associated with ischemic lesions and frank infarcts,[160,389] whereas renal involvement leads to the development of hypertension.[160] Emboli have been reported in the cerebral circulation on many occasions[247,333] and the manipulation of an ulcerated carotid sinus would definitely seem to be a hazardous procedure.[333] In view of the frequency in the aortic arch of ulcerated atheromatous plaques, the incidence of old small cortical softenings in the aged at autopsy, the not uncommon finding of such emboli in random sections of the brain, and the slight likelihood of finding them on a single section of a cortical infarct, it seems highly probable that a thorough study of such infarcts by the serial section technique would reveal a much higher incidence of atheromatous embolism than is generally accepted.

Foreign bodies, depending on size, introduced into the cerebral circulation during major or minor surgical procedures either become impacted and induce thrombosis locally or pass through the cerebral circulation via the capillary bed or arteriovenous shunts. The thrombus undergoes organization or lysis to a variable extent, whereas the reaction induced by the foreign body varies according to its nature. Cotton fibrils from gauze swabs induce a foreign-body giant cell reaction,[314] which should be differentiated from atheromatous embolism and giant cell arteritis.

Other ischemic lesions

Lacunar softenings (état lacunaire). Lacunes are deep areas of softening (Fig. 4-36) ranging from 0.5 mm. to lesions up to 1.5 cm. in diameter, caused by the occlusion of penetrating arteries chiefly from the middle cerebral, posterior cerebral, and basilar arteries to the basal ganglia or pons. Although extremely frequent on account of their size, they are often either overlooked or ignored. Their size and shape are irregular. They tend to be less than 5 mm. in diameter and old, rather than recent or in a state of colliquative resolution and sometimes contain trabeculae. Usually they are pale, but a brown pigmentation may be noticed.

Clinically, they are manifested by relatively minor neurological disturbances, which Fisher[125] called lacunar strokes, manifesting themselves as (1) a pure motor hemiplegia or hemiparesis,[129] (2) a pure sensory stroke,[124] (3) a syndrome combin-

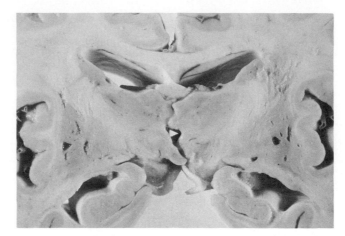

Fig. 4-36. Multiple lacunar softenings mostly in the putamen of each side. Such a finding is highly suggestive of preexisting hypertension.

ing cerebellar ataxia with weakness of the corresponding leg,[128] and (4) dysarthria and clumsiness of one hand caused by a small lacune deep in the upper part of the basis pontis near the midline.[125] Some lacunes are clinically silent[124] and other clinicopathological correlations can be determined, but in view of the variable size and position, the clinical picture is probably variable too.

Sites of predilection include the lenticular nucleus, especially in the putamen, the thalamus, pons, the central white matter, the internal capsule, centrum ovale, corpus callosum, and rarely the cerebellum (Table 4-5). No lesions were found in the cortex, cerebral peduncles, or medulla. A horizontal section a little below the genu of the corpus callosum displays the majority of lacunes.[114]

Ferrand[114] estimated that 90% of hemiplegias in subjects over 60 years of age were caused by lacunar softenings. Fisher[124,126] found lacunes in 11% of 1042 consecutive postmortem examinations of the brain. Of the 114 persons, 71 were male and 43 female; only 8.7% were under 50 years of age and the peak incidence was in the seventh decade. Multiplicity of lesions is extremely frequent.

Microscopically, lacunes are small, irregular cavities and like other softenings may contain thin connective tissue strands projecting into or crossing the lumen. A few small blood vessels may lie within the cavity, the walls of which may be relatively smooth and exhibit gliosis. Residual lipophages and more seldom siderophages may be within the lacune or the perivascular space of neighboring vessels.

The *état lacunaire* is to be distinguished from the *état criblé* in which the perivascular spaces of perforating arteries are unduly enlarged without obvious change in the surrounding parenchyma except for a diminution in staining capacity. These spaces contain vessels and impart to the

Table 4-5. Distribution of lacunar softenings

Site	Number of lacunes according to site	
	Ferrand[114]	Fisher[124]
Lenticular nucleus	89	138
Thalamus	41	52
Internal capsule	26	46
Caudate nucleus	20	38
Pons	24	59
White matter	14	30
Corpus callosum	3	7
Cerebellum		6
Total number of cases	88	114
Total number of lacunes	217	376

brain the appearance of being riddled with small holes. The basal ganglia, thalamus, and white matter are affected.

Of 88 patients with lacunes,[114] 15 (17%) died from hemorrhage into the basal ganglia. In Fisher's series[124] of 114 patients, hemorrhage was found in 41 (35%). Large hemorrhages (more than 2 cm. in diameter) occurred in 24 patients (putamen 17, thalamus 4, pons 1, cerebellum 3) and smaller hematomas alone or in combination were present in 24 patients. Multiple small hemorrhages were relatively frequent. Superficial infarction of the cerebral cortex was present in 30 subjects (26%), being major in 25, minor in five, and multiple in 12. Cerebral atherosclerosis is usually severe, with hypertension in 97.3% of Fisher's series. Foley[136] asserts that in the aged cerebral atherosclerosis and normotension may coexist. Fisher[124] found diabetes mellitus in 11%.

Obstruction of the small perforating vessels at their origin from the major cerebral arteries does not appear to be a factor.[124] Emboli may be responsible but rarely. Occluded vessels deep in the cerebral parenchyma are not uncommon, but they exhibit hyaline obliteration at times and the occlusion is believed to result from thrombosis of miliary aneurysms. Fisher[126] found total occlusion of the perforating artery supplying 45 of 50 lacunes. "Segmental arterial disorganization" often with localized enlargement of the vessel and evidence of local hemorrhage was responsible for 40 lacunes. Two were obviously thrombosed microaneurysms. In one, homogeneous pink-staining material lay within a thin partially disorganized wall. In all probability, these lesions cause cerebral hemorrhage, and it is therefore not surprising that hemorrhage was customary in the series with lacunes reported by Ferrand[114] and Fisher.[124] In two other instances, foam-cell lesions allegedly occluded the lumen. Of the remaining five lacunes in which no obstruction was found, arteriosclerotic changes were present in three, one was attributed to compression of a neighboring

vessel by a microaneurysm, and the remaining lacune was unexplained. Antegrade and retrograde thromboses with organization were found in many of the occluded vessels.

Circulatory arrest. A characteristic of brain tissue is pronounced susceptibility to anoxia or ischemia, which, when sufficiently prolonged, results in infarction. Milder degrees exhibit selective necrosis of specific areas.

Complete arrest of the circulation in the cat is possible only for 3 minutes 10 seconds without neurological disturbance. An additional 15 seconds of arrested circulation leads to permanent behavioral and psychic changes and areas of cortical softening. Circulatory arrest for 6 minutes brings about widespread cortical necrosis and dissolution. After an arrest of from $7\frac{1}{2}$ to 8 minutes, the animals could be maintained alive for only a few hours.[374,375] The brain stem and spinal cord were not damaged by periods of circulatory arrest incompatible with survival of the animal. The most vulnerable gyri were cortical areas 5, 7, 18, and 19, and then areas 3, 6, and frequently 29. The orbital, olfactory, and temporal lobes and a portion of the parietal lobe did not undergo necrosis until the circulatory arrest lasted for $7\frac{1}{2}$ minutes. The basal ganglia became necrotic after an arrest of 6 to 7 minutes. The Purkinje cells were next to the cortical nerve cells in susceptibility. Within the cortex, the most vulnerable laminae were III and IV, and the least affected I and II.

Pathological changes in the brain after cardiac arrest in man have been reviewed by Steegman.[324] Anoxic encephalopathy occurred after cardiac arrest of 2 to 3 minutes' duration. Extensive generalized convolutional atrophy was found with widening of the sulci, especially in the frontal, parietal, and occipital regions and in the cerebellum. The cerebral cortex was thinned or exhibited extensive laminar necrosis. The deep white matter was slightly gray and the ventricles were slightly dilated. In some subjects, softening of the caudate nucleus and putamen was observed with considerable variation from subject to subject. In severe cases, the entire gray matter was damaged or necrotic.

Brain stem ischemia and raised supratentorial pressure. Secondary hemorrhages in the brain stem are known to complicate rapidly increasing supratentorial pressure, but ischemic lesions also occur in this location under similar circumstances.[383] Dott and Blackwood[100] described such ischemia and Wolman[383] reported eight cases, but usually these lesions are seldom reported. Edema and vascular engorgement are more readily observed,[230] and the vascular damage often leading to the extravasation of blood initially causes stasis, which if prolonged can result in irreversible ischemia. Hemorrhage, as well as softening, is to be found. Wolman suggested that ischemia is the outcome when the supratentorial pressure increases relatively slowly in contradistinction to cases with hemorrhage when the pressure increase is rapid.

Lindenbergh[230] reviewed the infarcts and ischemic lesions that result from brain shift secondary to space-occupying lesions. They include compression of (1) the posterior cerebral artery and its branches by the tentorial margin (ischemic or hemorrhagic), (2) the anterior choroidal by the tentorial edge, (3) the anterior cerebral artery by the falx cerebri, (4) the middle cerebral artery by the lesser wing of the sphenoid bone, and (5) cerebellar arteries by the tentorial margins or the rim of the foramen magnum.

Granular atrophy of the cerebral cortex. The rare condition of granular atrophy of the cerebral cortex, which is bilateral and usually limited to the middle frontal gyrus and the parieto-occipital convolutions,[39] results from severe focal ischemia and has been likened to the granular atrophy of kidneys. On stripping the meninges from the cortex, the gyri are narrowed with multiple irregular depressions, which histologically are caused by many small areas of infarction and gliosis within the cortex.

Miscellaneous causes of ischemia. In an autopsy study of 38 patients dying as the result of blunt head injury, there was ischemic brain damage in 21 cases (55%), but in only four was the vascular lesion apparent.[151] It was hypothesized that post-traumatic reduction in cerebral blood flow was instrumental in producing the ischemia. In other cases, thrombotic occlusion of traumatized vessels results in infarction.

Day[88] reported the death of a 36-year-old man from massive hemorrhagic infarction (with small secondary pontine hemorrhages) after multiple wasp stings.

Cerebral thrombosis and oral contraceptives. Women taking oral contraceptives have been found to have an unduly high incidence of thromboembolic disorders, including cerebral arterial and massive venous sinus thrombosis.[15,364] Thromboembolic disorders tend to be more frequent in patients with blood groups A, B, and AB. They are even more pronounced in those on oral contraceptives and with pregnancy.[224] Causes of death among these women have not always been confirmed by autopsy. In two autopsies, arterial thrombosis was unaccompanied by significant pathology in the underlying vessel walls.[20] In another case with a hemorrhagic cerebral infarct, thrombosis of both internal carotid arteries together with fibrinoid swelling of intracerebral arterioles was described.[13] Segmental narrowing or occlusion of multiple small vessels and irregularity of the carotid siphon on angiography have been observed.[141] The risk appears greatest in those contraceptives with high doses of estrogen,[15,189] but the long-term metabolic effects of contraceptive steroids on metabolism are not entirely clear. Estrogens have been linked with other ill-effects such as hypertension, diabetes mellitus, and hyperbetalipoproteinemia, all of which may affect cerebrovascular disease. However, their apparent enhancement of (cerebral) thrombogenesis may be mediated by an effect on platelets[110] or by the formation of high molecular weight complexes with fibrinogen.[134] Users of oral contraceptives have often been found to have cryofibrinogenemia[276] so often associated with thrombotic disorders. Unusual levels of the plasma proteins have also been observed,[178] but the significance of such findings awaits elucidation.

Puerperal hemiplegia and strokes. The sudden onset of hemiplegia in a young healthy woman during pregnancy or the puerperium is a rare complication of childbearing. In the past, it has been attributed to cerebral venous thrombosis,[330] an assumption only in many cases.[73] Cross and associates recently analyzed 31 cases, all of which were associated with hemiplegia of varying degree. One instance occurred during the first trimester, six in the second trimester, nine in the third trimester, and 15 in the puerperium (1 to 16 days after birth). In age, the range was from 22 to 37 years. Cross and associates alleged that occlusion of the middle cerebral or internal carotid arteries was responsible for many of the lesions, with venous occlusion accounting for only the minority of cases.[73] This thesis requires verification.

The prevalence of cerebral infarction during pregnancy and the puerperium is unduly high.[73,222] The enhanced tendency for thrombosis may be related to hormonal factors and has an underlying mechanism similar to that associated with oral contraceptives.

"Multiple progressive intracranial arterial occlusions." Taveras[349] reviewed "multiple progressive intracranial arterial occlusions," a syndrome occurring predominantly in young adults and children and distinct from infantile hemiplegia. There is unilateral or bilateral occlusion of the intracranial segments of the internal carotid arteries of the middle and anterior cerebral arteries and sometimes of the basilar and posterior cerebral arteries as well. The occlusions are thought, perhaps incorrectly, to be chronic because of the prominent collateral circulation via (1) the unaffected leptomeningeal arteries, (2) transdural anastomoses between leptomeningeal vessels and branches of the external ca-

rotid, and (3) a very prominent network of vessels in the basal ganglia and upper brain stem at times filling the anterior and middle cerebral arteries. Comparable cases have been reported primarily in the Japanese[218] as examples of "moyamoya" disease, rete mirabile (Chapter 1), or hemangiomatous malformations of the base of the brain. The etiology is speculative for insufficient pathological material has been adequately examined. Prensky and Davis[280] considered that the occlusive process could occur in uterine life. The cause of primary occlusion is not known.

Fisher[121] reported occlusion of the internal carotid artery in early life in two subjects who died many years later of intracranial hemorrhage believed to have originated from the unusual collateral circulation.

Blood diseases. In primary hematological diseases, thrombosis (either arterial or venous) can be found within the cranium. Thus in polycythemia rubra vera, Lucas[238] found softenings in the brain and cord in four subjects from 23 autopsies on patients with this disease. Transient paralysis and sensory disturbances are also prevalent.[199]

In patients dying of sickle cell anemia, capillary hyperemia and thrombosis are usually pronounced. Sickle cells are seen in the lumen of vessels in the subarachnoid space, at the margin of hemorrhages, and particularly in vessels in the depth of the sulci. Small foci of softening without specific localization and areas of demyelination in the white matter are prevalent. Large areas of old and recent infarction are less frequent. There may be some arteriolar thickening and siderosis of the cerebral vessels. Lipid globules may be found within and sometimes occluding cerebral vessels, thus resembling fat embolism.[379]

Microcirculatory occlusion. By definition,[380] aggregation of the cellular constituents of the blood within the microcirculation can produce thrombi of sufficient size to occlude vessels. The behavior of the leukocytes, erythrocytes, and platelets in vivo studied under experimental condi-

tions[315,326,328] serves to explain how parenchymal ischemia can result from microthrombi and sludging of the erythrocytes.[327,329] Associated with their formation,
there is usually severe stasis, and for restoration of the circulation several hours may
be required. Histological sections do not
readily reveal all of these changes. They
can be sufficiently severe to cause frank
necrosis.[323] Particulate matter and bacteria
can initiate severe microcirculatory disturbances, though virulence and immunological factors play a role.[328,329] Cerebral
ischemia because of severe sludging[327] may
also participate in collapse associated with
anaphylaxis. Disseminated microthrombi
have been observed with bacteremia,[329] possible viremia,[249] and even parasitemia.[214,220]
Most of the experimental work on this subject has been performed on the extracranial tissues and circulation. It is reasonable
to assume that the cerebral circulation is
affected similarly, though confirmation has
not been provided.

Microthrombi consisting of platelet
masses incorporating some leukocytes and
red cells have received much emphasis, but
in some cases red cell aggregation may be
considerably more damaging. It is associated with an increased sedimentation rate
and hyperviscosity of the blood. Sluggish
blood flow through cerebral vessels and
neurological symptoms frequently occur
concomitantly. Similarities exist between
these reactions and those associated with
large molecular weight substances, bacterial endotoxins, and particulate matter, referred to as the "macromolecular hematologic syndrome" by Hueper.[179] Individual differences exist.[327]

Intravascular aggregation of red cells
and sometimes platelet clumping occurs
after the administration of fatty meals.[75,337]
The effect is more pronounced with fats
containing a high percentage of saturated
fatty acids.[339] In the brain, oxygen availability is reduced[342] and convulsions have
been induced in hamsters after meals of
cream.[343] Infusion of commercial fat emul-
sion produces effects[326] corresponding to
those of postprandial lipemia, and such
states may aggravate an already impoverished cerebral circulation.

In macroglobulinemia in mice, sludging
of erythrocytes with greatly reduced velocity has been observed in the cerebral microvasculature[295] and manifestations that
are analogous account for some features
of Waldenström's macroglobulinemia in
man.[234] The hemorrhagic diathesis of Waldenström's macroglobulinemia may correspond to the apparently enhanced tendency for bleeding seen in rabbits under
some of the above experimental conditions.

Disseminated intravascular coagulation
(consumption coagulopathy) is now recognized as an aspect of a number of clinical
conditions such as fat embolism, septicemia, and endotoxin shock.[105] It has been
suggested[105] that the activation of factor
XII (Hageman factor) may be the single
primary factor responsible for this condition, which also closely resembles Hueper's macromolecular hematologic syndrome, in which an anemia, sometimes
hemolytic in type, may become manifest.[326]

Pathological states in which there are
microthrombi of platelets and possibly
fibrin give rise to hemolytic anemia, the
so-called microangiopathic hemolytic anemia, which occurs in its most pronounced
form in diseases of small blood vessels such
as fibrinoid necrosis, necrotizing arteritis,
and microthrombi and emboli (polyarteritis nodosa, malignant hypertension,
lupus erythematosus, metastatic adenocar-
cinomatous emboli in small vessels, thrombotic thrombocytopenic purpura).[44] These
conditions affecting the central nervous
system may cause multiple small vessels to
be occluded and multiple small ischemic
infarcts may be found in association with
them.

Embolic encephalitis. The chief cause
of embolic encephalitis is bacterial endocarditis, which in both the acute and subacute forms is accompanied by neurological involvement in upwards of 30% of
cases,[202,216] but the percentage affected is

probably higher than is clinically apparent. In many cases, the first indication is a major embolic episode. The classical features of bacterial endocarditis are changing because of the declining incidence of rheumatic fever, the increase in cardiac surgery, and the longer life of the population. The frequency of bacterial endocarditis caused by *Streptococcus viridans* is declining and that of *Staphylococcus aureus* and *Streptococcus fecalis* is increasing. Calcific disease of the aortic valves or valvular atherosclerosis may underlie the endocarditis.

Neurological manifestations of bacterial endocarditis are protean. First, embolic episodes of varying severity are frequent and may be a terminal event or the cause of presentation. The episodes are often multiple and evidence of extracranial embolism is frequent. Such emboli involve the carotid system more often than the vertebrobasilar and, like other emboli, lodge most frequently in the middle cerebral artery. Transient ischemic attacks, no doubt embolic in nature, not infrequently precede the cerebral embolism. Morgan and Bland[261] found 30 such instances in 92 autopsies in bacterial endocarditis. Cates and Christie[59] reported major embolism in 35% of their cases and, of these, 17.9% were of the brain. Infected emboli, once the artery is obstructed, can cause an acute arteritis with rupture and fatal hemorrhage. This leads to the second group in which hemorrhage results from either an acute arteritis or a bacterial aneurysm (Chapter 9). In most reported cases in the literature, bacterial aneurysms at autopsy are associated with hemorrhage into the subarachnoid space or ventricular system. The subarachnoid hemorrhage may also be caused by septic thrombophlebitis. The commencement of antibiotic therapy does not preclude the occurrence of embolism nor the rupture of a preexisting bacterial aneurysm.[59]

In bacterial endocarditis, a small group of cases involves development of meningitis, which can be the presenting manifestation.[202] Abscesses, whether single or large,

rarely complicate the disease. Apart from the above, the brain usually exhibits edema and foci of pink discoloration or petechial hemorrhages at the junction of cortex and white matter in the cerebrum or in the gray matter in the brain stem. The foci may be numerous and microscopically they are small embolic lesions with septic thrombi or bacterial plugs filling the vessels (Fig. 4-37). Several vessels may be filled with thrombi or polymorphs, which also infiltrate the surrounding parenchyma of these affected vessels sometimes forming microabscesses. Perivascular hemorrhages and microinfarcts are not infrequent, and the subarachnoid space reflects the changes in the underlying brain. The cerebral cortex reveals the often patchy toxic nerve cell damage, and proliferation of astrocytes and microglia accompanies organization of the thrombi and healing.

Embolic encephalitis may also occur in pulmonary or systemic infections and pyemic states, but widespread microemboli are less likely.

Merchant and associates[252] reviewed 34 cases of fungal endocarditis. Fungi implicated were *Candida, Blastomyces, Coccidioides, Aspergillus, Cryptococcus, Histoplasma* and *Mucor. Candida* and *Histoplasma* are the two most common causes of fungal endocarditis and of 19 subjects with clinical or pathological evidence of major embolism, cerebral involvement occurred in seven cases (37%). *Candida* was the cause in five instances. In the single instance of *Mucor* infection, the meningeal vessels were involved.

Cerebral fat embolism. Cerebral fat embolism is only one aspect of a generalized disease, but is probably the major factor in the death of patients with fat embolism (usually after 2 to 4 days). Fat embolism is only an occasional cause of death after trauma, particularly after fractures of long bones. In such cases, the embolism is constantly present and was the principal cause of death in 5.5% of autopsies on patients dying of trauma[140] and a secondary cause in 10.8%.

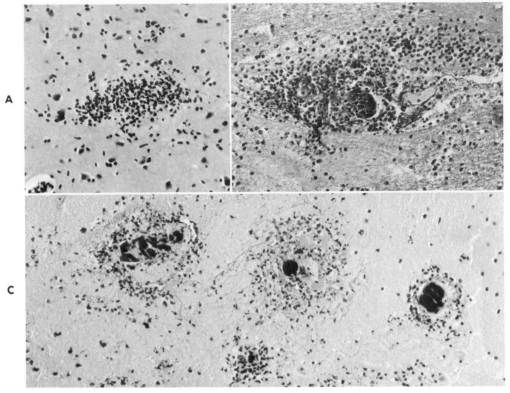

Fig. 4-37. Embolic lesions from cases of bacterial endocarditis. **A,** Small aggregate of polymorphonuclear leukocytes suggests a neighboring embolic focus. **B,** Thrombosed and possibly necrotic vessels are associated with intense perivascular leukocytic infiltration. **C,** Multiple emboli containing bacterial clumps in disorganized vessels surrounded by leukocytes, some of which are necrotic. (Hematoxylin and eosin, ×110.)

In another study of autopsies on accident victims, it was found that 80% of those who died at the scene of the accident or during transportation to hospital had fat embolism (severe in 15%). Of those surviving for 6 hours, 96% had fat embolism and every victim surviving 12 hours was affected. The prevalence of massive embolism was greatest at 12 hours, and thereafter it diminished presumably as the fat was eliminated slowly. Nevertheless, it was still found in 65% of victims who survived 15 days.[270] Massive fat embolism was not found in those with soft tissue injuries alone, but one or multiple fractures were present. However, evidence of fat embolism at autopsy should not implicate it as a cause of death for it may have been subclinical only.

Clinically, fat embolism is characterized by cerebral and respiratory disturbances and petechial eruptions. The clinically significant cerebral form occurs in 3.2% to 6% of subjects with fractures of the long bones and is fatal in 2% to 4.2%.[293]

At autopsy, petechial hemorrhages may be visible on the upper trunk and face, or beneath the conjunctiva. Fat emboli may be demonstrable in all viscera and the lung is severely affected. At autopsy, the microscopic examination of air bubbles expressed from a piece of lung immersed in distilled water revealed fat globules in pulmonary fat embolism.[351] The brain exhibited a varying degree of congestion with some patchy or confluent areas of mild subarachnoid hemorrhage.[240] On sectioning of the brain and cord, multiple small petechiae

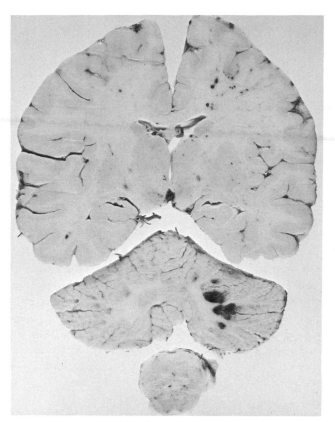

Fig. 4-38. Sections of a brain exhibiting fat embolism. Multiple petechiae or ecchymoses are present in cerebrum, cerebellum, and pons.

pepper the white matter of the brain and cord (Fig. 4-38), especially the centrum ovale.[362] The hemorrhages may be grouped (four to twelve per group), and occasionally are extremely numerous.[362] Larger hemorrhages are infrequent. Histologically, fat emboli are demonstrable in arterioles and capillaries throughout the brain in both cortex and gray matter. The characteristic lesion has been described as an embolus of fat in an arteriole that is surrounded by a zone of necrosis and then a further zone of red cells derived from neighboring capillaries.[362] Perivascular or ring hemorrhages occur particularly in the gray matter. Foci of anemic softening are not uncommon. Microthrombi also occur and stasis is probably severe. Fat droplets may be found in the perivascular tissues,

which are ultimately phagocytosed. Fat embolism in the choroid plexus of the ventricles is often conspicuous. It is most unlikely that the fragments of bone marrow frequently recognized in the lung will reach the brain. Extensive demyelination of the cerebral white matter was found in a patient who had cerebral fat embolism clinically 7 years previously.[251]

Fat droplets and foamy macrophages may be demonstrable in the lung, and lipuria is variable. Retinoscopy has revealed the presence of fat emboli, and fat droplets were found in the cerebrospinal fluid in 62% of patients with hip fractures and much less often in some chronic diseases.[167] An increase in the serum levels of lipase and tributyrinase follows bone trauma and is proportional to the severity of the injury.[351] The lipase level may be of prognostic value.[351] The drop in hemoglobin, often noted, suggests red cell damage, which also follows an infusion of lipid emulsions.[326]

There is abundant evidence that trauma precipitates fat embolism. The most common associated fractures are those involving the femur and tibia.[293] However, skeletal fractures or orthopedic surgery are not essential for soft-tissue trauma or surgery on subcutaneous fat[240] and even cardiac massage[270] can produce it. There is an ever-growing list of diverse nontraumatic causes of fat embolism including necrotizing pancreatitis,[240] alcoholic fatty liver, carbon tetrachloride poisoning, sepsis, phlegmonous gastritis, chronic tuberculosis, hepatitis, diabetes, burns, cardiovascular disease,[351] intoxications from phosphorus, alkalis, ether, and Salvarsan, and sickle cell crises.[379] Though fat embolism is not common in children, in one series three of the nine children had an associated systemic collagen disease.[101] The amount of fat said to be lethal to experimental animals varies within wide limits (12 gm. to 120 cc.),[371] but much depends on the physical state and the composition of fat or oil administered. It has been generally believed that fat from adipose tissue in the medullary cavity enters the damaged veins and thus causes fat embolism, a concept substantiated by the finding of bone marrow cells in the pulmonary vessels. Furthermore, oil injected into the medullary cavity of a long bone can be recovered soon after from the inferior vena cava and the lung, suggesting rapid absorption from the medulla via the Haversian veins.[362] It is unlikely that significant amounts of fat reach the blood by means of the lymphatics.[362]

It has been estimated that the quantity of fat droplets in the bloodstream exceeds by far the total fat content of the medulla of the injured bone.[372] On the other hand, the total blood lipid level need not exceed the normal limit.[371] The presence of large amounts of fat in the lungs and brain after mild trauma or fractures of the smaller bones of the body has raised doubts concerning the validity of this theory. Lehman and Moore[225] considered it unlikely that fat would enter the damaged veins in sufficient quantity or that the trauma is very often so severe as to liberate such large quantities of fat. Consequently, there is growing belief that an instability of blood lipids results in the formation of intravascular globules of fat that may grow and coalesce to obstruct small blood vessels. Posttraumatic lipemia and fat embolism may be produced experimentally, a tendency accentuated by alimentary hyperlipemia.[31] In the microcirculation, microthrombosis and embolism and red cell aggregation or sludging with diminution in flow have been observed.[31] This state of affairs is basically similar to microcirculatory changes after the intravenous infusion of lipid emulsions[305,326] and postprandial lipemia.[75,340] Consequently, not only will emboli of fat and platelet-leukocyte thrombi cause focal cerebral ischemia, but so also will the sluggish flow and sludging of the blood. Controversy still persists over these two opposing views, and it seems that a combination of the two mechanisms is distinctly possible except where fat embolism results directly from the inadvertent intravascular injection of oil. It has also been suggested that emboli arise directly from fatty livers, in poisoning with carbon tetrachloride, phosphorus, alcohol, and aviation fuel.[240,354]

More recently, it has been demonstrated in the experimental animal that the composition of the triglycerides in pulmonary fat emboli occurring after trauma is similar to that of marrow fat and dissimilar to that of plasma.[209] This suggests that the source of emboli is predominantly adipose tissue. No similar studies have been performed in nontraumatic fat embolism, but fat mobilization occurring after shock[331] could well explain some apparent contradictions in the experimental evidence.

Clearance of the fat from the blood takes place via the lungs, liver, kidney, and reticuloendothelial system and by the action of blood lipases.

Controversy over the pathogenesis continues. The pathologist faces a difficult and practical problem, that is, evaluation of the contribution that fat embolism makes in each instance to the demise of the patient.

Air embolism. Air embolism may be venous or less frequently arterial in type. In the case of pulmonary or venous air embolism, experimental animals tolerate surprisingly large amounts of air, presumably because of the filtering effect of the pulmonary capillary bed. The effect depends on the quantity injected, the speed of administration, posture, and the efficacy of the respiratory excretory mechanism.[102,103] In man, air enters the systemic veins under varying circumstances, including (1) operations involving the veins of the neck, dural sinuses,[288] or intravenous catheters, (2) diagnostic or therapeutic injections of air (intrapleural, intraperitoneal, perirenal, or into the joints or bladder)[102,103] or tubal and vaginal insufflation, (3) obstetrical procedures and uterine curettage, (4) injuries of the chest wall or lung, and (5) lavage of nasal sinuses. Obstruction of vessels and particularly interference with the function of cardiac valves by air or frothy blood can be fatal. Small quantities pass unnoticed. The diminution of cardiac output that results can cause a degree of systemic hypotension. A patent foramen ovale may permit the passage of air to the left side of the heart, and this possibility is no doubt enhanced by the pulmonary hypertension and systemic hypotension that follow venous air embolism. Some air will, like as not, reach the systemic circulation. Thrombi, some containing fat, have been found experimentally in the terminal pulmonary arteries.[165]

In arterial air embolism, air gains entrance to the circulation via the pulmonary veins or is injected directly into a systemic artery. Air from the pulmonary vein enters the systemic circulation and its distribution is determined by gravity and hence by posture. Embolism of the heart or brain will cause rapid death. With assumption of the upright position, air passes to the brain and small quantities may be tolerated in the cerebral capillaries without ill effect. However, animals can tolerate much less air in the systemic circulation than in the venous circulation and less again in the head-up position.[361] Cerebral air embolism can be demonstrated radiologically if sufficient air outlines cerebral and meningeal vessels, particularly in the temporoparietal regions. At autopsy, there is vascular engorgement, subarachnoid hemorrhage, and a few cortical petechiae. Hemorrhages stem from capillaries and small veins. The microvascular response to experimental mesenteric air embolism has been described by Chase,[61] and de la Torre and associates[90] described the pathological (ischemic) changes in the brain of animals surviving cerebral air embolism for periods of time.

Caisson disease. The too-hasty decompression of divers working under raised atmospheric pressure results in the formation of bubbles, chiefly of nitrogen, in the circulation. A similar event may occur in pilots subjected to subatmospheric pressures.[168] Bubbles simultaneously appear throughout the circulation and coalesce to form even larger bubbles. The brain is congested with petechial hemorrhages and possibly some subarachnoid perivascular hemorrhages, foci of edema, and subcortical demyelination. The spinal cord exhibits multiple focal lesions. Cerebral fat embolism occurred in four of the five cases studied by Haymaker and Davison.[168]

Embolism of brain tissue. Under very rare circumstances and usually attended by severe head injury, fragments of brain tissue may be forced into lacerated veins or venous sinuses with the emboli so formed lodging in the lung.[215,268] McMillan[250] estimated that this occurs in 2% of necropsies for severe head injury. The mechanics are somewhat obscure and the pulmonary embolism is a curiosity rather than a serious complication. Potter and Young[279] reported the presence of ectopic brain tissue in the lung in two anencephalic monsters, and attributed its presence to embolism during the development of the brain. This is in accord with Gruenwald's[153] case of a severe head injury during the second month in utero. The embolic brain tissue was invaded by bronchi.

Thrombosis of cerebral veins and dural sinuses

Thrombosis of intracranial veins and dural sinuses is an uncommon disease, though mild undiagnosed cases could occur more often than is currently appreciated.[26] The incidence is difficult to estimate, but it is probably less than early in the century[244] for antibiotics and greater attention to the fluid balance of sick patients have wrought change. In the preantibiotic era, German figures indicate that sigmoid sinus thrombosis was a significant factor in 0.3% of all deaths and that 0.55% of patients with otitis media developed thrombosis of the sigmoid sinus,[198] a rarity nowadays.

Intracranial venous thrombosis was the primary cause of 21.7 deaths annually in England and Wales between 1952 and 1961. Of the cases, 33.1% were less than 1 year of age, 44.7% under 5 years, 34.1% between 5 and 65, and the remainder were over 65 years.[205] Unquestionably, the peak incidence falls in the first year of life.

Etiology. Thrombosis of the veins and dural sinuses is customarily grouped into (1) primary or medical cases—a heterogeneous group in which local inflammation is not the precipitating cause—and (2) secondary, surgical, or septic cases in which thrombosis is secondary to a local inflammation. This classification is difficult to justify and serves little purpose since the causes of these thromboses are multiple.

Marantic thrombosis is found in extremely wasted and debilitated children in whom it has been thought a reduction in blood flow associated with cardiac insufficiency and severe toxemia results in cerebral venous thrombosis as a terminal event. Consequently, malnutrition, infectious disease, and chronic wasting diseases have been considered as predisposing factors, but

it seems that severe dehydration plays the major role.[50] Martin and Sheehan[245] pointed out that puerperal venous thrombosis was most likely in patients who had severe vomiting and diarrhea, yet cerebral venous thrombosis may complicate severe wasting diseases such as tuberculosis, neoplasms, and leukemia in the young and in adults.

Intracranial venous thrombosis also compounds heart disease both congenital and acquired. The feature common to most of the patients is severe right-sided cardiac insufficiency with chronic venous congestion.[26]

A variety of other causes is at times responsible, including trauma[39] from an accident or from birth injuries, surgery, compression or invasion by a tumor, paroxysmal nocturnal hemoglobinuria,[201] and blood dyscrasias, such as sickle cell anemia,[303] polycythemia rubra vera, leukemia,[208] and in the past, chlorosis. In infants and children, it is an occasional complication of infectious fevers in the absence of a local inflammatory lesion.[205] A possible association with hyperpyrexia has also been suggested.[26] Local inflammatory diseases, once a common cause of dural venous sinus thrombosis, are seldom the cause now and accounted for only two of the 31 cases reviewed by Kalbag and Woolf.[205] The most common site is the sigmoid sinus as a result of the spread of infection from an acute or chronic mastoiditis. Thrombosis of the cavernous sinus follows the spread of infection along veins draining the upper lip, the nose, and the orbital and frontal regions. The superior longitudinal sinus may be thrombosed secondarily to infectious lesions in the scalp, nose, and paranasal air sinuses, osteomyelitis of the skull, meningitis, encephalitis, and septicemia.

Thrombosis of cerebral veins or dural sinuses can materialize with recurrent thrombosis in the veins of the lower limbs or viscera[74] or in the clinical state labeled thrombophlebitis migrans.[49,205] In tropical primary phlebitis, thought to be a syndrome of phlebitis and thrombosis of large veins accompanied by hyperpyrexia in East Africa, thrombosis of a dural sinus was recorded in two subjects out of 71 cases. The thrombosis was considered to be secondary to an acute phlebitis that could not be attributed to an infectious agent.[120] In general, thrombophlebitis is used erroneously and synonymously with phlebothrombosis. When the thrombosis is secondary to a local inflammatory lesion, thrombophlebitis is the correct term.

These venous thromboses may occasionally be associated with cerebral arterial occlusion[39] and two instances of cavernous sinus thrombosis have been encountered occurring after rupture or leakage of an aneurysm of the cavernous sinus of the internal carotid artery.[244] It may arise spontaneously in a carotid cavernous fistula. Martin[244] theorized that embolism to the cerebral venous circulation could arrive via the vertebral venous system from the pelvic veins.

Currently, one of the commonest types of cerebral venous thrombosis affects healthy young women either during pregnancy or in the puerperium. The reported prevalence varies from once in 1500 to once in 3000 pregnancies.[53] In a review of 158 cases related to pregnancy,[53] more than 90% had reached the third trimester and in 113 of the remaining 140 subjects the thrombosis occurred during the puerperium (Table 4-6). In the first trimester, cerebral venous thrombosis usually follows a complication of pregnancy, such as abortion or threatened abortion. A few have arisen in the early stages of an apparently normal pregnancy. In some instances, a coincidental infection is responsible.[208] Thromboses in the puerperium have been attributed to increases in blood fibrinogen, platelets, and platelet adhesiveness known to occur post partum, especially from the fourth to fourteenth day. A relationship to eclampsia or a low-grade infection has been suggested but not substantiated. Cross and associates[73] recently suggested that many cases labeled as cerebral venous thrombosis are

Table 4-6. Time of occurrence and mortality of 158 cases of cerebral venous thrombosis related to pregnancy*

Time of occurrence	Number	Deaths
First trimester	13	7 (53.8%)
Second trimester	5	1
Third trimester	21 ⎫	
Intrapartum	6 ⎬	44 (31.4%)
Post partum	113 ⎭	
Total	158	52 (32.9%)

*Modified from Carroll, J. D., Leak, D., and Lee, H. A.: Cerebral thrombo-phlebitis in pregnancy and the puerperium, Quart. J. Med. **35**:347, 1966.

likely to be arterial occlusions. Thorough angiographic studies of such patients in the future should clarify the issue.

Young women taking oral contraceptives suffer from cerebral venous thrombosis[21,48] and the prevalence appears to be unduly high. Although the pathogenesis is unknown, it is believed that the metabolic effects of the hormones are ultimately responsible as with thromboses related to pregnancy and the puerperium. Irey and associates[190] assert that intimal thickenings associated with thrombi in both arteries and veins are possibly induced by the steroid therapy, but the cause and effect relationship to the thrombi is as yet uncertain.

Stasis, local injury, or a hypercoagulable state are the three classic factors held to be responsible for the initiation of thrombosis. Such factors cannot be invoked in some instances and the cases are classified as idiopathic. Phlebosclerosis occurs in extracranial veins, but little is known about phlebosclerosis within the cranium except when it is associated with long-standing arteriovenous shunts, which can be complicated by thrombosis.

Pathology. The commonest site of an intracranial venous thrombosis is the superior longitudinal sinus, and it is usually nonseptic in type. Those associated with sepsis are most often observed in the sigmoid and transverse sinuses. In 31 instances unattributable to local infection or surgical procedures, Bailey and Hass[23] found the superior longitudinal sinus thrombosed in 31, the superior cerebral veins in 15, the lateral sinus in 17, the straight sinus in 10, the great vein of Galen in seven, and the cavernous sinus in two. They considered it reasonable to suppose that the other sinuses were involved secondarily by propagation of a thrombus formed initially in the superior longitudinal sinus[23] though thrombosis can occur at two distinct sites. Thrombosis of dural venous sinuses may or may not be associated with thrombosis of the venous tributaries. Irish[191] asserted that cerebral veins alone are affected in only 10% of instances. More frequently, they are thrombosed concomitantly with occlusion of the posterior three-fifths or all of the superior longitudinal sinus[50] and the opposite side is likely to be involved secondarily.

The superior longitudinal sinus is the commonest site for most of the noninflammatory cases, such as those associated with pregnancy, the puerperium, trauma, marasmus, cachexia. However, it can be involved in the extension of infection from the nose or scalp, or by a secondary extension from the transverse sinuses or cortical veins. The Rolandic veins are often involved so that motor and sensory disturbances result. The transverse sinus is thrombosed secondarily to that of the sigmoid sinus and extension to the internal jugular vein is likely. In many instances, the thrombus extends to involve the torcular and beyond. The anatomy of the torcular and the extent of propagation of this sinus is of importance in otitic hydrocephalus. Long-standing idiopathic bilateral sigmoid sinus thrombosis has been reported in a boy (4½ years old) with mild hydrocephalus and congenital aortic stenosis. Very prominent tortuous veins were visible over his forehead and scalp as drainage apparently occurred via emissary and orbital veins though no doubt the vertebral veins assisted.[319]

The inferior petrosal sinus is associated with infections of the middle ear.[45] The superior petrosal sinus is involved by the spread of infection through the tegmen tympani from the middle ear, or by spread from the inferior petrosal or the cavernous sinus.

The cavernous sinus thrombosis is generally secondary to infection in the "danger area" of the face, the nose, and orbits. Spread to the cavernous sinus may come from the inferior or superior petrosal sinuses. Usually septic, only occasionally is it bland or unilateral. The venous tributaries are usually also thrombosed with resultant edema and congestion of the orbits and proptosis. Suppurative leptomeningitis is almost invariably present and infarction of the pituitary may occur.[376]

Thrombosis of the straight sinus or vein of Galen is more likely to be associated with or caused by the extension of a thrombus from the superior longitudinal or transverse sinus. Otherwise, it is in association with an arteriovenous aneurysm as in the aneurysm of the vein of Galen or due to birth trauma or neonatal infection. Thrombosis of the vein of Galen is rare after the neonatal period.

Most thrombi have the usual macroscopic and microscopic features of bland thrombi, with a varying degree of propagation and involvement of tributaries. Evidence of organization is quite frequent at autopsy. It may be present at one site and not at another, suggesting recent terminal propagation. In long-standing occlusion, the veins or sinuses may be recanalized.[241]

In cases associated with sepsis, the local inflammatory lesion, usually suppurative, can be found either in the middle ear and mastoid air cells, the orbit, face, paranasal air sinuses, skull, or scalp. Infection can readily spread by emissary and anastomotic veins to the dural sinuses without there necessarily being direct spread. There may be suppuration within the thrombus, which leads to its further propagation or to pyemia. With pyogenic infections, meningitis or cerebellar abscess may follow. Commonly, the thrombosis is secondary to acute or chronic mastoiditis and local inflammatory changes in the wall of the sinus without necessarily bacterial invasion. Thrombi so induced are frequently bland rather than septic. In rare instances, tumor tissue is found in the thrombus.[241]

The effect of the thrombotic occlusion on the brain is variable. In view of the plentiful anastomoses between the superficial cerebral veins and the sinuses, there may be thrombotic occlusion of a limited number of veins and even of the superior longitudinal sinus without untoward developments. The rapidity of the occlusion is crucial. In the series examined by Byers and Hass,[50] approximately half of the brains exhibited no changes. In other patients, the brain exhibits a variable amount of infarction, which may be very extensive and involve the whole of one or both cerebral hemispheres. At surgery, the cortex is gray rather than pink with firm, blue-black thrombosed veins.[244] At autopsy, the dura and arachnoid may be tense and the gyri very flattened with obvious evidence of considerable increase in intracranial pressure. Vessels are congested and thrombosed veins are prominent. Subarachnoid hemorrhage is usual and at times bilateral and severe. A few instances of mild subdural bleeding have occurred.[23] On section, areas of infarction are usually edematous and hemorrhagic. The hemorrhages are usually not confined to the cortex, but involve the white matter at times to a greater extent than the cortex. There may be petechiae throughout the white matter or an actual frank subcortical hematoma. Despite evidence of considerable swelling of the infarcted area, secondary hemorrhages in the brain stem are infrequent.

Thrombosis of the superior longitudinal sinus anteriorly may not produce much damage, but in the posterior half of its course it often involves the tributaries bilaterally and is associated with extensive red softening in both cerebral hemispheres. The parietal lobes are infarcted most frequently, although the frontal and occipital lobes are involved almost as often and the temporal lobes least frequently. Occlusion of the vein of Galen results in hemorrhagic infarction in the midline structures in the drainage area of the vessel. Consequently, there is extensive bilateral softening in the basal ganglia and perhaps intraventricular hemorrhage. The brain stem and cerebellum are rarely affected. Organization continues in the usual manner, and in the chronic stages, apart from organization of the thrombosed venous channels, enlarged collaterals may be apparent. The meninges can be opaque with an accumulation of xanthochromic fluid over an area of shrunken, atrophic, brownish yellow cortex, which microscopically reveals old cystic and laminar softenings. The lesions usually involved the third to the sixth layers of the cortex,[22] the superficial rim of cortex being gliotic. The deeper structures in the infarct are shrunken and cystic with complete demyelination of the affected zone. Much pigment may still be present in the spongy gliotic scar tissue.

Laboratory findings. There is occasionally a polymorph leukocytosis and pyrexia. In septic cases, the blood and cerebrospinal fluid may yield positive cultures. The cerebrospinal fluid may be clear or xanthochromic or bloodstained with hemorrhagic infarction. The pressure may be normal or elevated as in the otitic hydrocephalus in which the cells and protein content are usually not raised. The cellular content may reach 1000 cells per cu. mm., many being polymorphs particularly in the presence of infection.

Otitic hydrocephalus. Symonds[345,346] introduced the term "otitic hydrocephalus" for a syndrome principally affecting children with a history of acute or chronic mastoiditis, in whom there is weakness or paralysis of both lateral recti muscles (sixth nerve palsy), headache, and greatly increased cerebrospinal fluid pressure with no appreciable increase of cells or protein. Many had a thrombosis of the lateral sinus.[344,346] It is a benign condition in which bilateral optic nerve atrophy may develop unless the intracranial pressure is relieved. Autopsy material is rare, but in the five necropsies reviewed by Symonds[344] thrombosis of the transverse sinus had extended to involve the torcular and the posterior part of the superior longitudinal sinus in three instances and in the remaining two cases, occlusion of one transverse sinus was present, but no mention of the torcular pattern nor the size of the opposite transverse sinus was made. In another patient, Kinal and Jaeger[212] demonstrated angiographically that the transverse sinus was occluded by a thrombus that did not extend as far as the torcular. In other cases studied similarly, the evidence strongly suggested that an increase in intracranial pressure was restricted to cases in which the major transverse sinus was occluded or seriously stenosed (by a mural thrombus or atresia),[211,212] and it is pertinent that otitic hydrocephalus is more frequent with occlusion of the right transverse sinus than with the left. Alternatively, it seems that if the middle ear infection does not lead to occlusion of the major transverse sinus, then the thrombus must needs extend to the torcular and thereby dam up most of the blood draining the brain by also occluding the superior longitudinal, and straight and contralateral transverse sinuses as was the case in yet another autopsy described by Kalbag and Woolf.[205] It appears that increased intracranial pressure in such cases is the result of increased venous pressure.[211,212] Some degree of ventricular dilatation occurs in patients with this variety of hydrocephalus and it is pertinent that Bering and Salibi[32] produced increased intracranial and cerebral venous pressure and some ventricular enlargement in 74% of 21 dogs subjected to experimental occlusion of cerebral venous drainage.

The increased intracranial pressure has been attributed to venous congestion and edema of the brain, the ventricular dilatation possibly caused by some cerebral atrophy.[205] The sixth nerve palsy has been attributed to compression of the nerve by thrombus in the inferior petrosal sinus.[344] There is, however, need for still more postmortem or angiographic studies in these cases, and also perhaps some physiological investigations of cerebrospinal fluid mechanics in patients with this disease.

Prognosis. Major dural sinus thrombosis can be associated with hemorrhagic cerebral infarction and edema, intracranial hypertension, and death, but may not necessarily be immediately fatal. The prognosis is usually given to be about 30%, but much depends on the site. For instance, cavernous sinus thrombosis has been estimated to have a mortality of 72.8% and a morbidity among survivors of 65.3%, both figures probably being conservative.[385]

Ischemic lesions of the spinal cord

Ischemic lesions of the spinal cord are rare. During the past 15 to 20 years, there has been an enhanced awareness of these pathological states but little increase in our knowledge of the pathogenesis.

Occlusion of the medullary portion of the anterior spinal artery is more often than not an extension of and overshadowed by more serious obstruction of the vertebral and perhaps the basilar artery.[85,86] Occlusion of the spinal portion of the spinal arteries is seen more often than that of the medullary portion and is associated with a distinct syndrome (sudden paraplegia, anesthesia of syringomyelic type, disturbances of urination and defecation). Occlusion of the posterior spinal artery occurs less often.

Etiology. The causes of these occlusions are varied.

Trauma. The trauma may be associated with damage sufficiently severe to cause thrombosis of the spinal vessels, which may be associated with vertebral dislocation.[38,152] Ischemic lesions can extend for several segments above or below the site of a cord injury.[170] Trauma involving segmental vessels in the thorax or abdomen rather than the spine may obstruct or even avulse an intercostal or lumbar artery and produce secondary effects on the cord.

Compression of the spinal arteries. Although venous compression is likely to precede it, anterior spinal artery compression can conceivably result from a number of space-occupying lesions or bony spurs. Local compression or obstruction of the anterior spinal artery or of its central branches may be responsible for the dissociated sensory disturbances and motor loss associated with herniation of an intervertebral disc.[360] Mair and Druckman[242] presented three instances of herniation of the nucleus pulposus in the cervical region causing lesions suggestive of obstruction to the anterior spinal artery.

The medullary or radicular arteries can be compressed by osteoarthritic spurs or other lesions while coursing through the intervertebral foramina. However, there is doubt whether such skeletal changes can be entirely responsible for the spinal cord changes. Metastatic tumor of the vertebrae, even primary tumors locally[170] or a cold abscess can compress either segmental, medullary, or spinal arteries.

Postoperative complications. With the advance in and progressive complexity of modern surgical techniques, an increase in the prevalence of spinal cord ischemic lesions has become evident.[4] Ligation, intentional or otherwise, of segmental vessels can be associated with severe spinal cord ischemia, and the procedure is particularly critical in the region of the diaphragm where the great anterior medullary artery may be deprived of its blood supply. It is a hazard of aortic grafting and repair for aortic coarctation and aneurysm,[174] sympathectomy,[262] and major chest surgery.[4] Clamping of the aorta above the renal arteries for more than about 18 minutes[4] in the absence of hypothermia or a shunt is dangerous. The clamping procedure is used experimentally in studies of spinal cord ischemia, but the critical times vary with the animal, the vascular anatomy of the cord, and the level of the aorta clamped.[311,360] Thrombosis of the posterior spinal arteries has resulted from intrathecal phenol injections for intractable pain.[180]

Atherosclerosis. Blackwood[38] in 1958 reported that in the autopsy records of the previous 50 years at the National Hospital for Nervous Diseases, London, no cases of spinal cord infarction had arisen from primary disease of the spinal arteries. However, spinal arteries are but small vessels and atherosclerosis rarely involves them directly. A mild or moderate degree of intimal thickening is quite frequent and frank atherosclerosis extremely rare, again because of the small caliber of the vessels. When the anterior spinal artery is greatly enlarged in coarctation of the aorta, thrombosis may occur,[107] but the vascular changes are seldom those classified as atherosclerosis. Cases in the literature purporting to exemplify atherosclerotic occlusion of the spinal arteries[144,390] are unconvincing and may well be instances of atheromatous embolism.

Gruner and Lapresle[154] reviewed 58 cases of spinal cord softening of vascular origin, 21 of which were attributed to primary arteriosclerosis. In 14 subjects, the softening affected the area supplied by the anterior spinal artery. In only three cases was the territory of the posterior spinal affected. In the remaining four, distribution was atypical and difficult to attribute to a particular spinal artery. The nature of the vascular lesion was variable, and in 11 of the 21 cases, arteriosclerosis of the intraspinal vessels was noted. Other lesions found were aortic atherosclerosis (eight cases), aortic aneurysm (two cases), rupture of a splenic artery (one case), and aortic embolism (one case), but neither thrombosis nor frank atherosclerosis of the spinal arteries was observed. Although arteriosclerosis may impair blood flow, frank acute infarction is not usually a manifestation, unless it is a necrotizing vascular lesion. The spinal cord ischemia in a large number of these cases remains undetermined.

Pathological changes in the spinal cord caused by sclerosis of the spinal vessels (excluding syphilis) are less frequent in the cord than in the brain. Keschner and Davison[210] found but two instances of cord involvement in approximately 200 autopsied cases of cerebral arteriosclerosis. Both exhibited severe degenerative changes in the cord and were attributed to such vascular changes as arteriosclerosis, severe atherosclerosis, and hyaline changes of spinal vessels.

Whether ischemia is the cause of chronic progressive disease of the spinal cord is debatable. Irregular cavitation in elderly patients presenting with progressive atrophic paraparesis with similarities to a motorneurone disease may be of vascular origin,[197] but a cause-and-effect relationship has not been firmly established.

Garland and associates,[142] in a review of spinal cord infarction, recorded six instances. Although definite causes were found for several (dissecting aneurysm of the aorta, spinal thrombophlebitis, ligation of intercostal arteries during aortic grafting), others remained unexplained. Henson and Parsons[170] reviewed spinal cord ischemia, briefly reporting the histories of many patients. They asserted that atherosclerosis had replaced syphilis as the commonest cause of spinal cord ischemia and attributed the ischemia to the aorta and its branches, listing the ill effects as follows:

1. Intermittent claudication of the cord with an impoverished blood supply, ischemia of which can be brought on by exertion. Attributed to the inability of sclerotic vessels to dilate, ischemia has been reproduced experimentally in dogs by ligating medullary arteries[289] and has been associated with thrombosis of the abdominal aorta.[286]
2. Transient ischemic attacks in the cord, analogous to those of the brain, may occur in isolation or as a prelude to frank infarction.
3. Frank infarction of the spinal cord is the most severe manifestation.

The pathogenesis of these lesions remains obscure, and histological studies of the spinal cord have been of little assistance. A precise knowledge of the pathology of medullary and segmental arteries is not easy to obtain because of the difficult and laborious dissection necessary to examine all the small vessels but dissection in association with postmortem angiography would help in elucidating the pathology of many of these lesions. Just as cerebral infarction and ischemia may result from disease of the extracranial arteries supplying the brain, so too spinal cord ischemia may succeed obstructive lesions of segmental and medullary arteries. Whether these lesions are atherosclerotic or embolic remains to be determined. In view of the prevalence and severity of aortic ulceration in man, emboli therefrom must pass into the segmental arteries in greater numbers than is currently recognized. Atheromatous emboli, if infrequently, have been observed in the spinal cord[247,321] and atherosclerotic narrowing of intercostal and lumbar arteries has been demonstrated by selective angiography.[97]

Thrombosis of the proximal end of a segmental artery could readily go unobserved at autopsy. Grosser lesions affect the aorta. Osler[269] reported that aortic aneurysms, known to erode the vertebral column, can occasionally compress the spinal cord, rupture into the spinal canal, or cause paraplegia by blocking the aorta. Crucial segmental vessels are more probably involved by the lesion. Dissecting aneurysms are notorious for causing spinal ischemia when dissection occludes or avulses segmental vessels (Fig. 4-39).

Hypotension. Hypotension, a cause of ischemia, usually complicates aortic atherosclerosis or some other factor interfering with the blood supply to the spinal cord. It occurs in elderly patients or in those with frequent Stokes-Adams attacks. Shock or a hypotensive episode seem to accentuate an impoverished blood supply to the cord. Experimentally, it is said to precipitate paraplegia after uneventful ligation of medullary arteries in dogs.[367] Levy and Strauss[229] recorded a unique case. The aorta of a severely exsanguinated young woman with postpartum hemorrhage had been subjected to intermittent compression for 2 hours, which resulted in paraplegia within the first postoperative week.

Miscellaneous causes. Ischemia of the cord may occur in aortic coarctation. The portion of the spinal cord lying above the level of the coarctation is well supplied

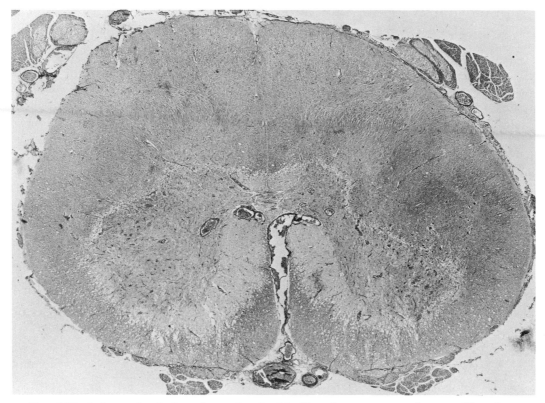

Fig. 4-39. Infarct of spinal cord associated with dissecting aneurysm of aorta. Note infarction of the two anterior horns and neighboring white matter. (Hematoxylin and eosin.)

with blood at a high pressure, but as with the lower limbs, the lower spinal cord, it is thought, occasionally suffers from a relative degree of ischemia. The symptoms and signs may be overshadowed by compression of the spinal cord by the enlarged and tortuous anterior spinal artery and rarely by a complicating aneurysm.

Emboli from endocarditic valves or occlusion of intraspinal vessels in malaria, caisson disease,[170] polyarteritis nodosa, and syphilitic arteritis have all been incriminated. Occlusion of the spinal arteries by tumor, possibly emboli, has been observed in several cases.[363]

Naiman and his colleagues[264] reported the case of a 15-year-old boy who died a little more than 3 hours after receiving an injury while engaged in sport. At autopsy, multiple arterial emboli of nucleus pulposus material, most numerous in the cer-

vical region and in the gray matter, were found involving a considerable segment of spinal cord and adjacent brain stem. The mode of access of the nucleus pulposus to the spinal arterial tree was obscure. It was suggested that the anterior spinal or anterior medullary artery was damaged and injected at the time of injury. The illustrations of arterial emboli were not convincing and the possibility that the lesions were caused by emboli via the vertebral venous system cannot be excluded.

Pathology of the infarct. Spinal cord infarction caused by these variable and often unexplained causes is usually pale, and the distribution may or may not correspond to the territory typical of the anterior or posterior spinal artery. Resolution of the infarcts is similar basically to that of the brain, and the softened area eventually becomes a cystic or collapsed gliosed area, possibly with a minor degree of encapsulation.

For reasons unknown, the anterior two-thirds of the spinal cord is implicated more frequently than the posterior third. The small size and the plexiform nature of the posterior spinal arteries may be factors. The areas of the cord most susceptible to ischemia lie at the junction or overlap of the areas of supply of adjacent medullary arteries, that is, the "border zone." When the cause of the ischemia is remote (aorta, intercostal or anterior medullary artery), the most susceptible area is the central region of the cord at the junction or overlap of the territories of anterior and posterior medullary arteries.[174] Such lesions do not differ significantly from the typical spinal artery occlusion. Unexplained ischemic foci (six in all), found in the anterior horns of five elderly subjects with severe atherosclerosis, were considered to be ischemic lacunar softenings,[119] which are, no doubt, frequent in such patients.

Venous infarction. The effect of venous occlusion on the cord is different from arterial occlusion. Because of the plexiform nature of the venous drainage, numbers of veins would need to be occluded before lesions would arise. Such is the case in spinal thrombophlebitis[38,142] where many thrombosed, recanalized, and occluded veins are seen histologically.[142] The clinical picture is of cord transection,[170] but pathologically the cord is eventually shrunken and gliosed, the white matter being severely affected. The gray matter, particularly the anterior horn cells, tends to be spared.[170]

References

1. Acheson, J., and Hutchinson, E. C.: Observations on the natural history of transient cerebral ischaemia, Lancet 2:871, 1964.
2. Adams, C. W. M.: Vascular histochemistry, Chicago, 1967, Year Book Medical Publishers, Inc.
3. Adams, G. F., and Merrett, J. D.: Prognosis and survival in the aftermath of hemiplegia, Brit. Med. J. 1:309, 1961.
4. Adams, H. D., and Boyd, D. P.: Complications of thoracic surgery, Surg. Clin. N. Amer. 37:615, 1957.
5. Adams, J. H., and Graham, D. I.: Twelve cases of fatal cerebral infarction due to arterial occlusion in the absence of atheromatous stenosis or embolism, J. Neurol. Neurosurg. Psychiat. 30:479, 1967.
6. Adams, R. D., and Fisher, C. M.: Pathology of cerebral arterial occlusion. In Fields, W. S.: Pathogenesis and treatment of cerebrovascular disease, Springfield, 1961, Charles C Thomas, Publisher, p. 126.
7. Adams, R. D., and Vander Eecken, H. M.: Vascular diseases of the brain, Ann. Rev. Med. 4:213, 1953.
8. Agee, O. F.: Two unusual cases of subclavian steal syndrome, Amer. J. Roentgen. 97:447, 1966.
9. Aguayo, A. J.: Cerebral thrombo-embolism in malignancy, Arch Neurol. 11:500, 1964.
10. Alajouanine, T., Lhermitte, F., and Gautier, J. C.: Transient cerebral ischemia in atherosclerosis, Neurology 10:906, 1960.
11. Allen, A. C., and Sirota, J. H.: The morphogenesis and significance of degenerative verrucal endocardiosis (terminal endocarditis, endocarditis simplex, nonbacterial thrombotic endocarditis), Amer. J. Path. 20:1025, 1944.
12. Alpers, B. J., and Forster, F. M.: The reparative processes in subarachnoid hemorrhage, J. Neuropath. Exp. Neurol. 4:262, 1945.
13. Altshuler, J. H., McLaughlin, R. A., and Neuburger, K. T., Neurological catastrophe related to oral contraceptives, Arch. Neurol. 19: 264, 1968.
14. Alvarez, W. C.: The little strokes, J.A.M.A. 157:1199, 1955.
15. Annotation: Oestrogen content of oral contraceptives, Lancet 2:1345, 1969.
16. Antia, A. U., and Ottesen, O. E.: Collateral circulation in subclavian stenosis or atresia, Amer. J. Cardiol. 18:599, 1966.
17. Aring, C. D., and Merritt, H. H.: Differential diagnosis between cerebral hemorrhage and cerebral thrombosis, Arch. Intern. Med. 56: 435, 1935.
18. Aronson, S. M., and Aronson, B. E.: Ischemic cerebral vascular disease, N. Y. State Med. J. 66:954, 1966.
19. Aronson, S. M., and Rabiner, A. M.: Studies on vascular encephalomalacia: evaluation of clinical syndromes in five hundred consecutive cases studied pathologically, Arch. Neurol. Psychiat. 80:324, 1958.
20. Ask-Upmark, E., Glas, J., and Stenram, U.: Oral contraceptives and cerebral arterial thrombosis, Acta Med. Scand. 185:479, 1969.
21. Atkinson, E. A., Fairburn, B., and Heathfield, K. W. G.: Intracranial venous thrombosis as complication of oral contraception, Lancet 1: 914, 1970.
22. Bailey, O. T., and Hass, G. M.: Dural sinus thrombosis in early life: recovery from acute thrombosis of the superior longitudinal sinus and its relation to certain acquired cerebral lesions in childhood, Brain 60:293, 1937.
23. Bailey, O. T., and Hass, G. M.: Dural sinus thrombosis in early life. I. The clinical man-

ifestations and extent of brain injury in acute sinus thrombosis, J. Pediat. **11:**755, 1937.

24. Baker, A. B., Dahl, E., and Sandler, B.: Cerebrovascular disease, Neurology **13:**445, 1963.
25. Baker, R. N., Schwartz, W. S., and Ramseyer, J. C.: Prognosis among survivors of ischemic stroke, Neurology **18:**933, 1968.
26. Barnett, H. J. M., and Hyland, H. H.: Noninfective intracranial venous thrombosis, Brain **76:**36, 1953.
27. Barnett, H. J. M., Wortzman, G., Gladstone, R. M., and Lougheed, W. M.: Diversion and reversal of cerebral blood flow, Neurology **20:**1, 1970.
28. Barron, K. D., Siqueira, E., and Hirano, A.: Cerebral embolism caused by non-bacterial thrombotic endocarditis, Neurology **10:**391, 1960.
29. Battacharji, S. K., Hutchinson, E. C., and McCall, A. J.: Stenosis and occlusion of vessels in cerebral infarction, Brit. Med. J. **3:**270, 1967.
30. Bauer, R. B.: Evaluation of the stroke patient with respect to associated diseases. In Fields, W. S., and Spencer, W. A.: Stroke rehabilitation, basic concepts and research trends, St. Louis, 1967, Warren H. Green, Inc., p. 31.
31. Bergentz, S.: Studies on the genesis of posttraumatic fat embolism, Acta Chir. Scand. vol. 123, suppl. 282, 1961.
32. Bering, E. A., and Salibi, B.: Production of hydrocephalus by increased cephalic-venous pressure, Arch. Neurol. Psychiat. **81:**693, 1959.
33. Berry, R. G.: The vascular lesion in cerebral softenings, Trans. Amer. Neurol. Ass. **84:**49, 1959.
34. Berry, R. G., and Alpers, B. J.: Occlusion of the carotid circulation, Neurology **7:**223, 1957.
35. Berthrong, M., and Sabiston, D. C.: Cerebral lesions in congenital heart disease, Bull. Johns Hopkins Hosp. **89:**384, 1951.
36. Bickerstaff, E. R.: Aetiology of acute hemiplegia in childhood, Brit. Med. J. **2:**82, 1964.
37. Biemond, A.: Thrombosis of the basilar artery and the vascularization of the brain stem, Brain **74:**300, 1951.
38. Blackwood, W.: Discussion on vascular disease of the spinal cord, Proc. Roy. Soc. Med. **51:**543, 1958.
39. Blackwood, W.: Vascular disease of the central nervous system. In Blackwood, W., McMenemey, W. H., Meyer, A., Norman, R. M., and Russell, D. S.: Greenfield's neuropathology, ed. 2, Baltimore, 1963, The Williams & Wilkins Co., p. 71.
40. Blackwood, W., Hallpike, J. F., Kocen, R. S., and Mair, W. G. P.: Atheromatous disease of the carotid arterial system and embolism from the heart in cerebral infarction: a morbid anatomical study, Brain **92:**897, 1969.
41. Bladin, P. F.: A radiologic and pathologic study of embolism of the internal carotid–middle cerebral arterial axis, Radiology **82:**615, 1964.
42. Blakemore, W. S., Hardesty, W. H., Bevil-

acqua, J. E., and Tristan, T. A.: Reversal of blood flow in the right vertebral artery accompanying occlusion of the innominate artery, Ann. Surg. **161:**353, 1965.
43. Boldrey, E., Maass, L., and Miller, E.: The role of atlantoid compression in the etiology of internal carotid thrombosis, J. Neurosurg. **13:**127, 1956.
44. Brain, M. C.: Microangiopathic hemolytic anemia, Ann. Rev. Med. **21:**133, 1970.
45. Braun, A.: The pathology of sinus thrombosis, Ann. Otol. **27:**461, 1918.
46. Brice, J. G., and Crompton, M. R.: Spontaneous dissecting aneurysms of the cervical internal carotid artery, Brit. Med. J. **2:**790, 1964.
47. Bruetman, M. E., Fields, W. S., Crawford, E. S., and De Bakey, M. E.: Cerebral hemorrhage in carotid artery surgery, Arch. Neurol. **9:**458, 1963.
48. Buchanan, D. S., and Brazinsky, J. H.: Dural sinus and cerebral venous thrombosis, Arch. Neurol. **22:**440, 1970.
49. Bucy, P. C., and Lesemann, F. J.: Idiopathic recurrent thrombophlebitis with cerebral venous thromboses and an acute subdural hematoma, J.A.M.A. **119:**402, 1942.
50. Byers, R. K., and Hass, G. M.: Thrombosis of the dural venous sinuses in infancy and in childhood, Amer. J. Dis. Child. **45:**1161, 1933.
51. Callow, A. D., Moran, J. M., Kahn, P. C., and Deterling, R. A.: Patterns of atherosclerosis of extracranial cerebral arteries, Ann. N. Y. Acad. Sci. **149:**974, 1968.
52. Carpenter, S.: Injury of neck as cause of vertebral artery thrombosis, J. Neurosurg. **18:**849, 1961.
53. Carroll, J. D., Leak, D., and Lee, H. A.: Cerebral thrombo-phlebitis in pregnancy and the puerperium, Quart. J. Med. **35:**347, 1966.
54. Carter, A. B.: Ingravescent cerebral infarction, Quart. J. Med. **29:**611, 1959.
55. Carter, A. B.: Strokes, Proc. Roy. Soc. Med. **56:**483, 1963.
56. Carter, A. B.: Cerebral infarction, New York, 1964, The Macmillan Co.
57. Carter, A. B.: Prognosis of cerebral embolism, Lancet **2:**514, 1965.
58. Castaigne, P., Lhermitte, R., Gautier, J.-C., Escourolle, R., and Derouesné, C.: Internal carotid artery occlusion, Brain **93:**231, 1970.
59. Cates, J. E., and Christie, R. V.: Subacute bacterial endocarditis, Quart. J. Med. **20:**93, 1951.
60. Chase, T. N., Rosman, N. P., and Price, D. L.: The cerebral syndromes associated with dissecting aneurysm of the aorta, Brain **91:**173, 1968.
61. Chase, W. H.: Cerebral thrombosis, hemorrhage and embolism, pathological principles. In: The circulation of the brain and spinal cord, Ass. Res. Nerv. Ment. Dis. **18:**365, 1938.
62. Chason, J. L.: Brain, meninges and spinal cord. In Saphir, O.: A text on systemic pathology, New York, 1959, Grune & Stratton, Inc., vol. 2, p. 1798.
63. Chiang, J., Kowada, M., Ames, A., Wright,

R. L., and Majno, G.: Cerebral ischemia. III. Vascular changes, Amer. J. Path. **52**:455, 1968.

64. Chiari, H.: Über das Verhalten des Teilungswinkels der Carotis communis bei der Endarteriitis chronica deformans, Verh. Deutsch. Path. Ges. **9**:326, 1905. Cited by Fisher.[130]

65. Choi, S. S., and Crampton, A.: Atherosclerosis of arteries of neck, Arch. Path. **72**:379, 1961.

66. Clarke, P. R. R., Dickson, J., and Smith, B. J.: Traumatic thrombosis of the internal carotid artery following a non-penetrating injury and leading to infarction of the brain, Brit. J. Surg. **43**:215, 1955-1956.

67. Coder, D. M., Frye, R. L., Bernatz, P. E., and Sheps, S. G.: Symptomatic bilateral "subclavian steal," Mayo Clin. Proc. **40**:473, 1965.

68. Cone, W., and Barrera, S. E.: The brain and the cerebrospinal fluid in acute aseptic cerebral embolism, Arch. Neurol. Psychiat. **25**:523, 1931.

69. Connett, M. C., and Lansche, J. M.: Fibromuscular hyperplasia of the internal carotid artery, Ann. Surg. **162**:59, 1965.

70. Connor, L. A., and Holt, E.: The subsequent course and prognosis in coronary thrombosis, Amer. Heart J. **5**:705, 1929-1930.

71. Constantinides, P.: Pathogenesis of cerebral artery thrombosis in man, Arch. Path. **83**:422, 1967.

72. Courville, C. B.: Pathology of the central nervous system, Mountain View, Calif., 1937, Pacific Press Publishing Association.

73. Cross, J. N., Castro, P. O., Jennett, W. B.: Cerebral strokes associated with pregnancy and the puerperium, Brit. Med. J. **3**:214, 1968.

74. Cruickshank, A. H.: Venous thrombosis in internal organs associated with thrombosis of leg veins, J. Path. Bact. **71**:383, 1956.

75. Cullen, C. F., and Swank, R. L.: Intravascular aggregation and adhesiveness of the blood elements associated with alimentary lipemia and injections of large molecular substances, Circulation **9**:335, 1954.

76. Dalal, P. M., Shah, P. M., and Aiyar, R. R.: Arteriographic study of cerebral embolism, Lancet **2**:358, 1965.

77. Dalal, P. M., Shah, P. M., Aiyar, R. R., and Kikani, B. J.: Cerebrovascular diseases in west central India, Brit. Med. J. **3**:769, 1968.

78. Dalal, P. M., Shah, P. M., Deshpande, C. K., and Sheth, S. C.: Recanalisation after cerebral embolism, Lancet **2**:495, 1966.

79. Dalal, P. M., Shah, P. M., Sheth, S. C., and Deshpande, C. K.: Cerebral embolism, Lancet **1**:61, 1965.

80. Dardik, H., Gensler, S., Stern, W. Z., and Glotzer, P.: Subclavian steal syndrome secondary to embolism, Ann. Surg. **164**:171, 1966.

81. David, N. J., and Heyman, A.: Factors influencing the prognosis of cerebral thrombosis and infarction due to atherosclerosis, J. Chronic Dis. **11**:394, 1960.

82. David, N. J., Klintworth, G. K., Friedberg, S. J., and Dillon, M.: Fatal atheromatous cerebral embolism associated with bright plaques in the retinal arterioles, Neurology **13**:708, 1963.

83. Davie, J. C., and Coxe, W.: Occlusive disease of the carotid artery in children, Arch. Neurol. **17**:313, 1967.

84. Davis, D. O., Rumbaugh, C. L., and Gilson, J. M.: Angiographic diagnosis of small-vessel cerebral emboli, Acta Radiol. **9**:264, 1969.

85. Davison, C.: Syndrome of the anterior spinal artery of the medulla oblongata, Arch. Neurol. Psych. **37**:91, 1937.

86. Davison, C.: Syndrome of the anterior spinal artery of the medulla oblongata, J. Neuropath. Exp. Neurol. **3**:73, 1944.

87. Davison, C., and Spiegel, L. A.: The syndrome of the posterior inferior cerebellar artery resulting from a metastatic neoplasm, J. Neuropath. Exp. Neurol. **4**:172, 1945.

88. Day, J. M.: Death due to cerebral infarction after wasp stings, Arch. Neurol. **7**:185, 1962.

89. De Bakey, M. E., Crawford, E. S., Cooley, D. A., and Morris, G. C.: Surgical considerations of occlusive disease of innominate, carotid, subclavian, and vertebral arteries, Ann. Surg. **149**:690, 1959.

90. de la Torre, E., Meredith, J., and Netsky, M. G.: Cerebral air embolism in the dog, Arch. Neurol. **6**:307, 1962.

91. Denny-Brown, D.: The treatment of recurrent cerebrovascular symptoms and the question of "vasospasm," Med. Clin. N. Amer. **35**:1457, 1951.

92. Denny-Brown, D.: Recurrent cerebrovascular episodes, Arch. Neurol. **2**:194, 1960.

93. Denny-Brown, D., and Meyer, J. S.: The cerebral collateral circulation. 2. Production of cerebral infarction by ischemic anoxia and its reversibility in early stages, Neurology **7**:567, 1957.

94. Derrick, J. R.: Carotid kinking and cerebral insufficiency, Geriatrics **18**:272, 1963.

95. Derrick, J. R., and Smith, T.: Carotid kinking as a cause of cerebral insufficiency, Circulation **25**:849, 1962.

96. Dixon, K. C.: Ischaemia and the neurone. In Adams, C. W. M.: Neurohistochemistry, Amsterdam, 1965, Elsevier Publishing Co., p. 558.

97. Djindjian, R., Hurth, M., and Houdart, R.: Artériographie et ischémie médullaire dorsolombaire d'origine athéromateuse, Rev. Neurol. **122**:5, 1970.

98. Doniger, D. E.: Bilateral complete carotid and basilar artery occlusion in a patient with minimal deficit, Neurology **13**:673, 1963.

99. Dooley, J. M., and Smith, K. R.: Occlusion of the basilar artery in a 6-year-old boy, Neurology **18**:1034, 1968.

100. Dott, N., and Blackwood, W.: Communication to the Society of British Surgeons, 1952. Cited by Wolman.[383]

101. Drummond, D. S., Salter, R. B., and Boone, J.: Fat embolism in children: its frequency and relationship to collagen disease, Canad. Med. Ass. J. **101**:200, 1969.

102. Durant, T. M., Long, J., and Oppenheimer,

M. J.: Pulmonary (venous) air embolism, Amer. Heart J. **33:**269, 1947.

103. Durant, T. M., Oppenheimer, M. J., Lynch, P. R., Ascanio, G., and Webber, D.: Body position in relation to venous air embolism: a roentgenologic study, Amer. J. Med. Sci. **227:**509, 1954.

104. Editorial: A new vascular syndrome—"the subclavian steal," New Eng. J. Med. **265:**912, 1961.

105. Editorial: Consumption coagulopathy in septicemic shock, New Eng. J. Med. **279:**884, 1968.

106. Editorial: Cerebral ischaemia: need for a more active policy, Lancet **1:**743, 1971.

107. Edwards, J. E.: Pathology of anomalies of the thoracic aorta, Amer. J. Clin. Path. **23:**1240, 1953.

108. Eisenberg, H., Morrison, J. T., Sullivan, P., and Foote, F. M.: Cerebrovascular accidents, J.A.M.A. **189:**883, 1964.

109. Eliot, R. S., Kanjuh, V. I., and Edwards, J. E.: Atheromatous embolism, Circulation **30:**611, 1964.

110. Elkeles, R. S., Hampton, J. R., and Mitchell, J. R. A.: Effect of oestrogens on human platelet behavior, Lancet **2:**315, 1968.

111. Faris, A. A., Hardin, C. A., and Poser, C. M.: Pathogenesis of hemorrhagic infarction of the brain. 1. Experimental investigations of role of hypertension and of collateral circulation, Arch. Neurol. **9:**468, 1963.

112. Fazio, C.: Red softening of the brain, J. Neuropath. Exp. Neurol. **8:**43, 1949.

113. Fazio, C.: 'Haemodynamic' factors in pathogenesis of brain infarct, Europ. Neurol. **2:**76, 1969.

114. Ferrand, J.: Essai sur l'hémiplégie des vieillards. Les lacunes de désintégration cérébrale, Thesis, 1902, Paris. Cited by Fisher.[124]

115. Fields, W. S.: Reflections on "the subclavian steal," Stroke **1:**320, 1970.

116. Fields, W. S., Crawford, E. S., and De Bakey, M. E.: Surgical considerations in cerebral arterial insufficiency, Neurology **8:**801, 1958.

117. Fields, W. S., North, R. R., Hass, W. K., Galbraith, J. G., Wylie, E. J., Ratinov, G., Burns, M. H., MacDonald, M. C., and Meyer, J. S.: Joint study of extracranial arterial occlusion as a cause of stroke I. Organization of study and survey of patient population, J.A.M.A. **203:**955, 1968.

118. Fieschi, C., and Bozzao, L.: Transient embolic occlusion of the middle cerebral internal carotid arteries in cerebral apoplexy, J. Neurol. Neurosurg. Psychiat. **32:**236, 1969.

119. Fieschi, C., Gottlieb, A., and De Carolis, V.: Ischaemic lacunae in the spinal cord of arteriosclerotic subjects, J. Neurol. Neurosurg. Psychiat. **33:**138, 1970.

120. Fisher, A. C., Fisher, M. M., and Lendrum, A. C.: Tropical primary phlebitis, J. Path. Bact. **59:**405, 1947.

121. Fisher, C. M.: Early-life carotid-artery occlusion associated with late intracranial hemorrhage, Lab. Invest. **8:**680, 1959.

122. Fisher, C. M.: Observations of the fundus oculi in transient monocular blindness, Neurology **9:**333, 1959.

123. Fisher, C. M.: Clinical syndromes in cerebral arteries occlusion. In Fields, W. S.: Pathogenesis and treatment of cerebrovascular disease, Springfield, Ill., 1961, Charles C Thomas, Publisher, p. 151.

124. Fisher, C. M.: Lacunes: small deep cerebral infarcts, Neurology **15:**774, 1965.

125. Fisher, C. M.: A lacunar stroke, Neurology **17:**614, 1967.

126. Fisher, C. M.: The arterial lesions underlying lacunes, Acta Neuropath. **12:**1, 1969.

127. Fisher, C. M.: Occlusion of the vertebral arteries, Arch. Path. **22:**13, 1970.

128. Fisher, C. M., and Cole, M.: Homolateral ataxia and crural paresis: a vascular syndrome, J. Neurol. Neurosurg. Psychiat. **28:**48, 1965.

129. Fisher, C. M., and Curry, H. B.: Pure motor hemiplegia of vascular origin, Arch. Neurol. **13:**30, 1965.

130. Fisher, M.: Occlusion of the internal carotid artery, Arch. Neurol. Psychiat. **65:**346, 1951.

131. Fisher, M.: Transient monocular blindness associated with hemiplegia, Arch. Ophthal. **47:**167, 1952.

132. Fisher, M.: Occlusion of the carotid arteries, Arch. Neurol. Psychiat. **72:**187, 1954.

133. Fisher, M., and Adams, R. D.: Observations on brain embolism with special reference to the mechanism of hemorrhagic infarction, J. Neuropath. Exp. Neurol. **10:**92, 1951.

134. Fletcher, A. P., and Alkaersig, N.: Cerebral infarction and oral contraceptive agents. In Toole, J. F., Moosy, J., and Janeway, R.: Cerebral vascular diseases, Seventh Princeton Conference, New York, 1971, Grune & Stratton, Inc., p. 188.

135. Flory, C. M.: Arterial occlusions produced by emboli from eroded aortic atheromatous plaques, Amer. J. Path. **21:**549, 1945.

136. Foley, J. M.: Hypertensive and arteriosclerotic vascular disease of the brain in the elderly. In: The neurologic and psychiatric aspects of the disorders of aging, Ass. Res. Nerv. Ment. Dis. **35:**171, 1956.

137. Folger, G. M., and Shah, K. D.: Subclavian steal in patients with Blalock-Taussig anastomosis, Circulation **31:**241, 1965.

138. Ford, F. R.: Syncope, vertigo, and disturbances of vision resulting from intermittent obstruction of the vertebral arteries due to defect in the odontoid process and excessive mobility of the second cervical vertebra, Bull. Johns Hopkins Hosp. **41:**168, 1952.

139. Ford, F. R., and Clark, D.: Thrombosis of the basilar artery with softenings in the cerebellum and brain stem due to manipulation of the neck, Bull. Johns Hopkins Hosp. **98:**37, 1956.

140. Fuchsig, P., Brücke, P., Blümel, G., and Gottlob, R.: A new clinical and experimental concept on fat embolism, New Eng. J. Med. **276:**1192, 1967.

141. Gardner, J. H., Van Den Noort, S., and Horenstein, S.: Cerebrovascular disease in young

women taking oral contraceptives, Neurology **17**:297, 1967.

142. Garland, H., Greenberg, J., and Harriman, D. G. F.: Infarction of the spinal cord, Brain **89**:645, 1966.

143. Garland, H., and Pearce, J.: Carotid arteritis as a cause of cerebral ischaemia in the adult, Lancet **1**:993, 1965.

144. Garstka, M.: Atherosclerotic occlusion of nutrient branches of the anterior spinal artery, Ill. Med. J. **103**:305, 1953.

145. Garvin, C. F.: Mural thrombi in the heart, Amer. Heart J. **21**:713, 1941.

146. Gerber, N.: Congenital atresia of the subclavian artery, Amer. J. Dis. Child. **113**:709, 1967.

147. Gillilan, L. A.: The arterial and venous blood supplies to the cerebellum of primates, J. Neuropath. Exp. Neurol. **28**:295, 1969.

148. Gilroy, J., and Meyer, J. S.: Pituitary insufficiency with cerebrovascular symptoms, New Eng. J. Med. **269**:1115, 1963.

149. Gore, I., and Collins, D. P.: Spontaneous atheromatous embolization, Amer. J. Clin. Path. **33**:416, 1960.

150. Gore, I., McCombs, H. L., and Lindquist, R. L.: Observations on the fate of cholesterol emboli, J. Atheroscler. Res. **4**:527, 1964.

151. Graham, D. I., and Adams, J. H.: Ischaemic brain damage in fatal head injuries, Lancet **1**:265, 1971.

152. Grinker, R. R., and Guy, C. C.: Sprain of cervical spine causing thrombosis of anterior spinal artery, J.A.M.A. **88**:1140, 1927.

153. Gruenwald, P.: Emboli of brain tissue in fetal lungs, Amer. J. Path. **17**:879, 1941.

154. Gruner, J., and Lapresle, J.: Étude anatomo-pathologique des médullopathie d'origine vasculaire, Rev. Neurol. **106**:592, 1962.

155. Gull, W.: Thickening and dilatation of the aorta, with occlusion of the innominata and left carotid, atrophic softening of the brain, Guy's Hosp. Rep. (Series 3), **1**:12, 1855.

156. Gurdjian, E. S., Hardy, W. G., Lindner, D. W., and Thomas, L. M.: Analysis of occlusive disease of the carotid artery and the stroke syndrome, J.A.M.A. **176**:194, 1961.

157. Haas, J. E., Dekker, A., Perri, J. A., and Mankin, H. J.: Fat in cerebrospinal fluid: possible significance in the diagnosis of fat embolism, J. Trauma **8**:593, 1968.

158. Hain, R. F., Westhaysen, P. V., and Swank, R. L.: Hemorrhagic cerebral infarction by arterial occlusion, J. Neuropath. Exp. Neurol. **11**:34, 1952.

159. Hammes, E. M.: Reaction of the meninges to blood, Arch. Neurol. Psychiat. **52**:505, 1944.

160. Handler, F. P.: Clinical and pathologic significance of atheromatous embolization with emphasis on an etiology of renal hypertension, Amer. J. Med. **20**:366, 1956.

161. Hardin, C. A.: Vertebral artery insufficiency produced by cervical osteoarthritic spurs, Arch. Surg. **90**:629, 1965.

162. Hardin, C. A., and Poser, C. M.: Rotational obstruction of the vertebral artery due to

163. Harrison, M. T., and Gibb, B. H.: Electrocardiographic changes associated with a cerebrovascular accident, Lancet **2**:429, 1964.

164. Hart, M. N., and Cyrus, A.: Hyaline globules of the adrenal medulla, Amer. J. Clin. Path. **49**:387, 1968.

165. Hartveit, F., Lystad, H., and Minken, A.: The pathology of venous air embolism, Brit. J. Exp. Path. **49**:81, 1968.

166. Harvey, J., and Rasmussen, T.: Occlusion of the middle cerebral artery, Arch. Neurol. Psychiat. **66**:20, 1951.

167. Hass, W. K., Fields, W. S., North, R. R., Kricheff, I. I., Chase, N. E., and Bauer, R. B.: Joint Study of extracranial arterial occlusion. II. Arteriography, techniques, sites and complications, J.A.M.A. **203**:961, 1968.

168. Haymaker, W., and Davison, C.: Fatalities resulting from exposure to simulated high altitudes in decompression chambers, J. Neuropath. Exp. Neurol. **9**:29, 1950.

169. Heidrich, H., and Bayer, O.: Symptomatology of the subclavian steal syndrome, Angiology **20**:406, 1969.

170. Henson, R. A., and Parsons, M.: Ischaemic lesions of the spinal cord: on illustrated review, Quart. J. Med. **36**:205, 1967.

171. Hicks, S. P., and Warren, S.: Infarction of the brain without thrombosis, Arch. Path. **52**:403, 1951.

172. Hill, N. C., Millikan, C. H., Wakim, K. G., and Sayre, G. P.: Studies in cerebrovascular disease. VII. Experimental production of cerebral infarction by intracarotid injection of homologous blood clot, Proc. Staff Meet. Mayo Clin. **30**:625, 1955.

173. Hockaday, T. D. R.: Traumatic thrombosis of the internal carotid artery, J. Neurol. Neurosurg. Psychiat. **22**:229, 1959.

174. Hogan, E. L., and Romanul, F. C. A.: Spinal cord infarction occurring during insertion of aortic graft, Neurology **16**:67, 1966.

175. Hollenhorst, R. W.: Significance of bright plaques in the retinal arterioles, J.A.M.A. **178**:23, 1961.

176. Hollenhorst, R. W.: Carotid and vertebral-basilar arterial stenosis and occlusion: neuro-ophthalmologic considerations, Trans. Amer. Acad. Ophthal. Otolaryng. **66**:166, 1962.

177. Höök, O. Lidvall, H., and Åström, K.-E.: Cervical disk protrusions with compression of the spinal cord, Neurology **10**:834, 1960.

178. Horne, C. H. W., Weir, R. J., Howie, P. W., and Goudie, R. B.: Effect of combined oestrogen-progestogen oral contraceptives on serum-levels of α_2-macroglobulin, transferrin, albumin, and I_gG, Lancet **1**:49, 1970.

179. Hueper, W. C.: Arteriosclerosis, Arch. Path. **39**:117, 187, 1945.

180. Hughes, J. T.: Thrombosis of the posterior spinal arteries, Neurology **20**:659, 1970.

181. Hughes, J. T., and Brownell, B.: Traumatic thrombosis of the internal carotid artery in

the neck, J. Neurol. Neurosurg. Psychiat. **31:** 307, 1968.

182. Hultquist, G. T.: Über Thrombose und Embolie der Arteria carotis und hierbei vorkommende Gehirnveränderungen, Jena, 1942, Gustav Fischer Verlag. Cited by Fisher.[130]

183. Humphrey, J. G., and Newton, T. H.: Internal carotid artery occlusion in young adults, Brain **83:**565, 1960.

184. Hunder, G. G., Ward, L. M., and Burbank, M. K.: Giant-cell arteritis producing an aortic arch syndrome, Ann. Intern. Med. **66:**578, 1967.

185. Hunt, J. R.: The role of the carotid arteries, in the causation of the vascular lesions of the brain, with remarks on certain special features of the symptomatology, Amer. J. Med. Sci. **147:**704, 1914.

186. Hutchinson, E. C.: Little strokes, Brit. Med. J. **4:**32, 1969.

187. Hutchinson, E. C., and Yates, P. O.: The cervical portion of the vertebral artery: a clinicopathological study, Brain **79:**319, 1956.

188. Hutchinson, E. C., and Yates, P. O.: Caroticovertebral stenosis, Lancet **1:**2, 1957.

189. Inman, W. H. W., Vessey, M. P., Westerholm, B., and Engelund, A.: Thromboembolic disease and the steroidal content of oral contraceptives. A report to the committee on safety of drugs, Brit. Med. J. **2:**203, 1970.

190. Irey, N. S., Manion, W. C., and Taylor, H. B.: Vascular lesions in women taking oral contraceptives, Arch. Path. **89:**1, 1970.

191. Irish, C. W.: Sinus thrombosis. Part IV. Venous thrombosis: thrombosis of the superior cerebral vein, Ann. Otol. **47:**775, 1938.

192. Irvine, W. T., Luck, R. J., and Jacobey, J. A.: Reversed blood-flow in the vertebral arteries causing recurrent brain-stem ischaemia, Lancet **1:**994, 1965.

193. Irvine, W. T., Luck, R. J., Sutton, D., and Walpita, P. R.: Intrathoracic occlusion of great vessels causing cerebrovascular insufficiency, Lancet **1:**1177, 1963.

194. Janeway, R., Toole, J. F., Leinbach, L. B., and Miller, H. S.: Vertebral artery obstruction with basilar impression, Arch. Neurol. **15:**211, 1966.

195. Janon, E. A.: Traumatic changes in the internal carotid artery associated with basal skull fractures, Radiology **96:**55, 1970.

196. Javid, H., Julian, O. C., Dye, W. S., and Hunter, J. A.: Management of cerebral arterial insufficiency caused by reversal of flow, Arch. Surg. **90:**634, 1965.

197. Jellinger, K., and Neumayer, E.: Myélopathies progressives d'origine vasculaire, Rev. Neurol. **106:**666, 1962.

198. Jensen, A. M.: Sinus thrombosis and otogene sepsis, Acta Otolaryng. **55:**237, 1962.

199. Johnson, D. R., and Chalgren, W. S.: Polycythemia vera and the nervous system, Neurology **1:**53, 1951.

200. Johnson, H. C., and Walker, A. E.: The angiographic diagnosis of spontaneous thrombosis of the internal and common carotid arteries, J. Neurosurg. **8:**631, 1951.

201. Johnson, R. V., Kaplan, S. R., and Blailock, Z. R.: Cerebral venous thrombosis in paroxysmal nocturnal hemoglobinuria, Neurology **20:** 681, 1970.

202. Jones, H. R., Siekert, R. G., and Geraci, J. E.: Neurologic manifestations of bacterial endocarditis, Ann. Intern. Med. **71:**21, 1969.

203. Jörgensen, L., and Torvik, A.: Ischaemic cerebrovascular diseases in an autopsy series. Part I. Prevalence, location and predisposing factors in vertified thromboembolic occlusions and their significance in the pathogenesis of cerebral infarction, J. Neurol. Sci. **3:**490, 1966.

204. Joynt, R. J., Zimmerman, G., and Khalifeh, R.: Cerebral emboli from cardiac tumors, Arch. Neurol. **12:**84, 1965.

205. Kalbag, R. M., and Woolf, A. L.: Cerebral venous thrombosis, London, 1967, Oxford University Press.

206. Kane, W. C., and Aronson, S. M.: Cardiac disorders predisposing to embolic stroke, Stroke **1:**164, 1970.

207. Kapp, J., Cook, W., and Paulson, G.: Chronic brain syndrome, Geriatrics **21:**174, 1966.

208. Kendall, D.: Thrombosis of intracranial veins, Brain **71:**386, 1948.

209. Kerstell, J., Hallgren, B., Rudenstam, C.-M., and Svanborg, A.: The chemical composition of the fat emboli in the post-absorptive dog, Acta Med. Scand. Suppl. **499:**3, 1969.

210. Keschner, M., and Davison, C.: Myelitic and myelopathic lesions. III. Arteriosclerotic and arteritic myelopathy, Arch. Neurol. Psychiat. **29:**702, 1933.

211. Kinal, M. E.: Hydrocephalus and the dural venous sinuses, J. Neurosurg. **19:**195, 1962.

212. Kinal, M. E., and Jaeger, R. M.: Thrombophlebitis of dural venous sinuses following otitis media, J. Neurosurg. **17:**81, 1960.

213. Kleihues, P., Tehrani, M., and Tschangisian, H.: The distribution and effect on the brain of metallic microemboli following arterial and venous injection: In Meyer, J. S., Lechner, H., and Eichhorn, O.: Research on the cerebral circulation, Springfield, Ill., 1969, Charles C Thomas, Publisher, p. 286.

214. Knisely, M. H.: The settling of sludge during life, Acta Anat. **44:** Suppl. 41, 1961.

215. Krakower, C.: Pulmonary embolus containing cerebral tissue, Arch. Path. **22:**113, 1936.

216. Krinsky, C., N., and Merritt, H. H.: Neurologic manifestations of subacute bacterial endocarditis, New Eng. J. Med. **218:**563, 1938.

217. Kubik, C. S., and Adams, R. D.: Occlusion of the basilar artery—a clinical and pathological study, Brain **69:**73, 1946.

218. Kudo, T.: Spontaneous occlusion of the circle of Willis, Neurology **18:**485, 1968.

219. Kurtzke, J. F.: Epidemiology of cerebrovascular disease, Heidelberg, 1969, Springer-Verlag.

220. Lack, A. R.: The occurrence of intravascular agglutination in avian malaria, Science **96:** 520, 1942.

221. Lascelles, R. G., and Burrows, E. H.: Occlu-

sion of the middle cerebral artery, Brain **88:** 85, 1965.

222. Lavy, S., and Kahana, E.: Cerebral arterial occlusion during pregnancy and puerperium, Obstet. Gynec. **35:**916, 1970.

223. Lavy, S., Stern, S., Herishianu, Y., and Carmon, A.: Electrocardiographic changes in ischaemic stroke, J. Neurol. Sci. **7:**409, 1968.

224. Leading article: Blood-groups and thromboembolism, Lancet **1:**561, 1969.

225. Lehman, E. P., and Moore, R. M.: Fat embolism, Arch. Surg. **14:**621, 1927.

226. Lehrich, J. R., Winkler, G. F., and Ojemann, R. G.: Cerebellar infarction with brain stem compression, Arch. Neurol. **22:**490, 1970.

227. Lehv, M. S., Salzman, E. W., and Silen, W.: Hypertension complicating carotid endarterectomy, Stroke **1:**307, 1970.

228. Levine, S.: Anoxic-ischemic encephalopathy in rats, Amer. J. Path. **36:**1, 1960.

229. Levy, N. A., and Strauss, H. A.: Myelopathy following compression of abdominal aorta for postpartum hemorrhage, Arch. Neurol. Psychiat. **48:**85, 1942.

230. Lindenberg, R.: Compression of brain arteries as pathogenetic factor for tissue necroses and their areas of predilection, J. Neuropath. Exp. Neurol. **14:**223, 1955.

231. Lindenberg, R.: Incarceration of a vertebral artery in the cleft of a longitudinal fracture of the skull, J. Neurosurg. **24:**908, 1966.

232. Lochaya, S., Kaplan, B., and Shaffer, A. B.: Pseudocoarctation of the aorta with bicuspid aortic valve and kinked left subclavian artery: a possible cause of subclavian steal, Amer. Heart J. **73:**369, 1967.

233. Loeb, C., and Meyer, J. S.: Strokes due to vertebro-basilar disease, Springfield, Ill., 1965, Charles C Thomas, Publisher.

234. Logothetis, J., Silverstein, P., and Coe, J.: Neurologic aspects of Waldenström's macroglobulinemia, Arch. Neurol. **3:**564, 1960.

235. Louis, S., and McDowell, F.: Stroke in young adults, Ann. Intern. Med. **66:**932, 1967.

236. Louis, S., and McDowell, F.: Age: Its significance in nonembolic cerebral infarction, Stroke **1:**449, 1970.

237. Low-Beer, T., and Phear, D.: Cerebral infarction and hypertension, Lancet **1:**1303, 1961.

238. Lucas, W. S.: Erythremia, or polycythemia with chronic cyanosis and splenomegaly, Arch. Intern. Med. **10:**597, 1912.

239. Luessenhop, A. J., Gibbs, M., and Velasquez, A. C.: Cerebrovascular response to emboli, Arch. Neurol. **7:**264, 1962.

240. Lynch, M. J. G., Raphael, S. S., and Dixon, T. P.: Fat embolism in chronic alcoholism, Arch. Path. **67:**68, 1959.

241. MacLean, A. R.: Primary thrombosis of the superior longitudinal sinus with chronic obstruction. Thesis, 1937, Graduate School of the University of Minnesota.

242. Mair, W. G. P., and Druckman, R.: The pathology of spinal cord lesions and their relation to the clinical features in protrusion of cervical intervertebral discs, Brain **76:**70, 1953.

243. Marshall, J.: The natural history of transient ischaemic cerebro-vascular attacks, Quart. J. Med. **33:**309, 1964.

244. Martin, J. P.: Venous thrombosis in the central nervous system, Proc. Roy. Soc. Med. **37:** 383, 1943-44.

245. Martin, J. P., and Sheehan, H. L.: Primary thrombosis of cerebral veins (following childbirth), Brit. Med. J. **1:**349, 1941.

246. Martin, M. J., Whisnant, J. P., and Sayre, G. P.: Occlusive vascular disease in the extracranial cerebral circulation, Arch. Neurol. **3:**530, 1960.

247. Maurizi, C. P., Barker, A. E., and Trueheart, R. E.: Atheromatous emboli, Arch. Path. **86:** 528, 1968.

248. McBrien, D. J., Bradley, R. D., and Ashton, N.: The nature of retinal emboli in stenosis of the internal carotid artery, Lancet **1:**697, 1963.

249. McKay, D. G., and Margaretten, W.: Disseminated intravascular coagulation in virus diseases, Arch. Intern. Med. **120:**129, 1967.

250. McMillan, J. B.: Emboli of cerebral tissue in the lungs following severe head injury, Amer. J. Path. **32:**405, 1956.

251. McTaggart, D. M., and Neubuerger, K. T.: Cerebral fat embolism: pathologic changes in the brain after survival of 7 years, Acta Neuropath. **15:**183, 1970.

252. Merchant, R. K., Louria, D. B., Geisler, P. H., Edgcomb, J. H., and Utz, J. P.: Fungal endocarditis: review of the literature and report of three cases, Ann. Intern. Med. **48:**242, 1958.

253. Merritt, H. H., and Fremont-Smith, F.: The cerebrospinal fluid, Philadelphia, 1938, W. B. Saunders Co.

254. Meyer, J. S.: Acute stroke, Minn. Med. **47:**265, 1964.

255. Meyer, J. S., and Denny-Brown, D.: The cerebral collateral circulation. I. Factors influencing collateral blood flow, Neurology, **7:**447, 1957.

256. Meyer, J. S., and Portnoy, H. D.: Localized cerebral hypoglycemia simulating stroke, Neurology **8:**601, 1958.

257. Millikan, C. H., Siekert, R. G., and Whisnant, J. P.: The clinical pattern in certain types of occlusive cerebrovascular disease, Circulation **22:**1002, 1960.

258. Moniz, E., Lima, A., and de Lacerda, R.: Hémiplégies par thrombose de la carotide interne, Presse Med. **45:**977, 1937.

259. Moosy, J.: Cerebral infarction and intracranial arterial thrombus, Arch. Neurol. **14:**119, 1966.

260. Moosy, J.: Cerebral infarcts and the lesions of intracranial and extracranial atherosclerosis, Arch. Neurol. **14:**124, 1966.

261. Morgan, W. L., and Bland, E. F.: Bacterial endocarditis in the antibiotic era with special reference to the later complications, Circulation **19:**753, 1959.

262. Mosberg, W. H., Voris, H. C., and Duffy, J.: Paraplegia as a complication of sympathectomy for hypertension, Ann. Surg. **139:**330, 1954.

263. Murphy, J. P.: Cerebrovascular disease, Chicago, 1954, Year Book Publishers Inc.

264. Naiman, J. L., Donohue, W. L., and Prichard, J. S.: Fatal nucleus pulposus embolism of spinal cord after trauma, Neurology **11:**83, 1961.

265. Najafi, H., Dye, W. S., Javid, H., Hunter, J. A., Ostermiller, W. E., and Julian, O. C.: Carotid bifurcation stenosis and ipsilateral subclavian steal, Arch. Surg. **99:**289, 1969.

266. Ng, L. K., and Nimmannitya, J.: Massive cerebral infarction with severe brain swelling, Stroke **1:**158, 1970.

267. North, R. R., Fields, W. S., De Bakey, M. E., and Crawford, E. S.: Brachial-basilar insufficiency syndrome, Neurology **12:**810, 1962.

268. Oppenheimer, E. H.: Massive pulmonary embolization by cerebral cortical tissue, Bull. Johns Hopkins Hosp. **94:**86, 1954.

269. Osler, W.: Aneurism (revised by Howard, C. P.). In Osler, W., McCrae, T., and Funk, E. H.: Modern medicine its theory and practice, Philadelphia, 1927, Lea & Febiger, vol. 4, p. 840.

270. Palmovic, V., and McCarroll, J. R.: Fat embolism in trauma, Arch. Path. **80:**630, 1965.

271. Patel, A., and Toole, J. F.: Subclavian steal syndrome—reversal of cephalic blood flow, Medicine **44:**289, 1965.

272. Peabody, C. N., and O'Brien, B.: Subclavian steal from the circle of Willis, Angiology **17:**149, 1966.

273. Penry, J. K., and Netsky, M. G.: Experimental embolic occlusion of a single leptomeningeal artery, Arch. Neurol. **3:**391, 1960.

274. Piazza, G., and Gaist, G.: Occlusion of middle cerebral artery by foreign body embolus, J. Neurosurg. **17:**172, 1960.

275. Pincock, J. G.: The natural history of cerebral thrombosis, Ann. Intern. Med. **46:**925, 1957.

276. Pindyck, J., Lichtman, H. C., and Kohl, S. G.: Cryofibrinogenaemia in women using oral contraceptives, Lancet **1:**51, 1970.

277. Poole, J. C. F., Sanders, A. G., and Florey, H. W.: The regeneration of aortic endothelium, J. Path. Bact. **75:**133, 1958.

278. Portnoy, H. D.: Transient "ischemic" attacks produced by carotid stenosis and hypoglycemia, Neurology **15:**830, 1965.

279. Potter, E. L., and Young, R. L.: Heterotopic brain tissue in the lungs of two anencephalic monsters, Arch. Path. **34:**1009, 1942.

280. Prensky, A. L., and Davis, D. O.: Obstruction of major cerebral vessels in early childhood without neurological signs, Neurology **20:**945, 1970.

281. Prineas, J., and Marshall, J.: Hypertension and cerebral infarction, Brit. Med. J. **1:**14, 1966.

282. Quattlebaum, J. K., Upson, E. T., and Neville, R. L.: Stroke associated with elongation and kinking of the internal carotid artery: report of three cases treated by segmental resection of the carotid artery, Ann. Surg. **150:**824, 1959.

283. Rainer, W. G., Cramer, G. G., Newby, J. P.; and Clarke, J. P.: Fibromuscular hyperplasia of the carotid artery causing positional cerebral ischemia, Ann. Surg. **167:**444, 1968.

284. Rainer, W. G., Guillen, J., Bloomquist, C. D., and McCrory, C. B.: Carotid artery surgery, Amer. J. Surg. **116:**678, 1968.

285. Ralston, B., Rasmussen, T., and Kennedy, T.: Occlusion of the middle cerebral artery, J. Neurosurg. **12:**26, 1955.

286. Ratinov, G., and Jimenez-Pabon, E.: Intermittent spinal ischemia, Neurology **11:**546, 1961.

287. Rees, J. E., Du Boulay, G. H., Bull, J. W. D., Marshall, J., Russell, R. W. R., and Symon, L.: Regional cerebral blood-flow in transient ischaemic attacks, Lancet **2:**1210, 1970.

288. Reichert, F. L.: The danger of air embolism when removing meningiomas along the superior sagittal or longitudinal sinus, J. Neurosurg. **8:**494, 1951.

289. Reichert, F. L., Rytand, D. A., and Bruck, E. L.: Arteriosclerosis of the lumbar segmental arteries producing ischemia of the spinal cord and consequent claudication of the thighs, Amer. J. Med. Sci. **187:**794, 1934.

290. Reivich, M., Holling, H. E., Roberts, B., and Toole, J. F.: Reversal of blood flow through the vertebral artery and its effect on cerebral circulation, New Eng. J. Med. **265:**878, 1961.

291. Rob, C.: Technique of surgical therapy. In Millikan, C. H., Siekert, R. G., and Whisnant, J. P.: Cerebral vascular diseases, New York, 1961, Grune & Stratton, Inc., p. 110.

292. Robinson, R. W., Cohen, W. D., Higano, N., Meyer, R., Lukowsky, G. H., and McLaughlin, R. B.: Life-time analysis of survival after cerebral thrombosis—ten-year experience, J.A.M.A. **169:**1149, 1959.

293. Rokkanen, P., Lahdensuu, M., Kataja, J., and Julkunen, H.: The syndrome of fat embolism: analysis of thirty consecutive cases compared to trauma patients with similar injuries, J. Trauma **10:**299, 1970.

294. Romanul, F. C. A., and Abramowicz, A.: Changes in brain and pial vessels in arterial border zone, Arch. Neurol. **11:**40, 1964.

295. Rosenblum, W. I., and Asofsky, R. M.: Malfunction of cerebral microcirculation in macroglobulinemic mice, Arch. Neurol. **18:**151, 1968.

296. Ross, R. S., and McKusick, V. A.: Aortic arch syndromes, Arch. Intern. Med. **92:**701, 1953.

297. Rundles, W. R., and Kimbell, F. D.: The kinked carotid syndrome, Angiology **20:**177, 1969.

298. Russell, R. W. R.: Observations on the retinal blood-vessels in monocular blindness, Lancet **2:**1422, 1961.

299. Russell, R. W. R.: Atheromatous retinal embolism, Lancet **2:**1354, 1963.

300. Russell, R. W. R.: The source of retinal emboli, Lancet **2:**789, 1968.

301. Samiy, E.: Thrombosis of the internal carotid artery caused by a cervical rib, J. Neurosurg. **12:**181, 1955.

302. Sammartino, W. F., and Toole, J. F.: Reversed vertebral artery flow, Arch. Neurol. **10:**590, 1964.

303. Schenk, E. A.: Sickle cell trait and superior longitudinal sinus thrombosis, Ann. Intern. Med. 60:465, 1964.

304. Schrire, V.: Arteritis of the aorta and its major branches, Aust. Ann. Med. 16:33, 1967.

305. Schulz, H., and Wedell, J.: Elektronenmikroskopische Untersuchungen zur Frage der Fettphagocytose und des Fetttransportes durch Thrombocyten, Klin. Wschr. 40:1114, 1962.

306. Schwartz, C. J., Mitchell, J. R. A., and Hughes, J. T.: Transient recurrent cerebral episodes and aneurysm of carotid sinus, Brit. Med. J. 1:770, 1962.

307. Sedzimir, C. B.: Head injury as a cause of internal carotid thrombosis, J. Neurol. Neurosurg. Psychiat. 18:293, 1955.

308. Shaw, C.-M., Alvord, E. C., and Berry, R. G.: Swelling of the brain following ischemic infarction with arterial occlusion, Arch. Neurol. 1:161, 1959.

309. Sheehan, S., Bauer, R. B., and Meyer, J. S.: Vertebral artery compression in cervical spondylosis, Neurology 10:968, 1960.

310. Shillito, J.: Carotid arteritis: a cause of hemiplegia in childhood, J. Neurosurg. 21:540, 1964.

311. Shimomura, Y., Hukuda, S., and Mizuno, S.: Experimental study of ischemic damage to the cervical spinal cord, J. Neurosurg. 28:565, 1968.

312. Siekert, R. G., and Millikan, C. H.: Studies in cerebrovascular disease. II. Some clinical aspects of thrombosis of the basilar artery, Proc. Staff Meet. Mayo Clin. 30:93, 1955.

313. Sights, W. P.: Incarceration of the basilar artery in a fracture of the clivus, J. Neurosurg. 28:588, 1968.

314. Silberman, J., Cravioto, H., and Feigin, I.: Foreign body emboli following cerebral angiography, Arch. Neurol. 3:711, 1960.

315. Silver, M. D., and Stehbens, W. E.: The behaviour of platelets in vivo, Quart. J. Exp. Physiol. 50:241, 1965.

316. Silverstein, A., and Hollin, S.: Occlusion of the supraclinoid portion of the internal carotid artery, Neurology 13:679, 1963.

317. Simeone, F. A., and Goldberg, H. I.: Thrombosis of the vertebral artery from hyperextension injury to the neck, J. Neurosurg. 29:540, 1968.

318. Skovborg, F., and Lauritzen, E.: Symptomless retinal embolism, Lancet 2:361, 1965.

319. Smith, K. R.: Idiopathic bilateral sigmoid sinus occlusion in a child, J. Neurosurg. 29:427, 1968.

320. Snyder, H. E., and Shapiro, J. L.: A correlative study of atheromatous embolism in human beings and experimental animals, Surgery 49:195, 1961.

321. Soloway, H. B., and Aronson, S. M.: Atheromatous emboli to central nervous system, Arch. Neurol. 11:657, 1964.

322. Spector, R. G.: Water content of the brain in anoxic-ischaemic encephalopathy in adult rats, Brit. J. Exp. Path. 42:623, 1961.

323. Stalker, A. L.: Histological changes produced by experimental erythrocyte aggregation, J. Path. Bact. 93:203, 1967.

324. Steegman, A. T.: The neuropathology of cardiac arrest. In Minckler, J.: Pathology of the nervous system New York, 1968, McGraw-Hill Book Co., vol. 1, p. 1005.

325. Stehbens, W. E.: Contentious features of coronary occlusion and atherosclerosis, Bull. Post-Grad. Comm. Med. Univ. Sydney 19:216, 1963.

326. Stehbens, W. E.: Microcirculatory changes in rabbit ear chambers following the infusion of fat emulsions, Metabolism 16:473, 1967.

327. Stehbens, W. E.: Effects of Adrenalin and anaphylaxis on the aggregation of the cellular constituents of the blood in vivo, Quart. J. Exp. Physiol. 54:41, 1969.

328. Stehbens, W. E., and Florey, H. W.: The behaviour of intravenously injected particles observed in chambers in rabbits' ears, Quart. J. Exp. Physiol. 45:252, 1960.

329. Stehbens, W. E., Sonnenwirth, A. C., and Kotrba, C.: Microcirculatory changes in experimental bacteremia, Exp. Molec. Path. 10:295, 1969.

330. Stevens, H.: Puerperal hemiplegia, Neurology 4:723, 1954.

331. Stoner, H. B., and Mathews, J.: Studies on the mechanism of shock, Brit. J. Exp. Path. 48:58, 1967.

332. Strassman, G.: Formation of hemosiderin and hematoidin after traumatic and spontaneous cerebral hemorrhages, Arch. Path. 47:205, 1949.

333. Sturgill, B. C., and Netsky, M. G.: Cerebral infarction by atheromatous emboli, Arch. Path. 76:189, 1963.

334. Sullivan, J. F., and Callow, A. D.: Unpublished data. Cited by Callow et al.[51]

335. Sundt, T. M., Grant, W. C., and Garcia, J. H.: Restoration of middle cerebral artery flow in experimental infarction, J. Neurosurg. 31:311, 1969.

336. Sundt, T. M., Waltz, A. G., and Sayre, G. P.: Experimental cerebral infarction: modification by treatment with hemodiluting, hemoconcentrating, and dehydrating agents, J. Neurosurg. 26:46, 1967.

337. Swank, R. L.: Changes in blood of dogs and rabbits by high fat intake, Amer. J. Physiol. 196:473, 1959.

338. Swank, R. L.: Blood viscosity in cerebrovascular disease, Neurology 9:553, 1959.

339. Swank, R. L.: Effects of large fat meals on the circulation and function of the hamster, Bibl. Anat. 1:281, 1961.

340. Swank, R. L., Glinsman, W., and Sloop, P.: The production of fat embolism in rabbits by feeding high fat meals, Surg. Gynec. Obstet. 110:9, 1960.

341. Swank, R. L., and Hain, R. F.: The effect of different sized emboli on the vascular system and parenchyma of the brain, J. Neuropath. Exp. Neurol. 11:280, 1952.

342. Swank, R. L., and Nakamura, H.: Oxygen availability after lipid meals, Amer. J. Physiol. 198:217, 1960.

343. Swank, R. L., and Nakamura, H.: Convulsions in hamsters after cream meals, Arch. Neurol. 3:594, 1960.

344. Symonds, C.: Otitic hydrocephalus, Neurology 6:681, 1956.

345. Symonds, C. P.: Otitic hydrocephalus, Brain 54:55, 1931.

346. Symonds, C. P.: Hydrocephalic and focal cerebral symptoms in relation to thrombophlebitis of the dural sinuses and cerebral veins, Brain 60:531, 1937.

347. Tatlow, W. F. T., and Bammer, H. G.: Syndrome of vertebral artery compression, Neurology 7:331, 1957.

348. Tatsumi, T., and Shenkin, H. A.: Occlusion of the vertebral artery, J. Neurol. Neurosurg. Psychiat. 28:235, 1965.

349. Taveras, J. M.: Multiple progressive intracranial arterial occlusions: a syndrome of children and young adults, Amer. J. Roentgen. 106:235, 1969.

350. Taylor, A. R., and Chakravorty, B. C.: Clinical syndromes associated with basilar impression, Arch. Neurol. 10:475, 1964.

351. Tedeschi, C. G., Walter, C. E, and Tedeschi, L. G.: Shock and fat embolism: an appraisal, Surg. Clin. N. Amer. 48:431, 1968.

352. Thierry, A., Vieville, C., Duquesnel, J., Fischer, G., Brunon, J., and Mansuy, L.: Hémodétournement vertébro-carotidien à la suite d'une ligature de la carotide primitive, Neurochirurgie, 16:33, 1970.

353. Thompson, J. E., Kartchner, M. M., Austin, D. J., Wheeler, C. G., and Patman, R. D.: Carotid endarterectomy for cerebrovascular insufficiency (stroke): follow up of 359 cases, Ann. Surg. 163:751, 1966.

354. Tonge, J. I., Hurley, R. N., and Ferguson, J.: Systemic fat embolism associated with the toxic effects of aviation-fuel inhalation and general anaesthesia, Lancet 1:1059, 1969.

355. Toole, J. F.: Discussion. In (Millikan, C. H., Siekert, R. G., and, Whisnant, J. P.: Cerebral vascular diseases, New York, 1961, Grune & Stratton, Inc., p. 31.

356. Toole, J. F.: Reversed vertebral-artery flow, Subclavian-steal syndrome, Lancet 1:872, 1964.

357. Toole, J. F., and Patel, A. N.: Cerebrovascular disorders, New York, 1967, McGraw-Hill Book Co.

358. Toole, J. F., and Tucker, S. H.: Influence of head position upon cerebral circulation, Arch. Neurol. 2:616, 1960.

359. Towbin, A.: Recurrent cerebral embolism, Arch. Neurol. Psychiat. 73:173, 1955.

360. Tureen, L. L.: Circulation of the spinal cord and the effect of vascular occlusion. In: The circulation of the brain and spinal cord, Ass. Res. Nerv. Ment. Dis. 18:394, 1938.

361. Van Allen, C. M., Hrdina, L. S., and Clark, J.: Air embolism from the pulmonary vein, Arch. Surg. 19:567, 1929.

362. Vance, B. M.: The significance of fat embolism, Arch. Surg. 23:426, 1931.

363. Van Wieringen, A.: An unusual cause of occlusion of the anterior spinal artery, European Neurol. 1:363, 1968.

364. Vessey, M. P., Doll, R., Fairbairn, A. S., and Globers, G.: Postoperative thromboembolism and the use of oral contraceptives, Brit. Med. J. 3:123, 1970.

365. Vost, A., Wolochow, D. A., and Howell, D. A.: Incidence of infarcts of the brain in heart disease, J. Path. Bact. 88:463, 1964.

366. Wade, J. G., Larson, C. P., Hickey, R. H., and Ehrenfeld, W. K.: Effect of carotid endarterectomy on carotid chemoreceptor and baroreceptor function, Surg. Forum 19:144, 1968.

367. Wagner, J. A., and Alvarez de Choudens, J.: Unpublished experiments. Cited by Mosberg et al.[262]

368. Wakim, K. G., and Fleischer, G. A.: The effect of experimental cerebral infarction on transaminase activity in serum, cerebrospinal fluid, and infarcted tissue, Proc. Staff Meet. Mayo Clin. 31:391, 1956.

369. Wallenberg, A.: Acute Bulbäraffection (Embolie der Art. cerebellar. post. inf. sinistr.?), Arch. Psychiat. Nervenkr. 27:504, 1895. (Translation, Arch. Neurol. 22:380, 1970.)

370. Waltz, A. G.: Red venous blood occurrence and significance in ischemic and nonischemic cerebral cortex, J. Neurosurg. 31:141, 1969.

371. Warren, S.: Fat embolism, Amer. J. Path. 22: 69, 1946.

372. Warthin, A. S.: Traumatic lipaemia and fatty embolism, Int. Clin. 4:171, 1913.

373. Weibel, J., and Fields, W. S.: Tortuosity, coiling, and kinking of the internal carotid artery. II. Relationship of morphological variation to cerebrovascular insufficiency, Neurology 15: 462, 1965.

374. Weinberger, L. M., Gibbon, M. H., and Gibbon, J. H.: Temporary arrest of the circulation to the central nervous system. I. Physiologic effects. Arch. Neurol. Psychiat. 43:615, 1940.

375. Weinberger, L. M., Gibbon, M. H., and Gibbon, J. H.: Temporary arrest of the circulation to the central nervous system. II. Pathologic effects, Arch. Neurol. Psychiat. 43:961, 1940.

376. Weisman, A. D.: Cavernous-sinus thrombophlebitis, New Eng. J. Med. 231:118, 1944.

377. Wells, C. E.: Cerebral embolism, Arch. Neurol. Psychiat. 81:667, 1959.

378. Wells, C. E., and Timberger, R. J.: Cerebral thrombosis in patients under fifty years of age, Arch. Neurol. 4:268, 1961.

379. Wertham, F., Mitchell, N., and Angrist, A.: The brain in sickle cell anemia, Arch. Neurol. Psychiat. 47:752, 1942.

380. Wessler, S., and Stehbens, W. E.: Thrombosis. In Bang, N. U., Beller, F. K., Deutsch, E., and Mammen, E. F.: Thrombosis and bleeding disorders, Stuttgart, 1971, Georg Thieme Verlag, p. 488.

381. Whisnant, J. P., Martin, M. J., and Sayre, G. P.: Atherosclerotic stenosis of cervical arteries, Arch. Neurol. 5:429, 1961.

382. Wisoff, H. S., and Rothballer, A. B.: Cerebral

arterial thrombosis in children, Arch. Neurol. 4:258, 1961.

383. Wolman, L.: Ischaemic lesions in the brainstem associated with raised supratentorial pressure, Brain 76:364, 1953.

384. Wood, M. W., and Murphey, F.: Obstructive hydrocephalus due to infarction of a cerebellar hemisphere, J. Neurosurg. 30:260, 1969.

385. Yarington, C. T.: The prognosis and treatment of cavernous sinus thrombosis, Ann. Otol. 70:263, 1961.

386. Yates, P. O.: Birth trauma to the vertebral arteries, Arch. Dis. Child. 34:436, 1959.

387. Yates, P. O., and Hutchinson, E. C.: Cerebral infarction: the role of stenosis of the extracranial cerebral arteries, Med. Res. Council Spec. Rep. (London) 300:1-95, 1961.

388. Yates, P. O.: Arterial pathology in cerebral infarction. In Chalmers, D. G., and Gresham, G. A.: Biological aspects of occlusive vascular disease, Cambridge, 1964, Cambridge University Press, p. 312.

389. Zak, F. G., and Elias, K.: Embolization with material from atheromata, Amer. J. Med. Sci. 218:510, 1949.

390. Zeitlin, H., and Lichtenstein, B. W.: Occlusion of the anterior spinal artery, Arch. Neurol. Psychiat. 36:96, 1936.

5 / Cranial and spinal extradural hematoma

Cranial extradural hematoma

An extradural (epidural) hematoma is an accumulation of blood assuming the proportions of a space-occupying lesion between the dura mater and the inner table of the skull. The hemorrhage causes a dramatic clinical syndrome after a fall or a blow to the head, the major clinical and pathological features being recognized in the last century.[19,40]

Incidence

Extradural hematoma is an uncommon lesion and accounts for 1% to 5% of all the cases of cranial trauma[32,43,55,64,75] generally seen in a neurosurgical unit. Freytag,[23] investigating 1367 cases of death attributed to blunt trauma from the Chief Medical Examiner's records (Baltimore) over a period of 10 years, reported 211 cases of epidural bleeding (15%). When only head injuries in which the skull is fractured are considered, the incidence is decidedly higher. In 504 cases, LeCount and Apfelbach[52] found 39.5% with an extradural hematoma, and Freytag[23] gives an incidence of 22% in 956 patients. Moody[67] found significant extradural hemorrhage in 100 of 547 patients who died with a fractured skull, and Vance[96] found 56 in 233 patients with fractures in the temporoparietal region.

Age and sex distribution

Extradural hematoma may occur at any age. Its distribution (in decades) is depicted in Table 5-1. Jamieson and Yelland[43] regarded it as a disease of youth with the

Table 5-1. Age distribution of extradural hematoma*

Authors	0-9 or 1-10	10-19 or 11-20	20-29 or 21-30	30-39 or 31-40	40-49 or 41-50	50-59 or 51-60	60-69 or 61-70	70 or over	Total
Vance (1927)[96]		2	13	18	17	7	2	2	61
Munro & Maltby (1941)[68]	1	7	6	9	7	5	2	1	38
Voris (1947)[90]		4	3	3	11	1			22
Rowbotham et al. (1954)[78]		2	11	5	5	4	1		28
Hooper (1959)[34]	14	12	20	15	9	7	6		83
McKissock et al. (1960)[64]	17	33	29	14	19	9	4		125
Mealy (1960)[66]	6	9	4	5	7	1	2		34
Freytag (1963)[23]	14	18	35	49	30	29	18	18	211
Heyser & Weber (1964)[32]	9	8	17	9	7	13	5	3	71
Jamieson and Yelland (1968)[43]	22	51	30	26	24	7	4	3	167
Total	83	146	168	153	136	83	44	27	840

*The cut-off period for each decade varied with the author.

peak incidence in the second decade, although Table 5-1 does not reflect this trend.

Although a few cases have been reported,[6,34] birth injuries are rarely a cause of extradural hematoma, and doubtless the type of injury incurred during labor explains its singularity at this age. There is confusion concerning the frequency of the lesion in childhood. Gallagher and Browder[24] stated that extradural hematoma rarely occurs at the extremes of life, yet Table 5-1 indicates a significant incidence during the first decade. Hooper[34] considered that from his figures it is rare in the first 2 years of life, but his cases were too few in number for the application of statistics to be meaningful. Ingraham and associates[37] found 11 of their 20 cases in infancy and childhood to be under 2 years of age. In 1136 consecutive head injuries admitted to the Children's Medical Center of Boston, there were 20 instances of extradural hemorrhage,[11] an incidence of 1.8%, which is comparable to the lower end of the range found in adults. Differences in the manner of the selection of material may account for the discrepancies.

Males are subject to greater risk of trauma and sustain more accidents than females. They are consequently better represented in most published series of extradural hematomas. Despite this overall preponderance of males, Jamieson and Yelland[43] found that among children, girls predominated, but in the children reported by Campbell and Cohen[11] such was not the case.

Precipitating factors

Trauma. Extradural hematoma is almost invariably associated with head injury, the most frequent type being that arising from traffic accidents involving the driver, the motorcycle or bicycle rider, or pedestrians and passengers. The next most frequent cause is occasioned by accidental or suicidal falls, the majority of falls in Hooper's series[34] being less than 8 feet. Table 5-2 contrasts the incidence of the various causes of extradural hematoma between 1886 and more recent times and reflects the serious increase in traffic accidents. Blows to the head may be incurred during fights, muggings, horseplay, sport, or accidental injuries, but in a percentage of cases the manner of injury is unknown.

The severity of the injury varies considerably, often it is major but it can be relatively slight.[19,40] Vance[96] found the calvarium to be unusually thin in many cases in which the skull had been fractured by comparatively trifling force. Indications of the severity of the impact can be gauged from observation of associated injuries of the scalp, skull, or brain and from the duration of the initial period of unconsciousness. In six of Hooper's 27 cases for which information was available, there was no loss of consciousness.[34] In eight there was a period of unconsciousness lasting less than 30 minutes (mean of 10 minutes). Other patients

Table 5-2. Causes of cranial injury responsible for extradural hematomas (in percentage)

Cause of injury	Jacobson (1886)[40]	Hooper (1959)[34]	McKissock et al. (1960)*[64]	Freytag (1963)[23]	Gallagher & Browder (1968)[24]
Traffic accidents	7	39	44	43	19
Falls	70	35	28	41	29
Blows to the head	18	16	13	14	13
Unknown causes	5	10	8	2	37
War injuries			6		
Injury during convulsions					2

*McKissock's figures total only 99%.

may remain unconscious until the time of treatment or until they die. McKissock and his colleagues[64] encountered 27 patients (21.4%) who sustained no initial loss of consciousness, and of these 10 remained conscious until treatment was instituted. Hooper[34] asserts that extradural hematoma is less likely with very severe cranial injuries and is rarely associated with a depressed fracture of the skull. The incidence of depressed fractures of the skull was 14% in the series reported by Jamieson and Yelland,[43] who asserted that this type of lesion attained its highest incidence in children. The injury is such that it leads to separation of the dura from the bone. Hooper[34] suggests that cerebral swelling and intradural hemorrhage or a depressed skull fracture all play a part in limiting this separation and that severe injury may lead to death before much extradural extravasation can occur. Toole and Patel[93] state that this lesion is infrequent with penetrating wounds presumably because of the adequate drainage of extravasated blood in such circumstances.

The susceptibility of the skull to fracture has been attributed to either undue thinness of the bone[30] or fragility of the skull as in Paget's disease.[75] Freytag[23] found in her series that no predominance for either white or black populations was exhibited. Gallagher and Browder[24] however asserted without providing statistics that a greater thickness of cranial bones in Negroes as distinct from Caucasians accounted for the reduced Negro susceptibility to skull fractures and hence extradural hematoma. Peet[75] suggested that in some subjects the attachment of the dura mater to the skull may be exceptionally feeble and that conversely a very adherent dura mater would largely confine a hematoma and limit intracranial pressure effects. Extradural hematoma may also complicate surgical procedures involving the skull[23,46] when meningeal vessels or dural venous sinuses are injured and bleed postoperatively.

Ventricular decompression. Schorstein[85] recorded the case of a 14-year-old girl with stenosis of the aqueduct and hydrocephalus. During suboccipital craniectomy, after a sudden gush of ventricular fluid from a ventricular catheter, there was profuse and widespread bleeding and the cerebellum bulged. The patient died 16 hours postoperatively and extensive extradural hemorrhage over both frontal lobes was demonstrated at autopsy. Schorstein's second patient was a 10-year-old girl with hydrocephalus caused by a tegmental astrocytoma blocking the aqueduct. Ventricular drainage was instituted after ventriculography was performed, but 6½ hours later the patient died from extradural hemorrhage over both frontal lobes. Similar instances were reported in 4 patients under 21 years of age,[29,33,75] and then Weiss[101] reported catastrophic hemorrhage during ventricular decompression in a male of 42 years. A successful craniectomy was performed and a massive epidural hematoma (400 ml.) was exposed and drained.

Fiskin and Kurze[20] reported the sudden onset of hemorrhagic engorgement and swelling of the cerebellum after ventricular drainage for hydrocephalus in association with a pontine angle neurinoma. It was impossible to attain complete hemostasis and, despite transfusions, the patient, a Negro woman of 37 years of age, died 36 hours postoperatively with a massive parieto-occipital extradural hematoma. Other reports included a calcified and an ossified extradural hematoma believed to have complicated ventricular decompression sometime previously.[92,102,108] More recently Frera[22] reviewed 15 cases. In each, the extradural hematoma was supratentorial and complicated ventricular decompression for hydrocephalus. The patients were predominantly children or young adults.

Miscellaneous causes. Bleeding disorders such as hemophilia[34,42] seldom cause extradural hematoma.[93] Exceptional cases of hemangiomas of the skull and dura bleeding extradurally have been reported.[24,48] Schneider and Hegarty[82] provided the history of a patient with recurrent suppurative middle ear infection. Death was caused by a large extradural hematoma after rupture of the middle meningeal or the internal carotid artery involved in the spread of the inflammation from the ear. Novaes and Gorbitz[72] recorded a case of extradural hemorrhage evolving more slowly in a male with a history of middle-ear infection. On the upper surface of the petrous bone a zone of pachymeningitis with venous bleeding was observed and treated at craniotomy, the hematoma being mainly basal. Another patient[82] had a furuncle in the nose complicated by acute osteomyelitis of the frontal bone, acute pachymeningitis, and an extradural hemorrhage. In yet another case, a boy of 11 years, suffered an acute frontal sinusitis with acute pachymeningitis, erosion of the meningeal vessels, and extradural hemorrhage.[45] Acute arteritis secondary to middle-ear or nasal infections is extremely rare and inflammatory aneurysms from such causes have not been reported.

Pathological findings

Extradural hematomas are most often acute and thus at surgery or autopsy consist of saucer-shaped accumulations of the typical "red currant jelly" blood clot. Size varies considerably, but large hematomas are usually not more extensive than 10 or 12 cm. in diameter and 4 or 5 cm. thick. Voris[99] encountered hematomas more than 5 cm. thick, and Ingraham and associates[37] have seen others up to 400 ml. in volume, whereas Youmans and Schneider[108] described a hematoma of 920 ml. in volume. Not all hematomas are of such gross proportions. In a series of 199 cases of extradural hematoma, 95 were small, the clot weighing only a few grams, whereas the remaining 104 ranged up to 246 gm.[52] In 63 cases clinically unrecognized, Moody[67] found that although the average weight of the extradural hematoma was 110 gm., the range was from 40 to 246 gm. Vance[96] stated that 45 of his 106 extradural hematomas were small and consequently of insignificant size. The weight of the extradural clot was available in only 25 cases and ranged

from 40 to 300 gm. with an average of 122 gm., which is about twice the weight of the average subdural hematoma. According to Vance[96] those in the temporal region were larger than those associated with laceration of the lateral sinus. Chason[12] contended that the weight of fatal hematomas fell between 75 and 100 gm. In the series of Gallagher and Browder,[24] the majority were between 100 and 150 gm., but the largest clot was 400 gm.

Most hematomas are less than 3 or 4 days old when treated surgically or viewed at autopsy. Some, often regarded as subacute, run a more protracted course of 4 to 10 days, and the neurological deficit may not be very great.[95] Slow venous bleeding may be responsible, but it is likely that in the absence of bleeding disorders bleeding will cease spontaneously. Guthkelch[28] reported the successful surgical removal of a large hematoma overlying the cerebellum some 17 days after injury. The hematoma was described as consisting of a black clot mixed with a brownish viscous fluid, with brown granulation tissue growing from the external aspect of the dura mater. Although evidence of organization is an expected finding,[89] few lesions reached this age. Intervals of 1 to 6 weeks between the injury and the time of diagnosis have been reported.[5,36,39,50,71,79] The contents were black and tarry but ultimately became more brownish, although some renewed extravasation of blood occurred from the granulation tissue. This is thought to have occurred in a patient reported by Olsen and Watson,[73] the bleeding and exacerbation of symptoms being precipitated by a pneumatic drill on one occasion and subsequently by a fall, which led to hospitalization, although the head had not been struck.

Grant[26] reported the unique case of a 6-year-old hematoma of the frontal lobe in a girl of 19 years. A head injury at the age of 13 was believed to have been responsible for a chronic extradural hematoma found over the right frontal lobe 6 years later. The hematoma was enclosed on all sides by a dense heavily pigmented fibrous capsule. Calcification was present on the dural aspect of the hematoma, which itself was separated on the frontal aspect from the bone by old liquefied (black syrupy) blood, suggestive of a second episode. Distortion of the anterior horn of the right lateral ventricle had resulted in blockage and dilatation with exacerbation of the symptoms and signs of raised intracranial pressure. As the dura mater acts as a periosteum on the inner surface of the calvarium, evidence of bone formation was expected, but the pathological report revealed only calcification. A thin bony shell forms over the dural surface of a chronic encapsulated extradural hematoma and is continuous with the inner table of the cranial bones.[102] The inner surface of the capsule may exhibit numerous bony spicules. It is entirely likely that small extradural hematomas may remain subclinical and undergo absorption, but the coincidental finding of organizing extradural hematomas at routine autopsy is exceedingly rare as is the occurrence of calcification and ossification in hematomas of long standing.

Microscopically, the acute inflammatory changes about hematomas in any situation are mild in degree and are also to be expected in the early stages of extradural hemorrhage. Only rarely has an histological examination been undertaken. Organization of the blood clot most likely proceeds from the dura mater because it acts as periosteum and so is similar to the organization of a subperiosteal hematoma elsewhere. The fibrous tissue capsule completely encloses the hematoma on all surfaces and contains much pigment, but calcification or bone formation is effected only on the dural aspect.[26, 102]

Location. The classical and most frequent site for extradural hematoma is temporal. The base is rarely involved, but no area is exempt. The localization of the hematomas is indicated in Table 5-3, and it should be appreciated that some 20% occur at sites other than in the temporal region.[64] Jamieson and Yelland[43] found only 70% of

Table 5-3. Localization of extradural hematomas

Site of hematoma	McKissock et al. (1960)[64]	McLaurin and Ford (1964)[65]
Temporal	100	40
Frontal	9	1
Parietal or parieto-occipital	11	4
Occipital		1
Posterior fossa	5	1
Total	125	47

their hematomas situated laterally (frontal and parietal); the remainder were frontal (11.3%), vertical (18%), basal (6.0%), occipital (7.2%), and in the posterior fossa (7.2%). Hematomas of the posterior fossa in their series were mostly in children and teen-agers and those frontally situated principally in teen-agers and young adults.

The old concept that the extension of extradural hematomas was limited by the attachment of the dura mater to the suture lines of the skull is fallacious. It is true that the dura is particularly adherent at suture lines and along the lines of attachment of the superior longitudinal sagittal and lateral sinuses.[15,21] However, mapping the outlines of extradural hematomas reveals that they are not always limited by suture lines nor by dural venous sinuses[63] and that some are not restricted to the sites listed in Table 5-3. For instance hematomas occur at the vertex straddling the superior longitudinal sinus[1] or overlie the cerebellum and occipital lobe, not necessarily being restricted to the posterior fossa[13,63] and may extend even to the parietal lobe. Temporal hematomas may spread to the frontal lobe and anterior cranial fossa, posteriorly to the parietal lobe or superiorly to the vertex. Only rarely do they reach the posterior cranial fossa.[63]

In recent years there have been several reports concerning extradural hematomas of the posterior cranial fossa.[7,35,47,51,69,77,81,83] That such hematomas are the most common traumatic space-occupying lesion in the posterior cranial fossa has been emphasized, and only clinical awareness of this uncommon lesion is likely to reduce its disturbing mortality. Wright[107] found that in some 50 cases in the literature, half of the reported patients died without the benefit of operation, and this occurred despite the slow development of the syndrome on account of the venous bleeding. Other authors draw attention to the occurrence of extradural hematomas of the anterior fossa for these too may be overlooked.[25,104] Delay or failure to diagnose extradural hematomas in sites other than in the classical temporal region is also due no doubt to their neglect in current textbooks of pathology.

Isolated cases of bilateral hematoma have been reported at times.[58,61,75,93] McKissock and colleagues[64] recorded three cases (one bitemporal, one bifrontal, and the third biparietal), whereas Jamieson and Yelland[43] found five instances (three bitemporal and two biparietal), incidences of 2.4% and 3.0%, respectively.

Source of the bleeding. With regard to the classic syndrome of extradural hematoma, the common assumption is that the bleeding stems from a branch of the middle meningeal artery at a site corresponding to the position of the pterion. The meningeal vessels at this locale may be enclosed by a bony tunnel or lie within a deep groove in the inner table of the calvarium. This deep grooving of the inner table by meningeal vessels has been held responsible for the vulnerability of both the veins and arteries in cranial fractures even though the feature is much less prominent in the skulls of children. There is controversy about whether the bleeding is more frequently venous or arterial in origin.[34] The fact is that the vascular grooves in the skull are mostly caused by the *venae comitantes* rather than by the middle meningeal arteries.[106] In view of the thinner walls of veins, one might expect venous bleeding to be more prevalent in injuries involving the meningeal vascular grooves.[34,74] Wood Jones[105] demonstrated that the source of bleeding in three of his cases was venous. Paul[74] asserted that in 33 consecutive cases of extradural hemorrhage the bleeding arose from meningeal veins or from the large dural sinuses and

that he had never encountered arterial bleeding. In hematomas of the posterior fossa, bleeding is usually the result of a laceration of the lateral sinus, although in the patient attended by Beller and Peyser,[7] the sigmoid sinus was damaged.

In 34 consecutive cases, Hooper[34] listed an arterial source of bleeding in 15, arterial and venous in 5, tears in the dural venous sinuses in 8, and uncertain in 6. In 22 patients, Voris[99] found the bleeding originated from the posterior branch of the middle meningeal artery in 7, the anterior branch in 5, and the main trunk in 2, whereas in 6 the source was unknown though thought to be venous. The lateral sinus was lacerated in two instances. Jacobson[40] found the posterior branch involved more often than the anterior, but mostly the particular branch was not specified. In a series of cases, LeCount and Apfelbach[52] attributed the bleeding to the anterior branch in 49 and to the posterior in 44. In three cases the superior longitudinal sinus was lacerated and in eight the lateral sinus.

Nowadays it is accepted that bleeding may be either arterial or venous and in some patients both the arteries and veins contribute. A reinvestigation of the longstanding controversy is warranted, but the investigation should be surgical rather than pathological. The interval between the moment of injury and the time of operation is shortest in cases where bleeding is attributable to arterial injury and maximal in cases in which the bleeding is of venous origin, although laceration of large venous sinuses may also cause a fairly rapid demise. Bleeding is from middle meningeal arteries and veins at the site of injury or from other meningeal arteries in the anterior or posterior fossa.[9] Massive extradural hemorrhage from traumatic laceration of the internal carotid artery at the foramen lacerum in association with a fracture through the base of the skull is rare.[31,103]

Diploic vessels may bleed through the fracture site or from separated suture lines[54] but not to any significant degree usually. The lateral or superior longitudinal sagittal sinuses, the torcular Herophili, emissary veins, or the pacchionian corpuscles, respectively, may bleed. Surgical evacuation notwithstanding, when the hemorrhage recurs postoperatively, the episode is often fatal.[34,68] Meningeal vessels predominantly supply the calvarium, so that once the extradural hematoma is initiated, further separation of the dura from the skull brings in its wake the tearing of vessels to the bone. Progressive enlargement of the hematoma and further dissection of the dura is associated with additional bleeding, and such secondary hemorrhages could account for cases that run a protracted course. A most unusual finding is a false traumatic aneurysm of a meningeal artery, especially of the middle meningeal (Chapter 9). Spontaneous aneurysms of the meningeal arteries of the berry type are perforce exceptionally rare, and an indubitable case has not yet been published.

Kessler and associates[48] reported in a child of 8 years of age a fatal spontaneous extradural hemorrhage from a cavernous hemangioma of the petrous portion of the right temporal bone. No details of the extent of the hematoma were provided. Gallagher and Browder[24] mentioned that in one of their fatal cases the hemorrhage came from a bleeding hemangioma in the dura. With the vessels torn or lacerated because of the physical violence to which the head is subjected, the dura mater itself may display tears. Flakes or chips of bone are perhaps responsible for tears or perforations, but the sharp edges of larger fragments of bones, particularly if there is much displacement, may bring about the vascular injuries. Perforating injuries of the skull are also occasionally responsible.

Blood loss. Bleeding from meningeal arteries or dural venous sinuses may at times be severe without the formation of a significant extradural hematoma. Bradley[9] tells of a boy who incurred a depressed fracture of the skull with bleeding from the middle meningeal artery. Blood escaped through the fracture line and accumulated beneath the galea aponeurotica. In compound fractures of the skull the blood may seep through the wound, and subsequent exsanguination is a hazard.[40] In children with closed head injuries, extradural hemorrhage may be severe, the quantity amounting to a significant fraction of the total blood volume. The extradural hemorrhage may initiate profound shock[37,60] even though the neurological disturbance is relatively slight.[64]

Associated lesions. Injuries to other parts of the body may be of vital importance and should not be overlooked. It is likely that lesions other than extradural bleeding will be found in the head.

Scalp. Most extradural hematomas are the consequence of injury. The evidence of trauma, be it bruising, lacerations, or abrasions of the scalp, usually overlie the extradural hematoma. Subepicranial and subpericranial hematomas are also likely to occur.[71] On external examination of the head slight swelling and "bogginess" overlying the fracture in the temporal region may be the only change noticeable.[24] Bleeding from the ear, nose, or pharynx and the presence of otorrhea are suggestive of a fractured skull.

Fractured skull. Fracture of the skull is not invariably found with extradural hematoma, and conversely fractures in the temporal lobe need not be associated with the extradural accumulation of blood. The incidence however of concomitant skull fractures is quite high. Freytag[23] found fractures in 98.1% of 211 cases, and McLaurin and Ford[65] reported an incidence of 87.5% in 40 cases. Jamieson and Yelland[43] found fractures in approximately two-thirds of their series, but in some instances the presence or absence of a fracture was not determined either radiologically or at surgery. Mealy[66] found no fractures in 6 of his 34 cases and asserted that an extradural hematoma without a fracture was most likely to be encountered in the young. Separation of suture lines may occur in lieu of fracture.[54] Some fractures, overlooked or not recognized radiologically, may be out of the operative field at surgery. Fractures of the inner table of the cranium have been incriminated,[40] and Munro and Maltby[68] allege that fracture is invariable. However this is overstating the facts, for extradural hematomas are not all traumatic in origin.

Radiologically linear fractures may be seen to intersect the meningeal vascular groove or venous sinuses, but this does not necessarily indicate an extradural hematoma. The fracture may be of any type, yet a thin linear fracture line with little displacement does not preclude serious damage to the meningeal vessels, for the displacement of the bony edges was probably greater at the moment of fracture than that apparent after admission to hospital. Quite apart from pineal shift, the displacement of the blood vessels, extravasation of contrast medium from the meningeal arteries (Fig. 5-1) into the hematoma,[49] and traumatic meningeal aneurysms may be demonstrated angiographically.[31]

Hemorrhage internal to the dura mater. A head injury sufficient to cause a skull fracture and extradural hemorrhage can produce subdural, subarachnoid, and intracerebral hemorrhage. In the autopsy series of LeCount and Apfelbach,[52] there were 73 large extradural hematomas caused by

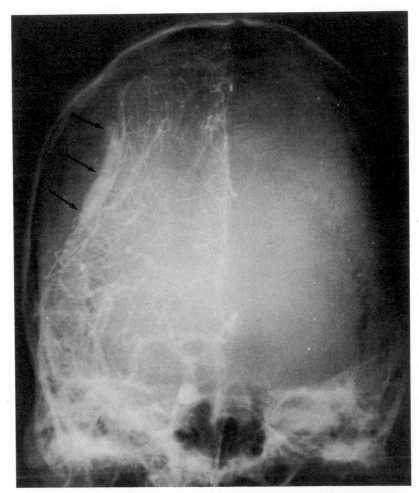

Fig. 5-1. Carotid angiogram showing displacement of vessels away from skull by an extradural hematoma. There is an extravasation of contrast medium (*arrows*) from a torn middle meningeal artery. Absence of a shift of midline structures is suggestive of bilateral hematomas. (Courtesy Dr. D. F. Weinman, Colombo, Ceylon.)

fractures of the middle cranial fossa and, of these, no brain injury was visible in 9, superficial bruising only in 33, 5 to 20 gm. of blood in the subdural space in 25, and large subdural hematomas (40 to 120 gm.) in 6. In all 15 subjects with extradural hemorrhage and fracture of the posterior fossa, the brain exhibited cerebral contusion mostly with a contrecoup injury. Gurdjian and Webster[27] found a subdural hematoma in 7 of their 30 patients with extradural hematoma. In 3 operative cases massive temporosphenoidal hemorrhage was encountered, and in 2 cases subdural accumulation of cerebrospinal fluid. In Hooper's 83 cases subdural hematomas were present in 27 subjects, but only 9 were large and the 6 that were small were less than 1 cm. thick.[34] In 20 patients the subdural hematoma was ipsilateral and contralateral in the remaining 7. In 15 subjects intracerebral hematomas were found, ipsilateral in 13, contralateral in 2, and usually in association with a subdural hematoma. In all there was a subdural or intracerebral hemorrhage in 32 patients (38.6%), excluding subarachnoid hemorrhage. Hooper[34] found no direct correlation between the advent of these complications and the severity of the injury.

In the 125 cases in McKissock's series,[64] there were subdural hematomas in only 12 (ipsilateral in 8, contralateral in 2, and bilateral in 2) and in 2 cases intracerebral hematomas were found in association with subdural hemorrhage. McLaurin and Ford[65] found an associated subdural hematoma in 7 of 47 patients with extradural hemorrhage, an incidence of 14.9%. Jamieson and Yelland[43] reported 79 cases with complications in their series of 167 patients. The complications included 35 with subdural hematoma alone, 30 with cerebral laceration and subdural hematoma, and 14 with intracerebral hematoma with or without a subdural hematoma. Subdural hematoma was the most frequent intradural complication, being present in 44% (74 patients) of the series.

Subarachnoid hemorrhage is frequently an added disorder in patients with extradural hematomas as evidenced by the occurrence of blood stained or xanthochromic cerebrospinal fluid on lumbar puncture,[24,46] despite the fact that this procedure is not generally recommended. The presence of blood in the subarachnoid space in most instances is probably indicative of cerebral contusion. Kennedy and Wortis[46] assert that most patients have an associated injury of the underlying brain seriously affecting the mortality.[65]

Secondary pressure lesions. Compression and distortion of the underlying brain may be considerable, and secondary pressure lesions because of a raised supratentorial pressure are both frequent and likely to be aggravated by a concomitant subdural hematoma or cerebral damage. Papilledema and subhyloid hemorrhages are also possibilities. In hematomas of the vertex there may be angiographic evidence of compression of the superior longitudinal sinus and venous lakes with delayed flow, believed to be the cause of cerebral engorgement and signs of a raised intracranial pressure.[1] The opposite cerebral peduncle is often affected, but midbrain and pontine lesions are usually terminal events. Lumbar puncture may precipitate the patient's demise. The third cranial nerve is frequently injured in this disease, a secondary pressure manifestation of the rapidly expanding supratentorial hematoma. In one case the third nerve had been avulsed from the brain stem as well as exhibiting bruising where it had been in contact with the posterior cerebral artery.[63]

Extradural hematomas of the posterior fossa may effect displacement of the cerebellum and brain stem. Anderson[3] attributed the moderate hydrocephalus in his case to secondary obstruction of the ventricular system, presumably at the level of the aqueduct. This would serve to aggravate the already jeopardized cerebral circulation. Hematomas in this site may also produce third-nerve involvement and much depends on the position and state of the anatomy of the posterior cerebral arteries as well as their pathological state. Wright[107] reported a large pontine hemorrhage in an 18-year-old male who died with a sizable extradural hematoma overlying one cerebellar hemisphere in the presence of only a few scattered contusions on the orbital surface of the frontal lobes. So the question is raised whether or not secondary or brainstem lesions can result from space-occupying lesions in the posterior fossa.

Browder and Hollister[10] found that extradural hematomas deformed the ventricular system and that ventriculography, in patients whose hematomas had been surgically removed 2 weeks to 5 years previously, revealed mild to moderate dilatation of the ventricles in many cases. Enlargement of the lateral ventricles when present may be asymmetrical, the large ventricle being on the side contralateral to that of the hematoma.

Mortality

Hooper[34] in 1959 reviewing the mortality for extradural hematoma found many reported rates exceeding 30% and ranging as high as 76%. Over a similar period several other mortalities below 30% were reported. Jamieson[41] recorded a rate of 8%, Ingraham and associates[37] 10%, and Hooper[34] himself reported a rate of 23%. The head injury may be so severe that survival is out of the question. The discrepancy in the above mortalities appears to be caused by the existence in most series of a variable number of patients who could have been saved but who died. McKenzie[63] stated bluntly that the most certain and obvious cause of death is failure to operate.

The prognosis of extradural hematoma depends on the following several factors:

The earliest possible recognition of the disease. Extradural hematoma causes a most dramatic clinical syndrome classically after a fall or a blow to the head, namely: (1) concussion with loss of consciousness for a variable period of time, (2) recovery, with a "lucid interval" lasting up to several hours or days, (3) the return of coma, possibly preceded by headache, drowsiness,

and vomiting, and finally (4) decerebrate rigidity and death. Variation in this clinical picture is the rule, and it is probably this very fact that accounts for the delay or failure in making a diagnosis.[97] In diagnosis, emphasis has been on the occurrence of a "lucid interval" rather than progressive impairment of the rate of consciousness or the deepening of the degree of unconsciousness.[43] Failure to suspect extradural hematoma in cases of minor trauma is a hazard.[84]

Rapid institution of adequate surgical therapy. Extradural hematoma is a surgical emergency. Delay increases the mortality and the incidence of serious neurological sequelae even in the event of survival. Evacuation of the hematoma and hemostasis in ideal cases result in rapid and dramatic recovery, but severe midbrain damage may have occurred prior to surgery if there has been undue delay. Air embolism may complicate lacerations to the venous sinuses, and postoperatively there may be recurrence of the hemorrhage.

The severity of the injury and associated lesions. The severity of the injury is of course a major factor in determining survival. Profuse hemorrhage will increase the rate of evolution of the clinical picture. Apart from injuries to other parts of the body, traumatic intradural lesions seriously affect the mortality. There was a mortality of 55% (7 cases) in 13 patients with concomitant cerebral contusion or laceration at autopsy or operation but only 33% (3 cases) in 9 subjects without macroscopic injury.[99] In a larger series (93 cases), Hooper[34] found a 48% mortality for extradural hematoma associated with intradural hematomas, four times higher than in uncomplicated cases (12.5%). Jamieson and Yelland[43] in their analysis of 167 cases indicated a similar increase in mortalities.

Miscellaneous factors. Other prognostic factors include (1) the level of consciousness, the mortality being highest among those in coma at the time of operation and in those comatose from the injury to the time of surgery, and (2) age, the mortality being least in patients under 7 years and greatest in those over 60 years.[64] Associated lesions internal to the dura greatly augment the mortality. Hooper[34] considered that an overall mortality of 10% was reasonable. Other authors concur.[43,64] A mortality greater than 28% was thought to indicate a poor institution or a low level of medical education. The number of avoidable deaths, therefore, even today, is considerable. The unavoidable mortality[100] has been rated at only 2.3%.

Neurological deficit may persist postoperatively and is dependent on the severity of the associated head injury and also on the severity of secondary pressure lesions. Recently ophthalmological and otological defects have been found in otherwise healthy patients who survived an extradural hematoma.[94] It is consequently of medicolegal importance.

Pathogenesis

The immediate cause of most cases of extradural hemorrhage is trauma of one sort or another to the head. It may or may not be associated with external evidence of injury. The mechanism by which trauma results in an extradural hematoma is however still obscure. Erichsen[19] related how Sir Charles Bell years before had found that a forceful blow with a mallet to the side of a cadaver's head detached the dura without occasioning a fracture of the bone. In a similar experiment Bell found that an arterial infusion resulted in an accumulation of the infusate in the extradural space. Paul,[74] repeating Bell's experiments, confirmed that severe grades of blunt force were needed to fracture the skull or to detach the dura mater from the overlying bone. Blows to the skull were unsuccessful when the head was unsupported.

Traumatic separation of the dura from the calvarium is thought to be too localized to account for the extensive extradural hematomas encountered in practice.[74] Hence the assumption that progressive dissection of the dura mater from the bone follows as the hemorrhage continues.

Through a trephine hole, Paul[74] submitted the dura mater to a pressure of 200 mm. Hg for half an hour. This pressure was insufficient to detach the dura and pulsatile pressure was not used. Paul found that direct finger pressure on the dura through a trephine hole would not detach the dura, but a shearing force applied by inserting the finger between the edge of the bone and the dura caused it to strip away readily with little force. He suggested that the blunt edge of the clot would act as a wedge shearing off the dura mater, but no measurements were attempted and the explanation of the mechanics is still open to question. Nevertheless it appears that at the time of injury, whether the skull fractures or not, the dura is separated from the skull. Campbell and Cohen[11] contend that separation is caused by the difference in coefficients of elasticity of dura and bone causing a shearing stress at the junction of the layers.

The strength of the adhesion of the dura to the skull varies from site to site and person to person. McLaurin and Ford[65] assert that the dura is less firmly attached in the temporal region than elsewhere. Inbending of the skull at the time of impact followed by outward rebound deflection of the skull strips off the dura mater. The dural separation, which is always centered about the point of impact, is accentuated by actual displacement of bone at fracture sites, especially in depressed fractures.

In dogs a steady force of 90 gm. applied to the dura mater will induce separation of the dura from the inner surface of the skull, but pulsatile pressure requires much less force, being in the range of 35 to 70 gm.[21] Ford and McLaurin[21] explained that with the initial separation of the dura mater at the time of injury, and a laceration of a meningeal artery, an extradural hematoma would form, which, then acting as an hydraulic press, would magnify the input arterial pressure accordingly and thus initiate further stripping of the dura. Venous pressure was considered to be too low unless the laceration of a sinus was accompanied by simultaneous wide separation of the dura and loss of intradural pressure. If the argument is valid, the vulnerability of the middle meningeal vein is of little import because relative pressures would inhibit significant bleeding in most cases and the development of an extradural hematoma would then require arterial rupture. Ford and McLaurin[21] considered that detachment occurs suddenly rather than progressively and under such circumstances the hematoma would approximate full size within a brief time of the injury. The clinical picture was thought to evolve not so much from recurrent or persistent hemorrhage but rather from the interplay of the following factors responsible for the adaptation of the intracranial contents to the pressure of the hematoma:

1. Volume of the hematoma compared with the volume of the supratentorial contents, and specifically the volume of the extracellular fluid (cerebrospinal fluid and venous blood)
2. Location of the hematoma
3. Rapidity of the formation of the mass
4. Individual tolerance

Other authors believe that pulsatile pressure fluctuations, being of considerable magnitude, progressively enlarge the extradural space, rupturing adhesions and vessels to augment the size of the hematoma.[11]

Dogs with experimentally induced extradural hematomas tolerate their intracranial mass remarkably well despite uncal herniation and midbrain distortion at autopsy.[21] Temporal hematomas, which would form rapidly because of the relatively loose attachment of the dura, are more likely, it is thought, to obliterate the aqueduct and so interfere with the compensatory removal of cerebrospinal fluid in adaptation to the intracranial mass, and herniation of the uncus is most prominent in these hematomas.[21] Paul[74] suggested that the loss of consciousness is caused by the distortion and displacement of the brain rather than by intracranial pressure, and in all probability it is in the brain stem that the crucial damage occurs.

The occurrence of massive extradural hemorrhage secondary to ventricular drainage is a relatively unknown complication of this neurosurgical procedure, which surgical trauma does not seem to explain. It has been suggested that the pull of the cerebral veins on the dura mater during decompression promotes detachment of the dura from the calvarium.[29] Haft, Liss, and Mount[29] noted that the dura is supposed to be less adherent to the calvarium anteriorly, but this type of hematoma is not limited to the anterior two-thirds of the cranium. It is possible that during the prolonged hydrocephalic state the attachment of the dura mater to the calvarium may become weaker in association with the thinning of the calvarium, which so often occurs. This could readily be tested in hydrocephalic skulls at autopsy. Pulling on the dura by the vessels is not an attractive concept, but it is possible that the weight of a deflated hydrocephalic cerebrum could effect some separation of a loosely adherent dura. It does not explain extradural hemorrhage in the posterior fossa in the case reported by Frera.[22] The fact that profuse spontaneous bleeding occurred in these brains at about the time the extradural hematoma seemed to be initiated could be an important etiological factor. In hydrocephalic skulls with impaired circulation, it could be that rapid decompression results in an abrupt reflex augmentation of flow within the cranium, which accounts for the profuse and at times uncontrollable spontaneous bleeding and extradural hemorrhage. At times subdural hematoma complicates ventricular decompression in hydrocephalics.[17,85,108] Anderson[4] contended that decompression probably resulted in tension on veins traversing the subdural space, but events in most of these cases moved more slowly than with extradural hemorrhages. Study of the pathogenesis of extradural hemorrhage complicating ventricular decompression for hydrocephalus in the experimental animal could be readily and profitably essayed.

Spinal extradural hematoma

Unlike its counterpart within the cranium, extradural hematoma of the spinal cord is not a well-known entity, yet there is the same urgent need for prompt recognition and immediate surgical intervention to obviate neurological sequelae. Extradural hemorrhage, though a most unusual cause of sudden compression of the spinal cord, may accompany severe back injuries such as spinal fractures and dislocations, direct blows or falls on the back, and penetrating injuries (gunshot and stab wounds). In such cases subdural and subarachnoid hemorrhage are likely to accompany the extradural hemorrhage. A traumatic lumbar puncture may also result in extradural extravasation of blood.[44] Hemorrhage into the spinal extradural space can complicate blood dyscrasias, hemangioma of a vertebra (usually thoracic), or even the rupture of an aortic aneurysm. The bleeding however is either minor or incidental to more widespread and serious manifestations of the primary disease.[44] Yet, on occasions when a spinal extradural hemorrhage occurs spontaneously or occurs after a rather minor injury or fall, the hematoma so formed causes compression of the cord and paraplegia. Although such lesions may be associated with some subarachnoid or subdural bleeding, the extradural hematoma is the major feature of the illness, and because of compression, the result is a severe neurological deficit (paraplegia, paraparesis, or quadriplegia).

Shenkin, Horn, and Grant[87] found three extradural hematomas in 54 extradural lesions compressing the spinal cord, an incidence of 5.6% of the extradural lesions, which in turn constituted 30% of the total number of mass lesions of the spinal canal. Markham and associates[59] collected 49 cases of spontaneous extradural hematoma in 1967, but other cases have also been reported, including some caused by anticoagulant therapy.[14,32,38,88] Little information is available to indicate the true incidence of the condition, and though regarded as being fairly rare,[44] it is doubtless more frequent than the literature would indicate.

Mostly these lesions occur in adults, and no sex preponderance is obvious, since Markham and associates[59] found 28 males and 21 females having the lesions in the series they analyzed. One instance during pregnancy (sixth month),[8] has been reported, and one case was of an infant of 14 months of age.[38] Although any segment of the vertebral canal may be involved, the thoracic segment is most frequently affected.[32] In the main the hematoma deranges only the length of two or three vertebrae, although Lowrey[57] reported one extending from the fifth cervical vertebra to the fifth thoracic vertebra in a 71-year-old woman who sustained minor injury to the right side of her head. Another hematoma extended from the base of the skull to the lower thoracic vertebrae,[2] and yet another extended from the third cervical vertebra to the lumbar region.[76]

The hematoma at autopsy or operation may be more than 1 cm. thick and may resemble a hematoma at any other site. It can completely encircle the cord or be limited to one aspect, such as the dorsal half of the space, and need not be symmetrical. If recent, it will be blackish red, and as the interval between onset and inspection increases, the color will progressively change from chocolate brown to orange brown. The cerebrospinal fluid is clear, xanthochromic, or blood stained, while the protein level, if tested, is generally elevated above 45 mg. and may be over 1000 mg. per 100 ml. Obstruction in the subarachnoid space may be demonstrated by myelography and less often by manometric testing.[59] In their series, Shenkin, Horn, and Grant[87] classified as chronic two hematomas that were cystic encapsulated masses easily separated from the dura. The capsules consisted of fairly dense vascular granulation tissue with many hemosiderin-laden macrophages toward the inner aspect. The description of the encapsulated hematomas does not appear to be consistent with the relatively short duration of the histories, and it is possible that like subdural hematomas, they may manifest themselves after a lag period.

The hematoma causes acute compression of the spinal cord or cauda equina sufficient to produce paraplegia, unless the pressure is relieved. Relief of pressure however is not measured in minutes as in ischemic lesions but in hours, suggesting that the flow of blood to the cord or cauda equina is never completely interrupted. The changes in the cord have not been described in any detail. The cord may be indented and has been said to appear so on external examination,[87] although hemorrhages might be expected because of compression of pial veins, and extensive softening was observed in one case.[2] Microscopically edema may be prominent in association with both a honeycomb appearance and demyelination.[18] Ultimately, compound granular corpuscles and gemistocytic astrocytes become prominent as repair proceeds. The prevalence of persistent paraplegia or paraparesis postoperatively is attributable to the degeneration of the long fiber tracts, which are particularly susceptible to compression.

The onset of pain in the back with the subsequent development (from 1 hour to 10 days) of symptoms and signs of cord compression may be spontaneous or may be apparently precipitated by straining, lifting, vomiting, or the valsalva maneuver (during defecation, urination, coughing,[38] and sneezing). Twisting in bed,[87] trivial falls,[91,98] or bumps on the head[57] have preceded the onset in some cases. The hemorrhage may occur even during sleep.[88] Cube[16] asserted that 13 of the 19 cases he reviewed were caused by extradural hemangiomas. This high incidence is not supported by the analysis of Markham and associates,[59] who found only one in 49 cases of extradural hemorrhage. Spurny and colleagues[88] found that 10 (or 23%) of the 43 cases of spontaneous extradural hematoma in the literature up to 1964 were attributable to anticoagulant therapy (cou-

marin derivatives). Furthermore, the hemorrhage occurred at levels of prothrombin time generally regarded as within the therapeutic range.[88] Instances have also been associated with polycythemia vera and hemophilia.[42,90]

The prognosis for this lesion in practice is bad. In the absence of other serious accompanying lesions, early surgical relief of the pressure minimizes the degree of permanent neurological damage. Early intervention may be followed by complete recovery,[88] and with delay in diagnosis some degree of paraplegia with incontinence persists in many cases. Only two of the 10 cases attributable to anticoagulant therapy made a good recovery and of Lowrey's 24 reviewed cases, only 11 patients recovered.[57] Several died some days after the onset from infection or other pathology. Maxwell and Puletti[62] reported a chronic hematoma in a young boy who made almost a complete recovery postoperatively, indicating that the duration is probably less important than the severity of the compression.

There has been no investigation into the conditions under which extradural hemorrhage produces spinal cord compression. The spinal dura mater is equivalent to the inner layer only of the intracranial dura and, unlike its intracranial counterpart, it is not firmly attached to the walls of the canal.[53] The spinal dura is firmly attached to the margin of the foramen magnum and to the second and third cervical vertebrae. Caudally it is protracted as a sheath about the filum terminale and fixed to the periosteum on the posterior surface of the coccyx. Tubular sheaths of dura extend outward about the spinal nerve roots into the intervertebral foramina. Loose fibrous strands, least prominent in the thoracic region, form attachments to the posterior longitudinal ligament of the vertebral column. The extradural space contains soft fatty tissue, plexiform thin-walled veins (the internal vertebral venous plexus), and arteries supplying the bones, ligaments, and structures within the canal. The anatomy of the spinal extradural space is thus vastly different from that of the cranium. An extravasation of blood into the extradural space permeates the soft extradural fat, and normally, clotting tends to localize the hematoma and to restrict pressure effects. The dura mater is easily displaced inward toward the cord. The expanding hematoma then exerts pressure on the subarachnoid space, pial vessels, and the cord.

The source of the bleeding, though generally believed to be venous, is uncertain.[44] Some instances are caused by a hemangioma,[16] whereas other cases are possibly arteriovenous aneurysms.[56,70] Recurrent symptoms[86] suggest a hemangioma or an arteriovenous aneurysm. However, except in the above-cited cases, there is no evidence that the veins are unduly varicose, even though this would be the most logical conclusion. No good reason exists for assuming the presence of a hypothetical weakness in the vessel walls. In those patients under anticoagulant therapy, excessive bleeding presumably occurs from small petechiae or ecchymoses, which normally pass unnoticed. Sadka[80] put forward the theory that spinal extradural hemorrhage could be akin to primary intracerebral hemorrhage, but there is no evidence to support this concept. The mechanisms involved in the production of cord damage await elucidation.

References

1. Alexander, G. L.: Extradural haematoma at the vertex, J. Neurol. Neurosurg. Psychiat. 24:381, 1961.
2. Amyes, E. W., Vogel, P. J., and Raney, R. B.: Spinal cord compression due to spontaneous epidural hemorrhage, Bull. Los Angeles Neurol. Soc. 20:1, 1955.
3. Anderson, F. M.: Extradural cerebellar hemorrhage, J. Neurosurg. 6:191, 1949.
4. Anderson, F. M.: Subdural hematoma, a complication of operation for hydrocephalus, Pediatrics 10:11, 1952.
5. Avol, M.: Chronic subdural hematoma, Bull. Los Angeles Neurol. Soc. 19:37, 1954.
6. Ballance, A. C., and Ballance, C. A.: Intracranial haemorrhage in the newborn, Lancet 2:1109, 1922.
7. Beller, A. J., and Peyser, E.: Extradural cerebellar hematoma, J. Neurosurg. 9:291, 1952.
8. Bidzinski, J.: Spontaneous spinal epidural hematoma during pregnancy, J. Neurosurg. 24: 1017, 1966.
9. Bradley, K. C.: Extra-dural haemorrhage, Aust. New Zeal. J. Surg. 21:241, 1952.
10. Browder, J., and Hollister, N. R.: Air encephalography and ventriculography as diagnostic aids in craniocerebral trauma. In: Trauma of the central nervous system, Ass. Res. Nerv. Ment. Dis. 24:421, 1945.
11. Campbell, J. B., and Cohen, J.: Epidural hemorrhage and the skull of children, Surg. Gynec. Obstet. 92:257, 1951.
12. Chason, J. L.: Brain, meninges, and spinal cord. In Saphir, O.: A text on systemic pathology New York, 1959, Grune & Stratton, Inc., vol. 2, p. 1798.
13. Coleman, C. C., and Thomson, J. L.: Extradural hemorrhage in the posterior fossa, Surgery 10:985, 1941.
14. Cooper, D. W.: Spontaneous spinal epidural hematoma, J. Neurosurg. 26:343, 1967.
15. Courville, C. B.: Pathology of the central nervous system, ed. 3, Mountain View, Calif., 1950, Pacific Press Publishing Association.
16. Cube, H. M.: Spinal extradural hemorrhage, J. Neurosurg. 19:171, 1962.
17. Davidoff, L. M., and Feiring, E. H.: Subdural hematoma occurring in surgically treated hydrocephalic children, J. Neurosurg. 10:557, 1953.
18. Davison, C.: Pathology of the spinal cord as a result of trauma. In: Trauma of the central nervous system, Ass. Res. Nerv. Ment. Dis. 24:151, 1945.
19. Erichsen, J. E.: Lectures on injuries of the head, Lancet 1:1, 1878.
20. Fiskin, R. D., and Kurze, T.: Acute epidural hemorrhage complicating resection of acoustic neurinoma, J. Neurosurg. 21:58, 1964.
21. Ford, L. E., and McLaurin, R. L.: Mechanisms of extradural hematomas, J. Neurosurg. 20: 760, 1963.
22. Frera, C.: Supratentorial extradural haematomas secondary to ventricular decompression, Acta Neurochir. 20:31, 1969.
23. Freytag, E.: Autopsy findings in head injuries from blunt force, Arch. Path. 75:402, 1963.
24. Gallagher, J. P., and Browder, E. J.: Extradural hematoma. Experience with 167 patients, J. Neurosurg. 29:1, 1968.
25. Gordy, P. D.: Extradural hemorrhage of the anterior and posterior fossae, J. Neurosurg. 5:294, 1948.
26. Grant, W. T.: Chronic extradural hematoma, Bull. Los Angeles Neurol. Soc. 9:156, 1944-1945.
27. Gurdjian, E. S., and Webster, J. E.: Extradural hemorrhage, Int. Abt. Surg. 75:206, 1942.
28. Guthkelch, A. N.: Extradural haemorrhage as a cause of cortical blindness, J. Neurosurg. 6:180, 1949.
29. Haft, H., Liss, H., and Mount, L. A.: Massive epidural hemorrhage as a complication of ventricular drainage, J. Neurosurg. 17:49, 1960.
30. Hawkes, C. D., and Ogle, W. S.: Atypical fea-

tures of epidural hematoma in infants, children, and adolescents, J. Neurosurg. **19:**971, 1962.

31. Helmer, F. A., Sukoff, M. H., and Plaut, M. R.: Angiographic extravasation of contrast medium in an epidural hematoma, J. Neurosurg. **29:**652, 1968.

32. Heyser, J., and Weber, G.: Die epiduralen Hämatome, Schweiz. Med. Wschr. **94:**2, 46, 1964.

33. Higazi, I.: Epidural hematoma as complication of ventricular drainage, J. Neurosurg. **20:**527, 1963.

34. Hooper, R.: Observations on extradural haemorrhage, Brit. J. Surg. **47:**71, 1959.

35. Hooper, R. S.: Extradural haemorrhages of the posterior fossa, Brit. J. Surg. **42:**19, 1954-1955.

36. Imler, R. L., and Skultety, F. M.: Subacute extradural hematomas, Ann. Surg. **140:**194, 1954.

37. Ingraham, F. D., Campbell, J. B., and Cohen, J.: Extradural hematoma in infancy and childhood, J.A.M.A. **140:**1010, 1949.

38. Jackson, F. E.: Spontaneous spinal epidural hematoma coincident with whooping cough, J. Neurosurg. **20:**715, 1963.

39. Jackson, I. J., and Speakman, T. J.: Chronic extradural hematoma, J. Neurosurg. **7:**444, 1950.

40. Jacobson, W. H. A.: Middle meningeal haemorrhage, Guy's Hosp. Rep. **43:**147, 1886.

41. Jamieson, K. G.: Extradural haemorrhage, Med. J. Aust. **1:**938, 1954.

42. Jamieson, K. G.: Extradural haematoma in a haemophilic child (complicated by diabetes insipidus), Aust. New Zeal. J. Surg. **24:**56, 1954.

43. Jamieson, K. G., and Yelland, J. D. N.: Extradural hematoma, J. Neurosurg. **29:**13, 1968.

44. Kaplan, L. I., and Denker, P. G.: Acute nontraumatic spinal epidural hemorrhage, Amer. J. Surg. **78:**356, 1949.

45. Kelly, D. L., and Smith, J. M.: Epidural hematoma secondary to frontal sinusitis, J. Neurosurg. **28:**67, 1968.

46. Kennedy, F., and Wortis, H.: "Acute" subdural hematoma and acute epidural hemorrhage, Surg. Gynec. Obstet. **63:**732, 1936.

47. Kessel, F. K.: Cerebellar extradural haematoma, J. Neurol. Neurosurg. Psychiat. **5:**96, 1942.

48. Kessler, L. A., Lubic, L. G., and Koskoff, Y. D.: Epidural hemorrhage secondary to cavernous hemangioma of the petrous portion of the temporal bone, J. Neurosurg. **14:**329, 1957.

49. Khatib, R., Gannon, W. E., and Cook, A. W.: Cerebral angiography in supratentorial epidural hematoma, N. Y. State J. Med. **68:**2547, 1968.

50. King, A. B., and Chambers, J. W.: Delayed onset of symptoms due to extradural hematomas, Surgery **31:**839, 1952.

51. Kosary, I. Z., Goldhammer, Y., and Lerner, M. A.: Acute extradural hematoma of the posterior fossa, J. Neurosurg. **24:**1007, 1966.

52. LeCount, E. R., and Apfelbach, C. W.: Pathologic anatomy of traumatic fractures of cranial bones and concomitant brain injuries, J.A.M.A. **74:**501, 1920.

53. Le Gros Clark, W. E.: Central nervous system. In Brash, J. C., and Jamieson, E. B.: Cunningham's textbook of anatomy, ed. 8, London, 1943, Oxford University Press, p. 803.

54. Lemmen, L. J., and Schneider, R. C.: Extradural hematomas of the posterior fossa, J. Neurosurg. **9:**245, 1952.

55. Lewin, W.: Factors in the mortality of closed head injuries, Brit. Med. J. **1:**1239, 1953.

56. Lougheed, W. M., and Hoffman, H. J.: Spontaneous spinal extradural hematoma, Neurology **10:**1059, 1960.

57. Lowrey, J. J.: Spinal epidural hematomas, J. Neurosurg. **16:**508, 1959.

58. MacCarty, C. S., Horning, E. D., and Weaver, E. N.: Bilateral extradural hematoma, J. Neurosurg. **5:**88, 1948.

59. Markham, J. W., Lynge, H. N., and Stahlman, G. E. B.: The syndrome of spontaneous spinal epidural hematoma, J. Neurosurg. **26:**334, 1967.

60. Matson, D. D.: Discussion, J. Neurosurg. **19:**978, 1962.

61. Maurer, J. J., and Mayfield, F. H.: Acute billateral extradural hematomas, J. Neurosurg. **23:**63, 1965.

62. Maxwell, G. M., and Puletti, F.: Chronic spinal epidural hematoma in a child, Neurology **7:**596, 1957.

63. McKenzie, K. G.: Extradural haemorrhage, Brit. J. Surg. **26:**346, 1938.

64. McKissock, W., Taylor, J. C., Bloom, W. H., and Till, K.: Extradural hematoma observations on 125 cases, Lancet **2:**167, 1960.

65. McLaurin, R. L., and Ford, L. E.: Extradural hematoma, J. Neurosurg. **21:**364, 1964.

66. Mealy, J.: Acute extradural hematomas without demonstrable skull fractures, J. Neurosurg. **17:**27, 1960.

67. Moody, W. B.: Traumatic fracture of the cranial bones, J.A.M.A. **74:**511, 1920.

68. Munro, D., and Maltby, G. L.: Extradural hemorrhage, Ann. Surg. **113:**192, 1941.

69. Munslow, R. A.: Extradural cerebellar hematomas, J. Neurosurg. **8:**542, 1951.

70. Nichols, P., and Manganiello, L. O. J.: Extradural hematoma of the spinal cord, J. Neurosurg. **13:**638, 1956.

71. Nora, P. F., and Rosenbluth, P. R.: Chronic extradural hematoma, Amer. J. Surg. **94:**628, 1957.

72. Novaes, V., and Gorbitz, C.: Extradural hematoma complicating middle-ear infection, J. Neurosurg. **23:**352, 1965.

73. Olsen, A. K., and Watson, J. R.: Chronic extradural hematoma, Guthrie Clin. Bull. **18:**14, 1948.

74. Paul, M.: Haemorrhage from head injuries, Ann. Roy. Coll. Surgeons Eng. **17:**69, 1955.

75. Peet, M. M.: Extradural hematoma, subdural hematoma, subdural hydroma, cephalhematoma. In Brock, S.: Injuries of the brain and

spinal cord and their coverings, Baltimore, 1949, The Williams & Wilkins Co., p. 136.

76. Reid, J., and Kennedy, J.: Extradural spinal meningeal haemorrhage without gross injury to spinal column, Brit. Med. J. 2:946, 1925.

77. Reigh, E. E., and O'Connell, T. J.: Extradural hematoma of the posterior fossa with concomitant supratentorial subdural hematoma, J. Neurosurg. 19:359, 1962.

78. Rowbotham, G. F., Maciver, I. N., Dickson, J., and Bousfield, M. E.: Analysis of 1,100 cases of acute injury to the head, Brit. Med. J. 1:726, 1954.

79. Rowbotham, G. F., and· Whalley, N.: Prolonged compression of the brain resulting from an extradural haemorrhage, J. Neurol. Neurosurg. Psychiat. 15:64, 1952.

80. Sadka, M.: Epidural spinal haemorrhage, with a report on two cases, Med. J. Aust. 2:669, 1953.

81. Saleeby, R. G., Le Fever, H. E., and Harmon, J. M.: Acute posterior fossa epidural hematoma, Ann. Surg. 140:748, 1954.

82. Schneider, R. C., and Hegarty, W. M.: Extradural hemorrhage as a complication of otological and rhinological infections, Ann. Otol. 60:197, 1951.

83. Schneider, R. C., Kahn, E. A., and Crosby, E. C.: Extradural hematoma of the posterior fossa, Neurology 1:386, 1951.

84. Schneider, R. C., and Tytus, J. S.: Extradural hemorrhage: factors responsible for the high mortality rate, Ann. Surg. 142:938, 1955.

85. Schorstein, J.: Fatal intracranial venous haematoma following ventricular drainage, J. Neurol. Psychiat. 5:142, 1942.

86. Schultz, E. C., Johnson, A. C., Brown, C. A., and Mosberg, W. H.: Paraplegia caused by spontaneous spinal epidural hemorrhage, J. Neurosurg. 10:608, 1953.

87. Shenkin, H. A., Horn, R. C., and Grant, F. C.: Lesions of the spinal epidural space producing cord compression, Arch. Surg. 51:125, 1945.

88. Spurny, O. M., Rubin, S., Wolf, J. W., and Wu, W. Q.: Spinal epidural hematoma during anticoagulant therapy, Arch. Intern. Med. 114:103, 1964.

89. Stevenson, G. C., Brown, H. A., and Hoyt, W. F.: Chronic venous epidural hematoma at the vertex, J. Neurosurg. 21:887, 1964.

90. Sumner, D. W.: Spontaneous spinal extradural hemorrhage due to a hemophilia, Neurology 12:501, 1962.

91. Svien, H. J., Adson, A. W., and Dodge, H. W.: Lumbar extradural hematoma. J. Neurosurg. 7:587, 1950.

92. Taveras, J. M., and Wood, E. H.: Diagnostic neuroradiology, Baltimore, 1964, The Williams & Wilkins Co.

93. Toole, J. F., and Patel, A. N.: Cerebrovascular disorders, New York, 1967, McGraw-Hill Book Co.

94. Troupp, H., Heiskanen, O., Tarkkanen, A., Koivusalo, P., Aho, J., and Tarkkanen, J.: The neurological deficit after extradural hematoma, Lancet 2:891, 1964.

95. Trowbridge, W. V., Porter, R. W., and French, J. D.: Chronic extradural hematomas, Arch. Surg. 69:824, 1954.

96. Vance, B. M.: Fractures of the skull, Arch. Surg. 14:1023, 1927.

97. Verbrugghen, A.: Extradural hemorrhage, Amer. J. Surg. 37:275, 1937.

98. Verbrugghen, A.: Extradural spinal hemorrhage, Ann. Surg. 123:154, 1946.

99. Voris, H. C.: The surgical treatment of extradural hematoma, J. Int. Coll. Surg. 10:655, 1947.

100. Weinman, D. F., and Jayamanne, D.: The role of angiography in the diagnosis of extradural haematomas, Brit. J. Radiol. 39:350, 1966.

101. Weiss, R. M.: Massive epidural hematoma complicating ventricular depression, J. Neurosurg. 21:235, 1964.

102. Whisler, W. W., and Voris, H. C.: Ossified epidural hematoma following posterior fossa exploration, J. Neurosurg. 23:214, 1965.

103. Whitehurst, W. R., and Christensen, F. K.: Epidural hemorrhage from traumatic laceration of internal carotid artery, J. Neurosurg. 31:352, 1969.

104. Whittaker, K.: Extradural hematoma of the anterior fossa, J. Neurosurg. 17:1089, 1960.

105. Wood Jones, F.: The vascular lesion in some cases of middle meningeal haemorrhage, Lancet 2:7, 1912.

106. Wood Jones, F.: On the grooves upon the fossa parietalia commonly said to be caused by the arteria meningea media, J. Anat. Physiol. 46:228, 1912.

107. Wright, R. L.: Traumatic hematomas of the posterior cranial fossa, J. Neurosurg. 25:402, 1966.

108. Youmans, J. R., and Schneider, R. C.: Posttraumatic intracranial hematomas in patients with arrested hydrocephalus, J. Neurosurg. 17:590, 1960.

6 / Subdural hematoma

Subdural hematoma, recognized since the days of Ambroise Paré,[62,113] is a localized accumulation of blood in the subdural space, which normally is only a potential cavity between the dura mater and the arachnoid. Actually chronic subdural hematoma has also been considered as intradural from its onset.[11] Like extradural hematoma, the manner of clinical presentation varies considerably.[140] It is usually classified acute, subacute, or chronic[43] according to the duration of the history of the lesion.

In the acute form, the subdural hematoma is manifested within a day or two of a head injury, and relatively continuous symptoms and signs appear fairly promptly. A few patients will not seek attention for 2 or even 3 weeks, and such cases are often classified as subacute. This form usually occurs after trauma that is often mild in degree and subsequently for a week or two the symptoms develop insidiously. Patients with chronic subdural hematoma may not recall any injury to the head, and the relatively mild symptoms progress slowly over a long period.[43] They are prone to misdiagnosis because of the atypical modes of clinical presentation.[10] A patient, often elderly, may exhibit unduly rapid mental deterioration, fall repeatedly, or become drowsy, or there is urinary retention. A reliable history may be difficult to elicit because of the rapidly deteriorating mental state, and only physical findings, radiological investigation, and surgical exploration preclude death or permanent mental damage.[7]

Incidence

With the progressive increase in trauma (accidental or otherwise), the aftereffects of injury to the head assume more importance. Subdural hematoma, it is said, occurs in 9% to 13% of all severe head injuries,[74] which is four times more frequent than that for extradural hemorrhage[50] and indicates the neurosurgical importance of the lesion. Leary[78] found that in 10% of several hundred fatal accidents in which there was an intracranial lesion, subdural hematoma accounted directly either for the death or the disability and mental deterioration. Munro[99] estimated that approximately 10% of all patients hospitalized with craniocerebral trauma had subdural hemorrhage. Freytag[50] reported subdural hematomas in 861 of 1367 subjects who died after head injuries caused by blunt force and only 211 cases with extradural hematoma. Wright[152] asserted that below the tentorium, subdural hematomas are probably less frequent than extradural hematomas, though no statistics to this effect are yet available. Browder[18] reported subdural hematomas in 1.6% of 18,272 patients with craniocerebral injuries. Many cases of subdural hematoma do not become apparent immediately after trauma and hence are classified as chronic hematomas. The incidence of the latter, and in particular of spontaneous hematomas unrelated to trauma, is difficult to gauge numerically.

Subdural hematomas infrequently are secondary to other pathological lesions such as tumors and infections. They can complicate the rupture of intracranial arterial aneurysms.[133,134] The incidence has been said to vary[134] from 1% to 8%, but Stehbens[133] recorded 35 (18.7%) in 187 subjects who died of a ruptured aneurysm. The incidence in primary intracerebral hemorrhage was 1.6%.[133]

Allen and associates[4] found evidence of subdural hemorrhage (varying in extent and duration) in 7.9% of 3100 autopsies at mental hospitals. It was the primary cause of death in only 1.1%.

Rare cases complicate ventricular drainage in hydrocephalus; Anderson[6] encountered three in 24 hydrocephalic children treated surgically and Epstein[43] found two in six microcephalic children. Still others complicate anticoagulant therapy. Wiener and Nathanson[149] reported that in six of 50 cases of subdural hematoma, anticoagulant therapy had been prescribed during the month prior to admission. The incidence of subdural hematoma as a complication of anticoagulant therapy, though difficult to assess, is sufficient to cause concern. Accidents are on the increase, and anticoagulant therapy is popular, and so subdural hematomas will no doubt become more common.

Sex and age distribution

The comparatively greater aggressiveness and activity of the male is thought to account for the higher trauma rate[4,50] and hence the preponderance of subdural hematomas in men. The ratio of males to females approximates 2:1 (Table 6-1). McKissock and associates[90] found a ratio of 3:1 among patients with a chronic subdural hematoma. In the combined acute and subacute cases (under 3 weeks' duration) it was only 1.4:1. Freed and Boyd[49] found a predominance of males among patients less than 1 year old.

The age distribution is demonstrated in Table 6-2. Apart from an early peak in the first decade, there is a steady increase to a maximum in the sixth decade before it declines. In McKissock's series[90] according to chronicity (Table 6-2), the incidence of acute and subacute hematomas increased to a maximum at and after 70 years. The more numerous chronic lesions reached a peak in the sixth decade, and the subsequent decline in the seventh decade and beyond was thought to be partly due to misdiagnosis, for with the absence in particular of a history of trauma, cerebrovascular disease might seem to be an adequate explanation for symptoms. Allen, Moore, and Daly[4] found the peak incidence among inmates of mental hospitals to be the seventh decade.

There is a high incidence of subdural hematoma in the first decade, and apart from the cases resulting from birth trauma, the others no doubt reflect the frequency of accidents, particularly of falls with this age group. Freytag,[50] for instance, found approximately 10% of her series of medical examiner's cases of head injuries fell within the first decade. More than half had a fractured skull. Ingraham and Matson[68] regarded subdural hematoma as a common lesion in the first 2 years of life, with the greatest incidence during the first 6 months of life. They estimated that from 1937 to 1943, an average of 17 cases per year were admitted to the Children's Hospital, Bos-

Table 6-1. Sex distribution of subdural hematoma

Author	Number of cases	Number of males	Number of females
Leary (1934)[78]	50	34	16
Allen, Moore, & Daly (1940)[4]	245	148	97
Ingraham & Matson (1944)[68]	98	61	37
Voris (1946)[146]	100	88	12
Vance (1950)[143]	102	69	33
Gurdjian & Webster (1958)*[60]	270	217	53
Mateos & Daly (1958)[88]	123	89	34
Freed & Boyd (1960)[49]	106	90	16
McKissock et al (1960)†[90]	393	265	128
Till (1968)‡[138]	116	70	46

*Including 47 cases of subdural hygroma.
†McKissock's figures include a small error, as his total number of cases cited here exceeds the number actually studied by 4.
‡Including subdural hygromas.

Table 6-2. Age distribution of subjects with subdural hematoma

Authors	0-9 or 0-10	10-19 or 11-20	20-29 or 21-30	30-39 or 31-40	40-49 or 41-50	50-59 or 51-60	60-69 or 61-70	Over 70	Total
Bowen (1905)[17]	2	3	5	6	4	6	3	1	30
Kennedy & Wortis (1936)[74]	2	3	11	17	16	15	4	4	72
Baker (1938)[11]	1	0	4	6	7	7	3	3	31
Allen, Moore, & Daly (1940)[4]	1	3	7	24	45	44	59	62	245
Voris (1946)[146]	0	1	11	21	29	18	16	1	97
Vance (1950)[143]	3	0	9	17	27	23	17	6	102
McKissock et al. (1960)[90]	23	13	19	29	42	100	84	79	389
Freytag (1963)[50]	85	32	91	130	127	160	128	108	861
Total	117	55	157	250	297	373	314	264	1827
McKissock et al. (1960)[90]									
Acute cases	1	4	6	5	9	15	13	29	82
Subacute cases	0	3	4	7	8	16	20	33	91
Chronic cases	22	6	9	17	25	69	51	17	216

ton. They concluded that the frequency with which subdural hematoma is found in infancy is related to the industry with which it is sought.

Precipitating factors

Many factors, in some instances multiple, have been incriminated in the etiology of subdural hemorrhage. Sherwood[127] reviews the amazing change in views on the etiology. In Gilmartin's series of 58 cases,[53] 42 (one doubtful) were attributed to trauma (75%). Of the remaining 15 cases, three were due to ruptured berry aneurysms, two complicated anticoagulant therapy, one occurred in thrombocytopenic purpura, two in intracranial tumor (one metastatic and one glioma), one was attributed to meningitis (7 years previously), and no cause was discovered in six.

Trauma. Trauma is the most frequent etiological factor in the production of subdural hematoma,[18,77,146] particularly in acute lesions, in which the trauma is severe[74] and associated with a cerebral laceration or contusion[58] whence bleeding originates.

Laudig and associates[77] found that in 133 cases of subdural hematoma precipi-

tated by trauma, the injury was to the occipital region of the head in 45 subjects (33.9%), lateral in 32, frontal in 24, multiple sites in 10, and unknown sites in 22.

McKissock and associates[90] analyzed the etiological factors responsible for subdural hematoma in 387 cases. Most were caused by trauma either major (sufficient to cause loss of consciousness) or minor (unaccompanied by loss of consciousness), and a significant proportion was unassociated with a known injury, whereas four cases were attributed rightly or wrongly to coughing (Table 6-3). Indirect trauma such as a fall on the buttocks is unusual, but several cases are on record[94] as well as blast and even whiplash injuries.[104,144] Multiple petechiae to gross hemorrhages transpire in the cranium as a result of blast injuries, and Abbott, Due, and Nosik[1] encountered 37 such cases with subdural hematoma. Trotter[140] emphasized the minor nature of the trauma sometimes responsible. On occasions it is so trivial it is forgotten readily, which possibly accounts for the absence of a history of trauma in many instances, especially with chronic subdural hematoma.[74] Closer interrogation after surgical evacuation of the hematoma may provide the history of a

Table 6-3. Type of injury responsible for subdural hematoma*

Type of subdural hematoma	Etiological factor responsible			
	Major trauma	Minor trauma	Cough	No recognized cause
Acute	52	30	0	0
Subacute	42	40	0	9
Chronic	51	73	4	86
Total	145	143	4	95

*Adapted from McKissock, W., Richardson, A., and Bloom, W. H.: Subdural haematoma: a review of 389 cases, Lancet **1**:1365, 1960.

causative injury. The so-called spontaneous hematoma, that is, unassociated with trauma, has been found in anything from 2% to 34% of reported cases (average about 26%).[58,70,146] It is possible that minor or moderate bumps or blows to the head could be incorrectly incriminated in the causation of a chronic subdural hematoma.

Jewesbury and Josse[71] reported bilateral subdural hematomas in each of two brothers. Neither sibling had a history of trauma considered responsible for the bleeding. The authors speculated upon a congenital diathesis being responsible, but statistically there is no support for such a hypothesis.

Ingraham and Matson[68] considered subdural hematoma to be a common condition in the first 2 years of life, with mental retardation an almost universal result of the cerebral deficit consequent upon the hematoma of this age group. Bleeding in the neonatal infant is believed to result not so much from a difficult labor but from molding of the head, possibly with tearing of the tentorium or of small communicating veins. Fatal subdural hematomas in stillborn and newborn infants may also arise from (1) rupture of the vein of Galen with extensive subdural hemorrhage extending between the cerebral hemispheres and over the surface of the brain and (2) superficial vessels over the cerebral hemisphere, usually a branch of the middle cerebral artery.[110] Chase[24] attributed the bleeding in most cases to stretching and rupturing of the small venous tributaries

of the great cerebral vein of Galen near its junction with the straight sinus.

Not all subdural hematomas in infancy are the result of birth trauma, for in the process of learning to walk and climb, the infant is subject to repeated injuries, including severe head trauma. Caffey[21] reported six nonscorbutic infants with chronic subdural hematoma and, in addition, 23 fractures and 4 contusions of long bones. There was no history of trauma and no clinical or radiological evidence of systemic or skeletal disease to predispose to the pathological fractures. The lesions are known to be traumatic, though pyrexia and leukocytosis in many patients are misleading. Specifically, the violent and repeated trauma is inflicted by the not-so-loving parents or custodians of the unfortunate children. The syndrome is now colloquially known as the "battered baby" syndrome.[56,150] Kempe and colleagues,[73] in a national survery of 71 hospitals in the United States of America, discovered records of 302 cases in 1 year. Approximately 11% were fatal and 28% suffered permanent brain damage. The true incidence is difficult to assess and is probably greater.

Alcoholism. Excessive intake of alcoholic beverages prior to accidents or injuries in general is a frequent finding. Acute alcoholism complicated 40 of the 72 cases of acute subdural hematoma studied by Kennedy and Wortis.[74] Alcohol was deemed to be involved in 27 of the 50 cases reported by Leary.[78] The chronic inebriate is more prone to head injuries, and Vance[143] regarded 74% of his 102 cases as chronic alcoholics.

Mental disease. For a long time chronic subdural hematoma has been considered to be a frequent complication of mental disorders,[132] particularly in respect to general paralysis of the insane and chronic alcoholism. Quite possibly untreated cerebral syphilis in many patients with chronic hematomas may have contributed to the belief that chronic subdural hematoma was primarily an inflammatory disease (hence the synonym pachymeningitis hemorrhagica interna) rather than the sequel of traumatic hemorrhage. Subdural hematoma is said to be more frequently encountered in asylums than in the general population, but there is no recent satisfactory statistical substantiation of this contention. Inmates may be subject to more frequent head trauma than the general population. Subdural hematoma itself may cause serious mental deterioration, for, in infancy, mental retardation and, in older individuals, dementia frequently complicate the disease.[7,121]

Ventricular decompression. Hydrocephalus predisposes the patient to extradural and to subdural hemorrhage, although bleeding is not the acute early complication in the latter. Schorstein[123] in 1942 reported two instances of extradural hemorrhage occurring after ventricular decompression for hydrocephalus. A hydrocephalic woman of 24 years of age, subjected to ventricular drainage, died within 24 hours, and at autopsy bilateral frontal subdural hematomas were found, with intracerebral hemorrhage along the track of the ventricular drain through the left occipital lobe. Anderson[6] reported the development of subdural hematomas in three of 24 hydrocephalic children operated upon for decompression, the hematomas being discovered from 3 days to 6 weeks postoperatively. Davidoff and Feiring[32] reported subdural hematomas in three hydrocephalic children. The hematomas were found 1 month, 2 years, and 3 years respectively after surgery. Difficulty was experienced in the treatment of bilateral hematomas in one patient because of recurrent hemorrhage. Youmans and Schneider[154] reported the development of a subdural hematoma in a hydrocephalic male of 34 years after a fall, and recurrence of the hematoma after surgical intervention. One of the cases of traumatic subdural hematoma reported by Putnam and Cushing[113] had hydrocephalus. There is the possibility that the hydrocephalic state may contribute a predisposition to traumatic subdural bleeding.

The ventricular system is dilated in microcephaly, usually in symmetrical fashion. The dilatation may be extremely prominent in advanced microcephaly,[43] and two instances of associated subdural hematoma have been reported and attributed to birth trauma. This association may not be significant, but the ventricular dilatation and enlargement of sulci and cisterns may predispose the subject to subdural hemorrhage because of the greater mobility of the brain within the skull.

The development of subdural hematoma in a patient with atrophic brain disease and moderate ventricular enlargement has been reported.[22] It is believed that the basic underlying mechanism is the traction on and thus tearing of veins crossing the subdural space when the brain separates from the dura after decompression. Similar events produce the subdural hemorrhage after pneumoencephalography and the passage of air into the subdural space.[20]

Pneumoencephalography. Subdural hematoma after pneumoencephalography in an adult is reported sporadically. Whittier[148] reported only six deaths in 2409 pneumoencephalograms with no instance of subdural hematoma, but Bucy[20] told of serious personality changes in a 66-year-old male on whom a lumbar pneumoencephalogram was performed, with 350 cc. of cerebrospinal fluid being replaced by air. No ventricular deformity was observed, but large collections of air entered the subdural spaces over the cerebral hemispheres. Abrupt deterioration in the patient's condition became evident, and bilateral hematomas were found and evacuated 3 months later with subsequent return to the clinical status preceding the air studies. Robinson[118] reported the history of a male of 48 years of age who had a head injury and was later subjected to pneumoencephalography, with 40 cc. of air being injected with normal results. The onset of severe headache after the investigation and subsequent somnolence led to the discovery of a large subdural hematoma, which was not present on previous angiograms. Khalifeh and associates[76] investigated a male of 52 years and 160 cc. of fluid was replaced by air, with the pneumoencephalogram revealing only cerebral atrophy with apparent recovery. About 2 months later it was found that frontal headaches had persisted since the air studies, and a chronic hematoma was removed.

In at least two of the cases severe cerebral atrophy was present and it is likely that the replacement of cerebrospinal fluid by air permits the brain to settle and separate unduly from the dura mater, with consequent stretching of vessels bridging the subdural space. Howard[64] was able to demonstrate without complications some of these corticodural attachments of the brain by subdural insufflation of air. Similar widening of the subarachnoid space in cerebral atrophy has been suggested as the reason for the high incidence of subdural hematomas in the elderly.[76] The escape of air through a tear in the arachnoid into the subdural space, a frequent occurrence in pneumoencephalography, is especially likely in those patients with cerebral atrophy and can accentuate undue stretching of the bridging vessels.[76] Thus, the cases of subdural hematoma seemingly precipitated by pneumoencephalography have a similar pathogenesis to that occurring after ventricular decompression.

Infective theory. During the nineteenth century, chronic subdural hematomas with their membranous capsules were often attributed to some infective process afflicting the insane especially. Inflammatory exudate and hemorrhage from newly formed hyperemic vessels of granulation tissue were supposed to result in encapsulated hematomas (pachymeningitis hemorrhagica interna).[113] The prevalence of chronic subdural hematomas in general paralysis of the insane was said to bear out the contention. There is no evidence that syphilis per se produces subdural hemorrhage. Tuberculosis, often included as an etiological agent,[125] could conceivably cause rare hemorrhages.

Barratt[12] did much to dispel the inflammatory theory by finding subdural hematomas to be consistently sterile, histologically free of demonstrable bacteria, and incapable of reproducing pachymeningitis hemorrhagica interna when portions of the wall were implanted subdurally in experimental animals. Bucy[20] found bilateral chronic hematomas in a male of 72 years with cystitis. The contents of one hematoma were purulent, the causative organism being identical to that in the urinary bladder and infection was believed to be secondary to the cystitis rather than primary. This complication is quite unique. Nine instances of subdural accumulation of xanthochromic fluid with encapsulation as with subdural hematoma have been found as complications in 23 cases of acute leptomeningitis caused by *Haemophilus influenzae*.[89] Uncertainty persists whether or not they represent hematomas or blood-stained exudates.

Hannah[61] and others[53,98] have attributed subdural hematoma to acute leptomeningitis, and in view of the acute arteritis that may sometimes occur, secondary hemorrhage, though rare, is a distinct possibility.

Nutritional factors. The role of a secondary bleeding defect in subdural hematomas of postnatal infants has been debated. Sutherland[135] in 1894 reported subdural hemorrhage in two infants suffering from rickets and scurvy and the presence of multiple bruises. In one there were also fractures of two long bones whereas the second was one of a family of 12 children, nine of whom died in early life. The bleeding was attributed in each case to scurvy, but the malnutrition like the fractures and bruises may have other explanations (such as the battered baby syndrome). Scorbutic changes have been thought to be present in the bones in some children, and Ingalls[65] concluded that a vitamin C deficiency was the underlying factor predisposing the majority of infants to subdural hemorrhage after insignificant trauma to the head. Ingraham and Matson[68] alleged that 20 of 98 infants exhibited some clinical evidence of vitamin C deficiency. However Griffith and Moynihan[56] considered that many cases purporting to illustrate the effects of scurvy on the skeletal system were probably instances of parental cruelty. The role of scurvy and vitamin K deficiency has probably been overestimated, and it is unlikely that such conditions are responsible nowadays for the intracranial bleeding. It has been noted that several of the children with subdural hematoma were living with foster parents or in institutions,[107,127] and there could have been a greater likelihood of trauma in such patients. Indeed one of Ingraham and Matson's infants[68] had two fractured limbs in addition to the subdural hematoma, and these are the classic features of the battered baby syndrome, in which poor nutrition is frequently manifest. Any incrimination of avitaminosis in the etiology nowadays would certainly need to be accompanied by laboratory evidence.

Blood dyscrasias. Secondary hemorrhages within the cranial cavity in blood dyscrasias are not frequent. Russell[119] in 1954 found only 36 instances among the 461 autopsy records of spontaneous intracranial hemorrhage from 1912 to 1952, and only one of 126 in such autopsies at another hospital was attributed to a bleeding disorder.[16] Russell[119] reported that 15 of the 36 cases were caused by acute leukemia, 13 were caused by thrombocytopenia, 3 by aplastic anemia, 3 by other anemias, 1 by erythrocythemia, and 1 by hemophilia. Instances where the hemorrhages were less than 3 cm. in diameter in the cerebrum and cerebellum and less than 1.5 cm. in the brain stem were excluded. However, of 23 cases of nontraumatic subdural hemor-

rhage, 11 were caused by blood dyscrasias. Massive subdural hemorrhage is not commonly caused by bleeding disorders or coagulation defects except after anticoagulant therapy. In many cases the hemorrhage may involve the dura[72] or the brain including the subarachnoid space with a little blood in the subdural space. Purpura is more likely to cause multiple small hemorrhages rather than massive hemorrhage, although Evans and Perry[45] recorded 22 deaths in 75 cases of thrombocytopenic purpura with half of the deaths being attributed to subdural hemorrhage. Subdural hematoma occurs in leukemia[61] and has been observed in each of three children with acute lymphocytic leukemia.[14] No cases were seen in another series.[57]

Intracranial hemorrhage is a leading cause of death in hemophilia,[75] and not surprisingly subdural hemorrhage sometimes complicates this disorder.[98,130] Ferguson and associates[46] reported such a hemorrhage in a hemophiliac treated surgically after the administration of cryoprecipitate to elevate the serum factor VIII. They reviewed the literature dealing with surgical treatment of intracranial bleeding, primarily extradural and subdural hematomas.

In this era of chemotherapy, intracranial hemorrhage as a complication of anticoagulant therapy for thromboembolic diseases is on the increase. Hypoprothrombinemia, induced by anticoagulants, is the most commonly encountered coagulation defect in clinical practice today. The complications are not specific to any particular anticoagulant. Wells and Urrea[147] investigated cerebrovascular accidents accompanying anticoagulant therapy, and of their 23 cases, five had a subdural hematoma, six intracerebral, one brain stem, and two subarachnoid hemorrhages. The apparent high incidence of subdural hematoma caused concern, and it is now recognized that this is a relatively frequent complication of anticoagulant therapy. Wiener and Nathanson[149] reviewed 50 cases of subdural hematoma at the Mount Sinai Hospital (New York). There was an overall incidence of coagula-

Table 6-4. Reported cases of subdural hemorrhage during anticoagulant therapy

Authors	Sex	Age in years	Subdural hemorrhage	Died	Indication for anticoagulation
Shlevin & Lederer (1944)[128]	Female	79	Multiple hemorrhages	Yes	Retinal vein thrombosis
Nathanson, Cravioto, & Cohen[102] (1958)	Male	61	Unilateral	Yes	Auricular fibrillation
	Male	64	Bilateral	No	Myocardial infarction
	Female	65	Bilateral	Yes	Phlebitis
Barron & Fergusson (1959)[13]	Female	60	Unilateral	Yes	Pulmonary embolism
Eisenberg (1959)[41]	Male	56	Unilateral	Yes	Myocardial infarction
Pan, Rogers, & Pearlman (1960)[105]	Male	75	Bilateral	No	Myocardial infarction
Wells & Urrea (1960)[147]	Male	67	Bilateral	No	Myocardial infarction
	Male	65	Bilateral	No	Myocardial infarction
	Female	50	Unilateral	Yes	Myocardial infarction
	Male	63	Unilateral	Yes	Myocardial infarction
	Female	70	Unilateral	Yes	Myocardial infarction
Wiener & Nathanson (1962)[149]	Male	67	Unilateral	No	Myocardial infarction
	Female	74	Bilateral	No	Recurrent pulmonary emboli
	Male	72	Bilateral	No	Myocardial infarction
	Male	80	Unilateral	Yes	Congestive cardiac failure, partial heart block, hypertension
	Male	64	Unilateral	Yes	Myocardial infarction, undiagnosed cerebral disorder
	Male	61	Unilateral	No	Myocardial infarction
Dooley & Perlmutter (1964)[37]	Male	43	Unilateral	No	Myocardial infarction
	Male	—	Unilateral	No	Myocardial infarction

tion defects in 22% (additional patients suffered from leukemia, thrombocytopenia, and liver disease). Six subjects (12%) had received anticoagulant therapy in the previous month. Most subdural hematomas so induced are associated with anticoagulant therapy of myocardial infarction (Table 6-4). Fluctuation will occur in the prothrombin time or index, and obviously continuous monitoring is impossible. It is believed that bleeding occurs at therapeutic levels varying with the patient, and the precise moment of onset of the hemorrhage is usually uncertain. The apparent lack of correlation between the prothrombin time and the onset of bleeding is a disturbing factor.[37] The problem is compounded by the recent discovery that the hypoprothrombinemic effect of warfarin, a commonly used anticoagulant, is potentiated by many drugs currently used, including chloral hydrate, which enhances the effect by 40% to 80%.[36,126] Other drugs can inhibit the effect of warfarin.[36] Chronic subdural hematomas have been recognized weeks or months after suspension of the anticoagulant therapy.

In many patients the hemorrhage appears to be spontaneous or some unduly mild trauma may suffice to precipitate bleeding. Wiener and Nathanson[149] noted that their patients were somewhat older than their general series of subdural hematomas, but Table 6-4 indicates that most are middle aged or elderly and the mortality is not inconsiderable.

Hemodialysis. Leonard and associates[82] reported subdural hematomas in three patients undergoing hemodialysis and thought this to be a complication of either acute or chronic hemodialysis. Del Greco and Krumlovsky[35] recorded yet another in a woman inadvertently subjected to dialysis with hyperosmotic dialysate with a very high sodium content. It was thought that the hemorrhage may have been caused by tearing of dural veins, consequent upon brain shrinkage caused by intense extra-cellular dehydration. However, the patient had also had systemic heparinization. Marshall and Hinman's patient[87] died with a subdural hematoma after the intravenous administration of a hypertonic urea solution; the bleeding was again attributed to tearing of dural veins consequent upon brain shrinkage. Luttrell and associates[84] found that intraperitoneal hypertonic urea or saline solutions resulted in brain retraction in cats, though the concentration was greater than usually given to man. Hyperosmolarity caused considerable reduction in cerebrospinal fluid, negative pressures of which reached −120 mm. of water after 60 to 80 minutes and −20 to −155 mm. of water after 4 hours. Stretching of veins bridging the subdural space does not seem to be the only possible mechanism because intradural, subdural, subarachnoid, and intracerebral hemorrhage occurred in their animals, the negative pressure no doubt playing an important role (no extracranial bleeding occurred). Brain shrinkage with associated negative intracranial pressure may account for subdural hemorrhage with inadvertent hypertonic hemodialysis or excessive urea shifts. Alternatively it may be systemic anticoagulation generally accompanying hemodialysis.[81,137] Leonard[81] found that in approximately 880 patients on maintenance hemodialysis, subdural hematoma had occurred in 14 patients (1.6%). In all, 27 cases were identified in the survey with this complication, and in only two was there suspicion of head trauma.

Miscellaneous factors. Subdural hematoma, usually acute, is often a manifestation of a ruptured intracranial arterial aneurysm,[133] and it also occurs with bacterial aneurysms.[27,119] Cases of subdural hemorrhage in the posterior fossa caused by a ruptured intracranial aneurysm have been encountered only twice; in one the sac arose from a vertebral artery[151] and in the other the aneurysm was on the posterior inferior cerebellar artery.[27] It has been seen

with primary intracerebral hemorrhage[133] and is associated with nontraumatic subarachnoid hemorrhage,[54] although in cases of the latter, many could be instances of unrecognized aneurysmal rupture. Subdural hematoma has also been found with a massive intracerebral hemorrhage in eclampsia[54] and more frequently with ruptured arteriovenous angiomatous formations.[18,27,77,146] Metastatic tumors have produced subdural hemorrhage,[18,77,120] with subcortical abscesses,[18] acute exanthemas,[74] and salicylism being less frequent causes.

Convulsions are known to be symptomatic of subdural hematoma, but several authors have reported subdural hematoma in epileptic patients. Cole and Spatz[29] reported on eight patients with a past history of convulsions apparently unrelated to the hematoma. Echlin and associates[40] found five chronic epileptics among 300 patients treated surgically for subdural hematoma and another four cases were reported by Arieff and Wetzel.[8] The association is rare and of uncertain significance. The most likely explanation is that the subdural hemorrhage is caused by trauma incurred during the grand mal seizure, and even a fractured skull has been disclosed.[8] Minor cerebral trauma occasioned by a fall at the commencement of the seizure might well result in considerable bleeding because of the Valsalva mechanism during the tonic phase of the convulsion. Alternatively the association could be coincidental.

Macroscopic appearance

Macroscopically hemorrhage into the subdural space varies considerably in extent. Sometimes it amounts to only a thin diffuse coating of blood, but unless it forms a localized accumulation, it is in most cases disregarded, though eventually these hemorrhages are recognized as a diffuse xanthochromic staining of the inner surface of the dura mater. Such findings are mostly coincidental and likely to be overshadowed by more serious damage.

In the infant a subdural hematoma of significant size need not be as thick as in the adult and is mostly less than 4 mm. thick. In the adult, acute hematomas may be as thick as 4 cm.[23] Acute and subacute hematomas tend to be somewhat ovoid and disc shaped, being concave on the arachnoidal surface. Chronic hematomas on the other hand are more localized, thicker and biconvex as is well demonstrated by angiography.[53] The hematomas of significant size range from 50 to 200 ml. in volume.[58] LeCount and Apfelbach[80] found that they weighed from 10 to 210 gm., most being about 40 gm. In another series,[77] the clots varied from 25 to 300 gm. Vance[142] in 1927, weighing the hematomas from 36 cases, found a range of 15 to 220 gm. and an average of 61 gm. In 1950, he[143] reported details of another 42 hematomas (weighing 30 to 250 gm.), averaging 125 gm., and noted that there was not necessarily a direct relationship between the severity of the underlying brain injury and the size of the hematoma.[142] The correlation between the size of the hematoma and the severity of the clinical manifestations is also frequently poor[140] possibly because of the advent and site of associated cerebral damage. Aronson and Okazaki[9] estimated that a hematoma of 50 cc. or more was invariably associated with some neurological deficit and psychiatric disturbance though individual tolerances varied. When the hematoma is more than 100 cc., the immediate cause of death is most likely due to the hematoma itself.

In the subdural hematoma of recent origin, the overlying dura mater is very tense and the typically red currant jelly type of subdural clot beneath imparts to it a bluish black or even purplish hue. When the dura is incised, soft gelatinous clot may be extruded under pressure through the opening. The hematoma is initially moist, soft, readily detached from the dura mater and generally confined to an area surrounding injury in the cerebral hemisphere. The hematoma within a few days becomes drier, firmer in consistency, and more adherent to the dura mater. The hematomas of considerable thickness are usually more extensive, covering a larger part of the cerebral hemisphere. The subdural space elsewhere may have a thin coating of blood. Shift of the brain and reduction in the size of the ipsilateral ventricle may be quite marked. The ipsilateral hemisphere exhibits flattened gyri and shallow sulci consistent with the increased intracranial pressure. Facing the arachnoid, the hematoma usually exhibits a relatively smooth concave surface.

In subacute hematomas the dura mater is tense and likely to be dark brown or coffee colored. The hematoma is a dark brown, relatively firm, saucer-shaped mass adherent to it. The innermost surface is fairly smooth and bloodstained or xanthochromic fluid may be present. In acute and subacute hematomas fluid has often been found in association with solid clots[77] and has been attributed to exudation, osmotic imbibition, or leakage of cerebrospinal fluid.

The completely encapsulated chronic hematoma is firmly adherent to the dura, which is deeply pigmented and occasionally greenish when viewed from the external surface.[113] The hematoma contains brownish or yellow-brown liquid although the inner and outer coverings may be in varying stages of fusion. The capsule applied to the dura is from 1 to 4 mm. in thickness and facing the dura it is generally less than 1 mm. Pigmentation is prominent. The arachnoid surface of the underlying brain often exhibits xanthochromia. Leary[78] asserts that siderophages invade the arachnoid and give rise to varying xanthochromic staining of the leptomeninges. However subarachnoid hemorrhage and some cerebral contusion may occur simultaneously with the subdural hemorrhage, and minor adhesions can intervene between the arachnoid and the capsule of the hematoma. Paul[106] found at operation that the pressure within a chronic subdural hematoma was 7 cm. of water in one patient and 8 cm. in another (with the skull opened). Compression and molding of the brain is associated with large hematomas and the underlying hemisphere may be greatly reduced in size.

Leary[78,79] divided subdural hematomas on pathological grounds in the following manner:

Group 1. Hemorrhages of recent origin, being of the typically moist, semifluid, red currant jelly clot, with death from ½ hour to 18 hours after the accident or onset of symptoms

Group 2. Hematomas of dark reddish black clots, firmer and drier than those of group 1 and tending to adhere to the dura; death is from 17 hours to 3 days after the accident

Group 3. Hematomas appearing in the form of chocolate-colored clot containing yellow fluid and adhering to the dura mater; organization with a neomembrane from the dural surface is evident but there is no inner membrane; the patients survived from a few to 15 days after the hemorrhage

Group 4. Hematomas completely encased by neomembranes enclosing chocolate-colored clot and brownish fluid; the completed membranous capsule takes more than a month and possibly years to develop

Group 5. Hematomas virtually absorbed, with only the fused pigmented neomembranes present and healing almost complete; duration of the lesion is considered longer than those of group 4

Chronic subdural hematomas, like those elsewhere, can undergo calcification[83] mostly after about 3 years but sometimes after an interval as short as 4 months.[97] Calcification in these lesions is rare, only 28 instances having been reported up till 1966.[92] The fibrous capsule of long-standing hematomas initially undergoes extensive hyalinization and then becomes liable to calcification. There is no evidence that a disorder of calcium metabolism is necessary. The mineral deposit may be merely in the capsule but can extend to the necrotic debris within. Calcification may be a feature of the bilateral lesions. In infants, distinctive bony changes with asymmetry of the skull can develop secondarily.[97] The calcification tends to appear in the frontal region particularly. McLaurin and Mc-Laurin[92] reported six instances in young children, three of them premature, and five suffering from serious mental retardation. This is however a complication of chronic subdural hematoma of infancy and so it should not be held peculiar to calcified

lesions per se. Calcified hematomas may be symptomless; compare the case of a 55-year-old male laborer who had a calcified hematoma 15 by 6 by 4 cm.[97] Chusid and his colleagues[26] reported not only calcification but ossification of the dural part of the capsule about a chronic subdural hematoma. The portion of the capsule removed surgically was 12 by 7 cm. and 3 to 4 mm. thick. The inner part of the capsule facing the arachnoid was not mentioned. These authors found only three previous authentic cases in which bone (distinct from calcification) had been demonstrated histologically. Other cases have since been reported.[3] No doubt it would be found more frequently in calcified hematomas if adequate histological searches were conducted. Baker[11] asserted that old hematomas may contain cartilage.

Pathological changes may be demonstrated radiologically, and though skull fracture or pineal displacement may be found at times, no abnormality is to be seen on plain films of the skull. Toole and Patel[139] state that no pineal displacement occurs if the hematoma is less than 100 ml. in volume or if it is subfrontal, temporal, or subtentorial in location. Calcification or ossification naturally are rare, but time permitting, hematomas can now be demonstrated by angiography,[53] echoencephalography, electroencephalography, and brain scanning. Pneumoencephalography frequently demonstrates shifting of the lateral ventricles to the opposite side, the contralateral ventricle often being dilated and the ipsilateral ventricle normal or reduced in size. A pathognomonic clear zone may be demonstrated between the subdural hematoma and the underlying brain when air enters the subarachnoid or subdural space.[39,139]

Location

The position of supratentorial hematomas of the subdural space is characteristically over the cerebral convexity, as they are generally frontoparietal. The site tends to be nearer the frontal than the occipital pole, although in very extensive collections of subdural blood clot, temporal and occiptal lobes are covered, as well as frontal.[78] The hematoma may also extend inferiorly onto the floor of the anterior and middle cranial fossas.[68] The occipital lobes are frequently covered in recent subdural hemorrhage in association with a fractured skull, but hematomas of long duration are extremely rare in this situation.[78] The propensity for the frontoparietal region may be allied with local differences in intracranial pressures and less resistance to the displacement of the brain in that area. Voris[146] held that as blood escapes into the subdural space, the brain settles to a more dependent part in the intracranial cavity, permitting blood to accumulate over the superolateral aspect of the cerebrum.

The falx and tentorium, it has been alleged, serve as a partition to limit the spread of blood. Leary disagrees[78] and indeed two frontal hematomas may be connected with each other under the falx.[95] Blood spreading beyond one hemisphere to the opposite side will no doubt produce bilateral hematomas. Alternatively blood accumulating on one side and clotting fairly rapidly, will, with pressure and by crowding the brain to the other side and against the tentorium and falx, serve to limit spread of the hematoma.[78] The source of the bleeding is an all important factor. When near the midline, bilateral accumulation of blood is more likely to ensue. Moreover supratentorial and subtentorial subdural hematomas can coexist.[47] Subdural hematomas may be found at other sites. One reported case was predominantly basal.[113] Others have been encountered over the occipital poles, the Sylvian fissure, the optic chiasm[60] and even between the two cerebral hemispheres.[51]

Subdural hematoma in the posterior fossa is infrequent at any age.[59] McKissock and associates[90] encountered only two in 389 cases of subdural hematoma, Freed and Boyd[49] none in 106 cases, Allen, Moore, and Daly[4] one in 245 cases, and Fisher, Kim, and Sachs[47] four in 296 cases with injuries

to the back of the head. To 1961 Estridge and Smith[44] were able to find only 15 cases involving the posterior fossa. Several cases have been reported subsequently.[117] The scanty records of subdural hematomas of the posterior fossa indicate a particularly low incidence, and at this site acute lesions are more frequent than long-standing chronic hematomas,[9,109] which are thus even more unusual. Nelson[103] contends that subdural hemtaomas of the posterior fossa in the newborn are more numerous than generally believed. Most are fatal because of the severity of the birth injury, and consequently the lesions are not included in clinical reports.

Subdural hematoma of the posterior fossa is usually occipital, overlying the cerebellum either unilaterally or bilaterally although it may be localized to the region of the pons and medulla alone.[47] In four cases involving the posterior fossa,[47] subdural hemorrhage was found in the anterior and middle fossas as well.

Unilateral hematomas show little predilection for one or the other side of the brain. Gurdjian and Webster[60] in 227 cases of unilateral subdural hematoma and hygroma found 120 on the left side and 107 on the right. Of unilateral lesions, Vance[143] found 36 on the left and 57 on the right; Allen, Moore, and Daly,[4] 58 on the left and 64 on the right, 36 being unspecified; and Laudig, Browder, and Watson,[77] 71 on the left and 62 on the right. Bilateral hematomas occur in up to 30% of cases of subdural hematoma (Table 6-5). In series of infants and children,[63,68] the incidence was 79% and 71% (Table 6-5). Chase[24] in a series of 32 subdural hematomas due to birth injuries found 66% to be bilateral, and Elvidge and Jackson[42] reported bilateral lesions in 37 of 55 cases (67%) of subdural hematomas and effusions. Thus, subdural hematoma in infants and children is more often bilateral than unilateral. Yet, Schreiber[124] found a bilateral hematoma only once in 17 newborn infants and alleged a distinct difference from the higher incidence seen in older infants.

Table 6-5. Prevalence of bilateral subdural hematomas

Author	Total number of cases	Unilateral	Bilateral
Adults			
Leary (1934)[78]	50	43	7
Kennedy & Wortis (1936)[74]	72	62	10
Baker (1938)[11]	31	21	10
Allen, Moore, & Daly (1940)[4]	209	122	87
Laudig, Browder, & Watson (1941)[77]	143	133	10
Voris (1946)[146]	100	86	14
Vance (1950)[142]	102	93	9
Gurdjian & Webster (1958)*[60]	223	193	30
McLaurin & Tutor (1961)[93]	90	76	14
Gilmartin (1964)[53]	58	48	10
Svien & Gelety (1964)[136]	69	58	11
Total	1147	935	212 (18.5%)
Infants			
Ingraham & Matson (1944)[68]	98	21	77
Hollenhurst et al. (1957)[63]	31	9	22
Total	129	30	99 (76.7%)

*These authors' figures include hygromas.

Bilateral hematomas are also usually in the characteristic location and hence are fairly symmetrical and unconnected. Exceptions occur such as in one subject[95] in whom were present three chronic subdural hematomas, two frontal hematomas connected with each other below the falx cerebri, and a third entirely separate lesion over the left parietal lobe.

Bilateral hematomas vary in size. Mostly they are unequal. Vance[143] found that each of the hematomas in one patient weighed 30 gm., in a second they weighed 40 and 60 gm., and in a third, 100 and 150 gm.

Microscopic appearance

In the early subdural hematoma, the blood resembles postmortem clot. The inflammatory reaction in the neighboring dura is mild and polymorphonuclear cells may be visible initially. Fibrinous exudate coating the hematoma, though emphasized by some authors,[100] is not prominent or universal. Red cells and leukocytes are well preserved and by the second and third days fibroblastic invasion has started forming a layer internal to the dura. Red cells may stain poorly and lose sharpness of contour.[100]

A subdural hematoma becomes organized from the dura mater. The lack of participation of the leptomeninges has been attributed to the absence of a capillary bed in the arachnoid,[78] although mobility of the brain itself may be a factor.

Christensen[25] asserted that histological assessment of the age of a hematoma is inaccurate, but it could be stated that the capsule is formed within the first 2 to 3 weeks. During the first week, a thin layer of young fibrous tissue forms along the dural surface of the hematoma with ingrowth of small blood vessels and increased cellularity of the neighboring dura mater. Macrophages containing red cells and blood pigment are prominent by the fourth or fifth day. In the second and third weeks the contents undergo progressive liquefaction and the capsule thickens and increases in its pigment content (Fig. 6-1). The inner surface of the hematoma becomes covered by a thin layer of relatively avascular fibrous tissue, extending in from the margins. Some authors have seen mesothelium covering the inner surface,[113] whereas others believe that such a lining does not exist. Variation in the thickness and density of the capsule is often noted. Inflammatory cells and newly formed vessels (some being sinusoidal) as well as numerous sider-

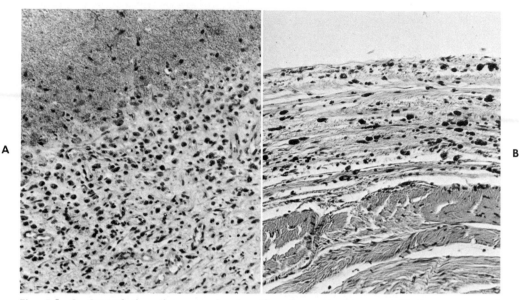

Fig. 6-1. A, Granulation tissue on dural surface is encroaching on old degenerate red cells (*above*) of a chronic subdural hematoma. **B,** Hematoma is organized, old dura is below, and all that remains is a newly formed layer of collagen. There are many siderophages in the granulation tissue of **A** and the healed lesion in **B.** (Hematoxylin and eosin, ×110.)

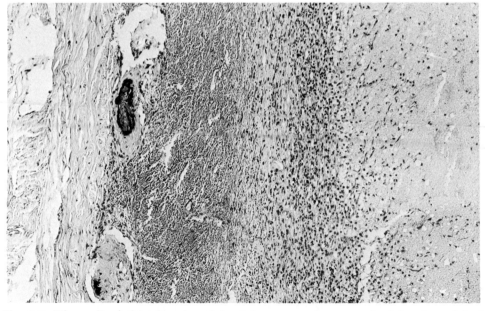

Fig. 6-2. The wall of this chronic subdural hematoma shows on the left, the original dura mater, two foci of early bone formation, a zone of recent hemorrhage, and a zone of granulation tissue and on the right the contents of the hematoma consisting of degenerate blood, invaded by fibroblasts, macrophages, and a few vessels. (Hematoxylin and eosin, ×65.)

ophages are present in the outer wall of the capsule or neomembrane, which still separates fairly readily from the dura. In the innermost part of the dura siderophages are found.

Hematomas of several months' duration are enclosed by heavily pigmented dense capsules, possibly with some degree of fusion of the inner and outer layers. There is liquefied blood and debris in the cavity. The capsule, containing numerous blood vessels, siderophages, and round cell infiltrations, becomes progressively more dense, and hyalinization of the fibrous tissue ensues. Vascularity may diminish, but the pigment often persists for years and healing has been found to be incomplete in one hematoma even after 12 years.[78] Calcification or ossification may be found microscopically (Fig. 6-2); however, erythropoietic activity in a hematoma of a very anemic infant is an oddity.[131]

Munro and Merritt[100] contend that evidence of fresh bleeding is infrequent. Putnam[113] stated that there is an apparent variation in the age of the blood in any particular hematoma. However, procedures for gauging the age of extravasated blood by its microscopic appearance are inexact at present and variation in fixation complicates the issue.

Some authors[113,114] emphasize the presence of large irregular spaces, lined by mesothelial cells generally near the junction of the capsule with the dura mater. The spaces may contain a few red cells, leukocytes, fibrin, or granular debris but are often empty and are probably artifacts or large sinusoidal blood vessels from which the blood has drained.

Little alteration occurs in the dura mater except that vessels beneath the mesothelium enlarge and are prominent. Siderophages are found in the dense fibrous tissue of its substance and continuity of the collagen accounts for the adhesion of the outer capsular wall or neomembrane.

Subdural hygroma

Subdural hygroma (or hydroma) is a subdural accumulation of xanthochromic or bloodstained fluid. Grossly there are no blood clots of any sort.[100] The phenomenon is believed to be the result of a small amount of bleeding and a large extravasation of cerebrospinal fluid into the subdural space[30,101,153] as a result of a cortical injury with tearing of the arachnoid. It is considered to be related to subdural hematoma. A variable quantity of cerebrospinal fluid may accrue to ordinary subdural hematomas at the time of the injury, but this is not usually regarded as being quantitatively significant. The volume of these hygromas varies from 50 to 100 ml. Munro and Merritt[100] believed that they slowly increased in size for the first month and then remained essentially unchanged. Their distribution and the structure of the capsule are similar to that of subdural hematomas. Hygromas of the posterior fossa also occur.[47] In traumatic cases, the fluid is predominantly cerebrospinal fluid of high protein content with some admixture of blood. In other cases altered permeability of the arachnoid is suspected.

Source of the bleeding

In subdural hemorrhage the source of bleeding is dependent on the etological factors involved. It is widely believed that when caused by trauma, bleeding stems from tearing or avulsion of thin-walled veins bridging the subdural space.[140] They are most often encountered in four locations:[79]

1. The lateral aspect of the frontal lobe, 1 to 4 cm. from the superior longitudinal sagittal sinus, and less usually over the parietal convexity where they tend to be larger
2. Traversing the space from the inferior surface of the temporal lobe to the tentorium and dura of the middle cranial fossa; apart from those to the sinuses, aberrant veins are found most often over the middle of the inferior surface of the temporal lobe
3. The apex of the temporal pole to the dura over the sphenoid bone
4. Numerous aberrant subtentorial veins (rarely involved in subdural hematoma)

Leary[79] emphasized their variability and their thin delicate walls. The inference is that they are weak, but histological architecture is a poor method of judging functional adequacy. Obviously the veins function adequately for such conditions of the cerebral circulation as are imposed by the unique requirements of the brain. The vessels are however subjected to singular and little understood stresses when head injuries are sustained, and the vessels may be avulsed from their arachnoidal or dural attachments. Leary believed that the small arteries responsible for bleeding were probably bridging arteries from the pial circulation to the dura and that the mechanism of their rupture was akin to the mode of venous rupture. Pudenz and Sheldon[112] demonstrated experimentally with transparent calvarial Lucite windows that blows to the head could cause subdural hemorrhage, the bleeding emanating not from veins traversing the subdural space to reach the superior longitudinal sinus but from veins in the region where the greatest convolutional glide was observed by high-speed cinematography. Rand[116] found several patients in whom the pia arachnoid overlying a thrombosed pial vein was adherent to the organizing hematoma. Such findings suggest that the vein that subsequently underwent thrombosis was the source of the hemorrhage.

Gross[59] attributed the rarity of subdural hematomas in the posterior fossa to the anatomy of the venous drainage of the cerebellum, where cortical veins do not bridge the subdural space to enter dural sinuses as frequently as the cerebral veins. The cranial cavity above the tentorium is more voluminous than that of the posterior fossa and would thus allow greater shift of brain tissue and brain shrinkage and a correspondingly greater tendency to place bridging veins on the stretch.

Vance[142] believed that these bridging veins were rarely responsible for subdural hematomas. In 87 of 90 cases of unilateral hematoma and in 40 of the 42 cases with bilateral hematoma, he asserted that the hemorrhage arose from a cerebral laceration caused by direct trauma or more frequently a *contrecoup injury*. When not caused by a cerebral laceration, the bleeding stemmed from a torn dural sinus or vein, from an injury of an old adhesion between the cortex and the dura, or from a dural tear with bleeding from the middle meningeal artery. Thus the sinus or bridging veins were incriminated only in the minority of cases. Drake[38] saw a spurting cortical artery at operation in 11 of 100 cases, all the injured vessels being in the region of the lateral aspect of the Sylvian fissure. In a second study, Vance[143] attributed the bleeding in 48 of 102 forensic cases of subdural hemorrhage[143] to ruptured blood vessels on the external surface of the cerebral hemisphere (parietal in 23 brains, temporal in 14, frontal in seven, occipital in one, uncertain in three). The torn blood vessel at times projected like a teat and was occluded by thrombus. In other instances, a conical clot was found over the torn artery or vein, and less frequently the vessel was open and oozed blood. In the remaining 54 cases no source of bleeding was found, presumably because they were subacute or chronic. In 15 cases the area of vascular rupture was sectioned histologically by the serial section technique. In five case, no sizable vessel was found ruptured, but of the remainder there was rupture of four pial veins and six pial arteries.

Bleeding may stem from dural vessels in tentorial tears during birth. Dural veins and sinuses may also be torn or damaged as the result of head injuries.[68] Thrombotic occlusion of dural sinuses and cerebral veins may result in subdural hemorrhage in association with hemorrhagic cerebral infarction.[125] Other causes include cerebral aneurysms, arteriovenous aneurysms, primary intracerebral hemorrhage, and bleeding intracranial tumors other than those infiltrating the dura mater. Subdural hematoma can complicate neoplastic invasion of the dura mater.[120] Russell and Cairns[120] concluded that neoplastic obstruction and invasion of the capillaries and veins of the outer dural network result in engorgement of and subsequent bleeding from large capillaries of the inner submesothelial network. The hematoma thus formed is similar to other varieties of subdural hematoma.

When healing has been initiated and is well advanced, little chance of determining the source of bleeding remains. In chronic hematomas it has been surmised that bleeding comes from ruptured dural vessels. Hannah[61] alleged that the hemorrhage was not subdural as is generally held, but intradural in location. Postmortem injection of blood into the dura raises small blebs on its inner surface, and Hannah[61] alleged that the innermost layer, split off in this manner, becomes the inner limiting membrane of the encapsulated hematoma. Study of two instances of intradural hemorrhage and a case of chronic subdural hematoma were offered in support. However, no study has been performed to determine the pressure required to dissect the dura over an area 10 cm. in diameter by the intradural injection of blood post mortem. Furthermore, Putnam and Putnam[114] demonstrated experimentally in dogs that the innermost layer of the artificially produced encapsulated hematoma consists of relatively mature fibrous tissue and forms rapidly, closely resembling that occurring in man.

Trumble[141] argued that a subdural hemorrhage is not likely to remain above the Sylvian fissure and that an intradural location of the hematoma is the only plausible explanation for their location on the superolateral aspect of the hemisphere. Neither theory adequately explains the localization of the subdural hematomas.

Trumble[141] considered that in any individual the formation of bilateral chronic subdural hematomas due to hemorrhage into the subdural space was an extremely remote possibility and it was more likely that bilateral intradural hematomas would form because of some "peculiar weakness" of the dura mater predisposing it to extensive hemorrhage. Invocation of a second hypothesis ("weakness" of the dura) to support the first is hardly convincing. Arguments discrediting this theory of intradural hemorrhage are the following:

1. No instance of acute massive intradural hematoma has yet been described and the mode of origin of a chronic subdural hematoma cannot be satisfactorily determined by a study of the advanced lesions alone.[79]
2. There is the practical difficulty of splitting the dura mater to accommodate up to 300 ml. of blood and more within the cavity.[79]
3. The progressive steps in the development of an encapsulated subdural hematoma of both man[66] and the experimental animal discredits the hypothesis that the massive hematoma is intradural.[79]

At the present time the evidence suggests strongly that chronic subdural hematomas are subdural rather than intradural from the outset.

Trauma 2 to 12 months prior to admission occurred in four cases of chronic subdural hematoma with the history of a severe injury some 5 to 11 years previously. The presence of long-standing deformity of the skull was interpreted as being indicative of a subdural hematoma acquired in the past, and a relapse of symptoms and signs was thought to be caused by a further hemorrhage occasioned by the second injury.[31]

Associated lesions

Trauma. The major cause of subdural hematoma is trauma. Consequently in patients dying of acute or subacute subdural hemorrhage, evidence of trauma is likely to be found about the face or neck. Vance[143] found external injuries of the face and scalp in 80 of 102 fatal forensic cases. In the remaining 22 cases of subdural hematoma, there were no external head injuries. Other traumatic lesions that may be found are legion.

Fractured skull. The incidence of a concomitant skull fracture is considerably lower than that associated with extradural hemorrhage, but in fatal cases with a fractured skull LeCount and Apfelbach[80] found subdural hemorrhage in approximately 77% at autopsy. They found hematomas in 115 of 136 fractures of the posterior cranial fossa (104 contrecoup, 11 homolateral), in 98 of 134 fractures involving the middle cranial fossa (66 contrecoup,

35 homolateral) in 21 of 48 fractures of the anterior fossa (13 homolateral, 8 contrecoup), in 43 of 50 extensively comminuted fractures, and in 38 of 40 fractures of the cranial vault. Vance,[142] in a study of fractures of the skull, found 132 deaths from cerebral compression because of subdural hematoma. Most subjects died within 24 hours. Others survived for several days but few lived 2 weeks. Analysis of the fracture sites revealed that most fractures occurred on the posterior or lateral aspects of the skull, and relatively few (10 of 32) involved the anterior or vault regions. Hematomas are more often bilateral when the skull is fractured.[78]

Freytag[50] reported fractures in 69.7% of 861 forensic autopsies on subjects who died with subdural hematomas. Several authors have reported a lesser incidence in clinical material[68,77] particularly in chronic subdural hematomas.[74] Ingraham and Matson[68] emphasized the mildness of the head injury necessary to cause subdural hematomas in infants as evidenced by the incidence of skull fracture in only 11 of their 98 patients (11.2%).

Extradural hematoma. Extradural hemorrhage is often associated with subdural hemorrhage. LeCount and Apfelbach[80] found subdural hemorrhage in 31 of 73 cases of large extradural hemorrhage and Gurdjian and Webster[60] found seven in 30, whereas McKissock and colleagues[91] found only 12 in 125 cases. Jamieson and Yelland[69] stated that subdural hematoma is the commonest intradural complication of extradural hemorrhage as it occurred in 44% of his patients. By contrast in 389 cases of subdural hematoma, McKissock[90] found only one instance of extradural hemorrhage.

Intracerebral hematoma. In acute subdural hemorrhage, damage to the brain is frequent. Thus subarachnoid hemorrhage may be caused by a cerebral contusion, laceration, or even a contrecoup lesion. In view of the frequency of bloodstained cerebrospinal fluid in acute subdural hemorrhage, involvement of the brain with subarachnoid bleeding is practically the rule in these cases. In subacute or chronic lesions the trauma is generally less severe and with the passage of time there may be little obvious evidence of hemorrhage. The damage to the brain may be derived from a combination of trauma and secondary effects of the hematoma. McKissock and associates[90] performed a lumbar puncture on six acute hematomas and 28 subacute lesions. The cerebrospinal fluid was blood stained or xanthochromic in six and 22 cases respectively. In 86 chronic lesions, the fluid was clear in 64 and xanthochromic in 22 instances. In hematomas caused by bleeding disorders, associated subarachnoid or intracerebral hemorrhage is to be expected.

Large intracerebral hemorrhages are infrequent. McLaurin and Tutor[93] encountered only 11 instances, mostly temporal lobe hematomas in 90 patients with acute subdural hemorrhage. Frank intracerebral hematomas were found in 11 acute lesions and three subacute lesions from a total of 82 and 91 cases respectively by McKissock and associates.[90] In many surgical cases, it is likely that a subdural hematoma could be evacuated without full appreciation of the existence or extent of intracerebral hemorrhage. Vance[142] found a cerebral laceration 87 times in 90 cases of unilateral hematoma and 40 in 42 cases of bilateral hematoma. His cases were all fatal and the injury recent. The lower incidence in other series[90] probably derives from the larger percentage of chronic lesions and to variations in the severity of the head injury.

Chronic changes in the skull and scalp. No constant changes have been described in concert with chronic subdural hematoma in adults,[113] though thinning, thickening, and roughening of the skull have been reported.[113] Extensive thinning of the skull and actual perforation of the bone and dura have been observed over a chronic subdural hematoma.[95] Chronic subdural hematomas in infants are associated with an enlargement of the head simulating that of a hydrocephalic but with the characteristic facies of the disease absent. The anterior fontanelle bulges and the fundi on ophthalmoscopy reveal increased intracranial pressure. Thinning of the calvarium is not unusual and, in addition, over a chronic hematoma it may bulge externally, producing considerable asymmetry of the skull.[95]

Miscellaneous associated lesions. Leukocytosis is a frequent finding. Papilledema was found in 54 of 72 acute cases[74] and fundal hemorrhages are often to be seen. The level of consciousness does not relate to the pressure at lumbar puncture. Aronson and Okazaki[9] noted an incidence of secondary brain-stem hemorrhage or softening in 28.8%. Although such secondary lesions were not present with hematomas less than 25 cc., their numbers increased with hematomas of greater volume, until in those of more than 100 cc. in volume when the incidence declined. This the authors attributed to the older age of the patients. However, the number of cases with such large hematomas was small. Vance[143] found a similar prevalence of brain-stem hemorrhage. Mateos and Daly[88] found hypertension in 33% of 123 cases. In view of the age distribution of the disease, the incidence does not appear unduly high, but no statistical analysis was made.

Maroon and Campbell[86] reported two patients with chronic subdural hematomas and concurrently the syndrome of antidiuretic hormone secretion with hyponatremia, decreased serum osmolality, and increased urine osmolality. The syndrome is known to occur after head injury. It was thought that the considerable degree of shift and distortion of the third ventricle and nearby hypothalamus may have been a significant factor in causing the syndrome, which was reversed in both instances by drainage of the hematoma.

Sequelae

Despite long survival of some individuals who live for years harboring a chronic subdural hematoma, the almost unanimous view concerning subdural hemorrhage is that the hematoma requires prompt diagnosis and surgical evacuation if death and mental deterioration are to be obviated. In acute subdural hematomas, the patient may die from the ill effects of the hemorrhage. Alternatively such patients may succumb from the associated lesions, depending on the etiology and precipitating factors.[99] Infection may be posttraumatic or postoperative. In chronic subdural hematomas, the patients, if vegetative, may die of intercurrent infections or of coincidental causes. The major causes of death in uncomplicated subdural hemorrhage will be found within the cranium. All are not necessarily always demonstrated, but the most important is cerebral compression.

Cerebral compression. Trotter[140] felt the onset of cerebral compression fell into three stages. Firstly, the extravasated blood displaces intracranial fluid (venous blood and cerebrospinal fluid) without interference of the circulation. The second stage is reached when enlargement of the hematoma reduces the capacity of the venous drainage system, thereby interfering with venous flow, the resultant engorgement of which causes "irritative" symptoms. In the third stage, the increasing intracranial pressure displaces fluid next highest in order of resistance to displacement, that is, the cerebral microcirculation, and consequently cerebral anemia follows, most marked in the vicinity of the space-occupying lesion. This results in cessation of function and paralytic symptoms. Slow enlargement of the hematoma allows physiological compensation to occur, there being increased tolerance to venous congestion with a reduction in irritative symptoms. No compensatory mechanism counteracts the anemia.

One of the early effects of acute compression of one cerebral hemisphere is often ipsilateral swelling of the white matter, no doubt caused by venous obstruction due to the presence of the space-occupying lesion in the subdural space.[9,140] This swelling is accounted for by interstitial edema and perivascular accumulations of fluid, especially in the centrum semiovale. This is accompanied by some loss of myelin, and acute phlebitis of the transcerebral veins has been noted.[9] Hemorrhagic infarction of the temporal and occipital lobes in the distribution of the posterior cerebral artery occurs in about 28% or 29% of those patients with a subdural hematoma greater than 25 cc. After a variable period of time the level of consciousness may become depressed suddenly and the pupils may become dilated and fixed with decerebrate rigidity. Such clinical manifestations are often portents of the occurrence of secondary hemorrhage or infarction of the midbrain and pons.[9]

Subsidence of the edema in the early stages of cerebral compression may permit the alteration of symptoms and the occurrence of a latent interval clinically until the hematoma, often suddenly, manifests itself as a chronic subdural encapsulated mass. At this time the hemiatrophy and molding of the brain may be quite extreme, there being gross cerebral atrophy, extensive neuronal loss, and gliosis, with loss of white matter as well. Complete destruction of the underlying brain may occur,[66] and cortical softening and status spongiosus with wrinkled and shrunken meninges[108] have been observed. The frequently severe damage to the brain accounts for the epilepsy[90] and the recognized high incidence of mental retardation in the infant and dementia in the adult.[7,33,129] Munro[99] generalized when he stated that if the subdural hematoma is not fatal, the patient will survive and later but inevitably be disabled because of the permanent structural changes in the brain.

In chronic subdural hematoma, failure to remove the inner and outer membranes (the capsule) as well as the contents is considered by many authors to impede the reexpansion of the brain[136] though simple evacuation has been found satisfactory in the hands of others.[48] Ingraham and Heyl[67] pointed out that the human infant brain doubles its volume within the first 3 months of life and doubles again within the subse-

quent 6 months and that in view of this enormous growth any constriction imposed by an organizing subdural hematoma could be detrimental. Svien and Gelety[136] concluded that leaving the capsule in situ has no deleterious effect and theoretically after surgical evacuation the hematoma should collapse and undergo resolution with shrinkage of the scar tissue. There is no record of calcification occurring in those chronic hematomas that have been merely evacuated.

Spontaneous resorption. The subdural space is a closed area, and absorption from it appears to be virtually ineffective[78,101,146] possibly because (1) it is the border zone of the cerebral and systemic circulations, (2) the dura is comparatively avascular, (3) the arachnoid is relatively impervious and there seems to be no lymphatic drainage of the brain, bone, and dura mater, and (4) Leary[78] held that cerebrospinal fluid is not absorbed from the subdural space and that blood or exudate can be removed by surgical evacuation or organization. Leary[79] later considered that the arachnoid has to be essentially intact as the prerequisite for the production of a chronic hematoma. In regard to subdural injections of blood, ample evidence in the literature attests to their frequent failure to result in a chronic encapsulated hematoma, though the inefficacy has been attributed to inadvertent subarachnoid injection rather than subdural.[114] It is probable however that just as experimentally produced subdural hematomas undergo spontaneous absorption at times, so do naturally occurring lesions. The process of removal no doubt is one of organization, for the lymphatics actively participate under normal conditions at other sites but are unavailable in the subdural space. Arseni and Stanciu[10] stated that in most cases, when the lesion remains undiagnosed, the progressive course of spontaneous subdural hematoma ends in death or surgery. The number of times a subdural hematoma will undergo complete and effective resorption is unknown, but its size is undeniably a factor if not the major limiting one. Small quantities of subdural blood are probably removed fairly readily. Larger clots may also undergo organization without serious progression of symptoms, though incorporation and constriction of the optic nerves by an organizing traumatic hematoma at the base are said to have occasioned bilateral optic atrophy.[10]

Several instances have been reported in which after trauma, patients developed symptoms and signs with angiographic verification of subdural hematomas.[5,15] After medical therapy, there was improvement and follow-up studies revealed that the space-occupying lesion had subsided. In the absence of autopsy or surgical verification, one wonders whether they were hygromas rather than subdural hematomas.

Hydrocephalus. Ingraham and Heyl[67] asserted that untreated subdural hematomas in infants in contradistinction to those in adults are frequently associated with hydrocephalus, allegedly caused by (1) pressure tending to obliterate the subarachnoid space and (2) hemogenic meningitis. Hydrocephalus may also occur after subdural hematomas in the posterior fossa, as a consequence of obstruction in the region of the fourth ventricle. There is recorded the history of a neonatal infant[28] whose head, because of hydrocephalus, enlarged rapidly within the first 2 weeks. A recent subdural hematoma in the posterior fossa with early encapsulation was discovered and evacuated, thus relieving the acute ventricular dilatation. Ventricular blockage was thought to have been caused by obstruction of the outflow of cerebrospinal fluid from the ventricles. A similar case with a communicating hydrocephalus has been reported by Nelson,[103] and in yet another neonate,[117] evacuation of the subdural hematoma caused by birth trauma relieved the hydrocephalus, a consequence of an obstruction at the level of the fourth ventricle.

Ingraham and Matson[68] asserted that the lateral ventricles may undergo considerable dilatation in the later stages of untreated subdural hematomas (supratentorial). However, this is due to extensive cortical atrophy and obstruction to spinal fluid absorption. Of their 28 patients, all of whom manifested some degree of hydrocephalus before treatment, only one with the cause uncertain showed progression postoperatively.

Subsequent to the removal of a relatively small subdural hematoma, gross shift of the lateral and third ventricles may persist for some time and even intensify,[19] presumably in association with edema and the altered cerebral circulation through the damaged brain. The ventricles return gradually to the midline with dilatation of the frontal and temporal poles of the ipsilateral ventricles. No changes may become evident in the ventricular system postoperatively. Browder and Hollister[19] were unable to correlate ventricular changes, often bizarre, with either the size or position of the hematoma. Meredith and Rinaldi[96] reported two cases of obstructive hydrocephalus after the treatment of chronic subdural hematomas, but the pathogenesis was obscure.

Secondary infection. Secondary infection of a subdural hematoma may eventuate, resulting from the spread of infection through a fracture site. The spread may be hematogenous as suggested by Bucy's case[20] in which the urinary bladder was believed to be the primary site. Alternatively, it may present itself as a postoperative complication after evacuation.

Hemorrhage. Secondary hemorrhage into a chronic hematoma may be extensive and rupture the inner wall of the capsule.[78] The precise role of small intermittent hemorrhage from the granulation tissue is uncertain. However postoperative hemorrhage whether it be acute, subacute, or chronic is a major complication of the surgical therapy of this disease,[145] and an evacuated hematoma may refill.

Pathogenesis of chronic subdural hematoma

A middle-aged or elderly man may suffer an accidental blow to the head and immediate symptoms may be trivial and the injury soon forgotten. Over the ensuing months, there may be headaches and the gradual development of pressure symptoms and progressive deterioration until death intervenes 6 to 9 months or so later. The precise explanation for the paucity of symptoms and signs in patients with these chronic hematomas is undetermined as is the reason for the insidious but progressive clinical deterioration that ultimately induces them to seek medical assistance. It is difficult to envisage the formation of a hematoma in the subdural space over the many weeks or even months, the happenstance of the slow seepage of blood.

At the turn of the century several authors attempted to clarify experimentally the pathogenesis of the chronic subdural hematoma. No detailed histological investigations were conducted and results were contradictory.[85,114,132] Putnam and Putnam[114] injected blood into the subdural space, but, when examined, the size of the coagulum was less than had been anticipated upon consideration of the amount injected. The clot was always adherent to the dura, and within 5 days mesothelium and a thin layer of fibrous tissue covered the arachnoidal surface. Vessels appeared in the capsule only in the second week. When the clot was removed, traces were still present after 50 days. At 3 months a scar covered by mesothelium was all that remained. The authors[114] regarded the organization of these experimental hematomas as being entirely analogous to those occurring naturally in man, and these findings have been confirmed.[55] Unexplained spherical spaces in the granulation tissue were thought to have been caused by paraffin from the syringe. None of the hematomas was complicated by secondary hemorrhage despite attempts to precipitate such bleeding.

Gardner,[52] impressed by the long latent interval before the lesion manifests itself, suggested a progressive augmentation in size after the injury. Several authors have supported his theory.[78,106,111] Slow and continuous or perhaps intermittent bleeding from the injured vessel of origin is not a feature of extracranial hematomas. Nevertheless growing and newly formed vessels in granulation tissue are known to bleed readily, and such an event could explain some increase in size of the hematoma. Secondary bleeding of this sort is generally mild in degree although multiple extravasations could be cumulative. Interestingly enough, secondary hemorrhage with rupture of the inner wall or neomembrane of a chronic hematoma was the cause of death in three of Leary's cases.[78] Munro and Merritt[100] attributed the increase in size to repeated hemorrhage in part and in subjects with dementia or chronic alcoholism who are prone to repeated head injuries, it is understandable that such could occur. The occasional appearance of lamination within the hematoma is thought to corroborate this view.

The hematoma is generally sterile[12] so that infection occurring secondarily in the subdural hematoma is a most unlikely cause of the progression. Gardner[52] demonstrated that the osmotic pressure of blood, kept at 37° C., caused the imbibition of cerebrospinal fluid across a cellophane membrane to such an extent that the blood had increased the weight by 93% after 66 hours. Similar imbibition of fluid occurred when small blood-filled cellophane sacs were inserted beneath the dura in experimental animals. Dialysis of blood against cerebrospinal fluid with use of a capsule from a subdural hematoma caused an increase of only 2.9% in volume of the blood after 16 hours, considerably less than when cellophane was used in vivo or in vitro. Nevertheless Gardner[52] concluded that the capsule behaved satisfactorily as a semipermeable membrane primarily because of the discrepancy in protein content between the blood and the cerebrospinal fluid. The absence of lymphatics in the bone and meninges and hence in the granulation tissue about the hematoma signifies that protein and breakdown products of blood may not be so readily removed as in extracranial sites and thus contribute to the enlargement of the hematoma by osmosis as Gardner suggested. However for cerebrospinal fluid to be imbibed it must cross the arachnoid, the subdural space, and often a relatively thick fibrous capsule or zone of granulation tissue. In view of the poor dialysing properties of the capsule as demonstrated by Gardner,[52] it appears feasible that if the breakdown products of the hematoma attract fluid, it will be more likely to materialize as an exudate from the vessels of the capsule. Munro and Merritt[100] believed that the arachnoid is the effective dialysing membrane, and though this may be so initially, the intervention and development of the innermost wall of the capsule (usually by the end of the third week but earlier in the experimental animals[114]) complicate the issue.

Zollinger and Gross[155] dialyzed blood within a chronic hematoma removed at autopsy against a solution containing 0.9 gm. of sodium chloride and 0.1 gm. of sodium oxalate per 100 ml. of water. They showed that the capsule behaved as a semipermeable membrane and prevented the egress of protein. They also demonstrated that hemolyzed blood exerted much greater osmotic pressure than non-hemolyzed blood.

Munro and Merritt[100] analyzed the fluid in the subdural hematoma and found that the protein content, which increased to a high peak at the end of the second week, commenced to fall fairly abruptly by the sixteenth day, continuing until the end of the first month, and then proceeded more slowly till the end of the third month. The shape of the graph led these authors to propose that the fall was caused by dilution of the protein, rapid at first but subsequently slower as the protein and breakdown products continued to be diluted. They concluded that in the absence of further bleeding, the hematoma increased in size only for a period of three months, thence remaining stationary or diminishing as the result of absorption. The development of progressive symptoms within the first 2 to 3 months is understandable in view of Munro and Merritt's analysis[100] of the protein content, but their contention does not explain so well the more chronic variety where organization of the hematomas must be well advanced and of many months' duration before symptoms appear. Zollinger and Gross[155] believed that the breakdown of red cells occurred over a much longer period of time (that is, greater than 3 months).

At present both basic theories, that is, recurrent hemorrhage and osmotic imbibition of fluid, with their indirect supportive evidence have much to recommend them, but neither should be accepted with finality in the absence of unassailable direct experimental evidence.

Mortality

Apart from a few cases in which conservative therapy is associated with apparent resolution of subdural hematomas,[5,15] it is generally considered essential for a subdural hematoma, whatever its duration, to be evacuated. The mortality for untreated acute subdural hematoma was 100% in a combined series of 53 patients.[74,98] Surgical evacuation of the hematoma improves this mortality. The surgical mortality has been estimated[98,136,146] as an average of 20% to 30% with a range from 2.5% to 43%. Browder[18] had a mortality of 97 in 227 cases of subdural hematoma treated surgically—an incidence of 42.7%. An additional 62 patients not subjected to surgery were diagnosed at autopsy, giving an overall mortality of 55.7% Obviously much depends on the state of the hematoma and its associated lesions. McKissock and his colleagues[90] had a mortality of 51% of 77 acute cases, 24% of 91 subacute cases, and only 6% of 212 chronic cases, the overall rate being 20%. The high incidence of partial or total disablement of the acute hematomas (Table 6-6) contrasts however with the satisfactory recovery reported in those subjects with subacute or chronic hematomas. Other factors that influence the mortality are the size of the hematoma, the level of consciousness at diagnosis, and, when treated,[90] the seriousness of associated lesions (extradural hemorrhage and cere-

Table 6-6. Mortality for surgically treated subdural hematoma*

	Acute	Subacute	Chronic
Total number of cases	77	91	212
Mortality	51%	24%	6%
Known survivors	32	59	179
Totally or partially disabled	14	6	29
No incapacitation	18 (56%)	53 (90%)	150 (84%)

*Adapted from McKissock, W., Richardson, A., and Bloom, W. H.: Subdural haematoma: a review of 389 cases, Lancet **1**:1365, 1960.

bral contusion and hemorrhage) and the age of the patient.

Shulman and Ransohoff[129] treated 53 children, and of these 13% died, 19% were retarded, 5.7% had persistent convulsions, and 63% were apparently normal. Of the 57 infants followed up for at least 6 months by Ingraham and Matson,[68] 23% were retarded, with some being fairly grossly defective, and 77% were classified as normal. Other factors influencing the prognosis are as follows:

1. Age influences the mortality adversely.[90]
2. The volume of the lesion does not relate to the prognosis;[77,90] though all other things being equal, the size of the hematoma will obviously affect the outcome.
3. The presence of additional changes in the brain reflecting the level of consciousness and the rate of the evolution of symptoms seriously affects the mortality (Table 6-6).
4. Chronic hematomas have a lower mortality than the acute lesions[77,90] and further analysis of the time interval between injury and surgery indicates a greater mortality when the interval[77] is shorter.
5. As in the case of extradural hematoma, early diagnosis and surgical evacuation of the clot is essential.[115] When surgical relief is unduly delayed, it has been estimated that three patients of every four either die or suffer from dementia.[7]

Spinal subdural hematoma

Subdural hematoma of the spinal canal is rare and less frequent than spinal extradural hemorrhage.[34] Trauma is the most frequent cause, and the hematoma is usually not of sufficient size to cause compression of the cord. Chronic spinal subdural hematoma is unknown, but the acute variety is likely to complicate bleeding states.

Schiller and associates[122] recorded the successful treatment of a hemophiliac with a spinal subdural hematoma.[130] Dooley and Perlmutter[37] mentioned cord compression occurring after lumbar puncture in two patients on anticoagulants, but the location of the hemorrhage was not mentioned.

References

1. Abbott, W. D., Due, F. O., and Nosik, W. A.: Subdural hematoma and effusion as a result of blast injuries, Bull. Amer. Coll. Surg. **28**:123, 1943.
2. Achslogh, J.: Hématome sous-dural chronique de la fosse cérébrale postérieure, Acta Neurol. Psychiat. Belg. **52**:790, 1952.
3. Áfra, D.: Ossification of subdural hematoma, J. Neurosurg. **18**:393, 1961.
4. Allen, A. M., Moore, M., and Daly, B. B.: Subdural hemorrhage in patients with mental disease, New Eng. J. Med. **223**:324, 1940.
5. Ambrosetto, C.: Post-traumatic subdural hematoma, Arch. Neurol. **6**:287, 1962.
6. Anderson, F. M.: Subdural hematoma, a complication of operation for hydrocephalus, Pediatrics **10**:11, 1952.
7. Annotation: The other falling sickness, Lancet **1**:1397, 1960.
8. Arieff, A. J., and Wetzel, N.: Subdural hematoma following epileptic convulsion, Neurology **14**:731, 1964.
9. Aronson, S. M., and Okazaki, H.: A study of some factors modifying response of cerebral tissue to subdural hematomata, J. Neurosurg. **20**:89, 1963.
10. Arseni, C., and Stanciu, M.: Particular clinical aspects of chronic subdural haematoma in adults, Europ. Neurol. **2**:109, 1969.
11. Baker, A. B.: Subdural hematoma, Arch. Path. **26**:535, 1938.
12. Barratt, J. O. W.: On pachymeningitis haemorrhagica interna, Brain **25**:181, 1902.
13. Barron, K. D., and Fergusson, G.: Intracranial hemorrhage as a complication of anticoagulant therapy, Neurology **9**:447, 1959.
14. Belmusto, L., Regelson, W., Owens, G., Hananian, J., and Nigogosyan, G.: Intracranial extracerebral hemorrhages in acute lymphocytic leukemia, Cancer **17**:1079, 1964.
15. Bender, M. B.: Recovery from subdural hema-

toma without surgery, J. Mount Sinai Hosp. N. Y. **27**:52, 1960.

16. Blackwood, W.: Vascular disease of the central nervous system. In Blackwood, W., McMenemy, W. H., Meyer, A., Norman, R. M., and Russell, D. S.: Greenfield's neuropathology, ed. 2, Baltimore, 1963, The Williams & Wilkins Co., p. 71.

17. Bowen, W. H.: Traumatic subdural haemorrhage, Guy's Hosp. Rep. **59**:21, 1905.

18. Browder, J.: A résumé of the principal diagnostic features of subdural hematoma, Bull. N. Y. Acad. Med. **19**:168, 1943.

19. Browder, J., and Hollister, N. R.: Air encephalography and ventriculography as diagnostic aids in craniocerebral trauma. In: Trauma of the central nervous system, Ass. Res. Nerv. Ment. Dis. **24**:421, 1945.

20. Bucy, P. C.: Subdural hematoma, Ill. Med. J. **82**:300, 1942.

21. Caffey, J.: Multiple fractures in the long bones of infants suffering from chronic subdural hematoma, Amer. J. Roentgen. **56**:163, 1946.

22. Calkins, R. A., Van Allen, M. W., and Sahs, A. L.: Subdural hematoma following pneumoencephalography, J. Neurosurg. **27**:56, 1967.

23. Chambers, J. W.: Acute subdural haematoma, J. Neurosurg. **8**:263, 1951.

24. Chase, W. H.: An anatomical study of subdural haemorrhage associated with tentorial splitting in the newborn, Surg. Gynec. Obstet. **51**:31, 1930.

25. Christensen, E.: Studies on chronic subdural hematoma, Acta. Psychiat. Neurol. **19**:69, 1944.

26. Chusid, J. G., and de Gutiérrez-Mahoney, C. G.: Ossifying subdural hematoma, J. Neurosurg. **10**:430, 1953.

27. Clarke, E., and Walton, J. N.: Subdural haematoma complicating intracranial aneurysm and angioma, Brain **76**:378, 1953.

28. Coblentz, R. G.: Cerebellar subdural hematoma in infant 2 weeks old with hydrocephalus, Surgery **8**:771, 1940.

29. Cole, M., and Spatz, E.: Seizures in chronic subdural hematoma, New Eng. J. Med. **265**:628, 1961.

30. Da Costa, D. G., and Adson, A. W.: Subdural hydroma, Arch. Surg. **43**:559, 1941.

31. Davidoff, L. M., and Dyke, C. G.: Relapsing juvenile chronic subdural hematoma, Bull. Neurol. Inst. N. Y. **7**:95, 1938.

32. Davidoff, L. M., and Feiring, E. H.: Subdural hematoma occurring in surgically treated hydrocephalic children, J. Neurosurg. **10**:557, 1953.

33. Davies, F. L.: Mental abnormalities following subdural haematoma, Lancet **1**:1369, 1960.

34. Davison, C.: General pathological considerations in injuries of the spinal cord. In Brock, S.: Injuries of the brain and spinal cord and their coverings, ed. 3, Baltimore, 1949, The Williams & Wilkins Co., p. 471.

35. Del Greco, F., and Krumlovsky, F.: Subdural haematoma in the course of haemodialysis, Lancet **2**:1009, 1969.

36. Deykin, D.: Warfarin therapy, New Eng. J. Med. **283**:801, 1970.

37. Dooley, D. M., and Perlmutter, I.: Spontaneous intercranial hematomas in patients receiving anticoagulation therapy, J.A.M.A. **187**:396, 1964.

38. Drake, C. G.: Subdural haematoma from arterial rupture, J. Neurosurg. **18**:597, 1961.

39. Dyke, C. G.: A pathognomonic encephalographic sign of subdural hematoma, Bull. Neurol. Inst. N. Y. **5**:135, 1936.

40. Echlin, F. A., Sordillo, S. V. R., and Garvey, T. Q.: Acute, subacute, and chronic subdural hematoma, J.A.M.A. **161**:1345, 1956.

41. Eisenberg, M. M.: Bishydroxycoumarin toxicity: some physiological aspects and report of a death from spontaneous subdural hematoma, J.A.M.A. **170**:2181, 1959.

42. Elvidge, A. R., and Jackson, I. J.: Subdural hematoma and effusion in infants, Amer. J Dis. Child **78**:635, 1949.

43. Epstein, B. S.: Pneumoencephalography and cerebral angiography, Chicago, 1966, Year Book Medical Publishers, Inc.

44. Estridge, M. N., and Smith, R. A.: Acute subdural hemorrhage of posterior fossa, J. Neurosurg. **18**:248, 1961.

45. Evans, H., and Perry, K. M. A.: Thrombocytopenic purpura, Lancet **2**:410, 1943.

46. Ferguson, G. G., Barton, W. B., and Drake, C. G.: Subdural hematoma in hemophilia; successful treatment with cryoprecipitate, J. Neurosurg. **29**:524, 1968.

47. Fisher, R. G., Kim, J. K., and Sachs, E.: complications in posterior fossa due to occipital trauma—their operability, J.A.M.A. **167**:176, 1958.

48. Fleming, H. W., and Jones, O. W.: Chronic subdural haematoma, Surg. Gynec. Obstet. **54**:81, 1932.

49. Freed, C. G., and Boyd, H. R.: Subdural hematoma, Rocky Mountain Med. J. **57**:51, Nov. 1960.

50. Freytag, E.: Autopsy findings in head injuries from blunt force, Arch. Path. **75**:402, 1963.

51. Gannon, W. E.: Interhemispheric subdural hematoma, J. Neurosurg. **18**:829, 1961.

52. Gardner, W. J.: Traumatic subdural hematoma with particular reference to the latent interval, Arch. Neurol. Psychiat. **27**:847, 1932.

53. Gilmartin, D.: Arteriography in diagnosis of subdural haematoma, Lancet **1**:1061, 1964.

54. Golden, J., Odom, G. L., and Woodhall, B.: Subdural hematoma following subarachnoid hemorrhage, Arch, Neurol. Psychiat. **69**:486, 1953.

55. Goodell, C. L., and Mealey, J.: Pathogenesis of chronic subdural hematoma, Arch. Neurol. **8**:429, 1963.

56. Griffiths, D. L., and Moynihan, F. J.: Multiple epiphyseal injuries in babies ("battered baby" syndrome), Brit. Med. J. **2**:1558, 1963.

57. Groch, S. N., Sayre, G. P., and Heck, F. J.: Cerebral hemorrhage in leukemia, Arch. Neurol. **2**:439, 1960.

58. Groff, R. A., and Grant, F. C.: Chronic subdural hematoma, Int. Abstr. Surg. **74**:9, 1942.

59. Gross, S. W.: Posterior fossa hematomas, J. Mount Sinai Hosp. N. Y. **22**:286, 1955.

60. Gurdjian, E. S., and Webster, J. E.: Head injuries, mechanisms, diagnosis, and management, Boston, 1958, Little, Brown and Co.

61. Hannah, J. A.: The aetiology of subdural hematoma, J. Nerv. Ment. Dis. **84**:169, 1936.

62. Hoessley, G.: Intracranial hemorrhage in the seventeenth century, J. Neurosurg. **24**:493, 1966.

63. Hollenhorst, R. W., Stein, H. A., Keith, H. M., and MacCarty, C. S.: Subdural hematoma, subdural hygroma, and subarachnoid hemorrhage amongst infants and children, Neurology **7**:813, 1957.

64. Howard, C.: Subdural pneumography, Amer. J. Roentgen. **55**:710, 1946.

65. Ingalls, T. H.: The role of scurvy in the etiology of chronic subdural hematoma, New Eng. J. Med. **215**:1279, 1936.

66. Inglis, K.: Subdural haemorrhage, cysts, and false membranes: illustrating the influence of intrinsic factors in disease when development of the body is normal, Brain **69**:157, 1946.

67. Ingraham, F. D., and Heyl, H. L.: Subdural hematoma in infancy and childhood, J.A.M.A. **112**:198, 1939.

68. Ingraham, F. D., and Matson, D. D.: Subdural hematoma in infancy, J. Pediat. **24**:1, 1944.

69. Jamieson, K. G., and Yelland, J. D. N.: Extradural hematoma, J. Neurosurg. **29**:13, 1968.

70. Jelsma, F.: Chronic subdural hematoma, Arch. Surg. **21**:128, 1930.

71. Jewesbury, E. C. O., and Josse, S. E.: Arteriography on diagnosis of subdural haematoma, Lancet **1**:1277, 1964.

72. Kaump, D. H., and Love, J. G.: "Subdural" hematoma, Surg. Gynec. Obstet. **67**:87, 1938.

73. Kempe, C. H., Silverman, F. N., Steele, B. F., Droegemueller, W., and Silver, H. K.: The battered-child syndrome, J.A.M.A. **181**:17, 1962.

74. Kennedy, F., and Wortis, H.: "Acute" subdural hematoma and acute epidural hemorrhage, Surg. Gynec. Obstet. **63**:732, 1936.

75. Kerr, C. B.: Intracranial haemorrhage in haemophilia, J. Neurol. Neurosurg. Psychiat. **27**:166, 1964.

76. Khalifeh, R. R., Van Allen, M. W., and Sahs, A. L.: Subdural hematoma following pneumoencephalography in an adult, Neurology **14**:77, 1964.

77. Laudig, G. H., Browder, E. J., and Watson, R. A.: Subdural hematoma, Ann. Surg. **113**:170, 1941.

78. Leary, T.: Subdural hemorrhages, J.A.M.A. **103**:897, 1934.

79. Leary, T.: Subdural or intradural hemorrhages? Arch. Path. **28**:808, 1939.

80. LeCount, E. R., and Apfelbach, C. W.: Pathologic anatomy of traumatic fractures of cranial bones and concomitant brain injuries, J.A.M.A. **74**:501, 1920.

81. Leonard, C. D.: Subdural hematoma and dialysis: survey of reprint requests, New Eng. J. Med. **282**:1433, 1970.

82. Leonard, C. D., Weil, E., and Scribner, B. H.: Subdural haematomas in patients undergoing haemodialysis, Lancet **2**:239, 1969.

83. Lusignan, F. W., and Cross, G. O.: Calcified intracerebral hematoma, Ann. Surg. **132**:268, 1950.

84. Luttrell, C. N., Finberg, L., and Drawdy, L. P.: Hemorrhagic encephalopathy induced by hypernatremia. II. Experimental observations on hyperosmolarity in cats, Arch. Neurol. **1**:153, 1959.

85. Marie, P., Roussy, G., and Laroche, G.: Sur la reproduction expérimentale des pachyméningites hémorrhagiques, C. R. Soc. Biol. **74**:1303, 1913.

86. Maroon, J. C., and Campbell, R. L.: Subdural hematoma with inappropriate antidiuretic hormone secretion, Arch. Neurol. **22**:234, 1970.

87. Marshall, S., and Hinman, F.: Subdural hematoma following administration of urea for diagnosis of hypertension, J.A.M.A. **182**:813, 1962.

88. Mateos, J. H., and Daly, R.: Subdural hematoma: analytical study of 123 cases, Southern Med. J. **51**:94, 1958.

89. McKay, R. J., Morissette, R. A., Ingraham, F. D., and Matson, D. D.: Collections of subdural fluid complicating meningitis due to *Haemophilus influenzae* (type B), New Eng. J. Med. **242**:20, 1950.

90. McKissock, W., Richardson, A., and Bloom, W. H.: Subdural haematoma a review of 389 cases, Lancet **1**:1365, 1960.

91. McKissock, W., Taylor, J. C., Bloom, W. H., and Till, K.: Extradural hematoma, observations on 125 cases, Lancet **2**:167, 1960.

92. McLaurin, R. L., and McLaurin, K. S.: Calcified subdural hematomas in childhood, J. Neurosurg. **24**:648, 1966.

93. McLaurin, R. L., and Tutor, F. T.: Acute subdural hematoma, J. Neurosurg. **18**:61, 1961.

94. Meredith, J. M.: Chronic or subacute subdural hematoma due to indirect head trauma, J. Neurosurg. **8**:444, 1951.

95. Meredith, J. M., and Gish, C. R.: Chronic subdural hematoma in an adult producing marked erosion and perforation of the overlying dura and skull, J. Neurosurg. **9**:639, 1952.

96. Meredith, J. M., and Rinaldi, I.: Obstructive internal hydrocephalus following operative removal of chronic subdural hematoma in infants, J. Neurosurg. **18**:19, 1961.

97. Mosberg, W. H., and Smith, G. W.: Calcified solid subdural hematoma, J. Nerv. Ment. Dis. **115**:163, 1952.

98. Munro, D.: The diagnosis and treatment of subdural hematomata, New Eng. J. Med. **210**:1145, 1934.

99. Munro, D.: Cerebral subdural hematomas, New Eng. J. Med. **227**:87, 1942.

100. Munro, D., and Merritt, H. H.: Surgical pathology of subdural hematoma based on a

study of one hundred and five cases, Arch. Neurol. Psychiat. 35:64, 1936.

101. Naffziger, H. C.: Subdural fluid accumulations following head injury, J.A.M.A. 82:1751, 1924.

102. Nathanson, M., Cravioto, H. and Cohen, B.: Subdural hematoma related to anticoagulation therapy, Ann. Intern. Med. 49:1368, 1958.

103. Nelson, T. Y.: Acute subdural haematoma in the posterior fossa, Med. J. Aust. 2:792, 1959.

104. Ommaya, A. K., and Yarnell, P.: Subdural haematoma after whiplash injury, Lancet 2: 237, 1969.

105. Pan, A., Rogers, A. G., and Pearlman, D.: Subdural haematoma complicating anticoagulant therapy, Canad. Med. Ass. J. 82:1162, 1960.

106. Paul, M.: Haemorrhages from head injuries, Ann. Roy. Coll. Surg. Eng. 17:69, 1955.

107. Peet, M. M., and Kahn, E. A.: Subdural hematoma in infants, J.A.M.A. 98:1851, 1932.

108. Phillips, J. Y.: Cerebral cortical damage incident to chronic subdural hematoma in infancy, Bull. Los Angeles Neurol. Soc. 20:30, 1955.

109. Picken, C. B.: A case of subdural haematoma, Guy's Hosp. Rep. 78:368, 1928.

110. Potter, E. L.: Pathology of the fetus and infant, ed. 2, Chicago, 1961, Year Book Medical Publishers, Inc.

111. Pringle, J. H.: Traumatic meningeal haemorrhage, with a review of seventy-one cases, Edinburgh Med. J. 45:741, 1938.

112. Pudenz, R. H., and Shelden, C. H.: The lucite calvarium—a method for direct observation of the brain. II. Cranial trauma and brain movement, J. Neurosurg. 3:487, 1946.

113. Putnam, T. J., and Cushing, H.: Chronic subdural hematoma, its pathology, its relation to pachymeningitis hemorrhagica and its surgical treatment, Arch. Surg. 11:329, 1925.

114. Putnam, T. J., and Putnam, I. K.: The experimental study of pachymeningitis hemorrhagica, J. Nerv. Ment. Dis. 65:260, 1927.

115. Pygott, F., and Street, D. F.: Unsuspected treatable organic dementia, Lancet 1:1371, 1960.

116. Rand, C. W.: Chronic subdural hematoma, Arch. Surg. 14:1136, 1927.

117. Reigh, E. E., and Nelson, M.: Posterior-fossa subdural hematoma with secondary hydrocephalus, J. Neurosurg. 19:346, 1962.

118. Robinson, R. G.: Subdural haematoma in an adult after air encephalography, J. Neurol. Neurosurg. Psychiat. 20:131, 1957.

119. Russell, D. S.: The pathology of spontaneous intracranial haemorrhage, Proc. Roy. Soc. Med. 47:689, 1954.

120. Russell, D. S., and Cairns, H.: Subdural false membrane or haematoma (pachymeningitis interna haemorrhagica) in carcinomatosis and sarcomatosis of the dura mater, Brain 57:32, 1934.

121. Russell, P. A.: Subdural haematoma in infancy, Brit. Med. J. 2:446, 1965.

122. Schiller, F., Neligan, G., and Budtz-Olsen, O.: Surgery in haemophilia: a case of spinal subdural haematoma producing paraplegia, Lancet 2:842, 1948.

123. Schorstein, J.: Fatal intracranial venous haematoma following ventricular drainage, J. Neurol. Psychiat. 5:142, 1942.

124. Schreiber, M. S.: Acute subdural haematoma in the newborn, Med. J. Aust. 1:157, 1959.

125. Scott, M.: Spontaneous nontraumatic subdural hematomas, J.A.M.A. 141:596, 1949.

126. Sellers, E. M., and Koch-Weser, J.: Potentiation of warfarin-induced hypoprothrombinemia by chloral hydrate, New Eng. J. Med. 283:827, 1970.

127. Sherwood, D.: Chronic subdural hematoma in infants, Amer. J. Dis. Child. 39:980, 1930.

128. Shlevin, E. L., and Lederer, M.: Uncontrollable hemorrhage after Dicoumarol therapy with autopsy finding, Ann. Intern. Med. 21: 332, 1944.

129. Shulman, K., and Ransohoff, J.: Subdural hematoma in children, J. Neurosurg. 18:175, 1961.

130. Silverstein, A.: Intracranial bleeding in hemophilia, Arch. Neurol. 3:141, 1960.

131. Slater, J. P.: Extramedullary hematopoiesis in a subdural hematoma, J. Neurosurg. 25: 211, 1966.

132. Spiller, W. G., and McCarthy, D. J.: A case of internal hemorrhagic pachymeningitis in a child of nine years, with changes in the nerve cells, J. Nerv. Ment. Dis. 26:677, 1899.

133. Stehbens, W. E.: Aneurysms and anatomical variation of cerebral arteries, Arch. Path. 75: 45, 1963.

134. Strang, R. R., Tovi, D., and Hugosson, R.: Subdural hematomas resulting from the rupture of intracranial arterial aneurysms, Acta Chir. Scand. 121:345, 1961.

135. Sutherland, G. A.: On haematoma of the dura mater associated with scurvy in children, Brain 17:27, 1894.

136. Svien, H. J., and Gelety, J. E.: On the surgical management of encapsulated subdural hematoma, J. Neurosurg. 21:172, 1964.

137. Talalla, A., Halbrook, H., Barbour, B. H., and Kurze, T.: Subdural hematoma associated with long-term hemodialysis for chronic renal disease, J.A.M.A. 212:1847, 1970.

138. Till, K.: Subdural haematoma and effusion in infancy, Brit. Med. J. 3:400, 1968.

139. Toole, J. F., and Patel, A. N.: Cerebrovascular disorders, New York, 1967, McGraw-Hill Book Co.

140. Trotter, W.: Chronic subdural haemorrhage of traumatic origin, and its relation to pachymeningitis haemorrhagica interna, Brit. J. Surg. 2:271, 1914.

141. Trumble, H. C.: Chronic subdural haematoma, so-called, Med. J. Aust. 2:106, 1947.

142. Vance, B. M.: Fractures of the skull, Arch. Surg. 14:1023, 1927.

143. Vance, B. M.: Ruptures of surface blood vessels on cerebral hemispheres as a cause of subdural hemorrhage, Arch. Path. 61:992, 1950.

144. Van Gijn, J., and Wintzen, A. R.: Whiplash

injury and subdural haematoma, Lancet **2:** 592, 1969.

145. Vieth, R. G., Tindall, G. T., and Odom, G. L.: The use of tantalum dust as an adjunct in the postoperative management of subdural hematomas, J. Neurosurg. **24:**514, 1966.

146. Voris, H. C.: Subdural hematoma, J.A.M.A. **132:**686, 1946.

147. Wells, C. E. and Urrea, D.: Cerebrovascular accidents in patients receiving anticoagulant drugs, Arch. Neurol. **3:**553, 1960.

148. Whittier, J. R.: Deaths related to pneumoencephalography during a six year period, Arch. Neurol. Psychiat. **65:**463, 1951.

149. Wiener, L. M., and Nathanson, M.: The relationship of subdural hematoma to anticoagulant therapy, Arch. Neurol. **6:**282, 1962.

150. Woolley, P. V., and Evans, W. A.: Significance of skeletal lesions in infants resembling those of traumatic origin, J.A.M.A. **158:**539, 1955.

151. Wright, J. R., Slavin, R. E., and Wagner, J. A.: Intracranial aneurysm as a cause of subdural hematoma of the posterior fossa, J. Neurosurg. **22:**86, 1965.

152. Wright, R. L.: Traumatic hematomas of the posterior cranial fossa, J. Neurosurg. **25:**402, 1966.

153. Wycis, H. T.: Subdural hygroma, J. Neurosurg. **2:**340, 1945.

154. Youmans, J. R., and Schneider, R. C.: Posttraumatic intracranial hematomas in patients with arrested hydrocephalus, J. Neurosurg. **17:** 590, 1960.

155. Zollinger, R., and Gross, R. E.: Traumatic subdural hematoma: an explanation of the late onset of pressure symptoms, J.A.M.A. **103:**245, 1934.

7 / Subarachnoid hemorrhage

The subarachnoid space is anatomically unique in that it not only surrounds the brain, spinal cord, and cauda equina but contains all the large and distributing arteries together with most of the veins and communicates with the ventricular system and the Virchow-Robin spaces. The pathological term "subarachnoid hemorrhage" merely denotes the presence of blood in the subarachnoid space, the bleeding being primarily intraspinal or more frequently intracranial. This blood, therefore, stems from (1) blood vessels within the subarachnoid space itself, (2) parenchymal hemorrhage with blood escaping through the cortex or via the ventricular system to reach the subarachnoid space, (3) the choroid plexuses within the ventricular system, the blood then escaping into the subarachnoid space, or (4) blood within the subdural space from whatever source, reaching the subarachnoid space via a deficient arachnoid.

With the introduction and clinical application of the lumbar puncture technique, and the eventual correlation of the pathological state of bleeding into the subarachnoid space with the clinical syndrome of primary subarachnoid hemorrhage,[218,219] the diagnostic criteria for such bleeding were firmly established. Lumbar or cisternal puncture readily reveals the presence of blood in the subarachnoid space. The finding is not, however, a diagnosis in itself, but merely a sign or indication of another pathological state. In this sense all subarachnoid hemorrhages are ultimately secondary, despite the use of the prefix "primary" or "spontaneous" to indicate cases in which nontraumatic bleeding comes from blood vessels within the subarachnoid space itself. The classification is pointless particularly since ruptured cerebral aneurysm, the most usual cause, is more often than not associated with considerable intracerebral and sometimes intraventricular hemorrhage. The history of subarachnoid hemorrhage is closely allied to that of intracranial arterial aneurysms and the reader is referred to Walton's review.[236]

Subarachnoid hemorrhage may be divided into two major types—traumatic and nontraumatic.

Traumatic subarachnoid hemorrhage

Trauma, the most common cause of subarachnoid hemorrhage,[156] encompasses a great variety of injuries to the head and spine, including homicidal, suicidal, accidental, and war injuries, most of which are outside the scope of this book. The reader is thus referred to textbooks of forensic pathology and to texts dealing specifically with injuries of the brain and cord.[13,30]

The primary pathological conditions caused by an acute head injury are fracture, contusions, lacerations, and intracranial hemorrhage (extradural, subdural, subarachnoid, or intracerebral)[90] and with each of these, blood in the cerebrospinal fluid is a common finding. With the exception of cerebral edema,[50] subarachnoid hemorrhage is the unremitting accompaniment of cerebral contusions and is usually more extensive than the actual zone of bruising. When a pial vessel or a bridging vein is torn, the extent of the hemorrhage may be considerable.

Subarachnoid hemorrhage is usually present in cases of severe cranial or intracranial damage caused by birth injuries. From 20% to 40% of deaths among stillborn and newborn infants have been attributed to intracranial injury.[6,170] Hemorrhage is least frequent in the natural cephalic delivery. Trauma is particularly likely to follow the abrupt changes in shape of the skull attendant upon breech delivery, precipitate delivery, or high application of forceps. Although subdural hemorrhage at birth has a high mortality, subarachnoid hemorrhage is usually mild. Some indication of its frequency may be gleaned from the studies of Sharpe and Maclaire,[194,195] who found blood-stained or xanthochromic cerebrospinal fluid in 46 of 500 babies (9.2%) within the first 2 days after birth. Roberts,[176] examining the cerebrospinal fluid in 423 babies within 24 hours of birth and excluding those in whom the presence of blood was due to a traumatic lumbar puncture, found blood microscopically in 60 (14.1%). Not all subarachnoid hemorrhages in the neonatal infant are mild. Among 391 cases of intracranial damage caused by birth injuries, Courville[50] found four cases of extradural hemorrhage, 223 of subdural hemorrhage (mostly as a result of tearing of the falx cerebri or tentorium cerebelli with six caused by tears through venous sinuses), 16 of intradural hemorrhage, three of chronic subdural hematoma, 82 of subarachnoid hemorrhage, and 36 of cerebral hemorrhage (petechial or gross), as well as 21 cases of intraventricular hemorrhage and several other miscellaneous injuries.

The subarachnoid hemorrhage in the newborn is generally attributed to anoxia.[170] Asphyxia causes venous congestion and increased venous and cerebrospinal fluid pressure. These changes in turn are believed to initiate edema and the rupture of small vessels, which results in multiple petechial hemorrhages not restricted to the brain and subarachnoid space. However, Windle[242,243] has reported that experimental asphyxia in monkeys and guinea pigs did not produce petechial hemorrhages. He found that asphyxia of less than 7 minutes produced no neurological deficit, but that if it persisted longer than 7 minutes, permanent nonhemorrhagic brain damage ensued, the most vulnerable areas being the inferior colliculus and the ventrolateral thalamic nuclei. Hemorrhage was observed as a consequence of traumatic delivery, experimentally increased intrauterine pressure (induced by oxytocin), postnatal distress, and other factors leading to a moribund state. To explain these hemorrhages as a terminal phenomenon, he invoked Cammermeyer's hypothesis[37] that the cerebral ring (perivascular) hemorrhages were agonal because of a mixture of anoxia and ischemia during the actual process of dying in association with the impact of venous back pressure after cardiac arrest.

Nontraumatic subarachnoid hemorrhage

Unless otherwise qualified, subarachnoid hemorrhage usually refers to bleeding traceable to causes within the cranium with hemorrhage into the subarachnoid space. Nontraumatic subarachnoid hemorrhage is caused by a heterogeneous group of diseases. In the classification of cerebrovascular diseases, primary intracerebral hemorrhage, a common cause of blood-stained cerebrospinal fluid, is generally excluded and, like trauma, is classified as secondary subarachnoid hemorrhage. Others,[136] because of the difficulty in differential diagnosis, include primary intracerebral hemorrhage, which would then account for a large percentage of the cases of subarachnoid hemorrhage. With trauma and primary intracerebral hemorrhage excluded, subarachnoid hemorrhage is most often caused by rupture of an intracranial arterial aneurysm of the berry type. Consequently, the history, pathology, and clinical manifestations of the two lesions are so closely interwoven that the two are often inferred to be virtually synonymous. However, it is preferable to classify clinical states strictly according to etiology. Ultimately, subarachnoid hemorrhage, like pyrexia of unknown origin, will become merely an important clinical syndrome or sign for investigation that subsequently leads to the diagnosis of the basic underlying disease. Similarly, there is no specific

Table 7-1. Estimated incidence and mortality for types of cerebrovascular disease*

Type of cerebrovascular disease	Estimated frequency during decade ending 1969	Estimated annual death rate per 100,000 population
Subarachnoid hemorrhage	12%	20
Primary intracerebral hemorrhage	16%	40
Cerebral thrombosis-embolism	62%	120
Miscellaneous	10%	20
Total	100%	200

*Adapted from Kurtzke, J. F.: Epidemiology of cerebrovascular disease, Berlin, 1969, Springer-Verlag.

treatment, and therapy should be directed to the causative disease when this can be determined.

Incidence

Walton[236] estimated that approximately 8% of cases of cerebrovascular disease are caused by subarachnoid hemorrhage. From the weighted mean of the frequencies in four population studies, Kurtzke[128] estimated that subarachnoid hemorrhage comprises approximately 12% of all cases of cerebrovascular disease and that its annual death rate is 20 cases per 100,000 of population. His comparative figures for primary intracerebral hemorrhage and the thrombosis-embolism group are given in Table 7-1.

The reported frequency of the causes of nontraumatic subarachnoid hemorrhage is given in Table 7-2.

Subarachnoid hemorrhage is a common intracranial cause of sudden or unexpected death,[101] but in such cases the etiology can usually be traced to an aneurysm.

Age and sex distribution

In the Cooperative Study of Intracranial Aneurysms and Subarachnoid Hemorrhage,[135] there were 4880 patients admitted with their first subarachnoid hemorrhage and they were classified into hemorrhages attributable to an aneurysm (54%), arteriovenous malformation (6%), or other miscellaneous causes (40%). The latter group is naturally a heterogeneous group, many of which were of undetermined etiology. It was found that only 19% occurred under the age of 40 years and the peak frequency fell between 55 and 60 years. Of those admitted with their first hemorrhage, 54.3% were female. This slight preponderance is, in all probability, a reflection of the predominance of females among those with aneurysms. Those with subarachnoid hemorrhage of undetermined cause exhibited no preponderance of either sex.

Precipitating factors

Physical and emotional stress are often invoked as precipitating factors in the onset. In the Cooperative Study,[135] approximately 33% of the cases occurred during sleep and as one-third of our lives is spent in sleep, the results suggest that the bleeding may be a random event. However, many factors such as defecation, urination, coitus, coughing, emotional strain, trauma, lifting and bending, etc., account for approximately one-third of the cases but do not account for a similar proportion of our day. This suggests that these are elements of some significance probably by means of the Valsalva effect and a rise in blood pressure. In cases where the underlying cause is a blood dyscrasia, mild trauma may initiate the hemorrhage.

Pregnancy is an associated finding in some cases of subarachnoid hemorrhage regardless of whether or not aneurysms, arteriovenous aneurysms, or vascular anomalies are found. Unlike those associated with aneurysms, the majority of cases of subarachnoid hemorrhage of other etiology in the Cooperative Study[136] related to pregnancy occurred during parturition or

Table 7-2. Causes of nontraumatic subarachnoid hemorrhage

Causes	Courville (1950)[50]	Odom et al. (1952)[158]	Dekaban & McEachern (1952)[54]	Walton (1956)[226]	McKissock et al. (1959)[145]	Levy (1960)*[131]	af Björkesten et al. (1965)[4]	Cooperative Study Locksley, 1966[135]	Trumpy (1967)†[227]	Pakarinen (1967)[162]	Richardson (1969)[174]
Intracranial arterial aneurysm	17.8%	32.3%	22.2%	20%	45%	39%	75%	51%	31.9%	76.1%	51.5%
Hypertension arteriosclerosis	40.1%	13.6%									
Primary intracerebral hemorrhage		2.5%	26%					15%	5.2%		24%
Arteriovenous aneurysms (angiomas)	0.2%	6.3%	9.6%	1.9%	5%	14%	5%	6%	5.6%	2.9%	4.5%
Hemorrhage caused by rupture of anatomically normal artery or vein	0.2%		0.7%	0.3%					1.3%		
Miscellaneous	29.7%			3.9%		0.7%		6%	3.1%		
Cause unknown	11.9%	45.3%	41.5%	73.7%	50%	46%	20%	22%	52.8%	21%	20%
Total number of cases	596	316	135	310	781	164	113	5,431	229	511	3,042

*Angiographic series and, in some instances, aneurysms were not demonstrated by arteriography.
†Instances of primary intracerebral hemorrhage with intraventricular rupture proved at autopsy were excluded from the series.

post partum (12 of 20 cases). Toxemia or preexisting hypertension was noted in four patients. Cannell and Botterell[38] analyzed 61 cases of subarachnoid hemorrhage occurring prior to, during, or subsequent to pregnancy but could not determine any positive relationship or effect of pregnancy on the bleeding.

Etiology

The causes of nontraumatic subarachnoid hemorrhage vary considerably from author to author (Table 7-2) with much depending on the type of institution and the nature and selection of material. It is obvious that clinical material of recent origin with improved ancillary investigative techniques will be of more value than older material. Accurate appraisal of the etiology from published reports is not easy, for the reliability of the information is sometimes open to question.

In general, it may be stated that any disease producing intracerebral hemorrhage can also cause subarachnoid bleeding by extension to the subarachnoid space either by the direct route or via the ventricular system. The causes of intracranial subarachnoid hemorrhage, exclusive of trauma and intracerebral hemorrhage, are as follows: arterial aneurysms, occlusive cerebrovascular disease, arteriovenous aneurysm or hemangiomas, nonaneurysmal arterial rupture, infections, hypersensitivity and necrotizing lesions of small vessels, intracranial neoplasms, blood dyscrasias, and miscellaneous causes.

Intracranial arterial aneurysms. The largest collection of cases of nontraumatic subarachnoid hemorrhage was assembled in the Cooperative Study,[135] in which 51% of cases were attributed to rupture of an aneurysm (Table 7-2), mostly of the berry type. It is probable that some of the cases of unknown cause were also of aneurysmal origin. Several authors have demonstrated that intracranial arterial aneurysms account for more than 50% of the cases of subarachnoid hemorrhage (Table 7-2). In Falconer's series[78] of 148 cases, 100 had aneurysms, 12 had angiomas, and, of 26 cases of uncertain cause angiographically, six subsequently died and four were found to have aneurysms. Walton's series,[236] on the other hand, included a smaller proportion of aneurysms, only 20%, as angiography was not in routine use during much of the period surveyed in his monograph. In Walton's autopsy series of cases of subarachnoid hemorrhage, there was an incidence of 71.7% of arterial aneurysms, and the series included but a small percentage of cases of primary intracerebral hemorrhage. Pakarinen[162] excluded intracerebral hemorrhage from his series and found that 69.6% of 207 clinical cases investigated by angiography were attributed to aneurysms, and in 270 necropsies, aneurysms caused the subarachnoid hemorrhage in 81.8%. Such results have led Walton and Pakarinen to conclude that subarachnoid hemorrhage, exclusive of trauma and primary intracerebral hemorrhage, is caused by a ruptured cerebral aneurysm in over 70% of cases. Aneurysms account for 60% of the collective series of subarachnoid hemorrhage in the Cooperative Study[136] when primary intracerebral hemorrhage is excluded. The aneurysms usually referred to are the berry type of aneurysm and very rarely are they of other varieties, although the literature, especially in the last century, contains many instances of ruptured bacterial aneurysms complicating bacterial endocarditis.

Occlusive cerebrovascular disease. Bloodstained cerebrospinal fluid occurs in hemorrhagic infarction, whether due to arterial or venous occlusion. Arterial occlusion, responsible for red softenings, is usually embolic, though it may arise from external compression as with the posterior cerebral arteries in raised supratentorial pressure. Thrombosis of the dural sinuses and cerebral veins occurs under varying conditions. These subjects are dealt with elsewhere, but the degree of bleeding associated with such softenings may be considerable[12,22,33,58,122] and sufficient at times to cause concern as to whether the lesion is primarily a hemorrhage or a softening.

Some patients will present clinically as acute subarachnoid hemorrhage.[220] In general, however, the bleeding is not sufficiently severe to cause staining of the cerebrospinal fluid. For instance, Kendall[116] reported 11 cases with the presumptive diagnosis of intracranial venous thrombosis, five associated with pregnancy, and six of infective origin, but red cells were found in the cerebrospinal fluid only twice.

Arteriovenous aneurysms and hemangiomas. For a long time, it has been known, that like intracranial aneurysms, arteriovenous aneurysms and hemangiomas are prone to bleed, and after so doing, subarachnoid hemorrhage is the common result although more than half have other symptoms prior to hemorrhage.[162] The small so-called cryptic angiomas tend to bleed into the parenchyma and not into the subarachnoid space. Hereditary hemorrhagic telangiectasia rarely affects the central nervous system, but Quickel and Whaley[172] recently encountered it in a male of 17 years. The reported overall incidence of these interesting vascular lesions as a cause of nontraumatic subarachnoid hemorrhage varies from 1% to 14%,[162,236] as indicated in Table 7-2. An intracranial arterial aneurysm is not uncommon in association with an arteriovenous aneurysm, and it may well be the saccular aneurysm rather than the arteriovenous malformation that has ruptured.

Nonaneurysmal arterial rupture. Several authors have attributed subarachnoid hemorrhage to rupture of an anatomically "normal" artery[54] or to arterial rupture without aneurysm formation.[222,236] Walton found four instances in 193 cases of subarachnoid hemorrhage from the literature, and in his own autopsy series of 173 cases, three were caused by a ruptured atherosclerotic artery, two caused by ruptured nonatherosclerotic arteries, and one allegedly caused by a ruptured "anomalous" posterior communicating artery. Russell[184] attributed four instances of intracranial hemorrhage (presumably subarachnoid as well) to rupture of cerebral arteries exhibiting medial defects without aneurysms. It is also sometimes maintained that sudden rupture of an intracranial aneurysm may tear off the whole sac, which is then lost in the hematoma and therefore unrecognized. Such instances as these are of doubtful validity and are probably caused in most cases by an aneurysm, which the pathologist overlooked. Suspected sites of leakage should be examined by the serial section technique. Rupture of a noninflamed artery in the absence of aneurysmal dilatation or dissecting aneurysm is an extremely rare occurrence. Bagley,[17] in what could be an authentic case, reported the death of a male of 40 years from renal hemorrhage of unknown cause. Sections of the left internal carotid artery were interpreted as representing healed rupture believed to have been responsible for a previous subarachnoid hemorrhage. With greater care being taken by the pathologist, this category should become even more exceptional in the future.

Infections. Infections account for relatively few cases of nontraumatic subarachnoid hemorrhage, in general, less than 1%. Embolism to the brain is extremely common in bacterial endocarditis and the clinical picture of an acute subarachnoid hemorrhage in this disease is a well-recognized entity.[208] Arteritis may also complicate other bacteremias and pyogenic infections in the lung or elsewhere. The resultant arteritis does not always cause aneurysmal dilatation, and the necrotic and softened wall may simply yield to the blood pressure, causing massive subarachnoid hemorrhage. The source of the bleeding may not be identified, but as it mostly occurs peripherally on the cerebral arteries, careful and extensive dissection is needed to exclude a bacterial aneurysm. Russell[184] found 28 bacterial aneurysms (6.5%) among 461 autopsies on patients with intracranial hemorrhage. The frequency is high but gives an indication of the prevalence of such embolic phenomena at autopsy.

Schonfield[190] reported the case of a child with pyelonephritis and perinephric ab-

scess who developed septic thrombophlebitis of the lateral sinus and a fatal subarachnoid hemorrhage. Other patients with acute leptomeningitis may succumb to subarachnoid bleeding, no doubt because of an acute arteritis of a sizable vessel with rupture.[136,184,235,236] Involvement of smaller vessels can give rise to multifocal bleeding. Subarachnoid hemorrhage in fulminating meningococcal septicemia may mask the diagnosis of Waterhouse-Friderichsen syndrome.[110] The bleeding in such cases is in all probability caused by multiple large extravasations as occur elsewhere in the body. A cerebral abscess might also involve a nearby artery or vein with serious bleeding therefrom.[136,186,236]

It is not generally recognized that severe hemorrhage may complicate the arteritis accompanying tuberculous meningitis. Hemorrhage may be massive because of the rupture of vessels affected by the inflammatory and necrotizing action of the tubercle bacilli, which are usually numerous. Alternatively, an aneurysmal dilatation may form and rupture, causing subarachnoid or even intracerebral hemorrhage. Smaller hemorrhagic extravasations are probably more frequent. Occlusion of involved vessels may lead to softening of extensive areas and secondary hemorrhage may occur therein. Goldzieher and Lisa[85] found hemorrhagic infarction to be responsible for the bleeding in their material although arteritis with incipient aneurysms was prevalent. Tubercle bacilli display a remarkable tendency to localize near and involve blood vessels in tuberculous meningitis.[100,173] Hektoen[100] reported intimal tubercles and a tubercle bacillus has been observed in an endothelial cell of an otherwise intact arteriole by Goldzieher and Lisa.[85] These observations explain the frequent occurrence of perivascular inflammatory response, and the prevalence of arteritis and phlebitis in tuberculous meningitis.

Literature of 30 and more years ago contains reports of meningovascular syphilis causing subarachnoid hemorrhage,[185,214,222] or cerebral aneurysms. Syphilis in any form is an extremely rare cause of intracranial hemorrhage, and most authors now doubt whether it is ever a cause of cerebral aneurysm. Unquestionably the same skepticism must be applied to syphilis as a cause of subarachnoid hemorrhage without aneurysm formation. The presence of a positive Wasserman reaction in heavily blood-stained cerebrospinal fluid may be a false reaction and, even if authentic, does not necessarily indicate a cause-and-effect relationship between syphilis and subarachnoid bleeding. Syphilis was incriminated in the etiology of subarachnoid hemorrhage in the Cooperative Study[136] and the high prevalance certainly warrants further analysis. Nevertheless, the conclusion was that syphilis was of inconsequential importance.

Dewar and Walmsley[56] reported a case of severe widespread subarachnoid hemorrhage in a man with relapsing fever and Rogers[180] estimated the evidence of such bleeding to be 1 in 6 autopsies on fatal cases of the disease.

In the Cooperative Study[136] of subarachnoid hemorrhage, infections of various types were thought to be of primary or secondary importance in the etiology of the bleeding in 32 patients. The infections were staphylococcal meningitis (one case), lobar pneumonia (one case), septicemia with meningitis (two cases), syphilis (20 cases), tuberculosis (three cases), herpes encephalitis (one case), staphylococcal pneumonia (one case), rubella encephalitis (one case), meningitis of unknown type (one case), and another case in which the diagnosis was either tumor or encephalitis. In another three cases, syphilis was an associated disease.

Subarachnoid hemorrhage has also been reported in association with fungal infections of the central nervous system such as mucormycosis[211] and aspergillosis.[143]

Hypersensitivity (autoimmune and necrotizing lesions of small vessels). Polyarteritis nodosa occasionally involves the central nervous system, and in accord with the frequency of hemorrhage from an acute

arteritis or a small aneurysm, subarachnoid hemorrhage sporadically complicates this disease.[60,105,238] Polyarteritis nodosa affects small arteries and arterioles predominantly, but Diaz-Rivera and Miller[57] recorded dilatation with rupture of the basilar artery just proximal to the bifurcation. The histological description was consistent with that of polyarteritis nodosa.

Gairdner[80] reviewed the Schönlein-Henoch syndrome (anaphylactoid purpura). In two cases, there were convulsive episodes. No subarachnoid hemorrhage was noted, but at autopsy of the single fatal case there was necrotizing arteritis of the meningeal and superficial cortical vessels. Miller[153] saw a case of subarachnoid hemorrhage in association with acute rheumatic carditis and a purpuric rash some 3 days after the appearance of measles. The ensuing cerebral catastrophe was attributed to purpura of the anaphylactoid type. Lewis and Philpott[133] reported other instances of subarachnoid hemorrhage.

Acute rheumatism, though listed as a rare cause of subarachnoid hemorrhage, is a very doubtful etiological factor. Sharpe[193] attributed a case of subarachnoid hemorrhage in a woman of 27 years of age to "rheumatic infection," but the bleeding rather than being caused by rheumatism was almost certainly caused by bacterial arteritis with or without aneurysm formation as *Streptococcus viridans* was cultured from the bloodstained cerebrospinal fluid. Easby[64] observed subarachnoid hemorrhage in a young girl (12 years old) with a history of rheumatic heart disease. The bleeding appeared to be the result of a bacterial aneurysm associated with bacterial endocarditis though the actual outcome and definitive diagnosis of the illness are unknown.

In diffuse lupus erythematosus necrotizing vascular lesions found in the central nervous system accounted for the subarachnoid hemorrhage reported by Tremaine.[225]

Walton[235] attributed subarachnoid hemorrhage in acute glomerulonephritis[164] to a general allergic vascular response. There is always the possibility that it was caused by a coincidental lesion.

Intracranial tumors. Hemorrhage into or about intracranial tumors is frequent, particularly in the case of glioblastoma multiforme (astrocytoma grade IV) and melanoma. Globus and Sapirstein[84] found evidence of blood in the cerebrospinal fluid in 22.3% of their 94 cases of intracerebral tumors (primary and secondary) that had not been subjected to surgery. However, it is only rarely that a tumor, either primary or secondary, causes gross bleeding into the subarachnoid space. Even more infrequently will the bleeding present the classical clinical picture of subarachnoid hemorrhage, and yet subarachnoid bleeding can be the first serious effect of a cerebral tumor.[36]

Oldberg[160] reviewed Cushing's 832 cases of glioma and found only 31 cases with hemorrhage. In seven, the clinical history was suggestive of subarachnoid hemorrhage. Globus and Sapirstein[84] reviewed an autopsy series of cases of cerebral tumor that had not been subjected to surgical interference and asserted that as a rule there is some degree of bleeding into the tumor. In 20 of their cases, there was evidence of subarachnoid bleeding. Glass and Abbott[83] selected from the literature and their own material 41 cases with sufficient detail to indicate clearly an association with subarachnoid hemorrhage. The bleeding varied in severity, being fatal on occasions even in the initial hemorrhage (three patients). Recurrent bleeding was not unusual and in 46.3% of the cases recurrent hemorrhages had arisen. Most of the tumors were supratentorial (34 cases). In 39 of the tumors, there were 20 gliomas, 11 cases of glioblastoma multiforme or astrocytoma grade IV, one case of astrocytoma grade III, four cases of astrocytoma grades I and 2, one case of medulloblastoma, one case of oligodendroglioma, one case of ependymoma, one case of perivascular sarcoma, 11 pituitary adenomas (eosinophilic and chromophobe), six vascular tumors (benign or malignant), one cerebel-

lopontine angle tumor, and one primary melanoma.

In the Cooperative Study[136] of 2092 cases of subarachnoid hemorrhage (excluding aneurysms and arteriovenous malformations), there were 12 cases of primary intracranial tumor, 12 metastatic tumors, and five suspected metastases. The primary tumors included a parasagittal meningioma, a papilloma of the choroid plexus, hemangiosarcoma of the floor of the middle cranial fossa, a chromophobe pituitary adenoma, and oligodendroglioma, and ependymoblastoma, three glioblastomas, and three tumors of unspecified type. The metastatic tumor most often encountered was a malignant melanoma (five cases), followed by bronchogenic carcinoma (four cases). Other metastases were hepatoma, myxoma of the heart with multiple tumor emboli (also anticoagulant therapy), and one tumor of unknown origin. Suspected metastatic tumors included two mammary cancers, two from the colon, and one from the cervix uteri.

Hemorrhage associated with gliomas of the brain is usually into the tumor and seen in its most typical form in the glioblastoma multiforme. The hemorrhage also arises from grade III astrocytomas and both types may produce massive subarachnoid hemorrhage.[55,65,183,214] Fatal massive intracerebral and subarachnoid hemorrhage can occur, and unless care is taken, the tumor may be overlooked at autopsy. Kalbag[115] reported a case in which an oligodendroglioma close to the ventricle caused subarachnoid hemorrhage. Angiography had given no indication of the diagnosis.

Very vascular meningiomas occurring at conventional sites may bleed. Askenasy and Behmoaram[11] reported two instances of meningioma in the lateral ventricle presenting with subarachnoid hemorrhage when cerebral aneurysms had been suspected. The authors encountered seven intraventricular meningiomas, and as two tumors presented as subarachnoid hemorrhage, they pondered that this might be a common mode of presentation.

Papillomas of the choroid plexus are now recognized as a cause of the escape of blood from the ventricular system into the subarachnoid space.[67,86] Clinically the patient may present as a typical acute subarachnoid hemorrhage.[2] Other symptoms and signs will result from local pressure and from some dilatation of the ventricular system because of a damming effect or to tamponade (acute hemocephalus).

Since Brougham and associates[32] reviewed the literature on hemorrhage into pituitary adenomas, interest in and awareness of pituitary apoplexy has increased. Wright and associates[246] found that approximately 85 cases had been reported. Pituitary adenomas are highly vascular tumors. In the main, the tumor manifests itself for months or years before sudden hemorrhage causes an acute exacerbation of pressure symptoms, but in 18 the hemorrhage was the first manifestation. Bloodstained or xanthochromic cerebrospinal fluid may be found on lumbar puncture and in some instances the hemorrhage closely resembles the clinical picture of subarachnoid hemorrhage as it is heralded by sudden headache, meningismus, etc. Death may occur within a few hours or a few days.[32,121] The bleeding may become intracerebral[134] or intraventricular[32] and recurrent. The hemorrhage has been attributed to retrogressive changes in the adenoma because the rapid growth outstrips the blood supply and necrosis is usually extensive. Thrombi may or may not be found.[32,134]

Simonsen[201] recorded the unusual case of a woman of 38 years of age who died suddenly from extensive subarachnoid hemorrhage, believed to have complicated a chordoma. Van Wagenen,[230] reporting another case of an intracranial chordoma and subarachnoid hemorrhage, found that the bleeding stemmed from a ruptured intracranial aneurysm.

Metastatic tumors in the central nervous system occasionally initiate subarachnoid bleeding,[136,184,235] and bronchogenic carcinoma,[140,212] hypernephroma, or other carcinomas may be diagnosed. Malignant melanoma, whether primary or secondary in the brain, is very disposed to bleed and thus promote subarachnoid hemorrhage, which may be recurrent.[81] Schnitker and Ayer[189] reviewed the rare primary melanomas of the central nervous system and found the cerebrospinal fluid in a few to be either bloodstained or xanthochromic. Metastatic malignant melanoma is considerably more prevalent than the primary variety and its perivascular extension and proclivity for bleeding are characteristic. Wortis and Wortis[245] concluded that whenever the cerebrospinal fluid is bloody or xanthochromic in patients with malignant melanoma, a diligent search for melanin pigment and melanoma cells in the fluid should be conducted. Loewenberg[137] discussed 14 cases of metastatic melanoma in the brain with the fluid bloody in several and xanthochromic in seven. In a review, Madonick and Savitsky[140] found the fluid either bloodstained or xanthochromic in 16 of 35 proved cases of metastatic melanoma and in 10 of 21 cases of primary melanoma of the brain (total incidence of 46%). By contrast, they found only two instances of bloodstained fluid in 56 cases of cerebral metastatic tumors of varied types.

Chorionepithelioma, notorious for its malignancy, predilection for vascular invasion, and hematogenous spread of metastases, not infrequently metastasizes to the central nervous system. The metastases are usually multiple, necrotic, and hemorrhagic, and as a result blood may reach the subarachnoid space. Evidence of tumor in blood vessels in the hemorrhagic and necrotic deposits may be caused by embolism[191] or vascular invasion. Massive intracerebral hemorrhage as well as subarachnoid and subdural hemorrhage were features in one young patient in whom multiple hemorrhagic metastases were probably caused by emboli of cerebral arteries.[233] One posterior cerebral artery was occluded and the area of supply was infarcted. Vaughan and Howard[233] briefly reviewed the incidence of metastases to the brain from chorionepithelioma and estimated it to be about 20%. From the literature in 12 cases of cerebral metastases with adequate clinical and pathological detail, five had bloodstained cerebrospinal fluid (two males, three females) and in eight, an acute apoplectic episode ushered in the signs of cerebral involvement.

Osteochondromas of the base of the skull are very rare.[235] King and Butcher[119] reported fatal subarachnoid hemorrhage in a young man with one of these tumors. No source of bleeding was determined.

Blood dyscrasias. Subarachnoid hemorrhage has been reported as a complication of many of the hematological diseases, which include hemophilia,[118] aplastic or hypoplastic anemia,[27,136] leukemia,[78,154] agranulocytosis,[186] thrombocytopenic purpura,[39,235] polycythemia rubra vera,[215] sickle cell anemia,[21] splenic anemia,[239] pernicious anemia,[136] and bleeding during anticoagulant therapy.[23]

In the Cooperative Study,[136] dyscrasias were incriminated (as primary or secondary factors) in subarachnoid bleeding in 17 cases. In two patients, myeloid leukemia was found, and sickle cell anemia in one case, polycythemia vera in one, aplastic or hypoplastic anemia four cases, dietary hypoprothrombinemia one case, salicylate poisoning one case, pernicious anemia four cases, hemorrhagic disease of the newborn one case, bleeding tendency in renal rickets one case, and chronic leukopenia secondary to marrow hypoplasia caused by anticancer therapy one case.

Upon examining 109 hemophiliac patients with bleeding symptoms, Ikkala[111] found five that had intracranial hemorrhage (three traumatic and two apparently spontaneous). Among fatal cases of hemophilia in Finland, intracranial hemorrhage was a common cause of death, with victims primarily under the age of 15 years. Not all of these episodes were necessarily subarachnoid hemorrhage and most were attributed to trauma. Recurrent subarachnoid bleeding may occur in hemophi-

lia.[14,197] Singer and Schneider[203] estimated that up to 1962 there were some 85 recorded cases of suspected intracranial hemorrhage and that subdural and subarachnoid hemorrhage were the most common sites. Hemorrhage into more than one site is not uncommon.[197] Kerr[118] asserts that intracranial bleeding is currently the most common cause of death in hemophilia in some countries. In 59 deaths from hemophilia, intracranial hemorrhage accounted for 6.8% between 1900 and 1940, and for 25.5% in 47 deaths between 1940 and 1962. Of 109 hemophiliacs investigated during a 5-year- period, 15 patients (13.8%) with a mean age of 23 years suffered one or more proved or probably intracranial hemorrhages and 5 died (33%). Of the 15 patients, 10 had a subarachnoid hemorrhage, and Kerr[118] cited the case of a severe hemophiliac with subarachnoid and intracerebral hemorrhage occurring after meningococcal leptomeningitis. Although injury is the major cause of intracranial bleeding in hemophilia, many of these patients can withstand considerable trauma to the head without ill effect. One notorious street fighter with factor IX deficiency had his promising career as a professional boxer cut short, not by posttraumatic bleeding, but by his inability to breathe through a flattened nose. Sudden changes in intracranial pressure may precipitate bleeding[118] and angiography via percutaneous puncture of the carotid arteries may be fatal.[202] External bleeding from the site of a lumbar puncture is rare.[197]

Intracranial bleeding is of frequent occurrence in leukemia either in the acute varieties or during acute exacerbations of a chronic form.[29,78] Moore and associates[154] analyzed 117 fatal cases of "acute" leukemia and found that 23 patients (20%) died of intracranial hemorrhage, and of these nine had subarachnoid hemorrhage. This was usually associated with intracerebral hemorrhage with extension to the subarachnoid space directly or via the ventricles. These authors noted that those with fatal intracerebral hemorrhage died predominantly during a blastic crisis with leukocyte counts above 300,000 per cu. mm., whereas fatal subarachnoid hemorrhage was not associated with a high terminal leukocyte count but appeared to bear a definite relationship to severe thrombocytopenia.[78] Acute hemorrhagic softening has been observed underlying subarachnoid hemorrhage in leukemia[78] and Belmusto and associates[25] suggested that hydrocephalus, which is not uncommon with leukemic involvement of the central nervous system, might be caused not by infiltration of the pia arachnoid but to hemogenic meningitis. Leukemic infiltrations of the subarachnoid space often exhibit a perivascular distribution and are generally associated with some local hemorrhage.[130]

Subarachnoid hemorrhage may occur in polycythemia vera, but it is not common.[114,215] The cerebrospinal fluid may also be bloodstained because of hemorrhagic softenings secondary to the thromboses so prevalent in this disease.

In primary thrombocytopenic purpura, intracranial hemorrhage is said to be the most common cause of death.[202] The hemorrhage may be purpuric or massive. Subarachnoid and subdural spaces are affected as often as the brain itself.[39] Hemorrhage occurs in secondary thrombocytopenic purpura also.[39,136,235] Brodie and associates[31] recently encountered fatal subarachnoid hemorrhage in association with thrombocytopenic purpura and bronchogenic carcinoma and considered the thrombocytopenia to be due to an immune mechanism. Thrombocytopenia in aplastic anemia accounts for the hemorrhage that may complicate the disease.[27] Russell[184] found such hemorrhage three times in 461 cases of nontraumatic intracranial bleeding.

Sickle cell anemia rarely manifests itself by intracranial hemorrhage. The patient described by Ballard and Bonder[21] was found unconscious and the bloodstained cerebrospinal fluid was under increased pressure. After clinical improvement, headache and meningismus became prominent symptoms. Other cases have been reported

and the red cells in the cerebrospinal fluid may exhibit sickling.[42,48,88]

Since their introduction, anticoagulants have been employed enthusiastically, both therapeutically and prophylactically for thromboembolic disorders, frequently in the absence of adequate clinical or laboratory control. Severe and often serious bleeding may eventuate, but such complications occur more often than not even with adequate laboratory control, possibly because of potentiation by other drugs of the hypoprothrombinemic effect of anticoagulants. Bleeding not infrequently is intracranial, subdural, subarachnoid, intracerebral, or intraventricular, or encompasses combinations of these. In some reports on the efficacy of anticoagulant therapy, intracranial hemorrhage is not found to be a complication. Russek and Zohman[182] found it to be the most common cause of death (45.1%), almost half of the hemorrhages being subarachnoid in location. In one patient reported by Barron and Fergusson,[23] clotted blood in the subarachnoid space was 1.2 cm. thick in the neighborhood of the middle cerebral artery. However, subarachnoid hemorrhage does not occur in isolation generally, but in association with intracerebral hemorrhage from which spread to the ventricles is likely. Although the intracerebral hemorrhage is frequently fatal, a few patients may have bloodstained cerebrospinal fluid apparently without extensive intracerebral bleeding and survive.[23,89] Anticoagulants have been found to enhance the risks of intracranial bleeding in patients with subacute bacterial endocarditis and also in those with a recent occlusive cerebrovascular lesion,[232] so that in these instances hemorrhage should be uncommon in future studies.

Abnormal bleeding occurs in at least two-thirds of the patients with Waldenström's macroglobulinemia, subarachnoid hemorrhage being one of the most common neurological manifestations of the disease.[138] The bleeding is usually purpuric, although fulminating intracerebral hemorrhage may arise due to thrombocytopenia, microcirculatory disturbances, and possibly secondary endothelial damage.

Miscellaneous. Subarachnoid hemorrhage has also been observed under several other circumstances. Bouquet[28] reported subarachnoid hemorrhage in a 14-year-old boy believed to have been suffering from sunstroke. It is known that a serious disturbance of the hemostatic mechanism occurs in heat stroke with a tendency to bleed. Subarachnoid hemorrhage may then occur but does not tend to be the dominant feature of the disorder.

Subarachnoid bleeding has been observed in patients subjected to insulin-induced hypoglycemic shock therapy.[77,163] Baker and Lufkin[19] recorded old and new intracerebral hemorrhages in patients dying of spontaneous hypoglycemia, whence it is understandable that blood could escape into the cerebrospinal fluid. Lawrence and associates[129] reviewed the literature on hypoglycemia. Gross hemorrhage was little in evidence in most cases. Psychiatric patients given pentylenetetrazol (Metrazol) shock therapy have died with intracerebral and subarachnoid hemorrhage,[175] and here the bleeding has been attributed to the toxic effects of the analeptic rather than the shock therapy per se. The characteristic observations in brains of animals dying after Metrazol and electric shocks were subarachnoid and intracerebral hemorrhage as in humans.[8,99,175] Subarachnoid hemorrhage has also been reported in a patient on cortisone therapy, but a ruptured aneurysm was discovered at autopsy.[103] The cortisone could possibly have contributed to the fatal outcome by inhibition of the repair processes. The administration of epinephrine has precipitated subarachnoid hemorrhage in a woman with urticaria 2 weeks post partum,[74] but the mechanism in such instances is obscure.

Kernohan and Woltman[117] recorded extensive subarachnoid hemorrhage in four patients within a few days of uncomplicated surgical operations. The bleeding was attributed to focal, nonseptic necrosis of the cerebral arteries. There is, however, a need for further information about these lesions, which do not conform to any other known disease entity.

The association of two factors may be coincidental and completely devoid of a cause-and-effect relationship. For example, patients with sickle cell anemia have been reported with subarachnoid hemorrhage, but the bleeding was caused by ruptured aneurysms.[42,88,240] Also Kerr[118] reported subarachnoid bleeding in a hemophiliac, but the hemorrhage was of aneurysmal origin, quite apart from the fact that the bleeding defect in this case was a serious complicating factor.

Subarachnoid hemorrhage of unknown etiology

There is an obvious but misleading tendency to associate the majority of subarachnoid hemorrhages with the rupture of aneurysms and even to use the two terms synonymously. However, rapid advances in angiographic techniques have enabled clinicians to determine the cause of subarachnoid hemorrhage in increasing numbers of cases.[4] The more thorough the investigation of the cerebral vascular tree, the larger is the percentage of cases of subarachnoid hemorrhage in which a cause for the bleeding is demonstrable.

Bilateral carotid angiography has virtually replaced unilateral angiography, and several authors[205,216] have demonstrated the value of vertebral angiography. Spatz and Bull[205] investigated by vertebral angiography 60 cases of subarachnoid hemorrhage in which bilateral carotid angiography had failed to disclose the source of the bleeding. In not one instance was there clinical suspicion of a posterior lesion, but in 16 cases (26.7%), vertebral angiograms revealed a demonstrable lesion (eight aneurysms and eight angiomas). Nevertheless, there were still 44 cases of subarachnoid hemorrhage without demonstrable cause. Even more significant is that Sutton and Trickey[217] were able to demonstrate lesions responsible for subarachnoid hemorrhage in 75% of 557 patients subjected to bilateral carotid angiography, but this incidence of positive findings was increased to 96% when four-vessel angiography was performed routinely. Table 7-2 reveals that the percentage of cases of subarachnoid hemorrhage of unknown etiology is considerable, varying from 12% to 74%, though naturally each series cannot be regarded as being of identical composition. It is the group of unknown etiology that can most justifiably be regarded as primary subarachnoid hemorrhage. The pathologist, accustomed to finding a demonstrable cause for the great majority of cases of subarachnoid hemorrhage, may attribute his failure to disclose aneurysms or perhaps cryptic angiomas to the limitations of angiography. Miliary aneurysms are prevalent in the cerebral cortex and if, like those more deeply situated, they are prone to bleed, they could be a cause of subarachnoid bleeding. The subarachnoid space could adapt more readily to the volume of extravasated blood than does the brain to an intracerebral hematoma. There is a considerable overlap in the age distribution of miliary aneurysms and idiopathic subarachnoid hemorrhage. Thrombosis of the small parent vessel is likely to occur, and consequently the incidence of recurrent hemorrhage would be less than in aneurysmal hemorrhage from a large artery. Such explanations at this stage, however, are sheer speculation. Some cases may also be due to undiagnosed primary intracerebral hemorrhage with survival. Nevertheless, it is possible that with the ever-improving clinical methods of investigating the cerebral vascular tree, this group of unknown etiology will be diminished.

Pathology of subarachnoid hemorrhage

In any case of subarachnoid hemorrhage, irrespective of the clinical diagnosis, the cerebral arteries should be most carefully inspected by the pathologist. Subarachnoid hemorrhage of aneurysmal origin frequently forms a thick layer of blood in the subarachnoid space. It tends to be most prominent about the anterior half of the circle of Willis, unless the sac is embedded in the brain and local adhesions prevent direct subarachnoid bleeding. In this case the blood is thickest in the posterior fossa if the aneurysm has ruptured into the ventricular system.

Primary intracerebral hemorrhage produces a subarachnoid hemorrhage in which blood escapes into the cisterns of the posterior fossa after ventricular rupture, unless the hematoma ruptures directly into the subarachnoid space, for then the blood is most prominent locally over the site of rupture. In general, the bleeding is not as gross as in the case of a ruptured aneurysm.

Most arteriovenous malformations are related to the middle cerebral artery and generally are to be seen over the cerebral hemispheres. Subarachnoid hemorrhage, therefore, is likely to be most extensive at this site though the blood extends to the basal cisterns. If intraventricular rupture takes place, the blood will appear in the posterior fossa about the foramina of Luschka and Magendie. The lesions are relatively uncommon and patients do not often die during the acute episode of bleeding. Cryptic hemangiomas and small varices rarely bleed into the subarachnoid space, but a massive hemorrhage can reach the subarachnoid space via the ventricular system.

In most cases of nontraumatic subarachnoid hemorrhage attributed to one of the rare causes of bleeding, the underlying disease usually manifests itself before the intracranial bleeding complicates the picture. However, at times the clinical picture may be indistinguishable from that of a ruptured aneurysm with the preceding symptoms and signs, namely, glioma, melanoma, osteochondroma, pituitary adenoma, purpura hemorrhagica, and subacute bacterial endocarditis insufficient to force the subject to seek medical attention.[236] Therefore, in any instance of subarachnoid hemorrhage, the less common causes must always be borne in mind. This admonition also holds true for the pathologist. When the clinical picture is acute and severe, the hemorrhage may be quite severe, and its location dependent primarily on the site of the causative lesion. In general, any subarachnoid hemorrhage that is atypical in location or is multifocal in distribution is strongly suggestive of bleeding secondary to one of the rarer causes. Diffuse and extensive hemorrhage may certainly occur in the blood dyscrasias, bacterial and fungal arteritis, and also with neoplasms occasionally.

The hemorrhage may not be severe and the patient may recover with appropriate therapy, with the blood being removed as in any other case of hemogenic meningitis. As time passes, dissection of the vessels is rendered more difficult, and though fibrosis becomes more evident, extensive fibrosis is unusual. As the blood is absorbed, the meninges appear yellowish orange or rust colored. Most of the pigmentation disappears but remnants are often found in the neighborhood of the source of bleeding many years later. Fibrotic encapsulation of extravasated blood in the subarachnoid space does not eventuate and consequently calcification and ossification as in hematomas elsewhere are not found.

Reaction to blood in the subarachnoid space

The subarachnoid space is lined by a continuous layer of flattened arachnoidal cells resembling mesothelium and it is from these arachnoidal cells that macrophages are believed to arise after the subarachnoid injection of particulate matter.[68] Macrophages are normally found within the pia[92] and in the arachnoid stroma also.[244] Blood injected into the serous cavities produces an aseptic inflammatory response[40] and a similar phenomenon occurs when blood enters the subarachnoid space. The reaction is referred to as a hemogenic meningitis.[113] Indeed subarachnoid hemorrhage has on occasions been mistaken for meningitis[82] with headache meningismus, pyrexia, leukocytosis, and possibly vomiting. The leukocytosis reaches as high as 20,000 per cu. mm. of blood.[159] The recurrence of such episodes enables the clinician

to eventually make the diagnosis of ruptured cerebral aneurysm.[219] Finlayson and Penfield[73] considered the syndrome of acute postoperative aseptic meningitis to be the result of bleeding into the subarachnoid space. They reproduced the meningitis by an intracisternal injection of blood or fluid from a subdural hematoma.

Evidence[190] suggests that, with the escape of blood into the subarachnoid space, a plasma factor becomes activated, with the subsequent generation of kinins. In turn, the kinins not only stimulate pain nerve endings, but also increase capillary permeability and appear to be responsible for other features of the hemogenic meningitis. Further investigation of the kininogen-kinin system and other enzymatic factors involved in the subarachnoid reaction to blood should prove to be enlightening. It is also pertinent that the kallikrein inhibitor in subarachnoid hemorrhage appears to be of therapeutic value.[196]

Several authors have been interested in this hemogenic meningitis,[7,18,94,113] which is akin to the reaction to extravasated blood elsewhere. Microscopically, the subarachnoid space is distended initially to a variable degree with fresh blood, which may seep into the sulci but rarely extends along the perivascular sheaths into the cortex. Sectioning of such thick layers of blood is difficult and artifacts are frequent. After 4 to 16 hours, occasional infiltrations with polymorphonuclear leukocytes may be found,[95] but this is frequently not particularly obvious and intense leukocytic infiltration should be suspected as having some other cause. After 1 to 3 days, lymphocytes are found and the leukocytes are at a peak about the third day.[95] Macrophages appear in the subarachnoid space within 2 days and siderophages are to be found by 5 [7,41] or 6 days.[213] By 3 days the polymorphonuclear leukocytes are overshadowed by lymphocytes and macrophages. Phagocytic activity at this stage is prominent and intact red cells may be observed in the cytoplasm of macrophages (Fig. 7-1). This reaction increases in intensity during

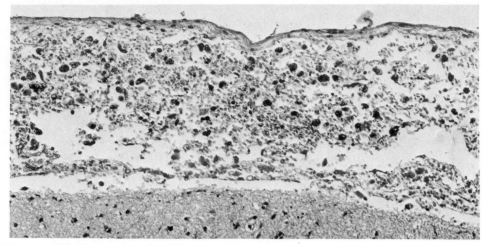

Fig. 7-1. Blood in subarachnoid space with numerous hemosiderin-laden macrophages, some of which at a higher magnification contain phagocytosed red cells. (Hematoxylin and eosin, ×110.)

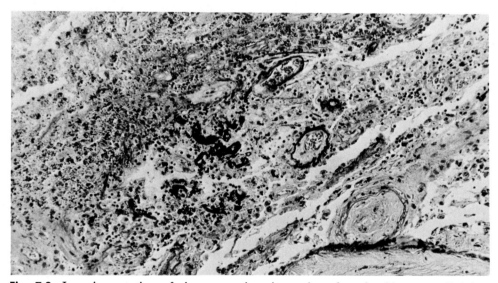

Fig. 7-2. Iron incrustation of the connective tissues in subarachnoid space adjoining a bleeding aneurysm. A few vessels have their elastic laminae outlined by purple-staining material (iron incrustation), simulating an elastic stain. No giant cell reaction was observed. There are many macrophages and some fibrosis. Note gross intimal thickening of small arteries. (Hematoxylin and eosin, ×110.)

the subsequent week. Hammes[95] asserts that fibrosis is first seen at 10 days. The amount of fibrosis is variable and fibroblasts are interspersed in the cellular reaction. Hematoidin may be found intracellularly but at times appears to impregnate the connective tissue or adventitia of vessels. It is seen particularly near the source of hemorrhage such as an aneurysm and it appears later than hemosiderin. In cerebral trauma, Strassman[213] did not find it till about 10 to 14 days, and even later according to Chason.[41] The adventitia of pial vessels may contain hemosiderin or be infiltrated by hematoidin. Iron incrustation of the connective tissues of pial vessels, probably of the elastica may be observed after severe hemorrhage (Fig. 7-2). Recurrent hemorrhage complicates the appearance, but in its absence the inflammatory reaction progressively subsides, leaving residual fibrosis in which are embedded many siderophages. Lymphocytes may be present in small numbers and occasionally a few perivascular siderophages may be found in the underlying cortex. The subarachnoid space may become obliterated because of fibrosis and approximation of the arachnoid to the pia. If the underlying cortex is damaged, the cellular reaction of the overlying subarachnoid space may be modified and eventually gliosis may merge with and adhere firmly to the fibrosis of the pia arachnoid.

Alpers and Forster[7] found that immediately after a subarachnoid hemorrhage, the erythrocytes were for the most part in a normal state, only a few being crenated. By 24 hours, the erythrocytes exhibited some clumping although this is difficult to appreciate and from 12 to 15 days they are entirely clumped, with few fresh or crenated cells. Bailey[18] agreed in the main with these findings.[7]

Schemm and associates[188] suggested that recurrent bleeding from a ruptured aneurysm may be caused by inadequate healing processes in the subarachnoid space. By implanting polyvinyl sponge in the subarachnoid space of goats, they found that new tissue growth and collagen production were slower than that in sponge implanted in muscle or subcutaneous tissue. The difference was, however, negligible after 4 weeks. The relationship this has to aneurysmal repair is of course dubious. Perhaps it would be better to compare intracranial aneurysm repair with that elsewhere. Furthermore, no investigation has been undertaken to determine whether extravasated blood is resolved more rapidly or less rapidly from the subarachnoid space than is the case elsewhere.

Recurrent subarachnoid hemorrhage irrespective of etiology may result in hydro-

cephalus. Ruptured intracranial aneurysms and trauma cause a communicating hydrocephalus in a small proportion of cases.[75,76,127,210] The degree of ventricular dilatation, however, is only of medium severity. Bagley[15-17] was able to produce hydrocephalus in dogs by injecting autogenous blood into the cisterna magna and this was more readily achieved in young pups than in adult animals. The hemogenic meningitis with fibrosis is the underlying cause although the raised intracranial pressure may enhance the likelihood of hydrocephalus by reduction of the subarachnoid space. It has also been suggested that fibrosis and siderosis of arachnoid villi secondary to subarachnoid hemorrhage might contribute toward the development of hydrocephalus.[66] Furthermore, hydrocephalus occurring after subarachnoid hemorrhage may in part be the consequence of impaired fibrinolytic activity of the cerebrospinal fluid and the meninges.[169]

There have been investigations of the time required to clear the subarachnoid space of extravasated blood. Sprong[206] observed that in both man and the experimental animal (dog) the cerebrospinal fluid became clear within 5 to 6 days, though microscopically red cells were still present. This time interval remained constant despite numerous lumbar punctures and repeated drainage of cerebrospinal fluid. Sprong[206] concluded that therapeutic drainage was a futile means of hastening the disappearance of blood. After 48 hours he was never able to retrieve more than 2% of the red cells injected into the animals. Meredith,[150] using a more efficient means of recovering all the available cerebrospinal fluid, found that after $2\frac{1}{4}$ hours only 31.4% of the injected erythrocytes could be recovered by complete subarachnoid drainage, and after 48 hours only 4.5% or less was retrieved. Histologically, there are still large numbers of red cells present in the subarachnoid spaces at this time, and so presumably some red cells are enmeshed in the subarachnoid space, possibly adhering to one another and to the meninges. Hammes[94] however considered that the removal of blood by spinal drainage decreases the incidence of permanent meningeal scarring.

Simmonds[198] demonstrated that only a small fraction of the red cells injected into the subarachnoid space of rabbits as in man and dog could be recovered at 48 hours. By labeling the red cells prior to injection, he found that a fairly large proportion disappeared from the subarachnoid space and were not trapped locally to be phagocytosed.[199,200] They entered the bloodstream at the rate of about 1% per hour for the first 16 hours, but plasma proteins returned to the circulation almost completely within 24 hours.

The meninges have no intrinsic lymphatics although there are routes by which material may drain to the lymphatic system: (1) in the head, the most prominent site being about the olfactory nerve sheaths to the nasal mucosa and thence to the cervical duct and (2) in the neighborhood of the posterior nerve root ganglia to the thoracic duct. Approximately 5% of injected protein was recovered by Simmonds[200] from the cervical duct within the first 4½ hours, but a more direct pathway accounted for some 15%. Approximately 6% of injected red cells could be recovered from the cervical duct and a lesser number through the thoracic duct. Lymphatic ligation did not alter absorption of red cells, which must be considerably more direct. Phagocytosis and hemolysis of the red cells in the subarachnoid space were believed to account for relatively little of the red cell removal and it is possible that the more direct route could be via the arachnoid villi and granulations. One week after intracranial surgery in monkeys, Shabo and Maxwell[192] found red cells beneath the endothelium of the arachnoid villi. No evidence of red cell passage to the circulation was obtained, but arachnoidal cells appeared and phagocytosed "trapped" erythrocytes. Conflicting evidence, however, has come to hand. Adams and Prawirohardjo[3] found that in the dog, 25% of labeled red cells injected were absorbed

directly into the bloodstream and that the remaining 75% could be explained by their becoming enmeshed in the subarachnoid space and then being cleared by the arachnoidal reaction. However, Dupont and associates[63] concluded from their investigations in dogs that red cells and colloidal particles are phagocytosed within the subarachnoid space, whereas albumin is cleared rapidly by some different mechanism. In view of the rapidity of red cell clearance, it is difficult to believe that most erythrocytes are removed by phagocytosis within 48 hours unless there is a species difference.

A group of 62 patients with subarachnoid hemorrhage was investigated to determine the rate of clearance of blood from the cerebrospinal fluid.[224] The clearance time varied from 6 to 30 days, slow clearing being associated with (1) old age, though rapid clearance is still consistent with advanced years, (2) past or family history of diabetes or vascular disease, (3) permanent neurologic deficit, and (4) possibly the size of the spontaneous hemorrhage.

Arterial spasm in subarachnoid hemorrhage, particularly in association with aneurysmal rupture and also trauma, is dealt with in Chapter 9.

The cerebrospinal fluid

In a recent subarachnoid hemorrhage, cerebrospinal fluid varies from colorless to a deeply bloodstained fluid. The extravasated red cells are found only by microscopic examination or they are numerous up to 3,500,000 red cells per cu. mm. with an appropriate leukocyte count. Siderophages together with macrophages containing red cells may be present. The fluid may appear to be uniformly bloodstained at lumbar puncture in contradistinction to its appearance at a traumatic tap, but the fluid within the subarachnoid space as a whole is much less uniformly contaminated with red cells than with plasma proteins.[200] The fluid, however, does not clot. On rare occasions it may be colorless, but this is more likely to be the case soon after the hemorrhage, since blood presumably is temporarily confined to a localized subarachnoid or intracerebral hematoma before further extension leads to contamination of the spinal subarachnoid space. The pressure varies from about 100 to 700 mm. of water or above[151] and is generally considerably raised.

In association with the inflammatory response to the presence of blood in the subarachnoid space, an increased vascular permeability will ensue together with the emigration of leukocytes. This exudation will increase the intracranial pressure, thus contributing further to the increase produced by the hemorrhage. McQueen and Jelsma[147] observed an increase in cerebrospinal fluid in dogs after the experimental injection of blood and blood fractions into the subarachnoid space. The most intense reaction followed the injection of red cell ghosts, and there was a moderate increase with blood or infusions of hemoglobin that lasted less than 24 hours and was attributed to mechanical blockage in the subarachnoid space. The replacement of cerebrospinal fluid in sheep by an equal quantity of fresh, cooled, autogenous blood increased the cerebrospinal fluid pressure to 300 to 400 or more over a period of 2 to 3 days[209] although inadequate controls were studied to exclude the possibility of a thermal effect.

The cerebrospinal fluid may be thought to be xanthochromic when the red cells are increased but not sufficiently numerous for the fluid to be pink. Then with definite bloodstaining and after centrifugation 2 to 4 hours after the bleeding commences, the supernatant is faintly yellow (xanthochromia). This xanthochromia increases in depth during the first week, persists despite clearance of the red cells from the fluid, and ultimately fades within about 3 weeks unless there has been a recurrence of the hemorrhage.

The cerebrospinal fluid protein is generally raised and may exceed 1000 mg. per 100 ml. The colloidal gold curve exhibits a variable pattern. The sugar and chloride levels are within normal limits or re-

duced.[151] The hydrogen-ion concentration of the fluid is increased in what Froman and Smith[79] refer to as a primary metabolic acidosis of the cerebrospinal fluid. It is associated with an increase in lactate concentration and a fall in bicarbonate.

Initially, the leukocyte count is proportional to the contamination of fluid with blood, but after about 24 hours the leukocyte count increases in association with the leukocyte infiltration of the subarachnoid space (hemogenic meningitis). Polymorphonuclear leukocytes at first predominate, but at the end of the first week are replaced by lymphocytes (up to 25 per cu. mm.), which may persist in reduced number for several weeks. The glucose level in the fluid is reduced 6 to 8 days after a subarachnoid hemorrhage sufficient to lead to the suspicion of meningitis.[226]

Bloodstained cerebral spinal fluid caused by a subarachnoid hemorrhage usually does not pose problems of differentiation from a traumatic lumbar puncture, which may occur concurrently. The traumatic tap usually does not provide three consecutive samples of fluid exhibiting equal admixture of blood, but rather the fluid progressively clears if it is allowed to flow. The red cell count of the first and last samples should be similar if it is an authentic subarachnoid hemorrhage. The traumatic tap may yield blood that will clot, or alternatively the supernatant fluid should not be xanthochromic. However, an early subarachnoid hemorrhage does not produce xanthochromia, which can nevertheless occur in an accidental hemorrhage (traumatic tap) under three conditions.[146] If the contamination of cerebrospinal fluid is heavy, with the red cell count exceeding 150,000 to 200,000 per cu. mm., the faintest coloration of fluid may result and be interpreted as xanthochromia. If for any reason, such as recurrent leakage from an aneurysm, the protein content exceeds about 150 mg. per 100 ml. prior to contamination, the supernatant fluid may appear tinted. Contamination of the collecting vial with a hemolytic agent such as a detergent can cause hemolysis sufficient to be confused with xanthochromia.

Xanthochromia, or yellow coloration of the cerebrospinal fluid before or after centrifugation, is not always evidence of bleeding and the following are well known exceptions:

1. Yellow spinal fluid with a very high protein content below a spinal subarachnoid block[232] gives a negative benzidine test.[178]
2. Yellow-green color is frequently seen in tuberculous meningitis.[232]
3. Xanthochromia associated with a high protein content in the spinal fluid occurs in occasional cases of cerebral tumor.[24,232]
4. Jaundice.[24,181]
5. Carotene is present in the spinal fluid in carotenemia.[52]

Barrows and associates[24] analyzed samples of xanthochromic cerebrospinal fluid from patients with various diseases and found that oxyhemoglobin, bilirubin, and methemoglobin were the pigments responsible for the color. In those with blood in the subarachnoid space, oxyhemoglobin was present in the xanthochromic supernatant fluid within 2 hours of the onset of clinical symptoms of hemorrhage and progressed to a maximum within the first few days, subsequently declining. Bilirubin appeared 2 to 3 days after the onset, increased within the first week, and gradually disappeared in the second and third weeks. However, the authors found one exception. Bilirubin was found in one patient within 6 hours and it was believed that a significant amount of serum bilirubin was introduced into the fluid from the blood. Methemoglobin can be identified in the cerebrospinal fluid from patients with subdural and intracerebral hematomas, craniopharyngiomas, and fluids near encapsulated blood. The protein is elevated and bilirubin is the predominant pigment where there is obstruction to the flow of cerebrospinal fluid and in cystic fluids and subdural effusions. In jaundiced patients, bilirubin is the only detectable pigment.

Physical laboratory methods to detect change in the cerebrospinal fluid will doubtless be utilized to a greater extent in future management of patients with subarachnoid hemorrhage. Van Der Meulen[229] has suggested using the xanthochromic index in following and evaluating the course of intracranial or intraspinal hemorrhage. The index is dependent on spectrophotometric readings of the optical density at wavelengths of 415 $m\mu$ and 460 $m\mu$, thus taking into account the coloration of the cerebrospinal fluid by oxyhemoglobin, bilirubin, and protein. Barrows and associates[24] suggested utilization of the following simple biochemical tests to study xanthochromic fluid when spectrophotometric methods are unavailable:

1. Benzidine reaction is positive whenever the oxyhemoglobin can be demonstrated spectrophotometrically. There are no false positives and it is negative in cases of "traumatic tap."
2. Modified van den Bergh reaction is positive when bilirubin is present in amounts of 0.08 mg. per 100 ml., except when the color reaction is marked by oxyhemoglobin or methemoglobin.
3. Potassium cyanide test is a test for methemoglobin and is positive only when significant quantities are present in the fluid.

Vastola[231] demonstrated that the normal cerebrospinal fluid of patients (mean age of 64 years) exhibited some coloration, mild when compared with normal saline at a similar wavelength (420 $m\mu$) to that of xanthochromia. The optical density did not relate to the total protein content of the fluid. In 184 patients with neurological diseases (nonhemorrhagic), the cerebrospinal fluid was tested for xanthochromia and significant degrees were found in 14% but in not one case was there a negative van den Bergh reaction, which fact, Vastola[231] considers, excludes the likelihood of the pigmentation being caused by hemorrhage. He attributed the color to active destruction of nervous tissue. Crosby and Weiland[52] found several lipidlike substances capable of producing xanthrochromia in patients with destructive lesions of the brain and spinal cord, but they have not been postively identified.

Associated findings

Superficial siderosis of the central nervous system. The deposition of large quantities of iron pigment in the leptomeninges and the subpial and subependymal tissues of the brain and spinal cord constitutes a rare pathological entity referred to as superficial siderosis (or hemosiderosis) of the central nervous system,[109,126,223] *Randzonensiderose,* hemochromatosis,[157] hemochromatotic pigmentation,[132] *surcharge férrique du système nerveux central,* subpial cerebral siderosis,[142] and *hémosidérose marginale.*[123] The earliest report is that of Hamill,[96] though the pigment was thought to be melanin.

The patients exhibit a clinical picture characterized by chronic but progressive dementia, nerve deafness, and cerebellar ataxia with neurological abnormalities being attributed to the widespread incrustation of the central nervous system with iron pigment. The cerebrospinal fluid may be variously xanthochromic, bloodstained,[223] or perfectly clear.[123] In more than 50% of the cases reported in the literature, there is an actual or potential source of bleeding and such lesions include intracranial arterial aneurysms, Sturge-Weber disease,[109] "venous malformation," angioma of the spinal cord, subdural hematoma, and primary (ependymoma and oligodendroglioma) and secondary neoplasms of the brain and cord.[123,142,223] It is considered that the infiltration of iron pigment in this disease is caused by often-repeated or long-sustained leakage of blood into the subarachnoid space. Koeppen and Barron[123] have reviewed the histochemical features of the pigment. It has also been thought that the disease is in reality hemochromatosis of the central nervous system, hence the alternative title "hemochromatosis." However, the distribution of iron within the brain in authentic systemic hemochromatosis differs from that in superficial hemosiderosis of the cen-

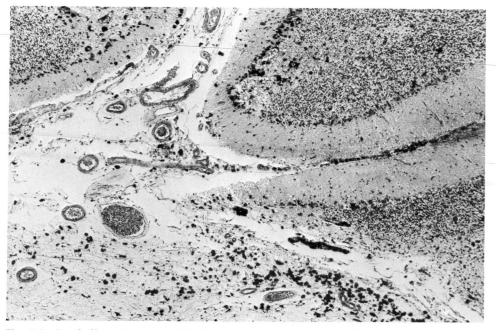

Fig. 7-3. Cerebellum in superficial siderosis showing numerous siderophages in subarachnoid space, which also exhibits some early fibrosis. Part of the cerebellar cortex has been completely destroyed; the remainder shows many siderophages, particularly in vicinity of Purkinje cell layer, though these cells themselves are widely destroyed. (Hematoxylin and eosin, ×45. From Koeppen, A. H. W., and Barron, K. D.: Superficial siderosis of the central nervous system, J. Neuropath. Exp. Neurol. **30**:448, 1971.)

tral nervous system.[141] In 18 cases of hemochromatosis, the only consistent change visible in the brain was pigmentation of the choroid plexuses particularly in the fourth ventricle. Coloration of the area postrema was also a general finding. Microscopically, hemosiderin was found in the choroid plexuses, the area postrema, the stalk and the posterior lobe of the pituitary, the adjacent tuberal part of the hypothalamus, the subfornical body, in siderophages that are in the perivascular spaces, and in the meninges and also the blood vessel walls of the lenticular and dentate nucleus. Consequently, the hemochromatosis theory is at present in disfavor.

On gross examination, the brain characteristically displays rusty brown pigmentation of the leptomeninges of the brain and cord, in particular over the base of the brain, the pons, medulla, and cerebellum. The meninges are thickened and the vessels more difficult to dissect. There is brown staining of the superficial layer (2 to 3 mm.) of the cerebral cortex and cord and in the subependyma.[223] The cerebellum is severely affected and may be reduced in size. The dura mater may disclose some pigmentation and the choroid plexus is usually unaffected.

Histologically, the leptomeninges are diffusely fibrosed and contain numerous siderophages (Fig. 7-3), though some pigment may appear to be free in the tissues.[123] In superficial layers of the brain and cord, siderophages are numerous in perivascular spaces and pigment has been observed in endothelium and in the media.[123] Hemosiderin is also present in the numerous and hypertrophied astrocytes within the cortex and considerably less is to be found in the subjacent white matter. Hyaline or ovoid bodies (Fig. 7-4) sometimes lie in the outer part of the cortex. They are round-to-oval well-defined granular bodies (15 to 50 μ in diameter) that are eosinophilic and often contain peripherally situated hemosiderin. Small quantities of fat may be demonstrable in these bodies on occasions. Although their origin is controversial, it has been postulated that they are degenerating macrophages,[223] neuroglia, and axons.[123] Numer-

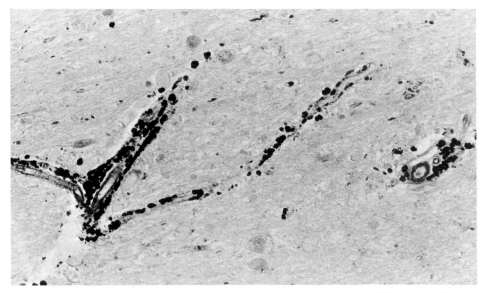

Fig. 7-4. Multiple ovoid bodies from a case of superficial siderosis. Note variation in size and staining intensity, and perivascular accumulation of siderophages. (Periodic acid—Schiff, ×110. From Koeppen, A. H. W., and Barron, K. D.: Superficial siderosis of the central nervous system, J. Neuropath. Exp. Neurol. **30:**448, 1971.)

ous in this disease, they are occasionally seen about old hemorrhagic softenings[223] or in regions of hemorrhage.[123]

In deeply pigmented areas in the cord and brain, degeneration of neurons and of glial cells is usually prominent. Neuronal loss in places may be extreme. Superficial demyelination occurs in the brain stem, spinal cord, and also the cranial nerves and nerve roots. The cerebellum is very severely damaged, with many convolutions virtually destroyed and exhibiting glial scars and demyelination of the underlying white matter.[132] Purkinje and granule cells are destroyed.

Although hydrocephalus of moderate degree has been observed[123,223] in this disease, in view of its chronicity and what is believed to be a chronic hemogenic meningitis, hydrocephalus might be expected to be a more prominent feature. Be that as it may, repeated experimental injections of blood, hemolyzed red cells, or iron preparations into the cisterna magna of dogs produce changes similar to the superficial hemosiderosis of the central nervous system of man even to the neuronal degeneration.[112] This evidence seems to be conclusive, and hence the current acceptance of the thesis that repeated or continuous bleeding of minor degree over prolonged intervals and the subsequent organization of the blood and diffusion of hemosiderin into the parenchyma with secondary changes will effect the clinical features of this disease.

Albuminuria and glycosuria. It has long been recognized that in patients with subarachnoid hemorrhage, albuminuria and glycosuria may be disclosed.[186,214,236,241] Experimentally, these signs may be caused by damage to the floor of the third ventricle. Walton[236] concluded that albuminuria and glycosuria suggest the presence of blood in the third ventricle but that the precise mechanism of their appearance is obscure. Buckell,[34] in a preliminary report of biochemical changes in patients with subarachnoid hemorrhage, reported that the blood sugar values were increased three times more in the comatose patients (45% were increased) than in the noncomatose subjects (15% increased), and particularly was this so among those patients with aneurysms of the middle cerebral artery. Otherwise, the author found that the biochemical changes indicated that dehydration was frequent in the comatose patient. In view of the possible serious significance of albuminuria and glycosuria, their presence should not be ignored, but renal disease and diabetes mellitus should be excluded.

Associated cardiac lesions. Gross abnormalities, simulating those of ischemic heart disease and even bundle-branch block,[207] may complicate cerebrovascular accidents, especially subarachnoid hemorrhage, and to a lesser degree intracerebral hemorrhage.[51,71] Fentz and Gormsen[71] found abnormal electrocardiographs in 15 (71%) 21 patients with intracranial hemorrhage. The abnormal electrocardiographic features return partly or wholly to normal except for a prolonged QTC interval, which frequently persists.[98] The cause of these changes is obscure. It has been suggested[51] that lesions of area 13 on the orbital surface of the frontal lobe might be responsible for the electrocardiographic changes because manipulation of the area induces multifocal ectopic beats in the electrocardiograph. Pool[168] found that manipulation of the circle of Willis in man induced arrhythmias and changes in the cardiac rate. Burch and associates[35] considered the changes were caused by "sympathetic storms," a result of the cerebral injury. One of their patients was found to have multiple areas of myocardial necrosis without demonstrable coronary occlusion. Koskelo and associates[125] found subendocardial hemorrhages in three cases of intracranial hemorrhage, and Connor[46] found myocytolysis in 8% of patients dying of intracranial lesions. The affected patients had died mostly from intracranial hemorrhage, though one succumbed to a cerebral infarct. However, cases have been reported with electrocardiographic abnormalities in association with subarachnoid hemorrhage but without myocardial damage[149,207] and vice versa.[87] Experimental intracerebral injection of blood in mice produces ultrastructural evidence of damage to the myocardial fibers similar to that of anoxia.[35] The probability undoubtedly exists that the changes are vasomotor effects, though the underlying mechanism remains uncertain. Greenhoot and Reichenbach[87] produced comparable lesions in cats by stimulating the midbrain reticular formation. They postulated that activation of sympathetic centers in the posterior diencephalon and upper midbrain results in sympathetic discharge with release of catecholamines from adrenergic endings in the heart and that these catecholamines cause myocardial necrosis. The pathogenesis may be similar to that underlying neurogenic peptic ulceration in association with subarachnoid hemorrhage. These cardiac lesions may be the source of a raised serum creatine kinase in patients with "stroke" and brain injuries.[46] Connor[47] has recently drawn attention to the importance of this neurogenic myocytolysis in donor hearts for cardiac transplantation, since it is thought that many of the donors have succumbed as the result of cerebrovascular accidents.

Miscellaneous. Subarachnoid hemorrhage is occasionally encountered with other diseases such as coarctation of the aorta[44,107] and polycystic disease of the kidneys.[236] In such cases, it is likely that hypertension with an aneurysm or primary intracerebral hemorrhage is responsible for the subarachnoid bleeding. Hypertension has been reported in as many as 66% of cases,[106] and in view of the age distribution of the patients and the frequency with which the bleeding is caused by a ruptured aneurysm or primary intracerebral hemorrhage, such a high incidence is not entirely unexpected. Then again, authors have been concerned with the familial incidence or the association with pregnancy or migraine. However, the incidence of these factors in such a heterogeneous group of cases seems to be of little consequence. Further analysis of possible related factors in cases of idiopathic subarachnoid hemorrhage is wanting.

Hemogenic meningitis or associated tissue damage has been held responsible for the presence of abnormalities in coagulation and fibrinolytic studies of patients with subarachnoid hemorrhage.[69]

Mortality and prognosis

In the Cooperative Study[136] of subarachnoid hemorrhage, after the exclusion of cases with aneurysms, arteriovenous aneurysms and angiomas, and also cases investigated by lumbar puncture alone, there were remaining 2092 cases studied by autopsy (14%), angiography (76%), or by both (10%). The overall mortality was 44% and of those reported dead when the study ceased, 76% had died within 6 weeks. However, the value of conclusions drawn from the perusal of such a miscellaneous group is extremely limited for the most frequent finding in the fatal cases was primary intracerebral hemorrhage, the inclusion of which was misleading as it only increased the mortality. In nonfatal cases, the most frequent diagnosis was merely subarachnoid hemorrhage of indeterminate cause, and it is this latter group that constitutes the clinical entity with the good prognosis.

Unlike intracranial arterial aneurysms, recurrence of the bleeding in subarachnoid hemorrhage in the absence of a demonstrable arterial lesion is not a particularly frequent complication.[5,62,221] Therefore, the initial hemorrhage is the serious consideration for those patients and, having survived this, they have a prognosis that becomes quite bright. The quality of survival is of no less importance. Walton[236] likened the sequelae of subarachnoid hemorrhage to those of severe head injury in regard to the incidence of epilepsy and mental symptoms.

The prognosis of subarachnoid hemorrhage is that of the underlying cause, be it aneurysm, neoplasm, blood dyscrasia, or infection. Odom and associates[158] found the mortality in their series of 316 cases of subarachnoid hemorrhage (Table 7-2) to be

100% for primary intracerebral hemorrhage and hypertensive cerebrovascular disease with arteriosclerosis, 90% for cerebral aneurysm, 33% for arteriovenous malformation and only 24% for the cases of unknown etiology. It is the idiopathic group that is the main concern here.

Walsh[234] in 461 cases of subarachnoid hemorrhage found no demonstrable cause in 124 (27%). Bilateral carotid angiography was performed in 93% of this group and vertebral angiography as well in 22 instances. In a follow-up for 1 to 11 years (average 3 years), only 15 had died (12.1%), six from aneurysmal hemorrhage, five from recurrent idiopathic subarachnoid hemorrhage, and four others from unrelated or unknown causes. Dunsmore and Polcyn[62] found a mortality of only 27% in a series of 71 patients with subarachnoid hemorrhage without angiographically demonstrable cause. Tappura[221] calculated that of his patients who survived the initial hemorrhage only 17% had a recurrence of the hemorrhage, 3% died, and the incidence of incapacitation among the final survivors was 33%. As in other series, the mortality and incidence of recurrent bleeding and of incapacitation was less than in the patients with a demonstrable aneurysm.[5,144,165] Of those who died, many died of cerebrovascular disease, including aneurysms, arteriovenous aneurysms, and intracerebral or subarachnoid hemorrhage. A prolonged follow-up including autopsy examination of the survivors is necessary, not only to disclose the prognosis but also the etiology.

Spinal subarachnoid hemorrhage

Subarachnoid hemorrhage originating in the spinal canal is a rare entity and is less widely recognized than its counterpart within the cranium. Clinical distinction between the two conditions is not always easy and no doubt some cases of spinal subarachnoid hemorrhage are occasionally overlooked when blood spreads to and infiltrates extensively the posterior cranial fossa. Characteristically, the patient complains of excruciating pain in the back or neck, often with a variable degree of radiation to the lower limbs and headache. Meningeal irritation perhaps with opisthotonos develops together with symptoms referable to sphincter control and very occasionally paraparesis or paraplegia may occur. The hemorrhage may be recurrent. Clinically, the features conveniently fall into the following groups: (1) the results of hemorrhage into the spinal subarachnoid space, (2) the results of intracranial extension of the hemorrhage, and (3) the results of damage to the spinal cord and nerve roots.

The onset of spinal subarachnoid hemorrhage may be entirely spontaneous or related to exertion or severe strain or bending of the back. Reported cases are too few at persent for any significant relationship with pregnancy or hypertension to have been determined. The causes of such hemorrhage are essentially similar to those of intracranial subarachnoid hemorrhage except that the incidence of cases associated with vascular degenerative changes is quite low. Many etiological factors are responsible.

Etiology

Arterial aneurysm. Examples of spinal subarachnoid hemorrhage of aneurysmal origin are rare because of the small caliber of the spinal arteries, the infrequency of degenerative changes, and consequently the low incidence of aneurysmal dilatation of spinal vessels. When coarctation of the aorta is present, the spinal arteries are comparatively enlarged and then aneurysms may occur.[187,247] Plotkin and associates[167] encountered a case of spinal subarachnoid hemorrhage in a 30-year-old man with coarctation of the aorta and a spinal block at the level of the sixth cervical vertebra. The exact cause of bleeding though not substantiated, could have been aneurysmal in origin. An additional nonfatal case in association with coarctation of the aorta was encountered by Watson,[237] but no aneurysm was demonstrated at laminectomy. Henson and Croft[102] encountered a bacterial aneurysm of a spinal artery in the lumbar sac in a baby with spina bifida and meningocele.

Arteriovenous aneurysms and hemangiomas. Arteriovenous aneurysms and related lesions, though not common, probably constitute the most frequent nontraumatic cause of spinal subarachnoid hemorrhage. The fragility of the vessels with or without some aneurysmal dilatation or varices makes them prone to bleeding[20,102,177,247] but hemorrhage is not the invariable complication. Henson and Croft[102] encountered bleeding in only two of their seven cases of spinal vascular malformations. The vessel not infrequently produce some local pressure symptoms and signs prior to the hemorrhage, and the occasional patient may have cutaneous hemangiomas over the trunk[102,228] involving the corresponding dermatome. The hemorrhage may cause extensive subarachnoid infiltration, and the cord is liable to be compressed by the hematoma locally, though there may be some direct damage and softening. Paraplegia is, therefore, not infrequent. Intraspinal angiomas may likewise bleed into the subarachnoid space, though the hemorrhage may be confined entirely to the cord itself. Henson and Croft[102] reported a case in which spinal subarachnoid hemorrhage from an angioma was thought to have been precipitated by an attack of herpes zoster. Clark[43] reported intramedullary and subarachnoid hemorrhage from an intramedullary cavernous hemangioma with calcification and in addition there was also aneurysmal dilatation of a vessel causing serious cord damage.

Cases of spinal subarachnoid hemorrhage caused by spinal telangiectasia have been reported by Walton[236] and Hieke.[104] Walton's patient[236] with hereditary telangiectasia suffered an intracranial hemorrhage some time before the onset of a spinal subarachnoid hemorrhage and paraplegia.

Polyarteritis nodosa. Polyarteritis nodosa rarely causes spinal subarachnoid hemorrhage, Russell[184] discussed one case, and Henson and Croft[102] reported a suspected case and two proved at autopsy.

Neoplasms. Subarachnoid hemorrhage may also arise from intradural spinal tumors.[1,179] The responsible neoplasms are of varying types, that is, meningioma,[155,179] neurospongioma,[179] neurofibroma,[72,91,171] ependymoma,[1,72,148,155] and a neuroglioma.[9] Prieto and Cantu[171] asserted that some 17 cases had been reported up to 1967 and, of these, five had an onset during some physical activity or after trauma. In the remaining 12 cases, the bleeding appeared to be spontaneous. Of the 17 tumors, there were nine ependymomas, five neurofibromas, and one each of meningoblastoma, neuroglioma, and neurospongioma.[171] Bhandari[26] told of a young girl of 3½ years who had a subarachnoid hemorrhage. At the age of 10 years, a complete spinal block caused by an astrocytoma was found and this was believed to be the source of the original bleeding. The age of most of these patients falls within the first four decades, and it is interesting that metastatic tumor and melanoma have not yet been incriminated in this type of hemorrhage.

Blood dyscrasias. Blood dyscrasias are usually listed among the causes of spinal subarachnoid hemorrhage,[235,236] although little attention has been paid to this complication in leukemia, hemophilia, hypoprothrombinemia, and the purpuras. As the source of bleeding is quite often difficult to determine, the hemorrhage, unless there is a localized hematoma, may often be mistaken for intracranial hemorrhage.

Anticoagulant therapy produces intracranial hemorrhage more frequently than bleeding into the spinal canal, but a few cases are on record of spinal subarachnoid hemorrhage.[61] Intraspinal hemorrhage with spinal cord damage occurring after lumbar puncture has been recorded.[166] A transient quadriplegia in a patient on excessive amounts of Dicumarol was described by Arieff and Pyzik.[10] Spastic paraplegia persisted after partial recovery but hemorrhage was not confirmed by operation. Cloward and Yuhl[45] reported extradural, subdural, and subarachnoid hemorrhage in a patient on anticoagulant therapy. Surgical intervention partially relieved the associated paraplegia. More recently a case of paraplegia due to spinal subarachnoid hemorrhage has been reported complicating anticoagulant therapy.[152] The clot was up to 1 cm. thick over the cord at laminectomy and the paraplegia persisted.

Trauma. Trauma accounts for spinal subarachnoid hemorrhage in the newborn as well as in the child and adult.[53] Trauma in these cases is usually a major feature of the presenting history. One unfortunate man of 63 years had a spinal anesthetic for cystoscopy. The lumbar puncture precipitated extensive spinal subarachnoid and subdural hemorrhage sufficient to cause paraplegia.[120] A few similar cases have been reported,[49,94] but despite the widespread use of this valuable technique, serious hemorrhage is exceptional. It is possible that an unusually large vein may be torn in such instances. Symptoms suffered by patients after a lumbar puncture could often be the result of a traumatic puncture.

Idiopathic spinal subarachnoid hemorrhage. These cases of spinal subarachnoid hemorrhage do not constitute a large group, but many are of unexplained etiology.[97,161,167,204] Hamby[93] referred to subarachnoid hemorrhage so caused by the rupture of a spinal artery but no mention of aneurysms was made and recurrent subarachnoid hemorrhage has been reported in association with typhoid fever.[59] One particularly unusual instance[139] was caused by endometriosis of the subarachnoid space at the level of the first and second lumbar roots. Radicular pain and repeated subarachnoid hemorrhages coincided with the menstrual period and symptoms were relieved by hormonal therapy.

Pathology

Spinal subarachnoid hemorrhage may be fairly mild and if the blood is well diluted, meningeal irritation and hemogenic meningitis will result. Irritation of the dorsal roots is common, resulting in pain particularly in the lower back and the legs.

The hemorrhage may be multifocal, especially in those caused by blood dyscrasias. A localized hematoma can occur, originating no doubt from brisk bleeding and clotting and thereafter causing spinal blockage and sometimes cord compression. In traumatic cases, bleeding is often found in an extradural or subdural position as well. The blood will be removed as in intracranial subarachnoid bleeding.

Though fatal cases have been reported,[108] spinal subarachnoid hemorrhage appears to be a rare cause of death, although the underlying disease or surgical interference may lead to a fatal outcome.

References

1. Abbott, K. H.: Subarachnoid hemorrhage from an ependymoma arising in the filum terminale, Bull. Los Angeles Neurol. Soc. **4:** 127, 1941.
2. Abbott, K. H., Rollas, Z. H., and Meagher, J. N.: Choroid plexus papilloma causing spontaneous subarachnoid hemorrhage, J. Neurosurg. **14:**566, 1957.
3. Adams, J. E., and Prawirohardjo, S.: Fate of red blood cells injected into cerebrospinal fluid pathways, Neurology **9:**561, 1959.
4. af Björkesten, G., and Halonen, V.: Incidence of intracranial vascular lesions in patients with subarachnoid hemorrhage investigated by four-vessel angiography, J. Neurosurg. **23:** 29, 1965.
5. af Björkesten, G., and Troupp, H.: Prognosis of subarachnoid hemorrhage, J. Neurosurg. **14:**434, 1957.
6. Alpers, B. J.: Cerebral birth injuries. In Brock, S.: Injuries of the brain and spinal cord and their coverings, ed. 3, Baltimore, 1949, The Williams & Wilkins Co., p. 229.
7. Alpers, B. J., and Forster, F. M.: The reparative processes in subarachnoid hemorrhage, J. Neuropath. Exp. Neurol. **4:**262, 1945.
8. Alpers, B. J., and Hughes, J.: Changes in the brain after electrically induced convulsions in cats, Arch. Neurol. Psychiat. **47:**385, 1942.
9. André-Thomas, Ferrand, Schaeffer, and de Martel: Syndrome d'hémorragie méningée réalisé par une tumeur de la queue de cheval, Paris Med. **20:**292, 1930.
10. Arieff, A. J., and Pyzik, S. W.: Paraplegia following excessive bishydroxycoumarin (Dicumarol) therapy, Arch. Neurol. Psychiat. **71:**517, 1954.
11. Askenasy, H. M., and Behmoaram, A. D.: Subarachnoid hemorrhage in meningiomas of the lateral ventricle, Neurology **10:**484, 1960.
12. Askenasy, H. M., Kosary, I. Z., and Braham, J.: Thrombosis of the longitudinal sinus, Neurology **12:**288, 1962.
13. Association for Research in Nervous and Men-

tal Diseases: Trauma of the central nervous system, Baltimore, 1945, The Williams & Wilkins Co., vol. 24.

14. Baer, S., Goldburgh, H. L., and Pearlstine, B.: Recurrent intracranial hemorrhages in a patient with hemophilia, J.A.M.A. **121**:933, 1943.

15. Bagley, C.: Blood in the cerebrospinal fluid: resultant functional and organic alterations in the central nervous system. A. Experimental data, Arch. Surg. **17**:18, 1928.

16. Bagley, C.: Blood in the cerebrospinal fluid: resultant functional and organic alterations in the central nervous system. B. Clinical data, Arch. Surg. **17**:39, 1928.

17. Bagley, C.: Spontaneous cerebral hemorrhage: discussion of four types, with surgical considerations, Arch. Neurol. Psychiat. **27**:1133, 1932.

18. Bailey, O. T.: The pathology of subarachnoid hemorrhage. In Fields, W. S.: Pathogenesis and treatment of cerebrovascular disease, Springfield, Ill., 1961, Charles C Thomas, Publisher, p. 398.

19. Baker, A. B., and Lufkin, N. H.: Cerebral lesions in hypoglycemia, Arch. Path. **23**:190, 1937.

20. Balck, C. A. J. A.: A case of angioma of the spinal cord, with recurrent haemorrhages, Brit. Med. J. **2**:1707, 1900.

21. Ballard, H. S., and Bondar, H.: Spontaneous subarachnoid hemorrhage in sickle cell anemia, Neurology **7**:443, 1957.

22. Barnett, H. J. M., and Hyland H. H.: Noninfective intracranial venous thrombosis, Brain **76**:36, 1953.

23. Barron, K. D., and Fergusson, G.: Intracranial hemorrhage as a complication of anticoagulant therapy, Neurology **9**:447, 1959.

24. Barrows, L. J., Hunter, F. T., and Banker, B. Q.: The nature and clinical significance of pigments in the cerebrospinal fluid, Brain **78**:59, 1955.

25. Belmusto, L., Regelsom, W., Owens, G., Hananian, J., and Nigogosyan, G.: Intracranial extracerebral hemorrhages in acute lymphocytic leukemia, Cancer, **17**:1079, 1964.

26. Bhandari, Y. S.: Subarachnoid hemorrhage due to cervical cord tumor in a child, J. Neurosurg. **30**:749, 1969.

27. Boon, T. H., and Walton, J. N.: Aplastic anaemia, Quart. J. Med. **20**:75, 1951.

28. Bouquet, H.: Hémorragie méningée curable chez un enfant, Prov. Med. Paris **19**:398, 1908.

29. Brandt, S.: Alterations leucémiques du système nerveux, Acta Psychiat. Neurol. **20**:107, 1945.

30. Brock, S.: Injuries of the brain and spinal cord and their coverings, ed. 3, Baltimore, 1949, The Williams & Wilkins Co.

31. Brodie, G. N., Bliss, D., and Firkin, B. G.: Thrombocytopenia and carcinoma, Brit. Med. J. **1**:540, 1970.

32. Broughan, M., Heusner, A. P., and Adams, R. D.: Acute degenerative changes in adenomas of the pituitary body—with special refer-

ence to pituitary apoplexy, J. Neurosurg. **7**:421, 1950.

33. Buchanan, D. S., and Brazinsky, J. H.: Dural sinus and cerebral venous thrombosis, Arch. Neurol. **22**:440, 1970.

34. Buckell, M.: Biochemical changes after spontaneous subarachnoid haemorrhage, J. Neurol. Neurosurg. Psychiat. **29**:291, 1966.

35. Burch, G. E., Sohal, R. S., Sun, S. C., and Colcolough, H. L.: Effects of experimental intracranial hemorrhage on the ultrastructure of the myocardium in mice, Amer. Heart J. **77**:427, 1969.

36. Burges, R. C. L.: Subarachnoid haemorrhage as the first effect of a cerebral tumor, Brit. Med. J. **2**:887, 1926.

37. Cammermeyer, J.: Agonal nature of the cerebral ring hemorrhages, Arch. Neurol. Psychiat. **70**:54, 1953.

38. Cannell, D. E., and Botterell, E. H.: Subarachnoid hemorrhage and pregnancy, Amer. J. Obstet. Gynec. **72**:844, 1956.

39. Chalgren, W. S.: Neurologic complications of the hemorrhagic diseases, Neurology **3**:126, 1953.

40. Chapman, J. S.: The reaction of serous cavities to blood, J. Lab. Clin. Med. **46**:48, 1955.

41. Chason, J. L.: Brain, meninges and spinal cord. In Saphir, O: A text on systemic pathology, New York, 1959, Grune & Stratton, Inc., vol. 2, p. 1798.

42. Cheatham, M. L., and Brackett, C. E.: Problems in management of subarachnoid hemorrhage in sickle cell anemia, J. Neurosurg. **23**:488, 1965.

43. Clark, J. M. P.: Traumatic haematomyelia from rupture of intramedullary angioma, J. Bone Joint Surg. **36(B)**:418, 1954.

44. Cleland, W. P., Counihan, T. B., Goodwin, J. F., and Steiner, R. E.: Coarctation of the aorta, Brit. Med. J. **2**:379, 1956.

45. Cloward, R. B., and Yuhl, E. T.: Spontaneous intraspinal hemorrhage and paraplegia complicating Dicumarol therapy, Neurology **5**:600, 1955.

46. Connor, R. C. R.: Heart damage associated with intracranial lesions, Brit. Med. J. **3**:29, 1968.

47. Connor, R. C. R.: Myocardial damage secondary to brain lesions, Amer. Heart J. **78**:145, 1969.

48. Cook, W. C.: A case of sickle cell anemia with associated subarachnoid hemorrhage, J. Med. **11**:541, 1930.

49. Courtin, R. F.: Some practical aspects of lumbar puncture, Postgrad. Med. **12**:157, 1952.

50. Courville, C. B.: Pathology of the central nervous system, ed. 3, Mountain View, Calif., 1950, Pacific Press Publishing Association.

51. Cropp, G. J., and Manning, G. W.: Electrocardiographic changes simulating myocardial ischemia and infarction associated with spontaneous intracranial hemorrhage, Circulation **22**:25, 1960.

52. Crosby, R. M. N., and Weiland, G. L.: Xanthrochromia of the cerebrospinal fluid.

II. Preliminary description of several new colored substances, Arch. Neurol. Psychiat. 69:732, 1953.

53. Davison, C.: Pathology of the spinal cord as a result of trauma. In: Trauma of the central nervous system, Ass. Res. Nerv. Ment. Dis. 24:151, 1945.

54. Dekaban, A., and McEachern, D.: Subarachnoid hemorrhage, intracerebral hemorrhage, and intracranial aneurysms, Arch. Neurol. Psychiat. 67:641, 1952.

55. De Saussure, R. L., Scheibert, C. D., and Hazouri, L. A.: Astrocytoma grade III associated with profuse subarachnoid bleeding as its first manifestation, J. Neurosurg. 8:236, 1951.

56. Dewar, H. A., and Walmsley, R.: Relapsing fever with nephritis and subarachnoid haemorrhage, Lancet 2:630, 1945.

57. Diaz-Rivera, R. S., and Miller, A. J.: Periarteritis nodosa: a clinicopathological analysis of seven cases, Ann. Intern. Med. 24:420, 1946.

58. Dickinson, L.: Spontaneous thrombosis of the cerebral veins and sinuses in chlorosis, Trans. Clin. Soc. 29:63, 1896.

59. Douglas-Wilson, H., Miller, S., and Watson, G. W.: Spontaneous subarachnoid haemorrhage of intraspinal origin, Brit. Med. J. 1:554, 1933.

60. Drury, M. I., Hickey, M. D., and Malone, J. P.: A case of polyarteritis nodosa treated with cortisone, Brit. Med. J. 2:1487, 1951.

61. Duff, I. F., and Shull, W. H.: Fatal hemorrhage in Dicumarol poisoning, J.A.M.A. 139:762, 1949.

62. Dunsmore, R. H., and Polcyn, J. L.: Subarachnoid hemorrhage: prognostic factors, J. Neurosurg. 13:165, 1956.

63. Dupont, J.-R., Van Wart, C. A., and Kraintz, L.: The clearance of major components of whole blood from cerebrospinal fluid following simulated subarachnoid hemorrhage, J. Neuropath. Exp. Neurol. 20:450, 1961.

64. Easby, M. H.: A case of rheumatic heart disease with subarachnoid hemorrhage, Med. Clin. N. Amer. 18:307, 1934.

65. Echols, D. H., and Rehfeldt, F. C.: Profuse subarachnoid hemorrhage caused by cerebral glioma, J. Neurosurg. 7:280, 1950.

66. Ellington, E., and Margolis, G.: Block of arachnoid villus by subarachnoid hemorrhage, J. Neurosurg. 30:651, 1969.

67. Ernsting, J.: Choroid plexus papilloma causing spontaneous subarachnoid haemorrhage, J. Neurol. Neurosurg. Psychiat. 18:134, 1955.

68. Essick, C. R.: Formation of macrophages by the cells lining the subarachnoid cavity in response to the stimulus of particulate matter, Contrib. Embryol. Carnegie Inst. (No. 42) 9:377, 1920.

69. Ettinger, M. G.: Coagulation abnormalities in subarachnoid hemorrhage, Stroke 1:139, 1970.

70. Falconer, M. A.: Surgical pathology of spontaneous intracranial haemorrhage due to aneurysms and arteriovenous malformations, Proc. Roy. Soc. Med. 47:693, 1954.

71. Fentz, V., and Gormsen, J.: Electrocardiographic patterns in patients with cerebrovascular accidents, Circulation 25:22, 1962.

72. Fincher, E. F.: Spontaneous subarachnoid hemorrhage in intradural tumors of the lumbar sac, J. Neurosurg. 8:576, 1951.

73. Finlayson, A. I., and Penfield, W.: Acute postoperative aseptic leptomeningitis, Arch. Neurol. Psychiat. 46:250, 1941.

74. Flexner, M., and Schneider, B.: Subarachnoid hemorrhage following injection of epinephrine, Ann. Intern. Med. 12:876, 1938.

75. Foltz, E. L., and Ward, A. A.: Communicating hydrocephalus from subarachnoid bleeding, J. Neurosurg. 13:546, 1956.

76. Fox, J. L., and Luessenhop, A. J.: Hydrocephalus secondary to hemorrhage from a basilar artery aneurysm. With a note on embolization technique, Acta Neurochir. 17:228, 1967.

77. Freed, H., and Wofford, C. W.: Subarachnoid hemorrhage during shock therapy for schizophrenia, Arch. Neurol. Psychiat. 39:813, 1938.

78. Freireich, E. J., Thomas, L. B., Frei, E., Fritz, R. D., and Forkner, C. E.: A distinctive type of intracerebral hemorrhage associated with "blastic crisis" in patients with leukemia, Cancer 13:146, 1960.

79. Froman, C., and Smith, A. C.: Metabolic acidosis of the cerebrospinal fluid associated with subarachnoid haemorrhage, Lancet 1:965, 1967.

80. Gairdner, D.: Schönlein-Henoch syndrome (anaphylactoid purpura), Quart. J. Med. 17:95, 1948.

81. Garin, C., Plauchu, M., and Masson: Nævocarcinome de la joue avec métastases cérébrales se traduisant par un tableau d'hémorragie méningée à allure paroxystique, Lyon Med. 149:803, 1932.

82. Gillies, S.: A case of cerebral aneurysm simulating meningitis, Med. J. Aust. 2:37, 1923.

83. Glass, B., and Abbott, K. H.: Subarachnoid hemorrhage consequent to intracranial tumors, Arch. Neurol. Psychiat. 73:369, 1955.

84. Globus, J. H., and Sapirstein, M.: Massive hemorrhage into brain tumor, J.A.M.A. 120:348, 1942.

85. Goldzieher, J. W., and Lisa, J. R.: Gross cerebral hemorrhage and vascular lesions in acute tuberculous meningitis and meningoencephalitis, Amer. J. Path. 23:133, 1947.

86. Graves, G. W., and Fleiss, M. M.: Neoplasm of the choroid plexus, Amer. J. Dis. Child. 47:97, 1934.

87. Greenhoot, J. H., and Reichenbach, D. D.: Cardiac injury and subarachnoid hemorrhage, J. Neurosurg. 30:521, 1969.

88. Greer, M., and Schotland, D.: Abnormal hemoglobin as a cause of neurologic disease, Neurology 12:114, 1962.

89. Groch, S. N., Hurwitz, L. J., McDevitt, E., and Wright, I. S.: Problems of anticoagulant

therapy in cerebrovascular disease, Neurology **9**:786, 1959.

90. Gurdjian, E. S., and Webster, J. E.: Experimental and clinical studies on the mechanism of head injury. In: Trauma of the central nervous system, Ass. Res. Nerv. Ment. Dis. **24**:48, 1945.

91. Halpern, L., Feldman, S., and Peyser, E.: Subarachnoid hemorrhage with papilledema due to spinal neurofibroma, Arch. Neurol. Psychiat. **79**:138, 1958.

92. Ham, A. W.: Histology, ed. 3, London, 1957, J. B. Lippincott Co.

93. Hamby, W. B.: Spontaneous subarachnoid hemorrhage of aneurysmal origin, J.A.M.A. **136**:522, 1948.

94. Hammes, E. M.: Hemorrhage in the cauda secondary to lumbar puncture, Arch. Neurol. Psychiat. **3**:595, 1920.

95. Hammes, E. M.: Reaction of the meninges to blood, Arch. Neurol. Psychiat. **52**:505, 1944.

96. Hamill, R. C.: Report of a case of melanosis of the brain, cord, and meninges, J. Nerv. Ment. Dis. **35**:594, 1908.

97. Harris, W.: Two cases of spontaneous hematorrhachis, or intrameningeal spinal haemorrhage—one cured by laminectomy, Proc. Roy. Soc. Med. (Neurol. Sect.) **5**:115, 1911-1912.

98. Harrison, M. T., and Gibb, B. H.: Electrocardiographic changes associated with a cerebrovascular accident, Lancet **2**:429, 1964.

99. Heilbrunn, G., and Weil, A.: Pathological changes in the central nervous system in experimental electric shock, Arch. Neurol. Psychiat. **47**:918, 1942.

100. Hektoen, L.: The vascular changes of tuberculous meningitis, especially the tuberculous endarteritis, J. Exp. Med. **1**:112, 1896.

101. Helpern, M., and Rabson, S. M.: Sudden and unexpected natural death. III. Spontaneous subarachnoid hemorrhage, Amer. J. Med. Sci. **220**:262, 1950.

102. Henson, R. A., and Croft, P. B.: Spontaneous spinal subarachnoid haemorrhage, Quart. J. Med. **25**:53, 1956.

103. Hickey, M., Coakley, J. B., Drury, M. I., and Moore, H.: Subarachnoid haemorrhage during cortisone therapy, Irish J. Med. Sci. **6**:284, 1953.

104. Hieke, L.: Über Hämatomyelie bei intramedullären Teleangiektasien, Beitr. Path. Anat. **110**:433, 1949.

105. Hiller, F.: Cerebral hemorrhage in hyperergic angiitis, J. Neuropath. Exp. Neurol. **12**:24, 1953.

106. Hirschfield, B. A., Tornay, A. S., and Yaskin, J. C.: Spontaneous subarachnoid hemorrhage: an analysis of fifty cases, Arch. Neurol. Psychiat. **49**:483, 1943.

107. Hodes, H. L., Steinfeld, L., and Blumenthal, S.: Congenital cerebral aneurysms and coarctation of the aorta, Arch. Pediat. **76**:28, 1959.

108. Huber, J., and de Massary, J.: Un cas d'hémorrhagie méningée d'origine spinale, Bull. Soc. Med. Hop. Paris, Series B **47**:916, 1923.

109. Hughes, J. T., and Oppenheimer, D. R.: Superficial siderosis of the central nervous system, Acta Neuropath. **13**:56, 1969.

110. Huskisson, E. C., and Hart, F. D.: Fulminating meningococcal septicaemia presenting with subarachnoid haemorrhage, Brit. Med. J. **1**: 231, 1969.

111. Ikkala, E.: Haemophilia: a study of its laboratory, clinical, genetic and social aspects based on known haemophiliacs in Finland, Scand. J. Clin. Lab. Invest. **12** (Suppl. 46): 1, 1960.

112. Iwanowski, L., and Olszewski, J.: The effects of subarachnoid injections of iron-containing substances on the central nervous system, J. Neuropath. Exp. Neurol. **19**:433, 1960.

113. Jackson, I. J.: Aseptic hemogenic meningitis: an experimental study of aseptic meningeal reactions due to blood and its breakdown products, Arch. Neurol. Psychiat. **62**:572, 1949.

114. Johnson, D. R., and Chalgren, W. S.: Polycythemia vera and the nervous system, Neurology **1**:53, 1951.

115. Kalbag, R. M.: Recurrent subarachnoid haemorrhage from paraventricular lesions with normal angiography, J. Neurol Neurosurg. Psychiat. **27**:435, 1964.

116. Kendall, D.: Thrombosis of intracranial veins, Brain **71**:386, 1948.

117. Kernohan, J. W., and Woltman, H. W.: Postoperative, focal, nonseptic, necrosis of vertebral and cerebellar arteries, J.A.M.A. **112**:1173, 1943.

118. Kerr, C. B.: Intracranial haemorrhage in haemophilia, J. Neurol. Neurosurg. Psychiat. **27**: 166, 1964.

119. King, L. S., and Butcher, J.: Osteochondroma of the base of the skull, Arch. Path. **37**:282, 1944.

120. King, O. J., and Glas, W. W.: Spinal subarachnoid hemorrhage following lumbar puncture, Arch Surg. **80**:574, 1960.

121. Kirshbaum, J. D., and Chapman, B. M.: Subarachnoid haemorrhage secondary to a tumor of the hypophysis with acromegaly, Ann. Intern. Med. **29**:536, 1948.

122. Klein, I. J., and Lederer, M.: Lateral sinus thrombosis complicating masked mastoiditis: report of a case with secondary subarachnoid hemorrhage, Amer. J. Dis. Child. **40**:1045, 1930.

123. Koeppen, A. H. W., and Barron, K. D.: Superficial siderosis of the central nervous system. A histological, histochemical and chemical study, J. Neuropath. Exp. Neurol. **30**:448, 1971.

124. Kolar, O., and Zeman, W.: Spinal fluid cytomorphology. Arch. Neurol. **18**:44, 1968.

125. Koskelo, P., Punsar, S., and Sipila, W.: Subendocardial haemorrhage and E.C.G. changes in intracranial bleeding, Brit. Med. J. **1**:1479, 1964.

126. Kott, E., Bechar, M., Bornstein, B., Askenasy, H. M., and Sandbank, U.: Superficial hemosiderosis of the central nervous system, Acta Neurochir. **14**:287, 1966.

127. Krayenbühl, H., and Lüthy, F.: Hydrozephalus als Spätfolge geplatzter basaler Hirnaneu-

rysmen, Schweiz. Arch. Neurol. Psychiat. **61:** 7, 1948.

128. Kurtzke, J. F.: Epidemiology of cerebrovascular disease, Berlin, 1969, Springer-Verlag.

129. Lawrence, R. D., Meyer, A., and Nevin, S.: The pathological changes in the brain in fatal hypoglycaemia, Quart. J. Med. **11:**181, 1942.

130. Leidler, F., and Russell, W. O.: The brain in leukemia, Arch. Path. **40:**14, 1945.

131. Levy, L. F.: Subarachnoid haemorrhage without arteriographic vascular abnormality, J. Neurosurg. **17:**252, 1960.

132. Lewey, F. H., and Govons, S. R.: Hemochromatotic pigmentation of the central nervous system, J. Neuropath. Exp. Neurol. **1:**129, 1942.

133. Lewis, I. C., and Philpott, M. G.: Neurological complications in the Schönlein-Henoch syndrome, Arch. Dis. Child. **31:**369, 1956.

134. List, C. F., Williams, J. R., and Balyeat, G. W.: Vascular lesions in pituitary adenomas, J. Neurosurg. **9:**177, 1952.

135. Locksley, H. B.: Report on the cooperative study of intracranial aneurysms and subarachnoid hemorrhage. Section V, Part I. Natural history of subarachnoid hemorrhage, intracranial aneurysms, and arteriovenous malformations, J. Neurosurg **25:**219, 1966.

136. Locksley, H. B., Sahs, A. L., and Sandler, R.: Report on the cooperative study of intracranial aneurysms and subarachnoid hemorrhage. Section III. Subarachnoid hemorrhage unrelated to intracranial aneurysm and A-V malformation, J. Neurosurg. **24:**1034, 1966.

137. Loewenberg, P. C.: Die Gehirnmetastasen der Melanome, Thesis, Berlin, 1939. Cited by Walton.[235]

138. Logothetis, J., Silverstein, P., and Coe, J.: Neurologic aspects of Waldenström's macroglobulinemia, Arch. Neurol. **3:**564, 1960.

139. Lombardo, L., Mateos, J. H., and Barroeta, F. F.: Subarachnoid hemorrhage due to endometriosis of the spinal canal, Neurology **18:** 423, 1968.

140. Madonick, M. J., and Savitsky, N.: Subarachnoid hemorrhage in melanoma of the brain, Arch. Neurol. Psychiat. **65:**628, 1951.

141. McDougal, D. B., and Adams, R. D.: The neuropathological changes in hemochromatosis, J. Neuropath. Exp. Neurol. **9:**117, 1950.

142. McGee, D. A., Van Patter, H. J., Morotta, J., and Olszewski, J.: Subpial cerebral siderosis, Neurology **12:**108, 1962.

143. McKee, E. E.: Mycotic infection of brain with arteritis and subarachnoid hemorrhage: report of a case, Amer. J. Clin. Path. **20:**381, 1950.

144. McKissock, W., Paine, K., and Walsh, L.: Further observations on subarachnoid haemorrhage, J. Neurol. Neurosurg. Psychiat. **21:**239, 1958.

145. McKissock, W., and Paine, K. W. E.: Subarachnoid haemorrhage, Brain **82:**356, 1959.

146. McMenemey, W. H.: The significance of subarachnoid bleeding, Proc. Roy. Soc. Med. **47:** 701, 1954.

147. McQueen, J. D., and Jelsma, L. F.: Intra-

148. Mendelsohn, R. A., and Mora, F.: Spontaneous subarachnoid hemorrhage caused by ependymoma of filum terminale, J. Neurosurg. **15:**460, 1958.

149. Menon, I. S.: Electrocardiographic changes simulating myocardial infarction in cerebrovascular accident, Lancet **2:**433, 1964.

150. Meredith, J. M.: The inefficiency of lumbar puncture for the removal of red blood cells from the cerebrospinal fluid, Surgery **9:**524, 1941.

151. Merritt, H. H., and Fremont-Smith F.: The cerebrospinal fluid, Philadelphia, 1938, W. B. Saunders Co.

152. Middleton, G. D., and Edwards D. H.: A case of spinal subarachnoid haemorrhage complicating anticoagulant therapy, Brit. J. Clin. Pract. **19:**414, 1965.

153. Miller, H.: Clinical consideration of cerebrovascular disorders occurring during the course of general diseases of an inflammatory or allergic nature, Proc. Roy. Soc. Med. **44:**852, 1951.

154. Moore, E. W., Thomas, L. B., Shaw, R. K., and Freireich, E. J.: The central nervous system in acute leukemia, Arch. Intern. Med. **105:**451, 1960.

155. Nassar, S. I., and Correll, J. W.: Subarachnoid hemorrhage due to spinal cord tumors, Neurology **18:**87, 1968.

156. Nathanson, M., Robins, A. L., and Green, M. A.: Blood in the subarachnoid space: a clinical evaluation of its occurrence in 190 consecutive cases, Neurology **3:**721, 1953.

157. Neumann, M. A.: Hemochromatosis of the central nervous system, J. Neuropath. Exp. Neurol. **7:**19, 1948.

158. Odom, G. L., Bloor, B. M., Golden, J. B., and Woodhall, B.: Acute subarachnoid hemorrhage: etiology and mortality, N. Carolina Med. J. **13:**624, 1952.

159. Ohler, W. R., and Hurwitz, D.: Spontaneous subarachnoid hemorrhage, J.A.M.A. **98:**1856, 1932.

160. Oldberg, E.: Hemorrhage into gliomas: a review of eight hundred and thirty-two consecutive verified cases of glioma, Arch. Neurol. Psychiat. **30:**1061, 1933.

161. Olsen, C. W.: Spinal meningeal hemorrhage, Bull. Los Angeles Neurol. Soc. **6:**139, 1941.

162. Pakarinen, S.: Incidence, aetiology, and prognosis of primary subarachnoid haemorrhage, Acta Neurol. Scand. **43:**Suppl. 29, 1967.

163. Pedersen, A. L.: Fatal case of subarachnoid hemorrhage under insulin-Cardiazol treatment of a psychotic patient, Acta Psychiat. Neurol. Scand. **19:**483, 1944.

164. Pedigo, G. W., and Nolan, D. E.: Subarachnoid hemorrhage, complicating hemorrhagic nephritis, Ohio State Med. J. **43:**743, 1947.

165. Petty, P. G.: Subarachnoid haemorrhage of undetermined aetiology, Med. J. Aust. **2:**1, 1966.

166. Phelps, E. T.: The dangers of Dicumarol therapy, Med. Clin. N. Amer. 34:1791, 1950.

167. Plotkin, R., Ronthal, M., and Froman, C.: Spontaneous spinal subarachnoid haemorrhage, J. Neurosurg. 25:443, 1966.

168. Pool, J. L.: Vasocardiac effects of the circle of Willis, Arch. Neurol. Psychiat. 78:355, 1957.

169. Porter, J. M., Acinapura, A. J., Kapp, J. P., and Silver, D.: Fibrinolysis in the central nervous system, Neurology 19:47, 1969.

170. Potter, E. L.: Pathology of the fetus and infant, ed. 2, Chicago, 1961, Year Book Medical Publishers Inc.

171. Prieto, A., and Cantu, R. C.: Spinal subarachnoid hemorrhage associated with neurofibroma of the cauda equina, J. Neurosurg. 27:63, 1967.

172. Quickel, K. E., and Whaley, R. J.: Subarachnoid hemorrhage in a patient with hereditary hemorrhagic telangiectasia, Neurology 17:716, 1967.

173. Rich, A. R., and McCordock, H. A.: The pathogenesis of tuberculous meningitis, Johns Hopkins Hosp. Bull. 52:5, 1933.

174. Richardson, A.: Subarachnoid haemorrhage, Brit. Med. J. 4:89, 1969.

175. Roback, H. N., and Miller, C. W.: Subarachnoid and intracranial hemorrhages due to Metrazol, Arch. Neurol. Psychiat. 44:627, 1940.

176. Roberts, M. H.: The spinal fluid in the newborn with special reference to intracranial hemorrhage, J.A.M.A. 85:500, 1925.

177. Robertson, E. G.: A case of arterial angioma of the spinal cord, Med. J. Aust. 2:384, 1938.

178. Robinson, F. H., and Miller, B. N.: On the differentiation of colored cerebrospinal fluids, Amer. J. Med. Sci. 191:538, 1936.

179. Roger, H., Paillas, J. E., and Duplay, J.: Hémorragie méningée spino-cérébrale révélatrice d'une tumeur de la queue de chevel chez deux jeunes sujets, Bull. Soc. Med. Hop. Paris 45:37, 1949.

180. Rogers, L.: Fevers in the tropics, ed. 2, London, 1910, Oxford Medical Publication.

181. Rosenberg, D. G., and Galambos, J. T.: Yellow spinal fluid, Amer. J. Dig. Dis. 5:32, 1960.

182. Russek, H. I., and Zohman, B. L.: Anticoagulant therapy in acute myocardial infarction, Amer. J. Med. Sci. 225:8, 1953.

183. Russel, C. K., and Kershman, J.: Spontaneous subarachnoid haemorrhage and brain tumor, Canad. Med. Ass. J. 36:568, 1937.

184. Russell, D. S.: The pathology of spontaneous intracranial haemorrhage, Proc. Roy. Soc. Med. 47:689, 1954.

185. Sands, I. J.: Subarachnoid hemorrhage as a clinical complication of neurosyphilis, Arch. Neurol. Psychiat. 24:85, 1930.

186. Sands, I. J.: Diagnosis and management of subarachnoid hemorrhage, Arch. Neurol. Psychiat. 46:973, 1941.

187. Sargent, P.: Haemangeioma of the pia mater causing compression paraplegia, Brain 48:259, 1925.

188. Schemm, G. W., Bentley, J. P., and Doerfler, M.: Wound healing in the subarachnoid space, Neurology 18:862, 1968.

189. Schnitker, M. T., and Ayer, D.: The primary melanomas of the leptomeninges, J. Nerv. Ment. Dis. 87:45, 1938.

190. Schonfield, W. A.: Renal calculi in an infant complicated by perinephritic abscess and subarachnoid hemorrhage, Amer. J. Dis. Child. 50: 686, 1935.

191. Seal, R. M. E., and Millard, A. H.: A case of chorionepithelioma presenting with subarachnoid haemorrhage, J. Obstet. Gynec. Brit. Emp. 62:932, 1955.

192. Shabo, A. L., and Maxwell, D. S.: Electron microscopic observations on the fate of particulate matter in the cerebrospinal fluid, J. Neurosurg. 29:464, 1968.

193. Sharpe, F. A.: Subarachnoid haemorrhage probably due to rheumatic infection, Brit. Med. J. 2:582, 1929.

194. Sharpe, W., and Maclaire, A. S.: Intracranial hemorrhage in the newborn, Amer. J. Obstet. Gynec. 9:452, 1925.

195. Sharpe, W., and Maclaire, A. S.: Further observations of intracranial haemorrhage in the newborn, Surg. Gynec. Obstet. 41:583, 1925.

196. Sicuteri, F., Fanciullacci, M., Bavazzano, A., Franchi, G., and Del Bianco, P. L.: Kinins and intracranial hemorrhages, Angiology 21: 193, 1970.

197. Silverstein, A.: Intracranial bleeding in hemophilia, Arch. Neurol. 3:141, 1960.

198. Simmonds, W. J.: The absorption of blood from the cerebrospinal fluid in animals, Aust. J. Exp. Biol. 300:261, 1952.

199. Simmonds, W. J.: The absorption of labelled erythrocytes from the subarachnoid space in rabbits, Aust. J. Exp. Biol. 31:77, 1953.

200. Simmonds, W. J.: The subarachnoid space: some experimental approaches to its pathology, Med. J. Aust. 2:452, 1953.

201. Simonsen, J.: Fatal subarachnoid haemorrhage originating in an intracranial chordoma, Acta Path. Microbiol. Scand. 59:13, 1963.

202. Simpson, D. A., and Robson, H. N.: Intracranial haemorrhage in disorders of blood coagulation, Aust. New Zeal. J. Surg. 29:287, 1959-1960.

203. Singer, R. P., and Schneider, R. C.: The successful management of intracerebral and subarachnoid hemorrhage in a hemophilic infant, Neurology 12:293, 1962.

204. Slavin, H. B.: Spontaneous intraspinal subarachnoid hemorrhage, J. Nerv. Ment. Dis. 86:425, 1937.

205. Spatz, E. L., and Bull, J. W. D.: Vertebral arteriography in the study of subarachnoid hemorrhage, J. Neurosurg. 14:543, 1957.

206. Sprong, W.: The disappearance of blood from the cerebrospinal fluid in traumatic subarachnoid hemorrhage, Surg. Gynec. Obstet. 58: 705, 1934.

207. Srivastava, S. C., and Robson, A. O.: Electrocardiographic abnormalities associated with subarachnoid haemorrhage, Lancet 2:431, 1964.

208. Starrs, R. A.: Subacute bacterial endocarditis presenting as subarachnoid haemorrhage (re-

port of a case with recovery), Ann. Intern. Med. **31**:139, 1949.

209. Stehbens, W. E.: Unpublished observations, 1954.

210. Stehbens, W. E.: Aneurysms and anatomical variation of cerebral arteries, Arch. Path. **75**: 45, 1963.

211. Stehbens, W. E.: Atypical cerebral aneurysms, Med. J. Aust. **1**:765, 1965.

212. Strang, R. R., and Ljungdahl, T. I.: Carcinoma of the lung with a cerebral metastasis presenting as subarachnoid haemorrhage, Med. J. Aust. **1**:90, 1962.

213. Strassman, G.: Formation of hemosiderin and hematoidin after traumatic and spontaneous cerebral hemorrhages, Arch. Path. **47**:205, 1949.

214. Strauss, I., Globus, J. H., and Ginsburg, S. W.: Spontaneous subarachnoid hemorrhage: Its relation to aneurysms of cerebral blood vessels, Arch. Neurol. Psychiat. **27**:1080, 1932.

215. Strauss, I., and Tarachow, S.: Prognostic factors in spontaneous subarachnoid hemorrhage, Arch. Neurol. Psychiat. **38**:239, 1937.

216. Sutton, D.: The diagnosis of intracranial vascular lesions by percutaneous vertebral angiography, Arch. Middlesex Hosp. **2**:228, 1952.

217. Sutton, D., and Trickey, S. E.: Subarachnoid haemorrhage and total cerebral angiography, Clin. Radiol. **13**:297, 1962.

218. Symonds, C. P.: Contribution to the clinical study of intracranial aneurysms, Guy's Hosp. Rep. **73**:139, 1923.

219. Symonds, C. P.: Spontaneous subarachnoid haemorrhage, Quart. J. Med. **18**:93, 1924.

220. Szancer, S.: Acute cerebral venous occlusion manifested by spontaneous subarachnoid hemorrhage, Neurology **5**:675, 1955.

221. Tappura, M.: Prognosis of subarachnoid haemorrhage, Acta Med. Scand. **173** (suppl. 392):1, 1962.

222. Taylor, A. B., and Whitfield, A. G. W.: Subarachnoid haemorrhage, Quart. J. Med. **5**:461, 1936.

223. Tomlinson, B. E., and Walton, J. N.: Superficial haemosiderosis of the central nervous system, J. Neurol. Neurosurg. Psychiat. **27**: 332, 1964.

224. Tourtellotte, W. W., Metz, L. N., Bryan, E. R., and De Jong, R. N.: Spontaneous subarachnoid hemorrhage: factors affecting the rate of clearing of the cerebrospinal fluid, Neurology **14**:300, 1964.

225. Tremaine, M. J.: Subacute Pick's disease (polyserositis) with polyarthritis and glomerulonephritis, New Eng. J. Med. **211**:754, 1934.

226. Troost, B. T., Walker J. E., and Cherington, M.: Hypoglycorrhachia associated with subarachnoid hemorrhage, Arch. Neurol. **19**:438, 1968.

227. Trumpy, J. H.: Subarachnoid haemorrhage.

Time sequence of recurrences and their prognosis, Acta Neurol. Scand. **43**:48, 1967.

228. Trupp, M., and Sachs, E.: Vascular tumors of the brain and spinal cord and their treatment, J. Neurosurg. **5**:354, 1948.

229. Van Der Meulen, J. P.: Cerebrospinal fluid xanthochromia: an objective index, Neurology **16**:170, 1966.

230. Van Wagenen, W. P.: Chordoblastoma of the basilar plate of the skull and ecchordosis physaliphora spheno-occipitalis, Arch. Neurol. Psychiat. **34**:548, 1935.

231. Vastola, E. F.: Non-hemorrhagic xanthochromia of cerebrospinal fluid, J. Neuropath. Exp. Neurol. **19**:296, 1960.

232. Vastola, E. F., and Frugh, A.: Anticoagulants for occlusive cerebrovascular lesions, Neurology **9**:143, 1959.

233. Vaughan, H. G., and Howard, R. G.: Intracranial hemorrhage due to metastatic chorionepithelioma, Neurology **12**:771, 1962.

234. Walsh, L. S.: Subarachnoid haemorrhage, Acta Radiol. **46**:321, 1956.

235. Walton, J. N.: Subarachnoid haemorrhage of unusual aetiology, Neurology **3**:517, 1953.

236. Walton, J. N.: Subarachnoid haemorrhage, Edinburgh, 1956, E. & S. Livingstone, Ltd.

237. Watson, A. B.: Spinal subarachnoid haemorrhage in patient with coarctation of aorta, Brit. Med. J. **4**:278, 1967.

238. Wechsler, I. S., and Bender, M. B.: The neurological manifestations of periarteritis nodosa, J. Mount Sinai, Hosp. **8**:1071, 1941.

239. Weill-Hallé, B., and Abaza, A.: Anémie splénomégalique et hémorragie méningée, Bull. Soc. Pediat. Paris **31**:340, 1933.

240. Wertham, F., Mitchell, N., and Angrist, A.: The brain in sickle cell anemia, Arch. Neurol. Psychiat. **17**:752, 1942.

241. Widal, F.: Le diagnostic de l'hémorragie méningée, Presse Med. **2**:413, 1903.

242. Windle, W. F.: Brain damage at birth, J.A.M.A. **206**:1967, 1968.

243. Windle, W. F.: Cerebral hemorrhage in relation to birth asphyxia, Science **167**:1000, 1970.

244. Wislocki, G. B.: The cytology of the cerebrospinal pathway. In Cowdry, E. V.: Special cytology, New York, 1928, Paul B. Hoeber, Inc., vol. 2, p. 1089.

245. Wortis H., and Wortis, S. B.: Metastatic melanoma involving the central nervous system, Arch. Neurol. Psychiat. **36**:601, 1936.

246. Wright, R. L., Ojemann, R. G., and Drew, J. H.: Hemorrhage into pituitary adenomata, Arch. Neurol. **12**:326, 1965.

247. Wyburn-Mason, R.: The vascular abnormalities and tumours of the spinal cord and its membranes, St. Louis, 1944, The C. V. Mosby Co.

8 / Intracerebral and intraventricular hemorrhage

Intracerebral hemorrhage

Hemorrhages into the brain parenchyma vary in size and causation and are best dealt with according to etiology.

Primary intracerebral* hemorrhage

Primary intracerebral hemorrhage is characterized by significant hemorrhage into the brain parenchyma in complete disassociation from such etiological factors as trauma, arterial aneurysms, inflammatory vascular lesions, arteriovenous or angiomatous formations, tumors, or blood dyscrasias. Thus the hemorrhages or hematomas have been designated as primary or spontaneous and not infrequently referred to as hemorrhagic or sanguineous apoplexy, apoplectic hemorrhage, or indeed as primary or hypertensive cerebral hemorrhage.

The term "apoplexy," more of a clinical term than a pathological diagnosis, is of Greek derivation.† Charcôt[41] emphasized that apoplexy, a clinical sign, is unfortunately often used synonymously with primary intracerebral hemorrhage. Expressions such as nervous apoplexy, pulmonary apoplexy (hemorrhagic pulmonary infarct), abdominal apoplexy (massive abdominal hemorrhage), and so on have increasingly compounded the meaning to the extent that "apoplexy" is best avoided even though other terms such as cerebral hemorrhage or primary intracerebral hemorrhage are far from ideal.

Spontaneous bleeding to the degree seen in primary intracerebral hemorrhage is virtually confined to the intracranial cavity.

Sudden, extensive bleeding in other parts of the body usually has a demonstrable cause such as aneurysm, blood dyscrasias, trauma, dissecting aneurysm, myomalacia cordis, or varices, etc. The few unexplained instances of sudden abdominal bleeding have been referred to as intra-abdominal apoplexy. Even conceding the existence of this not-very-convincing entity, its incidence is negligible when compared to that of primary intracerebral hemorrhage. The inescapable conclusion is that morphologically, functionally, or pathologically some very important peculiarity of the cerebrovascular system underlies the pathogenesis of the disease in man. At present this pathogenic factor, escaping detection, gives rise to speculation.

Yet another remarkable fact, possibly important etiologically, is the extreme rarity of the disease in animals other than man. Trauma is a common cause of bleeding in and about the brain and spinal cord of domestic animals and septicemic diseases such as hog cholera, anthrax, and leptospirosis are also oft-encountered causes. Cerebral tumors likewise may be associated with hemorrhage in other animals but not primary intracerebral hemorrhage. However hemorrhage associated with arteriosclerotic diseases of the brain and spinal cord has been reported in old parrots and ostriches.[201] The low incidence correlates well with the low incidence of degenerative vascular diseases among other animals.

Prevalence. Primary intracerebral hemorrhage is often fatal. Actuarial figures in most countries reveal cerebrovascular disease as the third most frequent cause of death. The incidence varies for reasons not apparent, and primary intracerebral hemorrhage is a major, contributary, mortality factor. In the U. S. 26% of deaths due to

---

*Cerebral is used here synonymously with encephalic.

† (Apo- means "away from"; plexis, "a stroke"; and -ia, "condition.") Apoplessein was used as long ago as the Galenic era to indicate the sudden loss of feeling and movement of the entire body excepting only respiration.[182]

cerebrovascular disease in 1965 were attributed to intracerebral hemorrhage[84] and in 1946 it was the fourth most common cause of death.[59] Kurtzke[136] estimated that in 1969 approximately 16% of all cerebrovascular deaths were caused by primary intracerebral hemorrhage (Table 7-1).

There has been variation in the frequency during this century in England and Wales. Deaths there from cerebral hemorrhage including subarachnoid hemorrhage (adjusted for change in age structure) actually diminished from 1932 to 1961, whereas the number of deaths from cerebral infarction rose during the same period.[271] Comparisons of the frequency of a necropsy diagnosis of cerebral infarction and the incidence of cerebral hemorrhage in three Manchester hospitals reflected the trend seen in the Registrar General's figures. In 1932 cerebral hemorrhage was almost three times more frequent at autopsy than cerebral infarction, whereas in 1961 the ratio had been very nearly inverted. Yates[271] suggested that the improved treatment of hypertension could account for the decline and that the steeper fall in the curve for females during the previous 10 years might be due to reduced parity and hence to less pyelonephritic hypertension. Improved and more critical diagnostic criteria for hemorrhage and infarction may have assisted.

The prevalence of primary intracerebral hemorrhage at autopsy was reported as 2.5% by Zimmerman[273] between 1927 and 1943 and by Stehbens[239] as 4.2%. In the Framingham Study, Kannel and his colleagues[131] found that during a 12-year observation period of 5106 men and women aged 30 to 62 years, only 4% of those with cerebrovascular disease had intracerebral hemorrhage, a very low frequency. Both subarachnoid hemorrhage (18%) and thrombotic brain infarction (63%) were considerably more prevalent. Intracerebral hemorrhage caused sudden, unexpected natural death in 6.5% of cases compared with 4.6% in subarachnoid hemorrhage.[113] Although a ruptured cerebral aneurysm can cause rapid death (within 5 minutes), primary cerebral hemorrhage rarely causes death within 1 hour, and so "sudden death" requires some modification here.

From the clinical viewpoint controversy exists about whether subarachnoid hemorrhage or cerebral hemorrhage is the more frequent.[257] In general primary intracerebral hemorrhage is believed to occur 1.5 to 2 times more frequently than subarachnoid hemorrhage.[136,164] Russell[203] analyzed 461 instances of spontaneous intracranial hemorrhage (from the autopsy records of the London Hospital [England] from 1912 to 1952), excluding traumatic and neonatal hemorrhages as well as hemorrhages less than 1.5 cm. in the brain stem and 3 cm. in the cerebrum or cerebellum. The number of "hypertensive" intracerebral hemorrhages was 232 (50% of the subjects). They were found much more often than aneurysmal hemorrhage (120 cases including 28 bacterial). Mutlu and colleagues[174] in a series of 222 cases of nontraumatic massive cerebral hemorrhage found 60% to have primary intracerebral hemorrhage. Many clinical cases of nontraumatic subarachnoid hemorrhage are due to primary intracerebral hemorrhage (Table 7-2). The frequency depends on the nature of the institution and the composition of the patient population. Some large teaching institutions only reluctantly admit patients with primary intracerebral hemorrhage whereas they are admitted with less difficulty at municipal hospitals.[257] The conclusion has to be that at autopsy primary intracerebral hemorrhage is more frequent than ruptured cerebral aneurysms, but hospital and autopsy data can provide very misleading information concerning true incidence. Cerebral hemorrhage as the diagnosis on death certificates (England and Wales, 1955), estimated officially, was overemployed by a ratio of 1.25:1.[271] In a U. S. study the official national mortality for cerebrovascular disease was said to represent only approximately 73% of the true mortality figure. The error for intracerebral hemorrhage was probably less.[84]

Familial incidence. No detailed statistical investigation of the familial occurrence of primary intracerebral hemorrhage has eventuated, but hypertension, the usual concomitant, has exhibited a distinct tendency to occur in families.[93] In a series of hypertensives[215] a family history of hypertension was found in 55%. The inheritance of hypertension is in all likelihood multifactorial,[185] and in view of the known frequency of primary intracerebral hemorrhage among hypertensives, the familial occurrence of intracerebral hemorrhage is not unexpected. Evidence is often vague, with the causes of deaths of near relatives being attributed to "stroke", and the terms "apoplexy" and "cerebral hemorrhage" not necessarily always indicating primary intracerebral hemorrhage. However, in some families the prevalence of such lesions is so great[93] that some instances of primary intracerebral hemorrhage appear to be included, though again definite statistical information on this subject has not been produced to date. In Dinsdale's series of pontine and cerebellar hemorrhages,[65] in 70 cases details of the parents were known. There was parental history of cerebral hemorrhage in two and a history of stroke in one parent of 12 of the cases. It would seem that the familial occurrence of this disease can be attributed to the hypertension.

Epidemiology. Fig. 13-1 reveals differences from country to country in the frequency of primary intracerebral hemorrhage. Explanations of these variations on ethnic, geographical, and sociological grounds are far from simple and have received little attention.

In the U. S. there are differences in the prevalence of cerebral hemorrhage between Caucasians and Negroes. Freytag[87] found a higher proportion of Negroes in her series than the composition of the local population warranted. Furthermore, the Negroes were on an average of 12 years younger than the Caucasians. Differences occurred at the extremes of age but the numbers were then such that the significance was minor. These ethnic differences have been attributed to the greater prevalence and younger age distribution of hypertension (benign and malignant) among American Negroes.[185]

Coronary artery disease and myocardial infarction predominate in the white population but lethal cerebral hemorrhage was found to be more common in the Negro.[130] Equivalent states of hypertension as judged by heart weight resulted in more disastrous hemorrhagic complications in the central nervous system in the Negro.

It is generally conceded that cerebral hemorrhage is extraordinarily high in Japan with the high mortality deriving from the prevalence of hypertension occasioned by a heavy salt intake. However evidence exists that the alleged prevalence of cerebral hemorrhage in the Japanese is the result of diagnostic fashion and the low autopsy rate.[136]

No satisfactory explanation has been advanced but hospital admissions with this lesion are higher in winter and spring.* In Freytag's series the phenomenon was not observed.

It has been held that cerebral hemorrhage is most likely to occur in broad, fat people with short necks and a florid complexion—the John Bull type of individual.[12] Correlation of body types with specific cerebrovascular diseases is not a popular avenue of investigation and any conclusions drawn from future investigations should be carefully analyzed statistically and cautiously interpreted.

Age and sex distribution. Table 8-1 demonstrates the age distribution of primary intracerebral hemorrhage. The mean age or peak incidence falls in the sixth decade.[114,273] Odom and associates[175] recorded a mean age of only 44 years in their 55 cases (range of 15 to 75 years), and Mutlu and colleagues[174] recorded a mean age of 55 years (57 years in men and 54 in women) with a range of 31 to 85 years. In the series of Aring and Merritt,[10] the mean age was 59 years, and in the series reported by

---

*In the U. S. the highest frequency is in March.[10,174]

Stehbens[238] the mean age for males was 56.2 years, 55.3 years for females, and 55.8 years when combined (range of 15 to 86 years). These figures are derived from hospital data that may not reflect the true peak of the incidence in the general community where the peak may occur later.

In her series, Freytag[87] noted both a high proportion of American Negroes and a peak incidence of 12 years before that of American Caucasians and observed that this age difference held true for each of the anatomical sites of primary intracerebral hemorrhage.

The age distribution according to sex is illustrated in Fig. 8-1. Most patients are

Table 8-1. Age distribution of primary intracerebral hemorrhage

Authors	0-9	10-19	20-29	30-39	40-49	50-59	60-69	70-79	80-89	Total
Aring & Merritt (1935)[10]	1	0	3	24	31	29	22	2		112
Richardson & Hyland (1941)[194]	2	0	7	30	35	37	18	2		131
Hicks & Black (1949)*[114]	1	3	6	24	35	12	15	1		97
Johansson & Melin (1960)[127]	1	4	9	36	38	45	28	1		162
Emblen (1961)[71]				3	7	13	7			30
Blackwood (1963)[27]		1	2	6	12	9	2			32
Stehbens (1963)[239]	2	6	27	74	119	107	38	7		380
Merritt (1967)[164]	1†	0	3	21	27	26	20	2†		100
Freytag (1968)[87]			44	88	117	79	48	17		393
Total	8	14	101	306	421	357	198	32		1437

*These figures may be in the wrong decade, but such a position would not significantly alter the results.

†Intraventricular and subarachnoid hemorrhage excluded.

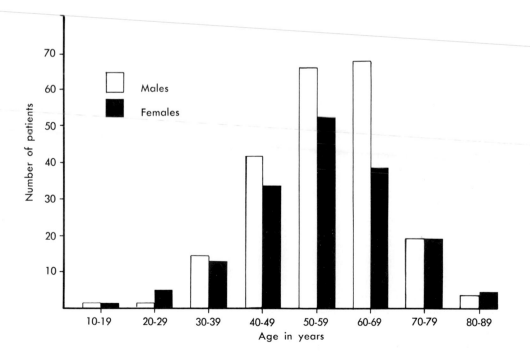

Fig. 8-1. Histogram of age distribution of primary intracerebral hemorrhage for males and females. (Adapted from Stehbens, W. E.: Aneurysms and anatomical variation of cerebral arteries, Arch. Path. **75**:45, 1963).

Table 8-2. Sex distribution in primary intracerebral hemorrhage

Authors	Number of males	Number of females	Total
Aring & Merritt (1935)[10]	53%	47%	116
Zimmerman (1949)*[273]	Equal		41
Johansson and Melin (1960)[127]	43%	57%	162
Mutlu et al. (1963)[174]	77	58	135
Stehbens (1963)[239]	214	166	380
Freytag (1968)[87]	244	149	393

*No definite figures or percentages were given, only that the sex distribution was equal.

between 40 and 75 years of age, but Table 8-1 reveals that 8.6% of the patients with primary intracerebral hemorrhage are under the age of 40 years. This type of hemorrhage in the young has been emphasized by several authors.[112,195,234] Intracerebral hemorrhage in the same age group is usually secondary rather than primary, and many unexplained hematomas have in recent years been attributed to cryptic arteriovenous aneurysms or hemangiomas. However primary intracerebral hemorrhage cannot be altogether excluded in the first four decades, for this age group is not immune from hypertension. A diagnosis of a primary hemorrhage in the young is permissible only after a thorough and unproductive search for and exclusion of all possible etiological factors. The subjects are not always hypertensive and inevitably some suspicion remains regarding the validity of the diagnosis.

In hospital series of primary intracerebral hematoma, males usually outnumber females.[87,120,238] Some authors assert that the sex difference (Table 8-2) is not significant.[136,273]

Pathology. Statistics on the pathological features of primary intracerebral hemorrhage are confusing. Interpretation is difficult, since criteria employed in the classification of lesions vary. Some authors include secondary pontine hemorrhage. Others refer to the lesions as hypertensive cerebral hemorrhage,[82,203] presuming incorrectly that this diagnosis cannot be made in the absence of hypertension. There is even a lack of detail concerning the size

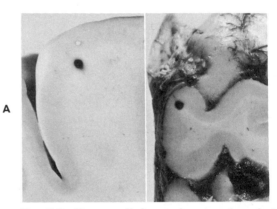

Fig. 8-2. Two small hemorrhages, subcortical in **A** and in the deep part of the cortex in **B**. The edge of an old cortical softening is present at lower aspect of **B**.

of the hematoma. The diagnosis of primary intracerebral hemorrhage has come to be associated pathologically with a hematoma of considerable or massive proportions and a clinical picture of an acute cerebrovascular accident of severe or grave nature. Russell[203] excludes all hematomas less than 3 cm. in size and less than 1.5 cm. for lesions of the brain stem. Small hematomas or those below these critical limits are disregarded for no better reason other than that they rarely contribute significantly to the cause of death.

Small hemorrhages up to 2 or 3 cm. in diameter occur at almost any site within the brain (Figs. 8-2 and 8-3). There is a predilection for the gray matter or the junction of the cortex and white matter (subcortical).[82] They are round or oval and frequently quite circumscribed dark red

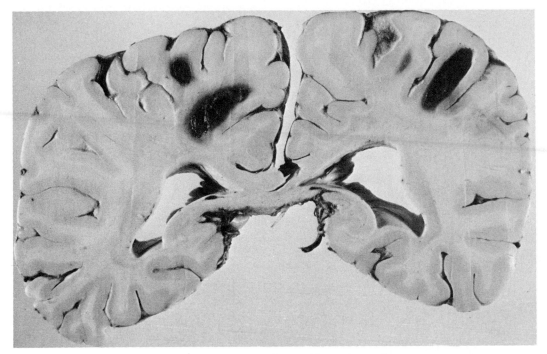

Fig. 8-3. Three subcortical hemorrhages in cerebrum.

Table 8-3. Distribution of massive primary intracerebral hemorrhage*

Authors	Region of basal ganglia (and thalamus)	Elsewhere in cerebrum	Brain stem (or pons)	Cerebellum	Total
Charcôt (1881)[41]	119		21	13	153
Zimmerman (1949)[273]	47	32	7	13	99
Courville (1950)[50]	938		124	73	1135
Odom, Bloor, & Woodhall (1952)[175]	41	6	5	2	54
Hyland & Levy (1954)[120]	543		61	31	630†
Russell (1954)[203]	151	25	32	18	226
Hudson & Hyland (1958)[118]	23		7	1	31
Adams & Vander Eecken (1959)[3]	112	17	12	21	162
Johansson & Melin (1960)[127]	107	36	11	8	162
Mutlu, Berry, & Alpers (1963)[174]	94	33	8		135
Stehbens (1963)[239]	274	27	53	26	380
Dinsdale (1964)[65]	429		30	52	511
Brewer et al. (1968)[34]	333	72	62	36	503
Freytag (1968)[87]	225	45	63	47	380
Total	3729 (81.6%)		496 (10.9%)	341 (7.5%)	4566 (100%)

*Omitting intraventricular and multiple hemorrhages.
†Hyland and Levy[120] gave the total as 630 cases, but there were 635 hemorrhages; so at least five multiple hemorrhages (possibly secondary pontine lesions) must have been present.

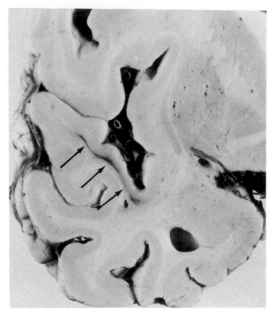

Fig. 8-4. Elongated slitlike cavity (*arrows*) with brown pigmented walls in temporal operculum. Cavity could have arisen from a hemorrhage similar to those in Fig. 8-3.

hematomas mostly without small punctate or satellite hemorrhages at the periphery. Their relationship with hypertension is close. They may occur in isolation, in association with similar lesions elsewhere, or with a more massive hemorrhage. The small size permits recovery and healing, whereas organization results in tiny slitlike softenings (Fig. 8-4) containing abundant macrophages laden with hemosiderin (Fig. 8-5) or hematoidin. These autogenously labeled macrophages (siderophages) probably persist for years, though they are thought to disappear eventually, in which case old softenings and hemorrhages may not be differentiated satisfactorily. Most reports on primary intracerebral hemorrhage exclude these minor lesions.

Seen very frequently at autopsy is the large or massive hemorrhage (Fig. 8-6). The reported distribution in the brain has varied considerably (Table 8-3). In a series of 380 cases collected from the autopsy records of the Royal Prince Alfred Hospital (Australia),[239] 79.9% occurred in the cerebrum, 14% in the pons, and 6.8% in the cerebellum. However some authors have recorded cerebellar hemorrhage to be more

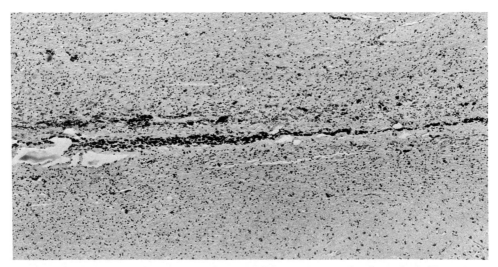

Fig. 8-5. Old but small slitlike hemorrhage exhibits numerous closely packed siderophages in a linear distribution with siderophages and some gliosis of neighboring tissue. Larger hemorrhages have a cleftlike cavity with gliotic and pigmented walls. (Hematoxylin and eosin, ×110.)

frequent than pontine hemorrhage, and in 135 cases, Mutlu, Berry, and Alpers[174] had not one instance of cerebellar hemorrhage. There is no significant sex difference in the distribution of the hemorrhages.

Hemorrhages in the basal ganglia and thalamus. On removal of the calvarium in patients who have died of massive primary hemorrhage into a cerebral hemisphere, the dura mater is frequently found to be tense. Upon opening the dura mater, one can see that the cerebrum has been under considerable tension and it bulges through the incision. Subarachnoid hemorrhage, if present, is usually not massive. The greatest degree of hemorrhagic coloration of the meninges is usually in the posterior fossa about the foramina of Luschka and Magendie. In some cases, especially shortly after the onset of bleeding, the cerebrospinal fluid at lumbar puncture does not contain blood and the external appearance of the brain reflects this fact. Subarachnoid

blood may be concentrated over the parietal lobe overlying a fluctuating hematoma, but this is relatively uncommon. The involved hemisphere may be visibly enlarged, with a fluctuating zone bulging in a localized area where the gyri are more flattened than elsewhere and where the sulci are shallow. The brain is often of a diminished consistency, flattening out when set on the dissecting board.[41] Excessive handling can lead to tearing of the cortex overlying the hematoma and extrusion of "red currant jelly" clot. To a variable degree signs of raised intracranial pressure are exhibited. The hematoma, if inspected in the fresh state, looks like a large mass of recently coagulated blood, which is readily removed from a ragged walled cavity up to 10 cm. or more in diameter. There are few fragments of cerebral tissue or debris in the macroscopically clotted mass and sometimes it appears that the neighboring brain has been pushed aside by the expand-

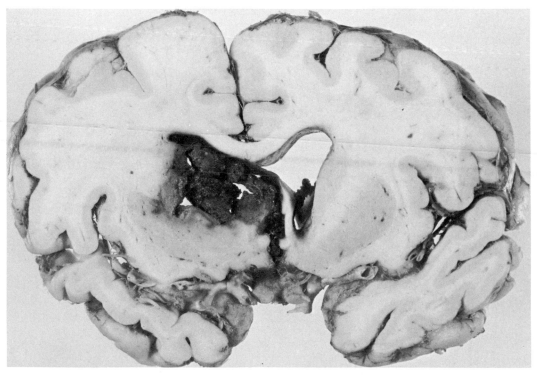

Fig. 8-6. Primary intracerebral hemorrhage involving caudate nucleus and internal capsule with extension into lateral ventricle.

ing hematoma rather than infiltrated and destroyed. The hematoma itself fixes poorly and a diffuse red staining can pervade the surrounding brain. Section of the wall of the hematoma reveals numerous small punctate hemorrhages of variable size. A communication with the ventricular cavity may be associated with an intraventricular blood clot, sometimes forming a cast of the ventricular system. Intraventricular rupture is much more frequent than rupture through the cortex into the subarachnoid space, but occasionally both occur.

It is rarely possible to ascertain the source of bleeding. Charcôt[41] found in the ragged hemorrhagic wall many small ruptured vessels with adherent clots, which could simulate miliary aneurysms. These miliary aneurysms, believed to be responsible for the hemorrhage, are also said to be readily demonstrated if the tissue and blood are washed away under running water.

The most frequent site for a massive intracerebral hemorrhage of this type is in the region of the basal ganglia and thalamus (Table 8-3), and hemorrhages there accounted for 72.1% of 380 cases.[239] Cour-

ville and Friedman[52] divided these hemorrhages into medial and lateral ganglionic hemorrhages. The dividing line passed anteroposteriorly between the putamen laterally and the globus pallidus medially. Lateral ganglionic hemorrhages occurred in the external capsule, putamen, and claustrum and frequently ruptured into the ventricular system, usually forward into the anterior horn or upward into the body of the lateral ventricle. Less frequently it was into the inferior horn of the temporal lobe or posteriorly into the junction of the body and posterior horn. Rarely is rupture through the subcortical white matter and cortex to the subarachnoid space. Lateral ganglionic hemorrhages are not always fatal and much of the clot gradually shrinks and disappears, leaving an old slit-like cavity with orange or rusty brown walls (Fig. 8-7). One of the large outermost vessels of the lateral group of lenticulostriate arteries, coursing near the outer surface of the putamen, has been designated the "artery of cerebral hemorrhage" ostensibly because it is responsible for most of the hemorrhages in this zone. Medial ganglionic hemorrhages involve structures medial to

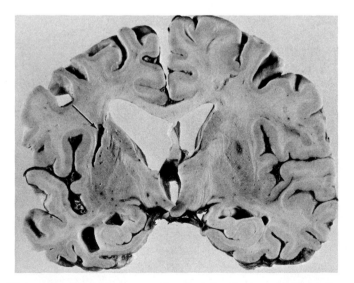

Fig. 8-7. Slit-like cavity (*arrow*) at outer border of putamen. Ipsilateral cerebral hemisphere is atrophic, and lateral ventricle is dilated. Walls of the cavity were pigmented. This was believed to be an old hemorrhage.

the division between the putamen and the globus pallidus and include the corpus striatum and thalamus. Almost invariably they are fatal because only recent hemorrhages are found.[52] The higher mortality was attributed to the proximity of the hypothalamic autonomic centers and secondary effects on the brain stem. No evidence suggests that these secondary effects on the brain stem are more numerous or more severe than with the lateral hemorrhages, and according to Fisher,[83] old hemorrhagic cavities more than 2 cm. in diameter are not infrequent.

Mutlu, Berry, and Alpers[174] analyzed the location of a large series of hematomas in the region of the basal ganglia and thalamus (94 hemorrhages) and divided them into four groups:

LATERAL HEMORRHAGES, the most common, account for one-third of all the hemorrhages in the region. They involve the external capsule grossly and at times the claustrum and the outer part of the putamen extending to the foremost portion of the outer limb of the internal capsule.

QUADRILATERAL HEMORRHAGES involved the entire basal ganglia from the ventricular wall to the insular cortex, including thalamus, internal capsule, external capsule, caudate nucleus, lenticular nucleus, and claustrum and accounted for 27% of the hemorrhages.

INTERMEDIATE HEMORRHAGES involved the putamen, globus pallidus, caudate nucleus, and sometimes part of the internal capsule and thalamus, tending to be restricted either anteriorly or posteriorly. They accounted for 27% of the hemorrhages.

MEDIAL HEMORRHAGES were the least common (12% of the 94). They were chiefly thalamic hemorrhages (Fig. 8-8) but could extend into the internal capsule and caudate nucleus.

Lateral hemorrhages were presumed to issue from a lateral lenticulostriate artery.[174] The other three varieties were interpreted as being etiologically secondary to an antecedent ischemic episode as propounded by Rochoux[200] and Globus.[94] The internal capsule was involved in 48% of the hemorrhages in the ganglionic re-

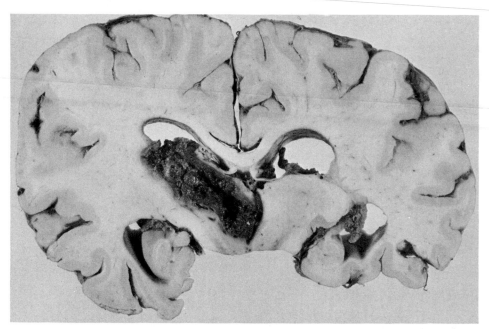

Fig. 8-8. Large thalamic hemorrhage with rupture into lateral ventricle and shift of midline.

gion,[174] with the frontal limb being most often involved and the genu least often. Complete involvement of the internal capsule was rare.

McKissock and associates[160] and other investigators found that hemorrhage arose most frequently in the region of the external capsule. They believed that extension therefrom damaged the basal ganglia and thalamus by distortion and compression of midline structures, or alternatively the hemorrhage burst into the frontal, temporal, or parietal lobes. The customary tabulation of hematomas according to site was held to be misleading. Most authors tend to localize the site of hemorrhage in rather vague terms only as in Table 8-3. The disparity in localization reported in the literature illustrates the difficulty in securing accurate detailed localization of massive destructive lesions. The commonest site of hemorrhage is held to be the external capsule.[160,174] Fisher[83] states that it is the putamen, and Zimmerman[273] contends that it is the internal capsule.

The supply of the external capsule and claustrum is attributed to the lateral lenticulostriate arteries. Stephens and Stilwell[244] however found them to be supplied by the perforating cortical vessels arising from branches of the middle cerebral artery distal to the origin of the striate vessels and they then penetrate the insula. Lateral lenticulostriate arteries were found to supply only as far as the lateral margin of the putamen.[244] As stated above, primary intracerebral hemorrhage is said to originate most frequently from the largest of the lateral lenticulostriate arteries (artery of cerebral hemorrhage), believed to supply the region of the external capsule. This concept of the "artery of cerebral hemorrhage" as such being the source of bleeding into the external capsule is at variance with the anatomical distribution of the striate arteries as described by Stephens and Stillwell,[244] who suggest that a hemorrhage in the external capsule or claustrum might represent a lateral extension of a hemorrhage from a lateral lenticulostriate

artery. Therefore, if the arteries supplying the external capsule are responsible for many of the hemorrhages in this area, the penetrating cortical branches are responsible and not lenticulostriate arteries.

Older hemorrhages demonstrate organization at their edges and change in the color of the blood. The hematoma takes on a brownish hue. The clotlike mass loses its gelatinous consistency, becomes semiliquid, and develops a distinct rusty brown color. Large hematomas may have a macroscopic capsule (Fig. 8-9), and smaller lesions occur less often. If the hematoma is close to the cortex, the overlying flattened gyri may exhibit rusty pigmentation.[181]

Between the capsule and the surrounding brain a loose zone of diminished consistency usually resembles a plane of cleavage (Fig. 8-9). The capsule proper rarely

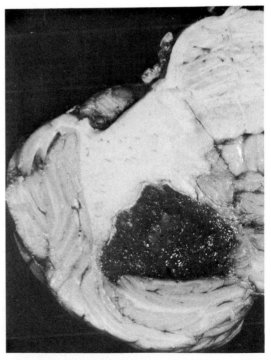

Fig. 8-9. An old hematoma of cerebellum. Contents were rust colored. Note capsule surrounding hematoma and narrow cleftlike zone between capsule and parenchyma.

merges externally with the surrounding brain as it will in very old hematomas. Calcification can be expected in some longstanding lesions, such as occur about old areas of encephalomalacia, and hematomas at other sites but very rarely as indicated by the low survival rate of these patients.

Old hematomas are usually subcortical, whereas softenings tend to leave only the residual superficial gliosed layers of the cortex, though the latter may be deficient. Softenings do not tend to be so pigmented, but old relatively depigmented hematomas could conceivably be mistaken for softenings in which a moderate amount of hemorrhage had occurred. Hemorrhages may be slitlike, whereas softenings tend to leave fibrils traversing the residual cavity. Softenings, unlike hemorrhages, tend to conform to the area of blood supply or venous drainage.

The disappearance of blood pigment, which may be found only on microscopic examination about hemorrhages,[52] has been emphasized. It is possible that slitlike cavities in the putamen or external capsule could be classified as old hematomas. Fisher[83] found that approximately 25% of hemorrhages over 2 cm. in diameter were of long standing and 33% of hemorrhages 0.5 cm. in diameter or larger quite old.

In another series Fisher[83] found 10 instances of primary intracerebral hemorrhage (over 2 cm. in diameter) in 200 autopsies from a chronic disease hospital. Five were recent. This inordinately high frequency leads to suspicion concerning the criteria used for the differentiation of aged hematomas from old cerebral softenings. McKissock and associates[160] contend that the mortality of primary intracerebral hemorrhage has been exaggerated by pathologists and found that, of 48 patients with primary intracerebral hemorrhage at autopsy, 13 had scars of old healed external capsular hemorrhages.

Antin, Prockop, and Cohen[8] recorded clinically a hemorrhage in the thalamic region in a normotensive woman of 64 years. Originally the mass was demonstrated radiographically to be indenting the third ventricle. A subsequent pneumoencephalogram revealed a diverticulum (1.5 cm. in diameter) of the third ventricle into the site of the previously demonstrated mass. The etiology of this presumed hematoma is uncertain, but resorption of the blood to produce a ventricular diverticulum is unusual and contrasts with Courville's "intracerebral hematoma" occurring after traumatic or spontaneous subependymal hemorrhage.[50] The ependyma was alleged to behave as a semipermeable membrane allowing the imbibition of fluid by the breakdown products of the blood—thus the enlargement of the hematoma, which acted as a growing space-occupying lesion. The occurrence of such a phenomenon is unconfirmed.

Intracranial arterial aneurysms are frequently overlooked at autopsy. The cerebral arteries should be carefully inspected in every case of intracranial hemorrhage. An intracerebral hematoma, especially if accompanied by hypertension and left ventricular hypertrophy and nephrosclerosis, has led many pathologists to believe they were dealing with primary intracerebral hemorrhage.[197] However, hematomas of many sites are common to both primary intracerebral hemorrhage and aneurysmal bleeding[57] and differentiation should be attempted despite the fact that the morphology of the cut surface of the brain may be identical in the two diseases. Thus the following facts appear:

1. Frontal and temporal hematomas are common with aneurysms and infrequent with primary intracerebral hemorrhage.
2. Hematomas of the parietal lobe or corona radiata are frequent with primary intracerebral hemorrhage and uncommon with aneurysms.
3. Hematomas of the occipital lobe are rare in both diseases.
4. Hematomas of the external capsule are frequent with both, and particularly with primary intracerebral hemorrhage.
5. Isolated hemorrhages into the thalamus or caudate nucleus are seen character-

istically in primary intracerebral hemorrhage.[57]

6. Caval, callosal, and bilateral frontal lobe hematomas usually indicate a ruptured aneurysm.

Crompton[57] reported a case of rupture of an aneurysm of the basilar bifurcation. It burst up between the cerebral peduncles, and blood tracked down the midbrain and pons between the tegmentum of these structures and the cerebral peduncles and basis pontis. Blood, it was thought, seeped down the perivascular sheaths of perforating vessels from the basilar and posterior arteries. In such a location it could be easily mistaken for midbrain hemorrhage.

The absence of identifiable brain tissue within the hematoma, the lack of conformity in site and shape of the hemorrhage to a definite arterial supply or area of venous drainage,[43] and the presence of obvious hemorrhagic softening of the adjoining brain are features that aid in the differentiation of primary intracerebral hemorrhage from recent hemorrhagic softening. It is also possible for the two lesions to coexist.

Hemorrhages in miscellaneous sites in the cerebrum. Primary intracerebral hemorrhages also develop in the cerebrum at sites other than the basal ganglia and thalamus (Table 8-3). They constitute anywhere from 7.1% to 32.3% of all primary hemorrhages in the brain.[239,273] The hemorrhage of significant size may occur in the frontal, parietal, occipital, or temporal lobes. According to Zimmerman[273] the most frequent site is the frontal lobe (Fig. 8-10). It is the temporal in Aring and Merritt's series,[10] yet these regions are frequently affected by intracerebral rupture of an aneurysm. Fisher[83] found four in the temporal and occipital lobes, three in the temporoparietal and parietal lobes, and five in the frontal lobes. Mutlu, Berry, and Alpers[174] found 36% in the occipital, 27% in the frontal, 19% in the temporal, and 18% in the parietal section and believe such hemorrhages to be basically consequent upon a preexisting softening. One case

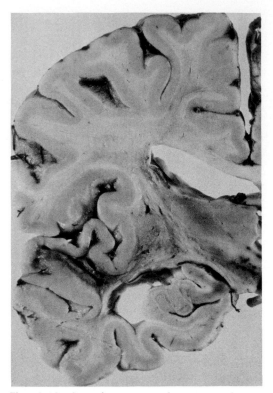

Fig. 8-10. Superior temporal gyrus and temporal operculum are the site of an old hemorrhage. Adjoining cortex is of slightly reduced width but collapsed and overlies a cavity with pigmented walls. Note that there appear to be trabeculae in the cavity. Lacunar softenings are present in the lenticular nucleus. Lateral ventricle is enlarged and thalamus is of reduced size.

they illustrated exhibited extreme hemorrhage in association with hemorrhagic cerebral infarction. This need not indicate that all hematomas in the white matter of the cerebrum are postinfarctional.

The hematomas occur in the central substance of the white matter, though not infrequently they come in proximity to cortical gray matter. They may be quite massive but in general do not tend to be as lethal as those related to the basal ganglia and thalamus. Absolutely massive hemorrhage can invade the white matter of the cerebrum, and the hematoma may extend from the frontal to the occipital pole at the level of the corona radiata.

In a woman of 58 years of age with migraine of 10 years standing, Pant and Drey-fus[179] described more than 100 old or recent hemorrhages, varying in size from petechiae to hematomas 5 cm. in diameter. Most large lesions were subcortical in position. Apart from one hypertensive episode the woman was normotensive and the cerebral arteries exhibited hyaline changes, some having been occluded and others recanalized. Feigin and Prose[76] reported a similar case. In a 57-year-old male Raeder[191] recorded multiple small hemorrhages not more than 1 mm. in diameter mostly in the cortex. All were attributed to multiple miliary aneurysms said to be caused by an arteritis, but no inflammatory vascular changes were seen. Multiple hemorrhagic foci such as these are usually secondary.

Primary brain stem hemorrhage. Primary pontine hemorrhages, generally considered to be more frequent than those of the cerebellum, constitute 10% to 16% of all primary intracerebral hemorrhages. A few reports show a higher frequency of cerebellar hemorrhage than those of the pons (Table 8-3). It has been suggested that the frequency of cerebellar hemorrhage is proportional to the weight of the cerebellum when compared with that of the cerebrum. The incidence of pontine hemorrhage allows of no such correlation.

The average age of patients dying of pontine hemorrhage is less than that for cerebellar or intracerebral hemorrhages, but the difference is too slight to be of practical diagnostic value. The mean age of 53 patients with hemorrhage into the pons was 52.8 years, for the cerebellum 54.1 years, and 56.4 years for the cerebrum.[239] Freytag[87] published similar results. Dinsdale[65] found 60% of the pontine hemorrhages occurred between 40 and 60 years of age, and a similar percentage of cerebellar hemorrhages occurred between 60 and 80 years. Differences in the peak incidence would have been 10 years at most. Freytag[87] recorded an unduly large proportion of Negroes among her cases of pontine hemorrhage. The presence of hypertension is the general rule[72] and pontine

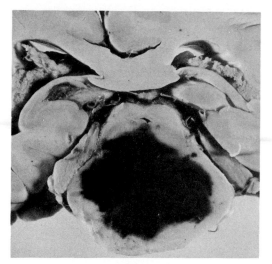

Fig. 8-11. Large recent pontine hemorrhage.

hemorrhage is likely when malignant hypertension is present.

Pontine hemorrhage evolves rapidly and the onset of coma is quite abrupt. The hemorrhage, usually moderately large, commences near the midlevel of the pons close to the junction of the basis pontis and the tegmentum.[65] The hemorrhage varies in degree and appears relatively symmetrical. When the hemorrhage is not symmetrical, the midline region is almost invariably involved (Fig. 8-11). The hematoma frequently extends upward into the cerebral peduncles and may reach the hypothalamus or even the thalamus.[65] Extension into the middle cerebellar peduncles for a short distance may occur, but it is rare in the medulla oblongata and only limited in extent. The hemorrhage usually involves a large part of the pons, displaying extensions along fiber tracts and satellite hemorrhages at the periphery. Remnants of brain tissue can be seen within the hematoma, especially bundles of transverse fibers. Some softness of the surrounding parenchyma may be noticeable, particularly if the hemorrhage is massive. There may be evidence of bleeding on the surface of the pons or cerebral peduncles, which are disposed to tearing during removal of the brain from the cranium. Alternatively, the pons may feel pulpy or fluctuant.

Frank rupture of the hemorrhage into the subarachnoid space is uncommon. Blood rarely penetrates the superficial transverse fibers of the pons. Though rupture into the fourth ventricle occurs frequently,[65,87] the onset of coma in subjects without ventricular rupture is equally rapid and profound.[65] The amount of subarachnoid blood varies from little to moderate in quantity and is found mostly in the posterior fossa. Acute hydrocephalus affects a few patients. On inspection of the brain the signs of raised intracranial pressure are unlikely to be in evidence.

Old hematomas of the pons are exceptional and, of necessity, quite small or the patient would not have survived.

Primary hemorrhage in the midbrain[218] is most unusual without extension to the pons, though petechial hemorrhages may occur here as well as in the medulla oblongata. Hemorrhages of significant size in the medulla, when not extensions from the pons, are in all likelihood associated with arteriovenous or angiomatous formations, or anticoagulant therapy.[18,74,157]

Cerebellar hemorrhage. Primary or spontaneous cerebellar hemorrhage is the most frequent cause of intracerebellar hemorrhage and is not the rare entity suggested by some authors. The reported frequency varies (Table 8-3). Michael[165] found that there were 1112 instances of cerebral hemorrhage in 17,257 autopsies and only 10 cases of cerebellar hemorrhage. Such a low frequency is hard to reconcile with other reports for it has been said to occur in up to 13% of all cerebral hemorrhages.[167] However some of the cases included were not primary. Cerebellar hemorrhage has been regarded as being less common than primary pontine or midbrain hemorrhage, but a few authors contend that cerebellar hematomas preponderate (Table 8-3). The frequency of cerebellar hemorrhage as indicated by hospital autopsy figures may be underestimated because of the "sudden" or rapid death of many of these patients and their transference to the jurisdiction of the medical examiner or coroner.

At autopsy the cerebellum may show secondary pressure phenomena caused by increased subtentorial pressure. There may be indications of subarachnoid hemorrhage in the posterior fossa and spinal canal, and the chances of the blood being more concentrated over the lesion are higher with cerebellar hemorrhage than with either cerebral or pontine hematomas. Although the cerebellum may feel rather fluctuant, this is not invariable, as much depends on the size and age of the hematoma. The bleeding has been assumed to originate in most instances from a branch of the superior cerebellar artery.

The hematoma varies in size, often being over 5 cm. in its largest diameter. Its appearance is similar to that of intracerebral hemorrhages and as is consistent with clinical data; most patients die early. However, a rapidly fatal outcome is not invariable and Fig. 8-9 demonstrates a large intracerebellar hematoma of several weeks' duration in the process of organization. The entire contents of this hematoma were rusty brown. The hemorrhage tends to arise in the region of the dentate nucleus and therefore affects one hemisphere in particular. Mitchell and Angrist[167] reviewed the literature up to 1942 and found that of 107 cases, 43 hematomas were in the left hemisphere, 49 in the right, and 15 in the vermis. Dinsdale[65] found only three of his 53 cerebellar hemorrhages in the vermis and 30 were in the left hemisphere and 19 in the right. Rey-Bellet[192] found eight in the left hemisphere, four in the right, six in both, two in the left hemisphere and the vermis, and one involving the vermis and both hemispheres (total of 21 hemorrhages). Six of the nine cerebellar hemorrhages investigated by Fisher[83] were on the left side. Dinsdale[65] regards this left-sided predominance as significant, but to be conclusive, a study of larger numbers and complete exclusion of all secondary hemorrhages is desirable. The hemorrhage may extend into a cerebellar peduncle and sometimes rupture into the brain stem.[162] Dinsdale[65] believes that the cerebellar hematoma is usually sufficiently large to cause death from medullary compression.

The hemorrhage reaches the subarachnoid space more often than intracerebral hematomas,[87] but intraventricular hemorrhage is less frequent. Mostly the hemorrhage extends into the subarachnoid space and/or the fourth ventricle.[65] In the latter the bleeding may be associated with clotted blood in the third ventricle, and blood-stained fluid in the lateral ventricles. Blood tends to escape into the cisterna magna. The enlarging hematoma may distort and ultimately occlude the aqueduct of Sylvius,[11] frequently causing internal hydrocephalus.[142] The foregoing features contribute to the raised intracranial pressure, which causes cerebellar coning. Upward transtentorial displacement of the cerebellum with large hematomas can occur, and uncal herniation is attributed to the acute internal hydrocephalus. McKissock and colleagues[162] performed ventricular drainage on several patients with cerebellar hemorrhage and acute hydrocephalus in an endeavor to relieve pressure. The hazard is fatal transtentorial herniation of the cerebellum, but all the patients were considered to be in extremis.

Intraventricular extension. The frequency of the extension of primary intracerebral hemorrhage to the ventricular system alters with the size of the hemorrhage, site, and proximity to the ventricles. Blood reaches the cerebrospinal fluid in a high percentage of cases mostly as a result of intraventricular rupture. Freytag[87] found that 75% of hematomas ruptured into the ventricular system filling all or part of the ventricular system. On occasions a secondary pontine or midbrain hemorrhage ruptured into it. Of 165 primary hemorrhages into the region of the basal ganglia, 143 ruptured into the ventricles (86.7%), whereas 96.7% of thalamic hematomas and only 39.5% of cerebellar hemorrhages extended into the ventricles. In the case of the pons, 65.1% ruptured into the ventricles. Crawford and Crompton[56] gave 93% as the overall frequency of intraventricular

rupture in their series of fatal cases of primary hemorrhage.

Varying degrees of intraventricular bleeding will be seen ranging from bloodstained ventricular fluid to acute hemocephalus in which the "red currant jelly" clot forms a cast of the ventricular system. Cappell[37] asserts that laceration with secondary hemorrhage may occur about the aqueduct. He did not state clearly if this was a complication of intraventricular hemorrhage nor did he discuss the relationship of this lesion to secondary brain stem hemorrhage.

Intraventricular hemorrhage, like that associated with a ruptured arterial aneurysm, may be associated with ventricular tamponade, for the rapid rise in intraventricular pressure causes laceration of the walls of the ventricles. Harris and associates[109] found three instances in which massive hemorrhage had occurred in the basal ganglia in association with acute hemocephalus and ventricular tamponade and with tears of the ventricular walls, particularly of the corners of the lateral ventricles. Similar lesions in the lateral ventricles were found in three more patients dying of massive cerebellar hemorrhage. The tears are probably overlooked in most cases.

In the past it was considered that death was inescapable after intraventricular rupture, but the evidence of extension of the hemorrhage to the ventricles in individuals surviving past intracerebral hemorrhage indicates that death is not invariably the sequel to this complication.

Subarachnoid hemorrhage. Blood reaches the subarachnoid space from primary intracerebral hemorrhage via the ventricular system, not by direct spread to the subarachnoid space. As a consequence, at autopsy a mild-to-moderate quantity of blood is to be found in the subarachnoid space, the greatest concentration being in the posterior fossa about the cerebellum and medulla. Direct extension from the hematoma to the subarachnoid space was found in only 15% of Freytag's series.[87] It is a likely outcome with massive hemorrhage into the cerebral white matter or into the cerebellum. Locally the hemorrhage is usually quite mild and is rarely massive.

The cerebrospinal fluid is almost universally blood stained if the bleeding is recent. Zimmerman[273] reported that the bloody fluid was found in 41 of the 45 cases of primary intracerebral hemorrhage in which the cerebrospinal fluid was examined, and McKissock and associates[161] reported the fluid to be clear and colorless in 20% of cases. The protein was raised in some and a few exhibited pleocytosis. The cerebrospinal fluid, clear initially, may become bloodstained at a subsequent lumbar puncture as the hematoma extends after secondary brain stem hemorrhage. There is danger in performing lumbar punctures in primary intracerebral hemorrhage, since the removal of much fluid from the lumbar sac can result in a further shift of brain tissue, aggravating the ill effects of herniation through the tentorium and foramen magnum.

Cytological examination of the cerebrospinal fluid can demonstrate a posthemorrhagic polymorphonuclear reaction with a peak on the second or third day. The fluid may also contain macrophages, possibly with ingested red cells and later hemosiderin.[232] Elevation of cerebrospinal fluid enzymes (creatine phosphokinase, aldolase, and lactic dehydrogenase) was a finding in each of 19 patients with intracerebral hemorrhage to a higher level then in nonhemorrhagic vascular lesions believed to be infarcts.[268] Xanthochromia is similar to that in any subarachnoid hemorrhage.

Subdural hematoma. Subdural hematoma complicates aneurysmal hemorrhage, but as a complication of primary intracerebral hemorrhage it is ever so much less frequent. Stehbens[238] found subdural hematoma in 1.6% of 380 cases of primary intracerebral hemorrhage in contrast to a frequency of 18.7% in association with a ruptured arterial aneurysm. In Stehbens' series an additional patient had an old subdural hematoma, which was excluded because chronologically it preceded the intracerebral hemorrhage. Freytag[87] reported

subdural hematomas in 6% of her series of primary intracerebral hematomas. It was found that cerebellar hemorrhages were most likely to involve the subdural space. Generally these subdural accumulations of blood are of minimal extent only. Close inspection of the head and scalp for evidence of trauma may reveal that the subdural hematoma is traumatic, occurring at the time of a fall when the subject lost consciousness.

Associated lesions of the central nervous system. It is not infrequent that additional lesions (softenings and hemorrhages other than secondary brain stem changes) are found in patients succumbing to primary intracerebral hemorrhage. They are often ignored once the major cause of death has been established but indicate the widespread and severe nature of the vascular disease that results in hemorrhage. Old softenings or lacunae are the most frequent lesions found with small accessory hemorrhages of secondary importance.

Greenacre[101] noted multiple hematomas in 24 of the 128 brains exhibiting primary intracerebral hemorrhage. The most usual combination was a massive hemorrhage into the region of the basal ganglia and a secondary pontine hemorrhage (15 brains or 11.7%). There were seven (5.5%) instances of bilateral symmetrical ganglionic hemorrhages. One brain contained hematomas in both the cerebrum and cerebellum. Another exhibited pontine and cerebellar hemorrhages. Fisher drew attention to the associated small hemorrhages and reported a frequency of 15.1%.

In 21 cases of cerebellar hemorrhage, Rey-Bellett[192] found old infarcts in the cerebral hemispheres in eight cases, a recent red infarct in the basal ganglia once, midbrain hemorrhage twice, basilar artery thrombosis with pontine softening once, and a small hematoma in one occipital pole once. In addition there was a chromophobe adenoma and an instance of lateral sclerosis.

Dinsdale[65] found old infarcts, previous hemorrhages, and lacunar states to be more frequent than the medical histories suggested. Indications of a previous disturbance were provided in 51% of cases with cerebellar hemorrhage and in only 26.4% of those with pontine hemorrhage. Dinsdale believed that the prevalence of advanced lacunar states was greater in his series than in a random series of hypertensives.

Freytag[87] found a lower frequency (25%) of previous vascular disturbances consisting of (1) old hematomas, mostly in the form of slitlike defects with xanthochromic walls (9%), and (2) old infarcts, small and usually multiple (16%). Crawford and Crompton[56] asserted that more than 25% of subjects dying from a recent primary intracerebral hemorrhage retain scars of old resolved brain hemorrhages, which are usually subcortical and in the external capsule and less often in the thalamus. There was evidence of rupture into the ventricular system in some.

Several softenings and small hemorrhagic foci should be expected in patients with primary intracerebral hemorrhage in view of age and long-standing hypertension. It is not known if the frequency is unduly high, as reliable detailed statistics are not available.

Circle of Willis. Saphir[206] suggested that certain variations of the circle of Willis could be associated with hemorrhage or softening within the cerebrum. Isolated cases were presented and the emphasis has since predominantly concerned ischemic lesions and arterial aneurysms. Fisher[83] found no relationship between (1) the size of the vertebral and cerebellar arteries, and (2) the configuration of the circle of Willis, and the side on which a cerebellar hematoma was found. He suggested that thalamic hemorrhages arose mostly in brains in which the supply to the posterior cerebral artery was predominantly from the internal carotid rather than from the basilar. It would be difficult indeed to study in detail the hemodynamic changes in blood flow through various areas of the brain engendered as a result of anatomical variations in the circle of Willis. A carotid-basilar anastomosis occurs as an incidental finding at autopsy and has been found with intracranial aneurysms, but they are apparently absent in cases of primary intracerebral hemorrhage.

Smith and associates[229] encountered a massive hemorrhage destroying the basal ganglia, thalamus, and internal capsule of the right cerebral hemisphere in a woman of 53 years with grossly idiopathic narrowing of both internal carotid arteries. Postmortem angiography revealed prominent proliferation of collateral channels through the basal ganglia of the left hemisphere. The blood for both hemispheres was derived predominantly from the vertebrobasilar system. Fisher[81] had previously reported two instances of hemorrhage on the same side as an occlusion of the carotid arterial system in early life. Hemorrhage was believed to originate from unusually large anastomotic and collateral vessels (secondarily formed).

Atherosclerosis of the cerebral arteries (moderate to severe) is usually though not always a feature in these patients. The severity however does not tend to be as prominent as in fatal cases in which cerebral softenings are found but is noticeably greater than in patients with cerebral aneurysms.

Yates and Hutchinson[272] contend that primary intracerebral hemorrhage in association with atherosclerotic stenosis or occlusion of large extracranial arteries was sufficiently rare to intimate that the obstructive lesion may afford a degree of protection to the brain distally. Reduction in blood pressure within the brain distal to the stenosis or occlusion could play a role in the phenomenon.

Frequency and age distribution of primary intracerebral hemorrhage are not dissimilar from those of intracranial arterial aneurysm, and in some hypertensive individuals the lesions coexist, as reported first by Moore[170] in 1880. Beadles[19] found 33 cases of unruptured cerebral aneurysm. In half, death had occurred after bleeding from a small central artery. Stehbens[235] recorded 11 cases of unruptured cerebral aneurysms in association with primary intracerebral hemorrhage. The hematoma may be intracerebral, pontine, or cerebellar, which illustrates the importance of a thorough examination of the cerebral arteries at autopsy in all cases of intracranial bleeding. Clinically the association of these two diseases adds to the recognized difficulty in the differential diagnosis, and angiography in such instances can mislead.

Secondary pressure complications. As with any rapidly enlarging supratentorial lesion, hemorrhages into the cerebrum, possibly accentuated by ventricular tamponade, cause secondary pressure complications in association with the herniation of the cerebrum through the tentorium and of the cerebellum into the foramen magnum. The rapidity with which intracerebral hematomas enlarge enhances the chances of secondary brain stem hemorrhage. The secondary changes are critical in determining the severity of the lesions, for singly or in conjunction they may substantially set the stage for or precipitate death. Attwater,[12] the first to describe the phenomenon, drew attention to its frequency with primary intracerebral hemorrhage. Multiple small hemorrhages that may become confluent one with another and with similar hemorrhages in the pons may be found in the elongated and flattened midbrain and may be so severe that the brain stem lesion is as massive as any primary pontine hemorrhage. Alternatively the hemorrhagic lesion in the brain stem may become confluent with the primary hemorrhage in the cerebrum. Freytag[87] reported secondary edema and hemorrhage in the brain stem in 54% of patients with intracerebral hemorrhages. In several others the midbrain was involved by direct extension from a thalamic hemorrhage, and if brain stem hemorrhage is caused by displacement of brain tissue from raised supratentorial pressure, one suspects that similar lesions may occur elsewhere. Fisher,[83] for example, found a hemorrhagic infarct adjacent to

an intracerebral hemorrhage in two subjects and considered the infarct secondary and the hemorrhage primary. No secondary vascular lesions have as yet been associated with herniation under the falx cerebri except locally in the herniated cingulate gyrus.

Greenacre[101] encountered a patient with a cerebellar hemorrhage in association with pontine hemorrhage. Rey-Bellett[192] reported a hemorrhage into the tegmentum of the midbrain in association with cerebellar hemorrhage, and another subject with a cerebellar hemorrhage exhibited hemorrhage about the aqueduct of Sylvius and the substantia nigra on one side. No indication of the sizes of the hematomas was provided. Whether or not cerebellar hemorrhage could, by means of distortion of the aqueduct of Sylvius and the production of acute hemocephalus, result in secondary brain stem lesions is unknown, and in these reports no reference was made to the extent of ventricular dilatation. The midbrain lesions in Rey-Bellett's two cases could have been caused by upward displacement of and pushing of the midbrain up through the tentorial opening.

Associated extracranial lesions. Subhyaloid hemorrhage can complicate massive intracerebral hemorrhages.[80] The association is less frequent than with ruptured intracranial arterial aneurysm.

The frequency of hypertension and obesity as well as the age distribution of patients with primary intracerebral hemorrhage is adequate explanation for the severity of aortic and coronary atherosclerosis associated with these lesions.[207] The severity of atherosclerosis however need not be unduly prominent in malignant hypertension. Primary intracerebral hemorrhage is but a complication of hypertensive cardiovascular disease, and consequently left ventricular hypertrophy, hypertensive nephrosclerosis, albuminuria, associated retinal changes, and myocardial lesions[127] are likely to be found. The associated pathological lesions will vary according to the cause of the hypertension if it is secondary.

Transient hyperglycemia[65] and glycosuria may be present[2,10] though the reasons are not clear. Because of the large hematoma, a neutrophil leukocytosis may eventuate with values of 12,000 to 25,000 and rarely up to 40,000 cells per cu. mm.[10] Many patients develop extensive pulmonary edema, and if the survival is prolonged, bronchopneumonia contributes to the causation of leukocytosis.

Sieber[222] surveying the literature on polycystic disease of the kidneys found that 10 of 212 patients died of "cerebral hemorrhage." This is to be expected[23,49] because polycystic kidneys are associated with hypertension in some 75% of cases.[208] The association of ruptured intracranial aneurysms with renal cystic disease[236] has been emphasized, but it is presumption pure and simple to suggest that all instances of intracranial hemorrhage in association with this disease are aneurysmal in origin, for some are quite definitely primary intracerebral hemorrhages. The latter can complicate coarctation of the aorta, although other secondary manifestations, for example, subarachnoid hemorrhage and ruptured intracranial aneurysm[236] have been stressed. Other congenital abnormalities and related lesions, differing in severity from the insignificant to deformities like pes cavus and talipes equinovarus, are seen in patients with primary intracerebral hemorrhages, but the association is not significant.[236]

Factors precipitating hemorrhage. Factors likely to precipitate primary intracerebral hemorrhage have not been positively ascertained. Some patients are found in bed in a comatose state. Others collapse suddenly during waking hours with few prodromal symptoms. Factors like injury, strenuous exertion, and severe emotional strain are often implicated.[54,59] The acute rise in blood pressure may be an important factor in precipitating the bleeding, but precisely how important is difficult to assess. However, as with aneurysmal bleeding, which is the end result of a chronic disease process, abrupt increases in blood

pressure are probably not prerequisite for the onset of the hemorrhage. Extremes of temperature have been incriminated in precipitating the hemorrhage,[59] but the significance of climatic factors is difficult to assess.

Primary intracerebral hemorrhage, as distinct from eclamptic hemorrhage, occasionally complicates pregnancy or labor,[16] but its association with menstruation, pregnancy, or parity is not significant.

The administration of vasopressor drugs has precipitated intracerebral hemorrhage but in atypical sites.[83] It is not known if the acute rise in blood pressure actually precipitates primary or secondary intracerebral hemorrhage.

Hypertension. Moser and Goldman[172] estimated that 8 to 10 million persons in the United States had significantly elevated blood pressure, a major contributory factor in a high proportion of deaths caused by cardiovascular, cerebrovascular, and renovascular disease. It has long been causally related to and incriminated in the early onset of cerebrovascular disease in general. With left ventricular hypertrophy it is the most characteristic feature found in association with primary intracerebral hemorrhage.[15] Some authors exclude nonhypertensives from their series by defining primary intracerebral hemorrhage as a disease exclusively of hypertensives. Although hypertension is found in a high percentage of the victims of the disease, a large series of cases, from which obviously secondary hemorrhages are excluded, will include a few subjects apparently normotensive and not infrequently senile.

Of 380 cases of primary intracerebral hemorrhage collected from autopsy records,[237,238] a description of the heart was available in 347 (193 males and 154 females). Left ventricular hypertrophy or a heart weight in excess of 420 gm. in the male and 400 gm. in the female (exclusive of valvular disease) was regarded as indicative of left ventricular hypertrophy probably in association with hypertension. Thus, 90.7% of males exhibited left ventricular hypertrophy and 85.7% of the females (88.5% of the combined series). Some of the remaining patients probably had hypertension, since it is difficult to be certain whether it existed during life when autopsy findings provide the only criteria. In 21 of the remaining patients the heart weight was below 320 gm. and, of these, 19 failed to exhibit any granularity of the renal subcapsular surface.

These subjects, if not hypertensive, are either examples of secondary hemorrhage or of primary intracerebral hemorrhage in normotensives. Johansson and Melin[127] consider that too much emphasis has been placed on the presence of hypertension in cerebral hemorrhage and that the incidence in many series was too high. In this disease where multiple factors in differing combinations are at work, a complete correlation between cerebral hemorrhage and hypertension should not be expected. They found that hemorrhage into the basal ganglia was four times more frequent in hypertensives than in nonhypertensives. Little difference in the frequency was noted when the hemorrhage was located elsewhere in the cerebral white matter. These authors recorded hypertension in only 62% of 162 cases, a very low incidence. Similar findings resulted from Johansson's study.[126] The consensus however is that hypertension exists in a considerably higher proportion of cases than he allowed. It may be primary (often labeled as essential) or secondary. The causes of secondary hypertension are numerous and include chronic pyelonephritis, chronic glomerulonephritis, polycystic disease of the kidneys, aberrant renal artery, coarctation of the aorta, pheochromocytoma, Cushing's syndrome, and lead poisoning. Nothing indicates that the incidence of primary intracerebral hemorrhages shows any variation when in association with a particular cause of hypertension. Russell[203] contends that pontine hemorrhage is more prevalent when the hypertension is of nephritic origin.

Cerebrovascular lesions, major or minor, hemorrhagic or ischemic, are the frequent complications of long-standing hypertension. Again the reported incidence varies from author to author. Bell and Clawson[24] studied the autopsies of 420 hypertensive subjects and found that although the primary cause of death was cardiac, apoplexy (encephalomalacia and hemorrhage) was responsible for 19.3% of the deaths. In a later report, Bell[22] asserted that 53% of the fatal cerebral lesions in hypertension were hemorrhages and 47% were softenings. Apoplexy was given as the cause of death in 13.7% of the fatalities in Janeway's hypertensive patients.[124] Once more one cannot be certain how many of these were caused by hemorrhage. Primary intracerebral hemorrhage was found in 11.9% at autopsy. Paullin and associates[180] reviewed the complications of 500 hypertensive patients clinically and found that 7.2% had suffered intracerebral hemorrhages. Smith and associates[227] studied the necropsy results of 376 hypertensive subjects, excluding those in which there was a recognized causative factor such as polycystic kidneys and glomerulonephritis. There were 56 cerebrovascular accidents (14.9%) including only primary intracerebral hemorrhage and encephalomalacia. An unspecified number were excluded because death was caused by a ruptured intracranial aneurysm, which would make the actual incidence of death from cerebral causes higher than indicated.

Hudson and Hyland[118] reviewed 100 fatal cases of hypertension, and in 16% the initial symptom was "stroke." Of the entire series 85% were conservatively estimated to have episodes of encephalomalacia or intracerebral hemorrhage. Death was caused by massive intracerebral hemorrhage in 31% and by terminal vascular occlusion in 11%. In addition 10% had had nonfatal hemorrhages (1 to 3.5 cm. in diameter) with half of these patients dying of new massive hemorrhages (excluding secondary brain stem lesions). There was mental deterioration varying from failing memory and mental lethargy to gross dementia necessitating institutional care in 18%.

Cole and Yates[48] found 51 of the 100 hypertensive patients dying in a general hospital had either ischemic or hemorrhagic lesions in their brains, but that only 24 of a similar though normotensive series (100 patients) were so afflicted. One normotensive patient had a massive intracerebral hemorrhage that was attributed to a "small vascular malformation." Of the hypertensive subjects, 20 had primary intracerebral hemorrhage. A similar predilection for hypertension was noted in the case of small hemorrhages, with 13 hypertensives affected but no normotensives.

Simpson and Gilchrist[224] in determining the prognosis of hypertensive vascular disease found that the 5-year mortality for 299 hypertensive hospital patients varied with the severity of the retinopathy: 75% with grade 1 retinal changes survived, with a gradation to only 1 survivor of 70 patients with the most severe retinal changes (grade IV). Cerebrovascular accidents accounted for 42% of deaths in the group with benign hypertension and 31% of the group with accelerated and malignant hypertension. Others[20,231] have also found that the mortality increases according to the severity of the retinal changes. No information concerning the frequency of intracerebral hemorrhage in relation to the differing grades of retinal change was provided. As primary intracerebral hemorrhage is virtually confined to hypertensive subjects, and the author is unaware of any reported instances in hypotensive subjects, the frequency of intracerebral hemorrhage might be expected to be more prevalent among those with the most severe grade of hypertension and retinal changes. No information is available on this aspect, and little is available concerning the location of cerebral lesions with this grade of hypertension and retinal change. Russell[203] found pontine hemorrhages predominant among patients with the severer grades of hypertension, and Dickinson and Thomson[63] found a significantly greater heart weight with hindbrain hemorrhages than with those in the forebrain. No significant difference was established in the heart weight between patients with cerebral and cerebellar hemorrhages.[34] The mean heart weight in females with primary pontine hemorrhage was significantly greater than in those with intracerebral hemorrhage without secondary pontine hemorrhage. No significant difference occurred in males. However no substantiated correlation between heart weight and the severity of hypertension has been proved, and it appears that heart weight relates more closely to the age of the patient and the duration of the hypertension.

Sokolow and Perloff[231] in a large series of hypertensive patients recorded death from intracerebral hemorrhage in 18% of males and 28% of females. In cerebral thrombosis it was 8% in the male and 14% in the female. Aring and Merritt[10] contend that hypertension is more severe among those dying of hemorrhage than among those who had encephalomalacia terminally. Dinsdale[65] found no correlation between the height of the blood pressure and the size of the hematoma, nor is there a known relationship between the length of survival after an intracerebral hemorrhage and the severity of the blood pressure.

In hypertensive patients dying of intracerebral hemorrhage, Fishberg[79] considered the intracerebral hemorrhage to be a constant danger threatening life. The evidence suggests that the hypertension, unless of the malignant variety, has been present for many years. Perera[183] noted that many individuals survive more than 25 years after the initial diagnosis of hypertension. Of the 150 subjects investigated, the peak age of onset was between 30 and 40 years and the peak age of death fell between 50 and 60 years, demonstrating a course of at least 20 years. In another study of subjects whose hypertension had a documented onset prior to the age of 25 years, 73% were still alive after 20 years.[184] The age of onset does not seem to influence the rate of the progression of the disease.

Fishberg[79] indicated that statistics concerning the causes of death in hypertension may be fallacious because of underestimation of the deaths from extraneous causes unrelated to heart, brain, and kidney. He believes that the deaths of many hypertensive patients in nonmedical wards are excluded from current statistics. This theory will become increasingly difficult to appraise because of the wide use of antihypertensive drugs.

The effect of antihypertensive therapy on cerebrovascular disease continues to be discussed. Many, if not most, hypertensive patients are not seen until rather late in the course of the disease when the effects of long-standing hypertension on the cerebral vasculature have already been well established. The earlier treatment is commenced the better the result is likely to be, and although complete restoration is improbable, progression and aggravation can be lessened.

Surgical treatment of hypertension by sympathectomy and adrenalectomy, it has been reported, prolongs the survival of patients with severe hypertension.[28]

Medical treatment, now supplementing surgical procedures, has rendered demonstrable improvement in mortality figures and survival rates for both benign and malignant hypertension. Indications then are that the complications of hypertension, including primary intracerebral hemorrhage, are beneficially influenced by such therapeutic measures[172] to the extent that Moser and Goldman[172] asserted that they had not seen in the previous 8 years cerebral hemorrhage in any patient under 55 years whose blood pressure had been controlled.

The overall frequency of intracerebral hemorrhage has declined drastically in treated hypertensives although it still occurs in patients in the older age groups. The decline in mortality is independent of the drug or combination of drugs used nor does the reduction in blood pressure so induced appear to precipitate ischemic change to any extent.[173]

Antihypertensive therapy has prolonged the life of patients with malignant or accelerated hypertension.[26] The impressive reduction in the frequency of renal failure has led to a change in the appearance of fatal complications, and cerebral and cardiac causes of death have become proportionately more frequent.[172]

There has been no controlled pathological study of the cerebral vasculature of hypertensive patients treated with antihypertensive drugs, though such an investigation is indicated.

Microscopic appearance. Microscopic examination of the extensive hemorrhage usually discloses a mass of clotted blood in which there are few parenchymal structures. The fixation, infiltration, and cutting of such large masses constitute quite a problem, as artifacts are difficult to avoid. The brain at the margin of the hematoma exhibits necrosis, edema, and multiple small extravasations of red cells, which are often perivascular.

The walls of small arteries may be necrotic and infiltrated with fibrin and red cells (Fig. 8-12), many being thickened and exhibiting diffuse hyperplastic sclerosis or arteriosclerosis. Arterioles may be thickened and hyaline, and there is a great range in the severity of the vascular changes. Indeed degenerative changes are at times inconspicuous. If a sufficient number of samples is selected from the edges of the hematoma, an occasional miliary aneurysm, dissecting aneurysm, or an apparently ruptured vessel will be found, but the search must be thorough. In the ordinary course of events in which only one or possibly two blocks are removed for histological examination, the vascular changes are usually missed. Aneurysmal dilatation can be better demonstrated upon examination of the vessel in three dimensions or by microangiography rather than by random histological sections.

With the patients surviving for varying periods of time, progressive histological changes in organization of the hematoma will be found at the periphery where edema and infiltration of polymorphonuclear leukocytes are easily seen and are succeeded by the infiltration and proliferation of microglia. As demyelination proceeds in necrotic brain tissue at the edge

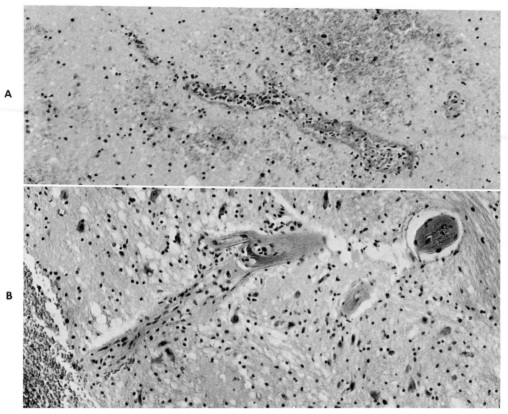

Fig. 8-12. Two vessels in **A** exhibit fibrinoid necrosis, and brain is necrotic and infiltrated with blood. **B,** Vessels neighboring a recent hematoma are infiltrated with fibrin or fibrinoid. (Hematoxylin and eosin, ×110.)

of the hematoma, lipid-laden macrophages accumulate. Hemosiderin appears in the macrophages by the sixth day according to Strassmann[245] and according to some authors earlier. Hematoidin, a canary yellow pigment, appears both intracellularly and extracellularly after 10 to 14 days. Mixing of the pigments is not uncommon, but zones of one or other pigment still occur in isolation. At this stage there commences gliosis and proliferation of vessels about the periphery, polymorphonuclear leukocytes are scanty or absent, but round cells occasionally cuff the vessels.

The appearance of the contents of the hematoma alters progressively from dark red currant jelly to dark chocolate and finally to an orange-brown gelatinous liquid. The leukocytes in the hematoma undergo necrosis, and the red cells ultimately hemolyze and disintegrate. No detailed morphological and chemical study of the age changes in the extravasated blood have been reported. Absorption of the breakdown products occurs, and eventually, if the hematoma is small, the cavity shrinks and a slitlike cavity, still containing a considerable quantity of blood pigment, manifests itself. The length of the period that hemosiderin-laden macrophages or siderophages remain in such a lesion is problematical but judging from indirect evidence at other sites, such pigment-laden cells may persist in situ for many years, possibly even indefinitely. Pigment is possibly removed completely or almost completely from small lesions and consequently differentiation from small softenings that may also contain siderophages can be difficult. Hematoidin is not present in old

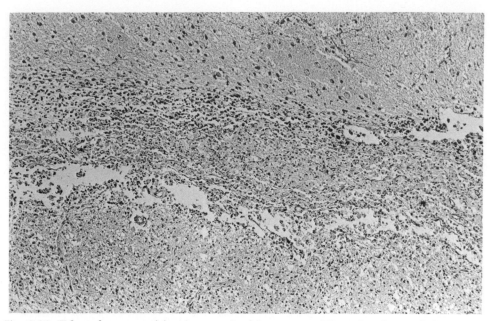

Fig. 8-13. Edge of an organizing intracerebral hematoma. There is a layer of degenerating lysed red cells at the top with a few invading macrophages, and then the capsule, a layer of granulation tissue, many siderophages, and a few fibroblasts above a loose zone or space. Finally at the bottom is the neighboring brain in which there is gliosis demyelination, vessel proliferation, and some lipophages and siderophages. (Hematoxylin and eosin, ×45).

hematomas, but iron incrustation of connective tissues can occur. The unusual bluish green blood pigments so often seen about aged splenic infarcts have not been described within the brain.

A distinct capsule ultimately walls off large hematomas (Fig. 8-13) after a month.[41] Microscopically the center of the encapsulated hematoma contains necrotic debris and disintegrating blood clot. At the periphery macrophages may be loose within the mass and contain red cells, debris, or altered blood pigment, though some have a foamy cytoplasm. The capsule itself consists of glial tissue, a variable quantity of fibrous tissue containing fibroblasts, newly proliferated vessels, and, in the interstices, numerous macrophages with a few round cells. Blood pigment is naturally prominent. Siderophages may be more obvious on the inner aspect and gitter cells in the outer portion (Fig. 8-13). External to this capsule is an indefinite zone of loose tissue containing macro-

phages. It separates the capsule macroscopically from the surrounding brain which also exhibits gliosis.

In very large, long-standing hematomas cholesterol clefts and calcification can be found but hematomas of this age and size are rare.

Mortality. Primary intracerebral hemorrhage is not one of the causes of sudden death,[199] though the onset of coma may be fairly sudden. Death rarely ensues within the first hour, and if it does, the case is generally referred to the coroner or medical examiner.[21] Thus the early deaths are not usually encountered in general hospitals.

Premonitory symptoms and signs, such as headache, vertigo, transient paresthesias, motor defects, and visual disturbances are frequent and may precede the loss of consciousness by a very variable time interval.[250] Symptoms such as sudden loss of consciousness, deepening coma, evidence of hemiplegia, and bloodstained cerebrospinal fluid under increased pressure usually indicate primary intracerebral hemorrhage. The outlook is usually regarded as hopeless to the extent that recovery casts doubt on the accuracy of the diagnosis. Survival however depends on both the site and the dimensions of the hematoma. If the hemorrhage is massive, a few patients may linger several weeks but the large hematomas are quite lethal, and authors tend to discuss the length of the survival rather than numbers surviving. Moreover, large encapsulated hematomas are extremely rare at autopsy.

In a series encompassing cases in which information was available concerning the duration of the illness,[239] of 368 cases 19% died within the first 6 hours, the shortest survival periods being 1½ to 2 hours. Within the first 24 hours, 51% had died, 64% within 48 hours, 74% in 3 days, 78% in 4 days, 87% by the end of the first week, and only five subjects survived longer than 1 month. The longest survival was 3 months. Freytag[87] reported a more rapid demise, with 65% dying within the first 24 hours, but 96% within the first week. All medical examiner's cases were included in Freytag's series,[87] and the disease is recognized as a cause of early and unexpected rather than sudden death.[113] Pontine and cerebellar hemorrhage tend to be rapidly fatal,[120,167] and in Freytag's series, 94% of those with pontine hemorrhage were dead within 24 hours and 83% of those with cerebellar hemorrhage died within this time, as against only 40% of cases with intracerebral hemorrhage. One of Dinsdale's 30 cases[65] of pontine hemorrhage did not die from the lesion. The patient recovered from the small hemorrhage but died shortly afterward from myocardial infarction. An old encapsulated pontine hematoma of significant size has not been reported.

An extremely poor prognosis has been established. Adams and Cohen[2] found only two "old" hematomas in an analysis of 69 cases of primary intracerebral hemorrhage, citing the low incidence as evidence of infrequent recovery. Fisher[83] reported 37 old hematomas among 102 autopsied cases of primary intracerebral hemorrhage, a frequency of 36%. In another study, Fisher[83] found 14 primary intracerebral hemorrhages among 200 autopsies and, of these, six were old and only eight were recent. Few pathologists would agree with Fisher's figures for apparent long survival and the criteria used in his study to distinguish an old hemorrhage from encephalomalacia remain in question. Furthermore, Fisher included small hemorrhages less than 3 cm. in diameter, although most authors would have excluded them,[203] for they are widely recognized as being not nearly so lethal.

Crawford and Crompton[56] indicated that over 25% of their cases of primary intracerebral hemorrhage exhibited evidence of old hematomas, some with intraventricular hemorrhage. They suggested that an appreciable number of people survive intracerebral hemorrhage despite intraventricular rupture. The view was put forward that recovery may be very satisfactory because it may be that little tissue damage is sustained with fiber-splitting hemorrhages.

It is not unusual certainly to find either small slitlike lesions heavily infiltrated with siderophages or tiny, slightly brown cystlike lesions or lacunae. Rightly or wrongly the brown lesions or lacunae are frequently presumed to be old hemorrhages, but their small dimensions are not comparable to those of the hematomas usually seen at autopsy and designated primary intracerebral hemorrhage. The current view of pathologists is that the prognosis of primary intracerebral hemorrhage as they know it, is grim in the extreme. According to the size of the lesion, the view can be modified. However, to discuss the frequency and mortality of small intracerebral hemorrhages, which cannot satisfactorily be diagnosed as such clinically, is not profitable. It is merely assumed that in a high percentage of cases the patients survive. McKissock and associates[160] asserted that the mortality of primary intracerebral hemorrhage (exclusive of pontine and cerebellar hemorrhage) is about 51% when patients are conservatively treated. This figure, astonishing as it is in view of current convictions of the almost inevitably fatal outcome of the disease, lends considerable support to the views of Fisher[83] and Crawford and Crompton.[56] Yet again no indication of the size of the hematomas under consideration is provided and to disregard this point is unsound, since it is the aspect with direct and totally unavoidable bearing on the results of the study of such series. Furthermore, in clinical studies the true etiology of the hemorrhage in the survivors cannot be said to be beyond doubt; so conclusions drawn may not be valid.

Etiology and pathogenesis. Primary intracerebral hemorrhage is a frequently seen, well-recognized complication of primary and secondary hypertension. As a topic it has been considered mundane, yet the etiology has been controversial.

General considerations. Although not absolutely essential, the most important predisposing factor is said to be hypertension. The associated arterial degenerative changes that inevitably accompany the elevated blood pressure can be regarded as indispensable. Changes occurring in specific parenchymal arteries appear to lead ultimately to rupture. They arise particularly in cases of long-standing hypertension but are not found in the larger arteries at the base of the brain nor in arteries elsewhere in the body. The only extracranial site at which hemorrhage is consistent in hypertension is the retina and the changes in retinal vessels may not be related to those responsible for primary intracerebral hemorrhage, for gross spontaneous bleeding does not occur in the eye as in the brain. A physical and functional characteristic of the cerebral circulation results in a predisposition to primary intracerebral hemorrhage, and attempts at the explanation have been made on morphological grounds. The thinness of intracranial arteries and veins and the unique architectural arrangement of elastic tissue have been invoked as etiological factors. The small arteries and arterioles within the brain and cord do not seem to develop frequently the degree of luminal narrowing and mural thickening found in the splanchnic circulation.

Greenacre[101] attributed the frequency of hemorrhage from the lateral lenticulostriate arteries to their angle of branching from the middle cerebral artery, believing that the pressure was unduly high when compared with that of other vessels of comparable diameter. Jain[123] maintains that in these vessels the tendency to rupture is caused by the ready reduction in intravascular blood pressure and flow due to their recurrent angle of origin. Stephens and Stilwell[244] point out that the recurrent artery of Heubner also arises at an obtuse angle from the side of the anterior cerebral artery and that its intracerebral course, somewhat more anteriorly situated, is otherwise identical to that of the lateral lenticulostriate arteries. Thus they affirm that when hemorrhage involves the putamen and external capsule, the assumption that the hemorrhage arises from a lenticulostriate vessel and not Heubner's artery is questionable. Friedman and Nielsen[90] allege that the relative infrequency of hemorrhage and lacunar sclerosis in the cerebellum had to do with the liberal anastomoses of cerebellar blood vessels and also lower pressure than in the basal perforating branches. Until direct physiological measurements of pressure and flow in such vessels are forthcoming, the opinions are speculative. Moreover, the reason for sites of special predilection for intracerebral hemorrhage may well depend on hemodynamic factors rather than vascular structural differences.

Capillary fragility, it has been reported, increases in some hypertensives.[104] Whether this holds true for the cerebral capillary bed is unknown. However it is generally thought that the intracerebral bleeding is not primarily from capillaries.

Scheinker[212] postulated that recurrent vasoparalytic episodes in hypertension lead to periods of stasis and congestion in veins and capillaries rather than in arteries. Ultimately permanent structural alterations ensue, namely, distension, thinning, atrophy, and necrosis of venous walls, and consequently these vessels become incapable of withstanding even transient increases in venous pressure. The prospect is rupture, the size of the hematoma being dependent on the caliber of the vein. This theory, not being corroborated, has largely been ignored, for the rapidity of the onset of the hemorrhage has led most authors to take for granted that the bleeding is arterial in origin.

Atherosclerosis of the major intracranial arteries is in general more severe in subjects with primary intracerebral hemorrhage than in control individuals. Though primary intracerebral hemorrhage has sometimes been loosely ascribed to atherosclerosis, the association of the two diseases seems to be attributed to the hypertension. Arteriosclerosis and long-standing hypertension have been accepted as etiological factors of importance and cannot be divorced from each other. In a brain containing such a hematoma, it is extremely difficult to demonstrate the site of the ruptured vessel. Many vessels are damaged and torn, some possibly in removal and handling of the brain and others from dissection by the enlarging hematoma. The small intracerebral arteries, from which the bleeding proceeds, are only occasionally observed to have collections of foam cells in the thickened intima. Infiltration of lipid droplets in the walls of miliary aneurysms and arteriosclerotic intracerebral arteries has been demonstrated[100] and is probably akin to similar phenomena in splanchnic vessels,[240] though such changes are not usually classified as atherosclerosis, even if related to it. It has been suggested that primary intracerebral hemorrhage results from the rupture of an atheromatous ulcer,[31] but conceding that the intracerebral vessels are atherosclerotic, one would find the severity not sufficient to cause ulceration to the degree seen in the aorta and other large arteries.

Degenerative changes in the intracerebral vessels are of signal import in the etiology of primary intracerebral hemorrhage. Whether these arteriosclerotic changes are related to atherosclerosis, or are the small vessel counterpart of this disease or even constitute an independent disease entity are matters for serious consideration. It has nevertheless been assumed outright that, as in atherosclerosis of larger arteries and in the aorta in dissecting aneurysm,[237,242] the vessel walls are of diminished tensile strength.

Lampert and Mueller[137] found that cerebral vessels were very difficult to rupture even with pressures as high as 1520 mm. Hg. Only two in a series of 30 brains revealed rupture of vessels. Both were syphilitic. In 10 hypertensive individuals the pressures caused rupture in two. Such abnormal pressures are never encountered during life and postmortem experiments are of course always open to indefensible criticism. The experiments are cited as evidence against hypertension alone causing the hemorrhage. Yet one might say that in practice a frequency of 20% among hypertensives correlates moderately well with that of intracerebral hemorrhage as a complication of hypertension. Certainly some pathological process bringing in its train weakening of the vessel wall is needed to produce hemorrhage. It is however the nature of the lesion responsible that has been the most controversial feature. In postmortem angiography the intracerebral vessels rupture, and leakage of the injected medium appears to occur fairly readily.[45,47,204] Extensive investigation of the tensile strength of the walls of intracerebral vessels in various pathological states is warranted.

Feigin and Prose[76] observed infiltration of the walls of small intracerebral arteries with fibrinlike material and termed the phenomena "fibrinoid arteritis." The changes were seen primarily in parenchymal arteries, most often in the basal ganglia, and less frequently in the cerebral cortex, cerebellum, and pons. Veins were affected rarely and several times the authors thought there was some focal aneurysmal dilatation. Hyaline thickening of vessels was frequently observed in such brains in association with vessels exhibiting fibrinoid changes. Thrombi were seen occasionally in the vessels. Inflammatory changes were often observed, with the cellular infiltrate consisting more often than not of lymphocytes, large mononuclear cells, fibroblasts, and infrequently of plasma cells, eosinophils, or multinucleated giant cells. In a few cases the polymorphonuclear leukocytes were predominant. Perivascular gliosis and small focal paravascular softenings containing appreciable numbers of pigment-laden macrophages were also found. The changes were observed only after careful intensive search in 15 hypertensive patients with massive intracerebral hemorrhage. But they also occurred in seven other patients, five of whom displayed cerebral softenings. During the same period of observation, normotensive individuals and 16 other patients with primary intracerebral hemorrhage were investigated, but the vascular changes were absent. Feigin and Prose[76] believed these vascular changes to be specifically related to the etiology of primary intracerebral hemorrhage.

Ikeda and colleagues[121] induced hypertension in rabbits by placing constricting clamps on the renal arteries and in some animals one kidney was extirpated. The severity of the hypertension so produced varied, and fibrinoid necrosis (recent and old) was observed in the small arteries and arterioles not only in the brain but in other organs. Significant cerebral hemorrhages were observed in 41.9% of 74 animals and visceral hemorrhages were also prevalent in rabbits with or without cerebral lesions. The bearing that results of such experiments has on the human problem is uncertain although the appearance of visceral hemorrhages as well as cerebral is more suggestive of a necrotizing vasculitis than malignant hypertension.

Prehemorrhagic softening. Rochoux[200] is credited with initiating the concept of prehemorrhagic softening of the brain as a precursor to primary intracerebral softening. This theory has enjoyed considerable popularity. Basically entailed is some vascular disturbance to an area of brain sufficient to alter the normal brain consistency, thereby reducing the natural tissue support of the adventitial surface of the blood vessels. This inequality in pressures has been thought to increase the susceptibility of the artery to rupture.

In view of the age distribution of primary intracerebral hemorrhage, it is inevitable that in some cases bleeding will by chance involve otherwise unrelated preexisting softenings or lacunae. But this cannot constitute proof of a theory excluding secondary pontine hemorrhage in which pontine softening secondary to a raised supratentorial pressure may accompany or precede the bleeding.

The theory has undergone modification. One popular variant has concerned angiospasm. [31,94] Vasospasm was thought to cause ischemia distally with stasis in the capillaries and venules, followed by massive diapedesis therefrom. Relief from the spasm, with restoration of the circulation, is associated with even further bleeding. Schwartz[216] believed that cerebral vessels, particularly in hypertension, were hyperirritable, that vasospasm of neurogenic origin resulted in ischemic changes with massive diapedesis of red cells to produce a confluent hematoma, and that infarction and primary intracerebral hemorrhage were the extremes of a range within the bounds of which all gradations lay. Currently the two diseases are regarded as separate and distinct entities.

Globus and his colleagues,[94-97] strong proponents of the theory, emphasized the frequency of clinical and pathological evidence of preceding ischemic episodes. Although these subjects often have evidence of old vascular lesions in the brain, it is usually not possible to demonstrate preexisting softenings in the region of massive hemorrhage. Globus and Epstein[95] placed clips on the middle cerebral artery about 2 to 3 mm. distal to the origin and in a few animals perivascular hemorrhages transpired. Some hemorrhages became confluent but their mode of formation remained obvious. Other animals were injected with Neo-Synephrine at varying intervals of the clipping procedure and sacrificed the following day. Hemorrhage was more massive and associated with subarachnoid hemorrhage and in two instances with intraventricular hemorrhage. Necrotic vessels were found, but it was not stated if evidence of the old infarction was obscured by the hemorrhage, and in some animals no hemorrhage was found. Scheinker[209] insists that these experimental lesions are classical hemorrhagic softenings rather than ganglionic hemorrhages (primary intracerebral hemorrhage), and a good many pathologists agree but some still espouse the concept.

Primary intracerebral hemorrhage superimposed on a preexisting softening is not necessarily proof of an etiological relationship. Then again the vascular changes responsible for the development of parenchymal softenings or lacunae are also those responsible for the hemorrhage, and coexistence of the lesions at times is very likely.

Miliary aneurysms (microaneurysms). In 1869 Charcôt and Bouchard[42] proposed that primary intracerebral hemorrhage was the result of the rupture of small aneurysms on the intracerebral arteries and called them miliary aneurysms. Thus the term, should not be used in allusion to the "berry" type of saccular aneurysm of the large arteries at the base of the brain. The conclusion was reached after study of brains of subjects dying of primary intracerebral hemorrhage and the miliary aneurysms were disclosed when the parenchyma was washed away with running water. The lesions had been described previously[107] but Charcôt and Bouchard in their papers popularized the theory.[30,41,42] Gull[107] had been the first to attribute such hemorrhage to a miliary aneurysm.

Charcôt and Bouchard[42] described miliary aneurysms as being 0.2 to 1 mm. in diameter on the intracerebral vessels and as

saccular, fusiform, and irregular dilatations, occurring most often in the thalamus and corpora striata, and with diminishing frequency also in the pons, cerebral cortex, claustrum, cerebellum, cerebellar peduncles, and lastly the centrum ovale. Charcôt[41] found miliary aneurysms quite readily on the surface of the cerebral cortex after stripping the pia arachnoid. The dilatations were attributed to a diffuse periarteritis unrelated to atheroma, and Charcôt and Bouchard[42] stressed that the miliary aneurysms were the direct cause of the primary intracerebral hemorrhage. Charcôt[41] observed the coexistence of intracerebral miliary aneurysms and saccular arterial aneurysms of the berry type at the base of the brain. Controversy regarding the nature of miliary aneurysms followed in the wake of their writings.

Miliary aneurysms were observed by Turner in 1882 in three patients who died of primary intracerebral hemorrhage, which he attributed to periarteritis.[253] The hemorrhages, he said, occurred independently of the miliary aneurysms.

Bramwell[32] agreed with Charcôt and Bouchard concerning the etiological role of miliary aneurysms in primary intracerebral hemorrhage. He found them in all but one instance. Robertson[198] did not believe the miliary aneurysms were caused by a periarteritis. He considered the infiltration with a few inflammatory cells to be a secondary phenomenon. Ellis[69,70] in 1909 investigated 31 cases of primary intracerebral hemorrhage and emphasized the frequency of arteriosclerosis in the vessels involved, the absence of "true" aneurysmal dilatation, and the frequency of false and dissecting aneurysms in association with perivascular hemorrhages in the neighborhood of primary intracerebral hematomas. The walls of the sacs consisted primarily of fibrin together at times with remnants of the adventitia. At the site of the disruption of the intima and media, pronounced degenerative changes were said to occur but no changes apart from arteriosclerosis were described. The macroscopic frequency of miliary aneurysms was generally in proportion to the severity of the atherosclerosis of the large arteries at the base. Ellis considered the hemorrhage arose from rupture of arteriosclerotic intracerebral vessels with or without the initial formation of false or dissecting aneurysms.

Shennan[220] contended that the rupture was from diseased arterioles that might have undergone preliminary dilatation, larger in most instances than the size customarily associated with miliary. Hemorrhage might stem from small dissecting aneurysms of the intracerebral arteries also, but miliary aneurysms, he contends, if they exist at all at sites of cerebral hemorrhage, are rare. He demonstrated very clearly, ruptured vessels occluded by thrombus, but it is difficult to know whether the lesions are causes or effects of the hematomas.

Authors have since confirmed the presence of miliary aneurysms with or without an associated primary intracerebral hemorrhage.[100,132,191] Not all agree about the association of miliary aneurysms and intracerebral hemorrhage, and Cappell[37] was unable to demonstrate the presence of miliary aneurysms in most cases of hemorrhage.

Matsuoka[158] on the other hand attributed cerebral hemorrhage to only two lesions—the miliary aneurysms and angionecrosis, both demonstrable by serial sections.

Ellis,[69,70] who is frequently misquoted, has erroneously been purported to have claimed that the perivascular hematomas, dissections, and false aneurysms accrued from the hemorrhage.[204] The misapprehension delayed further investigation of miliary aneurysms for a time, but recently Russell's[204,205] angiographic studies have kindled renewed interest. He demonstrated the presence of small saccular and irregular dilatations (Fig. 8-14) on intracerebral vessels of many hypertensive subjects and fewer normotensive individuals. Subjects with miliary aneurysms were always older than 50 years and stenotic lesions of the large basal arteries were more numerous and severe in subjects without miliary aneurysms. The miliary aneurysms (300 to 900μ in diameter) frequently occurred at points of branching and were often multiple on a single vessel. Moreover, they were not all false sacs, for their walls were often composed entirely of connective tissue. They were most abundant in the putamen, glo-

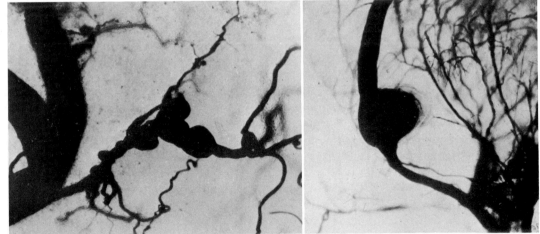

Fig. 8-14. Cleared specimens (made after postmortem arterial injection) displaying microaneurysms on intracerebral vessels, **A. B,** Miliary aneurysm (800 μ in diameter) on a long penetrating artery from the parietal cortex of a 71-year-old male who died of cerebral hemorrhage. (From Russell, R. W. R.: Observations on intracerebral aneurysms, Brain **86:**425, 1963.)

bus pallidus, and thalamus, but were also found in the caudate nucleus, internal capsule, centrum semiovale, and the cortical gray matter of the cerebrum.

Dinsdale,[65] using similar techniques, corroborated Russell's findings, observing miliary aneurysms both in the pons and cerebellum. He found early aneurysmal changes to be most prevalent near sites of branching and pointed out that the penetrating pontine arteries have their highest density of branchings at the junction of the basis and tegmentum pontis where pontine hemorrhages are most frequent.

Margolis[154] concluded that miliary aneurysms arise in the cerebral vascular bed secondarily to arterial and arteriolar fibrinoid necrosis. He was of the opinion that the vascular injury was caused by a prolonged and excessive myogenic reaction to the hypertension and that the cerebral vasculature was unusually susceptible because of inherent structural and physiological peculiarities. However the large series of miliary aneurysms studied histologically by Cole and Yates[45,46] demonstrated that not all such aneurysms form secondarily to fibrinoid necrotic lesions.

Cole and Yates,[45-47] examining the brains from 100 hypertensive and 100 normotensive patients (matched for age and sex), found 46 hypertensive and seven normotensive individuals with miliary or microaneurysms. Some were saccular, and others were very irregular dilatations. The lesions measured up to 2 mm. in diameter and in the main were concentrated on vessels below 250μ in diameter, but a few occurred on main lenticulostriate vessels of 500μ. The aneurysms were found in 86% of hypertensive individuals with primary intracerebral hemorrhage and in 35% of hypertensive individuals without hemorrhage. There was an increase in frequency with age. Within the cerebral hemispheres they were found to be most prevalent in the putamen, globus pallidus, and thalamus, occurring less often in the caudate nucleus and internal capsule. The subcortical white matter, particularly in posterior regions, dem-

onstrated a fairly high frequency. Pontine lesions were found in only 15 hypertensives and always in association with miliary aneurysms in the cerebrum. Of the hypertensives, four had cerebellar lesions that were always associated with both cerebral and pontine aneurysms. Peculiarly enough, there were no miliary aneurysms on the main trunk of the largest lenticulostriate artery. They[47] drew attention to two other types of lesion associated with intracerebral hemorrhage whether primary or secondary in origin, namely perivascular hemorrhages, the wall of which is composed of multiple eccentric laminae of fibrin, and hemorrhages into the perivascular space. Both types were believed to result from the hemorrhage and brain disruption. Cole and Yates[45,46] considered that the circumstantial evidence strongly indicated that these miliary aneurysms, though causally related to primary intracerebral hemorrhage, were also associated with the smaller subclinical hemorrhages that after resolution left only small cystic cavities. They did not believe like Green[100] that small softenings resulted from thrombotic occlusion of the aneurysm.

It would seem that the most likely cause of primary intracerebral hemorrhage is a degenerative change in the intracerebral arteries that we may call arteriosclerosis, and this, associated with reduced tensile strength of the connective tissues, results in rupture of the vessels. The rupture is incipient, with the vessel wall exhibiting considerable fibrin infiltration, or the result of a subclinical extravasation of blood. The bleeding may vary from an ecchymosis to gross and fatal hemorrhage with the disruption of brain tissue consequent upon the massive bleeding, possibly leading to secondary damage and bleeding from other vessels. Rupture may also be associated with dissection of the vessel wall, false aneurysm formation, or dilatation of the so-called true aneurysmal type. Misapprehensions regarding the term "false aneurysm" have delayed its acceptance and the further investigation of miliary aneurysms and underlying pathological changes in the intra-

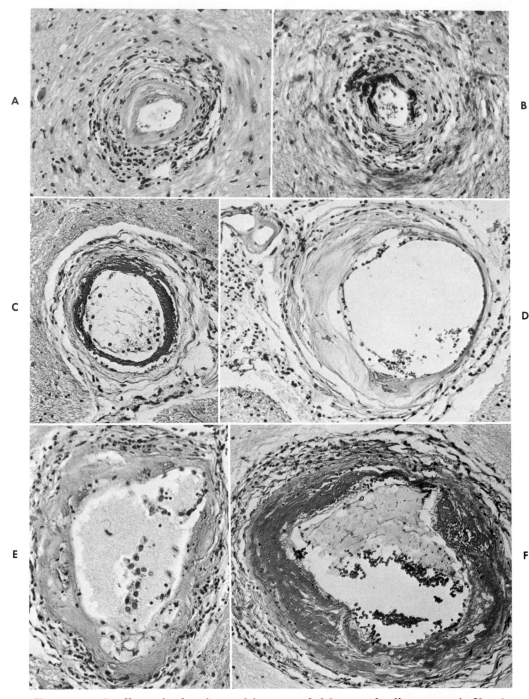

Fig. 8-15. A, Small arteriosclerotic vessel is surrounded by round cells, concentric fibrosis, and a few siderophages. **B,** Similar vessel is partially lined by fibrin that extends into the wall. **C,** Larger vessel or miliary aneurysm is completely lined with fibrin. **D,** Vessel with a hyaline wall of variable thickness is in all probability also a miliary aneurysm. **E** and **F,** Two miliary aneurysms, with the one in **F** being lined with fibrin. Both are surrounded by loose concentric collagen containing a few round cells and siderophages. In **E** there are lipophages in the sac wall. **(A, D** to **F,** Hematoxylin and eosin; **B** and **C,** phosphotungstic acid–hematoxylin; **A** to **E,** ×110; **F,** ×95.)

cerebral vessels. The aneurysmal dilatation of such vessels, whether of the false or true variety, still warrants the classification "miliary."

MICROSCOPIC APPEARANCE OF MILIARY AN-EURYSMS. Vessels bearing miliary aneurysms usually exhibit a severe degree of arteriosclerosis. Hyalinization is prominent and the media is thinned. The aneurysmal wall consists of hyaline and collagenous tissue, the media and internal elastic lamina in most cases terminating near the entrance to the sac. Red blood cells may be present within crevices in the hyaline sac wall. In small developing microaneurysms the elastica may be demonstrable within the sac wall and granularity and fraying are then usual. The adventitia and intimal tissue merge. Under ordinary circumstances such vessels will not be recognizable as aneurysmal in histological sections and will be regarded merely as large sclerotic and hyaline arteries (Fig. 8-15).

Green[100] drew attention to lipid in the arterial wall and also in the wall of the miliary aneurysm. He regarded the vascular changes as atheromatous. The lipid de-position appeared to be of greater severity than that usually encountered in renal vessels of comparable size, but unfortunately intracerebral vessels have not been extensively investigated for lipid content. Fig. 8-16 however demonstrates an aneurysm of a small cortical perforating vessel exhibiting many foam cells in its intima.

In some aneurysms a considerable amount of fibrin occurs in the thickened aneurysmal wall, and red cells and remnants of a hyaline or collagenous tissue are recognizable within the fibrin laminations. A few leukocytes and macrophages are not infrequent mostly within the outer half of the wall. Siderophages may be prominent and the surrounding brain exhibits some gliosis. These are the lesions that probably led Charcôt and Bouchard[42] to believe that miliary aneurysms were arteritic in nature. They are readily recognized in histological sections and should be distinguished from polyarteritis nodosa in which the inflammatory reaction is much more prominent and extracranial involvement predominant. The lesions could be false aneurysms if formed as the result of rupture of the wall

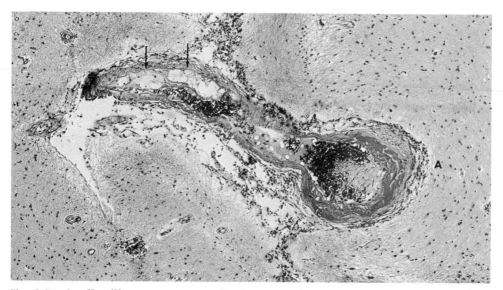

Fig. 8-16. Small miliary aneurysm, **A**, in the superficial layer of the cortex is lined internally with fibrin and arises from a small severely arteriosclerotic vessel with foam cells in its wall (*arrows*). There are a few round cells about the aneurysm and the vessels. (Hematoxylin and eosin, ×50.)

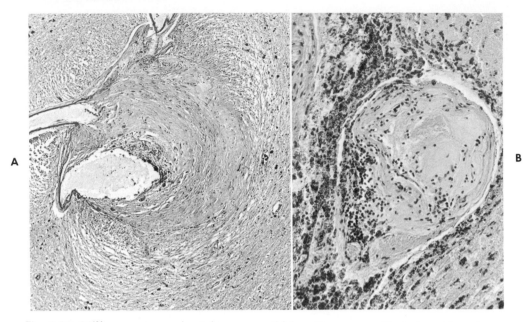

Fig. 8-17. Miliary aneurysm in **A** has a very thick collagenous wall. A few siderophages are in wall and surrounding parenchyma. Miliary aneurysms undergo partial or complete thrombosis and may eventually be replaced by a collagenous mass similar to that in **B,** which was found in an area of old hemorrhage. See Fig. 12-2. (Hematoxylin and eosin; **A,** ×45; **B,** ×110.)

rather than as a consequence of fibrin infiltration of a yielding vessel wall. They can nevertheless be regarded as demonstrating incipient rupture.

Russell[204] and Cole and Yates[45-47] noted that the endothelial layer is at times incomplete in the miliary aneurysms. This may well be the case, but in view of the frequent attenuation of endothelial cells and the limitations of light microscopy and wax embedding, this observation should be verified with a higher resolution.

Miliary aneurysms with walls of laminated fibrin may appear to be thrombosed if the plane of section does not pass through the lumen. In view of the size of the vessel, thrombosis is a likely sequel. Recanalization[45-47] may then ensue. However, in regard to the prevalence of these aneurysms, thrombosis with organization is probably more frequent than is at present recognized, and occluded vessels replaced by such hyaline structures as in Figs. 18-17 and 12-2 are probably the eventual outcome. A few siderophages can often be found, but vessel lumina associated with recanalization are not essential in vessels of this caliber. Though Cole and Yates[45,46] did not observe extension of the aneurysmal thrombus into the parent vessel causing infarction in the area of supply, it is still a possibility, for microangiography would not necessarily show the position of such lesions.

Russell[204] observed leakage from a thin-walled aneurysm on a lateral lenticulostriate artery during microangiography, and the frequent perianeurysmal collections of red cells, round cells, and siderophages were considered by Cole and Yates[45-47] to intimate previous leakage.

Problems in the etiology. The following several features of the etiology of primary intracerebral hemorrhage are problematical and worthy of further investigation:

1. The reason for the peculiar predisposition of intracerebral blood vessels to spontaneous hemorrhage and miliary aneurysms
2. To explain why 30% of all miliary aneurysms in the brain occur in the subcortical

white matter despite its lower frequency of primary hemorrhage

3. Why miliary aneurysms are apparently confined to the cerebral circulation (Kaufmann[132] indicated that miliary aneurysms occurred in extracranial vessels such as the lung and intestines)

4. To determine the prevalence of miliary aneurysms in midbrain, medulla oblongata, and spinal cord

5. Why miliary aneurysms so rarely occur before the age of 50 years

6. The prevalence of miliary aneurysms in countries like Japan that have an allegedly high mortality from primary intracerebral hemorrhage

7. Effects of antihypertensive agents on miliary aneurysms and their development

8. The prevalence of miliary aneurysms in young subjects with long-standing, untreated, benign hypertension

9. The importance of the duration and severity of hypertension in the pathogenesis of miliary aneurysms

10. The pathogenesis of the reduced tensile strength of intracerebral vessels resulting in rupture with or without aneurysm formation whether false, true, or dissecting

11. The rarity of primary intracerebral hemorrhage in animals other than man (with the possible exception of aged parrots[201]) and the importance of related factors such as hypertension, age, arteriosclerosis, and frequency of miliary aneurysms in lower animals

Therapy. Although the surgical therapy of primary intracerebral hemorrhage has been recommended by many neurosurgeons, the exact role of the surgery has not yet been determined. Evacuation of the hematoma, if the patient survives, merely reduces the quantity of blood and debris to be organized, and repair of the surrounding vessels and tissues proceeds in much the same manner as in any cerebral softening. The additional features likely to be encountered are foreign bodies and secondary infection. The frequency of recurrent hemorrhage and its survival rate await more extensive statistics than are at present available.

Secondary intracerebral hemorrhage

Traumatic hemorrhage. It is difficult to conceive of significant trauma befalling the brain in the absence of vas-cular injury, and there is little realization of just how susceptible to injury are the blood vessels and endothelium.[223,241] In transparent chambers in rabbits' ears, the mildest injury precipitates the formation of microthrombi and emboli and induces stasis. Almost certainly changes similar to these occur in the central nervous system where histologically stasis would be interpreted merely as congestion, and as for platelets, they are not readily distinguishable in paraffin sections. When the trauma results in edema, perivascular hemorrhages, and occlusive thrombi, the damage can be appreciated. More severe trauma can be recognized grossly primarily because of the hemorrhage though lacerations, and secondary necrosis may also be in evidence.

Penetrating injuries are more likely to be encountered in forensic pathology, and for information and description the reader is referred to texts in that field. Other head injuries occasioned by indirect or blunt forces applied to the skull may be divided into the following types: concussion, cortical contusions, intracerebral hemorrhages, delayed traumatic apoplexy, pituitary lesions, secondary lesions, and hemorrhages in infancy and the newborn.

Concussion. A patient, when stunned by a blow to the head, is usually comatose and paralyzed for a short time. Within minutes he recovers consciousness and mobility, though mild sequelae may persist. To such an episode has been applied the term "concussion"[248] which, according to Schneider,[213] is not synonymous with loss of consciousness. He grades concussion into mild, moderate, and severe degrees. The mild stage is characterized by immediate or transient impairment of neural function without unconsciousness but with variable degrees of amnesia, unsteady gait, dizziness, and mental confusion, with recovery being rapid. In the severe degree unconsciousness persists for longer than 5 minutes with profound retrograde amnesia (for several hours) and slow recovery. Cerebral concussion is usually regarded as being unassociated with permanent pathological sequelae, yet some permanent damage seems to be inevitable and the cerebrospinal fluid may be bloodstained.[248] Concussion has been considered in the past to be due to an arrest of the circulation causing temporary cerebral ischemia. This concept has become untenable, since the classical Witkowski experiment in which a frog with the heart removed, is stunned by a blow to the head.[62]

Denny-Brown and Russell[62] observed that the essential requirement in experimental concussion is that the head is free to move. In contending that the concussion is the result of excessive acceleration or deceleration of the brain within the skull, their concept is consistent with the preservation of consciousness in both crushing injuries of the skull sufficient to cause cranial fractures and penetrating wounds of the brain such as bullet wounds. It proved impossible to produce experimental concussion when an animal's head was prevented from moving at the instant of injury inflicted by a swinging pendulum.

Holbourn[115] asserted that the effects of head injury on the brain were dependent on the physical properties of the skull and brain, the most important of which were (1) the comparatively uniform density of the brain, (2) the extreme incompressibility of the brain, (3) its very small modules of rigidity, (4) the extreme rigidity of the skull, and (5) the shape of both the skull and the brain in respect to the site of injury.

He further deduced that injuries would be effected readily by shear strains, but that strains associated with compression and rarefaction would produce little damage to the brain. In a localized injury to the skull with distortion, only the underlying brain will be subjected to shear strains, and superficial bruising will be the result. If a fracture is sustained, shear strains will be maximal at the site of injury and brain damage superficial. However, when a large vessel crosses the fracture line, it may tear, causing serious hemorrhage. Shear strains, he explained, are minimal in changes of linear velocity and are beheld mostly in the neighborhood of the foramina. In contrast, shear strains from changes in rotational acceleration are dangerous and constitute the major cause of brain injury, sometimes at a distance from the site of impact. By using gelatin models of brains inside a paraffin skull, Holbourn[116] localized the maximal sites of shear strains by changes in color with the model viewed in a polariscope. He postulated that such shear strains might tear blood vessels, axons, synapses, and nerves and perhaps disrupt cells. The shear strain was found to be particularly great in the anterior part of the temporal lobe and comparatively absent in the cerebellum. In more severe rotational injury the model exhibited extreme fragmentation in the temporal and frontal lobes with a superficial layer of damage near the vertex. Changes in rotational velocity are usually greater at areas opposite the site of trauma,[116] and consequently the contrecoup is the result of the extreme shear stress at the site. It had been appreciated previously that the contrecoup effect was absent in crushing injuries of the skull.[138,256] Holbourn considers that the main motion at the periphery of the brain is between the pia and the arachnoid, because the dura is firmly attached to the calvarium.[115,116] Thus shear strains could lead to a tearing of the cortical veins crossing the subdural space to drain into the venous sinuses, which could bring about subdural and subarachnoid hemorrhage. Procedure and results of the experimental work of Denny-Brown and Russell[62] are consistent with Holbourn's theory of head injury, which in itself was substantiated by the experimental work of Pudenz and Shelden.[189] With high-speed cinematography during head injuries, they observed the rotational movement of the brain through transparent Lucite windows inserted in the skulls of monkeys. Immobilization of the head permitted little or no displacement of the brain when assailed with blows of comparable severity.

In association with the concussion is an

immediate but temporary rise in blood pressure and blood flow.[62] In cases of severe concussion there is sometimes local contusion of the brain, petechial hemorrhages, and bloodstained cerebrospinal fluid,[248] all of which are believed to be incidental to the concussion rather than its cause. The concussion itself is probably caused by actual nerve cell damage with tearing and stretching of nerve fibers caused by the rotational movements of the brain[246,248] at the time of the injury, just as postulated by Holbourn.[115] However associated with such damage, vascular stasis, diapedesis of red cells, and edema are likely to arise even though the effects are only temporary. In brains of patients dying a time after closed and apparently uncomplicated head injuries, Strich[246] found a few contusions, minute softenings, and occasional yellow punctate areas (old petechiae) in the hemispheres and brain stem. The old hemorrhages were often subependymal or where the cortex or basal ganglia joins with the white matter. In all cases hemorrhages into the corpus callosum were found and most had similar lesions in one or both superior cerebellar peduncles. The lesions were attributed to the shearing stresses and strains held responsible for the nerve fiber damage. Increased capillary permeability of vessels causing cerebral edema may be a factor in delayed recovery after injury[246] and may also cause secondary pressure lesions. Strich's observations[246] were made in cases of considerable severity, but conceivably milder injuries could be associated with corresponding mitigation of cerebral impairment. Symonds[248] believes that even in these mild degrees of concussion, irreversible damage, however small in extent, is effected, and can be cumulative. In all probability this is the explanation of the "punch-drunk" professional boxer.

Ommaya and associates[176-178] demonstrated experimentally in subhuman primates that without significant or direct head impact cerebral concussion as well as gross hemorrhages (subdural, subarachnoid, and intracerebral) and contusions over the surface of the brain and upper cervical cord could be produced with rotational displacement of the head and neck from a whiplash effect. They also demonstrated that a cervical collar designed to reduce rotational displacement of the head while permitting stretching of the neck and not reducing linear acceleration, raised the threshold for experimental concussion by head impact in 50% of animals. It has also been demonstrated that nondeforming rotational acceleration of the primate skull can cause traumatic lesions of the brain and the entire length of the cord. Lesions so produced included subdural and subarachnoid hemorrhage, and tearing and avulsion of vessels in the superficial part of the cortex with hemorrhages, areas of necrosis, and rhectic hemorrhages in cranial nerves.[254,255]

Individuals subjected to the blast of high explosives may suffer blast concussion, and in the past many were thought to suffer from psychoneuroses. It is now realized that an organic basis exists for many of their symptoms and abnormal electroencephalographic tracings.[55] The cerebral lesions are believed to be similar to those accruing from concussion from other causes such as shear stresses developing from rapid rotational acceleration of the head.

Controversy surrounds the acceptance of posttraumatic cerebral edema as an isolated lesion. Apfelbach[9] considered it a distinct entity, the affected patients dying at any time from several hours after the injury to the end of the third day when edema reaches its maximum. Although such posttraumatic edema contributes to the cerebral compression and secondary pressure manifestations, the edema is probably part of the cerebral and vascular injury incurred with the concussion. Careful macroscopic and microscopic examinations should reveal further manifestations of concussion.

Cortical contusions. Contusions of the brain occur either beneath the site of impact (the coup lesion) or at a distant focus

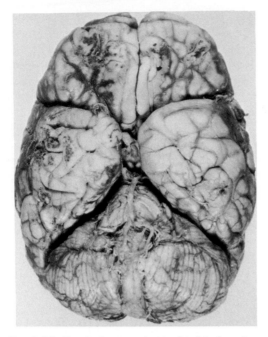

Fig. 8-18. Cortical contusions of orbital surface of each frontal lobe and lateral aspect of right temporal lobe after a head injury.

on the opposite side of the brain, that is, the contrecoup injury, which may be the more spectacular and is caused by mass movement of the brain.[146] Most cerebral contusions are located on the orbital surface of the frontal lobes, the anterotemporal lobe and the lateral aspect of the temporal lobe on one or both sides.[50] Fig. 8-18 illustrates this distribution. Contusions may affect other parts of the brain, including the cerebellum, but peculiarly enough the occipital lobes are less involved. Injuries to the back of the head cause a large number of contrecoup bruises; the sides have the next largest percentage of contrecoup bruises. Trauma to the front of the head is more frequently than not associated with a large direct contusion rather than a contrecoup.[138]

As a rule contrecoup injuries are more severe in adults than in children.[103] Freytag,[86] in her study of primary brain lesions in the fatal cases of head injury, found variation with age in the prevalence of cerebral contusions. Only 44% of infants under 1 year of age had contusions, whereas

between 1 and 10 years the frequency was 76% and rose thereafter to 90%. Contusions in very young babies consisted not of cortical bruising at the crest of the convolutions but of slitlike hemorrhagic tears in the white matter[147] in the regions of high predilection for contusions (gyri recti and the temporal lobes).

Bruising or a contusion located at or near the summit of the convolution or gyrus is wedge shaped with the apex directed into the white matter for a distance of some 1 to 1.5 cm. It consists of multiple, densely arranged petechial and streaklike hemorrhages mostly in the cortex and often arranged perpendicularly to the pia-arachnoid. Some occur in the cortex facing the sulcus. The subarachnoid hemorrhage, severe or minimal, and usually more extensive than the contusion, is related particularly to the frontal and temporal lobes. The color of the gray matter is accentuated because of vascular engorgement and small hemorrhages extending mostly no deeper than the subcortical white matter. Contusion necrosis[145] is often coexistent, the hemorrhages of which may coalesce to a variable extent. The whole wedge-shaped area may become infiltrated with blood and, while assuming the appearance of a massive hemorrhage, histologically is of confluent hemorrhages. Bleeding is profuse in the event of large vessel injury and is said to be aggravated by arteriosclerosis and hypertension.[145]

With survival for longer periods of time, the lesion undergoes resolution and a color change to rusty brown or yellow pigmentation in the contused area, which becomes excavated, forming circumscribed craterlike defects or some open trenches along the crest of the gyri somewhat like accessory sulci.[145] Yellow-brown pigmentation in the margin of these healed contusions persists for years. Larger hemorrhages are slow to organize and resolve, and the result is a cystlike structure. Gross connective-tissue scarring and encapsulation are infrequent.

The overlying meninges may be thickened, but adhesions to the dura mater are rare. Considerable parenchymal shrinkage occurs in association with contusions, which if large and deep may result in secondary expansion of the adjacent ventricular cavity.

Lindenberg and Freytag[145] differentiate between contusion hemorrhage and contusion necrosis. The wedge-shaped necrotic area is generally indicated by the presence of hemorrhages, but on occasions the necrosis occurs without hemorrhages and vice versa. The area of ischemic necrosis becomes swollen. The cortex, poorly demarcated from the white matter, takes on a translucent appearance. Contusions need not be divided into hemorrhage and necrosis, for the two usually occur concomitantly. Trauma induced in a rabbit ear chamber is, when sufficiently severe to cause hemorrhage, always associated with widespread vascular dilatation and stasis, and though it is not possible to distinguish arteriolar spasm, which is assumed to be the cause of the necrosis, the "sludging" or massive aggregation of red cells is a very prominent feature of the stasis and could well cause or contribute substantially to the ischemia. Assuming that the course of events is similar in any trauma of the central nervous system, one could expect necrosis in the damaged zone and only on rare occasions would the hemorrhage or necrosis occur independently. Smith, Ducker, and Kempe[228] observed virtually similar changes in the cerebral cortex of experimental animals after very mild injuries.

Microscopically the hemorrhages are perivascular and multiple. Tears of larger vessels entailing extensive hemorrhages are difficult to demonstrate, for in small vessels the extravasation can proceed from a small endothelial defect or gap. Many vessels, appearing engorged, are probably in stasis. Within 3 to 5 hours the necrotic cortex and white matter seem paler than the surrounding tissue in Nissl stains. The edges of the wedge-shaped zone may become well demarcated because of edema, and resolution is effected in much the same manner as about other areas of hemorrhage

and necrosis. The excavated area always communicates with the subarachnoid space.

The presence of a coup lesion is understandable, particularly when the skull is fractured and possibly depressed. The explanation of the contrecoup injury has always been controversial and few support Holbourn's theory of contrecoup lesions. Courville[50] considered that coup and contrecoup contusions were the result of abrupt movement (not necessarily centrifugal rotation) against the bony irregularities of the skull, the anatomy of the inner surface of the skull being particularly pertinent. His contention was that the contrecoup contusion had not been produced experimentally. Lindenberg and Freytag[146] reviewing the controversy over the mechanism of the contrecoup injury in some detail concluded with regard to the nature and site of the impact and the movement of the head as follows:

1. With blows to the movable head in the absence of a coup lesion, it seems that the blow has accelerated the head but has not indented the skull sufficiently to damage the underlying brain. The pressures resulting from the sudden acceleration of the skull are insufficient to cause contusions though extracerebral hemorrhage may occur.

2. The presence of a coup lesion after blows to the movable head indicates that, acceleration apart, considerable local depression of the skull and possibly a depressed fracture has been incurred at the site of impact. The coup lesion is caused by the positive acceleration pressure and the sudden local rise in pressure caused by depression of the skull. Sudden positive pressure at the site of impact, if severe enough, may force the brain toward the foramen magnum, causing "herniation contusions" of the cerebellar tonsils and medulla oblongata.

3. The presence of both coup and contrecoup lesions occurring after blows to the movable head indicates that severe depression of the skull transpired and caused a positive pressure throughout and exacerbations of the pressure over the contralateral aspect of the brain resulted in contrecoup. The contrecoup lesion in blows to the movable head is the result of the positive shifting pressure arriving at the contralateral side less the negative acceleration pressure due to inertia of the brain and so it is always less severe than the coup lesion.

4. In falls on the head, (a) the absence of

coup and contrecoup lesions suggests that no significant depression of the skull has been sustained, though extracerebral bleeding may occur; (b) the presence of coup but not contrecoup lesions indicates that a more circumscribed indentation of the skull, possibly a depressed fracture, has been incurred; (c) if, as in the majority of cases, the contrecoup lesion is extensive and the coup lesion absent or small, the pressure associated with depression of a larger part of the skull has been offset by negative acceleration pressure and has caused little or no coup injury but significant contrecoup damage.

5. In blows to the supported head, coup and contrecoup injuries are extremely rare because no significant acceleration occurs.

6. A sudden impulse-like shift of the brain along the line of direction of the impact is most severe beneath the site of impact and can produce intermediary coup lesions between the coup and the contrecoup injuries. "Intermediary coup" lesions occur mainly in falls on the forehead and vertex.

Attempting to analyze mechanical effects of trauma to the head, Lindgren[148,149] recorded pressure changes and accelerations during impact at significant sites within the movable skull of cadavers. The initial pressure wave at the site of impact was positive (1 to 3 atmospheres) and the contrecoup pressure was usually negative (barely −1 atmosphere). At the basal surface of the frontal lobe and laterally at the base of the temporal lobe, negative pressures developed as if a contrecoup site were in question. Associated with such pressure changes, the shear stresses imposed on the brain during trauma and movement of the brain must be more than considerable. Lindgren[149] believes that the injuries to the brain are the result of transmitted pressure changes and that contrecoup cavitation is an important factor. However animal experiments are of limited value in solving these mechanical problems. Given the advances of the past 30 years, it can be anticipated that future progress will resolve much of the present controversy.

Once again unusual fragility and hypoplasia of the cerebral vessels have been invoked as causative factors because the extent and severity of the hemorrhage appear to be out of all proportion to the minor degree of injury.[51] This belief, founded on subjective impressions alone, gains adherents only because of the present ignorance of the magnitude of shearing stresses incurred by trauma to the head.

Traumatic intracerebral hemorrhages. Small hemorrhages associated with cortical contusions are intracerebral and usually restricted to the cortex and often simulate red softening. More extensive hemorrhages form wedge-shaped necrotic lesions. Multiple small punctate or linear hemorrhages can appear in the white matter and basal ganglia or the brain stem, pons, and medulla. Usually perivascular, they may be called "ring hemorrhages" or "multiple concussion hemorrhages." They rarely involve the cerebellum and should not be confused with fat embolism.

Multiple traumatic hemorrhages in the medulla, upper spinal cord, and particularly the pons were often noted in the past.[12,39] Freytag[86] found primary lesions in the midbrain and brain stem in 23% of 1367 fatal head injuries. They are usually centrally located, 1 to 3 mm. in diameter, and demonstrate little tendency to coalesce. They have been attributed to a contrecoup effect and are associated as a rule with violent trauma to the back of the head,[256] being found in subjects dying almost immediately after the injury. Gurdjian and associates[108] considered that shear stresses consequent upon pressure gradients within the cranial cavity are concentrated in the region of the brain stem and that the damage therein is the prime cause of concussion. Secondary brain stem hemorrhages can complicate the rapidly rising supratentorial pressure, but this presupposes survival of the accident victim for some hours to a few days. In the experimental animal, petechial hemorrhages may be found in the roof of the fourth ventricle, in the medulla and upper cervical segments of the spinal cord, and occasionally in the pons, sometimes without other lesions but often with a coup injury.[62] Petechiae are more frequent in the upper cervical cord than in the medulla, though the medulla only is affected at rare intervals. Hemorrhages in the upper cervical cord varying from small petechiae to destructive hemorrhages (at times pronounced in the gray matter) can be produced experimentally by an impact at the vertex,[99] and in man similar lesions are occasioned by some football injuries.[214] The lesions are apparently caused by stretch injury of the upper cord consequent upon the disparity in mobility of the relatively mobile brain and the fixed spinal cord.

The tearing of vessels at the junction of the cortex and the white matter can produce small hematomas (diameter up to 1 cm.) without superficial bruising.[9] Similar hemorrhages, found by LeCount and Apfelbach[138] only 10 times in 504 fatal cases of skull fracture, were either in the basal ganglia or in the compressed cerebral hemisphere and associated with a large extradural hematoma.

Multiple hemorrhages in the basal ganglia were attributed to violent impacts near the zygomatic process of the frontal bone.[256] Bilateral multiple coalescing hemorrhages (into the right external capsule and left lenticular nucleus) with intraventricular rupture were recorded in an elderly male struck on the left temporal region.[51] Freytag[86] reported lesions in the corpus callosum and basal ganglia in 27% of her cases of fatal head injury.

Lindenberg and associates[144] found gross lesions of the corpus callosum in 16% of brains examined at autopsy from patients dying as the result of blunt mechanical trauma to the head. Although two-thirds of the cases had a fractured skull, this fact could not be correlated with the severity of the lesion in the corpus callosum. Early lesions consisted of areas of hemorrhage with disruption of tissue, the extent depending on the severity of the trauma. Within a few hours necrosis was apparent in the region of hemorrhage. Older lesions appeared as yellowish areas of softening coalescing at times till ultimately scar forma-

tion ensued. In some cases extensive anemic necrosis was seen with little in the way of hemorrhage. Twenty-one of the 51 cases exhibited small or multiple foci; in another 21 about one-third to two-thirds of the corpus callosum was involved; and in the remaining nine cases, the entire length was involved from knee to splenium, always excepting the rostrum and ventral portion of the genu. A plausible explanation for the pathogenesis of these lesions was considered to be the sudden stretching, pressure, and shearing forces associated with the traumatic impact, usually above the corpus callosum though occasionally at the lower occipital and always directed downward. Often in neighboring structures, like lesions, were found with subarachnoid hemorrhage in the callosal sulcus. Damage to the corpus callosum or neighboring cingulate gyrus by the free margin of the falx cerebri is another possibility.

Laceration of the vessels of the leptomeninges with hemorrhage into the subarachnoid space and the cortex of the brain constituted a frequent, important traumatic lesion within the cranial cavity in 82% of 309 autopsies of traumatic intracranial hemorrhage.[156] Mostly the fatal cases are associated with a fractured skull and the lacerations are caused by contrecoup more often than coup injuries. With trauma of more severe degree, larger cortical lacerations are encountered and subdural hemorrhage and arachnoidal tears are more often concomitant features. Severe lacerations of the brain may be 4 to 6 cm. in diameter extending 4 to 5 cm. into the brain with the defect filled with clotted blood and damaged brain tissue. Though most of the lacerations are contrecoup effects, direct laceration may be caused by the inward depression of the edge of the fractured bone, and it is then associated with a dural tear and subdural bleeding. Clot and pulped brain may herniate through defects in the dura and skull. LeCount and Apfelbach[138] in 504 autopsies of patients with fractured skulls encountered 54 cortical lacerations. In 15 the tear extended into one of the lateral ventricles. They noted that enlargement of the lateral ventricles made the frontal and lateral aspects more susceptible to tearing. In 39 cases a hematoma was found deep to the laceration and not in communication with the surface. Of the hematomas 36 were either frontal or temporal, and the remainder occipital. Vance[256] found most lacerations on the lateral surface of the temporal and parietal regions and a few on the lateral aspect of the occipital lobe. Comminuted fractures in the frontal region caused extensive contusions and lacerations of the orbital surface of the frontal lobes.

In 439 cases of craniocerebral injury, Courville and Blomquist[51] found 36 instances of gross intracerebral hemorrhage. The bleeding may be caused by a direct injury, which is usually a compound and comminuted fracture of the lateral aspect of the skull. The hemorrhage commonly can be traced to a lacerated branch of the middle cerebral artery. Recovery from such an injury brings in its train a more or less sharply defined cavity (traumatic porencephaly) in the brain, possibly communicating with the lateral ventricle.

Most large hemorrhages are caused by a contrecoup injury and tend to be deep in the lobe rather than superficial.[51] When large and without underlying contusion or brain laceration, they simulate primary intracerebral hemorrhages, in some instances, multiple and bilateral.[51] Angrist and Mitchell[7] in a series of 320 autopsies on subjects dying of head injury, found seven cases in which the hematoma involved the internal capsule, with no specific site of impact noted. Courville[50] drew attention to the tendency of these posttraumatic intracerebral hematomas to localize in the frontal and temporo-occipital regions.

Mosberg and Lindenberg[171] found multiple hemorrhages or a single large hematoma of the globus pallidus in 20 cases of head injury. The impact in most instances had been directed against the vertex. Most had other severe traumatic cranial or intracranial lesions. The hemorrhage was attributed to stresses on the branches of the anterior choroidal artery, closely related to the edge of the tentorium, and to tearing at the time of the concussive impact. Bruising of the uncus and hippocampal gyrus were seen in some.

Traumatic intracerebellar hemorrhage is not common. As in hematomas of the cerebrum there is the need to exclude primary nontraumatic hemorrhage in which the patient sustained a minor head injury and those cases in which the bleeding originated from small cryptic hemangiomas. The traumatic variety stems from a severe injury to the back of the head, frequently with a fractured skull and hemorrhage elsewhere. The cerebellum is usually severely contused or lacerated and severe supratentorial contrecoup injuries (contusions or intracerebral hematomas) complicate the subtentorial damage.

Shortly after the injury, the affected area is bright red. Edema is maximal within the first 2 or 3 days and can be complicated by secondary pressure changes, including brain stem softening or hemorrhage. The color of the blood changes progressively to brownish red, thence to brown, and finally to a rusty color at which time the injured, softened area has reduced in size. Finally scarring and cavitation ensue and surface pits and fossae are to be seen. Adhesions to the dura mater are limited and a degree of encapsulation may initiate a chronic encapsulated hematoma. Symonds[249] attributed symptoms suggestive of enlargement of the hematoma and evidence of increased intracranial pressure to recurrent hemorrhage into the hematoma because of additional trauma. The thick capsule of granulation tissue may not expand much. However, little is known of the shearing stresses at the junction of the brain and the capsule surrounding the hematoma, for here the brain is not of uniform density, and trauma from shear stress may then cause brain damage in the area. There may be calcification, sufficient for radiological detection,[186] in the capsule of such a long-standing encapsulated hematoma, but calcified intracerebral hematomas are extremely rare.

The relationship of trauma to intracerebral hemorrhage is not always easy to appraise. Patients are encountered in whom intracerebral hemorrhage of severe proportions has occurred apparently after trauma to the head[186] in the absence of extradural and subdural hematomas. The two events (trauma and hemorrhage) are possibly related fortuitously to each other in time. A cause-and-effect relationship has been propounded by many,[186] but the underlying mechanism is obscure. A head injury may follow the loss of consciousness caused by the primary intracerebral hemorrhage and it is conceivable that shearing stresses in the brain following trauma could contribute to the rupture or tearing of the wall of a miliary aneurysm.

Delayed traumatic apoplexy. Traumatic intracerebral hemorrhage at a prolonged interval after a head injury becomes of considerable medicolegal importance and has been the source of much controversy. Difficulties arise in substantiating a relationship between the trauma and the hemorrhage. Traumatic hemorrhage has been classified into three types.[17] The first is seen immediately at the time of injury, the second is produced a short time later as the result of intermediate factors, and the third type appears some time after the accident, even 3 or 4 weeks later. Symonds[249] and Courville and Blomquist[51] have reviewed the various arguments concerning these rather rare lesions. In the literature many alleged cases are in reality coincidental or unrelated hemorrhages. It is also theoretically possible that the trauma has contributed to the rupture of a preexisting lesion be it a miliary aneurysm, a cryptic angioma, or an arteriosclerotic vessel. Theories invoked to account for delayed posttraumatic hemorrhage are as follows:

1. Hemorrhage into a softened or necrotic zone as with "prehemorrhagic softening" in the case of primary intracerebral hemorrhage
2. Trauma to the vessel wall causing a *loci minoris resistentiae* or even a traumatic or false aneurysm
3. Recurrent hemorrhage from the previously damaged zone
4. Hemorrhage occurring after spread of infection (arteritis or phlebitis) in the trauma zone
5. Further head injury

In most instances of delayed posttraumatic hemorrhage, the possibility of a coincidental hemorrhage can be ignored, for authentic cases are generally and even invariably due to traumatic false aneurysms.

Pituitary lesions. Kornblum and Fisher[135] examined 100 pituitary glands from patients dying of cerebral injuries. There were 59 capsular hemorrhages, six hemorrhages into the stalk, one lacerated stalk, 42 lesions ranging from microscopic perivascular hemorrhages to large areas of hemorrhagic necrosis of the posterior lobe, and 22 instances of ischemic necrosis of the anterior lobe in a total of 62 of the glands examined. In patients with long survival, foci of gliosis or fibrosis were found in the posterior lobe, and infiltration of siderophages was indicative of old hemorrhage. The capsular hemorrhages were not considered to be specific, for extension of blood may occur down into the arachnoid of the pituitary capsule in subarachnoid hemorrhage of traumatic or nontraumatic origin. There was ischemic necrosis of the anterior lobe in victims surviving more than 12 hours, consistently only in cases of shock accompanied by severe swelling of the brain and pituitary. The appearance of posttraumatic pituitary dysfunction is understandable, though lesions in the hypothalamus are also a hazard.

Secondary lesions. Secondary pressure manifestations of craniocerebral trauma may cause brain stem lesions, edema, softening, or frank hemorrhages. In Freytag's material,[86] 24% of the brains exhibited such lesions. Compression of the posterior cerebral artery with hemorrhagic infarction in the field of supply complicates head injury and the associated supratentorial swelling and edema. Evans and Scheinker[73] recorded cases with hemorrhagic infarction of the middle cerebral and anterior cerebral arteries attributable to similar pressure phenomena associated with trauma. The compression of the anterior cerebral artery against the falx cerebri is feasible, but severe uncal herniation with compression of the middle cerebral artery is less so.

Posttraumatic hydrocephalus may result from a hemogenic meningitis, from compression and distortion of the aqueduct in cerebellar hematomas or from unusual herniation of the hippocampal gyrus.[86]

Trauma to cortical veins can cause thrombotic occlusion and hemorrhagic infarction, though pale infarcts may follow secondary thrombosis of small arteries.

Hemorrhages in infancy and the newborn. Intracerebral hemorrhage may precede the onset of labor. Small hemorrhages either recent or partially organized and 1 to 2 cm. in diameter are infrequently found in stillborn or newborn infants, the hemorrhage preceding the onset of labor. They may be the cause of small porencephalic areas seen in older children. The etiology is unknown and it has been assumed that sometimes the bleeding stems from abnormally weak or hypoplastic vessels.[188] Sheldon[219] reported the case of an infant harboring the remains of an old hemorrhage in the cerebrum thought to have been caused when the mother had been hit in the abdomen 3 months prior to delivery. He found three more cases of hemorrhage in utero in the literature. Trauma or even infection could cause such hemorrhages but actual proof is another matter.

In the newborn, intracerebral hemorrhage attributed to birth injury is not infrequent. Yagi[270] found intracerebral hemorrhage in five cases of 144 autopsies on newborn infants, whereas Weyhe[263] found 35 cases in 122 autopsies. The hemorrhages are either petechial or massive. Petechial hemorrhages are the more common and can arise anywhere within the cerebral white matter. Not infrequently they are subependymal or within the medulla, and microscopically they are perivascular.[6] Massive intracerebral hemorrhage seldom eventuates but can complicate very severe head trauma. There is no common or specific site.[6] Schwartz[216] considered many arose from injury to subependymal veins, most often the terminal veins. Hemorrhage also proceeds from multiple small vessels by diapedesis, and their confluence has resulted in massive hemorrhage and involvement of the basal ganglia. Hemorrhage into the midbrain and pons can complicate severe forceps injury.

Schwartz[216] attributed the hemorrhages to trauma although Potter[188] considered localized hemorrhage in the cerebrum or cerebellum of the newborn the result of anoxia rather than trauma. However Windle[267] could not produce cerebral hemorrhage by experimental asphyxia. Petechial hemorrhages were found implicating asphyxia and resuscitation, the hemorrhages being caused by an agonal state. In another monkey, bilateral hemorrhages into the globus pallidus were attributed to the oxytocin administration.

Posttraumatic thrombosis of veins (sinuses or cortical) may complicate parturition,[216] with hemorrhagic softening as the outcome.

As not all cases of cerebral birth injury are fatal, ill effects may cause serious incapacitation of the survivors. The incidence of these remote sequelae, which include congenital hemiplegia, cerebral diplegia, porencephaly, epilepsy, and mental deficiency[6] is difficult to estimate.

Cortical contusions are infrequent in the young infant (5 months old or younger). Blunt trauma produces slitlike hemorrhagic tears of the white matter.[147] Older tears consist of small smooth-walled clefts with little or no macroscopic pigmentation of the walls. Frequent in frontal and temporal lobes, they also appear beneath the site of impact. Cortical tears parallel to the pial surface are occasionally observed in these infants.

Secondary nontraumatic intracerebral hemorrhage. Intracerebral hemorrhage like subarachnoid bleeding has a variety of causes. Primary intracerebral hemorrhage is the most widely recognized type, but secondary nontraumatic intracerebral hemorrhages, sometimes unsuspected, constitute an important group, which the clinician as well as the pathologist should keep in mind. The causes of secondary hemorrhage encompass the following:

1. Secondary brain stem hemorrhage
2. Ruptured intracranial arterial aneurysms (Chapter 9)
3. Arteriovenous malformations and angiomas (Chapter 10)
4. Blood dyscrasias
5. Neoplasms (Chapter 11)
6. Infections, bacterial aneurysms
7. Inflammatory and necrotizing lesions of small vessels
8. Hemorrhagic infarction (Chapter 4)
9. Hypertensive encephalopathy (Chapter 12)
10. Miscellaneous causes

Secondary brain stem hemorrhage. The commonest cause of nontraumatic secondary hemorrhage into the pons and midbrain has a mechanical etiology—a raised supratentorial pressure, first described by Attwater[12] in 1911. He noted that many of the hematomas occurred simultaneously with, or as is more likely, immediately after a large intracerebral hemorrhage in the region of the basal ganglia, particularly when associated with intraventricular hemorrhage. In his review of 67 cases, 30% of the pontine hemorrhages were of this type. The phenomenon was observed with hematomas elsewhere in the cerebrum, with subarachnoid hemorrhage and gross traumatic supratentorial bleeding. Attwater[12] observed that it usually consisted of multiple small hemorrhages, and Greenacre[101] remarked on its tendency to be situated in the midline (Fig. 8-19) and attributed the hemorrhage to an unduly high intravascular pressure caused by the angle

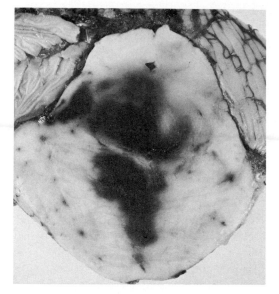

Fig. 8-19. Secondary pontine hemorrhage mainly in the midline but with some lateral spread.

of branching at which perforating pontine vessels arose from the basilar artery. Moore and Stern[169] recorded secondary vascular lesions in the pons and midbrain in 10.8% of 130 brains with expanding supratentorial lesions. Because of the midline position and the lateral spread to the sides of the aqueduct, they referred to a "fountain-like" hemorrhage in the midbrain.

Cannon[36] reviewed 122 cases of pontine hemorrhage of variable etiology. Most of the secondary pontine hemorrhages were in the tegmentum and followed perivascular spaces or fiber tracts, with the reticular substance and periaqueductal gray matter in particular being involved. When unilateral tentorial grooving of the basis pedunculi occurred, the hemorrhage within the brain stem was situated on the same side as the grooving and caudal to it. Poppen and associates[187] found 36 instances (14%) of brain stem hemorrhage among 258 subjects dying of supratentorial tumors. Over the same period the frequency of secondary brain stem hemorrhage in association with cerebral hemorrhage was 10.7%. Stehbens[239] found 15.3% in 301 cases of

Table 8-4. Frequency of secondary brain stem hemorrhage associated with supratentorial space-occupying lesions*

Lesion	Number of cases	Number with secondary brain stem hemorrhage	Frequency of brain stem hemorrhage
Intracerebral hemorrhage	168	96	57.1%
Cerebral encephalomalacia	266	24	9.0%
Cerebral glioblastoma multiforme	54	11	20.4%
Subdural hematoma	132	27	20.5%

*Adapted from Cohen, S. I., and Aronson, S. M.: Secondary brain stem hemorrhages: predisposing and modifying factors, Arch. Neurol. **19**:257, 1968.

significant primary hemorrhage into the cerebrum between 1910 and 1954, and the frequency was noticeably greater during the last 10 years of the survey. Fields and Halpert[77] found brain stem hemorrhage in 17 of 43 brains examined at the autopsy of subjects with raised supratentorial pressure. The supratentorial lesions responsible were variable and included intracerebral hemorrhage, subdural hematoma, extradural hematoma, traumatic hemorrhage, ruptured aneurysm, cerebral neoplasms (primary and secondary), cerebral abscesses, and massive cerebral softening. The commonest tumor causing secondary pontine hemorrhage is glioblastoma multiforme,[78] because of its rapid growth, hemorrhage, and necrosis.

Cohen and Aronson[44] analyzed 199 cases of secondary brain stem hemorrhage obtained from 7110 consecutive autopsies, a frequency of 2.8%. Their results confirmed once more that the advent of brain stem hemorrhage is dependent on an expanding supratentorial mass, and the larger and the more rapidly expanding the mass, the greater becomes the risk of secondary hemorrhage. In subdural hematomas there were no secondary brain stem hemorrhages when the volume of subdural blood was less than 25 cc. The frequency climbed to 42% when the volume was 76 to 100 cc., and 80% when it exceeded 100 cc. Similarly the magnitude of the infarcted brain associated with demonstrable vascular occlusion was directly proportional to the frequency of secondary brain stem hemorrhage, and this

was highest in cases of intracerebral hemorrhage (Table 8-4) and influenced by several factors. No significant sex difference was found, and no cases occurred in subjects under 25 years but the number of cases was very small. The frequency diminished progressively after 65 years of age. The presence of hypertension may influence the occurrence of these secondary hemorrhages, but heart weight, a rough index of the presence of raised blood pressure, could not be correlated with the frequency.

Freytag[86] asserted that secondary brain stem hemorrhage is practically unknown in infancy despite a severely raised supratentorial pressure.

PATHOLOGY. The hemorrhage in the brain stem is usually rostral and multiple, many extravasations often coalescing. In the midbrain the hemorrhages are usually in the tegmentum about the aqueduct. A hemorrhage characteristically elongated and extending anteroposteriorly in the midline may be seen in the midbrain and upper pons, but atypical pontine hemorrhages are frequent. Finney and Walker[78] found scattered petechial hemorrhages twice as often as midline infra-aqueductal hemorrhages. Multiple hemorrhages more laterally or asymmetrically placed may accompany these changes, and at times massive hemorrhage indistinguishable from primary pontine hemorrhage involves almost the whole pons. The hemorrhage does not usually extend superiorly above the tentorium and only seldom is it continuous with a supratentorial primary intracerebral hemorrhage. The reason the hemorrhages fail to extend below the pontomedullary junction is as yet unknown. A variable degree of edema and necrosis may accompany the hemorrhage. Survival is infrequent, and even when pressure from the initiating lesion is alleviated, secondary pressure changes may incapacitate. With survival the outcome is a cystic lesion in the necrotic areas, with evidence of the hemorrhage dependent on the severity of the extravasation of blood. Lindenberg[143] illustrated two cases in which the patients survived traumatic subdural hematomas for 2 and 3 months respectively.

Secondary pontine hemorrhages conjointly with infratentorial tumors were seen thrice in the series of Finney and Walker.[78] Each was attributed to operative trauma.

ETIOLOGY. These hemorrhages are associated with supratentorial lesions, particularly spontaneous or traumatic hemorrhage.[12] Cox[53] demonstrated that the brain stem hemorrhages occurred with supratentorial (20%) but not infratentorial tumors, and subsequently Dill and Isenhour[64] produced pontine hemorrhages experimentally in dogs by means of a supratentorial expanding mass. They thus demonstrated conclusively the importance of the transtentorial herniation. The bleeding was attributed to stretching and subsequent rupture of units of the vascular bed. Nevertheless the underlying pathogenesis and the actual source of the bleeding continue to be controversial.

The more rapid the increase in supratentorial pressure, the greater is the risk of brain stem hemorrhage. This accounts for the greatest frequency in massive intracerebral hemorrhage or in any hemorrhagic lesion including glioblastoma multiforme. Any increase in the differential pressure between that above and below the tentorium such as occurs with lumbar puncture[77] or jugular vein compression[78] may augment the herniation and precipitate the hemorrhage. Peculiarly enough, if the supratentorial pressure is alleviated, experimental brain stem hemorrhage is precipitated.[134] In association with the onset of the brain stem hemorrhage, a fairly sudden and severe exacerbation of symptoms and signs can be expected.

Moore and Stern,[169] impressed by the similarity of secondary pontine bleeding to primary hemorrhage, suggested that the underlying mechanism might be similar. Thus the rapidly increased supratentorial pressure was thought to cause a rise in blood pressure sufficient to induce hemorrhage in the brain stem.

Emphasis in recent years has been on the mechanical production of the hemorrhage. A considerable distortion of the midbrain and pons occurs with elongation (Fig. 8-20) and flattening from side to side (Fig. 8-21), with consequent increase in the anteroposterior diameter. Howell[117] stressed the actual buckling of the brain stem during transtentorial herniation, whereas Weinstein and colleagues,[259] using a vital dye, found that large arteries and veins were collapsed and the brain was ischemic in areas adjacent to their experimental space-occupying mass (inflated balloon). Ischemia was seen in remote areas of the brain such as the hypothalamus, but no ischemia was noted in the brain stem except as a direct extension of the ischemic zone around the balloon. However the vital dye in these experiments demonstrates only patency of the vessels and is no indication of the presence of flow or general stasis. With such severe distortion and compression of the brain stem, it seems highly likely that massive stasis in the microcirculation could come about even when not demonstrable at autopsy.

Venous obstruction (even of the vein of Galen) has been regarded by some authors as the underlying cause of the hemorrhage. Scheinker[210] asserted that the secondary hemorrhages in the brain stem were related predominantly to extremely congested medium-sized and small veins. In the center of some extravasations only the

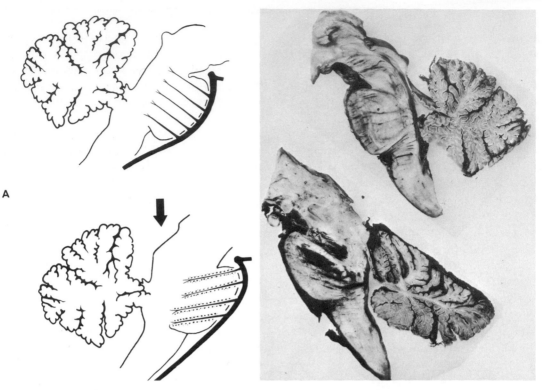

Fig. 8-20. A, Manner in which downward displacement of dorsal part of the brain stem causes distortion of the long penetrating arteries with rupture of their terminal branches. **B,** Specimens of brain stem corresponding to those in **A.** The lower specimen reveals elongation that the vessels undergo and associated hemorrhage. Normals above, and distorted brain stem below. (From Johnson, R. T., and Yates, P. O.: Brain stem haemorrhages in expanding supratentorial conditions, Acta Radiol. **46:**250, 1956.)

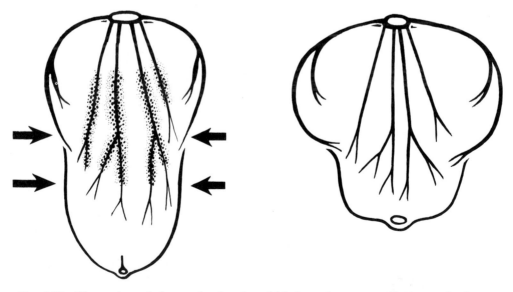

Fig. 8-21. Illustration of the mechanism by which lateral pressure, if appropriately applied even to an injected specimen post mortem, may cause elongation of the long penetrating arteries and extravasation of blood or injection medium, which runs back alongside the vessels. (From Johnson, R. T., and Yates, P. O.: Brain stem haemorrhages in expanding supratentorial conditions, Acta Radiol. **46:**250, 1956.)

"shadow" or "outline" of the venous wall was discernible and edema was said to be a notable feature in the parenchyma. As the transtentorial herniation progressed, the superficial draining veins over the brain stem became compressed and kinked and the venous obstruction caused severe congestion and stasis in the brain stem. Anoxic changes in the walls of the veins and overdistension were followed by the extravasation of blood. Poppen, Kendrick, and Hicks[187] believed that the secondary hemorrhages could be traced to mechanical distortion of arteries or more often of veins. The outstanding pathological change was described as fibrinoid necrosis of small arteries and veins with perivascular hemorrhage, rarely accompanied by thrombosis. Friede and Roessmann[89] examined by serial sections the pons, midbrain, and attached diencephalon of six patients with secondary brain stem hemorrhage. They considered that most of the hemorrhages were caused by focal necrosis and disintegration of medium-sized arteries, with occasional retraction of the stumps. Preexisting arterial disease was insignificant in the vascular changes, which they attributed to elongation of the midbrain in an anteroposterior direction. However, vascular necrosis is difficult to assess in the thin-walled vessels they illustrated. Johnson and Yates[128] did not find the severe degree of venous obstruction stressed by Scheinker[210] and attributed bleeding to venous rupture in rare cases only, that is, in cases where the hemorrhages were clustered beneath the ependyma of the aqueduct and fourth ventricle. Such periaqueductal hemorrhages were said to result from sudden internal hemocephalus.

Lindenberg[143] attributed the secondary bleeding in the brain stem to vascular compression, primarily of the arteries, with resultant necrobiosis. With mounting hypoxia, vessels exhibit increased permeability and diapedesis of red cells and with a restoration of flow hemorrhages increase and coalesce. He likened the lesions to the experimental model described by Globus and Epstein.[96] Lower pontine hemorrhages were thought to be caused by stretching of the small paramedian penetrating arteries of the basilar as the pons is displaced caudally and distorted.

Dott and Blackwood[67] suggested that the upper end of the basilar artery is anchored to the tentorial edge by the posterior cerebral arteries, and to the internal carotid artery by the posterior communicating arteries. Downward displacement of the brain stem thus causes lengthening and angulation of the penetrating branches of the basilar artery. Vasospasm or tearing of small vessels and active bleeding or infarction in the midbrain and pons is the result. Weintraub[260] believed that the stretching of the perforating vessels is aggravated by the taut, stretched oculomotor nerves supporting the posterior cerebral arteries, though it could be expected that the whole brain stem with attached nerves and vessels would be displaced downward. Johnson and Yates[128] did not consider this fixation of the basilar artery essential to the explanation of the secondary lesions.

Johnson and Yates[128] found the bleeding occurred in particular at sites of branching and explained the pathogenesis thus: Downward displacement of the brain stem elongates the penetrating arteries, causing them to run obliquely downward at a recurrent angle to the basilar (Fig. 8-20). The posterior part of the brain stem is thrust down farther than the anterior part. The resultant shift and distortion cause vasospasm or actually tear the small arterial branches. Postmortem angiography of brains with secondary pontine hemorrhages induced the injection medium to leak from the terminal branches. Flowing back and alongside the arteries, it mixed with the periarterial blood extravasated ante mortem, which suggests that the bleeding was arterial in origin. Arterial lesions were also observed in the anterior lobe of the cerebellum, the vascular supply of which is likewise derived from long attenuated vessels arising near the superior cerebellar arteries and seemingly is subjected to considerable tension in tentorial herniation. As to why the arteries are preferentially torn, Howell[117] explains that the veins are naturally very tortuous and therefore permit considerable stretching when the brain stem becomes distorted, whereas this does not apply with the arteries.

Johnson and Yates[128] pointed out that not all of the cases with hemorrhage into the pons and midbrain show marked downward displacement. They demonstrated that (1) the application of lateral pressure to the upper pons and midbrain during the injection brought about extravasation of the injection medium simulating brain stem bleeding (Figs. 8-21 and 8-22) and (2) with the application of lateral pressure to the midbrain during the injection only, the resultant extravasations from the torn vessels simulating actual hemorrhages were

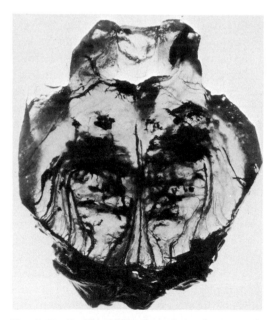

Fig. 8-22. Radiograph of section of pons subjected to lateral pressure during intra-arterial injection of silver iodide mixture at autopsy. The procedure caused extravasations into upper pons and midbrain, simulating secondary pontine hemorrhage. (Courtesy Dr. P. O. Yates, Manchester, England.)

restricted to this region alone. They believed that lateral pressure by temporo-occipital lobe herniation could flatten the midbrain and upper pons considerably while lengthening simultaneously by at least 1 cm. the anteroposterior diameter. Thus lateral compression alone was thought sufficient to cause arterial bleeding in some cases and in others to intensify the effects of the downward displacement. The disturbance of the blood supply to the midbrain and not actually the hematoma was said to cause the fatal damage. Johnson and Yates[128] thus demonstrated well how Dott and Blackwood's theory could work in practice. This is the most likely explanation of secondary brain stem hemorrhages (Fig. 8-23) although similar experiments during injection of the pontine veins are warranted.

Brewer and associates[34] found that in males with secondary pontine hemorrhage, the mean heart weight was significantly only slightly greater than in cases without brain stem hemorrhage. In females the difference was not significant. It is not known whether hypertension is a predisposing factor in the production of secondary brain stem hemorrhage and necrosis.

Blood dyscrasias. Hemorrhage into the central nervous system is a serious hazard with the heterogeneous group of diseases termed "blood dyscrasias."

LEUKEMIA. Intracerebral hemorrhage is not only the most frequent complication but the most serious manifestation of leukemia in the central nervous system. The intracerebral hemorrhages, like the extradural, intradural, and subdural hemorrhages, tend to be multiple and of small to moderate size. The cerebellum, midbrain, pons and medulla are each affected fairly frequently, but the hemorrhages are small and few in number. Primary intracerebral hemorrhage can conceivably occur in older patients with chronic leukemia; so large single hematomas require careful evaluation. Mostly the leukemic hemorrhages are associated with evidence of hemorrhage else-

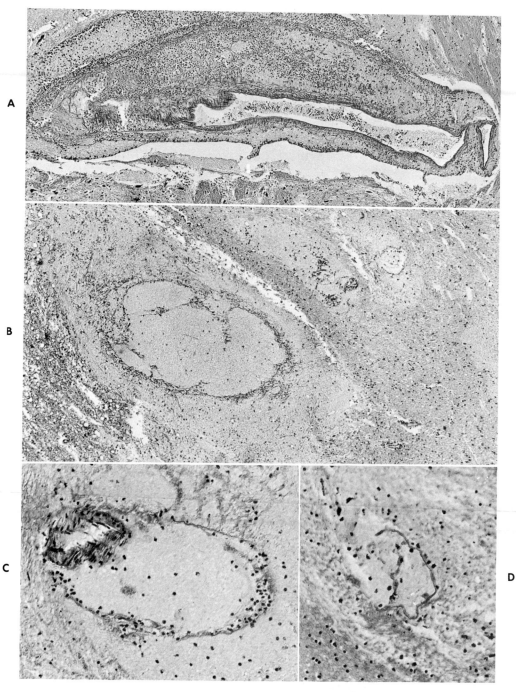

Fig. 8-23. Pontine vessels in secondary pontine hemorrhage. **A,** Periarterial hemorrhage appears to expand the adventitia or periarterial pia mater. **C,** Similar appearance in cross section. **B** and **D,** Perivascular hemorrhages are present, but it is uncertain what type of vessel is responsible in each instance. **D,** Vessel is ruptured and could be a vein. (Hematoxylin and eosin; **A** and **B,** ×45; **C** and **D,** ×110.)

where and occur in very ill patients. They usually end fatally within a few days. They complicate leukemia in the acute forms and during acute exacerbations of the chronic forms of the disease. Single hematomas like the pontine hemorrhage in acute lymphocytic leukemia described by Hawksley[111] are rare. Fried[88] found in the literature up to 1926 only 30 cases of leukemia in which the central nervous system had been examined and, of these, 13 had intracranial hemorrhage. Leidler and Russell[139] collected 67 cases of leukemia (with adequate detail of the central nervous system) and realized that the hemorrhages in the central nervous system were not prone to occur in the chronic forms of leukemia. Hemorrhage into the brain was observed macroscopically in 47 cases, in general associated with leukemic infiltration. The lesions were most often in the white matter, particularly the centrum ovale and rarely in the cortex. In 41 of 67 cases there were lesions in the cerebral hemisphere, in 21 the medulla and pons, in 31 the basal ganglia, in 19 the cerebellum, and in 10 the mesencephalon. Leidler and Russell[139] concluded however that approximately 80% of patients with leukemia have significant changes in the brain consisting of hemorrhages and leukemic infiltrations and that hemorrhage causes death in about 29% of patients.

Groch and associates[106] reported macroscopic hemorrhages in the brains of 49% of 93 leukemic patients and Brandt[33] found a frequency of 54% in 167 patients. Of all the cases with cerebral hemorrhage, 43% were caused by acute lymphocytic leukemia and the age distribution displayed a correspondingly high number of cases (22%) in the first decade of life.

Hunt and associates[119] found that the overall frequency of hemorrhage as a neurological complication was 10.6% in 815 leukemic patients (Table 8-5). This figure was regarded as conservative, for many patients die at home or in other institutions without the immediate cause of death being determined. Also encountered were a few terminal instances of hemorrhage in Hodgkin's disease (3 in 257 cases) and lymphosarcoma (3 in 87 cases). The bleeding was attributed to thrombocytopenia.

Williams and associates[265] found a high frequency of intracranial hemorrhage (mostly intracerebral) in a large series of patients with leukemia and drew attention to the secondary fungal invasion of the central nervous system (notably cryptococcosis) in these disorders. Such infections may be a cause of hemorrhage. As infiltration of the cranial nerves may occur, so could hemorrhage, although this aspect has not received much attention.

The leukemic hemorrhages appear to result from bleeding about gray round or oval infiltrations or nodules often recognized in the hematoma macroscopically.[85] Leidler and Russell[139] attributed the hemorrhage to thrombocytopenia and to leukemic infiltration. The infiltrations are closely related to blood vessels[33,139] and are thought to precede the hemorrhage and to

Table 8-5. Prevalence of intracranial or intraspinal hemorrhage in leukemia*

Type of leukemia	Number of patients	Hemorrhage	Percentage
Acute lymphatic	145	22	15.2
Chronic lymphatic	300	11	3.7
Acute myeloid	48	11	23.0
Chronic myeloid	170	18	10.6
Monocytic	152	24	15.8
Total	815	86	10.6

*After Hunt, W. E., Bouroncle, B. A., and Meagher, J. N.: Neurologic complications of leukemias and lymphomas, J. Neurosurg. **16**:135, 1959.

compress and probably cause necrosis of the vessel walls assisted by a deficiency of platelets. Jaffé[122] thought that hemorrhages resulted in the growth of leukemic infiltrations in the brain. Fried[88] considered that hemorrhages in leukemia were primarily caused by infiltration of the vessel walls and disruption of the mural constituents. A second factor was thought to be capillary stasis and thrombosis of small and large vessels due to the large number of leukocytes therein, the vascular walls at times forming small aneurysmal dilatations that proceed to rupture. Microangiography could prove or disprove the existence of such dilatations.

In a series of publications,[85,91,168] intracranial hemorrhage in leukemia has been correlated with the blood counts. Intracranial hemorrhage was the cause of death in 20% of 117 cases of acute leukemia, but the presence of leukocyte counts of over 300,000 per cu. mm. in some patients suggests that the authors also included acute crises of chronic leukemia.[168] Most cases of fatal intracerebral hemorrhage were associated with a notable prevalence of leukocytic stasis in cerebral blood vessels and leukemic nodules together with leukocyte counts greater than 300,000 per cu. mm., a high blast cell count, and a significantly high platelet population in the blood. In those patients with leukocyte counts below 300,000 per cu. mm., the frequency of intracranial hemorrhage was far less. In such patients the platelet count was low, subarachnoid infiltrations were frequent, and leukocytic stasis and leukemic nodules or infiltrations were sparse. The hemorrhage tended and to be subarachnoid of subdural with petechial hemorrhages or hemorrhagic softening in the neighbouring cortex in a few instances. However, most authors attribute intracerebral bleeding in acute or chronic leukemia to thrombocytopenia.[106]

HEMOPHILIA. Intracranial hemorrhage is a frequent complication of hemophilia.[190] Subdural and subarachnoid hemorrhage are said to be the most common.[225] Kerr[133] however found 14 instances of intracere-bral, intracerebellar, or midbrain hemorrhages in 19 episodes of intracranial hemorrhage. Trauma is the most frequent cause although one of Kerr's patients had a hemorrhage occurring after meningitis. Another died from a ruptured aneurysm of the vertebral artery. The mortality from intracranial hemorrhage in hemophilia is known to be high, but the availability of coagulation factor concentrates and plasma should lower the current rate. Quick[190] believed that the benefit of therapy was needed not so much for the initial traumatic bleeding, but for the seepage of blood associated with resolution of the traumatized tissue, because in some cases symptoms did not appear for days after the head injury.

THROMBOCYTOPENIC PURPURA. In essential thrombocytopenic purpura, bleeding as in all thrombocytopenic states is essentially a capillary hemorrhage and therefore mostly causes purpura. Intracranial bleeding is also essentially the same, but confluence of hemorrhages may occur so that lesions varying from petechial to massive hemorrhages, which destroy whole lobes of the cerebrum, may be present.[40] Intracranial hemorrhage is a major cause of death in this disease.[40,68] Subarachnoid and subdural bleeding also occur and may accompany the intracerebral hemorrhage. Retinal hemorrhages are frequent.[40] Similar hemorrhages occur in secondary thrombocytopenic purpura and the thrombocytopenia likewise accounts for the intracerebral hemorrhages that may appear in aplastic anemia. Boon and Walton[29] attributed a massive cerebellar hemorrhage in a woman of 35 years to aplastic anemia. Petechial hemorrhages within the brain also occur in the rare disease thrombotic thrombocytopenic purpura,[40] which is believed to be a disease primarily of small vessels.

A rare case of fatal cerebral hemorrhage from thrombocytopenia complicating infectious mononucleosis has recently been reported.[98]

HYPOPROTHROMBINEMIA. Intracerebral hemorrhage is a serious complication of anticoagulant therapy. Stephens[243] reported that of 181 patients with 221 thromboembolic episodes for which anticoagulants were administered, major bleeding occurred in 12 patients (7%) and minor bleeding in 36 patients (20%). Two patients died, one of them suffering from cerebral hemorrhage. Tulloch and Wright[252] analyzed 227 cases on long-term anticoagulant therapy (4 to 7 years). Forty-three patients (18.9%) suffered 70 hemorrhagic complications, of which 3 were intracranial (two intracerebral, one of uncertain site). MacMillan and Brown[152] analyzed the effects of anticoagulant therapy on 489 patients over a 2-year period. Of 28 patients with hemorrhagic complications, five deaths occurred. Three were attributed to hemorrhagic cerebral infarction, and another patient had an intracerebral hemorrhage. Other reports of anticoagulant therapy have listed intracerebral hemorrhage as a cause of death.[110,193,261] Suzman and associates[247] recorded one death from cerebral hemorrhage from each of two series of anticoagulant therapy (one of 82 patients on long term and one of 88 patients on short term). Both patients were hypertensive, as were many other patients succumbing to intracerebral hemorrhage.[261] The unavoidable fact is that some patients on anticoagulant therapy die or suffer from spontaneous bleeding from numerous sites including subdural hematoma, and these deaths have therefore all been accepted for the most part as a complication of the therapy. Russek and Zohman[202] give the incidence of major hemorrhages among patients treated with anticoagulants for acute myocardial infarction as from 0.25% to 10% with four deaths among 100 patients. In 122 deaths from anticoagulant therapy, 22 were attributed to subarachnoid hemorrhage (21.5%), and 24 to intracerebral hemorrhage (23.5%). Bjerkelund[25] reported the incidence of cerebral hemorrhage as 16.7% in causes of death of patients treated with anticoagulants for long terms. In the control group it was only 2.4%.

Reports of 32 deaths ascribed to Dicum-arol therapy were found by Wright and Rothman[269] in a review of literature to 1951. Their largest group consisted of patients with subacute bacterial endocarditis, all dying of cerebral hemorrhage. In the literature Barron and Fergusson[18] found 58 instances of intracranial hemorrhage during anticoagulant therapy and 27 in patients with bacterial endocarditis. The hemorrhages were intracerebral, intracerebellar, and subarachnoid, and of considerable significance is the fact that no bacterial aneurysms were found at autopsy in any of the patients. Thus, bacterial endocarditis is regarded as a contraindication to anticoagulant therapy.

Barron and Fergusson contend that two of their five cases of cerebral hemorrhage from anticoagulants were probably instances of massive hemorrhage into embolic infarcts. Experimental studies have demonstrated that anticoagulants aggravate the tendency to massive hemorrhage in areas of experimentally induced cerebral encephalomalacia in dogs.[221,264] Marshall and Shaw[155] after trials aimed at determining the efficacy of anticoagulant therapy in patients with acute nonembolic, nonhemorrhagic cerebrovascular disease concluded that anticoagulants were of no value and even hazardous. Others reached similar conclusions independently.[82]

Hypertension has also been considered a factor predisposing to intracerebral hemorrhage in anticoagulation, but in view of the age distribution of the patients likely to need anticoagulants and the absence of statistics, the contention continues as subjective impression only. Cole and Yates,[45] in discussing the pathological significance of miliary aneurysms in predominantly hypertensive subjects, suggested that anticoagulants could well initiate massive hemorrhage from these aneurysms.

Anticoagulant therapy may precipitate hemorrhage from or in a lesion not known to exist previously.[105] Thus if hemorrhage eventuates, it is necessary to consider the possibility of (1) some serious underlying pathology and (2) some unrelated lesion from which hemorrhage might be initiated, such as an aneurysm.

Hypoprothrombinemia from any other cause, be it hemorrhagic disease of the newborn, severe liver disease, inadequate intestinal absorption of vitamin K, salicylate therapy, or idiopathic (familial) hypoprothrombinemia may result in cerebral hemorrhage.[40]

Hypoprothrombinemia may cause multiple hemorrhages but the bleeding does not tend to be purpuric in type. As in hemophilia, a propensity to become a massive proportions usually atypical in site or distribution is demonstrated. In most cases it appears likely that trauma precipitates the bleeding.

SICKLE CELL ANEMIA. Multiple petechial hemorrhages may occasionally be encountered in sickle cell anemia[262] in association with capillary thromboses. Extensive focal hemorrhagic softenings or even a large hemorrhage may occur. In one case[262] there was a large, recent hemorrhage into the basal ganglia together with older hemorrhages. Another patient had cerebral encephalomalacia with a small secondary pontine hemorrhage, yet another a ruptured cerebral aneurysm. Fat embolism often occurs in this disease and this in itself may cause multiple petechial hemorrhages throughout the white matter. Siderotic pigment indicative of previous small hemorrhages is frequently seen in the adventitial or perivascular tissue of both small and large vessels.

POLYCYTHEMIA. In polycythemia rubra vera any involvement of the central nervous system has most likely been occasioned by arterial or venous thrombosis. Hemorrhagic softening can result in subarachnoid hemorrhage of varying severity. In 1912, Lucas[151] reviewed 179 cases of polycythemia, and of the 23 in which an autopsy was performed, softening of the cord and spinal cord were found in 4 cases (17.4%) and cerebral hemorrhage in three. Subarachnoid and even middle meningeal hemorrhage have been attributed to polycythemia as well as intracerebral bleeding.[226]

AFIBRINOGENEMIA. Congenital afibrinogenemia is an extremely rare disease. The afflicted patients are subject to episodes of recurrent bleeding including intracerebral hemorrhage.[40]

MACROGLOBULINEMIA. In about two-thirds of the patients with Waldenström's macroglobulinemia, a hemorrhagic diathesis is manifested though not often in the internal organs. In a review of 182 cases, two subjects died of cerebral hemorrhage (hypothalamic and cerebellar). In addition of course subarachnoid hemorrhage may occur in a few patients (intracranial or spinal) and also petechial hemorrhages within the brain.[150]

Infections. Infections from time to time cause intracerebral bleeding ranging from a petechial hemorrhage to a massive rapidly fatal intracerebral hematoma. Bacterial endocarditis immediately comes to mind, and the acute arteritis responsible may or may not have undergone aneurysmal dilatation. The increased risk of serious hemorrhage with anticoagulant therapy in this disease has already been mentioned. Hemorrhage may accompany almost any variety of acute leptomeningitis and is particularly common in tuberculous meningitis. Syphilis is a most unlikely cause, and even if there is some hemorrhage, it is likely to be incidental. Thrombotic occlusion of vessels may complicate any of the infections, producing hemorrhage of variable degree in the infarcted zone. Fungus infections of the central nervous system may occasionally be accompanied by hemorrhage, particularly mucormycosis (Chapter 12).

Capillary hemorrhage appears in the wake of viral infections of the brain and cord and the encephalitides. In acute hemorrhagic leukoencephalitis[102] the hemorrhages are particularly prominent, mostly petechial, and in the centrum semiovale. Microscopically, they are ring or ball type of hemorrhages, at times around thrombosed capillaries or necrotic venules.

Inflammatory and necrotizing lesions of small vessels. As in subarachnoid hemorrhage, the diseases of polyarteritis nodosa, diffuse lupus erythematosus, and other types of vasculitis may cause intracerebral hemorrhage, which is only rarely massive. In Schönlein-Henoch purpura (anaphylactoid purpura) the characteristic purpuric exanthem, the frequent occurrence of arthritis, abdominal colic, and melena, together with the possibility of renal damage and acute rheumatic carditis in young subjects, are well recognized. Serious neurological complications are rare. Several instances of subarachnoid hemorrhage have been reported[141,166] and in one case subarachnoid hemorrhage, convulsions, and a hemiplegia led to the presumptive diagnosis of intracerebral hemorrhage or thrombosis.[141] Headache is a symptom in up to 25% of cases, often in the absence of fever, hypertension, and renal pathology.[141] Convulsions are not infrequent and the cerebral symptoms seem to be the result of the necrotizing arteriolitis and arteritis, which involve other sectors of the body[92,140] as well as the cortical and pial vessels of the cerebrum.[92]

Other varieties are dealt with in Chapter 12.

Miscellaneous causes. Cerebral ring hemorrhages or small perivascular hemorrhages are seen in many diseases of the brain, such as fat embolism, concussion, blood dyscrasias, high altitudes, intoxications, acute hemorrhagic leukoencephalitis, and malaria.[35] The hemorrhages are confined to the cerebral white matter and histologically consist of a circular zone of extravasated red cells about a zone of perivascular necrosis.[35] The central vessel may contain an embolus or a hyaline red cell mass indicative of stasis. It may even be amorphous, sometimes with fibrin infiltration in the tissues. The vessel wall can be necrotic.

Although many small petechial hemorrhages are found in the cortex particularly, the preceding diseases typically involve the white matter. In some instances the petechial hemorrhages have a characteristic localization. In hemorrhagic leukoencephalitis they are mostly central in the white

matter, to a lesser extent in the cerebellum and brain stem, and slight or absent in the frontal, temporal, or occipital lobes. In arsenical or arsphenamine encephalopathy, there may be numerous petechiae in the subcortical white matter of the cerebrum with a striking predilection for the periventricular white matter, corpus collosum, and centrum semiovale.[212] Multiple petechiae in the cerebral white matter have also been described in sulfonamide therapy.[212] Similar petechiae in carbon monoxide poisoning may be observed in the corpus collosum and white matter, whereas larger hemorrhages may involve the basal ganglia or one of the lobes of the brain. The globus pallidus, which often exhibits ischemic necrosis, may also contain petechiae. In falciparum malaria, the petechia are studded throughout the white matter, particularly about the base and around the ventricles.

Cammermeyer[35] explains the pathogenesis of these ring hemorrhages thus: At the moment of cardiac arrest, the veins become engorged particularly in the neck, and increased venous pressure and venous backflow result. The stress on the venous system and the reduction in tissue support have been supposed responsible for the small amount of blood that is sometimes extravasated in the perivenous tissues. Essentially at fault is a hemodynamic imbalance occurring at the moment of death or shortly thereafter, the extravasation ceasing as the venous backflow diminished. On morphological grounds, Cammermeyer[35] said he could not accept the hemorrhages as being caused by stasis and diapedesis of red cells though this was possible, but stasis is difficult to appreciate in routine histological material. His hypothesis, being entirely too speculative, has not received much support. There is adequate explanation for the perivascular hemorrhages in thrombotic occlusion of small vessels and where there is necrosis of the vessel wall or stasis of its contents. Diapedesis of red cells, sufficient to cause petechial bleeding, readily occurs in such damaged and stagnant vessels.

Heat stroke is associated with a tendency to bleed because of a combination of hypoprothrombinemia, hypofibrinogenemia, thrombocytopenia, increased capillary permeability,[258] and endothelial damage.[230] The brain characteristically exhibits edema, congestion, and petechial hemorrhages.[153,258] Malamud and his colleagues[153] found such petechial hemorrhages in 65 of 125 cases and they were situated particularly in the walls of the third ventricle and the floor of the fourth ventricle. More extensive bleeding can occur, and microscopically, apart from severe neuronal and Purkinje cell damage, intravascular thrombi are found in small vessels. Experimentally in rats, heat stroke has caused subarachnoid or intracerebral hemorrhage or both in 50% of the animals. Bleeding into both the cerebrum and cerebellum was recorded.[5]

Massive hemorrhage may occur in the brain in association with eclampsia[125,196] Donnelly and Lock[66] found that on clinical grounds 89 women of 533 cases with toxemia or pregnancy had gross evidence of intracranial hemorrhage, such as hemiplegia or bloodstained cerebrospinal fluid on lumbar puncture. In a much smaller autopsy series, there were 5 massive hemorrhages in 13 cases studied post mortem. Petechial hemorrhages in the brain are more frequent than massive bleeding.

Cases of primary intracerebral hemorrhage in the absence of hypertension are kept apart as an idiopathic group. The present author does not feel any purpose is served with a separate classification. The etiology of massive intracerebral hemorrhage in children and youths has caused much controversy.[112,195] Sheldon[219] found only 50 cases of intracranial hemorrhage among 10,150 autopsies on children under 12 years of age, which indicates a low frequency in this age group. Of Sheldon's 50 cases, one was extradural, 11 subdural, 16 subarachnoid, 16 cerebral, four cerebellar, and two pontine and medullary. Death was attributed to a multiplicity of causes, including trauma, blood dyscrasias, endo-

carditis, varied infectious processes, and vascular thromboses. One additional case was associated with chronic nephritis.

Sheldon[219] reported intracerebral hemorrhage (in the vicinity of the internal capsule) in a child who fell against a cupboard 2 weeks previously. The interpretation given was traumatic hemorrhage. Another of Sheldon's cases was that of a boy who hit his head against a table 2 days before he died of a hemorrhage in the medulla oblongata with rupture into the fourth ventricle. On account of the rarity of spontaneous hemorrhage in children and the unusual location of the hemorrhage, trauma was said to have been responsible. Ritchie and Haines[195] presented eight cases in children 15 years or younger and reviewed 81 cases from the literature. Angiomas or arteriovenous malformations were the most common cause of hemorrhage with a few attributed to arterial aneurysms and a sizable group of undetermined cause. In many of these, inadequate clinical information was available, or the cause of the bleeding such as a small cryptic hemangioma or some other etiological factor was overlooked. Very thorough examinations of clinical information and autopsy material, particularly the brain, are mandatory. Normotensive adults under 40 years of age with an intracerebral hematoma must be regarded as having primary intracerebral hemorrhage, provided that secondary causes of the bleeding can be confidently excluded. Reluctance to accede to the possibility of such cases is based on an inability to accept that degenerative changes can occur in the blood vessels of young individuals.

Intraventricular hemorrhage

The frequency of intraventricular hemorrhage in the newborn has been estimated[6] as being between 2.2% to 8.5%. Yagi[270] found nine instances in 144 autopsies (6.3%) and Weyhe[263] 21 in 122 autopsies (17.2%). Alpers[6] attributes all these hemorrhages to trauma, conceding that some may be caused by a hemorrhagic diathesis or a hypothetical congenital defect in the vessel walls. The hemorrhage arises in one or both lateral ventricles, or forms a red currant jelly cast of the entire ventricular system. Being thought to stem from the choroid plexus, the internal cerebral, or one of the terminal veins, it can be so extentive as to form a cast of the ventricular system or part thereof. Small blood clots of recent origin on the surface of the choroid plexus are not unusual and are of little significance being attributed to anoxia.[188] Massive intraventricular hemorrhage in premature babies has also been considered a manifestation of hypoxia,[13] although Windle's experimental studies[266,267] do not support the theory.

Attwood and Stewart[13] found intraventricular hemorrhage in 3.5% of 2000 perinatal necropsies. Fedrick[75] determined that intraventricular hemorrhage in cases of stillbirth and neonatal death was associated with prematurity and growth retardation as indicated by body weight relative to the time of gestation with at times evidence of traumatic hemorrhage elsewhere within the cranium.

Primary intraventricular hemorrhage, a rare entity indeed, has been declared the result of bleeding from vessels in the choroid plexus,[251] although the initiating factor was not specified. Much more often the bleeding can be regarded as secondary in nature. Occasionally an intracranial arterial aneurysm may rupture into the ventricular system producing parenchymal damage so slight as to be readily overlooked. This is quite often the case with ruptured aneurysms of the anterior communicating artery and those at the bifurcation of the internal carotid or basilar arteries.[238] Thus a diagnosis of primary intraventricular hemorrhage should always be provisional unless irrefutable proof of its applicability has been provided.

Intraventricular hemorrhage frequently occurs with primary intracerebral hemorrhage and also follows rupture of intracranial arterial aneurysms associated with large intracerebral hematomas. Papillomas of the choroid plexus may bleed into the ventricular system while presenting clinically as an acute subarachnoid hemorrhage.[1] At times other intracranial tumors including pituitary adenomas bleed into the ventricles. Kalbag[129] reported three instances of a lesion (oligodendroglioma and two angiomas) close to the ventricle causing subarachnoid hemorrhage, with angiography not disclosing the diagnosis. The presence of small cryptic angiomas can be excluded if a very careful search for them has proved fruitless and when histological examination of any suspicious area has been nonproductive. Postmortem microangiography, though more valuable, is time consuming. Avol and Vogel[14] reported two instances of a large circumscribed encapsulated hematoma within the lateral ventricle, in each case simulating a tumor. In one of these cases a "vascular malformation" of the choroid plexus was found and incriminated in the pathogenesis of the hematoma.

There may be hemorrhage into the ventricles in blood dyscrasias though other evidence of hemorrhage within the cranium could be expected. Adeloye and colleagues[4] encountered a 3-month-old African male with hemophilia and intraventricular hemorrhage and some hydrocephalus.

McCarthy[159] cited an instance of intraventricular hemorrhage in a patient with fulminating tuberculosis, meningitis, and massive bleeding from the choroid plexus. Although such an event may theoretically occur in association with other infective and inflammatory lesions, in reality it is most exceptional.

Blood may also reach the ventricular system from the subarachnoid space, or a cerebellar or pontine hemorrhage. More frequently ventricular blood escapes into the subarachnoid space and is most dense in the subarachnoid space in the posterior fossa and initiates hemogenic meningitis.

Massive intraventricular hemorrhage with tamponade due either to obstruction by a blood clot or to distortion and compression of the aqueduct results in acute hemocephalus, with tears and lacerations of the ventricular walls being a possibility. Harris, Roessmann, and Friede[109] reported 11 cases, three cases from gunshot wounds involving the cerebral ventricles, 2 from ruptured cerebral aneurysms, and 4 from primary intracerebral and 2 from intracerebellar hemorrhage. The lacerations orientated in the parasagittal axis exhibited a predilection for the corners of the ventricle.

Intraventricular hemorrhage is usually a terminal event associated with deep coma, bilateral corticospinal tract signs, and decerebrate rigidity and hyperthermia,[251] although they are not invariable. The ventricular tamponade and the raised intracranial pressure attendant upon intraventricular hemorrhage cause serious herniation and compression of the brain stem and thus account for the serious and dire consequences that come in the train of massive bleeding into the ventricular system.[38]

Intraspinal hemorrhage

Intraspinal hemorrhage from whatever cause is rarely seen, but because of the infrequency with which the spinal canal and its contents are examined, it is likely that the entity is overlooked quite often.

Spinal arterial aneurysms (Chapter 9) have an extremely low incidence in direct contrast with their prevalence in the intracranial cavity. Arteriovenous malformations and angiomatous tumor masses are more prevalent than spinal arterial aneurysms and may bleed into the cord itself as well as between or external to the meninges. Just as a subdural or subarachnoid hemorrhage can cause a transverse lesion with paraplegia, so will intraspinal hemorrhage. Some fiber tracts, such as the more laterally placed spinothalamic fibers,[251] may be spared.

Hematomyelia has been reported in leukemia[33,119,265] and may be seen in other blood dyscrasias, but for such bleeding to be a major event in these clinical histories is unusual though it has been seen in caisson disease.[61]

Injury to the spinal cord differs considerably from cranial trauma. Head injuries may be associated with damage in the cord and even hemorrhages into the dorsal root ganglia and nerve roots[233] although there is some question as to whether the latter are caused by the head injury or raised intracranial pressure. However dislocations and fractures of the spine are the most frequent cause of spinal hemorrhage.[61] Less interest has been evinced in spinal concussion probably because of its lower incidence, but small perivascular or ring hemorrhages, hemorrhages, congestion (probably stasis), edema, and areas of necrosis have been described.[61] There can be association with gross intramedullary hemorrhage, but this is more likely to occur with contusion of the cord. The hemorrhage may extend upward or downward for a distance beyond the site of a crush injury. Bloodstained and necrotic tissue destroyed and crushed by the injury may be squeezed cranially or caudally in the posterior columns. McVeigh[163] demonstrated experimentally in dogs that digital compression of the cord after laminectomy caused the typical picture of hematomyelia, the squashed central pulp being forced to track up and down (for several centimeters) principally in the posterior white columns. Initially the trauma was accompanied by small hemorrhages and edema, with liquefaction of the pulp and affected cord after 48 hours. Animals with longer survival revealed the classic picture of hemorrhagic cavitation. Experimentation with a human spinal cord post mortem resulted in similar extension of the softened pulp into the anterior aspect of the posterior columns both above and below the site of compression.

The injury to the cord may be much more severe with transection in extreme cases. Resolution will occur in much the same manner as in the brain. In some instances there is delayed apoplexy and the patient develops neurological symptoms 1 or 2 weeks after a spinal injury.[60,61] In such cases thrombosis of the vessels may have supervened or otherwise essential information is lacking. Davison[61] refers to a condition called vasopathia traumatica in cases with progressive symptoms. The small arteries exhibit considerable intimal thickening with some medial thinning and also as appears from the illustration, significant elastic degeneration. In the absence of further detail, the appearance in the vessels is of arteriosclerosis or diffuse hyperplastic sclerosis.

Injury of the spinal cord at birth is rare but will transpire if sufficient force is applied to rupture or dislocate the spinal column.[58]

References

1. Abbott, K. H., Rollas, Z. H., and Meagher, J. N.: Choroid plexus papilloma causing spontaneous subarachnoid hemorrhage, J. Neurosurg. 14:566, 1957.
2. Adams, R. D., and Cohen, M. E.: Vascular diseases of the brain, Bull. New Eng. Med. Center 9:184, 222, 261, 1947.
3. Adams, R. D., and Vander Eecken, H. M.: Vascular diseases of the brain, Ann. Rev. Med. 4:213, 1959.
4. Adeloye, A., Seriki, O. Luzzatto, L., and Essien, E. M.: Intracranial ventricular haemorrhage as a first presentation of haemophilia, J. Neurol. Neurosurg. Psychiat. 32:470, 1969.
5. Allen, I. V.: Cerebral changes in experimental heatstroke, Irish J. Med. Sci. 6:413, 1964.
6. Alpers, B. J.: Cerebral birth injuries. In Brock, S.: Injuries of the brain and spinal cord and their coverings, ed. 3, Baltimore, 1949, The Williams & Wilkins Co., p. 229.
7. Angrist, A., and Mitchell, N.: Traumatic hemorrhage of the internal capsule, Arch. Surg. 46:265, 1943.
8. Antin, S. P., Prockop, L. D., and Cohen, S. M.: Transient hemiballism, Neurology 17:1068, 1967.
9. Apfelbach, C. W.: Studies in traumatic fractures of the cranial bones. I. Edema of the brain; II. Bruises of the brain, Arch. Surg. 4: 434, 1922.
10. Aring, C. D., and Merritt, H. H.: Differential diagnosis between cerebral hemorrhage and cerebral thrombosis, Arch. Intern. Med. 56: 435, 1935.
11. Aronson, H., Shafey, S., and Gargano, F., Intracerebellar haematoma, J. Neurol. Neurosurg. Psychiat. 28:442, 1965.
12. Attwater, H. L.: Pontine haemorrhages, Guy's Hosp. Ref. 65:399, 1911.
13. Attwood, H. D., and Stewart, A. D.: Perinatal mortality. A clinico-pathological study of 2,000 necropsies, Aust. New Zeal. J. Obstet. Gynaec. 8:33, 1968.
14. Avol, M., and Vogel, P. J.: Circumscribed intraventricular hematoma simulating an encapsulated neoplasm, Bull. Los Angeles Neurol. Soc. 20:25, 1955.
15. Baer, H.: Apoplexie und Hypertonie, Frankfurt. Z. Path. 30:128, 1924.
16. Bagley, C.: Spontaneous cerebral hemorrhage, Arch. Neurol. Psychiat. 27:1133, 1932.
17. Bailey, P.: Traumatic apoplexy, Med. Rec. 66: 528, 1904.
18. Barron, K. D., and Fergusson, G.: Intracranial hemorrhage as a complication of anticoagulant therapy, Neurology 9:447, 1959.
19. Beadles, C. F.: Aneurisms of the larger cerebral arteries, Brain 30:285, 1907.
20. Bechgaard, P.: The natural history of benign hypertension. In Bock, K. D., and Cottier, P. T.: Essential hypertension, Heidelberg, 1960, Springer-Verlag, p. 198.
21. Bedford, T. H. B.: The pathology of sudden death; a review of 198 cases "brought in dead," J. Path. Bact. 36:333, 1933.
22. Bell, E. T.: Renal diseases, Philadelphia, 1947, Lea & Febiger.
23. Bell, E. T.: Renal diseases, ed. 2, London, 1950, Henry Kimpton.
24. Bell, E. T., and Clawson, B. J.: Primary (essential) hypertension, Arch. Path. 5:939, 1928.
25. Bjerkelund, C. J.: The effect of long term treatment with Dicoumarol in myocardial infarction, Acta Med. Scand. 158 (suppl. 330):1, 1957.
26. Björk, S., Sannerstedt, R., Angervall, G., and Hood, B.: Treatment and prognosis in malignant hypertension: clinical follow-up study of 93 patients on modern medical treatment, Acta Med. Scand. 166:175, 1960.
27. Blackwood, W.: Vascular disease of the central nervous system. In Blackwood, W., McMenemey, W. H., Meyer, A., Norman, R. M., and Russell, D. S.: Greenfield's neuropathology, ed. 2, Baltimore, 1963, The Williams & Wilkins Co., p. 71.
28. Blakemore, W. S., Jeffers, W. A., Sellers, A. M., Itskovitz, H. D. Cooper, D. Y., Wolferth, C. C., and Zintel, H. A.: Sympathectomy and adrenalectomy in the treatment of hypertension. In Brest, A. N., and Moyer, J. H.: Hypertension, Philadelphia, 1961, Lea & Febiger, p. 619.
29. Boon, T. H., and Walton, J. N.: Aplastic anaemia, Quart. J. Med. 20:75, 1951.
30. Bouchard, C.: A study of some points in the pathology of cerebral haemorrhage (translated by Maclagan, T. J.), London, 1872, Simpkin, Marshall and Co.
31. Bouman, L.: Hemorrhage of the brain, Arch. Neurol. Psychiat. 25:255, 1931.
32. Bramwell, B.: Clinical and pathological memoranda, Edin. Med. J. 32:4, 97, 243, 911, 1886-1887.
33. Brandt, S.: Altérations leucémiques du système nerveux, Acta Psychiat. Neurol. 20:107, 1945.
34. Brewer, D. B., Fawcett, F. J. and Horsfield, G. I.: A necropsy series of nontraumatic cerebral haemorrhages and softenings, with particular reference to heart weight, J. Path. Bact. 96:311, 1968.
35. Cammermeyer, J.: Agonal nature of the cere-

bral ring hemorrhages, Arch. Neurol. Psychiat. **70:**54, 1953.

36. Cannon, B. W.: Acute vascular lesions of the brain stem. Arch. Neurol. Psychiat. **66:**687, 1951.
37. Cappell, D. F.: Muir's textbook of pathology, ed. 7, London, 1958, Edward Arnold (Publishers) Ltd.
38. Carpenter, S. J., McCarthy, L. E., and Borison, H. L.: Morphologic and functional effects of intracerebroventricular administration of autologous blood in cats, Neurology **17:**993, 1967.
39. Cassasa, C. S. B.: Multiple traumatic cerebral hemorrhages, Proc. N.Y. Path. Soc. **24:**101, 1924.
40. Chalgren, W. S.: Neurologic complications of the hemorrhagic diseases, Neurology **3:**126, 1953.
41. Charcôt, J. M.: Clinical lectures on senile and chronic diseases, London, 1881, The New Sydenham Society.
42. Charcôt, J. M., and Bouchard, C.: Nouvelle recherches sur la pathogénie de l'hémorrhagie cérébrale, Arch. Physiol. (Paris) **1:**110, 643, 725, 1869.
43. Chason, J. L.: Brain, meninges, and spinal cord. In Saphir, O.: A text on systemic pathology, New York, 1959, Grune & Stratton, Inc., vol. 2, p. 1798.
44. Cohen, S. I., and Aronson, S. M.: Secondary brain stem hemorrhages, predisposing and modifying factors, Arch. Neurol. **19:**257, 1968.
45. Cole, F. M., and Yates, P. O.: The occurrence and significance of intracerebral micro-aneurysms, J. Path. Bact. **93:**393, 1967.
46. Cole, F. M., and Yates, P. O.: Intracerebral microaneurysms and small cerebrovascular lesions, Brain **90:**759, 1967.
47. Cole, F. M., and Yates, P. O.: Pseudo-aneurysms in relationship to massive cerebral haemorrhage, J. Neurol. Neurosurg. Psychiat. **30:**61, 1967.
48. Cole, F. M., and Yates, P. O.: Comparative incidence of cerebrovascular lesions in normotensive and hypertensive patients, Neurology **18:**255, 1968.
49. Coombs, C.: Polycystic disease of the kidneys, Quart. J. Med. **3:**30, 1909.
50. Courville, C. B.: Pathology of the central nervous system, ed. 3, Mountain View, Calif., 1950, Pacific Press Publishing Association.
51. Courville, C. B., and Blomquist, O. A.: Traumatic intracerebral hemorrhage with particular reference to its pathogenesis and its relation to "delayed traumatic apoplexy," Arch. Surg. **41:**1, 1940.
52. Courville, C. B., and Friedman, A. P.: Hemorrhages into the lateral basal ganglionic region, Bull. Los Angeles Neurol. Soc. **7:**137, 1942.
53. Cox, L. B.: Haemorrhage of the brain stem as a significant complication of intracranial tumors, Med. J. Aust. **1:**259, 1939.
54. Craig, W. McK., and Adson, A. W.: Spontaneous intracerebral hemorrhage, Arch. Neurol. Psychiat. **35:**701, 1936.

55. Cramer, F., Paster, S., and Stephensen, C.: Cerebral injuries due to explosion waves—"cerebral blast concussion," Arch. Neurol. Psychiat. **61:**1, 1949.
56. Crawford, T., and Crompton, M. R.: The pathology of strokes. In Marshall, J.: The management of cerebrovascular disease, ed. 2, Boston, 1968, Little, Brown and Co., p. 26.
57. Crompton, M. R.: Intracerebral haematoma complicating ruptured cerebral berry aneurysm, J. Neurol. Neurosurg. Psychiat. **25:**378, 1962.
58. Crothers, B.: Birth injuries of the spinal cord. In Brock, S.: Injuries of the brain and spinal cord and their coverings, ed. 3, Baltimore, 1949, The Williams & Wilkins Co., p. 503.
59. Davidoff, L. M.: Intracerebral hemorrhage associated with hypertension and arteriosclerosis, J. Neurosurg. **15:**322, 1958.
60. Davison, C.: Pathology of the spinal cord as a result of trauma. In: Trauma of the central nervous system, Ass. Res. Nerv. Ment. Dis. **24:**151, 1945.
61. Davison, C.: General pathological considerations in injuries of the spinal cord. In Brock, S.: Injuries of the brain and spinal cord and their coverings, ed. 3, Baltimore, 1949, The Williams & Wilkins Co., p. 471.
62. Denny-Brown, D., and Russell, W. R.: Experimental cerebral concussion, Brain **64:**93, 1941.
63. Dickinson, C. J., and Thomson, A. D.: High blood-pressure and stroke: necropsy study of heart-weight and left ventricular hypertrophy, Lancet **2:**342, 1960.
64. Dill, J. V., and Isenhour, C. E.: Etiologic factors in experimentally produced pontile hemorrhages, Arch. Neurol. Psych. **41:**1146, 1939.
65. Dinsdale, H. B.: Spontaneous hemorrhage in the posterior fossa, Arch. Neurol. **10:**200, 1964.
66. Donnelly, J. F., and Lock, F. R.: Causes of death in five hundred thirty-three fatal cases of toxemia of pregnancy, Amer. J. Obstet. Gynec. **68:**184, 1954.
67. Dott, N., and Blackwood, W.: Communication to the Society of British Surgeons, 1951. Cited by Johnson and Yates.[128]
68. Elliott, R. H. E.: Diagnostic and therapeutic considerations in the management of idiopathic thrombocytopenic purpura, Bull. N. Y. Acad. Med. **15:**197, 1939.
69. Ellis, A. G.: The pathogenesis of spontaneous cerebral hemorrhage, Proc. Path. Soc. Philadelphia **12:**197, 1909.
70. Ellis, A. G.: The pathogenesis of spontaneous cerebral hemorrhage, Int. Clinics **2:**271, 1909.
71. Emblen, L.: Apoplexy—pathogenesis, Acta Psychiat. Scand. **36** (suppl. 150):22, 1961.
72. Epstein, A. W.: Primary massive pontine hemorrhage, J. Neuropath. Exp. Neurol. **10:**426, 1951.
73. Evans, J. P., and Scheinker, I. M.: Histologic studies of the brain following head trauma. III. Post-traumatic infarction of cerebral arteries, with consideration of the associated clinical picture, Arch. Neurol. Psychiat. **50:**258, 1943.

74. Façon, E., Schwarz, B., and Ionescu, S.: Das Spontanhämatom des Hirnstamms, Wien. Klin. Wschr. **74**:655, 1962.

75. Fedrick, J.: Comparison of birth weight/gestation distribution in cases of stillbirth and neonatal death according to lesions found at autopsy, Brit. Med. J. **3**:745, 1969.

76. Feigin, I., and Prose, P.: Hypertensive fibrinoid arteritis of the brain and gross cerebral hemorrhage, Arch. Neurol. **11**:98, 1959.

77. Fields, W. S., and Halpert, B.: Pontine hemorrhage in intracranial hypertension, Amer. J. Path. **29**:677, 1953.

78. Finney, L. A., and Walker, A. E.: Transtentorial herniation, Springfield, Ill. 1962, Charles C Thomas, Publisher.

79. Fishberg, A. M.: Hypertension and nephritis, ed. 5, Philadelphia, 1954, Lea & Febiger.

80. Fisher, C. M.: Cerebrovascular disease: pathophysiology, diagnosis, and treatment, J. Chronic Dis. **8**:419, 1958.

81. Fisher, C. M.: Early-life carotid-artery occlusion associated with late intracranial hemorrhage, Lab. Invest. **8**:680, 1959.

82. Fisher, C. M.: Anticoagulant therapy in cerebral thrombosis and cerebral embolism, Neurology **11**(4) (part 2):119, 1961.

83. Fisher, C. M.: The pathology and pathogenesis of intracerebral hemorrhage. In Fields, W. S.: Pathogenesis and treatment of cerebrovascular disease, Springfield, Ill., 1961, Charles C Thomas, Publisher, p. 295.

84. Florey, C. du V., Senter, M. G., and Acheson, R. M.: A study of the validity of the diagnosis of stroke in mortality data. I. Certificate analysis, Yale J. Biol. Med. **40**:148, 1967.

85. Freireich, E. J., Thomas, L. B., Frei, E., Fritz, R. D., and Forkner, C. E.: A distinctive type of intracerebral hemorrhage associated with "blastic crisis" in patients with leukemia, Cancer **13**:146, 1960.

86. Freytag, E.: Autopsy findings in head injuries from blunt force, Arch. Path. **75**:402, 1963.

87. Freytag, E.: Fatal hypertensive intracerebral haematomas: a survey of the pathological anatomy of 393 cases, J. Neurol. Neurosurg. Psychiat. **31**:616, 1968.

88. Fried, B. M.: Leukemia and the central nervous system with a review of thirty cases from the literature, Arch. Path. **2**:23, 1926.

89. Friede, R. L., and Roessmann, U.: The pathogenesis of secondary midbrain hemorrhages, Neurology **16**:1210, 1966.

90. Friedman, A. P., and Nielsen, J. M.: Cerebellar hemorrhage, Bull. Los Angeles Neurol. Soc. **6**:135, 1941.

91. Fritz, R. D., Forkner, C. E., Freireich, E. J., Frei, E., and Thomas, L. B.: The association of fatal intracranial hemorrhage and "blastic crisis" in patients with acute leukemia, New Eng. J. Med. **261**:59, 1959.

92. Gairdner, D.: Schönlein-Henoch syndrome (anaphylactoid purpura), Quart. J. Med. **17**:95, 1948.

93. Gates, R. R.: Human genetics, New York, 1946, The Macmillan Co., vol. 1 and 2.

94. Globus, J. H.: Massive cerebral hemorrhage. In: The circulation of the brain and spinal cord, Ass. Res. Nerv. Ment. Dis. **18**:438, 1938.

95. Globus, J. H., and Epstein, J. A.: Massive cerebral hemorrhage: spontaneous and experimentally induced, Proc. First Int. Congr. Neuropath. **1**:289, 1952.

96. Globus, J. H., and Epstein, J. A.: Massive cerebral hemorrhage: spontaneous and experimentally induced, J. Neuropath. Exp. Neurol. **12**:107, 1953.

97. Globus, J. H., and Strauss, I.: Massive cerebral hemorrhage, Arch. Neurol. Psychiat. **18**:215, 1927.

98. Goldstein, E., and Porter, D. Y.: Fatal thrombocytopenia with cerebral hemorrhage in mononucleosis, Arch. Neurol. **20**:533, 1969.

99. Gosch, H. H., Gooding, E., and Schneider, R. C.: Cervical spinal cord hemorrhages in experimental head injuries, J. Neurosurg. **33**:640, 1970.

100. Green, F. H. K.: Miliary aneurysms in the brain, J. Path. Bact. **33**:71, 1930.

101. Greenacre, P.: Multiple spontaneous intracerebral hemorrhages, Johns Hopkins Hosp. Bull. **28**:86, 1917.

102. Greenfield, J. G., and Norman, R. M.: Demyelinating diseases. In Blackwood, W., McMenemey, W. H., Meyer, A., Norman, R. M., and Russell, D. S.: Greenfield's neuropathology, ed. 2, Baltimore, 1963, The Williams & Wilkins Co., p. 475.

103. Greenfield, J. G., and Russell, D. S.: Traumatic lesions of the central and peripheral nervous systems. In Blackwood, W., McMenemey, W. H., Meyer, A., Norman, R. M., and Russell, D. S.: Greenfield's neuropathology, ed. 2, Baltimore, 1963, The Williams & Wilkins Co., p. 441.

104. Griffith, J. Q., and Lindauer, M. A.: Increased capillary fragility in hypertension: incidence, complications, and treatment, Amer. Heart J. **28**:758, 1944.

105. Groch, S. N., Hurwitz, L. J., McDevitt, E., and Wright, I. S.: Problems of anticoagulant therapy in cerebrovascular disease, Neurology **9**:786, 1959.

106. Groch, S. N., Sayre, G. P., and Heck, F. J.: Cerebral hemorrhage in leukemia, Arch. Neurol. **2**:439, 1960.

107. Gull, W. M.: Cases of aneurism of the cerebral vessels, Guy's Hosp. Rep. **5**:281, 1859.

108. Gurdjian, E. S., Hodgson, V. R., Thomas, L. M., and Patrick, L. M.: Significance of relative movements of scalp, skull, and intracranial contents during impact injury of the head, J. Neurosurg. **29**:70, 1968.

109. Harris, L. S., Roessmann, U., and Friede, R. L.: Bursting of cerebral ventricular walls, J. Path. Bact. **96**:33, 1968.

110. Harvald, B., Hilden, T., and Lund, E.: Longterm anticoagulant therapy after myocardial infarction, Lancet **2**:626, 1962.

111. Hawksley, J. C.: Lymphocytic leukaemia causing pontine haemorrhage, Arch. Dis. Child. **7**:29, 1932.

112. Hawthorne, C. O.: Cerebral and cerebellar haemorrhages in apparently healthy adolescents and children, Practitioner 109:425, 1922.

113. Helpern, M., and Rabson, S. M.: Sudden and unexpected natural death-general considerations and statistics, N. Y. State J. Med. 45:1197, 1945.

114. Hicks, S. P., and Black, B. K.: The relation of cardiovascular disease to apoplexy, Amer. Heart J. 38:528, 1949.

115. Holbourn, A. H. S.: Mechanics of head injuries, Lancet 2:438, 1943.

116. Holbourn, A. H. S.: Mechanics of head injuries, Lancet 1:483, 1944.

117. Howell, D. A.: Longitudinal brain stem compression with buckling, Arch. Neurol. 4:572, 1961.

118. Hudson, A. J., and Hyland, H. H.: Hypertensive cerebrovascular disease: a clinical and pathological review of 100 cases, Ann. Intern. Med. 49:1049, 1958.

119. Hunt, W. E., Bouroncle, B. A., and Meagher, J. N.: Neurologic complications of leukemias and lymphomas, J. Neurosurg. 16:135, 1959.

120. Hyland, H. H., and Levy, D.: Spontaneous cerebellar haemorrhage, Canad. Med. Ass. J. 71:315, 1954.

121. Ikeda, M., Fujii, J., Terasawa, F., Hosoda, S., Kurihara, H., and Kimata, S.: Cerebral hemorrhage in experimental renal hypertension Jap. Heart J. 5:466, 1964.

122. Jaffé, R. H.: Pathologic aspect (symposium on the recent progress of research in leukemia), Arch. Path. 18:763, 1934.

123. Jain, K. K.: Some observations on the anatomy of the middle cerebral artery, Canad. J. Surg. 7:134, 1964.

124. Janeway, T. C.: A clinical study of hypertensive cardiovascular disease, Arch. Intern. Med. 12:755, 1913.

125. Jewesbury, E. C. O.: Atypical intracranial haemorrhage with special reference to cerebral haematoma, Brain 70:274, 1947.

126. Johansson, S. H.: Hypertensive and normotensive intracerebral haemorrhage, Acta Psychiat. Neurol. Scand. 36 (suppl. 150):90, 1961.

127. Johansson, S. H., and Melin, H. S.: Spontaneous cerebral haemorrhage and encephalomalacia, Acta Psychiat. Neurol. Scand. 35:457, 1960.

128. Johnson, R. T., and Yates, P. O.: Brain stem haemorrhages in expanding supratentorial conditions, Acta Radiol. 46:250, 1956.

129. Kalbag, R. M.: Recurrent subarachnoid haemorrhage from paraventricular lesions with normal angiography, J. Neurol. Neurosurg. Psychiat. 27:435, 1964.

130. Kane, W. C., and Aronson, S. M.: Cerebrovascular disease in an autopsy population. I. Influence of age, ethnic background, sex, and cardiomegaly upon frequency of cerebral hemorrhage, Arch. Neurol. 20:514, 1969.

131. Kannel, W. B., Dawber, T. R., Cohen, M. E., and McNamara, P. M.: Vascular disease of the brain—epidemiologic aspects: the Framingham study, Amer. J. Public Health 55:1355, 1965.

132. Kaufmann, E.: Pathology for students and practitioners (Translated by Reimann, S. P.), Philadelphia, 1929, P. Blakiston's Son and Co., vol. 1, p. 141.

133. Kerr, C. B.: Intracranial haemorrhage in haemophilia, J. Neurol. Neurosurg. Psychiat. 27:166, 1964.

134. Klintworth, G. K.: The pathogenesis of secondary brainstem hemorrhages as studied in an experimental model, Amer. J. Path. 47:525, 1965.

135. Kornblum, R. N., and Fisher, R. S.: Pituitary lesions in cranio-cerebral injuries, Arch. Path. 88:242, 1969.

136. Kurtzke, J. F.: Epidemiology of cerebrovascular disease, Berlin, 1969, Springer-Verlag.

137. Lampert, H., and Müller, W.: Bei welchem Druck kommt es zu einer Ruptur der Gehirngefässe? Frankfurt Z. Path. 33:471, 1925-1926.

138. LeCount, E. R., and Apfelbach, C. W.: Pathologic anatomy of traumatic fractures of cranial bones and concomitant brain injuries, J.A.M.A. 74:501, 1920.

139. Leidler, F., and Russell, W. O.: The brain in leukemia, Arch. Path. 40:14, 1945.

140. Levitt, L. M., and Burbank, B.: Glomerulonephritis as a complication of the Schönlein-Henoch syndrome, New Eng. J. Med. 248:530, 1953.

141. Lewis, I. C., and Philpott, M. G.: Neurological complications in the Schönlein-Henoch syndrome, Arch. Dis. Child. 31:369, 1956.

142. Lichtenstein, R. S.: Spontaneous cerebellar hematomas, Johns Hopkins Med. J. 122:319, 1968.

143. Lindenberg, R.: Compression of brain arteries as pathogenetic factor for tissue necroses and their areas of predilection, J. Neuropath. Exp. Neurol. 14:223, 1955.

144. Lindenberg, R., Fisher, R. S., Durlacher, S. H., Lovitt, W. V., and Freytag, E.: Lesions of the corpus callosum following blunt mechanical trauma to the head, Amer. J. Path. 31:297, 1955.

145. Lindenberg, R., and Freytag, E.: Morphology of cortical contusions, Arch. Path. 63:23, 1957.

146. Lindenberg, R., and Freytag, E.: The mechanism of cerebral contusion, Arch. Path. 69:440, 1960.

147. Lindenberg, R., and Freytag, E.: Morphology of brain lesions from blunt trauma in early infancy, Arch. Path. 87:298, 1969.

148. Lindgren, S. O.: Studies in head injuries: intracranial pressure pattern during impact, Lancet 1:1251, 1964.

149. Lindgren, S. O.: Experimental studies of mechanical effects in head injuries, Acta Chir. Scand. Suppl. 360:1, 1966.

150. Logothetis, J., Silverstein, P., and Coe, J.: Neurologic aspects of Waldenström's macroglobulinemia, Arch. Neurol. 3:564, 1960.

151. Lucas, W. S.: Erythremia, or polycythemia

with chronic cyanosis and splenomegaly, Arch. Intern. Med. **10**:597, 1912.

152. MacMillan, R. L., and Brown, K. W. G.: Haemorrhage in anticoagulant therapy. Canad. Med. Ass. J. **69**:279, 1953.

153. Malamud, N., Haymaker, W., and Custer, R. P.: Heat stroke: a clinicopathologic study of 125 fatal cases, Milit. Surg. **99**:397, 1946.

154. Margolis, G.: The vascular changes and pathogenesis of hypertensive intracerebral hemorrhage. In: Cerebrovascular disease, Ass. Res. Nerv. Ment. Dis. **41**:73, 1966.

155. Marshall, J., and Shaw, D. A.: Anticoagulant therapy in acute cerebrovascular accidents: a controlled trial, Lancet **1**:995, 1960.

156. Martland, H. S., and Beling, C. C.: Traumatic cerebral hemorrhage, Arch. Neurol. Psychiat. **22**:1001, 1929.

157. Mastaglia, F. L.: Edis, B., and Kakulas, B. A.: Medullary haemorrhage: a report of two cases, J. Neurol. Neurosurg. Psychiat. **32**:221, 1969.

158. Matsuoka, S.: Histopathological studies on the blood vessels in apoplexia cerebri, First Int. Congress Neuropath. **3**:222, 1952.

159. McCarthy, D. J.: Exhibition of the different types of cerebral hemorrhage, Proc. Path. Soc. Philadelphia **12**:235, 1909.

160. McKissock, W., Richardson, A., and Taylor, J.: Primary intracerebral haemorrhage: a controlled trial of surgical and conservative treatment in 180 unselected cases, Lancet **2**:221, 1961.

161. McKissock, W., Richardson, A., and Walsh, L.: Primary intracerebral haemorrhage, Lancet **2**:683, 1959.

162. McKissock, W., Richardson, A., and Walsh, L.: Spontaneous cerebellar haemorrhage, a study of 34 consecutive cases treated surgically, Brain **83**:1, 1960.

163. McVeigh, J. F.: Experimental cord crushes with especial reference to the mechanical factors involved and subsequent changes in the areas of the cord affected, Arch. Surg. **7**:573, 1923.

164. Merritt, H. H.: A textbook of neurology, ed. 4, Philadelphia, 1967, Lea & Febiger.

165. Michael, J. C.: Cerebellar apoplexy, Amer. J. Med. Sci. **183**:687, 1932.

166. Miller, H.: Clinical consideration of cerebrovascular disorders occurring during the course of general diseases of an inflammatory or allergic nature, Proc. Roy. Soc. Med. **44**:852, 1951.

167. Mitchell, N., and Angrist, A.: Spontaneous cerebellar hemorrhage, Amer. J. Path. **18**:935, 1942.

168. Moore, E. W., Thomas, L. B., Shaw, R. K., and Freireich, E. J.: The central nervous system in acute leukemia, Arch. Intern. Med. **105**:451, 1960.

169. Moore, M. T., and Stern, K.: Vascular lesions in the brain-stem and occipital lobe occurring in association with brain tumours, Brain **61**:70, 1938.

170. Moore, N.: Notes of post-mortem examinations of cases of haemorrhage within the cranium, St. Bart's Hosp. Rep. **16**:241, 1880.

171. Mosberg, W. H., and Lindenberg, R.: Tramatic hemorrhage from the anterior choroidal artery, J. Neurosurg. **16**:209, 1959.

172. Moser, M., and Goldman, A. G.: Hypertensive vascular disease, Philadelphia, 1967, J. B. Lippincott Co.

173. Moyer, J. H.: Drug therapy of hypertension. IV. The indications and contraindications for antihypertensive drugs, Arch. Intern. Med. **98**:427, 1956.

174. Mutlu, N., Berry R. G., and Alpers, B. J.: Massive cerebral hemorrhage, Arch. Neurol. **8**:644, 1963.

175. Odom, G. L., Bloor, B. M., and Woodhall, B.: Intracerebral hematomas, Southern Med. J. **45**:936, 1952.

176. Ommaya, A. K., Di Chiro, G., and Doppman, J.: Ligation of arterial supply in the treatment of spinal cord arteriovenous malformations, J. Neurosurg. **30**:679, 1969.

177. Ommaya, A. K., Faas, F., and Yarnell, P.: Whiplash injury and brain damage, J.A.M.A. **204**:285, 1968.

178. Ommaya, A. K., Rockoff, S. D., and Baldwin, M.: Experimental concussion, J. Neurosurg. **21**:249, 1964.

179. Pant, S. S., and Dreyfus, P. M.: Multiple intracerebral hemorrhages of unusual nature, Neurology **17**:923, 1967.

180. Paullin, J. E., Bowcock, H. M., and Wood, R. H.: Complications of hypertension, Amer. Heart J. **2**:613, 1926-1927.

181. Penfield, W.: The operative treatment of spontaneous intracerebral hemorrhage, Canad. Med. Ass. J. **28**:369, 1933.

182. Pepper, O. H. P.: Medical etymology, Philadelphia, 1949, W. B. Saunders Co.

183. Perera, G. A.: Hypertensive vascular disease: description and natural history, J. Chronic Dis. **1**:33, 1955.

184. Perera, G. A.: The course of primary hypertension in the young, Ann. Intern. Med. **49**:1348, 1958.

185. Pickering, G. W.: High blood pressure, London, 1955, J. & A. Churchill Ltd.

186. Pilcher, C.: Subcortical hematoma: surgical treatment, with report of eight cases, Arch. Neurol. Psych. **46**:416, 1941.

187. Poppen, J. L., Kendrick, J. F., and Hicks, S. F.: Brain stem hemorrhages secondary to supratentorial space-taking lesions, J. Neuropath. Exp. Neurol. **11**:267, 1952.

188. Potter, E. L.: Pathology of the fetus and infant, ed. 2, Chicago, 1961, Year Book Medical Publishers Inc.

189. Pudenz, R. H., and Shelden, C. H.: The Lucite calvarium—a method for direct observation of the brain, II. Cranial trauma and brain movement, J. Neurosurg. **3**:487, 1946.

190. Quick, A. J.: Emergencies in hemophilia, Amer. J. Med. Sci. **251**:409, 1966.

191. Raeder, O. J.: Repeated multiple minute corticospinal hemorrhages with miliary aneurysms in a case of arteriosclerosis, Arch. Neurol. Psych. **5**:270, 1921.

192. Rey-Bellet, J.: Cerebellar hemorrhage, Neurology **10**:217, 1960.

193. Richards, R. L.: Anticoagulants in acute myocardial infarction. Brit. Med. J. 1:820, 1962.
194. Richardson, J. C., and Hyland, H. H.: Intracranial aneurysms, Medicine 20:1, 1941.
195. Ritchie, W. P., and Haines, G. L.: Spontaneous intracranial hemorrhage in children, Arch. Surg. 66:452, 1953.
196. Robb, J. P.: Neurologic complications of pregnancy, Neurology 5:679, 1955.
197. Robertson, E. G.: Cerebral lesions due to intracranial aneurysms, Brain 72:150, 1949.
198. Robertson, W. F.: A text-book of pathology in relation to mental diseases, Edinburgh, 1900, William F. Clay.
199. Robinson, G. W.: Encapsulated brain hemorrhages, Arch. Neurol. Psychiat. 27:1441, 1932.
200. Rochoux, J.-A.: Du ramollissement du cerveau et de sa curabilité, Arch. Gen. Med. 6:265, 1844.
201. Runnells, R. A., Monlux, W. S., and Monlux, A. W.: Principles of veterinary pathology, Iowa, 1960, Iowa University Press.
202. Russek, H. I., and Zohman, B. L.: Anticoagulant therapy in acute myocardial infarction, Amer. J. Med. Sci. 225:8, 1953.
203. Russell, D. S.: The pathology of spontaneous intracranial haemorrhage, Proc. Roy. Soc. Med. 47:689, 1954.
204. Russell, R. W. R.: Observations on intracranial aneurysms, Brain 86:425, 1963.
205. Russell, R. W. R.: Pathogenesis of primary intracerebral hemorrhage. In Toole, J. F., Siekert, R. G., and Whisnant, J. P.: Cerebral vascular disease, Sixth Conference of New York, 1968, Grune & Stratton, Inc.
205. Saphir, O.: Anomalies of the circle of Willis with resulting encephalomalacia and cerebral hemorrhage, Amer. J. Path. 11:775, 1935.
207. Sarner, M., and Crawford, M. D.: Ruptured intracranial aneurysm, Lancet 2:1251, 1965.
208. Schact, F. W.: Hypertension in cases of congenital polycystic kidney, Arch. Intern. Med. 47:500, 1931.
209. Scheinker, I. M., Discussion, J. Neuropath. Exp. Neurol. 8:114, 1949.
210. Scheinker, I. M.: Changes in cerebral veins in hypertensive brain disease and their relation to cerebral hemorrhage, Arch. Neurol. Psychiat. 54:395, 1945.
211. Scheinker, I. M.: Transtentorial herniation of the brain stem, Arch. Neurol. Psychiat. 53:289, 1945.
212. Scheinker, I. M.: Medical neuropathology, Springfield, 1951, Charles C Thomas, Publisher.
213. Schneider, R. C.: Craniocerebral trauma. In Kahn, E. A., Crosby, E. C., Schneider, R. C., and Taren, J. A.: Correlative neurosurgery, ed. 2, Springfield, Ill., Charles C Thomas, Publisher, 1969, p. 533.
214. Schneider, R. C., Gosch, H. H., Norrell, H., Jerva, M., Combs, L. W., and Smith, R. A.: Vascular insufficiency and differential distortion of brain and cord caused by cervicomedullary football injuries, J. Neurosurg. 33:363, 1970.
215. Schottstaedt, M. F., and Sokolow, M.: The natural history and course of hypertension with papilledema (malignant hypertension), Amer. Heart J. 45:331, 1953.
216. Schwartz, P.: Birth injuries of the newborn, New York, 1961, Hafner Publishing Co., Inc.
217. Schwartz, P.: Cerebral apoplexy, types, causes and pathogenesis, Springfield, Ill., 1961, Charles C Thomas, Publisher.
218. Scoville, W. B., and Poppen, J. L.: Intrapeduncular hemorrhage of the brain. Arch. Neurol. Psychiat. 61:688, 1949.
219. Sheldon, W. P. H.: Intracranial haemorrhage in infancy and childhood, Quart. J. Med. 20:353, 1927.
220. Shennan, T.: Miliary aneurysms, in relation to cerebral haemorrhage, Edinburgh Med. J. 15:245, 1915.
221. Sibley, W. A., Morledge, J. H., and Lapham, L. W.: Experimental cerebral infarction: the effect of Dicumarol, Amer. J. Med. Sci. 234:663, 1957.
221. Sieber, F.: Über Cystennieren bei Erwachsenen, Deutsch. Z. Chirurg. 79:406, 1905.
223. Silver, M. D., and Stehbens, W. E.: The behavior of platelets in vivo, Quart. J. Exp. Physiol. 50:241, 1965.
224. Simpson, F. O., and Gilchrist, A. R.: Prognosis in untreated hypertensive vascular disease, Scot. Med. J. 3:1, 1958.
225. Singer, R. P., and Schneider, R. C.: The successful management of intracerebral and subarachnoid hemorrhage in a hemophilic infant, Neurology 12:293, 1962.
226. Sloan, L. H.: Polycythemia rubra vera, Arch. Neurol. Psychiat. 30:154, 1933.
227. Smith, D. E., Odel, H. M., and Kernohan, J. W.: Cause of death in hypertension, Amer. J. Med. 9:516, 1950.
228. Smith, D. R., Ducker, T. B., and Kempe, L. G.: Experimental in vivo microcirculatory dynamics in brain trauma, J. Neurosurg. 30:664, 1969.
229. Smith, K. R., Nelson, J. S., and Dooley, J. M.: Bilateral "hypoplasia" of the internal carotid arteries, Neurology 18:1149, 1968.
230. Sohal, R. S., Sun, S. C., Colcolough, H. L., and Burch, G. E.: Heat stroke, Arch. Intern. Med. 122:43, 1968.
231. Sokolow, M., and Perloff, D.: The prognosis of essential hypertension treated conservatively, Circulation 23:697, 1961.
232. Sörnäs, R., and Müller, R.: The cytology of the CSF in cerebrovascular disease, Acta Neurol. Scand. 43 (suppl. 31): 118, 1967.
233. Spicer, E. J. F., and Strich, S. J.: Haemorrhages in posterior-root ganglia in patients dying from head injuries, Lancet 2:1389, 1967.
234. Sprofkin, B. E., and Blakey, H. H.: Acute spontaneous cerebral vascular accidents in young normotensive adults, Arch. Intern. Med. 98:617, 1956.
235. Stehbens, W. E.: Hypertension and cerebral aneurysms, Med. J. Aust. 2:4, 1962.
236. Stehbens, W. E.: Cerebral aneurysms and congenital abnormalities, Aust. Ann. Med. 11:102, 1962.

237. Stehbens, W. E.: Contentious features of coronary occlusion and atherosclerosis, Bull. Post-Grad. Comm. Med. Univ. Sydney **19**:216, 1963.

238. Stehbens, W. E.: Aneurysms and anatomical variation of cerebral arteries, Arch. Path. **75**:45, 1963.

239. Stehbens, W. E.: Unpublished data, 1963.

240. Stehbens, W. E.: Vascular changes in chronic peptic ulcer, Arch Path. **78**:584, 1964.

241. Stehbens, W. E.: Reaction of venous endothelium to injury, Lab. Invest. **14**:449, 1965.

242. Stehbens, W. E.: Blood vessel changes in chronic experimental arteriovenous fistulas, Surg. Gynec. Obstet. **127**:327, 1968.

243. Stephens, C. A. L.: Anticoagulant therapy in private practice, Circulation **9**:682, 1954.

244. Stephens, R. B., and Stilwell, D. L.: Arteries and veins of the human brain, Springfield, Ill., 1969, Charles C Thomas, Publisher.

245. Strassmann, G.: Formation of hemosiderin and hematoidin after traumatic and spontaneous cerebral hemorrhages, Arch. Path. **47**:205, 1949.

246. Strich, S. J.: Shearing of nerve fibres as a cause of brain damage due to head injury, Lancet **2**:443, 1961.

247. Suzman, M. M., Ruskin, H. D., and Goldberg, B.: An evaluation of the effect of continuous long-term anticoagulant therapy on the prognosis of myocardial infarction: a report of 82 cases, Circulation **12**:338, 1955.

248. Symonds, C.: Concussion and its sequelae, Lancet **1**:1, 1962.

249. Symonds, C. P.: Delayed traumatic intracerebral haemorrhage, Brit. Med. J. **1**:1048, 1940.

250. Taylor, R. D., and Page, I. H.: Signs and symptoms of impending cerebral hemorrhage, J.A.M.A. **127**:384, 1945.

251. Toole, J. F., and Patel, A. N.: Cerebrovascular disorders, New York, 1967, McGraw-Hill Book Co.

252. Tulloch, J., and Wright, I. S.: Long-term anticoagulant therapy: further experiences, Circulation **9**:823, 1954.

253. Turner, F. C.: Arteries of the brain from cases of cerebral haemorrhage, Trans. Path. Soc. London **33**:96, 1882.

254. Unterharnscheidt, F., and Higgins, L. S.: Pathomorphology of experimental head injury due to rotational acceleration, Acta Neuropath. **12**:200, 1969.

255. Unterharnscheidt, F., and Higgins, L. S.: Traumatic lesions of brain and spinal cord due to nondeforming angular acceleration of the head, Texas Rep. Biol. Med. **27**:127, 1969.

256. Vance, B. M.: Fractures of the skull, Arch. Surg. **14**:1023, 1927.

257. Walton, J. N.: Subarachnoid haemorrhage, Edinburgh, 1956, E. & S. Livingstone Ltd.

258. Weber, M. B., and Blakeley, J. A.: The haemorrhagic diathesis of heatstroke, Lancet **1**:1190, 1969.

259. Weinstein, J. D., Langfitt, T. W., Bruno, L., Zaren, H. A., and Jackson, J. L. F.: Experimental study of patterns of brain distortion and ischemia produced by an intracranial mass, J. Neurosurg. **28**:513, 1968.

260. Weintraub, C. M.: Bruising of the third cranial nerve and the pathogenesis of midbrain haemorrhage, Brit. J. Surg. **48**:62, 1960.

261. Wells, C. E., and Urrea, D.: Cerebrovascular accidents in patients receiving anticoagulant drugs, Arch. Neurol. **3**:553, 1960.

262. Wertham, F., Mitchell, N., and Angrist, A.: The brain in sickle cell anemia, Arch. Neurol. Psychiat. **47**:752, 1942.

263. Weyhe: 1889. Cited by Alpers.[6]

264. Whisnant, J. P., Millikan, C. H., Sayre, G. P., and Wakim, K. G.: Effect of anticoagulants on experimental cerebral infarction, Circulation **20**:56, 1959.

265. Williams, H. M., Diamond, H. D., and Craver, L. F.: The pathogenesis and management of neurological complications in patients with malignant lymphomas and leukemia, Cancer **11**:76, 1958.

266. Windle, W. F.: Brain damage at birth, J.A.M.A. **206**:1967, 1968.

267. Windle, W. F.: Cerebral hemorrhage in relation to birth asphyxia, Science **167**:1000, 1970.

268. Wolintz, A. H., Jacobs, L. D., Christoff, N., Solomon, M., and Chernik, N.: Serum and cerebrospinal fluid enzymes in cerebrovascular disease, Arch. Neurol. **20**:54, 1969.

269. Wright, L. T., and Rothman, M.: Deaths from Dicumarol, Arch. Surg. **62**:23, 1951.

270. Yagi, H.: Birth injuries in the newborn, Jap. J. Obstet. Gynec. **12**:130, 1929. Cited by Alpers.[6]

271. Yates, P. O.: A change in pattern of cerebrovascular disease, Lancet **1**:65, 1964.

272. Yates, P. O., and Hutchinson, E. C.: Cerebral infarction: the role of stenosis of the extracranial cerebral arteries, Med. Res. Council. Spec. Rep. **300**:1, London, 1961.

273. Zimmerman, H. M.: Cerebral apoplexy: mechanism and differential diagnosis, N. Y. State J. Med. **49**:2153, 1949.

9 / Intracranial arterial aneurysms

The word "aneurysm" is from the Greek *aneurysma,* which is derived from *ana,* meaning "across," and *eurys,* "broad,"[378] and exemplifies thus the phenomenon of widening or dilatation. Galen is considered to be the first to define and describe the lesion[468] though it has been averred that the ancient Egyptians knew of its existence.[315,450] By the term "aneurysm" may be understood a localized and persistent dilatation that results from the yielding of components of the wall of the heart or blood vessels. The wall may be altered and its constituent elements are not necessarily left intact. Hence a "true" aneurysm is one that is formed by dilatation of the components of the vessel wall, which frequently undergoes extensive structural change. In contradistinction, a "false" aneurysm is one resulting from the rupture of the vessel where the pulsatile hematoma so formed is walled off by organization and neighboring tissues and in which a functional communication with the parent artery persists.

The term "aneurysm" generally alludes to an arterial lesion and though cardiac and venous aneurysms are recognized, unless otherwise indicated, "aneurysm" will be used exclusively in reference to arterial dilatations. Those dilatations involving the whole vessel wall for a short distance are fusiform aneurysms and are termed "saccular" if only part of the wall is dilated. A pedunculated aneurysm is a saccular aneurysm with a relatively narrow or stalklike neck. Ectasia, a generalized dilatation of a considerable length of an artery, should not be confused with aneurysms. A cylindroid aneurysm, though it involves a longer segment than a fusiform aneurysm, is much more localized than ectasia.

In the correct sense an arteriovenous aneurysm (Chapter 10) is not an aneurysm at all, but rather an arteriovenous anastomosis or fistula, even though aneurysmal dilatation of vessels occurs at the site of the fistula.

The term "miliary" aneurysm, introduced by Charcôt and Bouchard,[87] refers to dilatations on the intracerebral arteries and has also been used with reference to the true saccular aneurysms of the basal arteries. To avoid confusion the term "miliary" should be restricted to the small lesions of Charcôt and Bouchard.[87]

Dissecting aneurysm has been defined as "a lesion produced by penetration of the circulating blood into the substance of the wall of a vessel with subsequent extension of the effused blood for a varying distance between its layers."[446] The term will be used exclusively for aneurysms fulfilling these conditions.

Types of cerebral aneurysm

Aneurysms of the intracranial blood vessels may be classified as follows: fusiform aneurysms, saccular arterial aneurysms, aneurysms of inflammatory origin (bacterial, syphilitic, mycotic; polyarteritis nodosa), dissecting aneurysms, miliary aneurysms (Chapter 8), arteriovenous aneurysms (Chapter 10), and traumatic aneurysms.

Fusiform aneurysms

Arteriectasis is commonly seen in advanced atherosclerotic cerebral arteries, often in association with tortuosity. Fusiform dilatation is a frequent complication, affecting the basilar and internal carotid arteries in particular. Fusiform aneurysms of the fourth or intracranial segment of the internal carotid artery are rarely of any consequential size and have their maximum diameter at the level of the origin of the posterior communicating artery. Those

351

of the cavernous segment are more prone to enlarge and cause pressure symptoms. Large fusiform dilatations on the vertebrobasilar system most often involve the basilar artery (Fig. 9-1) and affect all or part of the stem. In Fig. 9-2 is an early fusiform dilatation and in Fig. 9-3 is a longitudinal section through a fusiform dilatation affect-

ing the anterior wall of the artery, which has been convoluted.

These aneurysms are the direct result of severe atherosclerosis with loss of elasticity and are accepted as being atherosclerotic in nature. Rupture is rare. Pressure symptoms, basically similar to those associated with saccular aneurysms, depend on the

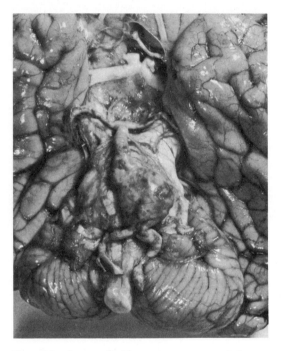

Fig. 9-1. Large fusiform aneurysm of lower two-thirds of basilar artery. Compare with Fig. 9-2.

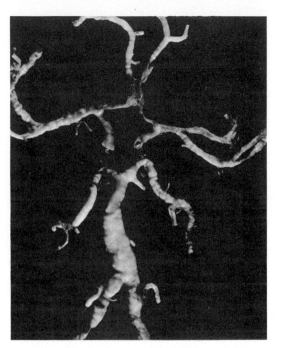

Fig. 9-2. Fusiform aneurysm of basilar artery of an atherosclerotic circle of Willis. Note irregular contour of arteries.

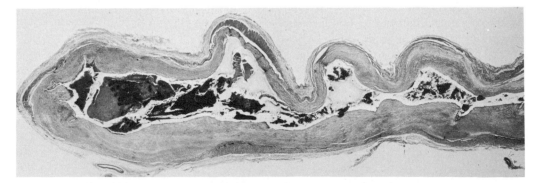

Fig. 9-3. Longitudinal section through upper end of a basilar artery that exhibited fusiform dilatation. Upper (anterior) wall is convoluted. Note considerable but irregular intimal thickening and extensive loss of elastica and media. (Verhoeff's elastic stain, ×10.)

size of the dilatation and the displacement due to the tortuosity and lengthening of the vessels. Associated lesions in the brain are the result of the severe atherosclerosis and hence acute and chronic ischemic changes are often in evidence.

Small fusiform aneurysms are also to be found low on the intracranial segments of the vertebral arteries. Frequently bilateral, the dilatations are less commonly cylindrical or saccular (Fig. 9-4). Stehbens[473] found an incidence of 10.8% of these dilatations in 185 circles of Willis from adult brains. Although their walls are thickened, more so than in the common saccular aneurysms of the cerebral arteries, they are not necessarily associated with gross atherosclerosis. Histologically fibrosis of the wall, medial thinning, severe elastic tissue degeneration with intimal thickening and prominent vasa vasorum are seen. These dilatations rarely progress to the saccular variety and

are probably poststenotic in type.[473] Enlargement of the external diameter need not be associated with dilatation, for because of atherosclerosis, the lumen may be narrowed.

Saccular arterial aneurysms

Saccular arterial aneurysms of noninflammatory origin are of two main types, those often erroneously called "congenital" or "developmental," which arise at the fork of bifurcations and those that are not associated with sites of branching. Usually both types of saccular aneurysm are grouped together despite differences in morphology, frequency of complications, and pathogenesis. Thus data and statistics appertain to combined totals.

Estimations of the prevalence of cerebral aneurysms at autopsy have varied considerably (Table 9-1). In many reviews the frequency in a general autopsy series has

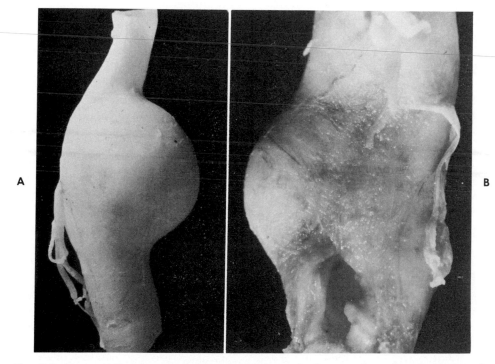

Fig. 9-4. Two small aneurysmal dilatations of vertebral artery just after it pierces the dura mater. **A,** Lower end is uniformly dilated and vessel then expands into a small dome-shaped aneurysm larger than that in **B.**

Table 9-1. The prevalence of intracranial arterial aneurysms at autopsy

Authors	Prevalence of aneurysms as a percentage
Pitt (1890)[383]	0.2
Turnbull (1918)[509]	0.64
Schmidt (1930)[429]	0.5
Richardson & Hyland (1941)[400]	0.87
Mitchell & Angrist (1943)[339]	1.1
Riggs & Rupp (1943)[403]	9
Brown (1951)[66]	1.3
Cohen (1955)[96]	3.6
Walton (1956)[523]	0.93
Housepian & Pool (1958)[254]	2.1
Chason & Hindman (1958)[89]	4.9
Stehbens (1963)[473]	5.6
McCormick & Nofzinger (1965)[323]	1.2
Berry et al. (1966)[42]	1.6

been given as 0.5% to 1.5%, but reference to Table 9-1 reveals decidedly higher figures on record. Gull[212] in 1859 commented upon the paucity of records of cerebral aneurysms in the literature and rightly adjudged the rarity of their occurrence to be only apparent. Even unruptured aneurysms at autopsy have been found to have an incidence[42,467,473] of 0.6% to 3.1% and the degree of care taken in the search for aneurysms directly affects the incidence affirmed. Other influences are geographic factors, the constitution of the autopsy material, and the individual pathologist's criteria for aneurysmal dilatation. Busse[70] claimed to have found aneurysms or early dilatations of the anterior "communicating" artery in almost 10% of 400 brains examined. When his doubtful cases are excluded, his figure still remains high, especially as the anterior communicating artery is but one of the common sites for the lesion. Stehbens[473] found aneurysms in 77 subjects (5.6%) in 1364 consecutive autopsies. Excluding autopsies in which no cranial examination was made, the incidence was 7.6%, and except for the fact that many stillborn and newborn infants were included in the series, the incidence would have been even higher. The very diverse nature of the au-

topsy material no doubt accounts in part for the variation in the reported prevalence of cerebral aneurysms and also, as Gull[212] indicated, much depends on the amount of care taken in examining the vessels. Stehbens[473] reported noninflammatory aneurysms of all extracranial arteries in only 2.6% of his autopsy series.

Although it is difficult to estimate the true incidence of cerebral aneurysms in the community, the preceding figures would suggest that cerebral aneurysms are the most common type of aneurysm occurring in man. The age distribution indicates that the prevalence of cerebral aneurysms will depend on the nature of the segment of the population under review. Their prevalence at autopsy serves only to illustrate the relative frequency of this disease as do the demographic mortality figures for subarachnoid hemorrhage, the principal cause of which is cerebral aneurysm.

Familial incidence. It is natural that a familial incidence should be sought in a lesion suspected of having a congenital or developmental fault underlying its pathogenesis (Table 9-2). A number of these patients have other pathological factors such as hypertension and arteriovenous aneurysms. Hypertension may account for the familial occurrence of cerebral aneurysms on sporadic occasions only.[83,381] Bannerman and associates,[24] reviewing the familial aggregation of cerebral aneurysms, included a 37-year-old woman with Ehlers-Danlos syndrome (cutis hyperelastica), multiple extracranial and intracranial aneurysms, and a carotid-cavernous fistula. This patient's illness was said to represent the arterial form of the familial and hereditary Ehlers-Danlos syndrome according to the classifications of Barabas.[25] Her brother had a spontaneous carotid-cavernous fistula but no definite evidence of a connective tissue disorder.

Dalgaard[123] tentatively included these cerebral aneurysms among the autosomal dominants in the catalog of Mendelian traits. An investigation of genealogy by Bannerman and associates[24] provided evi-

Table 9-2. Reported instances of familial occurrence of cerebral aneurysms

Authors	Relationship of victims
Ayer[19]	Two cousins
Chambers et al.[85]	Father, son
King et al.[284]	Mother, daughter
Stehbens*[467,473]	Brother, sister
Ross[414]	Mother, daughter
Ullrich & Sugar[511]	Two brothers
	Two brothers
	Uncle, nephew
	Brother, sister
Stark[464]	Three sisters
Matson[319]	Father, son, daughter
Phillips[381]	Two sisters
Chakravorty &	Brother, sister
Gleadhill[83]	Mother, son
	Mother, son
Graf[202]	Brother, sister
	Two sisters
Beumont[44]	Three sisters
Endtz[161]	Brother, sister
	Mother, son
Kak et al.[280]	Two brothers
	Two brothers

*Patients included in reported series but not specifically mentioned.

dence inadequate to allow any firm hypothesis. No single simple pattern of Mendelian inheritance can account for all the observations. Carroll and Haddon[78] made a study of the birth characteristics of a sample of persons under the age of 35 dying of cerebral aneurysm in New York State (exclusive of New York City) from 1949 through 1961 (excluding 1952 and 1953). No familial aggregation was detected. The authors concluded that there is no substantiated tendency to indicate a familial pattern. Jansen[266] had previously analyzed data from 147 patients with subarachnoid hemorrhage and 688 members of their families. Two relatives had aneurysms, but no patients had demonstrable aneurysms. Subarachnoid hemorrhage had occurred in 11 patients and 15 of their relatives. Endtz[161] deduced from Pakarinen's material[372] that eight patients and 11 of their relatives had had ruptured cerebral aneurysms and concluded that this familial relationship was too infrequent to substantiate the possible existence of a familial disorder of the vascular wall. He contended that the idea of a familial occurrence had evolved from the assumptions about a congenital origin of the aneurysms. It is well to remember furthermore that intracranial aneurysm is a common disease and that degenerative diseases such as coronory occlusion and spontaneous intracerebral hemorrhage are frequently found in family trees. The investigation of Carrol and Haddon[78] is the only known statistical evaluation of the familial occurrence of cerebral aneurysms. The results did not support the theory that a congenital or developmental defect underlies the formation of these lesions.

Ask-Upmark and Ingvar[15] advocated that women during the first trimester of pregnancy should avoid contact with victims of rubella as a prophylactic measure, but there is no evidence to support a relationship between cerebral aneurysm and German measles.

Epidemiology. Information on the prevalence of cerebral aneurysms in populations stems largely from Europe, Scandinavia, the United Kingdom, and North America and yet the frequency at autopsy varies considerably (Table 9-1). Estimates of the frequency of aneurysms in clinical material and pathological materials are often not comparable because of variation in the selection of cases and uncertain differences in base populations. Thus little of moment can be said at present concerning differences from country to country in the incidence of aneurysms.

The prevalence is thought to be lower in Oriental races than in Caucasians,[24] but no exhaustive, detailed epidemiological surveys similar in scope to those pertaining to atherosclerosis have yet been undertaken. Ramamurthi[392] has recently indicated a low incidence of clinically diagnosed intracranial aneurysms in his experience in Madras and in India in general, citing similar impressions from Iran and Japan, but no pathological evidence was provided. Sugai and Shoji[487] found small aneurysms (less than 2 mm.) in 50% of all cases of subarachnoid hemorrhage and in six of 28 cases of cerebral hemorrhage in Japan. These figures were above and beyond those for larger aneurysms. This suggests that cerebral aneurysms may well be more frequent in the Japanese than in peoples of Caucasian origin.

In North America where such a comparative investigation would be feasible, no statistical evaluation of the differences in the prevalence of cerebral aneurysms among those of Caucasian, Negro, and mixed origin has been embarked upon. So there is no certain evidence at present that geographic or ethnic factors are of decisive import in the pathogenesis.

Age distribution. The frequency of cerebral aneurysm in the young, particularly in the first 2 decades has been emphasized, probably because of the prominence of bacterial aneurysms in the literature of the last century.[212,383] The actual incidence indicates that the impression has little basis in established fact.

Although aneurysms in infancy have been reported,[132,178,185,265,352] considerable doubt has been cast upon the reliability of some accounts.[459,473] Smith and Windsor[459] assert that no conclusive instance of a noninflammatory cerebral saccular aneurysm occurring in an infant below the age of 2 years has been found. Riggs and Rupp[402,403] found no aneurysms in a group of 102 infants and children under 10 years of age, yet 9% of their 1437 consecutive adults had aneurysms at autopsy. Report-

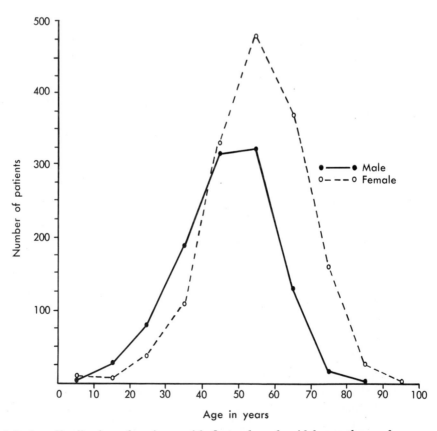

Fig. 9-5. Age distribution of patients with first subarachnoid hemorrhage of aneurysmal origin. Note predominance of males in the first three decades. (Adapted from Locksley, H. B.: Report on the co-operative study of intracranial aneurysms and subarachnoid hemorrhage, J. Neurosurg. **25:**219, 1966.)

ing an atypical case, Wagenvoort and his colleagues[516] detected multiple aneurysms including the intracranial segments of the internal carotid arteries in a boy of 34 months. Histologically giant cell arteritis was revealed, indicating the need for careful histological examination of aneurysms appearing at this unusual age. The histology of these aneurysms in the infant should be reviewed carefully for they may constitute a separate and distinct entity.

Housepian and Pool[254] found no cerebral aneurysms in the autopsy records of 3000 children and babies. At the Royal Alexandra Hospital for Children, Sydney, no non-inflammatory aneurysms of the cerebral vessels were found in approximately 4000 autopsies on children under 13 years of age during a period if 20 years.[398] Even conceding that a few of these aneurysms might have been overlooked, the incidence is virtually nil and not at all compatible with a congenital origin. In the Cooperative Study of Intracranial Aneurysms and Subarachnoid Hemorrhage 2627 patients with cerebral aneurysms were reported and only one was under 4 years of age.[302]

It is generally accepted nowadays that aneurysms are not present at birth and are in fact acquired lesions. Indeed the syndrome of subarachnoid hemorrhage before the age of 30 years is more likely to be caused by an arteriovenous aneurysm or a bacterial aneurysm. In the small series (81 subjects) of Taylor and Whitfield,[494] the average age was 39.7 years but in other large series of cerebral aneurysms, few individuals are under 20 years of age and the majority of patients with cerebral aneurysm at autopsy is between 40 and 70 years (Fig. 9-3) with a mean age of approximately 50 years.[473] Table 9-3 shows the age distribution of representative series of patients with cerebral aneurysms. Indeed only 21.1% of the subjects were younger than 40 years. Comparison of the age distribution of cerebral aneurysm and primary cerebral hemorrhage reveals that the differences are in no way remarkable.[473]

Sex distribution. Despite the predominance of cerebral aneurysms in the males of several series in the literature,[314,523] in most surveys females preponderated slightly (Table 9-4). The slight disparity in sex distribution contrasts with figures for aortic, coronary, and popliteal aneurysm in which conditions males outnumber females by a large margin.[60,65,126] Berry and associates[42] demonstrated a female preponderance even more significant in view of the greater number of males in their autopsy series. Ask-Upmark and Ingvar[15] decided that the predominance of females may be accounted for in part by the preponderance of females in the Swedish population, but the contention would not explain the higher figures of female involvement in the Austra-

Table 9-3. Age distribution of saccular intracranial aneurysms

Authors	0-9	10-19	20-29	30-39	40-49	50-59	60-69	70-79	80-89	90-99	Total
Dinning & Falconer (1953)[134]		4	8	21	34	57	71	45	10		250
Walton (1956)[523]	2	10	11	24	26	34	11	5	1		124
Housepian & Pool (1958)[254]		6	7	19	25	26	8	5	1		97
Stehbens (1963)[473]	1	2	20	33	61	58	60	11	3		249
Crompton (1964)[111]		1	4	21	36	53	40	3			158
Berry, Alpers, & White (1966)[42]	2	0	5	5	24	37	27	13	4		117
Freytag (1966)[181]		4	16	58	69	65	30	8			250
Locksley (1966)[302]	7	34	113	313	647	805	501	178	28	1	2627
Total	12	61	184	494	922	1135	748	268	47	1	3872

Table 9-4. Sex incidence in proved cerebral aneurysm (saccular)

Authors	Number of males	Number of females	Total
Dandy (1944)[125]	47	61	108
Hamby (1952)[216]	41	50	91
Dinning & Falconer (1953)[134]	91	159	250
Walker & Allègre (1954)[518]	17	22	39
Wilson, Riggs, & Rupp (1954)[538]	52	91	143
Walton (1956)[523]	73	51	124
Housepian & Pool (1958)[254]	59	54	113
Stehbens (1963)[473]	119	130	249
Du Boulay (1965)[147]	71	125	196
McCormick & Nofzinger (1965)[323]	53	100	153
Berry, Alpers, & White (1966)[42]	49	69	118
Crompton (1966)[114]	71	102	173
Freytag (1966)[181]	125	125	250
Hudson & Raaf (1968)[255]	72	120	192
Locksley (1966)[302]	1086	1541	2627
Total	2026	2800	4826
Percentage	42	58	100

lian population[473] in which males are more numerous.

Matson[320] reported a series of aneurysms in 13 children and, of these 12 were male. In the report of the Cooperative Study of Intracranial Aneurysms and Subarachnoid Hemorrhage, Locksley[302] reported the prevalence of females in 2627 instances of subarachnoid hemorrhage of aneurysmal origin to be 59%. In those below 40 years of age males predominated (Fig. 9-5), and the sex distribution was almost equal in the fifth decade. After 50 years, females preponderated. Locksley[302] found this similar to the sex distribution of hypertension in man but thought the preponderance of women afflicted with cerebral aneurysm could not be accounted for entirely by the incidence of hypertension.

Du Boulay[147] asserted that the female preponderance begins only after the age of 35 years and he considered that the sex differences supported the belief that atherosclerosis is of importance in the pathogenesis of cerebral aneurysms. Like Crompton[114] he attempted to correlate sex with the shape and behavior of aneuysms. However, the external configuration and the shape of the effective or functional lumen is dependent on many factors, and in any case the series was too small for productive

analysis.[147] Extensive investigations are needed before much of significance will be concluded from speculation on the shape of an aneurysm and its secondary or false sacs.

The reason for the female preponderance, though obscure, could be related to a predisposition to aneurysmal development attributable to hormonal influences, or to a deficiency in the repair processes. Not only do cerebral aneurysms afflict females somewhat more frequently than males, but recurrent bleeding is more common in the female.[15,521] Rupture during pregnancy has been emphasized, though the frequency of this event is not necessarily statistically significant.

Little is known concerning the underlying mechanism of the relationship of sex to the pathogenesis of cerebral aneurysms, but one must remember that (1) the coronary arteries of the female infant exhibit less intimal thickening, an apparent repair manifestation of hemodynamic injury,[470] than those of the male infant,[136] (2) the undetermined effect of recurrent pregnancies on the connective tissues of the pelvis, genital tract, perineum, and doubtless elsewhere, (3) the possibility that collagen proliferation and repair may be influenced by steroid hormones, and (4) the occur-

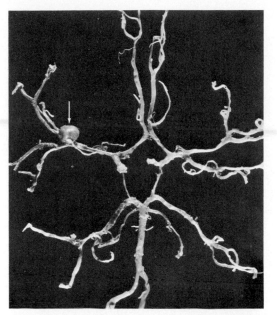

Fig. 9-6. Circle of Willis with a small saccular aneurysm on a middle cerebral artery (*arrow*). The appearance of this type of aneurysm and its similarity to a berry on a stalk led to the adoption of the term "berry aneurysm."

rence of spontaneous ecchymoses during the menstrual cycle in patients with the mild or varicose type of Ehlers-Danlos syndrome.[25]

Saccular berry aneurysms related to forks. This more common variety of saccular aneurysm is known generally as "berry" (Fig. 9-6), or congenital, aneurysm. Collier[97] introduced the term berry "because of the shining coats, and rounded outlines; they hang like berries on the arterial stalks and are often multiple." The term, however, inadvertently implies a pedunculated or polypoid dilatation with a narrow and readily accessible neck, conditions that very few aneurysms fulfill. Even Lebert[296] in 1866 realized that the aneurysms under discussion had wide necks, yet this fact is still not well known or widely accepted even today. Furthermore, like most analogies to foodstuffs, such a term is undesirable, but it appears to be firmly ensconced in the literature and will therefore be used in reference to those saccular aneurysms arising in the apical

region of forks. Congenital aneurysm is a misleading term, ineptly and too loosely used by pathologists. These aneurysms are rarely if ever congenital. In addition, by connotation the term implies defective development as an etiological factor in their pathogenesis, and such a belief has not at all been substantiated by fact.

Most of these aneurysms are less than 1 cm. in their largest diameter. When first recognizable, at about 1 mm. in diameter, they appear as little more than a filling out of the apical angle (Fig. 9-7, *A*) and are often more translucent than the surrounding vessel wall. The redundant area of the vessel wall can be better appreciated after perfusion or with the aid of a dissecting microscope. Small invaginations or dilatations, detectable only in serial histological sections, are early aneurysmal changes and will be dealt with separately. Increasing in size, sacs form dome-shaped swellings (Fig. 9-8) that, like the apertures of communication, are large in comparison with the diameter of the parent vessel. A few are relatively constricted at the base (Fig. 9-9), but most have a wide attachment to the parent vessel. A common misconception is that aneurysms are attached to the parent artery by a stalk. This fallacious impression is derived from the radiological appearance, which does not mirror the actual shape or configuration.[271]

Small aneurysms have thin, relatively transparent walls, but sacs of more than 3 mm. in diameter generally have thicker walls, which appear to be of the same consistency as the wall of the parent vessel. White or yellow atherosclerotic plaques are occasionally present, and usually a yellow zone can be demonstrated by sectioning the thickened opaque wall. Such atherosclerotic areas are sometimes more prominent in the sac than in the cerebral arteries themselves; their position is not constant, though most frequently they occur on the sides of the sac rather than at the fundus. The inner wall in most instances is smooth unless mural thrombosis has been initiated.

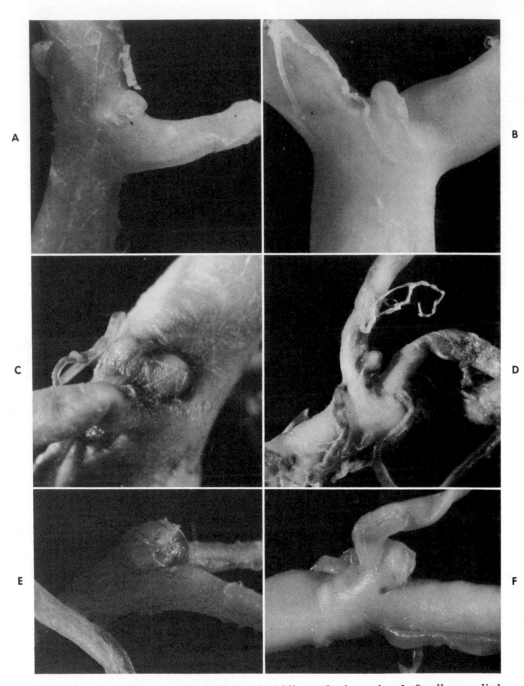

Fig. 9-7. Six small aneurysms in the forks of middle cerebral arteries. **A,** Small sac, a little more than a redundant wall. **B,** Somewhat larger sac. **C,** Two small sacs are developing in the fork, and bilocular aneurysms as in Fig. 1-4 probably form from such lesions. A small aneurysm has formed to the side of the actual apex in **D,** and one has formed near the facial aspect of the apex in **E.** Compare **D** and **E** with **F** in which a small dome-shaped aneurysm appears to be involving the center of the apex. These aneurysms are very easily overlooked at autopsy. (**A,** From Stehbens, W. E.: Aneurysms and anatomical variation of cerebral arteries, Arch. Path. **75:**45, 1963.)

These aneurysms arise in the apical angle of bifurcations. At times the sac takes origin from the distal side of one daughter branch (Fig. 9-7, *D*) rather than directly from the apex. Another site of origin is toward the dorsal or facial region of the apex. Occasionally two sacs are seen at the one fork (Fig. 9-7, *C*) and such lesions could conceivably develop into bilocular aneurysms (Fig. 1-4).

A comparison of the size of the aneurysm and the age of the patient evidences a trend toward larger aneurysms with increasing age[303] and suggests progressive aneurysmal enlargement, which is consistent with our knowledge of the behavior of aneurysms in general. By serial angiography it has been shown that cerebral aneurysms have enlarged during intervals ranging from 2 weeks to 10 years.[3] Very small aneurysms are not infrequently observed late in life, and such findings seem inconsistent with the concept that aneurysms are primordial at birth.[303] There is little evidence on the

rate of enlargement, but indications are that the sac tends to grow relentlessly at least until complications occur. Enlargement in the size of the sac need not be uniform and unequal expansion is illustrated by the numerous ovoid or irregular configurations. In addition to extending on to the face or dorsum of the fork, the enlarging basal attachment progressively encroaches upon and involves more of the distal side of one or both branches (Fig. 9-10). The arterial wall thus seems to have been "taken up" into the expanding sac. Eventually in extremely large aneurysms, the parent stem may enter the sac, with each of the two daughter branches leaving it at the sides at variable distances from the point of entry of the feeding vessel. With the exception of these vessels and small ves-

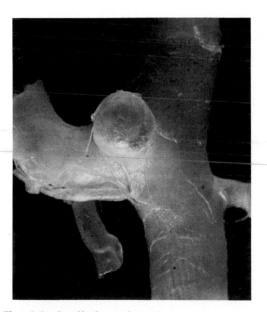

Fig. 9-8. Small dome-shaped aneurysm, eccentrically placed at fork of middle cerebral artery. Note transparent wall and wide base compared to diameter of the vessel of origin. (From Stehbens, W. E.: Aneurysms and anatomical variation of cerebral arteries, Arch. Path. **75:** 45, 1963.)

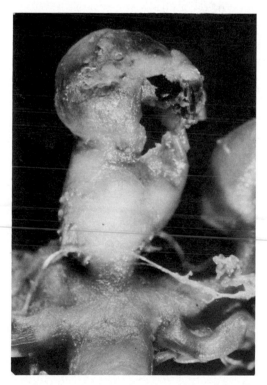

Fig. 9-9. Large hole in aneurysm of basilar artery. The sac appears relatively constricted at the base and the distal half or terminal knob is a false sac. Rupture has occurred through the false sac and line of junction with the true or previous sac.

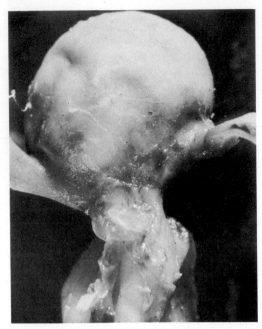

Fig. 9-10. Large unruptured aneurysm of middle cerebral artery. Flow is from below upward, and the aneurysm takes origin from wide segments of the two daughter branches.

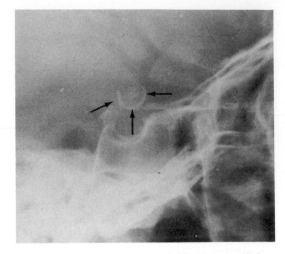

Fig. 9-11. Small ring of calcification outlining the wall of an aneurysmal sac (*arrows*) at upper level of sella turcica in the X-ray film. Though often called Albl's rings,[4] these shadows were first described by Heuer and Dandy.[243] (Courtesy Dr. S. Morson, Sydney, Australia.)

sels, which arise from the parent vessel near the neck of the aneurysm, no vessels issue forth from the sac wall. The surface of the sac is usually smooth and glistening, though from time to time, blood clot, meninges, brain tissue, or nerves adhere to it. Neighboring arteries too may be affixed to the surface of the sac. Serial sections of a large number of cerebral aneurysms indicate that despite appearances neighboring arteries do not arise from the aneurysm.[475]

In direct contrast to the case of splenic and renal aneurysms in which it is frequently a prominent feature macroscopically, calcification is rarely demonstrable in this type of aneurysm. However, mineralization sufficient to produce a radiological shadow (Fig. 9-11) may occur in the sac wall and is more likely to be encountered in large aneurysms.

Some aneurysms are distinctly bilocular (Fig. 1-4), being derived from two small primary sacs in the one fork (Fig. 9-7, *C*). Secondary lobulations, (6 or 7 mm. in diameter) may arise from the fundus of an aneurysmal sac and result in dumbbell-shaped aneurysms (Fig. 9-9) or even more rarely, complex lobulation. These secondary dilatations are usually false sacs, a consequence of the rupture of the primary dilatation, and are firmer in consistency than the primary sac when thrombosed. The false sacs, often only 1 to 2 mm. in diameter, impart a knobbled appearance to the aneurysm.[74] Previous leakage is also established by evidence of meningeal staining or an occasional brown granular mass adherent to the sac wall (Fig 9-12).

The aneurysm may lie within the subarachnoid space or in a depression in the brain substance. It may be surrounded by thickened, rust-colored meninges and is frequently embedded in blood clot.

Rupture usually occurs at the fundus of an aneurysm and less frequently at the side. Actual rupture at the neck of an aneurysmal sac is rare, unless occurring after surgical manipulation, although incipient rupture may occur. After the distal knob or false sac of a dumbbell-shaped aneurysm has thrombosed, the proximal or primary dilatation may rupture at the side, which

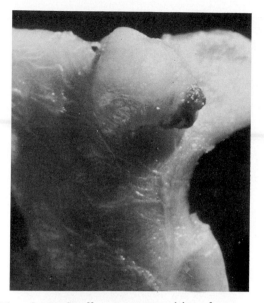

Fig. 9-12. Small aneurysm arising from an arterial fork. Small dark (rust-colored) granular nodule on the wall of sac indicates site of previous leakage.

is probably the explanation of the rupture in the proximal third of 2.7% of Crompton's aneurysms.[115] In ruptured aneurysms the aperture, often with ragged edges, varies in size and can be difficult to demonstrate because of the mass of blood clot. Perfusion of the parent vessel and tracing to the hole through which the liquid escapes often leads to a successful demonstration of the site of rupture. Tearing of the aneurysmal sac wall, irrespective of mild leakage or serious rupture, is the most likely lesion to initiate mural thrombosis within the sac. Lamination of the thrombus within the sac is similar to that known to occur in extracranial aneurysms and does not preclude fatal rupture. Aneurysms that rupture and cause death are usually more than 5 mm. in diameter. Most aneurysms with a lumen over 1 cm. in diameter contain a partially occlusive thrombus. In Bull's series[67] of large aneurysms, one extremely unusual sac with a functional lumen of some 6 by 4 cm. was demonstrated by angiography.

The assertion that with rupture of an aneurysm the sac wall may be torn off completely, leaving behind only a ragged hole in the parent artery, is patently false and has probably been used to excuse rough dissection of the vessels or failure to find the source of bleeding. The pathologist should not assume that the sac has been destroyed, and as a last resort serial sections of a small aneurysm will distinguish the sac wall proper from the thrombus and surrounding blood clot.

The prevalence of unruptured aneurysms found coincidentally at autopsy varies according to the care taken in the search. They are found to be not at all uncommon in middle-aged adults although unfortunately there is no means of estimating how long they have been present.[471] Attention has been drawn to the association of unruptured cerebral aneurysm with spontaneous intracerebral hemorrhage in 11 cases. This specific combination of lesions has been neglected and leads to serious difficulties in the clinical management of the patient.

Saccular aneurysms unrelated to forks. Saccular aneurysms not directly related to forks are by far the less common of the two types of saccular aneurysm. They are found invariably with severly atherosclerotic cerebral arteries and on the stems of the vertebral, basilar, and internal carotid arteries (cavernous and intracranial segments). These aneurysms probably occur at an age older than that of the berry aneurysms, but we await differentiation of the two varieties of saccular aneurysms according to age distribution.

These saccular aneurysms are not infrequently multiple along the vertebral and basilar (Fig. 9-13). The parent artery usually exhibits advanced atherosclerosis with fairly rigid walls, prominent vasa vasorum, and patchy rusty colorations of the adventitial surface (because of altered blood pigment). The artery may be tortuous, ectatic, and of irregular contour. The sacs are frequently more than 1 cm. in their largest diameter. They rarely rupture, tending to enlarge progressively until they either produce symptoms such as space-

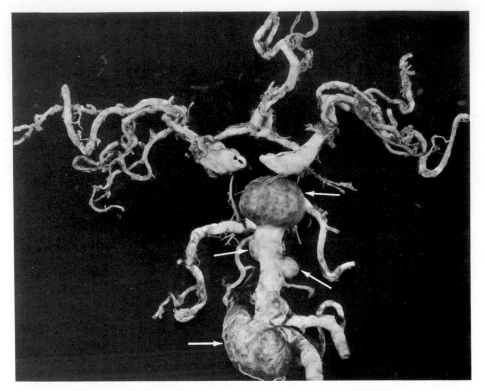

Fig. 9-13. Severely atherosclerotic circle of Willis with four aneurysms (*arrows*). Two large saccular aneurysms of the basilar artery, one at each end of the artery. There are also two dome-shaped aneurysms (*left* and *right*) below the upper sac. These aneurysms each contained thrombus and mural calcification. Note the fusiform dilatation of both internal carotid arteries.

occupying lesions or are fortuitously found at autopsy. Calcification occurs more often in the walls of these large aneurysms than in the berry variety of saccular aneurysm.

As a result of the progressive enlargement of a localized fusiform dilatation, the afferent vessel ultimately enters the sac, and the efferent vessel leaves the aneurysm on the side diametrically opposite. Alternatively, the sac springs from one side of the parent artery (Fig. 9-13), the type Dandy[125] alleged to be caused by the persistence of vestigial vessels, for it does not occur at sites of branching but arises (1) from weakness of a localized segment of the atherosclerotic vessel wall, or (2) like others in the aorta and iliac arteries, by ulceration or disruption of the atheromatous intima, with progressive excavation of the atheromatous wall and dilatation of the underly-

ing residual adventitia and media. Such was the type once thought to be caused by rupture of the inner coats of the artery.

Walton[523] believed that saccular aneurysms on the vertebrobasilar system rupture less often than those on the anterior part of the circle of Willis. However the two varieties of saccular aneurysm of the posterior half of the circle tend to behave differently from this point of view and combining them in the one group masks the difference in frequency of rupture.

Nontraumatic aneurysms of the cavernous segment of the internal carotid artery, a disease predominantly of women, either belong to this type of saccular aneurysm or are fusiform. A serpentine variety has been included but is usually ectasia or a cylindroid aneurysm. The aneurysms need not be confined solely to this segment, and their pathology at this site has been neglected for they have been assumed to be "congenital." A few small branches arise from this segment of the internal carotid, and the ophthalmic artery sometimes takes origin in the cavernous sinus, but the berry type of aneurysm, if it occurs on the cavernous segment, is very uncommon. In autopsy series they are infrequent,[473] but no doubt small sacs are overlooked because of the failure to dissect the cavernous sinus as a routine procedure. The incidence rises in angiographic studies, and Lombardi and colleagues[309] found them to comprise 11% of their cerebral aneurysms. They also constituted 1.9% of solitary aneurysms[302] and 14% of the unruptured aneurysms in the cooperative study of intracranial aneurysms.[303] They are confined to women in about 86% of cases.[303]

Aneurysms of the cavernous sinus appear as rounded swellings at the side of the pituitary fossa. Enlarging, they take up more of the medial aspect of the middle cranial fossa, stripping up the dura as they grow. They may be massive in size, but appear to be fairly slow growing. They are occasionally bilateral[215,309,441] and may be associated with supratentorial aneurysms.[533] Calcified shadows in X-rays may outline their position and size, and exophthalmos and a cranial bruit may be observed.[309,333]

Jefferson,[268] in a now classic paper, classified these aneurysms in groups according to whether they caused pressure symptoms in anterior, posterior, or middle zones of the cavernous sinus. Radiological evidence of bone erosion occurs very frequently[309] and hypophyseal symptoms and signs may result. Rupture of these aneurysms, though infrequent, causes a carotid-cavernous fistula unless the sac is sufficiently large to have obliterated the sinus. In which case the dural walls of the sinus will become applied to the sac, and rupture occurs into the cranial cavity and more frequently into the temporal lobe. Death may accrue from extracranial causes.

Multiple aneurysms. The occurrence of more than one cerebral aneurysm in a pa-

Table 9-5. The reported frequency of multiple cerebral aneurysms

Authors	Incidence as a percentage
Richardson & Hyland (1941)[400]	25
Dandy (1944)[125]	15
Hamby (1952)[216]	9.3
Dinning & Falconer (1953)[134]	6
Wilson, Riggs, & Rupp (1954)[538]	18.6
Bigelow (1955)[46]	15
Williams et al. (1955)[537]	17.2
Walton (1956)[523]	11.3
Housepian & Pool (1958)[254]	12
Crawford (1959)[105]	12.3
Poppen & Fager (1959)[386]	8.8
Stehbens (1963)[473]	20.6
McKissock et al. (1964)[328]	13.7
Du Boulay (1965)[147]	18.1
McCormick & Nofzinger (1965)[323]	25
Berry, Alpers, & White (1966)[42]	19
Crompton (1966)[115]	31
Freytag (1966)[181]	12
Hudson & Raaf (1968)[255]	13.5

tient is not unusual and consideration of the possibility of multiple sacs is fundamental in the clinical management of the patients. At autopsy the frequency of multiplicity varies (Table 9-5), for at the autopsy table even senior pathologists consistently miss aneurysms. In a thorough and deliberate search for aneurysms in 122 brains with cerebral aneurysms, the author found them to be multiple in 30.3%.[473] There is a higher incidence in patients with coarctation of the aorta, that is, 40%.[55] Bigelow[55] collected 2237 cases of intracranial aneurysms from the literature and of these 10.2% had more than one aneurysm. Locksley[302] reporting on the Cooperative Study of Intracranial Aneurysms and Subarachnoid Hemorrhage gave the incidence of multiplicity as 18.5% in subjects examined by angiography alone, as 22% in subjects examined by autopsy alone, and as 19% for those examined by both angiography and autopsy. He thought that 20% would be a reasonable estimate, but this figure is probably too low.

Stehbens[473] found more than 333 aneurysms in 251 brains. Only infrequently are more than three aneurysms found (Table

Table 9-6. Tabulation of the number of aneurysms in individual brains

Number of aneurysms found	Number of brains with aneurysms				
	Stehbens[473]	Courville*[100]	af Björkesten & Halonen[3]	McCormick[321]	Total
1	199	157	59	96	521
2	33	50	17	17	114
3	12	7	7	6	32
4	3	6		4	13
5	2	1	1		4
6				1	1
7	1	1		1	3
Several	1				1

*Ruptured aneurysms only.

9-6) and instances of eight, nine, and 10 aneurysms are quite exceptional. Stehbens[473] reported seven aneurysms in a woman of 59 years and eight in a chimpanzee.[474] Bigelow[55] recorded 10 in a woman of 52 years, with several occurring on small arteries only rarely involved.

No particular significance should be attributed to the multiplicity of cerebral aneurysms for it is a feature of "arteriosclerotic" aneurysms of extracranial arteries also. For example, Gliedman and associates[196] reported multiplicity in 23.4% of 68 patients with aneurysms of the abdominal aorta and its branches. Gifford and associates[192] found multiple popliteal aneurysms in 58% of their 69 patients, and in another report of aneurysms of the lower limb 70% were multiple.[102] Multiple cerebral aneurysms in man can as readily be attributed to widespread degenerative changes in the intima as to a multiplicity of hypothetical congenital factors, and it is of interest that Housepian and Pool[254] found arteriosclerosis more frequently associated with multiple than with single cerebral aneurysms.

Anatomical distribution of saccular arterial aneurysms. Aneurysms originating at the forks of the cerebral arterial tree do not appear to arise from the lateral angle. They are found at the apex of both large and small branchings of vessels but mostly occur at the origin of the larger forks. In the main they are found on the large arteries of the circle of Willis and proximally

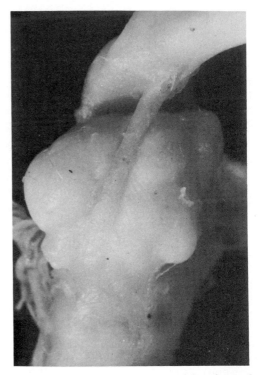

Fig. 9-14. An aneurysmal sac arising from the fork formed by an artery and a small branch that subsequently rejoins stem of parent artery.

on its main branches lying in the subarachnoid space unless embedded either partially or wholly within the cortical surface of the brain. Only infrequently are they detected on the peripheral branches of the cerebral or cerebellar arteries and never on intracerebral or intracerebellar vessels. In quite exceptional instances, an aneurysm has been found on an artery at the origin of a

Table 9-7. Location of saccular aneurysms

Authors	Middle cerebral	Internal carotid	Anterior cerebral and communicating	Basilar	Verte-bral	Cere-bellar	Posterior cerebral and communi-cating	Site not stated	Total
Primarily clinical data									
Hamby (1952)[316]	15	38	32	4		1	3		93
Harris & Udvarhelyi (1957)[229]	73	152	87	9	2	2	1		326
Hamilton & Falconer (1959)[217]	17	48	34	3				10+	112
Bull (1962)[68]	348	577	533	64				247	1769
Berry, Alpers, & White (1966)[42]	32	63	31	13	1	4	7		151
Locksley (1966)[302]	529	1104	895	77	25	20	22		2672
Pakarinen (1967)[372]	36	34	46					28	144
Total	1050	2016	1658	258				285	5267
Autopsy data									
Richardson & Hyland (1941)[400]	16	13	13	6	3		2		53
Dinning & Falconer (1953)[134]	127	5	90	52					274
Walker & Allègre (1954)[518]	6	18	13	1	2		3	2	45
Wilson, Riggs, & Rupp (1954)[538]	39	61	60	8	5		9		182
Williams et al. (1955)[537]	34	55	64	19					172
Walton (1956)[523]	51	34	35	3	14	3		5	145
Housepian & Pool (1958)[254]	17	50	31	5	1	1	10		115
Crawford (1959)[105]	54	31	66	7	1	1	3		163
Stehbens (1963)[473]	124	79	87	27	3		7		327
Freytag (1966)[181]	68	62	81	24	8	3	4		250
McCormick & Nofzinger (1966)[323]	66	68	60	4	2		6		206
Pakarinen (1967)[372]	99	37	43	14				26	219
Total	701	513	643	261				33	2151

small branch, which after a short course rejoined the parent stem (Fig. 9-14). Crompton[108] depicted two such instances, one on the basilar and the other on the anterior cerebral artery. Alternatively an aneurysm may arise from the angle formed by an anterior cerebral artery and one of two or more branches that constitute the anterior communicating artery. Such aneurysms still in effect arise from bifurcations.

If the circle of Willis is divided into anterior and posterior parts by a line through the posterior communicating arteries, it will be seen that 85% to 95% of these saccular aneurysms occur on the anterior and 5% to 15% arise on the posterior half of the circle. Last century aneurysms on the posterior half appeared more often than in recent years, probably because large atherosclerotic aneurysms are more common posteriorly, and the sac had to be large to be detected. Walton[523] considered the previously higher incidence of posteriorly situated aneurysms to be caused by an incorrect acceptance of vertebrobasilar ectasia as aneurysmal dilatation.

Table 9-7 sets forth the distribution of aneurysms on individual arteries and considerable variation from author to author is apparent. In recent years the fork formed by the anterior cerebral and the anterior communicating arteries is said to be the most frequent site affected with aneurysms, but at other branchings of the anterior cerebral artery it is infrequent. The aneurysms are usually found at one or the other end of the anterior communicating artery although its whole length may be involved eventually. These aneurysms often arise from a single bifurcation, a consequence of a considerable shunt of blood across the anterior communicating artery to the distal segment of the contralateral anterior cerebral artery[473] (Fig. 1-4). It is the only variation of the circle of Willis as yet positively correlated with the occurrence of an aneurysm of a cerebral artery. In McKissock's collection (published by Bull[68]), it was the most common site, and aneurysms of the internal carotid were more frequent than those of the middle cerebral artery. Frequently clinical and angiographic material[68,302] show a preponderance of aneurysms of the internal carotid and anterior communicating arteries, whereas investigation of autopsy material[473] tends to indicate that the middle cerebral artery is the usual location (Table 9-7).

Results of the Cooperative Study[302] indicate that the anterior communicating artery is the most usual single site, and when all aneurysms of the internal carotid are grouped together, this artery is the one most frequently involved. The value and reliability of the results obtained by such a cooperative study depend entirely on the value and reliability of the data collected and reported by each center. The vastness of the organization does not ensure rectitude of the results, and detailed, meticulous, though smaller, investigations from one or two individuals often produce more reliable information.[481] Autopsy studies of both ruptured and unruptured aneurysms are more likely to give accurate representations of the localization of aneurysms

than angiography. Nevertheless both methods are open to fallacies, human and otherwise. After long investigation I am convinced that the middle cerebral artery is the most frequent site for aneurysms of the cerebral arteries.

Small sessile aneurysms in the fork of a middle cerebral artery are readily masked by the overlapping shadows of the parent vessel and branches in anteroposterior and lateral angiograms, necessitating the use of the oblique view, a procedure not always implemented. Bull[68] stated that aneurysms less than 2 mm. in diameter on the middle cerebral artery cannot be diagnosed angiographically with any certainty. McKissock et al.[328] found that in 20% of 100 complete necropsies 27 aneurysms had been missed by angiography during life. The most common site for missed aneurysms was the middle cerebral artery. Pakarinen[372] provided additional evidence, for in his angiographic series of aneurysms, 32% were on the anterior cerebral (mostly the anterior communicating), 23.6% on the internal carotid, and only 25% on the middle cerebral artery. In contrast, his autopsy cases included 19.6% on the anterior cerebral and anterior communicating, 16.9% on the internal carotid, but 45.2% on the middle cerebral artery. The location of ruptured aneurysms was as follows: by angiography 34.7% occurred on the anterior cerebral and anterior communicating, 32.5% on the internal carotid, and 31.3% on the middle cerebral artery. In Pakarinen's autopsy series[372] only 21.9% of ruptured aneurysms were found on the anterior cerebral and anterior communicating, 18.3% on the internal carotid, and 48.4% on the middle cerebral artery. Only a remote possibility exists that variation in the location of aneurysms in Table 9-7 by different authors may be caused by geographic differences. An unfortunate omission in the Cooperative Study[302] was that the aneurysms were not subdivided by site into those found by autopsy and those localized by angiography or neurosurgery. The analysis of the localization of multiple aneurysms encountered clinically by McKissock and co-workers[328] supports the concept[481] that the middle cerebral artery is the prime site for aneurysmal formation. Among patients with two aneurysms the middle cerebral artery was involved once in 40% of the patients, there were two sacs in an additional 22%, the internal carotid artery was involved once in 27%, and twice in 14%, and the anterior cerebral and anterior communicating arteries had one aneurysm in 33% of subjects and two in 4%. Alternatively, of 624 aneurysms in 251 patients, 46% were on the middle cerebral artery, 31% on the internal carotid (including the posterior communicating artery), and 20% were found on the anterior communicating and anterior cerebral arteries. These figures are in direct contrast with the distribution McKissock and his colleagues[327] gave for 599 ruptured aneurysms found by angiography, that is, middle cerebral artery 17%, internal carotid 28%, anterior cerebral–anterior communicating 29%.

Aneurysms of the middle cerebral artery occur at the major bifurcation or trifurcation of this vessel 2 to 3 cm. from its origin. Alternatively three or four moderately large branches successively issue from the middle cerebral artery and the site of each branching is prone to aneurysm formation.

The internal carotid artery is also a common site; some authors credit this vessel with a higher incidence of involvement than the anterior communicating and middle cerebral arteries. Internal carotid aneurysms, which usually form a large proportion of the aneurysms treated by neurosurgeons, are often divided into supraclinoid and infraclinoid types, that is, those on the carotid artery after its emergence from the cavernous sinus and those in the cavernous sinus. This division, of value perhaps to radiologists, is not sufficiently precise and is losing favor. Most aneurysms on the internal carotid arise at the origin of the posterior communicating artery. Others are to be found quite frequently at the bifurcation of the internal carotid and the origins of the anterior choroidal and oph-

thalmic arteries.[142,143] At autopsy an aneurysm arising from the stem of the internal carotid can be partially damaged during removal of the brain and erroneously impart the appearance of not occurring at a bifurcation. Of such aneurysms, many probably have developed at the origin of the ophthalmic artery, which is left in situ, and consequently the true relationship of the aneurysm to the branch is not appreciated. Intracavernous aneurysms are much less frequent and may be bilateral. Several small branches are given off by the cavernous segment of the internal carotid but are not of any appreciable size, and aneurysms of this segment are probably independent of branchings. Aneurysms in the foramen lacerum[302] or in the carotid canal are rare.

Authors sometimes give the location of an aneurysm as the posterior communicating artery, but in reality it arises at the angle of origin of the above vessel from the internal carotid and is usually grouped with aneurysms of the internal carotid artery. The junction of the posterior communicating and posterior cerebral arteries is rarely the site of aneurysmal dilatation and requires histological examination to ensure its noninflammatory nature.

Aneurysms of the basilar artery most frequently are to be found at the bifurcation where this artery lies in close relationship to the floor of the third ventricle, which it may indent. A sac may be found at the origin of the anterior inferior cerebellar artery or the superior cerebellar arteries. Because of the proximity of origins of the posterior cerebral and superior cerebellar arteries, respectively, an aneurysm arising at the origin of the latter rapidly involves the adjoining surfaces of these two branches. Consequently a false impression of lateral expansion of the upper end of the basilar artery can be given rather than indications of a saccular aneurysm. Aneurysms at the junction of the vertebral and basilar arteries are not of this type and are of the obviously atherosclerotic variety.

The vertebral arteries are not usually involved by this type of aneurysm, which occurs at the origin of the posterior inferior cerebellar artery. One of these aneurysms seen by the author extended upward, involving a considerable part of the stem of the vertebral and thus imparting an unusual appearance because of its extensive, shallow base.

In the literature the incidence of aneurysms at different sites varies considerably. The clinician and the pathologist should keep in mind that aneurysms (1) at the bifurcation of the internal carotid, (2) at the carotid origin of the posterior communicating or anterior choroidal arteries, (3) of the first 2 to 3 cm. of the middle cerebral, (4) in the region of the anterior communicating, and (5) at the basilar bifurcation, account for about 90% to 95% of all saccular aneurysms of the cerebral arteries.

Locksley[302] indicated that (1) aneurysms of the internal carotid arteries occur more than twice as frequently in women as in men, (2) aneurysms on the middle cerebral artery are more prevalent in women than in men in the ratio of 3:2, and (3) those on the anterior communicating artery are more prevalent in males, who comprise 58% of the cases concerned with this site. Such figures are naturally of academic rather than of practical value in clinical prognostications.

From the results of the Cooperative Study, Locksley[302] explored the predictability of localizing a second aneurysm. His conclusions were as follows:

1. The location of a second aneurysm was not independent of the site of the first.

2. Of 449 cases with two aneurysms, both aneurysms were on the same side in 21%, on opposite sides in 47%, on one side plus a midline aneurysm in 29%, and both midline in 3%.

3. If an aneurysm was identified on the internal carotid, in 49% of cases a second aneurysm was also found on the internal carotid. The middle cerebral artery was the next most probable site (26%) followed by the anterior communicating artery (15%).

4. When a middle cerebral aneurysm was identified, the most probable site of the second aneurysm was the internal carotid artery (36%), either ipsilateral or contralateral, followed by the middle cerebral (27%) and anterior communicating (26%). When the second aneurysm was on the middle cerebral, there was a 4:1 chance that it would be contralateral.

5. When an aneurysm was identified on the anterior communicating artery, the most probable site of the second was the middle cerebral (48%) and then the internal carotid artery (38%).

6. The most likely site for a second aneurysm in the presence of an aneurysm of the vertebrobasilar system was the internal carotid artery (48%), followed by another on the posterior circulation in 22% or the anterior communicating artery in 22%.

7. When an aneurysm of the anterior part of the circle of Willis was present, the probability of the second aneurysm occurring on the vertebrobasilar system was from 3% to 5%.

8. Whatever the factors that determine the site and distribution of single aneurysms may be, they are greatly outweighed in cases of internal carotid and middle cerebral aneurysms by a tendency toward either symmetrical aneurysms or the development of a second aneurysm on the same vessel.[302]

Many authors[46,284,386] have stressed the importance and frequency of multiple cerebral aneurysms displaying a bilateral symmetry of location. Locksley[302] alleged that such symmetry implicates hypothetical congenital developmental factors in the pathogenesis of cerebral aneurysms. Bigelow[46] attributed the symmetry to the widespread nature of the degenerative changes in the arteries involved and drew attention to the occurrence of symmetrical fusiform atherosclerotic dilatations of the cervical segment of the internal carotid. Furthermore bilateral popliteal aneurysms are frequent[192] and the small fusiform aneurysms of the vertebral artery, believed to be poststenotic in type,[473] are also commonly bilateral. Many diseases, including atherosclerosis, manifest bilateral symmetry without congenital or genetic factors becoming implicated. Thus developmental factors should not be assumed to participate in the pathogenesis of cerebral aneurysms because some are bilateral and symmetrical.

Gowers[200] reported that aneurysms were more prevalent on the left side of the circle of Willis than on the right (4:3). McDonald and Korb[325] in a combined series of 1023 aneurysms of all sorts, recorded 385 on the left side and 368 on the right, exclusive of those on the midline. However, in many such series, a slight preponderance of aneurysms on the right side has been reported. Hamby[216] recorded 28 on the left side, and 48 on the right side, Williams and associates[537] had 67 on the left and 82 on the right, Walton[523] 57 and 66 respectively, and Stehbens[473] 126 and 140 respectively. Wells[532] on the other hand found vertebral aneurysms to occur predominantly on the left side, possibly because the left vertebral artery is usually larger than the right. Locksley[302] reported an overall right-sided incidence of 55% in the Cooperative Study. This he thought was attributed to the exclusion of some left-sided cases from referral to the reporting centers because of disheartening aphasia, compare the greatest right-sided preponderance (58%) with middle cerebral aneurysms. Locksley also pointed out that angiographers prefer to start on the right side, and many patients had right angiography only. For all that, the two reasons do not adequately account for the unequal distribution between left and right, and neither do they explain the autopsy distribution and a satisfactory explanation has not yet been presented.

Aneurysms at unusual sites. Aneurysms that occur at unusual sites or that are atypical in any feature, require histological confirmation of their nature.[479] Failure to provide adequate histology accounts for some bizarre aneurysms in the literature. It should be suspected that all peripherally placed aneurysms on the cortical branches of the cerebral and cerebellar arteries are inflammatory or even traumatic in etiology. Only a remote possibility exists that a berry aneurysm could occur at such sites.

Aneurysms of the ophthalmic artery beyond its origin reviewed by Jefferson[273] are very uncommon and may involve the orbital segment. An infective or inflammatory process or a connective tissue disease should be sought to explain them.

Aneurysms are often encountered at the origin of the anterior choroidal artery from the internal carotid artery.[143,473] Those of the distal portion of this artery are extremely rare. In Strully's case[486] of such an aneurysm in the posterior portion of the left lateral ventricle, at operation, it was 7 cm. in its largest diameter and attached to a "large blood vessel" in the choroid plexus. Quite possibly in this instance there may have been a small but unrecognized arteriovenous aneurysm in the choroid plexus of the lateral ventricle.

Lemmen and Schneider[298] discussed an 8-month-old child with advanced hydrocephalus and an aneurysm of the posterior cerebral artery causing occlusion of the posterior portion of the third ventricle and fed by branches from both posterior cerebral arteries. One efferent vessel from the anterior aspect coursed anteriorly along the right lateral wall of the third ventricle. For all intents and purposes this was an arteriovenous aneurysm. Schürmann and associates[436] found a small aneurysm in the thalamostriate sulcus within the lateral ventricle. It was fed exclusively by a small artery through the thalamostriate sulcus, and the sac had ruptured causing an intraventricular hemorrhage.

Aneurysms rarely occur on the internal carotid artery during its course in the carotid canal and only four such cases have been reported in the literature up to 1963.[230] These aneurysms cause considerable pain, unilateral cranial nerve lesions,[211] and erosion of the skull in the region of the foramen lacerum, extending partly into the apex of the petrous bone. They could be a cause of epistaxis, but Ehni and Barrett[159] reported bleeding from the ear in the case of an aneurysm similarly situated.

Aneurysms up to 1 cm. in diameter occasionally occur within the cerebral hemispheres or alternatively they may be classed as small encapsulated hematomas. One instance found incidentally at autopsy is seen in Fig. 9-15, *A.* The wall was irregular in contour as if partially collapsed and his-

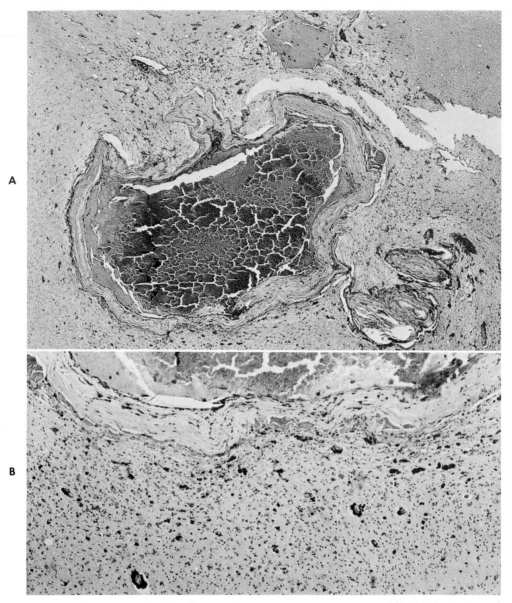

Fig. 9-15. A, Intracerebral aneurysm with irregularly convoluted wall of hyaline fibrous tissue. There is a large thin-walled vein above and sclerotic vessels below. The presence of numerous siderophages in and about the wall of the sac as well as in the parenchyma indicates previous hemorrhage. Although probably a large miliary aneurysm, postmortem microangiography is required to exclude the possibility of a small arteriovenous aneurysm. **B,** Part of the wall of sac in **A.** Note perivascular distribution of some siderophages in the parenchyma. The sac wall is quite hyaline but contains numerous siderophages and many vasa vasorum in its outer aspect. (Hematoxylin and eosin; **A,** ×20; **B,** ×45.)

tologically consisted of relatively acellular hyaline, fibrous tissue of variable thickness with some siderophages and round cell infiltration (Fig. 9-15, *B*). Closely associated with it were thick-walled hyalinized vessels and a greater vascularity of the brain in the immediate neighborhood. This lesion was probably a large miliary aneurysm although aneurysmal dilatation associated with a small cryptic arteriovenous aneurysm might account for some such lesions.

Aneurysms of the meningeal arteries over the cerebral convexities, the base of the skull or on the falx[539] are very rare. Charcôt[86] referred to an aneurysm of the middle meningeal artery in Durand's thesis but did not enlarge upon whether it was traumatic, inflammatory, or "spontaneous." Berk[41] reported the occurrence of a large saccular aneurysm of the middle meningeal artery in a hypertensive woman 73 years old with Paget's disease of the calvarium. The aneurysm had eroded through the temporal bone, was associated with a bruit, and arose from an enlarged meningeal artery, the enlarged vascular channels being the accompaniment of the Paget's disease. It was considered that this was a "congenital" aneurysm, despite the lack of histological examination, the arteriosclerosis that accompanies Paget's disease of bone, the patient's age, and the hypertension. No mention was made of any relationship between this aneurysm and an arterial fork nor was the idea of a traumatic origin entertained. Weibel and associates[528] reported bleeding from an aneurysm (2.5 by 1.8 cm.) arising from a terminal (presumably meningeal) branch of the left occipital artery and within the cisterna magna.

Such aneurysms on the meningeal arteries occurring in the absence of a history of trauma are extremely rare. The possibility of their being traumatic in origin has not been completely excluded. No detailed histopathological study of them has been performed. On account of the small size of the meningeal artery, we would not expect many saccular aneurysms of the berry type.

Rupture of saccular arterial aneurysms.
Rupture, the most frequent complication, is often the terminal event in the natural history of aneurysmal dilatations. Rupture of an aneurysm not related to arterial branchings is unusual. On the other hand, those arising at forks are exceedingly prone to rupture. As with aneurysms of extracranial sites, a warning of leakage varying in severity is often the prelude to subsequent severe hemorrhage. This characteristic feature, recurring subarachnoid hemorrhage, originally provided the clinician with the means of clinical diagnosis.

Of 252 autopsies of patients with cerebral aneurysms[473] a ruptured sac was found in 187 (or 74.2%). Furthermore the brains with ruptured aneurysms also contained unruptured sacs. Du Boulay[148] believes that aneurysms that never bleed constitute a group of formidable proportions, an unwise premise however on which to base clinical management. These unruptured aneurysms are probably in varying stages of development or growth and potentially progress to rupture in the absence of death from unrelated causes.

There is no way to predict clinically with certainty whether a cerebral aneurysm of this type will rupture. Reviewing aneurysms of the renal artery, Harrow and Sloane[231] found that rupture had not transpired in 69 radiologically calcified saccular aneurysms. In contrast 24 had ruptured in 100 cases of noncalcified aneurysm. In reviewing splenic aneurysm it appeared once more that predominantly the noncalcified aneurysm ruptured, but no precise incidence was provided. However, calcification of aortic aneurysms does not preclude rupture.[196] Radiologically calcified cerebral aneurysms are often of considerable size and have been regarded by some as unlikely to rupture. Yet there are varying degrees of calcification, and until there is statistical information concerning their natural history, calcified aneurysms should be regarded with some suspicion.

The Cooperative Study of cerebral aneurysms revealed that in general, aneurysms at a specific site do not tend to bleed earlier or later than those at other sites. Those above 6 mm. in diameter at the origin of the posterior communicating from the internal carotid artery are said to be at a stage where bleeding is imminent.[303] The incidence of rupture varies somewhat with the anatomical location, for aneurysms of the internal carotid artery constitute a much higher percentage among the unruptured aneurysms than in the series of ruptured sacs. The difference cannot be explained by subclinoid lesions.

Most ruptured aneurysms are between 5 and 10 mm. in diameter. Unruptured aneurysms are generally less than 6 or 7 mm. in external diameter.[115] In practice the risk of hemorrhage seems to be greater with increasing aneurysm size.[303] However large aneurysms over 3 cm. in diameter containing laminated thrombus and acting as space-occupying lesions do not commonly rupture, though, as with Fouché's patient,[179] fatal rupture cannot be excluded. Moreover in 88% of cases in which multiple aneurysms were present, Crompton[115] found the largest sac to have ruptured. It may be still that the size of the functional lumen is a more reliable guide.

Courville and Olsen[101] reported the simultaneous rupture of two cerebral aneurysms in a male of 55 years. Such a contingency is most unusual although at times incipient rupture may be observed in a second aneurysm upon histological examination. Turnbull and Dolman[507] reported a doubtful case of simultaneous rupture of at least four cerebral aneurysms. Greene and McCormick[207] reported concurrent rupture of cerebral and splenic aneurysms. Successive rupture of two aneurysms within 2 years was reported by Hyland,[258] with the patient dying from rupture of the second sac. Such events are always possibilities where multiple aneurysms are present.

It has long been accepted that hypertension is an aggravating factor in aneurysmal dilatation, although an increase in blood pressure accompanying exertion or other environmental events is not an essential antecedent factor precipitating rupture. Indeed the onset of subarachnoid hemorrhage may occur during sleep in as many as 36% of individuals and during physical effort such as lifting, bending, defecation, coughing, coitus, and parturition as well as emotional strain in less than 30% of cases.[302]

Freytag[181] noted that in 250 forensic autopsies, 50% of the patients appeared to have been engaged in some sort of activity when the rupture occurred. This author emphasized several cases of medicolegal interest in which the onset of bleeding appeared to be related to an injury, whether accidental or due to an altercation.

The aneurysm wall is often quite thin at the neck, yet rupture rarely occurs at this site, (Fig. 9-16) possibly because of support given by the adjacent wall of the parent vessel and branches. Although rupture of the sac usually occurs through a thin part of the wall, relatively thin walls are often intact (Fig. 9-17) when somewhat thicker walls have ruptured (Fig. 9-18). Indications are that some additional change in the connective tissues of the wall is necessary before tearing and bleeding transpire.

When fluid passes from a narrow tube into a wider one, according to Bernouilli's principle the velocity of flow decreases and the lateral pressure increases. This however is not the reason why aneurysmal dilatations "go from bad to worse," for the lateral pressure increase must be quite small.[543]

According to Laplace's formula for a hollow sphere:

$$P = 2\,T/r$$

where P is the internal pressure (excess over external pressure), T is the tangential tension in the wall, and r is the radius. For a cylinder, the formula is

$$P = T/r$$

Very great increases in tension may occur in the wall of dilated vessels though the blood pressure remains relatively unaltered. Wolf[543] likened an aneurysmal dilatation to a partially inflated tubular balloon. Air pressure within the balloon is everywhere equal, yet the taut dilated portion is under greater stretch and the rubber wall is thinner, in contrast to the flaccidity of the undilated segment. The tension in the wall at a given pressure is directly proportional to the radius of curvature, thus setting up a vicious cycle. The greater the tension, the more the sac wall is likely to yield and the more it expands, the greater the tension. With reduction in the cross-sectional thickness of the wall, because of dilatation, the

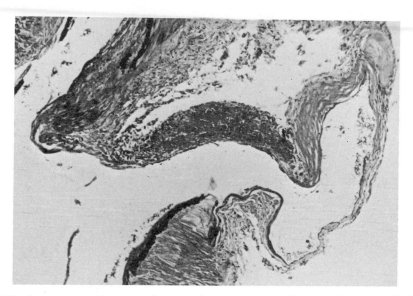

Fig. 9-16. Aneurysm with part of sac wall composed of fibrin with some cellular infiltration, suggesting imminent rupture. Location of the potential leak (that is, near the neck) is unusual. (Verhoeff's elastic stain, ×75.)

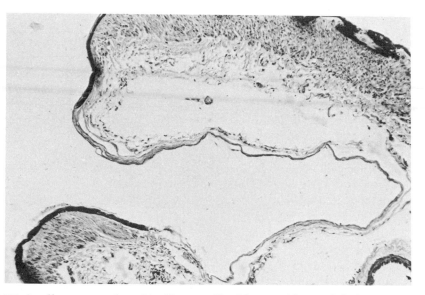

Fig. 9-17. Small aneurysm has thin flimsy wall without evidence of leakage or rupture. Media and elastic lamina are reflected into the sac on one side. On the opposite side, evagination does not commence where media ceases. (Verhoeff's elastic stain, ×75.)

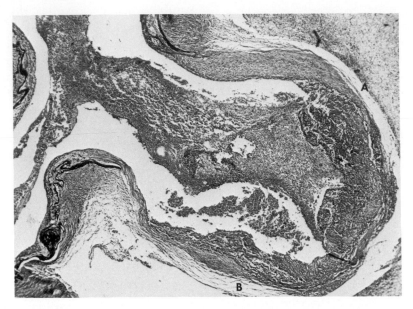

Fig. 9-18. Ruptured aneurysmal sac. Fundus is composed of thrombus that merges with the aneurysmal sac wall at **A** and **B** but continues on toward the neck as a lining on the inner surface. There is atherosclerosis of the intima of the artery near the entrance. The media and internal elastic lamina are reflected slightly into neck of sac. (Verhoeff's elastic stain, ×40.)

tension may increase even more than gauged by Laplace's proportionality between radius and tension.

German and Black[189] investigated the jet action in experimentally grafted vein-pouch aneurysms in dogs. The calculated velocities of the free jets ranged from 287 to 477 cm. per second and the theoretical force of such a "suppressed jet" was estimated to be almost 200 dynes. They concluded that the free jet action was a potent stress agent upon matter in its path. No consideration was given to the pulsatile nature of the jet. A jet may cause a small atheromatous plaque, but it is not the cause of dilatation and rupture in the poststenotic aneurysm.

The poststenotic dilatation of aortic coarctation, like an arteriovenous fistula, is associated with turbulence, thrill, bruit, and aneurysmal dilatation and hence has a propensity for rupture. Tearing and dissection of the wall with mural thrombosis under such conditions is thought to be the result of mechanical weakness or fragility (fa-

tigue) caused by hemodynamic stress.[480] The conditions in an aneurysmal dilatation appear analogous, for turbulent whirling of blood may be observed in small experimental saccular aneurysms. An audible bruit associated with cerebral aneurysms in man has been noted frequently[168,399] as well as a palpable thrill on palpation at surgical exposure.[74] Thus, the progressive dilatation and rupture of cerebral aneurysms has been attributed to mechanical fatigue consequent upon the altered hemodynamic stresses on the sac wall.[469]

Jain[265] in an experimental model of an aneurysm observed that pressure fluctuations associated with pulsatile flow caused it to rupture, and this he attributed to mechanical fatigue. The alternating stress was thought to be the pulse fluctuations visible in the aneurysm. No experiments were conducted with nonpulsatile flow to determine whether or not dilatation and rupture ensued. It is possible that the pressure fluctuations attendant upon turbulent flow in an aneurysmal dilatation, being of high frequency even though small, would contribute substantially to rupture of the aneurysm. In the case of pulsatile flow, the pulse pressure fluctuations would no doubt also contribute to the fatigue. Jain[265] noted too that the visible pressure fluctuations were considerably dampened distal to the aneurysm but not on the proximal side. A clamp proximal to the aneurysm could stop visible pulsations in the aneurysm if the lumen of the parent vessel were sufficiently narrowed, and flow remains undiminished. Injected dye did not wash out of the sac completely, in direct contradistinction to its rapid removal before the application of the clamp. When two identical aneurysms were inserted into the system, the distal aneurysm exhibited less pulsation than the proximal sac, which ruptured when pulsatile flow was increased. Likewise the tendency to poststenotic dilatation and rupture is greater beyond the first experimental stenosis than beyond second and third stenoses located distally to the first. With a static increase in intraluminal pressure in Jain's model, aneurysms of equal size were produced and distended to a greater size before rupturing. They tolerated pressures higher than those which aneurysms subjected to pulsatile flow could sustain without rupturing. The aneurysm's dampening effect on the pulse pressure distally was correlated with the rupture of the proximal of the two cerebral aneurysms on the internal carotid arterial tree in 12 of 18 cases. Crompton[115] confirmed this tendency on the internal carotid–middle cerebral artery (70% of cases) but not on the internal carotid–anterior communicating system.

The presence of leukocytic infiltration and some fibrin deposition on or permeation of the sac wall is not infrequent in unruptured aneurysms. On occasions the full thickness of portions of the wall of the sac may be replaced by thrombus. Such changes probably represent incipient rupture. Crompton[115] regarded these findings as fibrinoid necrosis and hence the cause of rupture. However, necrosis is little in

evidence and the changes are probably attendant upon the weakening and tearing of the wall.

When a cerebral aneurysm ruptures, the following pathological changes may be found at autopsy—subarachnoid hemorrhage, intracerebral hematoma and intraventricular hemorrhage, subdural hematoma, hemorrhage into unusual sites, perianeurysmal gliosis, ischemic lesions, secondary pressure lesions, degeneration of the granular layer of the cerebellum, spinal cord changes, arachnoidal adhesions and hydrocephalus, intraocular hemorrhage and papilledema, and neurogenic ulceration.

Subarachnoid hemorrhage. Because aneurysms arise from the large arteries in the subarachnoid space at the base of the brain, they generally bleed directly into this space. The bleeding is most profuse on the inferior surface of the brain, especially anteriorly. Blood may extend onto the convex surfaces of the cerebrum. Aneurysms on the middle cerebral and the anterior communicating arteries cause massive bleeding in the lateral fissure and between the two frontal lobes respectively. The aneurysm embedded in blood clot is generally easier to find before fixation of the brain, because the aneurysm itself and any false sacs can be damaged if dissection is performed after the blood clot has hardened. Fibrosis of the meninges, caused by organization of blood in the subarachnoid space, may localize the hemorrhage and produce a rapidly expanding, space-occupying hematoma. Alternatively, with the sac embedded in cerebral tissue, surrounding meningeal fibrosis may result in intracerebral and intraventricular hemorrhage. The blood in the subarachnoid space is then mostly in the cisterna magna and about the hindbrain.

Intracerebral hematoma and intraventricular hemorrhage. Massive bleeding into the brain and/or ventricles occurs in 55% to 70% of patients who die from a ruptured cerebral aneurysm.[400,410,523] The possibilities are (1) intracerebral hemorrhage, (2) intraventricular and intracerebral hemorrhage, or (3) intraventricular hemorrhage with minimal cerebral damage.

Tomlinson[503] described the perivascular extension of blood from the subarachnoid space into the brain at times in association with frank perivascular extravasation of blood in the neighborhood of the ruptured aneurysm. On occasions such hemorrhages, becoming confluent, result in a sizable hematoma. A bleeding aneurysm is known to tear or burrow deep into normal brain substance where, unless the aneurysm is embedded and sealed in the tissue, incipient softening of the adjoining and frequently gliosed cerebral tissue may precede the frank rupture, which gives rise to massive intracerebral hemorrhage. In any event premonitory leakage from the aneurysm[109,410] is the usual presage to the intracerebral hemorrhage.

Aneurysms of the anterior communicating artery rupture most frequently into one (Fig. 9-19) or both frontal lobes, effecting a secondary rupture into the frontal horn of a lateral ventricle. The resultant hematomas may be massive and extend posteriorly to the external capsule.[109] A large subarachnoid hematoma between the frontal lobes with distension of the sulci, sometimes resembles an intracerebral hema-

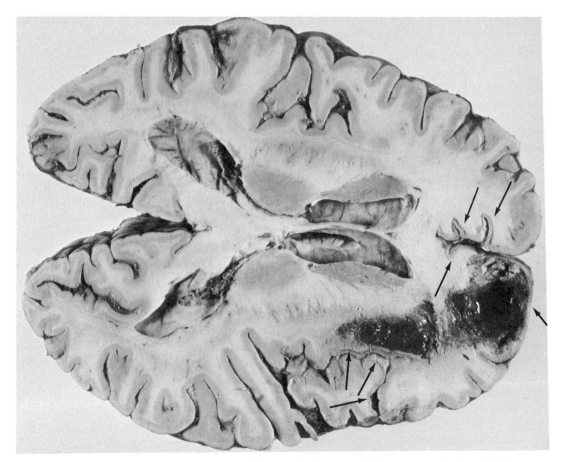

Fig. 9-19. Horizontal section of cerebrum displaying an old hematoma of frontal lobe extending posteriorly into external capsule. Cortical softening (*arrows*) is present on (1) the medial surface of both frontal lobes and (2) the frontal pole and in the distribution of the middle cerebral artery on the side of the hematoma. The hematoma originated from a ruptured aneurysm of the anterior communicating artery.

toma.[503] Adjoining brain tissue may be softened and superficial erosion of the brain is customary.

Anterior communicating aneurysms can damage the genu of the corpus callosum. Blood may pass through the rostrum of the corpus callosum into the cavity or cavum of the septum lucidum or burst through into a lateral ventricle. Crompton[109] believes the rostrum cannot be breached and that the blood passes behind these fibers into the cavum, but the blood can enter the lateral ventricle lateral to the septum lucidum with little parenchymatous damage. Thus the diagnosis would be primary intraventricular hemorrhage if the aneurysm and the fistulous track of the blood were both overlooked. Yet another contingency is the rupture of blood through the thin lamina terminalis directly into the third ventricle. Here it can also be mistaken for primary intraventricular hemorrhage. The subarachnoid hematoma has been said to[109] extend up over the corpus callosum to distend the cingulate gyrus from which it may burst laterally into the lateral ventricle, an extremely rare event when aneurysms of the anterior communicating artery are concerned. It is more likely to be encountered with those arising from the distal segment of the anterior cerebral artery.

Aneurysms of the cavernous segment of the internal carotid artery rarely rupture. If the aneurysm ruptures when small, a carotid-cavernous fistula will eventuate. If the aneurysm is large, and the cavernous sinus presumably obliterated, rupture is occasionally via the dural covering and causes subarachnoid and possibly subdural hemorrhage. Intracerebral hemorrhage is mostly into the temporal lobe but accompanying intraventricular hemorrhage can occur.

Aneurysms of the internal carotid artery at the origin of the posterior communicating usually produce hematomas of the temporal lobe severely damaging the hippocampal gyrus, the uncus, and dentate gyrus and rupturing into the temporal horn of the lateral ventricle.[245] Aneurysms at the bifurcation of the internal carotid artery, often embedded in the posteroinferior surface of the frontal lobe, rupture most frequently into the frontal lobe and thence into the frontal horn of the lateral ventricle. They may also produce hematomas in the thalamus and temporal lobe.[410]

Aneurysms of the middle cerebral arteries can cause, in the Sylvian fissure, a large hematoma that can be mistaken for intracerebral hemorrhage. Aneurysms on these arteries frequently rupture into the brain and involve the frontal or temporal lobes. Alternatively, rupture is into the insula involving the external capsule and even the basal ganglia, in which event secondary involvement of the ventricular system often takes place. Occasionally the hemorrhage extends well into the parietal lobe and may reach the occipital lobe.[410]

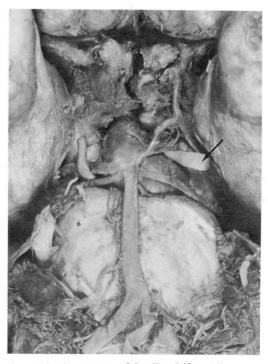

Fig. 9-20. Aneurysm of basilar bifurcation embedded in third ventricle into which rupture had occurred. Subarachnoid blood clot is present. Note displacement and apparent pinching of one oculomotor nerve (*arrow*).

Aneurysms of the basilar bifurcation (Fig. 9-20) tend to rupture through the floor of the third ventricle to produce massive intraventricular hemorrhage. Aneurysms at this site often bulge into the ventricle, which thereby is involved when rupture occurs.

Aneurysms of the posterior cerebral artery may rupture into the thalamus, occipital lobe, or posterior temporal lobe,[410] with damage to the posterolateral aspect of the cerebral peduncle being a further complication.

In concordance with the prevalence of anteriorly situated aneurysms, the common sites of cerebral hematoma secondary to rupture of aneurysms are the frontal, temporal, and parietal lobes and the insula. Parenchymatous involvement of the cerebellum, cerebral peduncles, and occipital lobe is unusual. Intracerebral hemorrhage occurs almost invariably close to the ruptured aneurysm rather than at a distance, and the hematoma can be attributed to an unruptured aneurysm and the ruptured aneurysm overlooked. Large intracerebral hematomas, especially when associated with a large accumulation of blood clot in the subarachnoid space, cause considerable compression and displacement of surrounding structures. In some surviving patients there is an old hemorrhagic cyst related to an aneurysm.

Massive bleeding into the ventricles can cause death within 6 hours. A lesser amount of intraventricular hemorrhage is associated with a somewhat longer survival period,[35] and associated cerebral damage may be minimal or extensive. The ventricular system distends with blood clot to several times its normal size (acute internal hemocephalus) on occasions and exerts pressure on pontine, medullary, and cerebellar structures.[503] Hemorrhages, edema, and sometimes infarction in the roof of the fourth ventricle are a likely result with less often lesions in the medulla and pons.[503] Tomlinson described subependymal hemorrhages in the lateral ventricles or about the aqueduct and in the anterior hypo-

thalamus. Acute necrosis of neurons has been observed[109] in subependymal nuclei such as the hypothalamic nuclei about the third ventricle, thalamic and caudate neurones around lateral ventricles, and hypoglossal and vagal nuclei beneath the fourth ventricle. In cases of rapid death histological evidence of necrosis will not be found.[109] The production of these lesions is thought to be bound up with acute distension of the ventricular system.

In two cases in which death was caused by a ruptured aneurysm of the right anterior cerebral artery, there was massive intraventricular hemorrhage with rapid dilatation of the ventricles in the presence of hemorrhagic tamponade of the aqueduct or of the third ventricle and tears in the walls of the lateral ventricles.[228] In one case the sac had burst into the third ventricle anteriorly with tamponade of the aqueduct, foramen of Monro, and the fourth ventricle. There was moderate, symmetrical ventricular dilatation in conjunction with bilateral tears (12 to 26 mm.) of the lateral corners and floors of the posterior horns of the lateral ventricles. In the second subject, the hemorrhage had been into the anterior horn of the right lateral ventricle with tamponade of the aqueduct and third and fourth ventricles. Marked ventricular dilatation had followed with tears (approximately 30 mm.) in both lateral and medial corners of the floor of the inferior horns and an additional tear in the sulcus at the lateral border of the left pulvinar. Such tears have been seen with massive spontaneous intracerebral hemorrhage and with gunshot wounds involving the ventricular system. They are associated with (1) petechial hemorrhages locally, (2) pallor of the white matter in the area, thought to be caused by permeation of the tissue with plasma or cerebrospinal fluid, (3) swollen axons and terminal clubs of Cajal with the Bodian stain, and (4) a short survival time of the patient (23 and 17 hours respectively).

Subdural hematoma. Subdural hematoma may result from rupture of a cerebral aneurysm. Clarke and Walton[93] reviewed subdural hematoma as a complication of intracranial aneurysm and angioma, giving the incidence as 1% to 2% of cases of subarachnoid hemorrhage. Walton[523] cited 5% in autopsied cases of cerebral aneurysm, Wilson and associates[538] reported subdural extension in 16.1% and Stehbens[473] found 35 instances (18.7%) among 187 subjects who died of a ruptured aneurysm. Schneck[430] provided a higher incidence, that is, 20% (21 cases in 105 autopsies). Subdural hematomas are usually overshadowed by more severe hemorrhage and damage elsewhere. The hematoma may be small and localized or extensive and bilateral but is rarely of sufficient severity to be clinically significant, and usually little organization of the blood is demonstrated.

Clarke and Walton[93] divided the cases of subdural hematoma associated with an "intracranial vascular anomaly" into the following groups: (1) cases with massive and rapidly fatal intracranial hemorrhage elsewhere in which the subdural hematoma is extensive but does not cause death, (2) cases in which there is only a trifling quantity of blood in the subdural space, and (3) cases in which a clinically significant subdural hematoma is not rapidly fatal and in which treatment is likely to alter the outcome of the disease.[57] The patient rarely presents with a primary subdural hematoma because bleeding solely into the subdural space is most uncommon. Hyland[259] has encountered only three such cases. Adhesion of the aneurysmal sac to the arachnoid after previous leakage may result in direct bleeding into the subdural space, and this is said to be frequently the reason why a subdural hemorrhage is associated with an aneurysm. The cerebrospinal fluid need not reveal evidence of hemorrhage, and in one such case the aneurysm was found on a cortical branch of the middle cerebral artery, which projected into the subdural hematoma.[55]

Table 9-8 gives the aneurysmal source of 130 cases with subdural hematoma in association with a ruptured aneurysm. Proximity of the aneurysmal sac to the subdural space is obviously not essential and few aneurysms if any lie exclusively in the subdural space. The problem of how blood from vessels of the subarachnoid space invades the subdural space is intriguing. Aneurysms are often sufficiently close to the subdural space to make perforation of the flimsy arachnoid conceivable. This is frequently difficult to demonstrate at autopsy. Other aneurysms, for example, those of the middle cerebral, anterior communicating, bifurcation of the posterior cerebral, and the distal segment of the anterior cerebral artery, are more deeply situated. When the aneurysm ruptures, the hematoma could become loculated because of arachnoidal adhesions and eventually rupture into the subdural space at some distance from the sac.

The onset of subarachnoid hemorrhage may be abrupt, with the patient losing consciousness and falling to the ground. Consequent trauma to the head may thus account for a few subdural hematomas. Bassett and Lemmen[29] believed that two of their cases each with an associated subdural blood clot were probably traumatic as was

Table 9-8. Sites of 130 aneurysms producing subdural hematomas

Site of aneurysm	Clarke & Walton[93]	Stehbens[473]	Freytag[181]	Total
Internal carotid	20	12	15	47
Middle cerebral	12	8	23	43
Anterior cerebral and anterior communicating	6	12	14	32
Vertebrobasilar system	2	3	3	8
Total	40	35	55	130

a further case presenting with a chronic subdural hematoma.

Hemorrhage into unusual sites. Ehni and Barrett[159] reported in a man of 26 years of age, severe recurrent hemorrhage into the ear from an aneurysm of the petrous segment of the internal carotid artery. The history indicated a chronic ear infection with mastoiditis since childhood. This aneurysm may have been caused by a low-grade bacterial infection that was not clinically apparent.

Aneurysms of the internal carotid in the cavernous sinus occasionally erode the wall of the sphenoid sinus into which they may either leak or bleed profusely, producing epistaxis and hemorrhage of varying severity into the nasopharynx.[269,515] Seftel and associates[440] emphasized the close anatomical relationship between the internal carotid artery and the sphenoid sinus and found 10 instances of aneurysmal hemorrhage into the sphenoid sinus in the literature. Other cases exist[247,269,515] but many if not most of these aneurysms are of traumatic origin.

Rupture of an aneurysm of the cavernous segment of the internal carotid artery, though uncommon, results in a carotid-cavernous fistula, which is readily detected because of bruit, pulsating exophthalmos, and gross facial disfiguration.

Perianeurysmal gliosis. Gliosis is frequently found around aneurysms that indent or are embedded in cerebral tissue and may be seen in patients who appear to have died as a result of their first subarachnoid hemorrhage.[503]

Ischemic lesions. It was not until Robertson's classic paper in 1949 that the importance of cerebral lesions, both hemorrhagic and ischemic, was fully appreciated.[410] Cerebral infarction (Fig. 9-19) in association with the rupture of a cerebral aneurysm has been confirmed repeatedly in subsequent publications.[111,306,538] These infarcts, with depressing regularity, are overlooked at autopsy or otherwise attributed to such factors as surgical intervention or superadded thrombosis. Logue[306] emphasized the role of vasospasm, which, while

possibly limiting the extent of the hemorrhage, produces the ischemic side effects likely to be aggravated by surgical intervention.

Bebin and Currier[35] state that subarachnoid hemorrhage in itself is not a cause of death, for the presence of brain damage is the essential factor and there will be histological confirmation of it unless death has occurred very soon after the rupture. This theory is supported in the Cooperative Study[303] by the relatively low incidence of subarachnoid hemorrhage pure and simple as the cause of early death.

Tomlinson[503] found areas of infarction, varying from small to massive in 25 of 32 brains examined, and accepted hypotension as a contributory factor. Birse and Tom[49] made a detailed study of eight brains associated with rupture of anterior communicating aneurysms. Areas of infarction were found in seven, but in only three were they demonstrable macroscopically. Of the eight cases, six exhibited the cytoplasmic eosinophilia of scattered cortical nerve cells suggestive of anoxia. Schneck[430] found infarcts associated with rupture of a cerebral aneurysm in 55% of 105 cases, and Arseni and Nash[14] recently reported an incidence of 45%. Logue and Smith[308] reported that in eight brains with subarachnoid hemorrhage of aneurysmal origin (without intracerebral hemorrhage or cerebral disruption) neuronal necrosis, arteriole-sized cortical areas of ischemia, and severe patchy pallor of the white matter were present. Some foci in the cortex were confluent and few were observed in the central gray matter, cerebellum, or brain stem. They considered the lesions sufficiently severe to cause coma and no doubt the lesions appear in lesser grades of severity than is currently suspected.

Crompton[111] found significant foci of cerebral infarction in 75% of 159 subjects who had died at least 24 hours after the initial ictus. A significant lesion was defined as (1) infarction of one third or more of the cortical distribution of one of the major arteries (anterior, middle, and posterior cerebral), or (2) ganglionic necrosis of 5 mm. or more. He found infarction in 80% of the women and in 69% of the males. Of the three most common sites for aneurysms, the incidence of infarction was highest among supraclinoid aneurysms of the internal carotid artery, followed by aneurysms of the middle cerebral artery, and least among anterior communicating aneurysms. In only two instances were intra-arterial thrombi incriminated in the infarction. The infarcts were by and large pale, sometimes involving the cortex alone and sometimes implicating the underlying white matter as well. The cortical softenings were laminar with relative sparing of the superficial layers or perivascular and poorly defined suggestive of a lesser degree of ischemia. The hemorrhagic infarcts were attributed to either (1) a hypertensive episode allowing the collaterals to fill the ischemic vessels from which perivascular hemorrhages are frequent, or (2) partial or intermittent compression of the posterior cerebral arteries against the tentorium cerebelli because of transtentorial herniation.[111] Gradations between the two types of infarct occur, but those involving the basal ganglia are pale.[111] In Crompton's series, arterial thrombi were found on only two occasions. One infarct was hemorrhagic and attributed to embolism, whereas the other was thought to have been aggravated by thrombus protruding from the neck of the aneurysm. In five instances a coincidental venous thrombus was found in the overlying cortex. This low incidence of vascular thrombi indicates that the cause of the infarction must be sought elsewhere. Old cerebral infarcts may be found with ruptured cerebral aneurysms and in some patients they may be associated with previous episodes of rupture. However in the age group under consideration, softenings may be coincidental and related to the accompanying severe atherosclerosis. Mostly the age of the softening was consistent with an onset at the time of rupture of the aneurysm, but multiple infarcts may be of different ages.

In Crompton's 119 cases with cerebral infarcts of significant size, cortical infarc-tion was found unaccompanied in 54 cases and ganglionic infarction was present in 16 cases.[111] Both were found in 49 cases. Infarcts occurred principally in the area of the brain supplied by the artery from which the aneurysm arose but not infrequently the area supplied by the contralateral vessel was ischemic as well. This was particularly so with aneurysms on or near the midline, such as those on the anterior cerebral or anterior communicating artery. However even aneurysms of the middle cerebral artery were associated with bilateral infarcts in 21% of Crompton's cases.[111] On other occasions, areas on the homolateral side but outside the territory of the aneurysm's parent artery were infarcted either in combination or less frequently as isolated lesions.

In addition, small foci less than 1 cm. in diameter or even microscopic in size also occur in the cortex.[49,503] They may be multiple and are particularly frequent on the medial aspect of the frontal lobes with aneurysms of the anterior communicating artery. Crompton found small foci of cortical softening in 79.2% of his series.[111] Lesions of similar size are not unusual in the white matter.[503]

Aneurysms arising at the bifurcation of the internal carotid artery may be embedded in the anterior hypothalamus and, together with those on the anterior communicating and the internal carotid arteries, are dangerously close to the small branches extending from the circle of Willis to the hypothalamus. Jefferson[271] reported damage to the hypothalamus and in a more recent series of 106 patients with ruptured cerebral aneurysms, 65 had demonstrable hypothalamic lesions mostly ischemic in type.[110] Such lesions occurred particularly in association with aneurysms of the internal carotid and anterior communicating arteries. The lesions were of three types: (1) most commonly areas of ischemic necrosis up to 8 mm. in diameter, (2) microhemorrhages, either blood tracking up the perivascular space, which it distended and ruptured (similar lesions occurring as far as the thalamus and the internal and external capsules), or microscopic hemorrhages (sometimes coalescing) in the supraoptic and paraventricular nuclei presumed to be caused by venous obstruction, and (3) least frequently the massive hemorrhage occurring in front of a ruptured sac. The ischemic lesions and microhemorrhages occurred frequently in combination with one another, and bilateral involvement of the hypothalamus was not uncommon. In 50% of the cases ganglionic infarction was also present, in one there was a perforated duodenal ulcer, and in two there was hemorrhage (gastrointestinal and pancreatic).

In eleven of 18 patients with ruptured aneurysms of the anterior communicating artery, abnormal diurnal variation in plasma cortisol levels were found and attributed to secondary lesions in the hypothalamus. In many patients after an interval of a month there was improvement in function.[274]

Pituitary necrosis has been found in 4 of 94 patients with ruptured cerebral aneurysms.[430] In all cases the anterior lobe was affected and in two, part of the posterior lobe as well. The necrotic lesions were out of all proportion to the amount of hemorrhage that was present in many cases in the capsule or extended into the stalk or the gland proper.[430]

The pathogenesis of infarcts associated with aneurysmal rupture is still indefinite. Thrombi are rarely found. Embolism from the aneurysmal sac is an unlikely cause of the infarction nor does it explain distant and contralateral infarcts. Infarction in the area of the posterior cerebral artery associated with rupture of aneurysms anteriorly situated is attributable to compression of the posterior cerebral artery by the tentorium because of raised supratentorial pressure, but this is the outcome in few of the cases. Large, localized subarachnoid hematomas distending the Sylvian or median longitudinal fissures could conceivably displace vessels therein to such an extent that the fine, mainly straight perforating arteries that enter the brain could be stretched, kinked, or narrowed.[112,503] Such

vessels in the Sylvian fissure impart a "clipped hedge" appearance angiographically.[112] Alternatively these small vessels or the parent artery may undergo reflex vasoconstriction attributed to mechanical stretching. Angiographically the circulation in such vessels is slowed and histologically (1) necrosis of the walls of small arteries and veins with secondary bleeding therefrom, (2) subendothelial leukocytic (polymorph) infiltration of arteries, and (3) sometimes edema and leukocytic infiltration of the entire arterial wall have been found.[112] The changes are indicative of interference with or at least temporary cessation of flow with, possibly, subsequent restoration.

Tomlinson[503] has suggested that because of excessive displacement of the parent vessel, small branches may be torn, the result being secondary hemorrhage into the subarachnoid space and ischemia in the field of supply.

At present there is no evidence to suggest that tearing or dissection of the wall of the sac causes vasoconstriction and nervi vasorum are not a prominent feature in the adventitia of the aneurysmal sac. Arseni and Nash[14] incriminate infiltration of the blood between the coats of the artery, but this seems unlikely. Although dissection of the sac wall may occur at the site of rupture, the escaping blood is limited mostly to the outer part of the adventitia of the parent and neighboring arteries.

Many authors ascribe ischemic infarcts to arterial vasospasm, which is peculiarly common after rupture of an intracranial aneurysm.[431] It is readily observed both by angiography[156] and craniotomy. There is reversion of the artery to normal caliber on follow-up arteriograms. In peripheral arteries, stretching of vessels, both large and small, is a potent stimulus of vasospasm. Florey[174] induced arterial contraction by mechanical stimulation and also observed spasm, which was however insufficient to stop the bleeding entirely, on either side of a point of rupture. The displacement with stretching of vessels is likely to contribute to the vascular constriction when an aneurysm ruptures. The vasospasm as noted by Echlin[154] was only a 30% to 70% reduction in diameter, and flow, though sluggish, did not cease altogether. Potter[387] estimated that the effect of spasm in patients with subarachnoid hemorrhage could be anything from a 28-fold to a 400-fold reduction in blood flow through a spastic anterior cerebral artery and a 25-fold to an 80-fold decrease in flow in a spastic internal carotid artery. These estimations were made from angiographic measurements in specific patients but collateral flow would have at least some effect on the incidence of ischemia. It is not known whether small (subclinical) leaks can initiate vasospasm.

Sudden carotid occlusion is often well tolerated especially in younger patients and almost-occlusive constriction may involve the carotid artery after puncture.[112] However infarction seldom follows and angiographically demonstrable spasm or constriction of cerebral vessels in the absence of an aneurysm does not usually result in cerebral infarction. It seems likely that the following factors[112,431] contribute to the effect of vasospasm in the causation of cerebral ischemia: (1) atherosclerosis of cerebral arteries, especially when stenotic, (2) bilateral small posterior communicating arteries or small divisional branches of the basilar arteries that provide a poor potential collateral flow between the internal carotid and basilar arteries, (3) intolerance of digital compression of the cervical common carotid artery on both sides, (4) vascular hypotension, (5) angiographically demonstrable vasospasm of the cerebral arteries, and (6) direct surgical attack on the aneurysm or carotid ligation in the neck. There is also the unrefuted possibility that contrast media used in angiography might at times contribute to either the vasospasm or the cerebral damage.[430]

Secondary pressure lesions. When a cerebral aneurysm ruptures, an expanding false sac can form and, with the involvement of a cranial nerve, (Fig. 9-21) cause local pressure symptoms. An expanding hematoma may also initiate pressure effects on cerebral

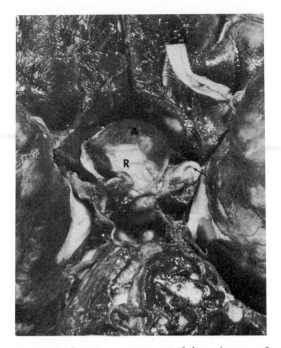

Fig. 9-21. Large aneurysm, **A,** lying above and anterior to the optic chiasm and right optic nerve, **R,** which is grossly flattened and adherent to the sac wall. Extensive subarachnoid hemorrhage had resulted from rupture of the aneurysm. There is hemorrhage into the left optic nerve (*arrow*).

areas and is likely to cause clinical symptoms and signs without necessarily bleeding into or inducing infarction of that area. However the enlarging hematoma, usually supratentorial and perhaps in association with acute internal hemocephalus in a cranial cavity in which the cerebrospinal fluid pressure is already elevated, results in secondary vascular lesions. The swelling of infarcted areas after aneurysmal bleeding may also usher in or contribute to the raised supratentorial pressure sufficient to cause secondary vascular lesions. Such lesions may be subdivided as follows:

1. Secondary hemorrhage or necrosis in the pons or cerebral peduncles like those in association with primary spontaneous cerebral hemorrhage or hemorrhage into a cerebral tumor
2. Compression of the posterior cerebral artery by the tentorium cerebelli with hemorrhagic infarction in the field of supply

3. Herniation of the uncus, or hippocampal gyrus and hippocampus into the incisura tentorii; this incisural herniation compresses the aqueduct of Sylvius producing secondary supratentorial obstructive hydrocephalus
4. Compression of the oculomotor nerve by the posterior cerebral artery, possibly with intraneural hemorrhage
5. Pressure on or indentation of the contralateral cerebral peduncle by the free edge of the tentorium cerebelli
6. Cerebellar tonsillar herniation perchance with actual hemorrhagic necrosis[531]
7. Subhyaloid hemorrhages and papilledema
8. Ruptured cerebral aneurysm and herniation of the cerebral cortex into pacchionian bodies and resultant hemorrhagic lesions of the motor cortex; the hernias occur in association with a greatly raised intracranial pressure

Degeneration of the granular layer of the cerebellum. Degeneration of the granular layer of the cerebellum is a little-recognized complication of ruptured cerebral aneurysm.[503] Tomlinson found four instances in 32 cases of ruptured aneurysm.[503] Crompton[113] confirmed it in 22 of 126 cases examined, and observed Purkinje cell necrosis in 18.

The cerebellar changes are similar to those described in association with visceral carcinoma and with diabetic or hypoglycemic coma by Leigh and Meyer,[297] who found similar lesions in a case of subarachnoid hemorrhage. Tomlinson's findings[503] varied from necrosis of all the cellular elements of the granular layer to patchy but severe destruction of the granular layer with survival of the Golgi type 2 cells[503] and in two cases the changes were widespread but restricted to the dorsomedial folia in the remaining two. In one case some Purkinje cells exhibited acute chromatolysis. There was no evidence of reaction to the necrotic foci, gliosis, or degeneration of myelin or neurofibrils suggesting that the changes are terminal.

Crompton[113] found no relation between the changes and the time elapsing between death and the autopsy but found a positive correlation between the frequency of the secondary cerebellar changes and cerebral infarction and evidence of cerebral anoxia. The cerebellar changes were therefore regarded as being associated with anoxia.

Spinal cord damage. Crompton[113] examined the spinal cord and cauda equina of eight subjects who had died of a cerebral aneurysm. Apart from blood about the subdural and extradural layers of the lumbar sac, thought to be the aftermath of a lumbar puncture, there was subarachnoid blood in the lumbar region. Blood was found in significant quantities in the interstitium of the nerve roots and dorsal root ganglia of the cauda equina or siderophages in the interstitial tissue when the subarachnoid hemorrhage was not of recent origin. Some nerve fibers were damaged in severe cases though no peripheral nerve lesion had been manifest and no neuronal damage was found. These changes were regarded as secondary effects of aneurysmal rupture at a remote distance from the site of bleeding, and a similar instance was found in one case of primary hypertensive parietal hemorrhage associated with subarachnoid hemorrhage. Such findings have not been confirmed as yet and the possible underlying mechanism defies elucidation.

Arachnoidal adhesions and hydrocephalus. Recurrent subarachnoid hemorrhage may result in obliteration of the subarachnoid space at the base of the brain large enough to cause internal hydrocephalus.[175] The hydrocephalus is infrequent and of moderate severity. Only one or two come to autopsy in most large series.[473] Hydrocephalus may, however, eventuate from a space-occupying aneurysm in the posterior fossa causing cisternal or ventricular (fourth) obstruction.[264]

Intraocular hemorrhage and papilledema. Subhyaloid hemorrhage, frequently regarded as pathognomonic of subarachnoid bleeding,[523] may be found in one or both eyes on ophthalmoscopic examination of patients with a ruptured cerebral aneurysm. By no means invariably present, Manschot[317] found it in one-fifth of the 225 patients with subarachnoid hemorrhage. Originally it was believed the blood extended along the optic nerve sheath through the lamina cribrosa of the sclera into the optic nerve head and retina. Riddoch and Goulden[401] demonstrated by serial sections in a case of ruptured cerebral aneurysm that the hemorrhage in the optic nerve sheath was contained within the prolongation of the subarachnoid space that surrounds the optic nerve in the optic foramen and the orbital cavity. To a lesser extent there was also blood in the prolongation of the subdural space that similarly extends and surrounds the optic nerve. There was no extension of the hemorrhage through the pial covering into the nerve itself. Retinal hemorrhages at some distance from the papilla were present but no continuity with the subarachnoid hemorrhage was observed. The findings, which support the earlier work of Doubler and Marlow,[138] attribute venous engorgement, papilledema, and retinal hemorrhages to compression of the central vein of the reina as it leaves the optic nerve to enter the subarachnoid space. Furthermore in such cases, edema of the optic nerve head and optic nerve ceased abruptly at the exit of the vein from the optic nerve.

Papilledema is a not infrequent finding in patients with severe hemorrhage from a ruptured intracranial aneurysm, occurring in approximately one-sixth of all patients. When severe, it is usually accompanied by retinal hemorrhages.[317] Walton[523] considered that it developed immediately as a result of direct compression of the venous return from the eye by a large effusion of blood into the optic nerve sheath (that is, the extensions of the subarachnoid and/or the subdural spaces about the optic nerve). When the onset of the papilledema was delayed for some 4 to 10 days, he attributed this delayed development to raised intracranial pressure consequent upon intracerebral hemorrhage or recurrent bleeding. The papilledema is caused by interference with venous return in much the same manner as occurs in the pathogenesis of the retinal hemorrhages. The obstruction appears to result from pressure locally by a hematoma

or alternatively to a generally raised intracranial pressure transmitted along the perineural extensions of the subarachnoid and subdural spaces.

Neurogenic ulceration. Neurogenic ulceration in the upper gastrointestinal tract (Chapter 2) has on several occasions complicated the rupture of cerebral aneurysms (Table 2-2).

Aneurysmal rupture during pregnancy. Cerebral hemorrhage, often extending to the subarachnoid space, can occur with eclampsia and toxemia of pregnancy. However all cases of subarachnoid hemorrhage in pregnancy, labor, or the puerperium cannot be attributed to this cause, for an arteriovenous aneurysm of the brain or spinal cord, spontaneous intracerebral hemorrhage, eclampsia, blood dyscrasias, neoplasms, or intracranial aneurysm may variously be implicated. Copelan and Mabon[99] consider the most common cerebrovascular complication of pregnancy to be subarachnoid hemorrhage of which the most frequent cause is cerebral aneurysm.

The incidence of ruptured intracranial aneurysm in pregnancy is reported as being 1 in 2000 deliveries.[76,99] This figure may be inflated because of institutional bias toward aneurysms. Daane and Tandy[122] gave an estimate of once in 8070 deliveries. Walton[522] reported two cases during pregnancy in a series of 312 cases of subarachnoid hemorrhage, and in a personal series of 252 cases of ruptured cerebral aneurysm at autopsy, only one patient was pregnant. In the Cooperative Study, the onset of subarachnoid hemorrhage of aneurysmal origin was related to parturition in 0.35% of cases.[302]

Various reports are available concerning ruptured cerebral aneurysms during pregnancy.[91,98,523] Cannell[76] reported a case in which a subarachnoid hemorrhage was sustained in each of two pregnancies. Several reviews discussing the association have been published[377,384,523] and the general conclusions reached can be summarized as follows:

1. Of 46 proved cases of cerebral aneurysm in pregnancy, 83% occurred during gestation, 4%

during labor, and 13% post partum. The maximum incidence (46%) occurred during the interval from 26 to 36 weeks.[99] The stress of labor is not a major precipitating factor, and the suggestion is that the hemodynamic changes inherent in pregnancy may predispose the aneurysm to rupture.[99,377]

2. The mortality does not differ materially from that of the nongravid state.[76]

3. The mean age of the collected cases of Pedowitz and Perell[377] and of Pool and Potts[384] is 30 years (approximately 20 years less than that for aneurysms at autopsy in the general population).

To date there is no statistical evidence indicating that the association of the rupture of a cerebral aneurysm with pregnancy is more frequent than one would expect, considering the age distribution of these aneurysms. Indications are that the interrelationship should be more thoroughly investigated. Heiskanen and Nikki[241] reporting seven instances of ruptured aneurysms during pregnancy, one of which occurred during the seventh and another during the tenth pregnancy, concluded that labor and gestation are of minor significance. The effect of multiple pregnancies has not been statistically examined.

Rupture of splenic aneurysms has also been reported, with the inference being that the association with pregnancy is more than fortuitous. Aneurysms of the splenic artery are for some unknown reason particularly prone to affect females, and "arteriosclerosis," sometimes restricted to this vessel, is singularly important in their pathogenesis.[369] Of all recorded cases of ruptured splenic aneurysm, 11% occurred in pregnant women.[213,368] Sherlock and Learmonth[477] asserted that of women with ruptured splenic aneurysms, 20% were pregnant. Rupture is also thought to complicate saccular aneurysm of the renal artery during pregnancy in an unusually high proportion of cases, but statistics are not available.[231,493] Pedowitz and Perell[377] found only 10 such reports in the literature in 1957. Of 19 instances of dissecting aneurysm of the renal artery, one occurred during gestation and there were seven instances of dissecting aneurysm of the coronary

arteries reported in the puerperium.[373] It has also been alleged that pregnancy predisposes to aortic rupture and dissection,[337,377,432] with approximately 49% of women under 40 years with dissecting aneurysm being pregnant or in the puerperium.

If indeed after further investigation it is found that pregnancy predisposes aneurysms, both cerebral and extracranial, to rupture, then the proclivity to rupture may well correlate with other known facts, such as the following:

1. The slight predominance of cerebral aneurysms in the female population
2. The tendency for other vascular disturbances (varices of the lower limbs, cutaneous spider nevi, the relapse and remission of symptoms related to spinal cord angiomas[169,353]) to occur during pregnancy
3. The greater development of the intima in the coronary arteries of males in comparison with females[136]
4. The effect of pregnancy on the connective tissues of the pelvis
5. The tendency for aneurysmal headache[269] and the occurrence of spontaneous ecchymoses in Ehlers-Danlos syndrome[25] during menstruation

It is unlikely that the hormonal effects on the connective tissue in the pelvic ligaments, genital tract, and perineum are restricted to these structures alone during pregnancy. The mechanism underlying the connective tissue changes is obscure nor is there information available on the nature, distribution, and degree of change. The increased laxity of the collagen fibers and elastic tissue may be considerable, for in the free-tailed bat, a mammal, the interpubic ligament stretches more than 15 times its original length.[106] Thus, if the connective tissues of the aneurysmal sac wall are influenced in like manner, then it is plausible to assume that the wall would at this time stretch and yield for any given tension and in doing so would greatly aggravate the hemodynamic stresses on the sac. The inevitable result appears to be that rupture is more prone to occur when women are in the gravid state. The mechanism by which gestation influences the other vascular lesions mentioned has not been determined though there is a possibility that steroid hormones might affect collagen proliferation adversely and consequently impair repair processes.[167,391]

Headache and migraine. The headache of subarachnoid hemorrhage of aneurysmal origin is usually occipital in location, sudden of onset, and high in intensity. A history of antecedent headache is not unusual before the onset of the hemorrhage. In the Cooperative Study, 85% of patients with single unruptured but symptomatic aneurysms complained of major headaches and 59% of orbital pain. In many of these patients the headache or periorbital pain was either recent or represented a significant change in the characteristics of a long-standing headache.[303] It is reasonable to assume that the headache and pain, apparently associated with the aneurysm but independent of subarachnoid hemorrhage, are caused either by stretching or compression of nerves as a consequence of aneurysmal dilatation.

The long-standing antecedent headache is often enough periodic in nature and migrainous in type.[314,544] Adie[2] believed migraine a not uncommon precursor of subarachnoid hemorrhage, and Magee,[314] in 150 cases of subarachnoid hemorrhage, found 2% with ophthalmoplegic migraine. Walton[523] had several cases of migraine in his series of patients with subarachnoid hemorrhage, the history varying in duration up to 32 years. The attacks of migraine varied in severity and, in nine of the 14 women, were worse at the menses. Many authors have mentioned migraine in histories of patients with cerebral aneurysm,[125,284,400] usually of the internal carotid artery.[125,180,523] The migraine has been known to cease after rupture or the onset of the subarachnoid hemorrhage.[523] Wolff[544] believed that the migraine in these patients is independent of the presence or absence of aneurysm and was not convinced that developing structural changes in the aneurysm were responsible for the migraine.

Walton[523] concluded that cerebrovascular accidents develop with unwonted frequency in patients with migraine, with various types of intracranial hemorrhage and bleeding into the orbit having been recorded. The association of migraine and subarachnoid hemorrhage of aneurysmal origin was regarded as being less definite than with migraine and ophthalmoplegia where the hemicrania was associated with a recurring cranial nerve palsy, most frequently of the oculomotor nerve and less frequently of the fourth or seventh cranial nerves. The nerve exhibits signs of pressure or irritation, and cure may be effected by carotid ligation in the neck.[523] However true ophthalmoplegic migraine associated with a cerebral aneurysm is uncommon. The headache in such instances is usually strictly unilateral and a distinct change in the character of the headache can be an ominous sign.[180] In the absence of an aneurysm this syndrome may be caused by the intermittent compression of the third nerve by an abnormally situated artery.[513]

Wolff[544] asserted that migraine headaches occur in persons who do not exhibit evidence of diffuse or local vascular disease and that the changes in the caliber of cranial vessels during the attacks of migraine or in the prodromal stage of preheadache are probably predisposing factors in vascular occlusions and hemorrhage. He also believed that the vasomotor changes associated with migraine could have an adverse effect on the aneurysm. Rupture could be precipitated and account for the onset of subarachnoid hemorrhage during the apparent attack of migraine.[544] Similarly, Wolff[544] and Frankel[180] believed, hemodynamic changes during a migrainous episode could contribute to the actual formation of the aneurysmal dilatation, particularly when factors of a labile blood pressure and arterial degenerative changes are superadded. However it seems that these hemodynamic stresses associated with attacks of migraine, like other episodes linked with changes in hemodynamics, are of contributory rather than primary etiological importance.

Mortality and survival. Rupture of a cerebral aneurysm is a serious event, with the mortality reported[423] varying from 33% to 64%. Ask-Upmark and Ingvar[15] postulated that without operation 20% of patients with subarachnoid hemorrhage of aneurysmal origin would recover well and resume previous occupations, 20% would remain crippled, and 60% would die sooner or later from subarachnoid hemorrhage. Symonds[490] was of the opinion that many patients who have subclinical subarachnoid hemorrhages are not admitted to hospital and subsequently recover. The exclusion of such cases from statistics may result in a somewhat more gloomy prognosis than is perhaps rightly deserved, but there is no way of corroborating the conjecture.

Crawford and Sarner,[103] in a community study of deaths from cerebrovascular disease, found that ruptured intracranial aneurysm accounted for 27.9%. Only 63% of the patients with ruptured intracranial aneurysms were diagnosed during life and they differed from those (37%) who died before admittance to a neurosurgical unit. The early deaths were more frequent in men than women, in those over 45 years of age than under, and in those with an aneurysm of the middle cerebral artery. The authors believed that a goodly proportion of patients who die of ruptured cerebral aneurysms either expire at home or prior to diagnosis and that this group is usually not taken into account in studies of intracranial aneurysm.

Death from rupture of a cerebral aneurysm is a notable cause of sudden unexpected death in apparently healthy men of military age. Martland[318] attributed 2% of all sudden or unexplained deaths to a ruptured cerebral aneurysm, The onset of coma may be sudden, but death rarely occurs within the first hour.

In the Cooperative Study,[302] 68% of 830 nonsurgical patients with their first subarachnoid hemorrhage (one aneurysm only) had died by the time the results were reported. Of those who died, 14% expired within 24 hours, 20% within 48 hours, 40% by 7 days, 56% within 14 days, 67% by the end of 3 weeks, and 93% by the end of the first year. Of the 562 known deaths, 88% were attributed to the cerebral aneurysm, 4% were unrelated, and the cause was not clearly established in 8%. The 252 patients with multiple aneurysms and their first subarachnoid hemorrhage displayed a similar mortality pattern except for a slightly higher overall mortality (70%). These figures, because of the selection of patients for nonsurgical management, may seem unduly pessimistic, but according to the community study of Crawford and Sarner,[103] approximately another 10% of individuals not included in the study would already have died at home.

Of the patients in the Cooperative Study dying within 72 hours, 90% had an intracranial hematoma (80% intracerebral, 9% intracerebellar, and subdural in 1%). Locksley[302] believes that this figure, higher than is usual for aneurysms, is attributed to the relatively high incidence of middle cerebral and distal anterior cerebral aneurysms, as aneurysms at such sites favor the production of intracerebral hematoma.

For aneurysms of the anterior part of the circle of Willis that remain at risk, the frequency of a second hemorrhage is 10% in the first week, 12% in the second, 6.9% in the third, and 8.2% in the fourth week. It falls after this to about 1.3% per week thereafter, except for aneurysms of the anterior communicating artery (2.6% per week). Within the first 2 weeks Locksley[303] indicated that 54% had had a second hemorrhage and 70% by the end of 4 weeks. Over 11% re-bled more than a year after the initial hemorrhage and the estimated mortality for the second hemorrhage is 41% to 46% for anteriorly located aneurysms. Intervals from 10 to more than 20 years between the initial and fatal hemorrhage as with aortic aneurysms[65,137,413] have been reported.

No follow-up study of unruptured asymptomatic aneurysms has been carried out but, of 34 untreated, unruptured, and symptomatic aneurysms, 26% of the patients died of a subarachnoid hemorrhage during the follow-up period.[303]

Pathologists are naturally concerned with the mortality of ruptured cerebral aneurysms but there is no detailed pathological follow-up of patients who have survived for long. Clinicians contend with the survivors as well and the quality of the survival is not always satisfactory, as surgical procedures not infrequently contribute to incapacitation. Clinical reports give an indication of the frequency of the ensuing severe cerebral damage. Ask-Upmark and Ingvar[15] estimated that only 20% can be expected to make a good recovery, despite having sustained some damage. Residual cranial nerve palsies and upper motor nerve neurone lesions, the most overt of the residual signs of damage, are frequent. Logue and co-workers[308] analyzed the physical, emotional, and intellectual state of a group of 79 (average age of 43.6 years) surviving the rupture of an aneurysm of either the anterior cerebral or anterior communicating arteries. Thirteen patients had been treated conservatively and the remaining 66 by intracranial clipping of the anterior cerebral proximal to the aneurysm. They were reexamined from 7 months to 8½ years later. Only 52 were found to be neurologically unimpaired and 44 had returned to their former occupations. Seventeen were working in an inferior occupation or working less competently, seven were unemployed but anticipated a return to work, five were disabled at home, and six were disabled in hospital. Seven patients suffered from occasional epilepsy, a lower proportion than that (10.4%) found by Rose and Sarner.[412] Of the 13 patients treated conservatively, six had died at the time of the follow-up, four from recurrent hemorrhage. Of the 66 treated surgically, 10 had died, four from hemorrhage. Changes in intellect (from mild impairment to dementia), emotion (euphoria in 25.3%, depression in 9.9%), and motor and

vegetative functions (diminished activity and interest, restlessness, irritability, tactlessness, outspokenness, and ready laughter and crying) were frequent. Impairment of memory was often disproportionate to the degree of intellectual impairment, and this phenomenon was believed to be related to the aneurysm's proximity to the base of the third ventricle where lesions affect new learning but leave other aspects of the intellect unimpaired. In patients who died, infarction and long-standing destructive lesions were found. There is obvious need for detailed assessment of the outcome of

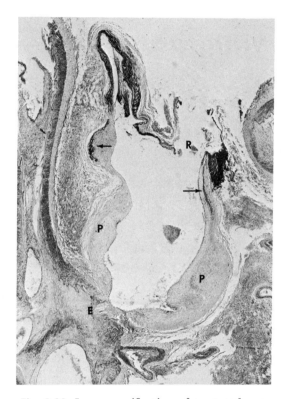

Fig. 9-22. Low magnification of ruptured aneurysm. The sac wall is of irregular thickness but is thin near entrance, **E,** has plaque-like structures simulating intimal pads, **P,** and is attenuated near site of rupture, **R.** Note the fibrin (staining very darkly) lining part of wall near rupture site, infiltrating the neighboring wall as by dissection (*arrows*), and forming fibrin tags at the margin of the hole. The parent artery exhibits considerable intimal thickening. (Mallory's phosphotungstic acid–hematoxylin, ×15.)

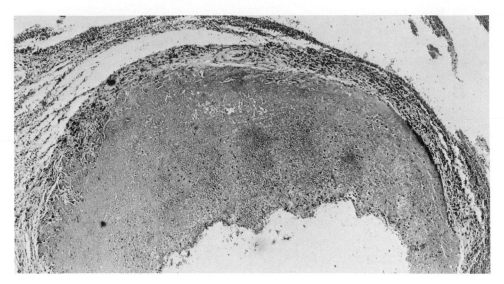

Fig. 9-23. False aneurysmal sac attached to ruptured fundus of a berry aneurysm. Inner layer consists of a thick layer of thrombus, the outer surface of which is being organized and is covered by a cellular layer of early granulation tissue and compressed arachnoidal trabeculae. (Hematoxylin and eosin, ×45.)

aneurysms at other sites with details of the various forms of treatment implemented.

Sequel to aneurysmal rupture. When an aneurysm ruptures, thrombus will form at the edges of the laceration and often appears to merge with the wall (Fig. 9-18). Frequently fibrin and red cell infiltration of the adjacent wall penetrate some distance (Fig. 9-22). The formation of a false sac occurs readily and the thrombus lining it, is directly continuous with edges of the true sac, though part of the latter may become lined with newly formed thrombus (Fig. 9-18). Organization commences on the outer aspect of the false sac (Fig. 9-23) and endothelialization begins on the inner surface nearest the true or primary sac. The wall of the false sac becomes progressively transformed into a hyalinized fairly acellular collagenous layer similar to any other well advanced aneurysmal wall, though evidence of previous leakage of blood, in the form of hemosiderin-laden macrophages, is repeatedly quite prominent. If a patient survives the rupture, the sac may enlarge with the successive layers of thrombus deposited in the sac producing lamination

characteristic of intra-aneurysmal thrombosis (Fig. 9-24). Organization of extravasated blood about the sac serves to reinforce the wall.

Most aneurysms over 10 mm. in diameter contain thrombus,[473] probably secondary to a tear or a leak of the sac wall. Some large aneurysms more than 2 cm. in diameter have a wide neck. They need not contain thrombus. They are not lobulated, and they are most unusual. Black and German[52] demonstrated that the presence of thrombosis in the sac of experimentally produced aneurysms was dependent on the mathematical relationship between the volume of the sac and the area of the orifice. Actually, the larger the sac or the smaller the orifice, the greater is the tendency to thrombosis.

It has been suggested that thrombosis within an aneurysmal sac might propagate in a retrograde manner so as to result in an occlusion of the parent stem.[276] The coexistence of these two lesions has been recorded.[165,256] but careful investigation of the cause of the thrombosis and the nature of the aneurysm is essential for verification,

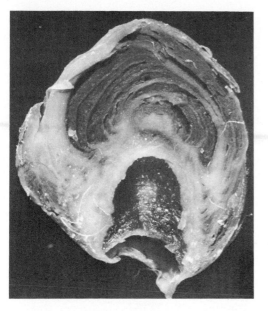

Fig. 9-24. Cerebral aneurysm (less than 2 cm. in diameter) bisected to display laminated thrombus in sac and residual functional lumen.

for the association may be coincidental and is quite rare in the case of noninflammatory aneurysms.

The thrombus in the false sac may progressively obliterate all of the false sac and much of the lumen of the primary sac as well. Maximal reduction in the functional lumen of the aneurysm is probably beneficial, being the aim of carotid ligation and medical hypotensive therapy. The factors governing the propagation of thrombi are ill understood. The thrombus undergoes organization and, in a small aneurysm (approximately 1 cm. in diameter or less), is eventually completely replaced. Large sacs (over 2 cm. in diameter) of long duration with laminated thrombus may exhibit only minimal evidence of organization. Complete organization of such a large thrombus has not been seen by the author and there is no report of such an occurrence. The reason for the slow or limited organization is not clear.

An aneurysm containing thrombus need not be healed, for a small residual functional lumen demonstrable radiologically,[147] histologically or on opening the sac usually persists (Fig. 9-24). Furthermore rupture of extracranial aneurysms may occur behind such a laminated thrombus. The reasons have not been explained, but there is adequate reason to doubt the safety of aneurysmal sacs almost filled by thrombus. Cronqvist and associates[118] contend that even partial thrombosis of an aneurysm is beneficial, and on theoretical grounds this is probably so but clinicopathological evidence indicates that, despite partial thrombosis of the sac, hemorrhage may still ensue. Mount and Taveras[344] followed 16 cases of ruptured cerebral aneurysm by angiography. The size of the sacs had either enlarged (3 cases) or remained unchanged (13 cases). Spontaneous thrombosis of the sac did not occur. Af Björkesten and Troupp[3] demonstrated enlargement in 10 cerebral aneurysms in an interval of one-half to 125 months, and 6 patients suffered recurrent hemorrhage. In eight patients, no enlargement was noted at intervals varying from 4 to 88 months. One sac could no longer be demonstrated in the second angiogram, but there had been an attempt at clipping and so the presumed thrombosis may not have been spontaneous. Lodin[305] reported a case in which a small residual diverticulum of the lumen persisted. Du Boulay[147] in an angiographic study of 252 aneurysms, reported dramatic or gradual enlargement of some aneurysmal sacs and reduction in the size of the functional lumen of others. No cases undergoing complete obliteration were mentioned.

One patient seen by the author had suffered a stroke 44 years before death at 69 years of age. The sac was collapsed and the lumen was partially obliterated by hyaline acellular tissue, the result of organization of the thrombus dating apparently from the time of rupture. A residual lumen was present (Fig. 9-25). Reinforcement of the wall from organization of the thrombus and reduction in the sac lumen had so strengthened the wall and reduced the hemodynamic stress that the aneurysm

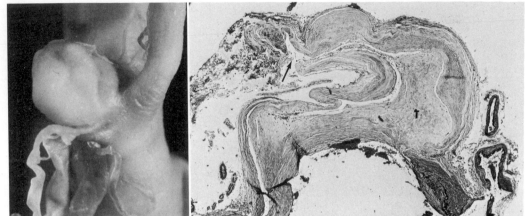

Fig. 9-25. A, Aneurysm on middle cerebral artery. Small vessels arise from the stem near the sac, which is white with a wrinkled surface. Pigmentation at old rupture site cannot be seen. **B,** Aneurysm in **A** thought to have ruptured 44 years before. Sac appears to be collapsed or shrunken. Site of old rupture is indicated by an arrow, and sac walls can still be recognized. Lumen is filled with acellular hyaline tissue, *T,* the result of organization of thrombus. Siderophages were present in the adventitia especially near rupture site. A small residual lumen is still present (*below*). (Verhoeff's elastic stain, about ×22. From Stehbens, W. E.: Histopathology of cerebral aneurysms, Arch. Neurol. **8:**272, 1963.)

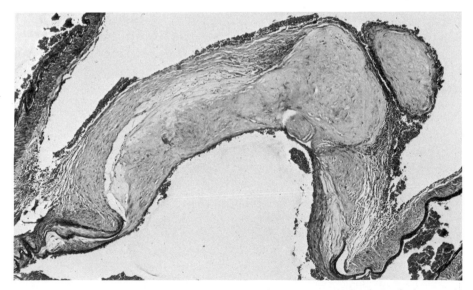

Fig. 9-26. Aneurysm previously ruptured with subsequent organization of the partially obliterating thrombus within sac. Small accessory nodule is probably the false sac at the rupture site. Note persistent lumen within the sac. (Verhoeff's elastic stain, ×36.)

withstood a blood pressure of 210 mm. Hg systolic and 150 mm. diastolic during the final illness. Another aneurysm, which appears to have ruptured previously with subsequent organization of the partially obliterating thrombus, is seen in Fig. 9-26. The secondary nodule looks like remnants of a false sac at the rupture site. Such aneurysms are infrequent, constituting between 0.5% to 1% of aneurysmal sacs found at autopsy. With a small but residual lumen, they probably should not be regarded as cured, and their clinical significance points to a need for detailed study of large numbers. Aneurysms like those depicted in Figs. 9-25, *B,* and 9-26 may be harmless.

From time to time cases of spontaneous cure are reported. Criteria for such claims whether firm or provisional and survival times are important in determining the adequacy and permanency of particular cures.[499] At the present time only with total and permanent anatomical obliteration of the lumen should the disorder be considered cured. Shumacker and Wayson[449] claimed eight spontaneous clinical cures, obviating the need for surgical intervention in 122 cases of aneurysm of the peripheral arteries. Their material was mostly traumatic in origin and the natural history of such lesions may well differ from those etiologically unrelated to injury. Spontaneous cure of a cerebral aneurysm is almost without precedent, but Stehbens[473] reported one instance in which the lumen appeared to be completely obliterated. The patient died of a ruptured cerebral aneurysm at another site. Dandy[125] "guessed" that spontaneous cure by thrombosis occurred in 15% to 20% of cerebral aneurysms but rarely in those of the cavernous segment of the internal carotid. He said that these always retained a functional lumen unless the artery was completely thrombosed.[124]

In the Cooperative Study,[303] untreated aneurysms, single or multiple, followed from the time of their first clinical rupture evinced a survival rate of 30% to 32% after more than 3 years. The pathological state of these aneurysms has neither been adequately defined nor was it resolved whether they had undergone spontaneous cure (complete obliteration) or only partial obliteration like those in Figs. 9-25, *B* and 9-26. Careful and long-term postmortem follow-up of such cases is necessary to provide a conclusive answer. Complete or partial fibrous obliteration is seen in such a small proportion of unruptured aneurysms at autopsy that one is skeptical of Dandy's guess and indeed of the feasibility of a complete cure.

Aneurysms as space-occupying lesions. Because of the progressive aggravation occasioned by hemodynamic stress on their walls, aneurysms have an inherent propensity to increase relentlessly in size, probably over a number of years. The result is a large aneurysmal sac usually containing laminated thrombus and acting as a space-occupying lesion. Almost without exception cerebral aneurysms of more than 2 cm. in diameter are partially filled by laminated thrombus. In the author's series of 333 aneurysms,[473] 19 measured more than 2 cm. in their largest diameter, four measured more than 4 cm., and five simulated intracranial tumors. Such large aneurysms occur on the vertebral, basilar, internal carotid, and middle cerebral or anterior communicating arteries and simulate pituitary adenomas, cerebral tumors, or posterior cranial fossa tumors including those in the cerebellopontine angle.[226] Bull[67] found these massive aneurysms to be more prevalent in the female than in the male.

Among the largest intracranial aneurysms on record are those reported by Kraus,[288] Stehbens,[467] and Cuatico and associates.[120] They measured 7 × 5 × 3.5 cm., 7.8 × 7 × 6.2 cm. (Fig. 9-27), and 8 × 5 × 5 cm. in diameter respectively. Several other large sacs have been reported.[33,67,462] In a man of 47 years, Sadik and associates[420] recorded a giant aneurysm (8.5 × 5.5 × 5 cm.) involving the

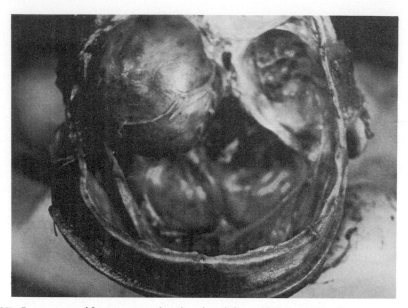

Fig. 9-27. Large carotid aneurysm in situ in right middle cranial fossa at autopsy.[467] Skull and scalp are seen below and floor of the posterior cranial fossa is out of focus. Middle cerebral artery is stretched over upper surface of large solid sac that contained laminated thrombus.

right middle cerebral artery. The parent artery exhibited a most extraordinary degree of ectasia and tortuosity. Sacs measuring up to 4 cm. are encountered sporadically but exceedingly large ones are curiosities. One large aneurysm seen by the author occurred in a hypertensive woman of 62 years. Ten years prior to her final admission to hospital she survived a subarachnoid hemorrhage with coma and was found to have a cerebral aneurysm of the right middle cerebral artery. The ipsilateral common carotid artery was ligated. Nine years later she experienced headache, facial pain, multiple cranial nerve palsies, and convulsions and died a day after admission to hospital from rupture of the same aneurysm (largest diameter 5 cm.) with intracerebral and intraventricular hemorrhage. Obviously the aneurysm had not been cured and in the interim had enlarged to form a massive space-occupying lesion in the middle cranial fossa. Cuatico and colleagues[120] reported a similar case.

Such large aneurysms cause symptoms and signs of raised intracranial pressure and the anatomical proximity of the cranial nerves to the circle of Willis explains the occurrence of local pressure symptoms and signs. In general the larger the sac, the more likely symptoms will be produced though variation occurs with the anatomical site of the aneurysm. In the Cooperative Study[303] no symptoms were produced by aneurysms smaller than 3 mm. in diameter. Aneurysms of the internal carotid artery have the greatest propensity for producing symptoms prior to rupture. Of those aneurysms at the origin of the ophthalmic artery, which produced visual symptoms, 75% were over 10 mm. and 50% were greater than 25 mm. in diameter. This also indicates a lesser tendency for aneurysms so placed to rupture because most aneurysms at other sites would have leaked before the sac attained such dimensions. Unruptured aneurysms at the origin of the posterior communicating artery and internal carotid have a critical size of 7 to 10 mm., above which they either produce symptoms or rupture. Aneurysms of the anterior communicating and middle cerebral arteries are less prone to produce symptoms prior to rupture. Ruptured aneurysms also produce cranial nerve involvement in one way or another and in most cases an episode of subarachnoid hemorrhage precipitates or precedes cranial nerve lesions.

The principal work on the involvement of cranial nerves by aneurysms was by Hyland and Barnett[260] who found 39 of 94 cases of cerebral aneurysm to have clinical nerve involvement. Forty-eight nerves were involved and of these the oculomotor was most frequently affected (73%) and the next in frequency was the abducent (19%). Lesions were of two types: (1) those in which the aneurysmal sac directly involved the nerve and (2) those in which the function of the nerve or its nucleus was disturbed by the secondary effects of hemorrhage from the aneurysmal rupture.

The first group accounted for 52% of the nerve lesions. The onset of functional impairment was in the main coincident with bleeding from the contiguous aneurysm. The cranial nerve exhibited morphological evidence of recent or past hemorrhage into its substance and varying degrees of fibrosis. Excluding unruptured aneurysms and those with terminal rupture, the nerve was generally adherent to the sac or incorporated into the wall of a false sac. In a few cases without evidence of bleeding, an abrupt onset of the nerve lesion suggested an episode of bleeding. When the onset of the palsy and hemorrhage was acute, evidence of previous damage to the nerve was apparent. The fibrosis was possibly caused by pulsations of the contiguous aneurysmal sac.[260] The chronic changes in the nerves could stand comparison with the unusually prominent perivascular fibrosis seen about experimental arteriovenous fistulas.

Most of the second group[260] were false localizing signs caused by the secondary effects of raised supratentorial pressure, often bilateral, usually terminal, and associated with severe hemorrhage with a poor prognosis. Such manifestations accounted for 48% of the nerve lesions in their series of cases. The oculomotor nerves were affected because of kinking or compression by the displaced posterior cerebral artery, compression by a herniated hippocampal gyrus or because of secondary midbrain hemorrhage involving either or both nuclei. Several other nerve lesions were attributed to secondary distortion and displacement of the brain stem, possibly with stretching of the nerve or impairment of the function of the nuclei. In only one case was there direct hemorrhage into the oculomotor nucleus.

In addition to changes outlined above, cranial nerves in proximity to aneurysms may be indented, grossly flattened and displaced (Fig. 9-21). They may lie on the frequently rust-colored floor of an aneurysm-caused depression in the adjoining brain. There is also the distinct possibility that there will be interference to the nerve's blood supply. Although solitary nerve involvement often of the oculomotor is not infrequent, multiple nerve lesions, especially with larger aneurysms are relatively common.[269,523]

No involvement of the first cranial nerve has yet been reported but optic nerves and pathways are often deranged.[273] Jefferson[268] stressed the close relationship between the circle of Willis and optic nerves, chiasm, and tracts and recorded involvement of the chiasm or visual pathways in about one in 10 cases of the Manchester series of 265 patients with aneurysms.[272] This incidence is high, but Walsh and King[520] indicated that an oculomotor nerve palsy and lack of cooperation by the patient often is the cause of small defects in the visual fields being overlooked. Optic nerve atrophy occurs with aneurysms of the internal carotid, anterior cerebral, and anterior communicating arteries and may be caused by direct involvement of the nerve[268] or is secondary to papilledema. Milliser and associates[338] recently described a small saccular aneurysm almost totally enclosed within the optic nerve. The origin of the sac was not determined. At autopsy the optic nerve appeared to have expanded into a fusiform mass and the nerve fibers reduced in number and size were severely compressed. The position of the internal carotid artery on the lateral side of the chiasm is such that monocular blindness or a junction hemianopia are most frequent.[268] Pure tract lesions caused by an aneurysm are rare and presage additional involvement of the chiasm, optic nerve, or both.[268]

The most common cranial nerve lesion associated with cerebral aneurysm is an oculomotor nerve palsy.[270,523] Fearnsides[166] reported it in 20% of cases, Richardson and Hyland[400] in 6%, Dandy[125] in 30%, and Walton[523] in 6%. The degree of involvement varies. In many cases the aneurysm is situated on the internal carotid artery at the origin of the posterior communicating artery, although aneurysms of the basilar may also be implicated. However oculomotor nerve palsy is a common false localizing sign occasioned by either (1) midbrain hemorrhage from rapidly increased supratentorial hemorrhage,[260] (2) kinking and compression of the contralateral third nerve, the effect of displacement of the posterior cerebral artery, (3) compression of the oculomotor nerve against the tentorial edge caused by uncal herniation, or (4) stretching or compression of the brain stem owing to sudden, severe, intracerebral and intraventricular hemorrhage.

The fourth (trochlear nerve) is occasionally affected. Paralysis of this nerve has been reported in a few instances,[125,523] usually in combination with the disorder of other cranial nerves.

The fifth (trigeminal) nerve can be involved. The sensory root is more frequently deranged than the motor[216,523] as is demonstrated in clinical histories by repeated references to facial pain, neuralgia, even typical tic douloureux, and sensory loss over the face.

The sixth (abducent) nerve is affected intermittently and less often than the oculo-

motor. The paralysis of this nerve is generally unilateral, occasionally bilateral, and sometimes a false localizing sign.

The seventh (facial) nerve is rarely damaged.[166,408,533] The eighth (auditory) nerve, though seldom affected, may when involved simulate an acoustic neurinoma.[68] It is quite unusual for the functions of the ninth, tenth, eleventh, and twelfth cranial nerves to be disturbed in patients with subarachnoid hemorrhage, but the nerves in question may be compressed by large aneurysms of the vertebral artery[71] or lower basilar.

Aneurysms in the cavernous sinus behave differently from other saccular aneurysms and rarely rupture.[124] Occasionally they are bilateral. Roe reported the association of paralysis of one or more of the third, fourth, fifth, and sixth cranial nerves with an intracavernous aneurysm and compression of the optic nerve or chiasm in 1851. It has become a well-recognized entity. Jefferson,[269] in a now classic paper, divided the clinical cases with such lesions into three groups on anatomical grounds and named them anterior, posterior, and middle cavernous syndromes. In the anterior cavernous syndrome, the ophthalmic division of the trigeminal nerve is involved and the other two divisions spared. The oculomotor nerve may be affected as well or alternatively all motor nerves to the extraocular muscles. In the middle cavernous syndrome, the least common, ophthalmic and maxillary divisions of the trigeminal nerve are affected and the third spared. There may also be paralysis of one or all three motor nerves to the extraocular muscles. In the posterior cavernous syndrome both the motor and sensory roots of the trigeminal nerve may be involved and the abducent nerve more frequently than the third and fourth cranial nerves. Compression of the oculomotor nerve in its course through the cavernous sinus by an aneurysm of the extracavernous segment of the internal carotid artery is not unknown.[82]

Aneurysms of the cavernous sinus may

cause nonpulsating exophthalmos, with chemosis of the conjunctiva and engorgement of retinal and conjunctival veins and sometimes ecchymoses and initiate fairly rapid obstruction of venous drainage from the orbit.[216,289,405]

Law and Nelson[294] reported an aneurysm of the supraclinoid segment of the internal carotid artery and an associated Raeder's paratrigeminal syndrome (type 2) consisting of ocular sympathetic paresis (ptosis and meiosis) and pain in the distribution of the trigeminal nerve. Another patient with this syndrome has been described but with the aneurysm on the extracranial segment of the internal carotid artery at the base of the skull.[127]

Hemiplegia and hemiparesis are readily produced when aneurysmal rupture initiates intracerebral bleeding and particularly is this so with aneurysms of the middle cerebral artery.[485] Subdural hematoma probably is the cause only rarely. Hemiplegia may arise with damage to a cerebral peduncle caused by raised supratentorial pressure. Associated vasospasm can contribute to the impairment. Large unruptured aneurysms may cause hemiplegia or hemiparesis by pressure effects on the motor tracts along a part of their course. Damage of the motor cortex is unlikely, but compression of the corona radiata, internal capsule, and cerebral peduncles are all possible. Involvement of pyramidal fibers in the pons or medulla oblongata is less frequent.

Hypopituitarism in concert with a large aneurysm is now well known but is rarely encountered. In consideration of the close vascular[206,227] and functional interrelationship[279] between the hypothalamus and pituitary gland, the pituitary dysfunction in cases of large parasellar aneurysms may not be caused simply by pressure on the gland but is perhaps the result of compression of the hypothalamus. Furthermore, acute hypothalamic lesions are frequent after rupture of an aneurysm.[110] Schneck[430] described pituitary hemorrhage and necrosis.

Such changes may contribute to the presence of hypopituitarism, for many of the aneurysms have probably given rise to an episode or two of subarachnoid hemorrhage.

The aneurysms compress the pituitary and usually slightly enlarge the pituitary fossa. Most frequently they arise from the internal carotid artery[183] and can displace the contralateral internal carotid. They may originate from the proximal segment of the anterior cerebral artery,[194] the anterior communicating,[137] or very rarely the bifurcation of the basilar.[400] Associated cranial nerve lesions are likely to be present with the aneurysm simulating a chromophobe adenoma, craniopharyngioma, or less frequently a meningioma. Kahana and colleagues[279] also found hypopituitarism in association with other lesions, that is, glioma of the optic chiasm, tumors of the third ventricle, arteriovenous angioma, and mucocele of the sphenoidal sinus. They reported two cases of cerebral aneurysm manifesting pituitary hypofunction but found three instances with overt radiological changes in the pituitary fossa in the absence of noticeable endocrine dysfunction. Van 'T Hoff and associates[512] recorded three such cases and stated that aneurysm and a chromophobe pituitary adenoma may coexist. Dandy[125] had reported the coexistence of a large hypophyseal tumor and bilateral internal carotid arterial aneurysms but did not mention pituitary dysfunction.

White and Ballantine[534] reviewed 35 instances. It had been considered originally that most of the patients were suffering from pituitary adenoma. In some, the aneurysm had expanded into the pituitary fossa and enlarged the sella turcica radiologically, although erosion is often only unilateral. Calcification of the sac may cast a shadow in the radiogram. Acute exacerbations, monocular blindness, and third, fourth, fifth, and sixth cranial nerve lesions are more characteristic of aneurysm than adenoma.

Mecklin[334] described the unusual case of an encysted hematoma overlying the pituitary fossa, considered to be the result of previous aneurysmal hemorrhage into the pituitary stalk. Curtis and Jimenez[121] reported hypopituitarism and pituitary atrophy caused by a cerebral aneurysm, but the patient died of the rupture of one of two aortic aneurysms. Pituitary atrophy is not essential. In one case[304] the pituitary gland was merely congested, though there was considerable softening of adjacent brain tissue. As indicated, the underlying mechanism of the pituitary disturbance is obscure and awaits further elucidation of the regulatory control of pituitary secretion. Furthermore, clinical signs other than hypopituitarism may appear. Aneurysms have been associated with acromegaly,[195,361] Cushing's syndrome,[252] and diabetes insipidus.[28,365]

Profound mental disturbances naturally occur at the time of or subsequent to bleeding from the aneurysm[523] but local or general disturbances to brain function are also apparent apart from rupture of the sac. Occasionally the first and only symptom of a cerebral aneurysm may be epilepsy[68] but severe psychiatric disturbances have been repeatedly reported in association with cerebral aneurysms.[269,400] The sacs are generally voluminous and the severe atherosclerosis has been regarded as insufficient to account for the dementia. Richardson and Hyland[400] reported two cases with progressive dementia for at least a year. One patient had multiple cranial nerve lesions, a hemiparesis, and hydrocephalus. Jefferson[269] stressed the association, believing the dementia to be etiologically related to the aneurysm and claiming that this relationship accounted for the frequency of aneurysms in inmates of mental asylums.

Considerable erosion of cranial bones may be associated with cerebral aneurysms, and it is more readily appreciated in radiograms than at autopsy when detailed skull changes are rarely sought. They have been described[268,384,461] and consist of (1) uni-lateral erosion of the sella turcica, especially of the anterior clinoids, (2) enlargement of the sella turcica, (3) unilateral enlargement of the optic foramen and superior orbital (sphenoidal) fissure, and (4) erosion of the margin of the carotid canal. Characteristically dense and narrow curvilinear shadows outline the wall of a small proportion of aneurysms of long standing. In addition, a displaced calcified pineal or choroid plexus and angiographic demonstration of the sac are other radiological features used in the diagnosis or investigation.

Variation of the circle of Willis. It is unfortunate that anatomical variations of the circle of Willis have been regarded as congenital anomalies. The assumption has led to the belief that they bear some causal relationship to cerebral aneurysms.[262] There is little to substantiate the supposition that anatomical variations (predominantly in external diameter) of the small cerebral arteries are developmental errors (Chapter 1). Several alleged "anomalies" of the circle of Willis must be regarded as fictitious because of the authors' obvious lack of anatomical knowledge of the cerebral vasculature and the completely unrealistic configuration portrayed.

Although anatomical variations may not be congenital abnormalities, there are other reasons why they occur in association with aneurysms. Lebert[296] first suggested that variation in the topography of the circle of Willis might bear a causal relationship to cerebral aneurysms. Jacques[262] reiterated the view and Slany reported 14 variations in 26 circles with aneurysms. Padget,[370] on whose work the perpetuation of the erroneous belief primarily depends, investigated circles of Willis with and without aneurysms. Stehbens[473] in analyzing Padget's work showed that her conclusions were dependent on misrepresentation of figures quoted in the literature. When corrected, her figures did not at all substantiate her contention that variations are significantly more frequent in patients with aneurysms than in those in whom aneurysms were not to be found. Wilson, Riggs, and Rupp[538] claimed to have found "anomalous" circles of Willis in 118 of 124 circles with aneurysms, assuming that this was a high incidence of correlation; however they provided no control series. Bigelow[46] found "anomalous" circles of Willis in one third of the cases in his series of aneurysms, whereas Walton reported an incidence of 26%. These figures are low according to Table 1-7. Riggs and Rupp[404] found atypical circles of Willis in at least 79% of specimens investigated. Chason and Hindman[89] found no differences in the prevalence of anatomical variations in those with and those without aneurysms. It appears indisputable that such figures do not provide evidence for the hypothesis that so-called anomalies of the circle are more prevalent in patients with cerebral aneurysms than in the general population. Moreover, it has become obvious that the incidence of anatomical variations in any given series of circles of Willis will depend on the exactitude and rigidity of criteria employed in defining a "normal" circle.

Wilson, Riggs, and Rupp[538] found inequality of the proximal segments of the anterior cerebral arteries in 40 of 47 circles with aneurysms on the anterior communicating artery. Stehbens[473] found inequality in 30 of 37 circles with aneurysm on that artery compared to only 18 with inequality of the anterior cerebral arteries in 59 brains with aneurysms of sites other than on the anterior communicating artery. This inequality of the proximal segments of the anterior cerebral artery (Fig. 1-4) results in a large shunt of blood across the anterior communicating artery and thus a veritable bifurcation forms. Such shunts vary in size. The arterial inequality is sometimes only moderate or otherwise the shunt is to a large median artery of the corpus callosum. For all that, it should not be assumed that this relationship is caused by congenital factors for it is probably hemodynamic in origin due to the compensatory

shunting of blood through the anterior communicating artery. This is the only known anatomical variation evincing a reliably definite correlation with aneurysmal site.

In an aneurysm series there is no statistically significant difference between the prevalence of duplicated arterial stems or plexiform communications about the anterior communicating artery and their prevalence in a control series.[473] Furthermore, no definite correlation of aneurysms with variations in the size of the posterior communicating arteries or of the internal carotid arteries has been forthcoming,[473] and the middle cerebral arteries rarely show inequality to a degree sufficient to be of import. Cases of aneurysms of the basilar bifurcation when both posterior communicating arteries supply the bulk of the blood to the posterior cerebral arteries have not been encountered.

Lagarde and associates[291] reported an instance of "hypoplasia" of an internal carotid artery, together with an aneurysm at the fork of the anterior communicating and the contralateral anterior cerebral artery. Lhermitte and associates[300] described the case of a woman of 63 years in whom the left internal carotid artery was of normal caliber in its first centimeter and the remainder of very small caliber. As a consequence the blood supply for the left anterior cerebral artery came predominantly from the right internal carotid and the basilar provided most of the blood for the left middle cerebral. An aneurysm was present at the junction of the right anterior cerebral and the anterior communicating arteries. In both patients, the aneurysm occurred when the anterior communicating artery was a large shunt, a compensatory formation caused by the small internal carotid and constituting a variation already discussed. However, most instances of so-called aplasia are in effect merely small vessels rather than a malformation. The abnormal vessels were not examined histologically and the "aplasia" could well have been from an acquired disease either in vitro or during postnatal life.

Moyes[345] recorded an aneurysm of the basilar artery in a woman of 37 years in whom he could not demonstrate the left internal carotid artery by angiography. He alleged that this was an instance of an aneurysm in association with agenesis of the internal carotid artery, but the exact reason for failure to demonstrate an artery by angiography is quite debatable.

Aneurysms have also been reported in association with persistent trigeminal (Table 1-3) and persistent hypoglossal arteries. Controversy surrounds the significance of these carotid-basilar anastomoses that are not generally related to any special pathological process. The anastomotic vessels are more prevalent than currently believed, for unless they are of large caliber, they are unquestionably often overlooked at autopsy or by angiography. Individual case reports render any precise estimation of the incidence of these vessels quite difficult. The association of the carotid-basilar anastomoses with cerebral aneurysms is not currently believed to be of statistical significance (Chapter 1).

McCormick[321] has argued that if persistent trigeminal artery occurs approximately once in 300 adult autopsies and cerebral aneurysm once in every 20 adults, both should be found in association once in every 6000 autopsies. However, he found two instances in 1600 autopsies. Thus the coexistence of the two findings appears to be unduly frequent, yet McCormick rightly considered the frequency too low for meaningful statistical analysis. Any conclusion to the contrary is unwarranted because of the following reasons:

1. The primitive trigeminal and hypoglossal arteries may be represented in the adult by small branches of the carotid and basilar arteries. Precise determination of how often they persist as very small vessels in adult life cannot be deduced and they could merely be exaggerations of commonly occurring anastomoses.

2. Such anatomical variations should not be regarded as developmental anomalies for no grounds exist to indicate that such variations are structurally or functionally inferior to any other vessel.

3. In horses, though the carotid-basilar anastomosis is almost always present,[147] to date no cerebral aneurysms have been found.

4. Atherosclerosis to a severe degree and arteriectasis are not uncommon in the anastomotic vessel.[541,545]

5. There is no information regarding any possible associated hemodynamic imbalance of flow, though stresses on the carotid because of its larger caliber are greater than in vessels without an anastomosis.

Hypertension. Cerebral aneurysms occur predominantly in that time of life when acquired degenerative diseases frequently become manifest. Of paramount importance is the influence of hypertension on the lesions. Walton[523] believed that the results of his study indicated a relationship between hypertension, atherosclerosis, and cerebral aneurysm. Indeed, the only two congenital diseases commonly associated with cerebral aneurysms, coarctation of the aorta and polycystic disease of the kidneys, are also the only two diseases frequently accompanied by hypertension.[472] Turnbull[508] claimed that the prevalance of hypertension in patients with spontaneous intracerebral hemorrhage was greater than with cerebral aneurysms. However, disparity in its frequency does not preclude the possibility of hypertension being more than a coincidental finding in subjects with aneurysm.

Magee[314] concluded that hypertension probably should not be implicated, for in a highly selected group of young people he found few patients with a raised blood pressure on admission to hospital with subarachnoid hemorrhage. Black and Hicks[50] found cardiac hypertrophy in 69 of 100 subjects with cerebral aneurysm, a ratio higher than in the general population when adjusted for age, sex, heart weight, and body weight. Fishberg[171] classified primary subarachnoid hemorrhage as a complication of essential hypertension and found that the correlation was not nearly as close as with primary intracerebral hemorrhage. In a small series (39 autopsy cases) with cerebral aneurysm, Walker and Allègre[518] disclosed an incidence of hypertension three times the expected rate calculated from a series of 500 consecutive autopsies adjusted for age, sex, and race. Generalized atherosclerosis approximated twice the expected rate. Wilson, Riggs, and Rupp[538] considered that any evaluation of the role of cardiovascular disease in elderly patients with aneurysm was quite difficult and would be inconclusive, but in 27 of 40 patients under 40 years of age, they found cardiac hypertrophy. The figure is undoubtedly high for that age group. Chason and Hindman[89] reported hypertension diagnosed clinically or at autopsy in almost 80% of 137 subjects with cerebral aneurysm. Sugai and Shoji[487] reported that in Japanese with cerebral aneurysms, the average heart weight increased with each decade and that the first part of the aorta was wider than that of control aortas.

The prevalence of preexisting hypertension in patients with subarachnoid hemorrhage of aneurysmal origin is difficult to determine chiefly because the aneurysm is rarely diagnosed prior to rupture, which entails a high mortality.[523] During the acute phase of the illness, high sphygmomanometric readings are not usually acceptable as evidence of hypertension, for blood pressure is thought to rise concomitantly with intracranial pressure although this is not invariably the case. In an effort to exclude possible fallacy, Stehbens applied very conservative criteria to investigate the pathological evidence for preexisting hypertension in a series of 215 necropsies in which cerebral aneurysms had been found.[471] Results indicated that hypertension was more prevalent in patients with aneurysms than in a control group of 839 patients. A conservative estimate is that at least 54% of patients found to have a cerebral aneurysm (ruptured or unruptured) at autopsy have hypertension. On theoretical grounds, it is apparent that hypertension, an aggravating factor in any degenerative vascular disease, must be regarded similarly

in cases of cerebral aneurysm. It has been demonstrated to have a size-augmenting effect on aneurysms.[303] Yet the absence of hypertension does not negate its general importance as a factor.[459] The difference in the frequency of hypertension in males and females is negligible as is the difference in its frequency between patients with multiple aneurysms and those with but a single lesion.[471]

Walton[523] was of the opinion that moderate or severe hypertension probably contributed to the death of patients with subarachnoid hemorrhage. However the prevalence of hypertension does not seem to be significantly greater when the aneurysm is the cause of death than when it is an incidental autopsy finding.[33,471] Cerebral aneurysms have been regarded as part of the hypertensive complex[171,244] and indeed unruptured cerebral aneurysms and primary intracerebral hemorrhage are found in association.[471]

Congenital abnormalities. Congenital abnormalities tend to occur together. The mere coexistence of such lesions and cerebral aneurysms has therefore been held to support the hypothesis that congenital factors are of basic importance in the etiology of cerebral aneurysms. However, in any large series of autopsies, numbers of congenital abnormalities should be expected, quite apart from those perhaps concerned in the production of the lesion under consideration. This is especially true of the saccular cerebral aneurysms of noninflammatory origin. In the only statistical analysis,[472] the prevalence of congenital abnormalities in a series of 215 subjects with cerebral aneurysms was compared with that in a control series of 849 subjects and in a series of 351 with primary nonaneurysmal cerebral hemorrhage. Completely at variance with and definitely contrary to the widely held belief, differences were found to be not statistically significant. On analyzing the incidence of individual congenital lesions, Stehbens[472] demonstrated that the frequency of their occurrence is lower than would be expected in the general population. However, polycystic disease of the kidneys and aortic coarctation are both associated with cerebral aneurysms with sufficient frequency for the association to be considered a clinical entity or syndrome.[472]

Cerebral aneurysms have also been reported in association with a congenitally deformed hand,[5] multiple meningiomas,[11] a cerebral arteriovenous aneurysm, undescended testis and an abdominal aortic aneurysm,[12] neurofibromatosis,[40] and Albers-Schönberg disease.[163] Isolated case reports do not constitute strong evidence. Stehbens[472] stressed that in the larger series the prevalence of individual congenital anomalies is usually lower in the aneurysm patients than in the estimates reported for the general population. Walker and Allègre,[518] though recording nine anomalies among 39 patients, did not distinguish among the different types. Yet in Stehbens' control series there was an incidence of 24.1%. It was concluded that the evidence for the high incidence of congenital lesions in patients with cerebral aneurysms is inadequate and provides no realistic basis for the postulation that a congenital factor participates in the pathogenesis of cerebral aneurysm.[472] Available figures do not completely disprove the possible participation of a congenital factor, but no assumptions regarding the applicability of the congenital theory should be advanced. An extremely detailed and exhaustive search for congenital anomalies in a large number of patients with cerebral aneurysms and in a control group would be necessary to finalize this question beyond all reasonable doubt.

Polycystic disease of the kidneys. The association of polycystic disease of the kidneys and cerebral aneurysm was first described[56] by Borelius in 1901. Many individual instances of the combination have since been reported,[77,460] but in many instances subarachnoid hemorrhage only and not aneurysms were found.[123,523] Dunger[150] recorded polycystic kidneys in a mother and daughter. The mother died of a ruptured cerebral aneurysm and the daughter of a pontine

hemorrhage. Ask-Upmark and Ingvar[15] found five instances of polycystic kidneys in 47 patients with ruptured cerebral aneurysms and Walton[523] recorded 10 in 173. The severity of the cystic change varied. Dalgaard[123] reported seven instances of subarachnoid hemorrhage in 173 autopsies of cases of polycystic kidneys, and it is likely that cerebral aneurysms were represented in this series.

Brown[66] recorded six instances of polycystic kidneys in 144 patients with proved cerebral aneurysms, Hamby[216] reported three in 86, and Sahs[421] four in 150, one of which had six cerebral aneurysms. Stehbens[472] found eight in a control series of 891 autopsies and two in 215 patients with cerebral aneurysm. Combining 314 patients with cerebral aneurysms from seven reports in the literature, Bigelow[45] found an incidence of 20 cases of polycystic kidneys in the series, which was higher than Bell[37] cited for the general population (once in 351 autopsies). Poutasse and associates[388] recorded three instances of the association and estimated that cerebral aneurysm occurs in 16% of patients with polycystic kidneys. Such a high estimate, if reliable, supports the contention that the association of the two diseases is more than fortuitous.

It is estimated that 75% to 80% of patients with polycystic disease of the kidneys develop hypertension.[427,451] These patients suffer from generalized vascular disease and often die of primary intracerebral hemorrhage. The factor in common is hypertension, and this also seems to be the common factor when cerebral aneurysm and polycystic kidneys occur concomitantly. In reports of the coexistence of these two diseases, hypertension is not always mentioned, but when relevant detail is included, hypertension is almost invariably present.[472] Hypertension moreover appears to be a predisposing factor in aneurysm formation and growth.

Bigelow[45] alleged that polycystic disease of the kidneys had not been found associated with aneurysms of other vessels, but polycystic kidneys may be associated with severe and widespread arterial disease. Among the complications in 70 cases of polycystic liver were 14 cases of myocardial infarction, nine cases of cerebral hemorrhage, two cases of ruptured aortic aneurym, four of cerebral aneurysm (each had polycystic kidneys), and one of coronary aneurysm.[335] Other instances of polycystic kidneys with aneurysms (saccular or dissecting) have been observed in extracranial arteries.[472] Thus the aneurysm formation in the disease is not specific to any arterial tree.[472] In the presence of advanced atherosclerosis and hypertension, the aortic aneurysms with polycystic kidneys would undoubtedly be classed as acquired lesions and one wonders why cerebral aneurysms have only recently come under the designation "acquired," and indeed how the "congenital theory" could have gained such credence.

Coarctation of the aorta. Coarctation of the aorta (adult type), met with only once in every 3000 or 4000 autopsies,[397] is frequently associated with cerebral aneurysms. The coexistence of the two lesions has been long recognized as a classical entity or syndrome.[1,397,472] Schwartz and Baronofsky[437] in 1960 found 32 such cases in the literature, and several cases have since been added, including some in which subarachnoid hemorrhage occurred but no cerebral aneurysms were found. Baker and Sheldon[23] reported a case of recurrent subarachnoid hemorrhage in a woman of 25 years with coarctation and an oculomotor palsy. No aneurysm was found and they agreed with Abbott[1] in assuming that all instances of spontaneous intracranial hemorrhage in patients with coarctation were caused by rupture of an aneurysm. No assumption of this kind should be made. In view of the long-standing hypertension that exists with coarctation, primary intracerebral hemorrhage could be the cause of many fatalities. Several cases in the literature are believed to be of such a nature.[1,75,472] Bacterial endocarditis is a frequent complication of aortic coarctation but no definite case of bacterial aneurysm on the cerebral arteries has been reported.

The concurrence of aortic coarctation and cerebral aneurysm may not be encountered so readily in the future because of the current propensity for surgical correction of the stenosis, although the damage already done to the arteries may not be repaired so readily as the coarctation. It is interesting that in the large number of cerebral aneurysms collected in the Cooperative Study, neither aortic coarctation nor polycystic kidneys were mentioned.[302,303]

Two patients with coarctation of the abdominal aorta have been recorded with cerebral aneurysms[172,281] whereas Hirano and associates recorded the association of a cerebral aneurysm and the infantile type of aortic coarctation with multiple cardiac abnormalities in a girl of 11 years.[245] Apart from these instances the coarctation has always been of the adult type and situated in the region of the ligamentum arteriosum.

Most patients with the untreated adult form of coarctation of the aorta die within

Table 9-9. Causes of death of patients with coarctation of the aorta*

Causes of death	Percentage of total deaths		Average age at death	
	Reifenstein et al.[397]	Abbott[1]	Reifenstein et al.[397]	Abbott[1]
Incidental causes	25.9	22.5	47	?
Rupture of aorta (nonbacterial)	23.1	20.0	27.7	22.2
Bacterial endocarditis	22.1	16.0	28.7	?
Congestive cardiac failure	18.3	29.0	39.3	?
Intracranial lesions	10.6	12.5	28.0	30.1

*From Stehbens, W. E.: Cerebral aneurysms and congenital abnormalities, Aust. Ann. Med. **11**:102, 1962, and adapted from Reifenstein et al.[397]

the first four decades.[1,209,397] The direct causes of death are to be seen in Table 9-9. At least 20% of patients with coarctation die from a ruptured aorta, the most common site of rupture being the ascending aorta, with the next most frequent site being immediately distal to the coarctation (poststenotic zone). The rupture is preceded by a saccular or fusiform aneurysm or associated with a dissecting aneurysm. Subacute bacterial aortitis may be responsible for rupture in some instances.

Hamilton and Abbott[218] described the autopsy findings in a boy of 14 years suffering from aortic coarctation. He had a saccular and early dissecting aneurysm of the ascending aorta with impending rupture. The aorta was atheromatous with early calcification and microscopically was thickened with gross hyalinization. The elastic tissue was seriously deficient in the media, and the intima displayed degenerative changes. The aneurysm however was not attributed to the severe and premature degenerative changes in the aorta but to congenital hypoplasia. The assumption that the aorta is hypoplastic in coarctation is frequently made, but Reifenstein and associates[397] assert that the histological changes on the aorta have been inadequately studied. Of cases of aortic rupture in general they wrote: "The media appeared somewhat decreased in thickness and showed varying amounts of necrosis, hyaline degeneration, fibrosis, elastic decrease and fragmentation, basophilic appearance, or cystic change. Atheromatosis was common and the vasa vasorum occasionally exhibited narrowing of lumina by intimal and/or medial thickening. Elastic destruction appeared to be the outstanding lesion. A few reports indicated that the various changes were more marked proximal to the coarctation." Such changes can be expected in an ectatic aorta or one associated with aneurysmal dilatation, and though the coarctation is congenital, other manifestations of this disease are acquired. The aorta proximal to the coarctation is subjected to the stress of a high pulse pressure in both naturally occurring[209,382] and experimentally induced coarctation.[313] Sloan and Cooley[456] found that in 32% of patients with coarctation, the proximal aorta displays tortuosity and ectasia when examined radiologically. It is a common site of rupture and the degenerative changes particularly of the elastica can be extreme even in the first decade[472] and are sufficient to account for the dilatation, aneurysm formation, and rupture. Because autopsy material of coarctation of the aorta is rare, there has been a lack of appreciation of the severity of the accompanying arterial degeneration. Moreover, it is now well recognized that many instances of dissecting aneurysm of the aorta are secondary to hemodynamic stress consequent upon aortic valvular stenosis,[239,331] and recently intimal tears with dissection have been experimentally induced in veins by chronic hemodynamic stress.[480] Moreover it is now widely recognized that the poststenotic dilatation or aneurysm is also acquired and caused by vibrational injury to the wall that is attributed to the disturbed hemodynamics[251] and can be readily produced experimentally in animals.[251,312]

The prevalence and severity of coronary atherosclerosis in coarctation has received little attention, yet its very gravity in young patients[472] probably hastens death by cardiac insufficiency in 18% to 29% of patients (Table 9-9). Death occurs at age 29 on an average.

Between 10% and 12% of the patients with coarctation of the aorta die from intracranial lesions (Table 9-9), although neurological signs and symptoms may be much more frequent.[510] These lesions are predominantly examples of hemorrhage, many of which are aneurysmal in origin. Atherosclerosis of the cerebral arteries is common. Even so Abbott[1] could not explain why the branches of the internal carotid arteries were often tortuous and atheromatous. Reifenstein and associates[397] noted that the systolic, diastolic, and pulse pressures tend to be unusually high in patients dying of intracranial lesions. The long-standing hypertension could well account for the prematurely severe atherosclerosis of the cerebral arteries and of the aorta and coronary arteries. Furthermore, fusiform aneurysms, also considered to be acquired and caused by atherosclerosis,[254] are found on the cerebral arteries in association with coarctation.[472,519] Walker and Livingstone[519] presented a case in which the left vertebral artery was tortuous and exhibited irregular saccular aneurysmal dilatations, one of which had apparently ruptured. Hence, saccular aneurysms that arise at the apices of the bifurcations should not be termed "congenital" merely because they occur in patients with coarctation of the aorta.

In coarctation of the aorta, collateral vessels are atherosclerotic even at a relatively young age.[472] The characteristic tortuosity of the intercostal arteries and the associated notching of the ribs are not usually demonstrable radiographically until after the first decade,[209] which indicates that these are acquired features stemming from the stenosis. No detailed histological study has been made of the tortuous collateral vessels in experimentally induced coarctation. The degenerative changes associated with loss of elasticity[209] probably augment the possibility of aneurysm formation, for they are occasionally seen on the collateral vessels in this disease.[456,472] Spinal vessels enlarge (Fig. 2-8) and participate in the collateral circulation and an aneurysm of the enlarged anterior spinal artery may complicate coarctation of the aorta.

Coarctation of the aorta is a disease of unknown pathogenesis. It is grouped with the congenital lesions of the heart and great vessels although it is neither the commonest occurring lesion nor the one with the highest incidence of extracardiac anomalies. Yet with one exception (a patient with a patent ductus arteriosus[43]) it is the only one associated with cerebral aneurysms and also the only one not characterized by systemic hypertension. Such circumstances suggest that cerebral aneurysm complicates coarctation of the aorta, not because of hypothetical congenital factors but indubit-

ably because of the associated hypertension and premature atherosclerosis of severe degree. A statistical reduction in the frequency of cerebral aneurysms in patients with surgically corrected coarctation of the aorta would support this concept. Furthermore, aortic coarctation of the infantile variety is associated with frequent abnormalities, with only one instance of an associated cerebral aneurysm,[245] and the adult type, with few other significant anomalies but much evidence of degenerative changes in the vessels, has a high incidence of aneurysms in general.

In the face of this evidence it is difficult to support the concept that because coarctation of the aorta is a congenital disease, associated cerebral aneurysms must therefore have a similar etiology. In coarctation, the duration of the hypertension is probably longer than that of the hyperpiesis of middle-aged patients presenting with cerebral aneurysm. Moreover the patients die of cerebral aneurysm at the time when the degenerative changes in the vessels have had ample time to develop. Certainly the evidence now available strongly suggests that cerebral aneurysms in cases of aortic coarctation are caused by acquired degenerative disease and, like polycystic disease of the kidneys, are most likely related to the associated hypertension.

Arteriovenous aneurysms. Cerebral aneurysm appears to be a relatively frequent complication of an intracranial arteriovenous fistula or aneurysm. An aneurysm may develop on one of the vessels directly involved in the arteriovenous aneurysm, on a feeding artery or a vessel apparently remote from the fistula. This association has been regarded as supporting a developmental factor in the pathogenesis of cerebral "berry" aneurysms, but it seems more likely that hemodynamic factors associated with the fistula are responsible (Chapter 10).

Cerebral aneurysms and miscellaneous pathological lesions. Intracranial arterial aneurysms of noninflammatory origin may be associated with almost any pathological lesion, including bacterial endocarditis, syphilis, meningitis, primary cerebral hemorrhage,[471] and severe cerebral atherosclerosis with cerebral ischemia and infarction. However certain lesions have attracted rather unwarranted attention when found in association with a cerebral aneurysm. For example, Raskind[394] reported a case of recurrent meningioma and an aneurysm not considered to be traumatic, although it appeared postoperatively. Obviously such aneurysms may be traumatic and present as a postoperative complication[496] or otherwise they are quite independent of the tumor and the surgery.[299] A further remote possibility is that a long-standing arteriovenous shunt associated with a tumor may influence the development of an aneurysm in much the same way as an arteriovenous aneurysm.

Aneurysms of the cerebral arteries are occasionally associated with extracranial aneurysms, either of the aorta (saccular and dissecting)[186] or of the splanchnic vessels.[145,250] Though extracranial aneurysms are occasionally attributed to congenital or developmental factors and likened to the cerebral berry aneurysm, other acquired factors should be carefully sought in explanation before there is recourse to such speculation.

Fibromuscular hyperplasia and cerebral aneurysms. Cerebral aneurysms have been found in several patients with fibromuscular hyperplasia of the extracranial arteries (Chapter 12). Although genetic factors have been incriminated in the association, it is much more likely that the severe hypertension, so frequently a complication of renal arterial stenosis, is of major etiological importance in the pathogenesis of the aneurysm formation. The subarachnoid hemorrhage and aneurysm then in this disease are more properly caused by the accompanying hypertension and not by the fibromuscular hyperplasia per se.

Familial hereditary connective tissue disorders. Intracranial arterial aneurysms have been found in association with hereditary connective tissue disorders and again the association has been considered to lend support to the congenital theory of cerebral aneurysms.[203] These connective tissue diseases are rare and only scanty information is available.

Ehlers-Danlos syndrome. The Ehlers-Danlos syndrome (or hyperelastosis cutis) is an inherited connective tissue disorder, believed to be transmitted as an autosomal dominant trait, although an X-linked form has been described.[204] Affected individuals characteristically have laxity of the skin, sufficiently striking to allow them to earn a living as circus curiosities. Thinness and fragility of the skin, hypermobility of joints, subcutaneous molluscous pseudotumors occurring after minor trauma over pressure points, skeletal and ocular abnormalities, and varied visceral manifestations have been described.[375] A propensity to bruising is a prominent feature of the disease,[488] but in many patients there are also lesions of large blood vessels,[326,375] including varicose veins,[25] dissecting aneurysm of the aorta,[375] spontaneous rupture,[326] and aneurysms of peripheral arteries.[25,36]

Barabas[25] classified the disease into three major types. The patients in his group 1 were of the classical type, many being born prematurely and having no varicose veins or arterial ruptures. The mildly affected patients in group 2 had moderate skin and joint manifestations and many had varicose veins. The patients in group 3 belonged to the arterial type, suffering from a tendency to bruising, spontaneous ecchymoses during menstruation, and severe and repeated arterial ruptures with or without aneurysm formation. More recently Barabas[26] has indicated that the third or arterial subgroup might be a separate but related entity. Some of these patients develop lesions of their cerebral arteries, and from available descriptions these vessels are just as friable as the extracranial arteries. This classification may be somewhat artifical but has served to focus attention on a group of patients prone to ecchymoses and the formation of arterial aneurysms.

Rubinstein and Cohen[416] reported the case of a woman of 47 years with a typical history of the Ehlers-Danlos syndrome. Her father, brother, and two deceased children were also afflicted. She had a saccular aneurysm at the origin of the left posterior communicating from the internal carotid, with a fusiform dilatation and two saccular aneurysms of the left vertebral artery. Cerebral arteries were fragile, and histologically there was little collagen in the adventitia. The subclavian artery was unexpectedly contused after only gentle manipulation, and the aorta histologically showed gross elastic tissue degeneration similar to that seen in aortic coarctation and dissecting aneurysm. In general the vessels had less than normal elastica and collagen.

Graf[201] reported spontaneous carotid-cavernous fistulas in two young women with Ehlers-Danlos syndrome. By angiography one patient exhibited gross and irregular dilatation of the entire left internal carotid artery. When the patient died, multiple extracranial aneurysms and additional unsuspected aneurysms were found on the internal carotid and basilar arteries.[24] The patient's 30-year-old brother developed a spontaneous carotid-cavernous fistula but without indubitable signs of the Ehlers-Danlos syndrome. Four other members of the family had suffered from subarachnoid or cerebral hemorrhage. Schoolman and Kepes[434] recorded bilateral spontaneous carotid-cavernous fistulas in a 39-year-old woman whose mother had died of a cerebrovascular accident of unknown type, and Taylor[495] encountered a large aneurysm of the vertebral artery (cervical segment) in a male of 28 years. These cases were thought to occur spontaneously, but trauma cannot be excluded, for so great is the fragility of the vessels, the injury need be only trivial. Tridon and associates[504] reported a cerebral aneurysm in a patient with Ehlers-Danlos syndrome and found a tortuous vertebral artery of irregular caliber. In six generations of the family, there were five instances of carotid-cavernous fistula and several of subarachnoid hemorrhage.

The defect in Ehlers-Danlos syndrome is still a matter for argument, as it is uncertain whether collagen or elastica is basically at fault. No ultrastructural defect has been demonstrated,[527] although histologically some architectural changes have been noted.[201,434] There is evidence that the collagen fibers in Ehlers-Danlos syndrome are fragmented, as well as being scanty and poorly organized, and as such may constitute the prime defect responsible for vascular fragility.[267,341,416] Nordschow and Marsolais[355] suggested that the primary defect rather than being molecular may be one of inadequate collagen production. Certainly in the case report of Rubinstein and Cohen[416] the adventitial collagen appeared to be defective and the occurrence of aneurysms in this syndrome is almost certainly attributed to the connective tissue disorder rather than to an inherited tendency to cerebral aneurysms per se. One can no more deduce from the limited material that the etiology of all cerebral aneurysms is based on a congenital deficiency of the arterial wall as Rubenstein and Cohen infer, than one can conclude that all venous varicosities are genetically determined because some are seen in this syndrome. Obviously aneurysms and varicose veins can be secondary manifestations of the disease.

From the study of Papp and Paley[375] it would seem that this syndrome is more prevalent than was once believed and many cases may not be diagnosed clinically because they represent *formes frustes*. In this regard, one also ponders upon the significance of hypermobility of the fingers, a not infrequent observation in otherwise healthy individuals.

Pseudoxanthoma elasticum. Pseudoxanthoma elasticum is a hereditary disease in which yellowish papules and plaques are distributed symmetrically in the very lax skin of the neck, axilla, groin, and the cubital and popliteal spaces (cutis laxa). Angioid streaks occur in the retina in about 50% of affected individuals.[7,428] The skin and retinal lesions are manifestations of the degenerative changes of the elastic tissue, and hypertension is said to be a frequent accompaniment.[157]

An important feature of this disease complex is the occurrence of clinical arterial disease. The arteries of the lower extremities are most frequently involved and exhibit varying degrees of occlusion and radiological evidence of calcification. There has been no detailed histological examination of the associated vascular changes, for material from this rare disease is extremely scanty. Aterman[16] encountered three male infants with a severe degree of cutis laxa in a Newfoundland family. Each of the infants died of the generalized connective tissue defect, with tortuous, elastic arteries and massive aneurysmal dilatation of the ascending aorta. No mention was made of involvement of cerebral arteries, but it is not surprising that cerebral aneurysms have been described in two patients suffering from pseudoxanthoma elasticum.[135,428] Another patient had bilateral aneurysms of the common carotid arteries.[428]

Unfortunately little is known of the nature of this disease and though prominent changes occur in the elastic tissue, it is believed to be a hereditary abiotrophy of collagen.[222]

Marfan's syndrome. Marfan's syndrome is an uncommon hereditary and familial disorder of connective tissue, somewhat better known than the two preceding syndromes. It is transmitted as a single autosomal dominant. The disease behaves as an abiotrophy of connective tissue,[329,330] is believed to be a metabolic disturbance of collagen formation, and exhibits remarkable similarities to experimental lathyrism. These patients with slender, tall, and elongated habitus, pectus excavatum, high arched palate, and arachnodactyly frequently have cardiovascular complications of a severe nature. There may be a dissecting or a diffuse aneurysm of the ascending aorta alone or a combination[329] and the central nervous system may then be secondarily affected. Cerebral aneurysms have not been described in association with this disease as have dissecting aneurysms of the common carotid arteries and aneurysms of the cervical segment of the internal carotid artery.[224]

Relationship of aneurysms to connective tissue disorders. The association of aneurysms and cerebral aneurysms in particular, with connective tissue disorders, is of intense interest. Naturally enough the concept that they are interrelated, because congenital defects tend to associate with one another, has been suggested,[416] but it seems to be an unlikely explanation. The evidence that these connective tissue disorders are familial because of an inherited defect in connective tissue is widely accepted but as yet no scientific evidence indicates that cerebral aneurysms are similarly determined. It is much more likely that cerebral aneurysms are occasional complications of Ehlers-Danlos syndrome and pseudoxanthoma elasticum because of the connective tissue deficiencies. Collagen and elastica are both essential for the strength of the arterial wall and also for its repair, and consequently it would be surprising if aneurysm formation was not a complication of each of these diseases. The aneurysm should be regarded as a secondary manifestation occasioned by a primary disorder of the connective tissue.

Histopathology of saccular aneurysms related to arterial forks

Small aneurysms. At the entrance to small aneurysmal sacs, the intima of the parent artery is invariably thickened slightly and sometimes elastic fibrils internal to the fragmented and degenerate elastic lamina are in evidence. The intima is continuous with the inner aspect of the sac wall and definite atherosclerosis of the facial and dorsal pads of the parent stem can be expected. The internal elastic lamina is reflected for a short distance into the neck or base of the aneurysm (Fig. 9-28).

Usually the media at the entrance ends more or less abruptly and often resembles the edge of a medial defect (Fig. 9-29). This feature is by no means invariable for the appearance of the media is not constant about the circumference of the neck. It sometimes tapers and extends for a short distance into the neck of the sac, becoming attenuated and disappearing or merging into the fibromuscular tissue of the sac wall. In Fig. 9-28, *B,* a small aneurysm with

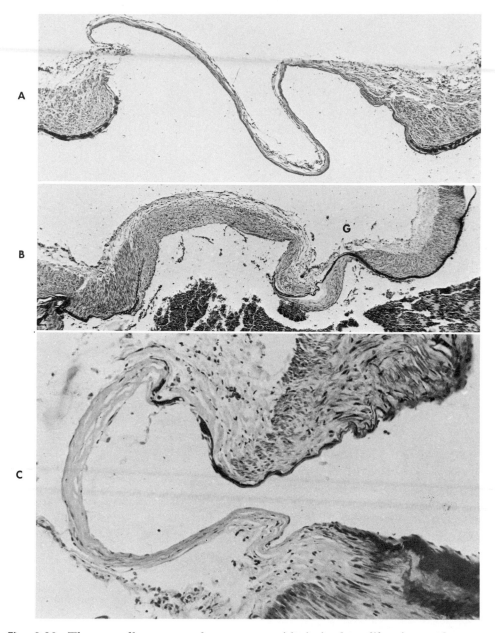

Fig. 9-28. Three small unruptured aneurysms with intimal proliferation and severe elastic tissue degeneration in the parent arteries at the entrance to the small sacs. Note medial fibrosis at the entrance to sacs **A** and **C** and the elastic tissue in the sac wall of **C. B,** Sac wall is moderately thick, the media merges with the sac wall on both sides, and a medial gap may have existed at *G* though it does not appear to have participated in the aneurysm formation. (Verhoeff's elastic stain; **A,** ×50; **B,** ×35; **C,** ×110. **B,** From Stehbens, W. E.: Histopathology of cerebral aneurysms, Arch. Neurol. **8:**272, 1963.)

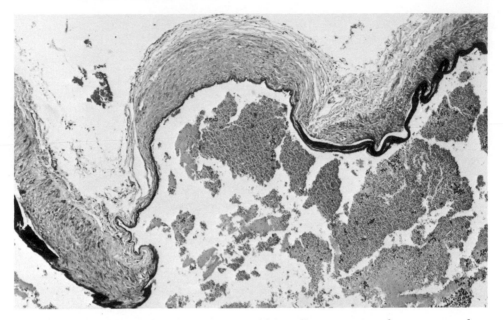

Fig. 9-29. Small aneurysm with moderately thick wall except near the entrance where it is thin. Note subendothelial elastica in the sac. Media of the parent stem terminates fairly abruptly and resembles the media at a medial gap. (Verhoeff's elastic stain, ×45.)

a moderately thick cellular wall has formed at a short distance to the side of the medial defect. On both sides the media merges with the fibromuscular tissue of the aneurysm and the adventitia covering the sac is continuous with that on the parent artery. The adventitia at the neck not infrequently contains a few small round cells.

Small aneurysms tend to have very thin walls consisting of little more than a thin layer of fibrous tissue in which a few remnants of the elastica may be found at the neck. The wall may be thicker and more cellular because of the apparent proliferation of plain muscle fibers and fine elastic fibrillar laminae on the inner aspect of the wall. This musculoelastic proliferation is not uniform in thickness and morphologically resembles the intimal pads or cushions (Fig. 9-30) seen in the intima of cerebral arteries.[470] Fibrous tissue in the external aspect of the wall looks like stretched adventitia in which a few pale-staining elastic fibrils have persisted. Metachromasia occurs particularly in the cellular and thicker portions of the wall where active prolifer-

ation, intimal in type, is well underway. No vessels have been found arising from these small sacs.[475]

Large aneurysms. The intimal thickening on the lateral aspects of the entrance to large aneurysmal sacs is always present, is thicker than in smaller sacs, and often contains foam cells (Fig. 9-18) and occasionally some calcification. The elastic lamina generally ends fairly abruptly at the entrance or extends for a short distance into the neck and varies in thickness, in staining, and in fragmentation. Frequently thinner accessory laminae with less intense staining characteristics fan out into the base of the sac from the internal elastic lamina. The intima tends to be directly continuous with the inner portion of the sac wall (Figs. 9-25, *B,* and 9-26).

The media generally ends abruptly especially when the angle of reflection of the sac wall is sharp, and at times it simulates a medial gap. A fairly sudden fibrous tissue replacement of the media is quite frequent.

The adventitia is reflected onto the outer

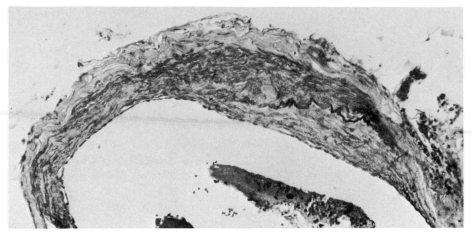

Fig. 9-30. Small aneurysmal sac wall. The thick portion resembles intimal proliferation. Note elastic fibrils in wall. (Verhoeff's elastic stain, ×110.)

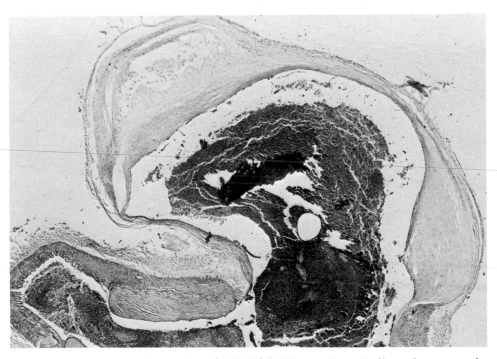

Fig. 9-31. Aneurysm with a wall of variable thickness. Note hyaline plaque on the right and atheromatous plaque on the left near the fundus. (Hematoxylin and eosin, ×25.)

surface of the sac wall and rapidly becomes stretched out, with the fine elastic fibrils normally seen in the adventitia usually lost. A few lymphocytes are occasionally found in the adventitia near the neck of large aneurysms.

The thickness of the sac wall even within the same aneurysm varies considerably (Fig. 9-31). Some aneurysms have fairly cellular walls, the cellularity being due to plain muscle fibers, which can be large and stellate as in the arterial intima. These cel-

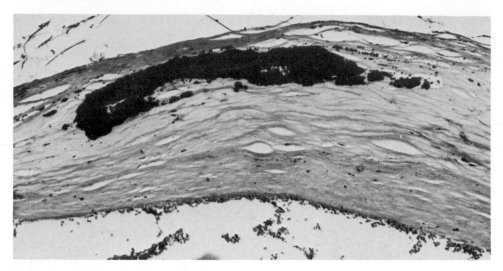

Fig. 9-32. Acellular hyaline wall of an aneurysm with calcification. (Hematoxylin and eosin, ×110.)

lular areas often form localized plaque-like thickenings of the sac wall and, except for the paucity of elastica in the aneurysms, are similar to those occurring at arterial bifurcations. Metachromasia particularly is seen in these cellular zones with the thickenings often at the sides of the sac and rarely at the neck. When the sac wall is reflected upon the parent vessel, the thickening appeared to be located, like lateral pads at arterial forks, in the stagnation area.

Larger and presumably older sacs usually have less cellular walls in which acellular hyaline fibrous tissue is the major constituent (Fig. 9-32). Lipophages or calcific stippling occur and ossification is rare. Occasionally small numbers of polymorphonuclear leukocytes are seen in the inner part of the wall.

The outer surface of the sac is covered by a thin layer of loose fibrous tissue corresponding to and continuous with the adventitia of the parent artery. In very old aneurysms with hyaline walls, distinctive adventitial tissue may be barely discernible. At times a few lymphocytes and vasa vasorum may be seen in or on the surface of this tissue. Meningeal reaction to extravasated blood may lead to considerable perianeurysmal fibrosis in which blood pigment is prominent.

Remnants of degenerate elastic tissue, though found mostly in the neck, can occur elsewhere in the sac wall. Pale staining elastic tissue has been observed beneath the endothelium and also close to the adventitial layer. As many as 3 or 4 laminae may be discernible but sometimes the elastica lies in irregularly curled masses or curlicues. Thin elastic fibrils are usually too pale-staining to photograph satisfactorily and the elastic tissue is never as extensive or prominent as in the intima of cerebral arteries.

Lipid is present in all large aneurysms examined for fat appearing as a diffuse fine stippling with lipid-laden macrophages prominent in the heavier deposits (Fig. 9-33). It is found particularly in the plaque-like thickenings. In some instances, large necrotic pultaceous areas of atheroma may be found in the walls (Fig. 9-31); these areas are then indistinguishable from very atheromatous arteries in which the normal architecture is completely destroyed. In older sacs containing organizing thrombus, lipid is also found in lipophages of the granulation tissue.

Atherosclerosis, indicated by the presence of foam cells or lipophages and/or cholesterol clefts, has been found histologically in 96% of 100 cases in which arterial forks

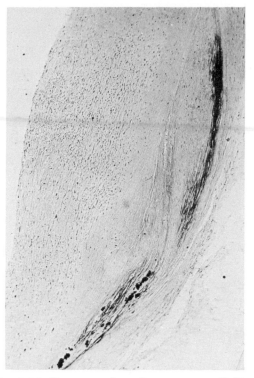

Fig. 9-33. Frozen section of aneurysm wall displaying lipid in the laminated wall. Note similarity to the intimal thickening seen in arteries. (Hematoxylin and oil red O, ×35.)

with aneurysms were serially sectioned. This criterion for atherosclerosis is of course quite conservative, for considerable amounts of lipid could precede the lipophages and cholesterol clefts. The examination of material using fat stains probably would have increased the frequency. The overt atherosclerosis indicates that the cerebral arteries of these patients have been the site of acquired degenerative changes.

Aneurysms from patients with polycystic disease of the kidneys and coarctation of the aorta are the same histologically as those in older patients.

Rupture of the aneurysm. The wall is usually thin and tapering at the site of rupture. Fibrin tags usually adhere to the edges and patchy fibrin infiltration is common in the neighboring sac wall, particularly on the inner aspect, where it sometimes forms a definite layer of thrombus (Fig. 9-22).

In small sacs, part of the wall may consist of thrombus (mostly fibrin), indicating that at this probably still vulnerable site there has been the possibility of rupture (Fig. 9-16). In larger aneurysms, small nodules are merely false sacs in which rupture is often imminent. Rupture tends to occur near the fundus. Recent thrombosis within the sac is always found to be associated with evidence of rupture or infiltration of part of the wall with blood and fibrin. The latter suggests impending rupture. The mural thrombus in the sac may become endothelialized and eventually organized. Moderate numbers of inflammatory cells may be present if such organization is underway, but large aneurysms presumably of long duration and containing laminated thrombus in abundance generally exhibit little effective organization. Small vessels participating in the repair process or organization may take origin from the luminal surface of the aneurysm[475] as they would from any other blood vessel. Intracellular blood pigment is to be seen in the wall. False sacs may equal the primary sac in size and their walls consist of an internal layer of thrombus mostly of fibrin, another layer of quite cellular connective tissue with large plump fibroblasts, many inflammatory cells, and pigment-laden macrophages that merge externally with meningeal tissues and vessels with evidence of hemogenic meningitis (Fig. 9-23).

Histopathology of saccular aneurysms unrelated to arterial forks. The parent artery exhibits advanced atherosclerosis, the media often being barely discernible. Calcification and vasa vasorum may be prominent, with round cell infiltrations in the adventitia and advanced elastic tissue destruction. The sac wall may join the parent artery at a reflected angle or in a direct line, depending on the plane of section and the size of the sac. The sac wall is composed of hyalinized fibrous tissue of variable thickness and is often considerably thinned near the fundus. The adventitia is compressed, thin, and devoid of elastic fibrils. Atheroma, vasa vasorum, calcification, hemosiderin-laden macrophages, and round cell infiltrations may be seen in the wall. Laminated mural thrombus is frequent within the sac and tends to merge with the wall, and thrombus organization is very limited. Calcification in the wall is frequent.

Early aneurysmal changes. Early aneurysmal changes at arterial forks are of the following three types: (1) funnel-shaped dilatations, (2) areas of thinning, and (3) microscopic evaginations. It is believed that these lesions ultimately develop into the small saccular aneurysms that occur in the apex of bifurcations.[475]

Funnel-shaped dilatations. Funnel-shaped dilatations[236,468,475] most frequently affect the origin of small branches such as the posterior communicating arteries from the internal carotid (Fig. 9-34). The dilatations are shaped like a steer horn, with the greatest curvature on the distal side of

their attachment to the main trunk. There are gradations to the stage of overt aneurysmal dilatations, which may be bilateral. Stehbens[473] found these lesions in 10% of 96 circles of Willis with saccular aneurysms, though they also occur independently of aneurysms.

Histologically there is considerable thinning in the area of greatest convexity (apical region).[475] The wall is attenuated, with the media often gradually tapering and finally disappearing but never ending abruptly. The intima is slightly thickened and the internal elastic lamina grossly degenerate, fragmented, or deficient over large areas, and to the greatest degree in the area of thinning. Evidence of an apical defect may or may not be found. The wall can be so thin as to consist of little more than fibrous tissue. Aneurysmal dilatation is obviously imminent. As the commence-

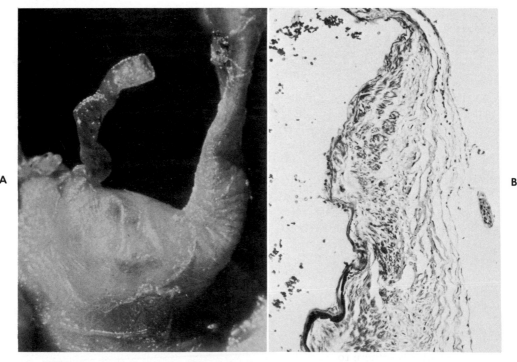

Fig. 9-34. A, Funnel-shaped dilatation at origin of posterior communicating artery from internal carotid artery. Wall at site of maximum curvature is thin and tends to buckle readily. **B,** Histologically, the thinning is associated with attenuation and fibrosis of the media, elastic tissue degeneration, and thinning of the adventitia. (**B,** Verhoeff's elastic stain, ×120.)

ment of the vessel is already dilated, theoretically it is aneurysmal though not saccular.

Areas of thinning. Macroscopically areas
of thinning either small or extensive are
found involving the apical region and adjacent aspect of the distal side of the
daughter branches of large bifurcations
(Fig. 9-35). The thin area is transparent
and contrasts with the opacity and atherosclerosis of the vessel wall nearby. The
lesions, which are closely related to the
funnel-shaped dilatations, are readily found
at the bifurcations of the middle cerebral
and internal carotid arteries,[475] though
they are seen elsewhere.

Histologically, the outstanding feature
of the lesion is gross thinning of the wall.
The early aneurysm may be found adjacent to but not involving the apex (Fig.
9-36). When the apex is involved, the adventitia is thinned and no longer forms the
connective tissue wedge of Forbus' medial
gaps[177]; the adventitial elastic fibrils stain
poorly and may have partially disappeared.
As in the funnel-shaped dilatations, the

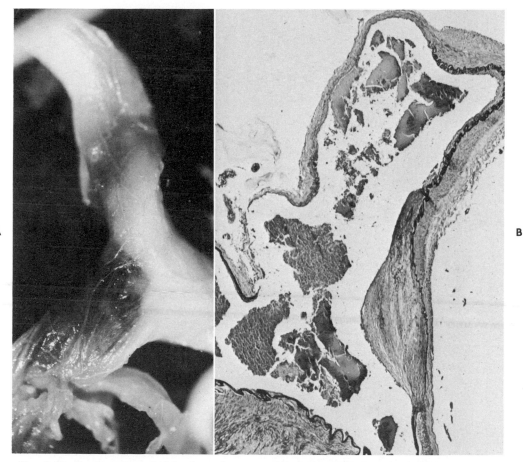

A

B

Fig. 9-35. A, An area of thinning of an arterial fork. Wall is quite transparent and
contrasts with the opacity of the thicker wall elsewhere. **B,** Fork exhibits considerable
thinning of media and adventitia with gross loss of elastica along the distal side of
daughter branch. Media is still visible along most of the wall except for one area,
which bulges. Note lateral pad and medial gap and its extension along proximal side
of the branch. (**B,** Verhoeff's elastic stain, ×32. **B,** From Stehbens, W. E.: Histopathology
of cerebral aneurysms, Arch. Neurol. **8:**272, 1963.)

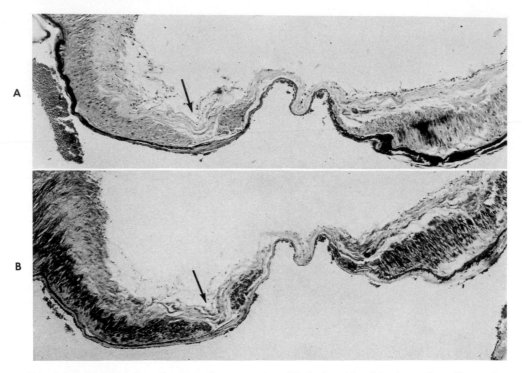

Fig. 9-36. Neighboring sections from an arterial fork with thinning of wall to the side of the apex (*arrow*). Thinning of the media and elastic loss are not inconsiderable. This early aneurysm formation involves the wall to the side of the apex rather than the medial gap. (**A,** Verhoeff's elastic stain; **B,** Mallory's phosphotungstic and hematoxylin, ×45. **B,** From Stehbens, W. E.: Histopathology of cerebral aneurysms, Arch. Neurol. 8:272, 1963.)

media at the edges is attenuated and fibrotic and the intimal elastica grossly deficient. The wall may be as thin and convoluted in sections as if redundant. In some instances the apex with its apical pad and medial gap (defect) are to be seen to the side of the thin zone with an intervening segment of media (Fig. 9-36). An aneurysm seems to be forming and the apex is either uninvolved or likely to be involved secondarily as the neck enlarges and takes up more and more of the adjacent arterial wall.

In Fig. 9-35 the area of thinning extends for a considerable distance along the distal side of the daughter branch. The contrast in the proximal and distal sides of the wall in this fork is quite striking. There is a large lateral pad with extension along the proximal side of the branch, whereas the distal side exhibits gross loss of elastica and

thinning of both media and adventitia. Part of this area, to the side of the apex, is extremely thin and resembles a small aneurysmal sac wall.

Carmichael[77] was under the misapprehension that areas of thinning were but larger examples of Forbus' gaps, some of which are known to be present at birth. Areas of thinning and funnel-shaped dilatations have been differentiated from Forbus' medial gaps or discontinuities as follows:

1. Forbus' medial gaps are much more common.
2. Forbus' defects are prevalent in the posterior half of the circle of Willis, whereas these lesions and aneurysms are much less common posteriorly.[77]
3. The lesions occur at or to the side of the apex and can coexist with the medial defects of Forbus.[475]
4. These lesions do not occur at the lateral

angle where Forbus' defects are prevalent.[469]

5. These lesions bulge when perfused under a pressure of 30 cm. of water,[77] whereas Forbus' defects do not bulge under a pressure of 60 cm. of mercury.[197]

6. They have not been seen in the cerebral arteries of infants or fetuses, nor have they been observed in the limited study of extracranial vessels. Forbus' ubiquitous defects on the other hand are present in all humans (both intracranially and extracranially) including fetuses and infants and also in all mammals studied. Carmichael[77] found a few lesions in the first decade, but his figures indicated an increase in incidence with age. Hassler[234] found similar lesions to be most prevalent in elderly subjects. In Stehbens' investigation,[475] the youngest subject with such a lesion was a man of 23 years with aortic coarctation; there were only 3 under 40 years of age, and the remainder were middle-aged or elderly.

7. There are considerable differences in the morphology. Forbus' gaps are smaller, being areas of partial or complete medial discontinuity, and the media ends fairly abruptly. The intervening gap is filled with collagen and elastic fibrils, that is, apparently normal adventitial tissue. On the other hand in the areas of thinning and funnel-shaped dilatations the media is grossly attenuated and may be deficient. The adventitia is thin and attenuated with loss of elastica, and the intima is associated with degenerative changes and loss of elastica more so than with Forbus' gaps. Moreover the thin segments of wall often display folding histologically intimating redundancy.

The areas of thinning and funnel-shaped swellings are related to aneurysm formation.[77,475] Carmichael[77] presumed them to be areas of hypoplasia or aplasia of the vessel wall, but their absence in the infant and fetus repudiates his conjectures. Carmichael* viewed elastic tissue degeneration as an essential part of aneurysm formation, believing that its occurrence at the apical angle was fortuitous. This is not substantiated by the study of serial histological sections of several hundred arterial forks of fetuses, infants, adults, and other animals (without aneurysms). In such forks, elastic tissue degeneration occurs at the apex and is less severe than in forks with early aneurysmal changes. The destruction of the elastic lamina appears to play an important role in initiating the aneurysm.

Small evaginations. The small evaginations are microscopic in size.[475] They do not extend beyond the adventitia and are not visible from the external surface, being found only by serial or random sections primarily in acute-angled forks. The apex is often slightly blunt and the evagination frequently involves only part of the medial discontinuity or gap (defect), or only the facial extension is involved and the remainder of the medial gap does not bulge despite extensive elastic tissue degeneration (Fig. 9-37). The evagination may commence at the side of the medial defect with an intervening segment of media, part of which may be incorporated in the side wall of the sac. The herniation therefore appears to be into rather than of the medial gap or defect, and the adventitia is stretched only in the neighborhood of the evagination.

Forbus[177] illustrated two small evaginations, both of which involved only portion of the medial gap or defect. In one, the media was stretched around the side of the evagination as if it too had been involved and elastic degeneration was prominent in both. Richardson and Hyland[400] illustrated one. Hassler[234] demonstrated two seemingly similar lesions and both had prominent elastic tissue changes. Stehbens[475] discovered 14. In two forks the elastic lamina was fairly complete despite fragmentation, duplication, and variation in thickness with intimal thickening at the entrance. The wall of one of these two sacs was extensively infiltrated with fibrin, red cells, and leukocytes, all extending through an apparent tear in the internal elastic lamina and continuous with a mural thrombus in the lumen of the small sac. In the remaining forks there was gross loss of elastica even beyond the confines of the medial gap. The full extent of the elastic tissue deficiency can be appreciated only by serial sections. Proliferation of fibrillary elastic lam-

---

*Carmichael[77] made no systematic study of the elastic tissue changes in his material, since his methods did not include elastic stains. Therefore he was unable to appreciate the frequency and severity of the elastic tissue degeneration.

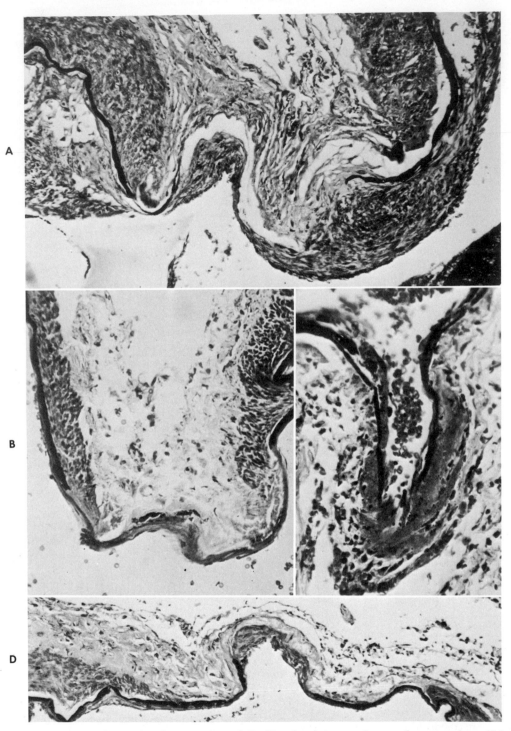

Fig. 9-37. Small evaginations. **A, B** and **D,** Evaginations are into only part of medial gap and are associated with severe elastic tissue degeneration. There is blunting of the apex in **A,** intimal proliferation (muscle) in the evagination in **A** and **D,** and in **C** there is fragmentation of the elastic lamina and infiltration of the wall with fibrin and red cells. In a section adjoining **C,** a small tear was found and the fibrin infiltration was continuous with a small mural thrombus in the sac. (Verhoeff's elastic stain; **A,** ×110; **B,** ×225; **C,** ×300; **D,** ×100.)

inae or of fibromuscular tissue has been described in a few sacs.[475]

Forbus[177] thought these small evaginations evidence of weakness of the medial defect, but involvement does not necessarily signify causation. Only part of the defect was involved in both of the evaginations he demonstrated, and the media was incorporated in one, suggesting that the media and defect are only secondarily affected. It has been explained[475] that if defects were areas of weakness, one would expect that the whole gap would be affected and that similar lesions would also occur at lateral angles, but such is not the case. Forbus also alleged that the intima bulged into the medial gap, which he had assumed was an area of weakness. He believed that the internal elastic lamina subsequently underwent degeneration secondary to the strain of overdistension. However, the elastic tissue degeneration is often considerably more extensive than either the evagination or the medial defect and may occur either in the absence of or at some distance from a medial gap, indicating that important alterations of adventitial tissue and/or media must precede the evagination.

The presence in the sac of the internal elastic lamina, though fragmented and duplicated in places, may be attributed to the persistence or regeneration of the original lamina. However, the histological appearance of tissues, both collagen and elastica, gives no indication of their functional state, and tensile strength in particular.[407,475] It is highly likely that in a few instances evagination precedes the histological loss of the elastic lamina, but in most instances the evagination occurs subsequent to the disappearance of the elastic tissue.

Except in the fork illustrated in Fig. 9-40, *C*, associated with a mural thrombus and fibrin infiltration of the sac, there is no evidence that inflammatory change or fibrinoid necrosis occurs in the early lesions or plays a role in the pathogenesis. It is highly likely that these three varieties of preaneurysmal change are acquired and

form early stages of aneurysm formation.[475]

Ultrastructure of saccular arterial aneurysms. Barely adequate ultrastructural studies of these aneurysms have been made, since the material is difficult to obtain. Nyström[358,359] and Lang and Kidd[293] have contributed little more than was available from light microscopy.[475] Detail was insufficient and technical difficulties had not been mastered. Nyström[358] described a beaded connective tissue fiber that he regarded as atypical collagen, but this was not confirmed by Lang and Kidd.[293] The occurrence of endothelium, plain muscle fibers, and collagen, together with a paucity of elastic tissue, can be seen by light microscopy. Lang and Kidd also found fibroblasts, which however may be modified plain muscle cells as seen in the venous walls of experimental arteriovenous fistulas.[482] Intensive study of small aneurysms and early aneurysmal changes should provide information of significance, especially when compared with changes in vessel walls subjected to similar hemodynamic stresses.

Aneurysms of extracranial arteries of comparable size. As indicated elsewhere saccular cerebral aneurysms are common in man but rare in extracranial arteries of comparable size, such as the splanchnic arteries and those of the musculoskeletal system. Excluding traumatic, bacterial, and mycotic aneurysms and polyarteritis nodosa, the two most frequent causes commonly cited are atherosclerosis and "congenital factors." Criteria used in diagnosis have usually been inadequate. Most such aneurysms arise from the apex of the arterial forks and have been likened to those of the cerebral arteries, but they have a thicker media and adventitia, and abundant elastica in the adventitia. The medial gaps (defects) have much more elastic tissue in the adventitial wedge and a thicker wall. Perivascular tissue around the splanchnic arteries will add strength and support, but about the cerebral arteries there is only displaceable fluid and flimsy arachnoidal filaments. Extracranial aneurysms therefore because of structural differences may occur less frequently.

Cerebral aneurysms of animals other than man. Despite the apparent universal occurrence of medial gaps in mammalian cerebral arteries and histological similarity to human cerebral arteries, cerebral aneurysms are almost exclusively restricted to *Homo sapiens.* The rarity of spontaneous subarachnoid hemorrhage and apoplexy[418] suggests that cerebral aneurysms are uncommon lesions in lower animals. Goldberg[199] found that cerebrovascular disease was not once the cause of death in approximately 2000 domestic animals. Atherosclerosis occurs in lower animals but generally to a considerably milder degree, whereas intimal thickening about their cerebral arterial forks is found if diligently sought by serial section.[477-479]

A cerebral aneurysm, parasitic in nature, was reported by Köppen[287] in a colt. Ask-Upmark and Ingvar[15] reported one in a llama without details of etiology. Hassler[234] reported what he believed was a minute aneurysm in a cow, but uncertainty existed because of inadequate sectioning. Stehbens[474] recorded a subarachnoid hemorrhage in an 8-year-old female chimpanzee *(Pan troglodytes).* Bleeding was caused by a ruptured aneurysm and eight cerebral aneurysms were found. These were histologically identical to those that occur in man, and atherosclerosis was a very prominent feature of the cerebral arteries (Fig. 3-21) and the walls of several sacs. Unruptured aneurysms were found in the bifurcations of middle cerebral arteries of two chimpanzees receiving a high coconut oil cholesterol diet[10] and were not attributed to the experimental diet.

Stehbens[474] found four minute or early evaginations in cerebral arterial forks of a young gorilla *(Gorilla gorilla gorilla)* but no frank aneurysm formation was observed. In a series of 122 sheep, no aneurysms were found except for one instance of polyarteritis nodosa.[474] A study of aged primates, particularly the chimpanzee, might be more fruitful.

Crompton[116] attributed the difference in the incidence of cerebral aneurysms between man and lower animals to cerebral size, arterial hypertension, longevity, and structural differences in the arteries. Brain size is probably not as important per se as is the caliber of the vessels, for in man the berry type of aneurysm rarely occurs on very small vessels. Hypertension is prevalent in patients with cerebral aneurysms and certainly seems to be a contributing, though not an essential, factor in the etiology. Little is known of hypertension in other animals. Crompton[116] asserted that medial defects were smaller in lower animals than in man. His investigation did not include the use of serial sections and neither the age nor comparative differences in the size of the arteries were considered. There is little difference in the structure of cerebral arteries from man and lower animals, though in some animals, such as the steer, the walls appear to be slightly thicker. It is possible that the mode of slaughter of the animal may be a factor in provoking vasoconstriction.

Cerebral aneurysms are then rare in lower animals because of the comparatively short life-span, the smaller caliber of the cerebral arteries, and the lesser incidence of atherosclerosis.

Etiology of saccular arterial aneurysms. The etiology of cerebral aneurysms, though fundamental, has been a controversial subject for many years. There are currently two basic views. The first is that they are the result of maldevelopment of the cerebral arteries—the so-called congenital theory. The second is that they are caused by acquired degenerative changes in the arterial wall—the degeneration theory. Proponents of a third concept contend that the etiology can be ascribed to factors from both theories in combination.

The congenital theory. In 1859 Gull[212] analyzed 62 cases collected mostly from the literature and he stated that an aneurysm "may be a simple pouch of all the coats [of the vessel wall], the pouched portion being as transparent and normal in appearance as the rest of the vessel, [and] giving the impression that it might have been some original deformity." At a loss to explain the pathogenesis in a young person in the absence of an evident macroscopic disease, he alluded to the possibility of a congenital origin of cerebral aneurysms, although Lancisi[202] was probably the first to infer that a congenital defect may be the cause of extracranial aneurysmal dilatation.[469] Lebert[296] noted that the cerebral arteries of some patients with a cerebral aneurysm did not exhibit atherosclerosis macroscopically, and Eppinger[164] arbitrarily labeled them congenital, stating that they were caused by an inborn defect of the elastic properties of the arterial wall. This theory, virtually a conjecture and based exclusively on a hypothetical congenital weakness of the arterial wall, the existence of which is difficult to prove or disprove, became popular and dominated thinking on this subject henceforth. However, the validity of this congenital or developmental theory is dependent on a certain amount of circumstantial evidence most of which will not withstand scientific or statistical analysis. Tenacious proponents usually proffer the following criteria in substantiation: age, multiplicity of aneurysms, variations of the circle of Willis, persistence of vestigial vessels, familial occurrence, medial gaps, associated congenital abnormalities, and associated cerebral arteriovenous aneurysms.

AGE. It is accepted, even by most protagonists of the congenital theory, that the aneurysms are not present at birth, being in fact acquired lesions, nor are they frequent in young children.[398,403] Their incidence in young adults has been emphasized probably because of the chance prominence of bacterial aneurysms in the literature of the last century.[212,383] The age distribution of cerebral aneurysms quite decidedly does not support a congenital theory; the mean age of patients with cerebral aneurysms is approximately 50 years, the majority occurring between 40 and 70 years, an age when complications of atherosclero-

sis are likely to be manifest. The occasional report of an aneurysm in a young person is no basis for a "congenital" theory. Furthermore, age cannot be used as a criterion in distinguishing "congenital" in the young from "acquired" aneurysms in the aged because on histological or other grounds they cannot be differentiated and it is erroneous to assume that degenerative diseases do not occur in the young.

MULTIPLICITY OF ANEURYSMS. The incidence of multiplicity of cerebral aneurysms in individual brains lends no support to the congenital theory because it is also associated with extracranial aneurysms reliably regarded as arteriosclerotic in origin.[101]

VARIATIONS OF THE CIRCLE OF WILLIS. Unfortunately anatomical variations of the circle of Willis have been called congenital abnormalities, yet vascular variability is a frequent feature of the cerebral arterial tree in man and other animals (Chapter 1). Regarding minor differences in size or symmetry as congenital anomalies is remarkable presumption. There is little to substantiate the supposition that anatomical variations of the small cerebral arteries are congenital anomalies and certainly there is no evidence that such variations indicate the presence of diverse underlying weaknesses of the arterial wall. Arterial variation is usual in the cerebral arterial tree of other animals.[473] Yet if these arterial variations indicate an underlying developmental defect that is the cause of cerebral aneurysms, one would expect aneurysms to occur frequently in such animals. This is not the case, and the lack of correlation in other animals suggests that the anatomical variations have no direct bearing on the pathogenesis of these aneurysms.

Neither are variations of the circle of Willis more prevalent with aneurysms than in the general population,[117,473] a belief based falsely on Padget's study of the posterior communicating and the divisional branch of the basilar artery. Her corrected results[473] contradicted her contention that variations are significantly more frequent in patients with aneurysms than in those without, and therefore little reliance should be placed on her conclusions.

One anatomical variation, that is, inequality of the proximal segments of the anterior cerebral arteries, is the only anatomical variation that has been correlated with the location of the aneurysm, and this relationship could be caused by hemodynamic factors rather than hypothetical congenital factors.

PERSISTENCE OF VESTIGIAL VESSELS. Drennan[145,146] postulated that the origin of a small vessel from the apex of a fork might constitute a site for potential aneurysm formation and that minor hypothetical defects in vascular plumbing whether degenerative, developmental, or infective might induce an aneurysm at such a site. Drennan's hypothesis has not been substantiated. In several hundred arterial forks studied by serial sections for medial defects,[468,469,475] small vestigial vessels were never found to arise directly from the apex, irrespective of whether an apical defect was present or not. Some middle cerebral arteries divide abruptly into three large branches, but this is not the configuration implied by Drennan. Moreover small vessels were never found to take origin from early aneurysmal lesions or small aneurysms, nor was there any evidence that the lesions arose from structures that could be interpreted as abnormal vestiges of the primitive capillary anlage. Diffuse early aneurysmal changes could conceivably involve the origin of small vessels and it is possible that small vessels arising from large aneurysms could be obliterated. However a vessel has been found to arise from the lumen of an aneurysm only in the organization of a false sac.[475] Occasionally vasa vasorum are seen in thick atheromatous aneurysm walls but their origin has not been traced to the lumen of the sac.

Busse[70] described small knoblike or club-shaped dilatations of small vessels in the vicinity of the anterior communicating artery. Bremer[62] reported dilatations on small arteries at the same site in an infant. Neither of the authors investigated the histological appearance of the structures. Bremer[62] considered that aneurysms might result if vessels of the primitive capillary plexus failed to atrophy and disappear.[62] However, if this were so, small vessels would arise from the sac wall. None has been found. Padget[370] and others[262,402,455] believed that Bremer's contention was favored by the prevalence of anatomical variations of the circle of Willis, but their sanguine expectations have a poor foundation. The only structures resembling that which Bremer[62] wrote of were found by Stehbens[474,479] in one adult patient and in one sheep. In both instances the arteries revealed polyarteritis histologically. Bremer's hypothesis in the absence of histological evidence cannot be seriously considered as in any way convincing despite the dogmatic affirmation of its validity by some authors.[30]

Moreover, there is no basis for believing that any of the primitive vascular plexus atrophies. The vascular bed has to increase in the growing brain, and all such endothelial tubes are probably incorporated into the vascular system. A number of facts appears to have been overlooked. Firstly, all arteries throughout the body in man and other animals arise from a primitive capillary plexus, and yet the aneurysms are rare except on the large cerebral arteries of man. Secondly, the property of endothelial tubes or capillaries to proliferate and dwindle as required is retained throughout life and is one of the fundamental features of inflammation and repair. It is also evident in atherosclerotic plaques. Therefore, if the hypothesis holds, the aneurysms could well be acquired, and there is not a shred of evidence to indicate that components of the primitive capillary plexus fail to be incorporated into the circulation as arteries, veins, or capillaries. Thirdly, such hypothetical vestiges of the capillary plexus would acquire arterial coats because the vascular system maintains its ability to develop these mural constituents. Lastly, the proliferation of muscle, elastic tissue, and collagen in the aneurysm wall after its formation tends to negate the possibility of origin from vestigial capillary tubes incapable of acquiring adequate connective tissue support. In the absence of any positive evidence to sustain the theory that aneurysms arise from vestiges of the primitive capillary network, it should be discarded.

FAMILIAL OCCURRENCE. The occasional report of a familial case of cerebral aneurysms lends little support to the congenital theory. In view of the familial occurrence of diseases such as spontaneous cerebral hemorrhage, essential hypertension and coronary occlusion, isolated case reports cannot be seriously considered. A very large scale investigation would have to be performed to confirm any significant hereditary tendency apart from those patients who have a hereditary connective tissue disorder that may or may not be complicated by aneurysm formation.

MEDIAL GAPS (DEFECTS). There has been considerable misconception concerning the nature of medial gaps (defects) at the bifurcations and branchings of cerebral arteries. Forbus[177] unfortunately called them defects of congenital origin and linked the presence of defects at the site of the fork where aneurysms occur with the absence of a distinct media in the sac wall. Later authors have generally accepted them as *loci minoris resistentiae* where aneurysms are prone to occur. Their anatomical distribution and significance are discussed in Chapter 2.

Detailed study of a large number of arterial forks by the serial section technique has demonstrated that the anatomical distribution of cerebral aneurysms differs from that of medial gaps because of the following reasons:

1. The prevalence of medial gaps at apices of cerebral arterial forks increases with age, and so all defects cannot be held to be congenital.[469]

2. Lateral angles, where aneurysms never occur, are common sites for medial gaps, almost all of which are acquired after birth (Chapter 2).

3. There is variation in the prevalence of the gaps with the angle of bifurcation, which sug-

gests the influence of a mechanical factor in the localization (Chapter 2).

4. Medial gaps are common in both large and small cerebral arteries, yet aneurysms are restricted to the larger vessels.[469,473]

5. Medial gaps are probably universal in the cerebral arteries of man, in contrast to the lower frequency of aneurysms.

6. Indications are that medial gaps are universal in the cerebral arterial forks of other animals, despite the rarity of aneurysms in other animals (Chapter 2).

7. Medial gaps appear to be universal in extracranial arterial forks of other animals and man, a distribution contrasting with the low frequency of aneurysms in these vessels.[474,476]

8. Medial gaps occur at the forks of human meningeal and spinal arteries, whereas aneurysms of these vessels are exceedingly rare.

9. No more reason exists for believing medial gaps are developmental abnormalities than for believing intimal pads are of a similar origin.

It can be concluded only that the role of medial gaps or discontinuities is not of prime importance in the etiology of cerebral aneurysms. This thesis is supported by the fact that the thinning or early evagination sometimes affects the medial gap and sometimes the neighboring distal wall of the daughter branch. Medial gaps at times are not at all involved in the early aneurysmal change. The gaps are secondarily incorporated rather than causative factors of the thinning or evagination.

The abrupt termination of the media at the entrance to cerebral aneurysms has been emphasized and has led authors to conclude that aneurysms result from bulging of the defect. The improbable assumption is that an abrupt termination of the muscle must be congenital. As most gaps are acquired after birth (Chapter 2), a similar histological appearance at the mouth of cerebral aneurysms could surely be an acquired feature also. Moreover, the entrances to most cerebral aneurysms are considerably wider than medial defects, and fairly abrupt terminations of the media are seen even in aneurysms with necks wider than medial gaps. Hence secondary widening of the sac entrance must eventuate. When the enormous local expansion of the lumen with the ensuing architectural alteration of the dilated vessel wall is considered, it is not surprising that the normal appearance of the media ceases fairly abruptly at the entrance to localized saccular aneurysms. Authors have had difficulty in understanding the transition from arterial to aneurysmal wall. They have been unaware that extreme proliferation of tissue must occur concomitantly with the great expansion of the involved segment of the wall, the architecture of which is retained in neither extracranial nor intracranial aneurysms. The absence of a distinct media in the sac wall does not denote a developmental origin any more than does the absence of a media in advanced atherosclerosis. The histological appearance of the advanced lesion does not necessarily indicate from which coats of the arterial wall the sac was derived, many of its features being secondary and acquired after inception. Emphasis has been placed on the absence of a media, and this has been correlated with Forbus' gaps.[177] Yet there is a virtual absence of elastica and in many aneurysms no distinct intima or adventitia exists. Moreover, aneurysms do not always develop through the defects.

According to one variant of the congenital theory, the aneurysm at the fork may arise from defective tissue, which may or may not be the medial defect. Such defective tissue might not be able to differentiate into the connective tissues of the arterial wall. However, detailed histological studies of cerebral aneurysms[475] indicate that the sac wall retains the reactions of the arterial wall, that is, the proliferation of endothelium, muscle, elastic tissue, and collagen. The development of advanced atherosclerosis even with vasa vasorum, and the ability to organize and repair are still retained by the sac wall, all of which leads to the conclusion that it is unlikely that defective tissue constitutes that portion of the wall from which the early sac develops.

ASSOCIATED CONGENITAL ABNORMALITIES. The coexistence of congenital abnormalities with cerebral aneurysms has no statistical significance. However, cerebral aneurysms frequently occur with polycystic disease of the kidneys and coarctation of the aorta, the only two congenital diseases commonly associated with hypertension. The coexistence of the lesions is in all probability due to the concomitant hypertension and premature atherosclerosis rather than to hypothetical congenital factors.

ASSOCIATED CEREBRAL ARTERIOVENOUS ANEURYSMS. The coexistence of arteriovenous aneurysm and saccular aneurysms of the cerebral arteries has been regarded as an instance of the association of two congenital abnormalities. Underlying hemodynamic factors in all probability are responsible for the development of cerebral aneurysms in patients with arteriovenous aneurysms (Chapter 10).

In conclusion, it can be stated categorically that the theory attesting to the congenital weakness as either the cause or a contributory factor in the etiology of cerebral aneurysms is based on feeble and unscientific evidence. The undeserved respectability of the congenital theory brings to mind Bean's words[34] concerning the perpetuation of another erroneous belief, that is, it "illustrates the ratio between the small work of making a positive but wrong assertion and the effort needed to demonstrate its invalidity, since science never proves a negative. Someone with authority and enthusiasm makes an uncontrolled observation, or an eager assistant makes it for him. It becomes established in what with innocent euphemism we call 'the literature.' It carries the mystical potency of the written word in an age when mere literacy exposes the uncritical to the hazard of believing whatever they read." The congenital theory, born of opinion, has enjoyed a comparable longevity.

The degeneration theory. The proponents of the degeneration theory assert that aneurysms occurring in the forks of cerebral arteries are the result of degenerative changes in the arterial wall and are thus acquired, in the true sense of the word.[197,475] Mounting evidence in support of this concept is becoming quite formidable; it depends on age, hypertension, congenital abnormalities, early aneurysmal changes, atherosclerosis, and intimal changes.

AGE. Cerebral aneurysms occur at an age when acquired degenerative diseases are known to become manifest.

HYPERTENSION. The evidence suggests, though not conclusively, that hypertension is unduly prevalent in patients with cerebral aneurysms.

CONGENITAL ABNORMALITIES. Cerebral aneurysms frequently complicate coarctation of the aorta and polycystic disease of the kidneys, the only two congenital diseases outside the cranium that are generally associated with hypertension. Study of the relationships suggests that the association is attributable to the concomitant hypertension and premature, severe arterial degenerative disease. Both diseases are also known to be associated with extracranial aneurysms, most of which are indubitably acquired, and there is no reason for doubting that cerebral aneurysms are of similar etiology.

EARLY ANEURYSMAL CHANGES. More reliance must be placed on the characteristics of early or preaneurysmal lesions than on those of advanced aneurysms. Early aneurysmal changes occur at a mean age of 56.5 years when degenerative vascular disease becomes manifest.[473]

ATHEROSCLEROSIS. There is indirect evidence that severe atherosclerosis is prevalent among subjects with cerebral aneurysms. Investigations by Crawford[105] and Du Boulay[147] produced evidence indicating that atherosclerosis is severe and of high incidence in victims of cerebral aneurysms. In an epidemiological survey,[426] hypertension, coronary artery, and ischemic heart disease were prevalent in patients with cerebral aneurysms. Crompton[114] noted an undue prominence of medial fibrosis. Atherosclerosis microscopically, as indicated by the presence of lipophages and/or cholesterol clefts, was present in the cerebral arteries of the large majority of patients with cerebral aneurysms sectioned serially.[475]

INTIMAL CHANGES. Serial sections indicate that intimal proliferation occurs at the mouths of all aneurysms and at the sites of early aneurysmal changes and thickens as the sac enlarges.[475] Early aneurysmal changes seem to be intimately associated with degenerative changes occurring about the fork, particularly of the elastica. The thinning of the wall and the elastic tissue destruction appear to be accentuations of alterations usually occurring at the apex of the forks, which change, as indicated,[470, 475,478] is an integral part of the atherosclerotic disease process.

Apical regions of arterial forks are not affected by chance alone as Carmichael suggested, but are the usual sites for intimal thickening and elastic tissue degeneration.[470] Hassler[234] and Crompton[114] found breaches in the elastic lamellae more frequently in subjects with cerebral aneurysms than in other individuals, and Glynn,[197] Carmichael,[77] and Walker and Allègre[518] regard the elastic tissue changes concerned with aneurysm formation as being degenerative. The elastic tissue degeneration is probably caused by the same factor that produces the thinning of the arterial wall at that site. Recent evidence has shown that these intimal changes about forks are integrally related to atherosclerosis. Moreover, in experimental arteriovenous fistulas, intimal thickening, destruction of elastic tissue, gross thinning of the media, and aneurysmal dilatation occur in the artery proximal to the anastomosis,[480] indicating the changes may be induced hemodynamically. Hence it is believed that cerebral aneurysms are acquired lesions, their etiology being closely related to that causing intimal proliferation and elastic tissue degeneration, which in turn appear to be intimately concerned with atherosclerosis.

Combined congenital and acquired factors. Eppinger[164] attributed these saccular cerebral aneurysms to an inborn defect in the elastic properties of the arterial wall or to a combination of congenital defects with subsequent degenerative or atheromatous processes. Forbus[177] considered the elastic tissue degeneration and intimal changes at the apex as an integral part of aneurysm formation but nevertheless secondary to dilatation of the allegedly defective arterial wall. Carmichael[77] concluded that both developmental and degenerative factors were concerned in the genesis of cerebral aneurysms, but mistakenly accepted medial gaps as early aneurysmal changes.[475] Authors[105,117,518] have also attributed them to a combination of factors without doubting the validity of the hypothetical congenital factors. Crawford[105] indicated that developmental faults, atherosclerosis, and hypertension played roles of varying importance according to the age at which the aneurysms developed despite their histological similarity at all ages. His concept ignores the young age at which overt atherosclerosis develops and the age at which degenerative intimal changes can occur microscopically. In essence it seems inaccurate to invoke the participation of hypothetical congenital factors.

MISCELLANEOUS FACTORS. Trauma has not been seriously regarded as a factor in the pathogenesis of this variety of aneurysm.

Handler and Blumenthal[221] postulated that cerebral aneurysms were the result of an inflammatory process, caused by an allergic phenomenon or an inapparent infectious agent, such as a virus or *Rickettsia*. In an extensive histological investigation of cerebral aneurysms and preaneurysmal lesions, no evidence for an inflammatory factor is to be found,[475] and the thesis cannot be supported.

CONCLUSION. Cerebral aneurysms are adjudged as being acquired degenerative lesions, and the age of the patient is incidental only. The development of early aneurysmal changes appears to be dependent on the following phenomena:

1. Naturally occurring degenerative changes in the walls of arterial forks, such changes being intimately related to atherosclerosis and etiologically related to the hemodynamic stresses at arterial forks (Chapter 3).

2. A tendency or its accentuation for a lesser compensatory formation of intimal thickening at the apex and distal side of the daughter branches in comparison with elsewhere at the fork[470,475] despite severe elastic degeneration.

3. Focal failure in either the tensile strength or the cohesive properties of the vessel wall in the region of the apex and adjoining distal surfaces of the daughter branches.[469] This permits the development of microscopic evaginations or thinning and slight dilatation. The loss of tensile strength also admits of further expansion of the aneurysm, incipient or frank rupture of the aneurysmal wall, and incidentally dissecting aneurysms and atherosclerotic ulceration and thrombosis. The histological appearances do not indicate where the vessel wall will yield or be broached, for the loss of tensile strength is evident only after the event.

Further information pertaining to the degenerative changes and hemodynamic stresses at arterial forks is the prerequisite for a more detailed outline of the pathogenesis of cerebral aneurysms.

Experimental production of saccular aneurysms. German and Black[188] successfully produced small saccular aneurysms of the common carotid artery in dogs by the insertion of a vein pouch. A segment of vein was removed, one end was sutured, and the other was anastomosed to a hole made in the artery. Such aneurysms were used to study flow and pressure within the sac.[52,189] No attempt has been made to use this technique within the cranial cavity, and it would be a formidable task, if one uses the smaller brain and arteries of the experimental animal.

McCune and associates[324] injected nitrogen mustard into the wall of dogs' aortas to produce experimental aneurysms. White and associates[535] succeeded in producing in dogs five lesions of the cerebral arteries that histologically resembled cerebral aneurysms of man. Four were produced by an intramural injection of hypertonic aqueous sodium chloride and the fifth by an injection of nitrogen mustard. However in another study[415] it was found that false aneurysms consistently formed after the cerebral artery was punctured. Long-term results were not studied.

Troupp and Rinne,[505] in an experimental study of the use of methyl-2-cyanoacrylate (Eastman 910) in closing an arterial wound, unexpectedly found that 16 of the 50 rabbits used had developed an aneurysm at the site of the arteriotomy. Presumably the lesions were false sacs, and it was suggested that this technique might be used in the production of intracranial aneurysms.

Such techniques as the above could conceivably be used to produce cerebral aneurysms for the investigation of hemodynamics, for the appraisal of various therapeutic procedures, and for the study of the secondary changes in the wall of aneurysms resembling intimal proliferation. They throw no light on the etiology.

Hassler[235] ligated the internal carotid artery in the neck of a series of rabbits and found that the altered hemodynamics had resulted in an increase in the size of some medial gaps. He alleged that there were aneurysm-like bulgings of the medial gaps in six animals. No distinct aneurysms resulted. This common surgical procedure does not cause aneurysms in man.

Obviously if a technique were available for inducing the development in experimental animals of saccular arterial aneurysms of the cerebral arteries, not only could the efficacy of therapeutic procedures and possibly of prophylactic measures be investigated, but the etiology and pathogenesis of cerebral berry aneurysms would be elucidated. The three experimental procedures most likely to be successful are the production of (1) experimental hypertension of severe degree, (2) coarctation of the aorta, and (3) cerebral arteriovenous fistulas. Experimental aortic coarctation was produced in a number of sheep, initially with the aim of producing aortic (other than poststenotic) or cerebral aneurysms. The changes in the aorta have been reported,[312] but no aneurysms were found macroscopically in the cerebral vessels.[482] It is likely that the experiment was terminated prematurely (at 6 years) and

that the sheep was an unsuitable animal since it has a rete mirabile proximal to the cerebral circulation. The most promising investigation in all probability is the production of experimental cerebral arteriovenous fistulas in a series of chimpanzees, provided that it is a long-term study.

Pathological results of treatment of saccular berry aneurysms. There have been numerous approaches to the treatment of intracranial arterial aneurysms, and changes, both beneficial and otherwise, will follow the application of these techniques. Basically the procedures are concerned with (1) the local reduction of blood pressure by induced hypotension or by Hunterian ligation, that is, ligation of the common carotid or internal carotid in the neck, (2) promotion of thrombosis within the sac in order to obliterate the lumen, (3) clipping or ligation of the base of the aneurysm, and (4) external reinforcement of the sac wall.

Carotid occlusion. Occlusion of the cervical portion of the carotid artery has been employed since 1855 for intracranial arterial aneurysm and for what was probably a posttraumatic carotid cavernous fistula.[95] Sweet and Bennett[489] demonstrated that in the cervical segment of the internal carotid artery distal to the ligature, the systolic pressure fell to about 50% and the pulse pressure to about 25% of the original level. It has since been confirmed that the intraarterial pressure intracranially can be reduced effectively by proximal internal or common carotid arterial occlusion.[21,499,547] Pressure reductions in arteries beyond the bifurcation of the internal carotid artery, that is, the intracranial internal carotid and middle and anterior cerebral arteries, are similar to those in the neck.[21,500] The fall in pressure and flow in vessels beyond the ligature or clamp will depend on the topography of the arterial tree and in particular upon the collateral circulation. The effect will thus vary with the individual, and in a total of 58 patients, the reduction in mean intracarotid pressure beyond the occlusion was less than 30% in six patients, from 30% to 40% in 14, from 41% to 50% in 18, from 51% to 60% in 13, and greater than 60% in 7 subjects.[500] Although the reduction in pressure within intracranial arteries (31% to 66%) is not sustained, it has been demonstrated in follow-up investigations that a significant pressure reduction is maintained in many instances (25% to 37%).[360,500] Ophthalmodynamometric retinal artery pressures substantiate these findings by indicating that between the two eyes the average difference in systolic pressures is 30% and in diastolic pressures 23%.[500] Christiansson[91] recorded a maintained reduction in pressure of 20% to 25% on the side of carotid occlusion several years postoperatively. In other words, the collateral circulation does not always restore the pressures to initial levels.

Wright[548] made direct pressure measurements within three aneurysms located on the middle cerebral artery, the results of which are documented in Table 9-10. In two of the patients the intra-aneurysmal pressures were suprisingly low before carotid occlusion. Spasm may have accounted for the low-pressure recordings in the third patient, and Wright attributed those in the second patient to a narrow aneurysmal neck. However, these results are at variance with those of Bakay and Sweet[21] whose figures provide a better correlation with Wright's first patient than with the other two. More intensive studies of intra-aneurysmal hemodynamics can be anticipated.

One major reason for carotid ligation is to reduce the stress on the aneurysmal wall and so enable beneficial healing processes to gain control over the adverse effects of the deranged pressure and flow within the sac. In discussing the stress factors after carotid ligation in the neck, Black and German[51] concluded that (1) a significant reduction in hydrostatic pressure occurs in the intracranial segment of the internal carotid artery, (2) the systolic pressure wave or water-hammer effect is materially reduced in the internal carotid artery, (3) the effects on the jet action would be to reduce the jet velocity by lowering the hydrostatic pressure head, whereas (4) the factor of turbulent flow would be difficult to assess. However, if, as seems very plausible, mechanical fatigue is responsible for rupture, reduction in pressure would delay the onset of fatigue and so healing processes may gain the ascendency. In addition a relative degree of stasis in the sac has been demonstrated by angiography.[155]

Shenkin and colleagues[445] regarded the two objectives of carotid ligation, both the reduction of the pressure head at the site of the aneurysm and the avoidance of neurological sequelae, as being mutually antagonistic and dependent on the resistance in the circulation by the circle of Willis. In practice the effects of carotid ligation on the aneurysm have been (1)

Table 9-10. Tabulation of pressure changes after temporary occlusion of common carotid artery*

| | Pressure readings in mm. Hg | | | |
| | Cervical carotid artery | | Aneurysmal sac (middle cerebral) | |
Patient and age	Before occlusion	After occlusion	Before occlusion	After occlusion
Female, 66 years	100/70	34/25	93/67	48/45
Male, 51 years	110/75	68/50	35/30	25/22
Female, 54 years	90/70	55/46	35/30	22/20

*Data from Wright, R. L.: Intraaneurysmal pressure with carotid occlusion, J. Neurosurg. **29**:139, 1968.

a reduction in the size of the aneurysmal sac,[277,354] with the very few aneurysms examined having been described as reduced in size and sclerotic,[114,277] (2) angiographic reduction in the size of the functional lumen,[155] which appears to shrink concentrically,[191] (3) greater firmness of the sac after an interval, presumably because of thrombosis within the lumen, (4) nonvisualization of the aneurysm by angiography in a small proportion of cases, (5) the development of radiological calcification in the sac,[385] said to be curvilinear opacities,[190] and (6) reduction in pressure symptoms but very rarely complete clinical regression.[310]

There is no proof that thrombosis within the sac is enhanced, for it occurs after leakage or rupture quite independently of carotid ligation and any advantage derived may be attributed solely to the reduced hemodynamic stress. No pathological study of these aneurysms has yet been made, despite the survival of many such patients for 10 to 15 years and more. It is possible that the aneurysms in question have progressed to a latent or quiescent stage as illustrated in Figs. 9-25, *B,* and 9-26.

Nonvisualization of aneurysmal sacs by angiography should be interpreted cautiously, for angiography has its limitations and complete obliteration of the sac is extremely rare. An aneurysm, which after therapeutic carotid occlusion could not be visualized by angiography, has been known to bleed again.[343]

Considerable discrepancy exists in the reported advantages of carotid ligation.[271,354,500] Recurrent hemorrhage occurs in a number of cases either from the original aneurysm or from a second unsuspected sac,[343,435] and the bleeding from a previously unruptured aneurysm may not be prevented by carotid occlusion.[343,354] Angiographically no alteration in the sac may occur postoperatively and in a few instances enlargement may ensue. Growth to the size of a space-occupying lesion occasionally results when presumably a collateral

circulation is responsible for restoring adequate flow and pressure to the aneurysm. As a consequence of ligation, the hemodynamics of the contralateral vessels are altered, and an increase in systemic pressure has been noted.[445] Accommodating these changes, aneurysms of the contralateral arteries have ruptured, although the cause-and-effect relationship is not clear. In a few instances aneurysms have developed on contralateral vessels that angiographically were previously clear.[190]

Ligation or compression of a carotid artery in the neck will cause slight local thrombus formation due to intimal damage. In most cases clinically flow can be reestablished by prompt removal of the clip. The thrombus may be more extensive and even propagate as far as the intracranial segment of the internal carotid.[354,435] Possible embolism from the thrombus at the site of ligation has been an unsubstantiated source of concern.[435] Gross and Holzman[210] recorded a traumatic aneurysm at the site of partial ligation of the common carotid artery, and ligatures or metal clips on large arteries may only slowly cut through the wall to reestablish the circulation at least in part. Such exigencies have not been a feature of carotid occlusion, and though it is a likely complication of such a procedure, no instances of poststenotic dilatation have been recorded after partial occlusion.

No pathological study has yet been made of either the arterial "atrophy," with its morphological changes in the cellular and connective tissue constituents of the wall or of the severity of atherosclerosis distal to the ligated segment. The frequent reduction in caliber of the internal carotid artery can be demonstrated readily by angiography.[191]

The principal danger of carotid occlusion is cerebral ischemia. Measurements of blood pressure changes, angiographic assessment of the cross-circulation, and electroencephalographic and other studies of blood flow alterations have been undertaken with a view to predicting the development of this complication. Schorstein[435] believed that preoperative impairment of the circulation precipitated cerebral damage after ligation. Certainly there is more risk with ligation in the first few days after the aneurysmal hemorrhage,[354] and vasospasm and space-occupying hematomas may impair the circulatory readjustments so essential after carotid ligation. The incidence of ischemia is lower in those patients who have had no subarachnoid bleeding than in those who have had a hemorrhage and is lower with common carotid ligation than with occlusion of the internal carotid artery. Most ischemic complications occur within the first 2 days and 95% within the first week.[354] However some may be very much delayed.[364] Clinically, the symptoms after carotid occlusion vary from transient paresthesias and episodes of dysphasia to gross mental confusion, convulsions, coma, hemiplegia, and death. Pathologically the lesions vary both in severity and extent. In milder cases patchy necrosis and gliosis may result in the territory of the middle cerebral artery. In fatal cases, the infarction is not necessarily restricted to the territory of the middle cerebral as Schorstein[435] stated. In the Cooperative Study,[354] in 35 autopsies on patients who died after carotid occlusion, the infarct was restricted to the area supplied by the middle cerebral artery in 17 cases, 11 of which had pale infarcts and six had hemorrhagic softenings. In 14 cases the infarct was in the territory of the anterior and middle cerebral arteries (eight pale and six hemorrhagic infarcts) and in one case there was a pale infarct of the area of the middle and posterior cerebral arteries. Three patients exhibited infarction of the entire homolateral hemisphere (one pale, one hemorrhagic, and one not stated). It is surprising there has been no correlation of the distribution of the encephalomalacia with the anatomy of the circle of Willis. Secondary vascular lesions resulting from raised supratentorial pressure may also appear.

Welch and Eiseman[530] performed reconstructive surgery on a common carotid artery that had been ligated 2 years previously for subarachnoid hemorrhage and were of the opinion that carotid ligation could be disadvantageous when subsequent atherosclerosis impairs the cerebral circulation.

Voris[514] recorded two fatal cases of aneurysm of the internal carotid artery in which thrombus was said to have propagated from the completely thrombosed aneurysm until it occluded the anterior and middle cerebral arteries.

Bakay and Sweet[22] measured distal blood pressures after occlusion of the vertebral artery, but there was no reduction in pressure of practical value. Consequently vertebral ligation is not in vogue.

Induced hypotension. Slosberg[457,458] used pharmacologically induced hypotension in the therapy of intracranial aneurysms. The rationale is similar to that of reducing the distal blood pressure by carotid ligation, that is, to reduce the hemodynamic stresses in the aneurysmal wall. The method obviates the risks associated with surgical procedures and the effects are not local but general. Consequently it is of value for multiple aneurysms, those on the vertebrobasilar system or those difficult of access. Drake,[140] using hypotension in association with direct surgical attack on an aneurysm, noted that the sac wall was soft, presumably because of reduced tension. On theoretical grounds this form of therapy should prove to be of considerable merit, but results of hypotensive therapy from the Cooperative Study[422] were disappointing. The long-term effects of this medical therapy on the ruptured aneurysm, the prevalence of previously undemonstrable aneurysms and the severity of atherosclerosis require investigation. The possibility exists that hypotension might precipitate ischemia in an already jeopardized circulation.

Promotion of intra-aneurysmal thrombosis. In the last century foreign material was introduced into aneurysmal sacs to promote thrombosis, and a similar therapeutic approach has been made to cerebral aneurysms. Small segments of hog or horse hair are fired into the aneurysm by means of a pneumatic gun, the procedure being called "pilojection."[182] Recently intra-aneurysmal thrombosis has been induced by the introduction of iron powder into the sac, with a magnet holding the particles in position.[6] Foreign material readily attracts platelets. Thrombosis will thus be initiated and organization of the thrombus will ensue. Macrophages were observed in large numbers in the thrombi experimentally induced by iron microspheres in dogs, and much of the foreign material was removed.[6] However, some foreign materials, such as hairs, tend to stimulate a foreign body reaction with giant cells, and the problem is compounded because superadded infection is an ever-present risk.

Drake and Vanderlinden[141] treated a large unruptured aneurysm of the basilar artery by pilojection and virtually occluded the lumen, but the sac ruptured 3 months later. The thrombus within the sac was initiated but was not adequately controlled.

Mullan and colleagues[347] have electrically induced thromboses of intracranial aneurysms. In some patients, hemiplegia or hemiparesis occurred, possibly because of embolism or thrombosis of an adjacent vessel. Refilling of the sac either in part or in whole was demonstrated in follow-up angiograms in several patients. The problem of fibrinolytic action on the thrombus is raised, but unfortunately little information on this aspect is at hand. Mullan and Dawley[346] treated patients with an antifibrinolytic substance in the belief that recurrent hemorrhage from an aneurysm is in part caused by the dissolution of the thrombus by circulating fibrinolysins.

Clipping or ligation of the base of the aneurysm. Clipping or ligature of the base of the aneurysm has been a popular method, but direct manipulation of the aneurysm is fraught with both the danger of rupturing or tearing of the thin-walled sac and damaging the neighboring brain. Although the procedure may be hazardous, effective reduction in size can be achieved. The facile tearing of the sac wall during manipulation may indicate that the wall is of reduced tensile strength. Furthermore, inadequate or incomplete closure of an aneurysmal neck or base by ligature or clip may still result in extensive thrombosis in the sac.[54] In addition there is the danger that a significant residual sac may enlarge, causing serious and fatal bleeding months or years later.[54,141]

Clipping an intracranial artery at some short distance proximal to the aneurysm has resulted in a reduction in the size of the lumen and considerable thickening of the wall of the sac.[114]

The foreign-body reaction to ligatures is well recognized but metal too may induce a tissue reaction. Silver clips have been in popular usage, yet experimentally they have induced an intensive inflammatory reaction with necrosis progressing to the formation of much fibrous tissue,[32,153] whereas several other metals invoked no reaction or one that was only minimal.

External reinforcement of the sac wall. The aneurysmal sac was reinforced by the application of hammered muscle to the exterior of the sac by Dott.[137] The muscle readily acts as a hemostatic and will stimulate a mild inflammatory reaction leading to the organization of the necrotic tissue. Such granulation tissue formation closely applied to the aneurysm will add considerably to the thickness and presumably the strength of the wall but will not ensure immunity from rupture.[141] Wrapping gauze about an aneurysmal sac on the middle cerebral artery has effected a reduction in size of the aneurysm and considerable fibrosis of the sac wall merging into a foreign-body reaction to the gauze. The parent artery in this case displayed some thickening of the wall and the lumen was still patent.[114] Muslin[193] and also gelfoam[465] have been utilized in a similar manner.[454] These will induce a foreign-body reaction and the formation of granulation tissue.

Various plastic coating methods have recently been employed with the aim of forming a plastic jacket about the sac. Dutton[151,152] used methyl methacrylate and this led to considerable interest in the possible use of rapidly hardening plastics. Selverstone[442,443] utilized a double coating technique (polyvinyl–polyvinylidene chloride copolymer and the hard two-component epoxy-polyamide resin). Silicone rubber has been used[501,502] and Eastman 910 Adhesive (monomer) has also been introduced into the neurosurgeons' armory.[79,80] Such substances are believed to be relatively inert, but Meacham[332] reported briefly the occurrence of an acute sterile inflammatory reaction that had progressed by 6 weeks to a marked fibrosis in the neighborhood of the plastic. Unfortunately the type of plastic was not specified. Dutton[151,152] asserted that the use of methyl methacrylate caused little reaction, only a mild proliferation of astrocytes and microglia in the molecular layer of the cortex after 7 weeks. Minimal response has been confirmed in long- and short-term experiments.[219,237]

Selverstone and colleagues[443] found no thrombosis and no inflammatory response after 2 years when they used the double coating technique. Carton and associates[79,80] illustrated a giant cell reaction with round cells and fibrosis in response to Eastman 910 monomer, but experimentally with application to extracranial arteries of 3 to 5 mm. in diameter, the result was fusiform dilatation, and when applied to vessels of 0.5 to 2 mm. in diameter, dilatation was a hazard, though 44% of the vessels underwent thrombosis. The adhesive caused muscle necrosis, though the internal elastic lamina was not disrupted. No mention was made of the endothelium.

A similar destruction of the muscle elements of an aneurysmal wall with an acute inflammatory reaction was observed in a patient on whom this adhesive had been used. Coe and Bondurant[94] reported an instance of thrombosis within an aneurysm and of the parent middle cerebral artery within 5 weeks of operation. Tsuchiya and associates[506] investigated seven different plastic materials and concluded that all produced the same type of change, but the response varied in intensity and duration. They confirmed the severe inflammatory reaction of Eastman 910 adhesive or monomer and admitted that the mildest reaction was caused by Biobond. They mentioned the carcinogenic effect of Eastman 910 monomer and other synthetic substances in rats. Long-term carcinogenic effects of such substances in man are unknown as yet, and adequate follow-up of patients so treated is essential at this stage of our knowledge.

Dissecting aneurysms

Lesions of the central nervous system may be produced by dissecting aneurysms of both extracranial and intracranial arteries.

Dissecting aneurysms of the aorta. Dissecting aneurysm of the aorta is two to three times more common in the male than in the female and most prevalent between 40 and 70 years of age.[248] There is autopsy evidence of hypertension in some 86% of cases, and though clinical evidence of hyperpiesis may not indicate an equally high incidence, the fact is that shock may be present when the patient is admitted to the hospital. Normotension is likely among patients under 40 years of age or in association with pregnancy or Marfan's syndrome (arachnodactyly). Hypertension is the most consistent pathological accompaniment of the disease.[248] Aortic dissection is a complication of coarctation of the aorta, Marfan's syndrome, aortic valvular stenosis,[239,331] and bicuspid aortic valve. It can occur with the *formes frustes* of Marfan's syndrome[248] and has been found in association with pregnancy on a significant number of occasions.[248,432] The presence of hypertension seems to be the common denominator in cases of dissecting aneurysm attendant on endocrine disorders.[248]

Dissecting aneurysm of the aorta is caused by mucoid degeneration of the media with extensive elastic tissue degeneration, which in some cases is a consequence of hemodynamic injury associated with aortic stenosis. Giant cell aortitis is seldom the cause and trauma is not a precipitating factor in the onset.

Most patients live for only a short period of time, during which evidence of neurological disturbances is often manifest and is caused by the reduction in circulatory flow through the aortic branches. The reduction has been ascribed to (1) compression of the small intercostal or lumbar arteries at their point of origin with little extension of the dissection along their walls,[248] (2) tearing of intercostal and lumbar arteries at their origin,[340,446] often with superadded thrombosis,[214] (3) obstruction of larger branches (such as the great vessels of the arch) by the intramural dissection. When these vessels are sectioned transversely, the intramural hematoma or false lumen is situated toward the outer part of the media or at the junction of media and adventitia. The inner portion of the wall is frequently pushed to one side and collapsed on itself. Often it appears contracted, thus reducing the true lumen to a fraction of its original size. The blood in this hematoma is likely to clot,

although a reentry tear in the branch may relieve the ischemia distally.[248] Hirst, Johns, and Kime[248] consider that a superadded thrombosis may convert the partial obstruction to complete obstruction.

The dissection can involve the aortic branches and produce neurological lesions, which may involve the brain, the spinal cord, or the peripheral nerves (Table 9-11). The lesions may be multiple.

Brain. In about 90% of cases mural tears through which arterial blood enters the aortic wall are found either in the ascending aorta or in the aortic arch. With peripheral dissection, the great vessels of the aortic arch are often implicated. In 505 cases of dissecting aneurysm, the innominate artery was involved 67 times, one or both common carotid arteries 75 times, and one or both subclavian arteries on 71 occasions. The internal carotid and vertebral arteries were not specifically mentioned.[248]

Neurological manifestations in dissecting aneurysm of the aorta, regarded as an important aid to diagnosis, have been recorded in 18% to 46% of cases.[248,340,529] Some patients die too rapidly for a detailed neurological examination to be performed, but neurological findings, which are hemiplegia, monoplegia, periods of stupor or loss of consciousness, and convulsions, denote ischemia of varying severity and extent because of carotid occlusion however incomplete. Much depends on the severity of the occlusion, the availability of collateral vessels, and the duration of the ischemia. The involvement of vertebral arteries in this disease and pathologi-

Table 9-11. Types of neurological disturbances associated with dissecting aneurysm of the aorta

Authors	Type of neurological lesion			
	Cerebral	Spinal cord	Neuropathy	Unclassified
Weisman & Adams[529]	1	1	9	
Moersch & Sayre[340]	8	3		1
Scott & Sancetta[439]	26	22	41	
Total	35	26	50	1

cal lesions of the nervous system have not been well investigated at autopsies of patients with dissecting aneurysms, for the main focus of attention has been the aorta. Interest has been evinced in the clinical symptomatology and signs, even though clinicopathological correlation in this disease is often difficult.

Chase and associates[88] analyzed 16 cases of nontraumatic dissecting aneurysm of the aorta presenting with associated cerebral dysfunction. They defined two distinctive syndromes. The first comprised patients having a precipitous onset of coma or semiresponsive state with pronounced focal neurological signs (hemiparesis, hemisensory deficits, and conjugate gaze palsies) caused by the dissecting aneurysm obstructing the great vessel in the neck. Some patients do not survive sufficiently long for neuropathological changes to be demonstrable. The second group presented with syncope or coma without persisting focal neurological signs and in the absence of significant obstruction of the major vessels in the neck. The neurological signs were attributed to transient or persistent hypotension complicating the aortic dissection, although multiple foci of recent cerebral infarction and acute hypoxic changes were present in the cerebrum and cerebellum of the illustrative case.

Neurological lesions are likely to occur early in the illness. In a few instances there is a late onset of cerebral ischemic lesions caused by emboli from cardiac mural thrombi associated with a myocardial infarction secondary to the aortic dissection. In the absence of myocardial damage, the origin of thrombi in the cerebral vessels is unresolved. Moersch and Sayre[340] found multiple arteriolar thrombi in the pons and medulla in one case and a thrombus of a middle cerebral artery in another. Embolism from thrombi formed in association with the aortic laceration and dissection might be responsible for such lesions, but two of their patients had massive cerebral hemorrhage. Such lesions are prob-

ably incidental to the associated hypertension.

Spinal cord. When a dissecting aneurysm involves the descending aorta, the intercostal and lumbar vessels become stretched and narrowed as the media dissects and the two layers of the aortic wall separate.[340] Complete occlusion follows and further stretching can lead to rupture of the vessel with reconstitution of the flow from the false lumen into segmental vessels.[340] Thrombosis can complicate such vessel damage. The resultant ischemia, whether temporary or persistent, may cause spinal cord damage. However, if the interference with blood flow in the segmental arteries has been of very short duration, there will be no sequelae.

Dissection of several intercostal arteries in the absence of clinical evidence of spinal cord damage is a possibility and difficulty is often experienced in explaining the mechanism of neurological lesions.[248] Clinically, numbness and tingling of the legs, weakness, or even paraplegia (lower limbs), may occur and differentiation between spinal cord ischemia and obstruction of the iliac artery is quite perplexing. Either one of these complications may initiate paraplegia (lower limbs), which occurred in 27 of 505 cases of dissecting aortic aneurysm.[248]

The upper part of the spinal cord (cervical and upper thoracic) is seldom affected, for its blood supply is mainly dependent on the vertebral and to a lesser extent on the ascending deep cervical and costovertebral arteries. The portion of the cord most frequently involved is the middle (from the fourth, fifth, and sixth thoracic segments) and lower thoracic segments. These segments are dependent on intercostal arteries for their blood supply. In addition, this portion of the cord is often the one most severely affected.[498] Lumbosacral portions of the cord are involved when the aortic dissection is extensive and severe.

The affected region of the spinal cord may be palpably softer than normal and the demarcation between gray and white matter indistinct and accompanied in mild cases by a few perivascular hemorrhages. Hemorrhagic infarction with spinal subarachnoid hemorrhage has been described by Scott and Sancetta.[439] The order in decreasing vulnerability of regions of the cord is (1) the gray matter, (2) the adjacent white matter, and (3) the peripheral or subpial white matter. The entire cord can be necrotic but usually this is not the case. Weisman and Adams[529] described a cord with variation in the extent of the disorder at the several levels cross-sectioned and a distinct tendency for the anterior portion of the cord to be more severely affected than the posterior, and at many levels the anterior horns and adjacent white matter were found to be softened whereas the posterior horns and posterior columns were more frequently spared.

Histologically the ischemic zone is necrotic and edematous initially with a variable amount of extravasated blood and leukocytic infiltration. If the patient survives, organization occurs and the central softened area is replaced by a yellowish honeycombed cavity. Secondary degeneration of ascending tracts and anterior roots is a likely event.[340]

Peripheral nerves. Ischemic necrosis of a peripheral nerve is of frequent occurrence (Table 9-11). The early symptoms are primarily sensory, and the limb is pulseless, weak or paralyzed, and discolored. Since the iliac arteries are the branches of the aorta most frequently involved by the dissection,[248] the lower limbs (unilateral or bilateral) are more frequently affected than the upper.

Dissecting aneurysms of the carotid arteries in the neck. Primary dissecting aneurysms of the cervical carotid arteries, though hardly ever seen, are most conveniently classified according to whether they are of spontaneous or of traumatic origin.

Spontaneous. Jentzer[275] reported a dissecting aneurysm of the left internal carotid artery in the neck of a woman of 31

years. The description was inadequate, and the plane of the dissection was not given. The patient died several years later with multiple cerebral aneurysms. At the original operation both the external and internal carotid arteries were fragile, but no mention was made of a coexisting connective tissue disorder.

Anderson and Schechter[9] discussed a hypertensive man of 41 years who developed right-sided hemiparesis with aphasia over several hours. Angiography revealed a localized filling defect (5 cm. in length) in the cervical segment of the internal carotid artery and there was extensive cerebral softening. The cervical segment of the internal carotid artery exhibited significant narrowing with opposing atherosclerotic plaques 1 cm. above its origin. About 1.5 cm. beyond this stenotic area was a dissecting aneurysm 3 to 4 cm. in length with a mural tear at both proximal and distal limits. The dissection was in the outer part of the media and the lumen was almost occluded, yet the contrast medium gained access to and filled the carotid siphon. Histologically the affected artery was said to demonstrate an unusual amount of metachromasia and excessive elastic tissue deterioration. The dissection may have been poststenotic in type similar to that developing in the aorta as a complication of aortic stenosis.[239,331]

Austin and Schaefer[18] reported dissection of the media of the terminal portion of the right innominate and first third of the right common carotid artery together with a similar dissection (2 cm. long) in the left common carotid artery. The patient was a male of 25 years with typical arachnodactyly.

Brice and Crompton[63] reported three spontaneous dissecting aneurysms of the cervical internal carotid artery in three normotensive individuals. The aneurysms had been responsible for sudden occlusion either partial or complete close to the origin of the artery. The first case was a woman of 40 with an occlusion of the left internal carotid artery caused by a dissecting aneurysm that commenced 1 cm. above the origin of the artery and extended to the base of the skull. The mural tear was near the lower extremity of the aneurysm, and occlusive thrombi, possibly embolic, were found in the three large branches of the homolateral middle cerebral artery. The second case alluded to was a man of 35 years with a small dissecting aneurysm at the origin of the right internal carotid artery and thrombi in large branches of the homolateral middle cerebral artery. The third case was that of a woman of 38 years with a dissecting aneurysm commencing 2.5 cm. above the origin of the left internal carotid artery and extending to the base of the skull. The lumen of the artery was occluded by thrombus, which extended up into the left middle cerebral artery and its branches. Histologically there was a recent dissection deep in the media in the left middle cerebral artery. In each case the dissection had arisen between the media and adventitia and was attributed to cystic medial degeneration.

Hardin and Snodgrass[225] successfully treated their patient, a male of 51 years who complained of a squirting noise in the left ear and a thrill in front of the left ear. Angiography revealed the double lumen of a dissecting aneurysm of the left internal carotid artery reaching from 4 cm. above the origin of the artery and involving the major portion of the vessel in its petrous segment.

Boström and Liliequist[58] described an old dissecting aneurysm (1 and 1.5 cm. in length respectively) of the internal carotid artery a short distance below the skull in each of two hypertensive patients. Yet another fatal case has been reported in a 35-year-old male.[497] Dissecting aneurysms characteristically occur in the outer media or at the junction of the adventitia and media, and in this connection resemble dissecting aneurysms of other peripheral but extracranial vessels. Moreover such lesions in vessels of this caliber are usually associated with a superadded thrombosis at the site of the tear. These cases are too few in number for generalizations to be made, although it would appear that hypertension is not a prominent feature of the lesion. Thrombi were found in peripheral cerebral arteries in three instances.[9,63] Possibly these are embolic phenomena complicating the mural tears and dissection proximally. This raises the question whether neurological lesions complicating aortic dissecting aneurysms are ever etiologically embolic in nature.

In the etiological interpretation of such lesions in the carotid arteries in the neck one must exercise caution in the quantitative estimation of the metachromasia and elastic tissue changes, for most pathologists do not examine a sufficient quantity of adequate control material.

Traumatic. The most important surgical risk of cerebral angiography appears to be the production of a dissecting aneurysm at the site of the arterial puncture. If a needle is inserted into the wall of an artery and fluid, whether blood, saline, or contrast medium, is forcibly injected, intramural dissection ensues, which explains why on occasions attempts at carotid angiography result in traumatic dissecting aneurysms of the artery.[104] Medial degeneration and sclerotic atherosclerotic thickening of the wall, even if present, are probably not essential predisposing factors.[176] In a case reported by Fleming and Park,[173] the patient was 4 months pregnant.

At autopsy, in any instance of dissecting aneurysm of the carotid arteries in the neck, the vessels should be carefully inspected for the presence of puncture wounds and the relationship to the site of the initiating tear determined.

Angiography may reveal the traumatic dissection with contrast medium in the false lumen, and though minor degrees of dissection may occur frequently, the extensive lesions of up to 7 cm. in length with considerable narrowing of the lumen are rare.[61] Sirois and associates[453] described a valvelike flap, 1 cm. long, occluding the lumen with its valvelike action. Gannon[184] recorded four cases studied by angiography and in each, it was believed that a comparable valvelike obstruction had been produced by percutaneous arteriography. In at least one case there was also a filling defect for a length of several centimeters. The distinction between such lesions and more extensive dissections, which are unquestionably dissecting aneurysms, is a moot point. In that they may mechanically impede the flow of blood through the external carotid, which brings superadded thrombosis in its wake, lies their importance.

Boyd-Wilson[61] reported dissecting aneurysms in 1% of his series of 900 carotid angiograms and DeGrood[129] found one instance in 400 cerebral angiograms. The dissection may be subintimal, but in general it is medial and frequently close to the junction of media and adventitia.[61,176] The initiating tear may be where the needle entered or on the diametrically opposite wall. The angiographic appearance is characteristic and diagnosis usually poses no problem.[61] Recovery is a possibility, but not infrequently the outcome is fatal because of cerebral ischemia.

Most of the contrast medium will be washed out and the blood invading the mural tear is prone to extend the dissection. If the patient survives, the intramural hematoma will undergo organization. Small experimental lesions of this kind leave a medial scar or no histological evidence at all.[525] In man, such severe dissections are frequently associated with a residual filling defect in the artery if the patient does not die of extensive encephalomalacia.

Traumatic dissecting aneurysms of the common and internal carotid arteries can complicate injuries to the neck in the absence of a perforating injury to the vessels and injuries to the head alone.[301] Northcroft and Morgan[357] described a dissecting aneurysm of the internal carotid artery of a 31-year-old male accidentally dragged for a short distance with a rope around his neck. The skin of the neck was not lacer-ated though the sternomastoid was partially severed. Coma appeared after an initial lag period. The internal carotid artery exhibited a circumferential tear with intramural dissection for 1.5 inches in the outer third of the media. The lumen was narrowed and the upper flap, consisting of intima and media, completely occluded the lumen like an inverted valve. The lumen was also occluded by thrombus, which had propagated distally along the full length of the internal carotid and extended into the middle cerebral artery. The victim died of massive cerebral infarction. Whether the atherosclerosis of such notable severity was a predisposing factor is uncertain and at present beyond our ken. Just why a closed neck injury should cause such tearing and dissection is difficult to understand. The arterial wall may have been rigid and brittle. It has also been suggested that in young subjects the internal carotid artery sustains a stretch injury because of being stretched over the bony prominences of the atlas and axis when the head is hyperextended and rotated toward the injury or laterally flexed away from the side of the injury.[301] A similar phenomenon is probably at times the cause of thrombosis of the vertebral artery and initiated by manipulation of the head and neck.

Boyd and Watson[59] reported a similar case in a man of 42 years who had a severe crushing injury of the chest and right side of the neck with medial dissection of the common, internal, and external carotid arteries and propagation of the thrombus into the middle and anterior cerebral arteries. Occlusive thrombi inevitably develop in these traumatic dissecting aneurysms but are not invariable in those complicating arteriography, and the explanation is probably based on the more severe mural laceration in the former condition. Severe nonpenetrating injury to the neck is a recognized though infrequent cause of occlusion of the cervical segment of the internal carotid artery. Houck and colleagues[253] found 15 cases in the literature up to 1964 and gave details of two additional instances.

Lesions ranging from contusions of the artery to frank dissecting aneurysms seem to be responsible for such traumatic occlusions. Hockaday[249] reported several cases of traumatic thrombosis of the internal carotid artery (cervical and intracranial segments) in which all the subjects recovered and angiographic demonstration of the blockages was made at a later date. Hence the underlying arterial lesions could well have been dissecting aneurysms, the distinction between the two lesions being one of degree. The prognosis for all these cases is bad, with severe neurological deficit resulting in most of the survivors.

Dissecting aneurysms of the vertebral arteries in the neck. Traumatic aneurysms of the extracranial segment of the vertebral artery may be the consequence of penetrating injuries, but dissecting aneurysms of the neck whether of spontaneous or traumatic origin are encountered exceedingly rarely.

Ouchi and colleagues[366] observed a small dissecting aneurysm of the right vertebral artery beyond its origin from the subclavian artery. It was attributed to a head injury sustained several months before. The depth of the mural tear and dissection was not given, but the outer sheath to the intramural hematoma was apparently somewhat dilated. The sac contained thrombus that might have been a source of embolism. Histologically the artery exhibited medial fibrosis and panarteritis.

Boström and Liliequist[58] described small dissecting aneurysms of both vertebral arteries at the level of the second, third, and fourth cervical vertebrae, findings incidental at autopsy. A similar lesion was found in one renal artery, the intramural hematoma being at the outer part of the media.

Renal ischemia was present, but no cerebral damage appeared to accrue from the injury to the vertebral arteries.

Dissecting aneurysms of the cerebral arteries. Primary dissecting aneurysms of the peripheral or pulmonary arteries occur much less frequently than those of the aorta. Watson[526] reviewing the literature up to 1956 found 23 acceptable cases of dissecting aneurysm of peripheral vessels. Foord and Lewis[176] found 48 in all, of which eight involved intracranial arteries and six affected the innominate or the carotid arteries in the neck. Involvement of the other splanchnic vessels is even more unusual and so are the lesions of the arteries in the neck. Those of the cerebral arteries are of more frequent incidence and a nonexhaustive compilation of 35 dissecting aneurysms of the cerebral arteries is seen in Table 9-12. However, in all cases details are not available.

Exact comparison between elastic and muscular arteries is not possible, but dissecting aneurysms of the splanchnic arteries are in general remarkably similar to those of the aorta. However dissecting aneurysms of the cerebral arteries differ from those of the aorta, splanchnic vessels, and cervical carotid arteries in several important respects, for they occur primarily in the second, third, and fourth decades (Table 9-12). The mean age of cerebral dissecting aneurysms is 26.5 years, with a range from 6 months to 47 years. Sex distribution is relatively equal (17 males and 13 females) and no cases in females occurred during pregnancy. One patient[379] was 15 days post partum, but this is an isolated case that cannot be regarded as in any way significant.

Macroscopic appearance. The cerebral

Abbreviations to Table 9-12:

AC	Anterior cerebral	MC	Middle cerebral
AntChor	Anterior choroidal	PC	Posterior cerebral
Bas	Basilar	PCom	Posterior communicating
F	Female	R	Right
IC	Internal carotid	SupCer	Superior cerebellar
L	Left	V	Vertebral artery
M	Male		

Table 9-12. Dissecting aneurysms reported in the literature

Authors	Sex	Age in years	Artery involved	Site of dissection	Cerebrospinal fluid	Possible and suggested etiological factors
Turnbull (1915)[508]			RMC			Syphilitic arteritis
Scholefield (1924)[433]	M	47	Bas, RV		Clear	
Hyland (1933)[257]	M	42	Bas	Media	Clear	Medial mucoid degeneration
Hassin (1933)[232]		31	Bas	Subintima with tearing of media and adventitia		Legal electrocution
Stern (1933)[484]	M	24	Bas, PC, P Com, Ant Chor	Subintima	Clear	
Szabo (1939)[492]	F	35	RV			Syphilis
DeVeer & Browder (1942)[131]	M	42	RIC, RMC	Subintima	Clear	Trauma
Dratz & Woodhall (1947)[144]	F	21	LIC, LMC LAC	Subintima	1950 red cells per mm.[3]	Trauma
Ramsey & Mosquera (1948)[393]	M	47	RMC	Media	Subarachnoid hemorrhage found at autopsy	Arteriosclerosis and cystic medial degeneration
Poppen (1951)[385] (two cases)			MC			
DeBusscher (1952)[120]	M	45	LV	Subintima		
Sinclair (1953)[452]	F	27	RMC	Subintima	Microscopic red cells	Associated with migraine
Bigelow (1955)[47]	F	46	RMC	Media		Surgical trauma
Watson (1956)[526]	M	32	Bas	Subintima	Clear	Medial degeneration
Norman & Urich (1957)[356]	M	½	RMC	Probably subintima		
Wolman (1959)[546]	M	16	RMC, RAC	Subintima	Clear	Tear occurred at site of medial defect and early small aneurysm
	F	19	LMC	Subintima	Clear	Medial gap or defect
	F	33	Bas, Proximal PC	Subintima	Clear	Medial gap or defect
Scott et al. (1960)[438]	F	29	LIC, LMC LAC	Subintima		
Crosato & Terzan (1961)[119]	M	30	Bas, RPC, LPC, SupCer	Subintima	Clear	
Ritchie (1961)[406]	M	17	LIC, LMC	Subintima	No blood	Trauma in history
Wisoff & Rothballer (1961)[542]	F	11	RIC, RMC RAC	Subintima	Microscopic red cells only	Necrosis of media
Spudis et al. (1962)[463]	F	30	RIC, RMC	Subintima	Clear	
Duman & Stephens (1963)[149]	M	21	LMC	Subintima		
Nedwich et al. (1963)[350]	F	30	RMC	Subintima		
Dourov et al. (1964)[139]	M	15	LMC	Subintima	Blood stained	
Perier et al. (1964)[379]	F	22	Bas	Subintima	Clear	
Robert et al. (1964)[409]	F	20	RMC	Subintima	Clear	
Crompton (1965)[113]			RV			
Hayman & Anderson (1966)[238]	M	16	Bas	Media	Clear	
Engeset et al. (1967)[162]	M	6	AC			Mild trauma
Walb et al. (1967)[517]	F	30	LV, Bas	Subintima	Clear	
Nelson & Styri (1968)[351]	M	5	LAC	Subintima	Clear	Trauma 2 days previously
Shaw & Foltz (1968)[444]	M	32	RMC	Subintimal in parts, possibly media also	Xanthochromic	Trauma

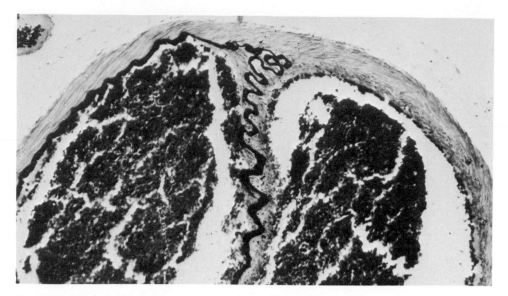

Fig. 9-38. Healed dissecting aneurysm of middle cerebral artery. Intima has been dissected away from media about part of the circumference and formed a septum in the vessel, with blood flowing through both true and false lumens. The elastic lamina is intact and no new elastic lamina has formed about the false lumen. (Verhoeff's elastic stain, ×110. Courtesy Norman, R. M., and Urich, H.: Dissecting aneurysm of the middle cerebral artery as a cause of acute infantile hemiplegia, J. Path. Bact. **73:**580, 1957.)

arteries, conforming with the pattern of age distribution, display little obvious macroscopic atherosclerosis. Their thin walls and collapsed state contrast with the involved segment, which is distended and dark red or brownish, closely simulating and often being mistaken for a fairly recent thrombus. Parts of the dissected wall may appear hemorrhagic. Where healing has taken place, the segment deranged may be smaller and more opaque than normal,[444] but in any event it is dependent on whether flow through the segment is reestablished. In the dissecting aneurysm reported by Norman and Urich,[356] no macroscopic abnormality was detected, for flow had been reestablished. In one branch of the middle cerebral artery, both the false and true lumens were functional and the vessel was divided by a septum (Fig. 9-38). In other branches of the middle cerebral the internal elastic lamina was incorporated in the wall on one side of the vessel and the true lumen was obliterated. In DeBusscher's unusual case of dissecting aneurysm of a

vertebral artery with the formation of a new false lumen, there was dilatation of the wall in the region of the dissection.[128] A long-standing sizable saccular dilatation that contained laminated thrombus and resembled a cerebellopontine angle tumor resulted.

In older, more aged individuals atherosclerosis is decidedly in evidence, and if syphilis is the underlying etiological factor precipitating the dissection, indications of a tertiary luetic infection will be present.

In angiograms, the radiological shadow of the lumen of the affected vessel ends abruptly and may simulate an aneurysmal pouch from which a faint linear shadow, eccentric in position, continues in the line of the vessel.

In at least 57% of cases a middle cerebral artery with or without the distal part of the internal carotid and/or the proximal segment of the anterior cerebral artery is involved (Table 9-12). For a yet-to-be-explained reason, the right middle cerebral artery is affected more frequently than is

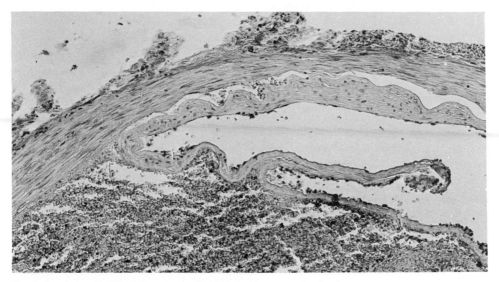

Fig. 9-39. Recent dissecting aneurysm of middle cerebral artery. The dissection is immediately external to the internal elastic lamina and the true lumen is much reduced in size. (Van Gieson stain, ×110. From Sinclair, W.: Dissecting aneurysm of the middle cerebral artery associated with migraine syndrome, Amer. J. Path. 29:1083, 1953.)

the left. The basilar arteries are also frequently affected and the superior portion of one vertebral or the proximal end of a posterior cerebral artery can be involved as well. The vertebral artery alone was affected three times. The dissected segment varied in length from 1 to 5 cm., with the dissection often extending into the branches.[356] The thickness of the linear shadow is dependent on the dimensions of the collapsed and displaced true lumen. The branches beyond the obstructed vessel may be outlined in normal fashion and dimensions.[436] This radiological appearance, thought to be pathognomonic of dissecting aneurysm,[409] is readily explained in view of the pathology of the lesion.

No instances of multiple dissections of the cerebral arteries have been reported, although extracranial arteries are known to be so affected.[176]

The brain in the territory of the dissected arteries is usually swollen and infarcted, in most cases the softening is pale or anemic in type as evidenced by the frequency with which the cerebrospinal fluid is not found to be bloodstained at lumbar puncture (Table 9-12). Occasionally small hemorrhagic zones occur, and in one instance, at least,[393] intracerebral and subarachnoid hemorrhage resulted from external rupture of the aneurysm. Secondary manifestations from raised intracranial pressure may be evident but secondary midbrain or brain stem lesions have not been described. If the dissecting aneurysm is of many years' duration, the damaged brain will have undergone shrinkage and resorption in a manner similar to other areas of encephalomalacia.

Microscopic appearance. Histologically the dissection is almost invariably between the internal elastic lamina and the media, (Fig. 9-39) whereas dissection in the case of the aorta and splanchnic arteries is usually deep in the media or even between the adventitia and media. The overlying intima exhibits little thickening except about orifices of branches, and if there is intimal proliferation, it too is stripped. Occasional smooth muscle cells from the media may continue affixed to the elastic lamina, which remains attached along at least part of the vessel's circumference. The detached intima is generally convoluted and pushed against one side of the vessel wall by the intramural hematoma, whereas the true lumen is often not much more than a thin cleft. The elastic lamina may be fragmented, and to demonstrate intimal tears with certainty, the serial section technique must be employed. An entrance is frequently found and on occasions a second and distal tear, the site of reentry, may be demonstrated. The media can be partially torn or disrupted in places, particularly in Hassin's dissecting aneurysm[232] caused by legal electrocution. Even in lesions without external rupture, some extravasation of blood may have reached the adventitia. In a few instances the dissection lies within the media.

When the intima tears, dissection in the cerebral vessels usually involves at least 50% of the circumference. Pressures within the false lumen and the true lumen are equal, and it is easy to imagine how the loose intimal sheath would fold over when caught in the stream and like a functional valve almost completely occlude the lumen. Indeed, obstruction to flow seems to be well nigh invariable. The deposition of thrombus on the newly exposed surfaces of the false lumen is likely to hinder the tendency for the true lumen to be restored to its original size and position. It can be readily appreciated how thrombosis of the false lumen and cerebral ischemia would ensue. Blood in the false lumen is usually thrombosed, and probably because of the absence of through flow, which would accompany an external rupture or a reentrance tear, the thrombus frequently resembles postmortem clot rather than antemortem thrombus. However with a careful histological examination, laminated fibrin and platelet aggregation may be found.

When reentry is made via a second, distal tear in the intima, through flow can be reestablished, and healing and the lining of the false lumen will result if the patient survives. With the development of a distal reentrance tear, as in the aorta, the prognosis can be better, and the event explains the long survival of Norman and Urich's patient[356] although a large cerebral softening had originally occurred causing infantile hemiplegia. In the subject reported by Shaw and Foltz,[444] the artery would have been thrombosed and recanalized, with the new blood channels being multiple and small.

Pathogenesis. Unlike patients with aortic dissecting aneurysms in which, except in those under 40 years of age, hypertension is the rule, patients with dissecting aneurysms of the cerebral arteries are almost invariably normotensive. Diastolic pressure of 90 mm. Hg in two patients[517,526] is not significant, and hyperpiesis cannot be regarded as a contributing causative factor although Watson[526] believes that blood pressure fluctuations might be involved in the etiology.

Cerebral dissecting aneurysms have occurred in direct relation to trauma of the head. Bigelow reported a case as a complication of operative trauma[47] but in the other instances the trauma has been blunt. Only once has the skull been known to be fractured,[444] and as the dissecting aneurysm involved the middle cerebral artery, it cannot be classed as a direct injury. The mechanism by which trauma indirectly causes disruption of the vessel wall is quite unknown, but the mechanical effects of head injuries on the brain and blood vessels are little understood. Electrocution seems to produce a similar pathogenesis. Hassin[233] described the detachment of the intima from a basilar artery in a case of accidental electrocution. No blood (intramural hematoma) was found in the subintimal space and so the case was not accepted as a dissecting aneurysm. Separation of the intima from the media is not infrequent in the cerebral arteries as a postmortem change, possibly accentuated by excessive physical manipulation.

Dissection has been attributed to syphilitic arteritis in two instances,[492,508] and it readily follows that such a lesion could appear in an inflamed and necrotic vessel wall.

Degenerative changes are severe in an aorta involved by a dissecting aneurysm, but the media of cerebral arteries so affected exhibits little alteration. Watson[526] and Hyland[257] have attributed dissecting aneurysms to medial degeneration, but the degenerative changes observed need not be dissimilar from those expected in the cerebral arteries of a corresponding age group. The dissection is essentially subintimal and degenerative changes, unless specifically subintimal in location, are not necessarily related to the tearing and stripping up of the intima. Watson's case[526] is illustrative, for the media seems to be relatively normal. In the case reported by Ramsey and Mosquera, of a 47-year-old male, the dissection was medial and the illustrations reveal extremely severe atherosclerosis.[393] In an 11-year-old girl, Wisoff and Rothballer[542] reported focal areas of unexplained necrosis in several arteries and to this attributed the dissecting aneurysm. No medial degeneration was found in the arteries of another patient[238] even though the dissection was in the media. Wolman[546] attributed each of three dissecting aneurysms to the existence of medial gaps or defects at the arterial forks but the observation is of doubtful significance.

A goodly proportion of dissecting aneurysms appears to be spontaneous (Table 9-12) with no explanation for the abrupt tearing of the intima. One might presuppose this disease to be a complication of arachnodactyly, but no such association has been reported.

In aortic dissecting aneurysm, the vessel wall is of reduced tensile strength. In some patients this has been attributed to a nonspecific hemodynamic injury associated with aortic stenosis. Whether the intima and the internal elastic lamina in particular are also of reduced tensile strength in patients with cerebral dissecting aneurysm is uncertain, but it appears likely though we know little of the reason or the underlying mechanism.

The relationship of mural dissection to thrombosis is of interest, for tears or "ulceration" of the vessel walls are frequently associated with a variable degree of dissection and superadded thrombosis. This holds true for the aorta, experimental mural thrombi,[480] and cerebral arteries, whether the underlying lesion is atherosclerosis. In Fig. 3-22 is a thrombosed cerebral artery: the internal elastica is torn, partially stripped from the underlying media and reflected and embedded in thrombus remarkably similar to dissecting aneurysm of the cerebral arteries. Actually if dissection had been more prominent, the diagnosis would surely have been dissecting aneurysm. There appears to be overlap between dissecting aneurysm and nonatherosclerotic thrombotic arterial occlusion. Several authors[131,257,542] included their cases of dissecting aneurysm with cases of thrombosis of intracranial arteries. Duman and Stephens[149] went so far as to suggest that dissecting aneurysms with thrombosis may be the cause of posttraumatic cerebral artery occlusion.

Aneurysms of inflammatory origin

Cerebral aneurysms of inflammatory origin occur but sporadically and are of several types: bacterial aneurysms (nonsyphilitic), syphilitic aneurysms, aneurysms caused by mucormycosis or other fungi (mycotic aneurysms), and aneurysms associated with polyarteritis or giant cell arteritis.

Bacterial aneurysms. Bacterial aneurysms are usually referred to by such inappropriate terms as "mycotic," "septic-embolic," and "embolomycotic." The term "mycotic" implies a lesion of fungal origin and should be restricted to aneurysms of this nature for they have been encountered. Furthermore, not all bacterial aneurysms are of embolic origin, thus neither the term septic-embolic nor embolomycotic is apt.

Turnbull,[509] in a survey of 6829 necropsies, discovered 42 cases of cerebral aneurysm and, of these, 13 patients had 15 bacterial aneurysms. Stengel and Wolferth[483] gathered 217 recorded cases of bacterial aneurysm of all arteries. The most frequent site of involvement was the aorta followed by splanchnic vessels in which bacterial infection constitutes an important cause of aneurysmal dilatation. Intracranial aneurysms were found in 44 of the cases

Table 9-13. Distribution of bacterial aneurysms in the circulation

Site of aneurysm	Stengel and Wolferth[483]	Chamberlain[84]	Goadby et al.[198]	Shnider and Cotsonas[448]
Aortic aneurysms	88	8	119	5
Aneurysms of lower limb	32	3	44	15
Cerebral aneurysms	86*	2	42	16
Mesenteric aneurysms	38	3	38	14
Aneurysms of upper limb	20	—	24	4
Hepatic aneurysms	19	2	20	2
Pulmonary aneurysms	37	3	18	2
Splenic aneurysms	15	—	15	—
Coronary aneurysms	22	—	14	—
Iliac aneurysms	11	2	12	5
Miscellaneous sites	14	2	26	6
Total	382+	25	372	69

*Includes three aneurysms of the internal carotid and one vertebral; they may be intracerebral or extracerebral.

(20.3%). Only 187 cases were associated with an infectious endocardial lesion.

McDonald and Korb[325] garnered from the literature 1125 cases of saccular aneurysm of the cerebral arteries of which aneurysms of embolic origin constituted 12.2% of the series. Of these patients, 44% were 20 years of age or younger. Mitchell and Angrist[339] in 36 cases of cerebral aneurysms found 10 to be bacterial, attributing the prevalence to the careful microscopic examination of small hemorrhagic foci in cases of infection. Brown[66] reported the occurrence of five bacterial aneurysms in 154 cases of proved intracranial aneurysm, and Hamby[216] found three in 86 such cases. Russell[419] attributed to the presence of bacterial aneurysms 28 out of 462 cases of non-traumatic intracranial hemorrhage (6.5%). Recently in 191 patients with proved ruptured intracranial aneurysm admitted to a neurosurgical unit in a period of 12 years, Roach and Drake[408] found five cases and regarded the frequency as startlingly high. This frequency is probably inflated because of the nature of the institution. Bacterial endocarditis is not a common malady, and by no means do all patients develop cerebral complications clinically, and even fewer will have bacterial aneurysms.[278]

The cerebral arteries are a common site for bacterial aneurysms (Table 9-13). Not all are embolic or metastatic in origin, and, just as many bacterial aneurysms of the aorta are caused by local spread, so too are some of the cerebral bacterial aneurysms, and this necessitates their subdivision into two distinct etiological types—those of embolic or metastatic origin and those caused by local infection.

Bacterial aneurysms of embolic or metastatic origin. In the past, these aneurysms have predominantly been associated with bacterial endocarditis and less often with a severe pulmonary inflammatory lesion or septicemia. The present upsurge of cardiac and vascular surgery, and the attendant increase in bacterial endocarditis as a complication may well bring about an increase in their prevalence.

A series of 125 cases of bacterial aneurysm of the cerebral arteries was collected from the literature.* The series, though not all-encompassing, includes only cases in which some detail was available. There may be some overlap with Stengel and Wol-

---

*The sources include two groups: (1) 70 cases listed by McDonald and Korb,[325] with the exception of those considered questionable, and (2) cases prior to 1938 excluded from the latter publication and others recorded since 1938, the reference numbers of which are 13, 27, 38, 46, 73, 92, 125, 177, 205, 208, 216, 278, 283, 286, 316, 320, 336, 339, 342, 374, 376, 384, 395, 408, 410, 454, 482, 491, 540.

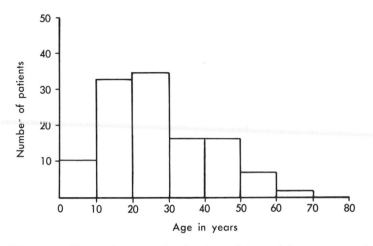

Fig. 9-40. Histogram illustrating age distribution of bacterial aneurysms (embolic or metastatic) of cerebral arteries.

ferth's series, since they did not specify their sources.

Of the 125 cases, 63 were males, 52 were females and, in the remaining 10, the sex was not specified. Age was available in 116 instances, the arithmetic mean age was 25.9 years and the age distribution is illustrated in Fig. 9-40. In contrast with cases of non-inflammatory saccular aneurysms of the cerebral arteries (Fig. 9-5), over 80% of these subjects were under 40 years of age, which fact is consistent with the age incidence of bacterial endocarditis. Many of the females were of child-bearing age and so the possibility existed that bacterial aneurysms would complicate pregnancy, but this does not often eventuate.[76]

Usually small, the aneurysms are less than 1 cm. in diameter (Fig. 9-41) and only occasionally are they 2 or even 3 cm. in their largest dimension. They are saccular or spherical, though fusiform dilatations are known and may be related to a fork or branching. When the aneurysm arises from the apical region of an arterial fork, the lesion is most likely to be of the berry type. Frequently the wall appears to be hemorrhagic, thin, or perhaps grayish white and friable and the sac may disintegrate if handled excessively. A saccular dilatation may actually be a false sac that can be

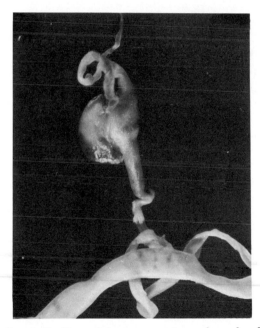

Fig. 9-41. Bacterial aneurysm on a branch of anterior inferior cerebellar artery. Note fusiform dilatation of the parent stem and hemorrhagic appearance of the saccular dilatation. (From Stehbens, W. E.: Atypical cerebral aneurysms, Med. J. Aust. 1:765, 1965.)

superimposed on a fusiform dilatation. A bilocular aneurysm is unusual.[92,408]

Frequently there is friable or even purulent thrombus in the sac occluding most if not all of the lumen. Evidence of leakage

Table 9-14. Distribution of bacterial aneurysms of embolic origin in the cerebral circulation

Artery	Number of aneurysms at each location	
	Stengel & Wolferth[483]	Present series
Internal carotid	3	5
Middle cerebral	23*	63*
Anterior cerebral	3	8
Anterior communicating	—	4
Posterior communicating	2	2
Vertebral	1†	1
Basilar	4	8
Posterior cerebral	1	8
Cerebellar	—	—
Ophthalmic	—	1
Perforating arteries	—	1
Small unspecified pial arteries	49+‡	13*
Site not specified	—	19
Total	86*	133*

*Additional aneurysms of uncertain number.
†Uncertain whether aneurysms were on intracranial or extracranial segments.
‡Numerous in two cases.

may be apparent, and at autopsy there are usually indications of rupture.

Table 9-14 gives the distribution of bacterial aneurysms of embolic or metastatic origin. The middle cerebral artery is unquestionably the most common site of involvement and although these aneurysms also involve the large arteries at the base of the brain as do the noninflammatory saccular berry aneurysms, they are often more distally situated. Thus their location seems to be confined to small unspecified arteries, pial or arachnoidal vessels or small branches of major trunks. Even perforating arteries may be affected. The peripheral location of the aneurysms is well demonstrated by angiography,[278,408] and any unusual location is adequate reason for suspecting their presence and indicating a need for histological investigation.[479] Roach and Drake[408] reported a case in point. The patient was quite well until suddenly, while pitching silage, he experienced a severe headache and fell to the ground. Angiography revealed an aneurysm on the surface of the left parietal lobe arising from a peripheral branch of the middle cerebral artery. The unusual location was suspect and subacute bacterial endocarditis was subsequently confirmed.

In 43 instances the aneurysm was located on the right side and in 37 the left. The remainder were either midline or the side was not specified. Twelve patients had multiple lesions. Bigelow[46] contended the incidence of multiplicity varied from 14% to 50%, but each series reviewed was small and the overall incidence was 22%. Occasionally bilateral symmetry is seen, and bacterial aneurysms of extracranial arteries may coexist.[46] Unfortunately there has been no detailed investigation of the early stages of aneurysm formation in cases of this nature.

Most bacterial aneurysms are of embolic origin, the infection originating in either the vegetations of a bacterial endocarditis or in an extracardiac septic lesion of the lung in particular. They may also complicate septicemia or bacteremia. Previously the so-called subacute bacterial endocarditis (endocarditis lenta) was the common cardiac lesion and hence *Streptococcus viridans* the commonest causative organism.[311] The heart exhibits the features of a subacute endocarditis, with evidence of preexisting rheumatic or congenital heart disease and associated embolic phenomena. An instance of coarctation of the aorta with bacterial endocarditis in association with a bacterial aneurysm of a small pial artery has been reported.[396] Other causative organisms include *Staphylococcus aureus, Staphylococcus albus,* pneumococcus, *Streptococcus faecalis,* and *Haemophilus influenzae.* The recent change in the clinical picture of bacterial endocarditis and a resurgence of the postcardiotomy endocarditis frequently caused by a penicillin-resistant staphylococcus suggest that bacterial aneurysms can be expected after cardiac surgery.

The pathogenesis of bacterial aneurysms of embolic origin is obscure, and no detailed study of the early stages of bacterial aneurysm formation exists. The role of fibrinolysins and migration of the embolus in the pathogenesis remain conjectural. It has generally been considered that a sizable septic embolus from the left atrium, mitral valve, or aortic cusps becomes impacted in a cerebral artery, perhaps near a fork. An acute arteritis of the vessel rapidly ensues, with softening and yielding of the wall. Superadded thrombus is likely to become occlusive and may propagate. The protective thrombus is not always adequate and the softened area of the wall may rupture without dilating further. Alternatively it expands and ultimately ruptures, with the formation of a false sac a further possibility. The propensity to thrombosis may at any time interrupt the aforementioned process. Alternatively a small embolus may become impacted in the entrance to a small branch and then acute arteritis affects both the branch and the parent vessel. Mural but not occlusive thrombus may be deposited in the parent vessel, the wall of which may then commence to expand. Another contingency is that the embolus may become impacted, an acute arteritis may result, and the thrombus may undergo lysis or soften as the result of leukocytic activity and break up with the lumen being reestablished. The weakened wall would then progressively dilate. Bacteria may lodge in vasa vasorum,[349] with the infection in effect commencing from without. Secondary infection of an atheromatous ulcer in the cerebral arteries is theoretically possible but unlikely.

The infrequency of these bacterial aneurysms is such that histological material is hard to come by and there is a need for further investigation of their pathogenesis. An alternative method of resolving the pathogenesis would be to study it in the experimental animal by injecting artificially prepared septic thrombi into a given arterial bed. This procedure would also provide estimates of the time required for such an aneurysm to form.

Histologically the artery exhibits an acute and severe arteritis with the architecture of the wall in places completely destroyed (Fig. 9-42). Subendothelial exudate and remnants of the media and internal elastic lamina may lie in a dense mass of polymorphonuclear leukocytes, which in places is frankly suppurative. Colonies of bacteria are frequently found. The contour of the wall may indicate dilatation and the lumen is often filled with exudate and septic thrombus. Alternatively the wall may merge with that of a false aneurysm perchance also showing evidence of sepsis. In some instances calcification has been seen in the original embolus from the cardiac valves.

The gross destruction of the vessel wall from the histological viewpoint provides adequate basis for the development of an aneurysm and also for rupture with subarachnoid hemorrhage even without prior arterial dilatation. Subacute aneurysms exhibit evidence of healing in the form of an intimal proliferation consisting of loose connective tissue and spindle cells with an infiltration of inflammatory cells. Macrophage activity is generally prominent.

In the surrounding meninges and brain, inflammatory changes vary in severity and small neighboring vessels are liable to be plugged with thrombus. Evidence of previous leakage and of recent frank hemorrhage into the subarachnoid space or brain is not exceptional, and the underlying brain may be infarcted, hemorrhagic, or in the process of abscess formation.

The effect of antibiotics on these lesions has not yet been documented, but, under treatment, the inflammatory lesion may heal, and if thrombosis of the parent vessel does not occur, it would be feasible for the aneurysm to persist though this is speculative. The focus of arteritis may heal with the aid of chemotherapy and the resultant scar eventually dilate, but this is not very probable unless there is already some dilatation. However, one should keep in mind that bacterial aneurysms containing demonstrable organisms may manifest themselves not only before or during treatment but

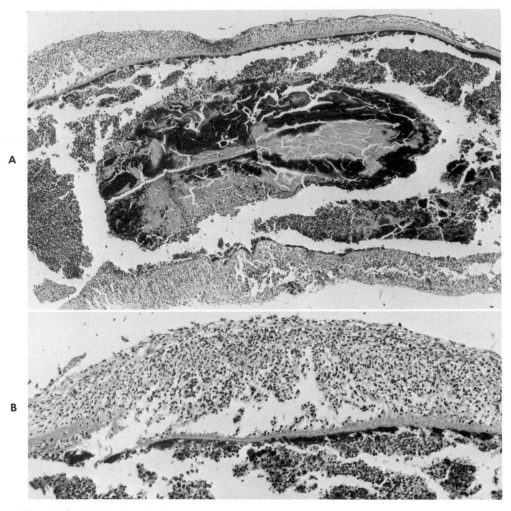

Fig. 9-42. Wall of embolic aneurysm (fusiform) segment of Fig. 9-41. Embolic plug with bacterial masses (dark-staining material in lumen in **A** and along internal elastic lamina in **B** and acute arteritis. Note gross destruction of mural architecture and elastic tear in **B**. (Hematoxylin and eosin; **A,** ×45; **B,** ×110.)

even months after alleged bacteriological cure.

Ray and Wahal[396] reported two cases in which saccular berry aneurysms at arterial bifurcations were believed to have been infected secondarily to a bacterial endocarditis. Rupture of the sac had occurred in both instances.

When considering aneurysms caused by septic emboli, it must be stressed that, with the exception of neoplasms, no evidence exists to indicate that bland, nonseptic emboli can result in aneurysm formation.

Bacterial aneurysms caused by local infection. Bacterial aneurysms of the cerebral arteries caused by a local infective process involving the vessel from outside are much less frequent than those caused by septic embolism or metastatic infection. The arteritis is secondary, and if the vessel is sufficiently damaged, aneurysmal dilatation is the outcome unless superadded, protective, and occlusive thrombus supervenes.

Examples of this type of lesion include the following:

1. Brown[66] reported a patient with a large aneurysm of the basilar and another of the

left superior cerebellar artery. Both aneurysms were attributed to tuberculous involvement of the arterial wall. There was no mention of histological confirmation.

2. One of the 10 patients with bacterial aneurysms reported by Mitchell and Angrist[339] developed the aneurysm secondarily to influenzal meningitis. The site of the aneurysm was not stated.

3. Barker[27] provided a history of a man of 32 years with acute sphenoidal sinusitis that spread to the cranial cavity causing thrombosis of the right cavernous sinus and bacterial aneurysms of both internal carotid arteries. One aneurysm ruptured fatally. In a similar case reported by de Rougemont and associates,[130] a male of 17 years suffered an injury to the left sub-orbital region, which became infected with a staphylococcus. Secondary cavernous sinus thrombosis resulted and an aneurysmal dilatation of the cavernous segment of the carotid artery developed. An earlier angiogram had revealed no deformity of outline.

4. Ojemann and associates[363] demonstrated radiologically four fusiform aneurysms of cingulate branches of the pericallosal artery in a 46-year-old woman with pneumococcal meningitis secondary to otitis media. Angiography after 5 weeks revealed only a slight residual dilatation at the site of one of the previously demonstrated aneurysms that were attributed to the meningitis although metastatic spread attributed to bacteremia cannot be excluded.

5. An 18-year-old male sustained a fractured skull in a motorcycle accident. Meningitis developed after surgical treatment of the skull and dura. The patient died and four aneurysms were found at sites regarded as unusual for the common variety of saccular cerebral (berry) aneurysm at forks.[240]

6. Hansmann and Schenker[223] reported melitensis meningoencephalitis in a 24-year-old male. There was a bacterial aneurysm of the proximal part of the basilar artery.

Such aneurysms caused by local infection might be found more frequently in instances of meningitis if postmortem angiography were used.

Syphilitic aneurysms. Syphilis affects blood vessels with unremitting frequency and there was once a time when this disease entity was regarded as the most common single cause of aortic aneurysm. Differentiated from atherosclerosis only about the turn of the century, syphilitic arteritis is now less prevalent at autopsy than in previous years. Yet even today syphilis of the aorta continues to be overdiagnosed, because the presence of perivascular lymphocytes and plasma cells in the adventitia of severely atherosclerotic aortas is misleading. In the case of the cerebral arteries also, considerable difficulty has been experienced in evaluating the role of syphilis in the etiology of cerebral aneurysms, the dilemma arising no doubt from the presence of chronic inflammatory cells in the adventitia of atherosclerotic vessels and inexact serological techniques.

In earlier centuries, syphilis was regarded as a not infrequent cause of aneurysm of the cerebral arteries. Investigators such as Fearnsides[166] and Turnbull[509] asserted that they could not find evidence of syphilis in the etiology of the lesions although other authors continued to ascribe their formation to luetic infection.[187,536] In a review of 1125 cases from the literature by McDonald and Korb,[325] 32 cases (in patients 20 to 75 years of age) were allegedly caused by syphilis. Richardson and Hyland[400] were of the opinion that it was conceivable that an active luetic process in the brain could precipitate rupture of a coexisting berry aneurysm. Bassoe[31] asserted that syphilis, though an uncommon cause of the small berry aneurysms, was less rare as a cause of the more infrequent large aneurysms of the basilar and vertebral arteries, sites repeatedly given for aneurysms thought to be syphilitic in origin.

Most authors currently writing on the etiology of cerebral aneurysms express the view that syphilis is not a cause, but at best a rare etiological factor in the formation of aneurysms.[216,523] However, Mitchell and Angrist[339] reported aneurysms said to be caused by gummatous inflammation of the arteries. Many of the aneurysms reported in the past as being syphilitic were probably not inflammatory in origin at all. The chance coexistence of syphilis and a cerebral aneurysm of other etiology must be borne in mind and also that false serological positives can be reduced to a minimum with improved present-day techniques. Furthermore spirochetes have yet to be demonstrated in the walls of these aneurysms.

One can only conclude that syphilitic aneurysms of the cerebral arteries are exceptionally rare, and with better chemotherapeutic control of the disease, chance encounters with such a case should become even more remote.

Aneurysms of the spinal arteries have been attributed to syphilitic arteritis,[549] and as with those of the cerebral vessels their authenticity must be regarded as doubtful.

Other aneurysms of inflammatory origin. Aneurysms may also arise as the result of other varieties of inflammation, such as fungal infections, polyarteritis nodosa, Wegener's granulomatosus, and giant cell arteritis, but they are uncommon (see Chapter 12).

Trauma and intracranial aneurysms

The relationship of trauma to the etiology and pathology of intracranial aneurysms is of considerable medicolegal importance. The trauma may be related to (1) either the onset of subarachnoid hemorrhage or aneurysmal rupture, (2) the pathogenesis of strictly traumatic aneurysms, (3) the development of traumatic arteriovenous fistula, and (4) the etiology of dissecting aneurysms.

Trauma and aneurysmal rupture. In many forensic cases of ruptured cerebral aneurysm, Freytag[181] emphasized the history of trauma. In the Cooperative Study,[302] a history of minor trauma preceding the onset of subarachnoid hemorrhage was established in 2.8% of the cases of cerebral aneurysm compared to an incidence of 4.4% in cases with arteriovenous aneurysms. The difference was attributed to the youthfulness and attendant greater vigor and activity of the patients with arteriovenous aneurysms, factors of less import with older victims of cerebral aneurysms.

The patient with a sudden rupture of an aneurysm may lose consciousness without warning and, in falling, suffer a head injury of varying severity. Such cases should be regarded as belonging to a category quite distinct from those in which a blow to the head preceded the onset of bleeding, despite extreme difficulty in ascertaining the primary lesion. The chance of the trauma and rupture occurring simultaneously is fairly remote.

The exact relationship of trauma to the rupture of cerebral aneurysms is unresolved, and it is difficult to prove that head injuries predispose an already existing aneurysm to rupture. It may be that trauma is the final stress demanded of an already weak, fragile sac wall in which rupture is imminent. We know little of the stresses and strains imposed on the large arteries at the base of the brain at the moment of impact. However, as trauma occasionally lacerates the internal carotid artery or a peripheral vessel, it seems logical to conclude that stresses on the sac wall of a degree sufficient to precipitate rupture can be derived from head injuries. Pool and Potts[384] reported one instance, but even so one cannot rule out that the simultaneous occurrence of trauma and aneurysmal rupture could be fortuitous.

Traumatic aneurysms of cerebral arteries. Trauma is a cause of saccular aneurysm of the intracranial arteries only extremely rarely as is to be expected in view of their protective bony encasement. In the pathogenesis of a traumatic aneurysm,[348] one constant condition must be met: the injury to the vessel must cause partial rupture only because retraction and clotting are likely if the vessel is completely severed. In view of the arterial lesions associated with electrocution[64,232] and the traumatic origin of some cerebral dissecting aneurysms, partial rupture of a cerebral artery with dilatation of the adventitia is at least plausible. A clot temporarily sealing a leak from a damaged extracranial artery may give way some days later. Such an event could transpire in the cranial cavity. Small leaks may seal off spontaneously without progressing to aneurysm formation. Yet again, a false sac may develop at the site of injury, forming in much the same manner as when an aneurysm ruptures. Bleeding is said to cease when pressure in the extracranial hematoma equals the arterial pressure within the involved vessel.[348] Indeed the tension in the tissues locally may be very great. It is not known if this holds true within the cranium, but extravasated blood remains sufficiently localized to form a pulsating hematoma in the complete absence of fascial sheaths and inappreciable amounts of resilient connective tissue, which limit spread. Contrary to expectations the blood in the hematoma does not coagulate. The central portion remains liquid or otherwise undergoes lysis. Histologically it is identical to other false sacs associated with ruptured berry aneurysms. Multiple traumatic aneurysms may also occur.[417]

Traumatic saccular aneurysms of peripheral cerebral arteries are exceptionally rare and the injuries responsible have varied. At least 20 such cases in the literature justified inclusion in the category.[69,417] The mortality was over 50%. Of particular interest were two cases in which postoperative complications[170,496] were attributed to trauma rather than infection. Such complications are most likely in patients with Ehlers-Danlos syndrome or a related disorder. Several cases were caused by bizarre penetrating wounds,[82,107] some were associated with a fractured skull, others resulted from indirect injury.[417] A subdural, or an intracerebral, hematoma or both are usually present. A 9-month-old infant[367] developed such an aneurysm on a pial artery after therapeutic needling through the anterior fontanelle, and more recently it has been a complication of trephination of the skull for subdural hematoma.[160]

Birley and Trotter[48] described severe recurrent epistaxis several weeks after a skull fracture in a young man of 23 years of age. A saccular aneurysm of the cavernous segment of his internal carotid artery was suspected in the vascular sheath and was thought to have enlarged, causing multiple cranial nerve palsies and bleeding from the aneurysm into the sphenoid sinus. An intracranial bruit was audible and disappeared only slowly after carotid ligation, but no carotid-cavernous fistula was in evidence. Similar cases have since been described,[72,220,380] and in some a saccular aneurysm of the intracavernous portion of the internal carotid artery has been demonstrated. Extensive erosion in the region of the sella turcica and roof of the sphenoid sinus can occur,[440] and the aneurysm may rupture into the sphenoid (or ethmoid) sinus causing exsanguination. Twenty proved cases of ruptured aneurysms of the cavernous portion of the internal carotid artery with epistaxis were found in 1964[322] and in 10 cases of probable aneurysm with epistaxis. Of the proved cases, 16 were associated with head injury and 6 of the 10 possible cases were associated with trauma. So it appears that trauma is a significant factor in the pathogenesis of most of these aneurysms, which are false in nature. Nontraumatic aneurysms in the cavernous sinus infrequently involve the paranasal air sinuses and consequently rarely cause epistaxis.

Seftel and associates[440] emphasized that epistaxis by erosion into the sphenoid sinus was the most common. It can also result from a traumatic aneurysm of the carotid artery within the carotid canal, which is separated from the eustachian tube by only a thin, bony cribriform barrier, through which rupture causes pharyngeal bleeding and epistaxis.

Kinley and Leighninger[285] reported a traumatic aneurysm of the ophthalmic artery that arose from the cavernous segment of the internal carotid artery. The sac presented in the sphenoid sinus, causing epistaxis and simulating a traumatic aneurysm of the internal carotid. Jefferson[269] believed that some fusiform or saccular aneurysms of the cavernous segment of the internal carotid were traumatic in origin, presenting apparently anew years after a forgotten accident. Aneurysms appearing to be nontraumatic occur predominantly in women. Those directly related to trauma are mostly confined to males.

The anatomy of the cavernous segment of the internal carotid artery is such that the vessel is peculiarly vulnerable to trauma. Fractures through the middle cranial fossa commonly involve the sphenoid sinus and hence the internal carotid is liable to damage. It has been assumed that this segment of the internal carotid has a congenital weakness, but there is no evidence in support. The concept is a convenient carry-over from the ill-founded "congenital" theory of saccular berry aneurysms. It may be pertinent that this carotid siphon frequently exhibits ectasia and augmented tortuosity in the adult.

Patients presenting with a cerebral aneurysm and a history of head injury long past, pose difficult medicolegal problems. Most of these aneurysms will probably be nontraumatic and the anatomical location of the sac aids in clarifying the issue.

Traumatic aneurysms of the meningeal arteries. Trauma to the meningeal arteries has long been known to cause extradural hematoma, often with a rapid course of some 6 to 48 hours. In recent years it has been shown that trauma to the meningeal arteries results in a traumatic or false aneurysm, often with an extradural hematoma of subacute course.[371] Eight had been reported up to 1964[290] and others have come to light since.[246,261,390] The frequency of traumatic meningeal aneurysms is difficult to gauge for recent improved angiographic techniques have resulted in an increase in clinical case reports. A similar increase from pathological material has not transpired and many are probably overlooked at autopsy.

The clinical picture of these lesions is characterized[290] by (1) a history of suspicion of head injury with (2) delayed neurological recovery or fairly abrupt deterioration in clinical status, (3) usually a linear fracture line crossing vascular markings on the meningeal arteries, and (4) a classic pattern on external carotid angiography or delayed filling and emptying on serial common carotid angiography.[133]

The most common site for these false sacs is on a branch of the middle meningeal artery and, when the sac is found on the fractured orbital roof, the anterior meningeal. One traumatic aneurysm was reported on the posterior meningeal artery.[390] These sacs are usually small and may project into the subdural space. An associated extradural hematoma of varying proportions can be expected and extravasated blood and altered blood pigment is likely to be found in the dura mater with sometimes evidence of trauma in the underlying brain and a subdural hematoma. Rupture of the false aneurysm produces extradural, subdural, or intracerebral hemorrhage.[389]

Histologically the lesions are characteristically false sacs, the wall consisting of blood clot, laminated fibrin, and granulation tissue. If the sac is not recent, the dense fibrous wall may resemble the berry variety of aneurysm. A merging of the arterial wall into the granulation tissue of the false sac can make the aneurysm appear to be a preexisting lesion.

The meningeal arteries because of their anatomical location are particularly vulnerable to trauma when the skull is fractured. The artery may be completely severed or sustain only a lateral tear of the wall with again variation in the degree of injury. Dissecting aneurysms readily occur in cases of trauma to the carotid and cerebral vessels, and it would not be surprising if the meningeal vessels were affected likewise. No instances of this have been recorded, even though Irachi and associates[261] used the term "dissecting aneurysm" as a synonym of traumatic aneurysm.

Several cases have been reported in which the clinical aspects were those of traumatic meningeal aneurysms whereas the arterial lesions were considered preexisting aneurysms of the berry type. In each case the histological picture was unconvincing.[8,17,524] Pallais and associates[371] encountered a false aneurysm of a small transdural anastomotic artery, and Salmon and Blatt[424] illustrated in one case the simultaneous occurrence of a middle meningeal and an internal carotid aneurysm of traumatic origin.

In a study of traumatic aneurysms of the aorta, the maximum danger period lasted

3 weeks.[39] This should apply to traumatic aneurysms both cerebral and meningeal with the danger of rupture diminishing as time passes and as the wall is reinforced or the vessel becomes thrombosed.

Saccular aneurysms of the large arteries of the neck

Ectasia, tortuosity, looping, and kinking are frequent in the carotid arteries in the neck. Frank aneurysmal dilatation, however, is not a common event. Aneurysms of the internal carotid usually arise close to its origin. Occasionally they are bilateral and relatively symmetrical. Those occurring spontaneously are most often caused by severe atherosclerosis. Stenotic lesions of these arteries are complications. Traumatic aneurysms are not infrequent and are caused by blunt trauma as well as perforating or penetrating injuries. Syphilis is a rare cause and "congenital factors" have occasionally been invoked. Apart from hemorrhage and symptoms referable to a visible or pharyngeal pulsating tumor, the victim not infrequently experiences neurological ischemic episodes attributed to emboli from the sac or associated ulcerated atheromatous plaques. Aneurysms of the vertebral artery are almost entirely caused by trauma.

Aneurysms of the spinal arteries

Physiological environment and histological structure are similar in spinal and cerebral arteries. Developmentally both arise from a primitive capillary plexus and considerable anatomical variation is demonstrable. Yet aneurysms of spinal arteries, in contrast to those of intracranial vessels, are rarities, and the paucity in their numbers seems to be related to the small caliber of the spinal vessels in conjunction with the infrequency of atherosclerosis of a significant degree in vessels of such limited size.

Garland[187] had one spinal arterial aneurysm in 167 patients with aneurysms at autopsy, but it was said to be of doubtful pathology. Bassett and Lemmen[30] reported

an aneurysm of the anterior spinal artery near its origin from the left vertebral artery. Henson and Croft[242] found an aneurysm of the posterior spinal artery, a branch of the posterior inferior cerebellar artery. The sac was lying between the right cerebellar tonsil and the adjacent posterolateral aspect of the medulla oblongata. These aneurysms within the cranial cavity, like any other dilatation of small peripheral vessels, should be examined histologically for they are rarely of the berry type, being most frequently of inflammatory origin. By angiography Weibel and associates[528] demonstrated on the left fifth cervical radicular (medullary) artery a small aneurysm that had caused spinal subarachnoid hemorrhage in a female of 59 years, but again no pathological details were available.

In coarctation of the aorta, the spinal arteries actively participate in the collateral circulation, and as a result, the anterior spinal artery, especially in the cervical and thoracic regions of the cord, becomes considerably enlarged and tortuous (Fig. 2-8). As a result, complications that include the anterior spinal artery syndrome (because of spinal artery thrombosis[198]), compression myelitis, and even saccular aneurysms may occur.

Sargent[425] described an aneurysm of the anterior spinal artery, but no mention was made of coarctation of the aorta although it was probably present[549] because of the presence of numerous large tortuous collateral vessels in the neck, about the spine, and on the spinal cord. This deduction seems to be reasonable. The patient had had progressive spinal cord compression for 2 years terminating with a complete transverse lesion at the level of the seventh cervical segment.

Wyburn-Mason[549] reported two spinal aneurysms in association with aortic coarctation, making three in all. Wyburn-Mason's first case was that of a girl who at 14 years of age experienced subarachnoid hemorrhage, diplopia, and weakness of the legs progressing to paraplegia, with sensory loss to the level of the nipple.* At 18 years she died postoperatively after an exploratory laminectomy at which time profuse bleeding was encountered. At autopsy aortic coarctation was confirmed and at the level of the first thoracic segment a hard round aneurysm was found compressing the cord. At the sixth cervical segment, a large anterior medullary artery joined the anterior spinal artery, which entered the aneurysm. A vessel of similar size emerged at the lower end of the sac, ran a tortuous course, and divided into two branches, which left the spinal canal as medullary arteries. It was thought that the aneurysm was probably a false sac formed at the time the patient had suffered a spinal subarachnoid hemorrhage.

The second case of Wyburn-Mason[549] concerned a man of 42 years with aortic coarctation and a history of progressive motor and sensory loss to the level of the fourth thoracic segment. This patient also died postoperatively, and an aneurysm of an enlarged and tortuous anterior spinal artery at the level of the third thoracic segment was found to be compressing the spinal cord.

Babonneix and Widiez[20] reported the occurrence of an aneurysm of the anterior spinal artery in its lower cervical segment. This aneurysm was attributed to syphilis. No coarctation was disclosed at autopsy. Intracranial saccular aneurysms, which are neither inflammatory nor traumatic in nature, are found very rarely if ever on small vessels of the caliber of the anterior spinal artery. This generalization can be applied equally satisfactorily to the spinal cord. Therefore it would seem that saccular aneurysms of the spinal arteries not accompanied by coarctation and the associated changes in the collateral circulation, should be suspect, and careful histological study is needed to identify the cause. Syphilis must remain a rare cause of the few alleged instances[20,549] but other causes should be sought. Another atypical aneurysm was

reported by Kinal and Sejanovich[282] in a woman of 41 years. An encapsulated intramedullary hematoma without definite arterial connections was removed from the spinal cord at the level of the first thoracic segment. The histological features of the wall were not clear, and the lesion may have been an aneurysm associated with a small undetected arteriovenous angiomatous formation.

Spontaneous spinal subarachnoid hemorrhage is much rarer than intracranial subarachnoid hemorrhage and aneurysms are a very infrequent cause. Henson and Croft[242] recorded two cases due to polyarteritis nodosa, and Russell[419] reported another instance but no distinct aneurysm was present. Moreover, in vessels of this size, bacterial aneurysm would be expected to occur spasmodically though such has not been the case, for descriptions are lacking.

References

1. Abbott, M. E.: Coarctation of aorta of adult type, statistical study and historical retrospect of 200 recorded cases with autopsy, of stenosis or obliteration of the descending arch in subjects above the age of two years, Amer. Heart J. **3:**381, 574, 1928.
2. Adie, W. J.: Permanent hemianopia in migraine and subarachnoid haemorrhage, Lancet **2:**237, 1930.
3. af Björkesten, G., and Troupp, H.: Changes in the size of intracranial arterial aneurysms, J. Neurosurg. **19:**583, 1962.
4. Albl, H.: Aneurysma der Carotis interna, einen Hypophysentumor vortaüschend, ein Beitrag zur Diagnose intrakranieller Aneurysmen, Fortschr. Roentgenstr. **39:**890, 1929.
5. Albright, F.: The syndrome produced by aneurysm at or near the junction of the internal carotid artery and the circle of Willis, Bull. Johns Hopkins Hosp. **44:**215, 1929.
6. Alksne, J. F., Fingerhut, A. G., and Rand, R. W.: Magnetic probe for the stereotactic thrombosis of intracranial aneurysms, J. Neurol. Neurosurg. Psychiat. **30:**159, 1967.
7. Allen, A. C.: Skin. In Anderson, W. A. D.: Pathology, ed. 5, St. Louis, 1966, The C. V. Mosby Co., vol. 2, p. 1231.
8. Ameli, N. O.: Aneurysms of the middle meningeal artery, J. Neurol. Neurosurg. Psychiat. **28:**175, 1965.
9. Anderson, R. McD., and Schechter, M. M.: A case of spontaneous dissecting aneurysm of the internal carotid artery, J. Neurol. Neurosurg. Psychiat. **22:**195, 1959.
10. Andrus, S. B., Portman, O. W., and Riopelle, A. J.: Comparative studies of spontaneous and

---

*This case was also reported by Blackwood.[53]

experimental atherosclerosis in primates. II. Lesions in chimpanzees including myocardial infarction and cerebral aneurysms, Progr. Biochem. Pharmacol. 4:393, 1968.

11. Arieti, S.: Multiple meningioma and meningiomas associated with other brain tumors, J. Neuropath. Exp. Neurol. 3:255, 1944.

12. Arieti, S., and Gray, E. W.: Progressive multiform angiosis; association of cerebral angioma, aneurysms, and other vascular changes in the brain, Arch. Neurol. Psychiat. 51:182, 1944.

13. Aring, C. D.: Neurological clinical pathological conference of the Cincinnati General Hospital, Case No. 249534, Dis. Nerv. Syst. 14: 282, 1953.

14. Arseni, C., and Nash, F.: Cerebral ischemia in the course of ruptured aneurysms, Europ. Neurol. 1:308, 1968.

15. Ask-Upmark, E., and Ingvar, D.: A follow-up examination of 138 cases of subarachnoid hemorrhage, Acta Med. Scand. 138:15, 1950.

16. Aterman, K.: Cutis laxa seen in 3 infants born to Newfoundland family, Hosp. Tribune 3:2, Aug. 25, 1969.

17. Auld, A. W., Aronson, H. A., and Gargano, F.: Aneurysm of the middle meningeal artery, Arch. Neurol. 13:369, 1965.

18. Austin, M. G., and Schaefer, R. F.: Marfan's syndrome, with unusual blood vessel manifestations, Arch. Path. 64:205, 1957.

19. Ayer, W. D.: So-called spontaneous subarachnoid hemorrhage, Amer. J. Surg. 26:143, 1934.

20. Babonneix, L., and Widiez, A.: Sclérose combinée; lesions diffuses et inflammatoires du névraxe: Anévrysme de l'artère spinale antérieure. Syphilis probable, Rev. Neurol. 1: 1214, 1930.

21. Bakay, L., and Sweet, W. H.: Cervical and intracranial intra-arterial pressures with and without vascular occlusion, Surg. Gynec. Obstet. 95:67, 1952.

22. Bakay, L., and Sweet, W. H.: Intra-arterial pressures in the neck and brain, J. Neurosurg. 10:353, 1953.

23. Baker, T. W., and Sheldon, W. D.: Coarctation of the aorta with intermittent leakage of a congenital cerebral aneurysm, Amer. J. Med. Sci. 191:626, 1936.

24. Bannerman, R. M., Ingall, G. B., and Graf, C. J.: The familial occurrence of intracranial aneurysms, Neurology 20:283, 1970.

25. Barabas, A. P.: Heterogeneity of the Ehlers-Danlos syndrome: description of three clinical types and a hypothesis to explain the basic fect(s), Brit. Med. J. 2:612, 1967.

26. Barabas, A. P.: Discussion, Proc. Roy. Soc. Med. 62:735, 1969.

27. Barker, W. F.: Mycotic aneurysms, Ann. Surg. 139:84, 1954.

28. Bartal, A., Schiffer, J., and Weinstein, M.: A successful case of basilar bifurcation aneurysm surgery, Acta Neurochir. 19:163, 1968.

29. Bassett, R. C., and Lemmen, L. J.: Subdural hematoma associated with bleeding intracranial aneurysm, J. Neurosurg. 9:443, 1952.

30. Bassett, R. C., and Lemmen, L. J.: Intra-

cranial aneurysms. II. Some clinical observations concerning their development in the posterior circle of Willis, J. Neurosurg. 11: 135, 1954.

31. Bassoe, P.: Aneurysm of the vertebral artery, Arch. Neurol. Psychiat. 42:127, 1939.

32. Bates, J. I., Lewey, F. H., and Reiners, C. R.: The reaction of cerebral tissue to silver, tantalum, and zirconium, J. Neurosurg. 5:349, 1948.

33. Beadles, C. F.: Aneurisms of the larger cerebral arteries, Brain 30:285, 1907.

34. Bean, W. B.: Vascular spiders and related lesions of the skin, Springfield, Ill., 1958, Charles C Thomas, Publisher.

35. Bebin, J., and Currier, R. D.: Cause of death in ruptured intracranial aneurysms, Arch. Intern. Med. 99:771, 1957.

36. Beighton, P.: Lethal complications of the Ehlers-Danlos syndrome, Brit. Med. J. 3:656, 1968.

37. Bell, E. T.: Renal diseases, ed. 2, London, 1950, Henry Kimpton.

38. Bell, W. E., and Butler, C.: Cerebral mycotic aneurysms in children, Neurology 18:81, 1968.

39. Bennett, D. E., and Cherry, J. K.: The natural history of traumatic aneurysms of the aorta, Surgery 61:516, 1967.

40. Bergouignan, M., and Arne, L.: A propos des anévrysmes des artères cérébrales associés à d'autres malformations, Acta Neurol. Psychiat. Belg. 51:529, 1951.

41. Berk, M. E.: Aneurysm of the middle meningeal artery, Brit. J. Radiol. 34:667, 1961.

42. Berry, R. G., Alpers, B. J., and White, J. C.: The site, structure, and frequency of intracranial aneurysms, angiomas, and arteriovenous abnormalities, Res. Publ. Ass. Res. Nerv. Ment. Dis. 41:40, 1966.

43. Berthrong, M., and Sabiston, D. C.: Cerebral lesions in congenital heart disease. A review of autopsies on one hundred and sixty-two cases, Bull. Johns Hopkins Hosp. 89:384, 1951.

44. Beumont, P. J. V.: The familial occurrence of berry aneurysm, J. Neurol. Neurosurg. Psychiat. 31:399, 1968.

45. Bigelow, N. H.: The association of polycystic kidneys with intracranial aneurysms and other related disorders, Amer. J. Med. Sci. 225:485, 1953.

46. Bigelow, N. H.: Multiple intracranial arterial aneurysms, Arch. Neurol. Psychiat. 73:76, 1955.

47. Bigelow, N. H.: Intracranial dissecting aneurysms, Arch. Path. 60:271, 1955.

48. Birley, J. L., and Trotter, W.: Traumatic aneurysm of the intracranial portion of the internal carotid artery, Brain 51:184, 1928.

49. Birse, S. H., and Tom, M. I.: Incidence of cerebral infarction associated with ruptured intracranial aneurysms, Neurology 10:101, 1960.

50. Black, B. K., and Hicks, S. P.: The relation of hypertension to arterial aneurysms of the brain, U. S. Armed Forces Med. J. 3:1813, 1952.

51. Black, S. P. W., and German, W. J.: The treatment of internal carotid artery aneu-

rysms by proximal arterial ligation, J. Neurosurg. **10**:590, 1953.

52. Black, S. P. W., and German, W. J.: Observations on the relationship between the volume and the size of the orifice of experimental aneurysms, J. Neurosurg. **17**:984, 1960.

53. Blackwood, W.: Vascular disease of the central nervous system. In Blackwood, W., McMenemey, W. H., Meyer, A., Norman, R. M., and Russell, D. S.: Greenfield's neuropathology, ed. 2, Baltimore, 1963, The Williams & Wilkins Co., p. 71.

54. Bonnal, J., and Stevenaert, A.: Thrombosis of intracranial aneurysms of the circle of Willis after incomplete obliteration by clip or ligature across the neck, J. Neurosurg. **30**: 158, 1969.

55. Boop, W. C., Chou, S. N., and French, L. A.: Ruptured intracranial aneurysm complicated by subdural hematoma, J. Neurosurg. **18**:834, 1961.

56. Borelius, J.: Zur Genese und klinischen Diagnose der polycystischen Degeneration der Nieren, Nord. Med. Arkiv. **34**:Afd. 1, Nr. 27, 1901.

57. Bornstein, M. B., and Bender, M. B.: Subarachnoid hematoma complicating ruptured intracranial arterial aneurysm, Arch. Intern. Med. **100**:50, 1957.

58. Boström, K., and Liliequist, B.: Primary dissecting aneurysm of the extracranial part of the internal carotid and vertebral arteries, Neurology **17**:179, 1967.

59. Boyd, J. F., and Watson, A. J.: Dissecting aneurysm due to trauma, Scot. Med. J. **1**:326, 1956.

60. Boyd, L. J.: A study of four thousand reported cases of aneurysm of the thoracic aorta, Amer. J. Med. Sci. **168**:654, 1924.

61. Boyd-Wilson, J. S.: Iatrogenic carotid occlusion medial dissection complicating arteriography, World Neurol. **3**:507, 1962.

62. Bremer, J. L.: Congenital aneurysms of the cerebral arteries, Arch. Path. **35**:819, 1943.

63. Brice, J. G., and Crompton, M. R.: Spontaneous dissecting aneurysms of the cervical internal carotid artery, Brit. Med. J. **2**:790, 1964.

64. Brihaye, J., Mage, J., and Verriest, G.: Anévrysme traumatique de la carotide interne dans sa portion supraclinoïdienne, Acta Neurol. Psychiat. Belg. **54**:411, 1954.

65. Brindley, P., and Stembridge, V. A.: Aneurysm of the aorta. A clinicopathologic study of 369 necropsy cases, Amer. J. Path. **32**:67, 1956.

66. Brown, R. A. P.: Polycystic disease of the kidneys and intracranial aneurysms: the etiology and inter-relationship of these conditions: review of recent literature and report of seven cases in which both conditions coexisted, Glasgow Med. J. **32**:333, 1951.

67. Bull, J.: Massive aneurysms at the base of the brain, Brain **92**:535, 1969.

68. Bull, J. W. D.: Contribution of radiology to the study of intracranial aneurysms, Brit. Med. J. **2**:1701, 1962.

69. Burton, C., Velasco, F., and Dorman, J.: Traumatic aneurysm of a peripheral cerebral artery, J. Neurosurg. **28**:468, 1968.

70. Busse, O.: Aneurysmen und Bildungsfehler der Arteria communicans anterior, Virch. Arch. **229**:178, 1920.

71. Cadman, E. F. B., and Baker-Bates, E. T.: A case of vertebral artery aneurysm, Med. Illust. **7**:243, 1953.

72. Cairns, H.: The vascular aspects of head injuries, Lisboa Med. **19**:375, 1942.

73. Campbell, E., and Burkland, C. W.: Aneurysms of the middle cerebral artery, Ann. Surg. **137**:18, 1953.

74. Campbell, E., Perese, D., and Bigelow, N. H.: Excision of multisaccular supratentorial aneurysm of infratentorial origin, J. Neurosurg. **11**:422, 1954.

75. Campbell, M., and Baylis, J. H.: The course and prognosis of coarctation of the aorta, Brit. Heart J. **18**:475, 1956.

76. Cannell, D. E.: Subarachnoid haemorrhage in pregnancy, Proc. Roy. Soc. Med. **52**:950, 1959.

77. Carmichael, R.: The pathogenesis of noninflammatory cerebral aneurysms, J. Path. Bact. **62**:1, 1950.

78. Carroll, R. E., and Haddon, W.: Birth characteristics of persons dying of cerebral aneurysms, J. Chronic Dis. **17**:705, 1964.

79. Carton, C. A., Heifetz, M. D., and Kessler, L. A.: Patching of intracranial internal carotid artery in man using a plastic adhesive (Eastman 910 adhesive), J. Neurosurg. **19**:887, 1962.

80. Carton, C. A., Kennady, J. C., Heifetz, M. D., and Ross-Duggan, J. K.: The use of a plastic adhesive (methyl-2-cyanocrylate, monomer) in the management of intracranial aneurysms and leaking cerebral vessels: a report of 15 cases: In Fields, W. S., and Sahs, A. L.: Intracranial aneurysms and subarachnoid hemorrhage Springfield, Ill., 1965, Charles C Thomas, Publisher, p. 372.

81. Chadduck, W. M.: Intracavernous compression of the third nerve by an extracavernous carotid aneurysm, J. Neurosurg. **30**:501, 1969.

82. Chadduck, W. M.: Traumatic cerebral aneurysm due to speargun injury, J. Neurosurg. **31**:77, 1969.

83. Chakravorty, B. G., and Gleadhill, C. A.: Familial incidence of cerebral aneurysms, Brit. Med. J. **1**:147, 1966.

84. Chamberlain, E. N.: Bacterial aneurysms, Brit. Heart J. **5**:121, 1943.

85. Chambers, W. R., Harper, B. F., and Simpson, J. R.: Familial incidence of congenital aneurysms of cerebral arteries. Report of cases of ruptured aneurysm in father and son, J.A.M.A. **155**:358, 1954.

86. Charcôt, J. M.: Clinical lectures on senile and chronic diseases (translated by Tuke, W. S.), London, 1881, New Sydenham Society.

87. Charcôt, J. M., and Bouchard, C.: Nouvelle recherches sur la pathogénie de l'hémorrhagie cérébrale, Arch. Physiol. (Paris) **1**:110, 643, 725, 1869.

88. Chase, T. N., Rosman, N. P., and Price, D. L.: The cerebral syndromes associated with dis-

secting aneurysm of the aorta. A clinicopathological study, Brain **91**:173, 1968.

89. Chason, J. L., and Hindman, W. M.: Berry aneurysms of the circle of Willis, Neurology **8**:41, 1958.

90. Christensen, E., and Larsen, H.: Fatal subarachnoid haemorrhages in pregnant women with intracranial and intramedullary vascular malformations, Acta Psychiat. Neurol. Scand. **29**:441, 1954.

91. Christiansson, J.: On the late effect of carotid ligation upon the human eye, Acta Ophthalmol. **40**:271, 1962.

92. Church, W. S.: On the formation of aneurysms, and especially intracranial aneurysms in early life, St. Barth. Hosp. Rep. **6**:99, 1870.

93. Clarke, E., and Walton, J. N.: Subdural haematoma complicating intracranial aneurysm and angioma, Brain **76**:378, 1953.

94. Coe, J. E., and Bondurant, C. P.: Late thrombosis following the use of autogenous fascia and a cyanoacrylate (Eastman 910 monomer) for the wrapping of an intracranial aneurysm, J. Neurosurg. **21**:884, 1964.

95. Coe, R. W.: Case of aneurism of the left internal carotid artery within the cranium diagnosed during life, and treated successfully by ligature of the left common carotid artery, Ass. Med. J. **2**:1067, 1855.

96. Cohen, M. M.: Cerebrovascular accidents: study of 201 cases, Arch. Path. **60**:296, 1955.

97. Collier, J.: Cerebral haemorrhage due to causes other than arteriosclerosis, Brit. Med. J. **2**:519, 1931.

98. Conley, J. W., and Rand, C. W.: Spontaneous subarachnoid hemorrhage occurring in non-eclamptic pregnancy, Arch. Neurol. Psychiat. **66**:443, 1951.

99. Copelan, E. L., and Mabon, R. F.: Spontaneous intracranial bleeding in pregnancy, Obstet. Gynec. **20**:373, 1962.

100. Courville, C. B.: Intracranial lesions secondary to congenital (saccular) aneurysms, Bull. Los Angeles Neurol. Soc. **30**:1, 1965.

101. Courville, C. B., and Olsen, C. W.: Miliary aneurysms of the anterior communicating artery, Bull. Los Angeles Neurol. Soc. **3**:1, 1938.

102. Crawford, E. S., Edwards, W. H., DeBakey, M. E., Cooley, D. A., and Morris, G. C.: Peripheral arteriosclerotic aneurysms, J. Amer. Geriat. Soc. **9**:1, 1961.

103. Crawford, M. D., and Sarner, M.: Ruptured intracranial aneurysm, Lancet **2**:1254, 1965.

104. Crawford, T.: The pathological effects of cerebral arteriography, J. Neurol. Neurosurg. Psychiat. **19**:217, 1956.

105. Crawford, T.: Some observations on the pathogenesis and natural history of intracranial aneurysms, J. Neurol. Neurosurg. Psychiat. **22**:259, 1959.

106. Crelin, E. S.: Interpubic ligament: elasticity in pregnant free-tailed bat, Science **164**:81, 1969.

107. Cressman, M. R., and Hayes, G. J.: Traumatic aneurysm of the anterior choroidal artery, J. Neurosurg. **24**:102, 1966.

108. Crompton, M. R.: The pathology of ruptured middle-cerebral aneurysms with special reference to the differences between the sexes, Lancet **2**:421, 1962.

109. Crompton, M. R.: Intracerebral haematoma complicating ruptured cerebral berry aneurysms, J. Neurol. Neurosurg. Psychiat. **25**:378, 1962.

110. Crompton, M. R.: Hypothalamic lesions following the rupture of cerebral berry aneurysms, Brain **86**:301, 1963.

111. Crompton, M. R.: Cerebral infarction following the rupture of cerebral berry aneurysms Brain **87**:263, 1964.

112. Crompton, M. R.: The pathogenesis of cerebral infarction following the rupture of cerebral berry aneurysms, Brain **87**:491, 1964.

113. Crompton, M. R.: Subtentorial changes following the rupture of cerebral aneurysms, Brain **88**:75, 1965.

114. Crompton, M. R.: Recurrent haemorrhage from cerebral aneurysms and its prevention by surgery, J. Neurol. Neurosurg. Psychiat. **29**:164, 1966.

115. Crompton, M. R.: Mechanism of growth and rupture in cerebral berry aneurysms, Brit. Med. J. **1**:1138, 1966.

116. Crompton, M. R.: The comparative pathology of cerebral aneurysms, Brain **89**:789, 1966.

117. Crompton, M. R.: The pathogenesis of cerebral aneurysms, Brain **89**:797, 1966.

118. Cronqvist, S., Lundberg, N., and Troupp, H.: Temporary or incomplete occlusion of the carotid artery in the neck for the treatment of intracranial arterial aneurysms, Neurochirurgia **7**:146, 1964.

119. Crosato, F., and Terzian, H.: Gli aneurismi dissecanti intracranici; Studio di un caso con interessamento dell'arteria basilare, Riv. Path. Nerv. Ment. **82**:450, 1961.

120. Cuatico, W., Cook, A. W., Tyshchenko, V., and Khatib, R.: Massive enlargement of intracranial aneurysms following carotid ligation, Arch. Neurol. **17**:609, 1967.

121. Curtis, J., and Jimenez, J. A.: Intracranial aneurysm with panhypopituitarism, J.A.M.A. **203**:982, 1968.

122. Daane, T. A., and Tandy, R. W.: Rupture of congenital intracranial aneurysm in pregnancy, Obstet. Gynec. **15**:305, 1960.

123. Dalgaard, O. Z.: Bilateral polycystic disease of the kidneys, Acta Med. Scand. **158** (suppl. 328):1, 1957.

124. Dandy, W. E.: Intracranial arterial aneurysms in the carotid canal, Arch. Surg. **45**:335, 1942.

125. Dandy, W. E.: Intracranial arterial aneurysms, New York, 1944, Comstock Publishing Co., Inc.

126. Daoud, A. S., Pankin, D., Tulgan, H., and Florentin, R. A.: Aneurysms of the coronary artery, Amer. J. Cardiol. **11**:228, 1963.

127. Davis, R. H., Daroff, R. B., and Hoyt, W. F.: Hemicrania, oculosympathetic paresis, and subcranial carotid aneurysm: Raeder's paratrigeminal syndrome (Group 2). Case report, J. Neurosurg. **29**:94, 1968.

128. DeBusscher, J.: Anévrysme de l'artère verté-

brale gauche chez un homme de 45 ans, Acta Neurol. Belg. 52:1, 1952.

129. DeGrood, M. P. A. M.: Anévrysme disséquant carotidien comme complication de l'angiographie carotidienne, Rev. Neurol. 90:661, 1954.

130. de Rougemont, J., Nivelon, J. L., Lamit, J., and Thierry, A.: Anévrysme bactérien du segment intra-caverneux de la carotide interne consécutif à des lèsions endartéritiques observées au cours d'une thrombo-phlébite des sinus caverneux, Lyon Med. 210:341, 1963.

131. deVeer, J. A., and Browder, J.: Post-traumatic cerebral thrombosis and infarction, J. Neuropath. Exp. Neurol. 1:24, 1942.

132. Dial, D. L., and Maurer, G. B.: Intracranial aneurysms, Amer. J. Surg. 35:2, 1937.

133. Dilenge, D., and Wuthrich, R.: L'anévrysme traumatique de la méningée moyenne, Neurochirurgia 4:202, 1962.

134. Dinning, T. A. R., and Falconer, M. A.: Sudden or unexpected natural death due to ruptured intracranial aneurysm. Survey of 250 forensic cases, Lancet 2:799, 1953.

135. Dixon, J. M.: Angioid streaks and pseudoxanthoma elasticum with aneurysm of the internal carotid artery, Amer. J. Ophthal. 34:1322, 1951.

136. Dock, W.: The predilection of atherosclerosis for the coronary arteries, J.A.M.A. 131:875, 1946.

137. Dott, N. M.: Intracranial aneurysms: cerebral arterio-radiography: surgical treatment, Edinburgh Med. J. 40:219, 1933.

138. Doubler, F. H., and Marlow, S. B.: A case of hemorrhage into the optic-nerve sheaths as a direct extension from a diffuse intra-meningeal hemorrhage caused by rupture of aneurysm of a cerebral artery, Arch. Ophthal. 46:533, 1917.

139. Dourov, N., Locoge, M., Themelin, G., and De Rede, J.: Étude anatomo-clinique et radiologique d'un cas d'hématome disséquant d'une artère cérébrale chez un sujet jeune, Rev. Belge. Path. 30:265, 1964.

140. Drake, C. G.: Further experience with surgical treatment of aneurysms of the basilar artery, J. Neurosurg. 29:372, 1968.

141. Drake, C. G., and Vanderlinden, R. G.: The late consequences of incomplete surgical treatment of cerebral aneurysms, J. Neurosurg. 27:226, 1967.

142. Drake, C. G., Vanderlinden, R. G., and Amacher, A. L.: Carotid-ophthalmic aneurysms, J. Neurosurg. 29:24, 1968.

143. Drake, C. G., Vanderlinden, R. G., and Amacher, A. L.: Carotid-choroidal aneurysms, J. Neurosurg. 29:32, 1968.

144. Dratz, H. M., and Woodhall, B.: Traumatic dissecting aneurysm of left internal carotid, anterior cerebral and middle cerebral arteries, J. Neuropath. Exp. Neurol. 6:286, 1947.

145. Drennan, A. M.: Aneurysms of the larger cerebral vessels, New Zeal. Med. J. 20:324, 1921.

146. Drennan, A. M.: Discussion, Edinburgh Med. J. 40:234, 1933.

147. Du Boulay, G. H.: Some observations on the natural history of intracranial aneurysms, Brit. J. Radiol. 38:721, 1965.

148. Du Boulay, G. H.: The natural history of intracranial aneurysms, Amer. Heart J. 73:723, 1967.

149. Duman, S., and Stephens, J. W.: Post-traumatic middle cerebral artery occlusion, Neurology 13:613, 1963.

150. Dunger, K.: Lehre von den Cystenniere, Beitr. Path. Anat. 35:445, 1904.

151. Dutton, J.: Acrylic investment of intracranial aneurysms, Brit. Med. J. 2:597, 1959.

152. Dutton, J. E. M.: Intracranial aneurysm, Brit. Med. J. 2:585, 1956.

153. Dymond, A. M., Kaechele, L. E., Jurist, J. M., and Crandall, P. H.: Brain tissue reactions to some chronically implanted metals, J. Neurosurg. 33:574, 1970.

154. Echlin, F. A.: Spasm of basilar and vertebral arteries caused by experimental subarachnoid hemorrhage, J. Neurosurg. 23:1, 1965.

155. Ecker, A., and Riemenschneider, P.: Deliberate thrombosis of intracranial arterial aneurism by partial occlusion of the carotid artery with arteriographic control, J. Neurosurg. 8:348, 1951.

156. Ecker, A., and Riemenschneider, P. A.: Arteriographic demonstration of spasm of the intracranial arteries, J. Neurosurg. 8:660, 1951.

157. Eddy, D. D., and Farber, E. M.: Pseudoxanthoma elasticum, Arch. Dermatol. 86:729, 1962.

158. Edwards, J. E.: Pathology of anomalies of the thoracic aorta, Amer. J. Clin. Path. 23:1240, 1953.

159. Ehni, G., and Barrett, J. H.: Hemorrhage from the ear due to an aneurysm of the internal carotid artery, New Eng. J. Med. 262:1323, 1960.

160. Eichler, A., Story, J. L., Bennett, D. E., and Galo, M. V.: Traumatic aneurysm of a cerebral artery, J. Neurosurg. 31:72, 1969.

161. Endtz, L. J.: Familial incidence of intracranial aneurysms, Acta Neurochir. 19:297, 1968.

162. Engeset, A., Nelson, J. W., and Munthe-Kaas, A. W.: Acute cerebral vascular insufficiency in young patients, Acta Neurol. Scand. 43:(suppl. 31):122, 1967.

163. Enticknap, J. B.: Albers-Schönberg disease (marble bones), J. Bone Joint Surg. 36:123, 1954.

164. Eppinger, H.: Pathogenesis (Histogenesis und Aetiologie) der Aneurysmen einschliesslich des Aneurysma equi verminosum, Arch. Klin. Chir. 35:Suppl. I, 1887. Cited by Fearnsides.

165. Epstein, B. S.: The roentgenographic aspects of thrombosis of aneurysms of the anterior communicating and anterior cerebral arteries, Amer. J. Roentgen. 70:211, 1953.

166. Fearnsides, E. G.: Intracranial aneurysms, Brain 39:224, 1916.

167. Feldman, S., Behar, A. J., and Samueloff, M.: Effect of cortisone and hydrocortisone on piarachnoid adhesions, Arch. Neurol. Psychiat. 74:681, 1955.

168. Ferguson, G. C.: Turbulence in human intracranial saccular aneurysms, J. Neurosurg. 33:485, 1970.

169. Fine, R. D.: Angioma racemosum venosum of spinal cord with segmentally related angiomatous lesions of skin and forearm, J. Neurosurg. **18**:546, 1961.

170. Finkmeyer, H.: Ein säckchenförmiges Aneurysma der A. cerebri media als postoperative Komplikation, Zbl. Neurochir. **15**:302, 1955.

171. Fishberg, A. M.: Hypertension and nephritis, ed. 5, Philadelphia, 1954, Lea & Febiger.

172. Fisher, E. R., and Corcoran, A. C.: Congenital coarctation of the abdominal aorta with resultant renal hypertension, Arch. Intern. Med. **89**:943, 1952.

173. Fleming, J. F. R., and Park, A. M.: Dissecting aneurysms of the carotid artery following arteriography, Neurology **9**:1, 1959.

174. Florey, H.: Microscopical observations on the circulation of the blood in the cerebral cortex, Brain **48**:43, 1925.

175. Foltz, E. L., and Ward, A. A., Jr.: Communicating hydrocephalus from subarachnoid bleeding, J. Neurosurg. **13**:546, 1956.

176. Foord, A. G., and Lewis, R. D.: Primary dissecting aneurysms of peripheral and pulmonary arteries, Arch. Path. **68**:553, 1959.

177. Forbus, W. D.: On the origin of miliary aneurysms of the superficial cerebral arteries, Bull. Johns Hopkins Hosp. **47**:239, 1930.

178. Forster, F. M., and Alpers, B. J.: Aneurysm of the circle of Willis associated with congenital polycystic disease of the kidneys, Arch. Neurol. Psychiat. **50**:669, 1943.

179. Fouché, C. H.: Aneurysm of the anterior communicating artery of the brain, Proc. Roy. Soc. Med. **24**:1471, 1931.

180. Frankel, K.: Relation of migraine to cerebral aneurysm, Arch. Neurol. Psychiat. **63**:195, 1950.

181. Freytag, E.: Fatal rupture of intracranial aneurysms, Arch. Path. **81**:418, 1966.

182. Gallagher, J. P.: Pilojection for intracranial aneurysms, J. Neurosurg. **21**:129, 1964.

183. Gallagher, P. G., Dorsey, J. F., Stefanini, M., and Looney, J. M.: Large intracranial aneurysm producing panhypopituitarism and frontal lobe syndrome, Neurology **6**:829, 1956.

184. Gannon, W. E.: Valves of the common carotid artery during angiography, Amer. J. Roentgen. **86**:1050, 1961.

185. Garcia-Chavez, C., and Moossy, J.: Cerebral artery aneurysm in infancy: association with agenesis of the corpus callosum, J. Neuropath. Exp. Neurol. **24**:492, 1965.

186. Gardner, E., and Hardwick, S. W.: Dissecting aneurysm of the aorta associated with intracranial aneurysm and cerebral haemorrhage, J. Path. Bact. **58**:289, 1946.

187. Garland, H. G.: The pathology of aneurysm: a review of 167 autopsies, J. Path. Bact. **35**:333, 1932.

188. German, W. J., and Black, S. P. W.: Intraaneurysmal hemodynamics: turbulence, Trans. Amer. Neurol. Ass. **79**:163, 1954.

189. German, W. J., and Black, S. P. W.: Intraaneurysmal hemodynamics—jet action, Circulation Res. **3**:463, 1955.

190. German, W. J., and Black, S. P. W.: Cervical ligation for internal carotid aneurysms, J. Neurosurg. **23**:572, 1965.

191. Gibbs, J. R.: Effects of carotid ligation on the size of internal carotid aneurysms, J. Neurol. Neurosurg. Psychiat. **28**:383, 1965.

192. Gifford, R. W., Hines, E. A., and Janes, J. M.: An analysis and follow-up study of one hundred popliteal aneurysms, Surgery **33**:284, 1953.

193. Gillingham, F. J.: The management of ruptured intracranial aneurysm, Ann. Roy. Coll. Surg. Eng. **23**:89, 1958.

194. Gilman, S., Braverman, L. E., Starr, A., Horenstein, S., and Tilles, J. G.: Intracranial aneurysm causing panhypopituitarism, blindness, seizures and dementia, Ann. Intern. Med. **57**:639, 1962.

195. Girard, P. F., Guinet, P., Devic, M., and Mornex, R.: Anévrisme de la carotide interne et syndrome acromégaloïde, Rev. Neurol. **89**:279, 1953.

196. Gliedman, M. L., Ayers, W. B., and Vestal, B. L.: Aneurysms of the abdominal aorta and its branches, Ann. Surg. **146**:207, 1957.

197. Glynn, L. E.: Medial defects in the circle of Willis and their relation to aneurysm formation, J. Path. Bact. **51**:213, 1940.

198. Goadby, H. K., McSwiney, R. R., and Rob, C. G.: Mycotic aneurysms, St. Thomas Hosp. Rep. **5**:44, 1949.

199. Goldberg, S. A.: Arteriosclerosis in domestic animals, J. Amer. Vet. Med. Ass. **69**:31, 1926.

200. Gowers, W. R.: A manual of diseases of the nervous system, ed. 2, London, 1893, J. & A. Churchill.

201. Graf, C. J.: Spontaneous carotid-cavernous fistula: Ehlers-Danlos syndrome and related conditions, Arch. Neurol. **13**:662, 1965.

202. Graf, C. J.: Familial intracranial aneurysms, report of four cases, J. Neurosurg. **25**:304, 1966.

203. Graf, C. J.: On the origin of intracranial aneurysm. Thesis prepared for the American Neurological Association, 1967.

204. Grahame, R., and Beighton, P.: Physical properties of the skin in the Ehlers-Danlos syndrome, Ann. Rheum. Dis. **28**:246, 1969.

205. Green, F. H. K.: "Congenital" aneurysm of the cerebral arteries, Quart. J. Med. **21**:419, 1928.

206. Green, J. D.: The comparative anatomy of the hypophysis with special reference to its blood supply and innervation, Amer. J. Anat. **88**:225, 1951.

207. Greene, J. L., and McCormick, W. F.: Concurrent rupture of intracranial and intraabdominal aneurysms, J. Neurosurg. **29**:545, 1968.

208. Greenfield, W. S.: Cases of aneurysm of the cerebral and brachial arteries, Trans. Path. Soc. London **29**:91, 1878.

209. Gross, R. E.: Coarctation of the aorta, surgical treatment of one hundred cases, Circulation **1**:41, 1950.

210. Gross, S. W., and Holzman, A.: Aneurysm of

common carotid artery in the neck, J. Neurosurg. 11:209, 1954.

211. Guirguis, S., and Tadros, F. W.: An internal carotid aneurysm in the petrous temporal bone, J. Neurol. Neurosurg. Psychiat. 24:84, 1961.

212. Gull, W. M.: Cases of aneurism of the cerebral vessels, Guy's Hosp. Rep. 5:281, 1859.

213. Guy, C. C.: Aneurysm of the splenic artery, Surgery 5:602, 1939.

214. Halliday, J. H., and Robertson, J. S.: Dissecting aneurysm of the aorta, Proc. Roy. Aust. Coll. Phys. 1:3, 1946.

215. Hamby, W. B.: Intracranial aneurysms of the internal carotid artery and its branches, J. Int. Coll. Surg. 5:216, 1942.

216. Hamby, W. B.: Intracranial aneurysms, Springfield, Ill., 1952, Charles C Thomas, Publisher.

217. Hamilton, J. G., and Falconer, M. A.: Immediate and late results of surgery in cases of saccular intracranial aneurysms, J. Neurosurg. 16:514, 1959.

218. Hamilton, W. F., and Abbott, M. E.: Coarctation of the aorta of adult type. I. Complete obliteration of the descending arch at insertion of the ductus in a boy of fourteen: bicuspid aortic valve, impending rupture of the aorta; cerebral death, Amer. Heart J. 3:381, 1928.

219. Hammon, W. M.: Intracranial aneurysm encasement, J. Neurol. Neurosurg. Psychiat. 31:524, 1968.

220. Handa, J. Kikuchi, H., Iwayama, K., Teraura, T., and Handa, H.: Traumatic aneurysm of the internal carotid artery, Acta Neurochir. 17:161, 1967.

221. Handler, F. P., and Blumenthal, H. T.: Inflammatory factor in pathogenesis of cerebrovascular aneurysms, J.A.M.A. 155:1479, 1954.

222. Hannay, P. W.: Some clinical and histopathological notes on pseudoxanthoma elasticum, Brit. J. Derm. 63:92, 1951.

223. Hansman, G. H., and Schenken, J. R.: Melitensis meningo-encephalitis; mycotic aneurysm due to Brucella melitensis var. porcine, Amer. J. Path. 8:435, 1932.

224. Hardin, C. A.: Successful resection of carotid and abdominal aneurysm in two related patients with Marfan's syndrome, New Eng. J. Med. 267:141, 1962.

225. Hardin, C. A., and Snodgrass, R. G.: Dissecting aneurysm of internal carotid artery treated by fenestration and graft, Surgery 55:207, 1964.

226. Harel, D., Lavy, S., and Schwartz, A.: Aneurysm of basilar artery simulating a cerebellopontine angle tumor, Confin. Neurol. 29:360, 1967.

227. Harris, G. W.: Central nervous control of gonadotrophic and thyrotrophic secretion, Acta Endocr. 34 (suppl. 50):15, 1960.

228. Harris, L. S., Roessman, U., and Friede, R. L.: Bursting of cerebral ventricular walls, J. Path. Bact. 96:33, 1968.

229. Harris, P., and Udvarhelyi, G. B.: Aneurysms arising at the internal carotid-posterior communicating artery junction, J. Neurosurg. 14:180, 1957.

230. Harrison, T. H., Odom, G. L., and Kunkle, E. C.: Internal carotid aneurysm arising in carotid canal, Arch. Neurol. 8:328, 1963.

231. Harrow, B. R., and Sloane, J. A.: Aneurysm of renal artery: report of five cases, J. Urol. 81:35, 1959.

232. Hassin, G. B.: Changes in the brain in legal electrocution, Arch. Neurol. Psychiat. 30:1046, 1933.

233. Hassin, G. B.: Changes in the brain in accidental electrocution, J. Nerv. Ment. Dis. 86:668, 1937.

234. Hassler, O.: Morphological studies on the large cerebral arteries with reference to the aetiology of subarachnoid haemorrhage, Acta Psychiat. Neurol. Scand. 36 (suppl. 154):1, 1961.

235. Hassler, O.: Experimental carotid ligation followed by aneurysmal formation and other morphological changes in the circle of Willis, J. Neurosurg. 20:1, 1963.

236. Hassler, O., and Saltzman, G. F.: Histologic changes in infundibular widening of the posterior communicating artery, Acta Path. Microbiol. Scand. 46:305, 1959.

237. Hayes, G. J., and Leaver, R. C.: Methyl methacrylate investment of intracranial aneurysms, J. Neurosurg. 25:79, 1966.

238. Hayman, J. A., and Anderson, R. McD.: Dissecting aneurysm of the basilar artery, Med. J. Aust. 2:360, 1966.

239. Heath, D., Edwards, J. E., and Smith, L. A.: The rheologic significance of medial necrosis and dissecting aneurysm of the ascending aorta in association with calcific aortic stenosis, Proc. Staff Meet. Mayo Clin. 33:228, 1958.

240. Heidelberger, K. P., Layton, W. M., and Fisher, R. G.: Multiple cerebral mycotic aneurysms complicating posttraumatic pseudomonas meningitis, J. Neurosurg. 29:631, 1968.

241. Heiskanen, O., and Nikki, P.: Rupture of intracranial arterial aneurysm during pregnancy, Acta Neurol. Scand. 39:202, 1963.

242. Henson, R. A., and Croft, P. B.: Spontaneous spinal subarachnoid haemorrhage, Quart. J. Med. 25:53, 1956.

243. Heuer, G. J., and Dandy, W. E.: Roentgenography in the localization of brain tumors, based upon a series of one hundred consecutive cases, Bull. Johns Hopkins Hosp. 26:311, 1916.

244. Hicks, S. P., and Black, B. K.: The relation of cardiovascular disease to apoplexy, Amer. Heart J. 38:528, 1949.

245. Hirano, A., Barron, K. D., and Zimmerman, H. M.: Ruptured aneurysms of the supraclinoid portion of the internal carotid and of the middle cerebral arteries, J. Nerv. Ment. Dis. 129:35, 1959.

246. Hirsch, J. F., David, M., and Sachs, M.: Les

anévrysmes artériels traumatiques intracraniens, Neurochirurgie **8**:189, 1962.

247. Hirsch, O.: Pathology of the sphenoidal sinus, Arch. Otolaryng. **67**:85, 1958.

248. Hirst, A. E., Johns, V. J., and Kime, S. W.: Dissecting aneurysm of the aorta: a review of 505 cases, Medicine **37**:217, 1958.

249. Hockaday, T. D. R.: Traumatic thrombosis of the internal carotid artery, J. Neurol. Neurosurg. Psychiat. **22**:229, 1959.

250. Hoehn, J. G., Bartholomew, L. G., Osmundson, P. J., and Wallace, R. B.: Aneurysms of the mesenteric artery, Amer. J. Surg. **115**:832, 1968.

251. Holman, E.: On circumscribed dilation of an artery immediately distal to a partially occluding band: post-stenotic dilatation, Surgery **36**:3, 1954.

252. Höök, O., and Norlén, G.: Aneurysms of the middle cerebral artery, Acta Chir. Scand. vol. 116, suppl. 235, 1958.

253. Houck, W. S., Jackson, J. R., Odom, G. L., and Young, W. G.: Occlusion of the internal carotid artery in the neck secondary to closed trauma to the head and neck: a report of two cases, Ann. Surg. **159**:219, 1964.

254. Housepian, E. M., and Pool, J. L.: A systematic analysis of intracranial aneurysms from the autopsy file of the Presbyterian Hospital 1914 to 1956, J. Neuropath. Exp. Neurol. **17**:409, 1958.

255. Hudson, C. H., and Raaf, J.: Timing of angiography and operation in patients with ruptured intracranial aneurysms, J. Neurosurg. **29**:37, 1968.

256. Humphrey, J. G., and Newton, T. H.: Internal carotid artery occlusion in young adults, Brain **83**:565, 1960.

257. Hyland, H. H.: Thrombosis of intracranial arteries, Arch. Neurol. Psychiat. **30**:342, 1933.

258. Hyland, H. H.: Prognosis in spontaneous subarachnoid hemorrhage, Arch. Neurol. Psychiat. **63**:61, 1950.

259. Hyland, H. H.: Discussion, Trans. Amer. Neurol. Ass. **78**:28, 1952.

260. Hyland, H. H., and Barnett, H. J. M.: The pathogenesis of cranial nerve palsies associated with intracranial aneurysms, Proc. Roy. Soc. Med. **47**:141, 1954.

261. Irachi, G., Carteri, A., and Galligioni, F.: Dissecting aneurysms of the middle meningeal artery: a case report, Med. Times **93**:840, 1965.

262. Jacques, L.: Aneurysm and anomaly of the circle of Willis, Arch. Path. **1**:213, 1926.

263. Jain, K. K.: Mechanism of rupture of intracranial saccular aneurysms, Surgery **54**:347, 1963.

264. Jamieson, K. G.: Aneurysms of the vertebrobasilar system, J. Neurosurg. **21**:781, 1964.

265. Jane, J. A.: A large aneurysm of the posterior inferior cerebellar artery in a 1-year-old child, J. Neurosurg. **18**:245, 1961.

266. Jansen, J. J.: De subarachnoidale bloeding, Thesis Utrecht, Utrecht, N. V. A. Oosthoek, 1963. Cited by Endtz.[161]

267. Jansen, L. H.: The structure of the connective tissue, an explanation of the symptoms of the Ehlers-Danlos syndrome, Dermatologica **110**:108, 1955.

268. Jefferson, G.: Compression of the chiasma, optic nerves, and optic tracts by intracranial aneurysms, Brain **60**:444, 1937.

269. Jefferson, G.: On the saccular aneurysms of the internal carotid artery in the cavernous sinus, Brit. J. Surg. **26**:267, 1938.

270. Jefferson, G.: Isolated oculomotor palsy caused by intracranial aneurysm, Proc. Roy. Soc. Med. **40**:419, 1947.

271. Jefferson, G.: Discussion, Proc. Roy. Soc. Med. **45**:300, 1952.

272. Jefferson, G.: Chiasmal lesions produced by intracranial aneurysms, Arch. Neurol. Psychiat. **72**:111, 1954.

273. Jefferson, G.: Further concerning compression of the optic pathways by intracranial aneurysms. In Congress of Neurological Surgeons: Clinical neurosurgery, Baltimore, 1955, The Williams & Wilkins Co., p. 55.

274. Jenkins, J. S., Buckell, M., Carter, A. B., and Westlake, S.: Hypothalamic-pituitary-adrenal function after subarachnoid haemorrhage, Brit. Med. J. **4**:707, 1969.

275. Jentzer, A.: Dissecting aneurysm of the left internal carotid artery, Angiology **5**:232, 1954.

276. Johnson, H. C., and Walker, A. E.: The angiographic diagnosis of spontaneous thrombosis of the internal and common carotid arteries, J. Neurosurg. **8**:631, 1951.

277. Johnson, R.: Discussion, Proc. Roy. Soc. Med. **45**:301, 1952.

278. Jones, H. R., Siekert, R. G., and Geraci, J. E.: Neurologic manifestations of bacterial endocarditis, Ann. Intern. Med. **71**:21, 1969.

279. Kahana, L., Lebovitz, H., Lusk, W., McPherson, H. T., Davidson, E. T., Oppenheimer, J. H., Engel, F. L., Woodhall, B., and Odom, G.: Endocrine manifestations of intracranial extrasellar lesions, J. Clin. Endocr. **22**:304, 1962.

280. Kak, V. K., Gleadhill, C. A., and Bailey, I. C.: The familial incidence of intracranial aneurysms, J. Neurol. Neurosurg. Psychiat. **33**:29, 1970.

281. Kaufman, S. F., and Markham, J. W.: Coarctation of the abdominal aorta with death from rupture of an aneurysm of a cerebral artery, Ann. Intern. Med. **43**:418, 1955.

282. Kinal, M. E., and Sejanovich, C.: Spinal cord compression by an intramedullary aneurysm, J. Neurosurg. **14**:561, 1957.

283. King, A. B.: Successful surgical treatment of an intracranial mycotic aneurysm complicated by a subdural hematoma, J. Neurosurg. **17**:788, 1960.

284. King, G., Slade, H. W., and Campoy, F.: Bilateral intracranial aneurysms, Arch. Neurol. Psychiat. **71**:326, 1954.

285. Kinley, G. J., and Leighninger, D. S.: Aneurysm of anomalous ophthalmic artery, J. Neurosurg. **9**:544, 1952.

286. Koch, V. W., and Nuzum, T. O.: Mycotic aneurysm; report of one case, Ann. Intern. Med. 14:522, 1940.

287. Köppen: Kleine Mitteilungen aus der Praxis, Berlin. Tierarztl. Wschr. 43:346, 1927.

288. Kraus, H.: Ein besonders grosses intrakranielles Aneurysma der Arteria carotis interna, Wien. Z. Nervenheilk. 5:23, 1952.

289. Krayenbühl, H.: Intracranial aneurysm, Arch. Neurol. Psychiat. 47:848, 1942. (Abstract.)

290. Kuhn, R. A., and Kugler, H.: False aneurysms of the middle meningeal artery, J. Neurosurg. 21:92, 1964.

291. Lagarde, C., Vigouroux, R., and Perrouty, P.: Agénésie terminale de la carotide interne anévrysme de la communicante antérieure, J. Radiol. Electrol. 38:939, 1957.

292. Lancisi, G. M.: De aneurysmatibus opus posthumum (revised and translated by Wright, W. C.), New York, 1952, The Macmillan Co.

293. Lang, E. R., and Kidd, M.: Electron microscopy of human cerebral aneurysms, J. Neurosurg. 22:554, 1965.

294. Law, W. R., and Nelson, E. R.: Internal carotid aneurysm as a cause of Raeder's paratrigeminal syndrome, Neurology 18:43, 1968.

295. Leading article: Popliteal aneurysms, Brit. Med. J. 1:625, 1966.

296. Lebert, H.: Ueber Aneurysmen der Gehirnarterien, Berlin. Klin. Wschr. 3:60, 209, 229, 249, 281, 336, 345, 387, 402, 1866. Cited by Charcôt,[86] Fearnsides,[166] and Jacques.[262]

297. Leigh, A. D., and Meyer, A: Degeneration of the granular layer of the cerebellum, J. Neurol. Neurosurg. Psychiat. 12:287, 1949.

298. Lemmen, L. J. and Schneider, R. C.: Aneurysm in the third ventricle, Neurology 3:474, 1953.

299. Levin, P., and Gross, S. W.: Meningioma and aneurysm in the same patient, Arch. Neurol. 15:629, 1966.

300. Lhermitte, F., Gautier, J.-C., Poirier, J., and Tyrer, J. H.: Hypoplasia of the internal carotid artery, Neurology 18:439, 1968.

301. Little, J. M., May, J., Vanderfield, G. K., and Lamond, S.: Traumatic thrombosis of the internal carotid artery, Lancet 2:926, 1969.

302. Locksley, H. B.: Report on the Cooperative Study of Intracranial Aneurysms and Subarachnoid Hemorrhage, Section 5, Part 1. Natural history of subarachnoid hemorrhage, intracranial aneurysms, and arteriovenous malformations, J. Neurosurg. 25:219, 1966.

303. Locksley, H. B.: Report on the cooperative study of intracranial aneurysms and subarachnoid hemorrhage, Section 5, Part 2. Natural history of subarachnoid hemorrhage, intracranial aneurysms and arteriovenous malformations, J. Neurosurg 25:321, 1966.

304. Lodge, S. D., Walker, G. F., and Stewart, M. J.: Aneurysm of the left internal carotid artery simulating pituitary tumour, Brit. Med. J. 2:1179, 1927.

305. Lodin, H.: Spontaneous thrombosis of cerebral aneurysms, Brit. J. Radiol. 39:701, 1966.

306. Logue, V.: Surgery in spontaneous subarachnoid hemorrhage, Brit. Med. J. 1:473, 1956.

307. Logue, V., Durward, M., Pratt, R. T. C., Piercy, M., and Nixon, W. L. B.: The quality of survival after rupture of an anterior cerebral aneurysm, Brit. J. Psychiat. 114:137, 1968.

308. Logue, V., and Smith, B.: Cerebral pathology in ruptured intracranial aneurysms, J. Neurol. Neurosurg. Psychiat. 25:393, 1962.

309. Lombardi, G., Passerini, A., and Migliavacca, F.: Intracavernous aneurysms of the internal carotid artery, Amer. J. Roentgen. 89:361, 1963.

310. Luessenhop, A. J., Mora, F., and Sweet, W. H.: Subarachnoid hemorrhage, intracranial aneurysms and arterio-venous anomalies; treatment by cervical carotid occlusion. In Sahs, A. L.: Pathogenesis and treatment of cerebrovascular disease, Springfield, Ill., 1961, Charles C Thomas, Publisher, p. 516.

311. MacCallum, W. G.: Mycotic aneurysms, Trans. Coll. Physicians Phila. 51:6, 1929.

312. Magarey, F. R., Roser, B. J., Stehbens, W. E., and Sharp, A.: Effects of experimental coarctation of the aorta on atheroma in sheep, J. Path. Bact. 90:129, 1965.

313. Magarey, F. R., Stehbens, W. E., and Sharp, A.: Effects of experimental coarctation of the aorta on the blood pressure of sheep, Circulation Res. 7:147, 1959.

314. Magee, C. G.: Spontaneous subarachnoid haemorrhage, Lancet 2:497, 1943.

315. Major, R. H.: A history of medicine, Springfield, 1954, Charles C Thomas, Publisher, vol. 1.

316. Mallory, T. B., Castleman, B., and Parris, E. E.: Case records of the Massachusetts General Hospital, Case 33122, New Eng. J. Med. 236: 445, 1947.

317. Manschot, W. A.: Subarachnoid hemorrhage: intraocular symptoms and their pathogenesis, Amer. J. Ophthal. 38:501, 1954.

318. Martland, H. S.: Spontaneous subarachnoid hemorrhage and congenital "berry" aneurysms of the circle of Willis, Amer. J. Surg. 43:10, 1939.

319. Matson, D. D.: Personal communication. Cited by Phillips.[381]

320. Matson, D. D.: Intracranial arterial aneurysms in childhood, J. Neurosurg. 23:578, 1965.

321. McCormick, W. F.: Problems and pathogenesis of intracranial arterial aneurysms. In Toole, J. F., Moosy, J., and Janeway, R.: Cerebral vascular diseases, Seventh Princeton Conference, New York, 1971, Grune and Stratton, Inc., p. 219.

322. McCormick, W. F., and Beals, J. D.: Severe epistaxis caused by ruptured aneurysm of the internal carotid artery, J. Neurosurg. 21:678, 1964.

323. McCormick, W. F., and Nofzinger, J. D.: Saccular intracranial aneurysms. An autopsy study, J. Neurosurg. 22:155, 1965.

324. McCune, W. S., Samadi, A., and Blades, B.: Experimental aneurysms, Ann. Surg. 138:216, 1953.

325. McDonald, C. A., and Korb, M.: Intracranial aneurysms, Arch. Neurol. Psychiat. 42:298, 1939.

326. McFarland, W., and Fuller, D. E.: Mortality in Ehlers-Danlos syndrome due to spontaneous rupture of large arteries, New Eng. J. Med. 271:1309, 1964.

327. McKissock, W., Paine, K. W. E., and Walsh, L. S.: An analysis of the results of treatment of ruptured intracranial aneurysms, J. Neurosurg. 17:762, 1960.

328. McKissock, W., Richardson, A., Walsh, L., and Owen, E.: Multiple intracranial aneurysms, Lancet 1:623, 1964.

329. McKusick, V. A.: The cardiovascular aspects of Marfan's syndrome: a heritable disorder of connective tissue, Circulation 11:321, 1955.

330. McKusick, V. A.: The genetic aspects of cardiovascular diseases, Ann. Intern. Med. 49:556, 1958.

331. McKusick, V. A., Logue, R. B., and Bahnson, H. T.: Association of aortic valvular disease and cystic medial necrosis of the ascending aorta, Circulation 16:188, 1957.

332. Meachem, W. F.: Discussion, J. Neurosurg. 19:895, 1962.

333. Meadows, S. P.: Intracavernous aneurysms of the internal carotid artery, Arch. Ophthal. 62:566, 1959.

334. Mecklin, B.: A case of fatal subarachnoid hemorrhages, congenital aneurysms of the brain, adrenal dysfunction, and pituitary cachexia, N. Y. State J. Med. 50:1272, 1950.

335. Melnick, P. J.: Polycystic liver, Arch. Path. 59:162, 1955.

336. Middleton, W. S., and Burke, M.: *Streptococcus viridans* endocarditis lenta, Amer. J. Med. Sci. 198:301, 1939.

337. Milazzo, S.: Dissecting aortic aneurysm, Med. J. Aust. 1:807, 1952.

338. Milliser, R. V., Greenberg, S. R., and Neiman, B. H.: Congenital or berry aneurysm in the optic nerve, J. Clin. Path. 21:335, 1968.

339. Mitchell, N., and Angrist, A.: Intracranial aneurysms—a report of thirty-six cases, Ann. Intern. Med. 19:909, 1943.

340. Moersch, F. P., and Sayre, G. P.: Neurologic manifestations associated with dissecting aneurysm of the aorta, J.A.M.A. 144:1141, 1950.

341. Mories, A.: Ehlers-Danlos syndrome with a report of a fatal case, Scot. Med. J. 5:269, 1960.

342. Moritz, A. R., and Zamcheck, N.: Sudden and unexpected deaths of young soldiers, Arch. Path. 42:459, 1946.

343. Mount, L. A.: Results of treatment of intracranial aneurysms using the Selverstone clamp, J. Neurosurg. 16:611, 1959.

344. Mount, L. A., and Taveras, J. M.: The results of surgical treatment of intracranial aneurysms as demonstrated by progress arteriography, J. Neurosurg. 13:618, 1956.

345. Moyes, P. D.: Basilar aneurysm associated with agenesis of the left internal carotid artery, J. Neurosurg. 30:608, 1969.

346. Mullan, S., and Dawley, J.: Antifibrinolytic therapy for intracranial aneurysms, J. Neurosurg. 28:21, 1968.

347. Mullan, S., Raimondi, A. J., Dobben, G., Vailati, G., and Hekmatpanah, J.: Electrically

induced thrombosis in intracranial aneurysms, J. Neurosurg. 22:539, 1965.

348. Nabatoff, R. A., Cordice, J. W. V., and McCown, I. A.: Traumatic (false) aneurysms, Arch. Surg. 72:277, 1956.

349. Nakata, Y., Shionoya, S., and Kamiya, K.: Pathogenesis of mycotic aneurysm, Angiology 19:593, 1968.

350. Nedwich, A., Haft, H., Tellem, M., and Kauffman, L.: Dissecting aneurysm of cerebral arteries, Arch. Neurol. 9:477, 1963.

351. Nelson, J. W., and Styri, O. B.: Dissecting subintimal hematomas of the intracranial arteries: report of a case, J. Amer. Osteopath. Ass. 67:512, 1968.

352. Newcomb, A. L., and Munns, G. F.: Rupture of aneurysm of the circle of Willis in the newborn, Pediatrics 3:769, 1949.

353. Newman, M. J. D.: Racemose angioma of the spinal cord, Quart. J. Med. 28:97, 1959.

354. Nishioka, H.: Report on the cooperative study of intracranial aneurysms and subarachnoid hemorrhage, Section VIII, Part 1. Results of the treatment of intracranial aneurysms by occlusion of the carotid artery in the neck, J. Neurosurg. 25:660, 1966.

355. Nordschow, C. D., and Marsolais, E. B.: Ehlers-Danlos syndrome: some recent biophysical observations, Arch. Path. 88:65, 1969.

356. Norman, R. M., and Urich, H.: Dissecting aneurysm of the middle cerebral artery as a cause of acute infantile hemiplegia, J. Path. Bact. 73:580, 1957.

357. Northcroft, G. B., and Morgan, A. D.: A fatal case traumatic thrombosis of the internal carotid artery, Brit. J. Surg. 32:105, 1944-1945.

358. Nyström, S. H. M.: Development of intracranial aneurysms as revealed by electron microscopy, J. Neurosurg. 20:329, 1963.

359. Nyström, S. H. M.: Cytological aspects of the pathogenesis of intracranial aneurysms. In Fields, W. S., and Sahs, A. L.: Intracranial aneurysms and subarachnoid hemorrhage, Springfield, Ill., 1965, Charles C Thomas, Publisher, p. 40.

360. Odom, G. L., Woodhall, B., Tindall, G. T., and Jackson, J. R.: Changes in distal intravascular pressure and size of intracranial aneurysm following common carotid ligation, J. Neurosurg. 19:41, 1962.

361. Offret, G., and Aron, J. J.: Syndrome acromégalique et anévrysme de l'artère communicante antérieure, Bull. Soc. Ophtal. France 3:228, 1959.

362. Ogle, J. W.: On the formation of aneurism in connexion with embolism or with thrombosis of an artery, Med. Times Gazette, Feb. 24, p. 196, 1866.

363. Ojemann, R. G., New, P. F. T., and Fleming, T. C.: Intracranial aneurysms associated with bacterial meningitis, Neurology 16:1222, 1966.

364. Oldershaw, J. B., and Voris, H. C.: Internal carotid artery ligation, Neurology 16:937, 1966.

365. Olivecrona, H.: Personal communication, 1959. Cited by White and Ballantyne.[534]

366. Ouchi, H., Ohara, I., Iwabuchi, T., and Suzuki, J.: Dissecting aneurysm of the extra-

cranial portion of the vertebral artery, Vasc. Dis. **2**:340, 1965.

367. Overton, M. C., and Calvin, T. H.: Iatrogenic cerebral cortical aneurysm, J. Neurosurg. **24**: 672, 1966.

368. Owen, O. E., Holmes, J. A., and Scannell, T. J.: Massive spontaneous intraperitoneal haemorrhage in late pregnancy, Lancet **2**:325, 1957.

369. Owens, J. C., and Coffey, R. J.: Aneurysm of the splenic artery, including a report of 6 additional cases, Int. Abst. Surg. **97**:313, 1953.

370. Padget, D. H.: The circle of Willis, its embryology and anatomy. In Dandy, W. E.: Intracranial arterial aneurysms, New York, 1944, Comstock Publishing Company, Inc., p. 67.

371. Paillas, J. E., Bonnal, J., and Lavieille, J.: Angiographic images of false aneurysmal sac caused by rupture of median meningeal artery in the course of traumatic extradural hematoma, J. Neurosurg. **21**:667, 1964.

372. Pakarinen, S.: Incidence, aetiology, and prognosis of primary subarachnoid haemorrhage, Acta Neurol. Scand. **43** (suppl. 29):1, 1967.

373. Palomino, S. J.: Dissecting intramural hematoma of left coronary artery in the puerperium, Amer. J. Clin. Path. **51**:119, 1969.

374. Pankey, G. A.: Acute bacterial endocarditis at the University of Minnesota Hospitals, 1939-1959, Amer. Heart J. **64**:583, 1962.

375. Papp, J. P., and Paley, R. G.: Ehlers-Danlos syndrome incidence in three generations of a kindred, Postgrad. Med. **40**:586, 1966.

376. Paul, O., Bland, E. F., and White, P. D.: Bacterial endocarditis experiences with penicillin therapy at the Massachusetts General Hospital, 1944-1946, New Eng. J. Med. **237**:349, 1947.

377. Pedowitz, P., and Perell, A.: Aneurysms complicated by pregnancy. Part I. Aneurysms of the aorta and its major branches, Amer. J. Obstet. Gynec. **73**:720, 1957.

378. Pepper, O. H. P.: Medical etymology, Philadelphia, 1949, W. B. Saunders Co.

379. Perier, O., Demanet, J. C., Henneaux, J., and Vincente, A. N.: Existe-t-il un syndrome des artères spinales postérieures? Rev. Neurol. **103**:396, 1960.

380. Petty, J. M.: Epistaxis from aneurysm of the internal carotid artery due to a gunshot wound, J. Neurosurg. **30**:741, 1969.

381. Phillips, R. L.: Familial cerebral aneurysms, J. Neurosurg. **20**:701, 1963.

382. Pickering, G. W.: High blood pressure, London, 1955, J. & A. Churchill Ltd.

383. Pitt, G. N.: On cerebral embolism and aneurysm, Brit. Med. J. **1**:827, 1890.

384. Pool, J. L., and Potts, D. G.: Aneurysms and arteriovenous anomalies of the brain, New York, 1965, Harper & Row, Publishers.

385. Poppen, J. L.: Specific treatment of intracranial aneurysms, J. Neurosurg. **8**:75, 1951.

386. Poppen, J. L., and Fager, C. A.: Multiple intracranial aneurysms, J. Neurosurg. **16**:581, 1959.

387. Potter, J. M.: Redistribution of blood to the brain due to localized cerebral arterial spasm, Brain **82**:367, 1959.

388. Poutasse, E. F., Gardner, W. J., and McCormack, L. J.: Polycystic kidney disease and intracranial aneurysm, J.A.M.A. **154**:741, 1954.

389. Pouyanne, H., Leman, P., Got, M., and Gouaze, A.: Anévrysme artériel traumatique de la méningée moyenne gauche: rupture un mois après l'accident: hématome intracérébral temporal intervention, Neurochirurg. **5**:311. 1959.

390. Raimondi, A. J.: Yashon, D., Reyes, C., and Yarzagaray, L.: Intracranial false aneurysms, Neurochirurg. **11**:219, 1968.

391. Ragan, C., Howes, E. L., Plotz, C. M., Meyer, K., and Blunt, J. W.: Effect of cortisone on production of granulation tissue in the rabbit. Proc. Soc. Exp. Biol. Med. **72**:718, 1949.

392. Ramamurthi, B.: Incidence of intracranial aneurysms in India, J. Neurosurg. **30**:154, 1969.

393. Ramsey, T. L., and Mosquera, V. T.: Dissecting aneurysm of the middle cerebral artery, Ohio State Med. J. **44**:168, 1948.

394. Raskind, R.: An intracranial arterial aneurysm associated with a recurrent meningioma, J. Neurosurg. **23**:622, 1965.

395. Rathmell, T. K., Mora, G., and Pessel, J. F.: Mycotic aneurysm of the circle of Willis, J.A.M.A. **150**:555, 1952.

396. Ray, H., and Wahal, K. M.: Subarachnoid hemorrhage in subacute bacterial endocarditis, Neurology **7**:265, 1957.

397. Reifenstein, G. H., Levine, S. A., and Gross, R. E.: Coarctation of the aorta, Amer. Heart J. **33**:146, 1947.

398. Reye, R. D. K.: Personal communication, 1961.

399. Richardson, C., and Kofman, O.: Cranial bruit with intracranial saccular aneurysms, Trans. Amer. Neurol. Ass. **76**:151, 1951.

400. Richardson, J. C., and Hyland, H. H.: Intracranial aneurysms, Medicine **20**:1, 1941.

401. Riddoch, G., and Goulden, C.: On the relationship between subarachnoid and intraocular haemorrhage, Brit. J. Ophthal. **9**:209, 1925.

402. Riggs, H. E., and Rupp, C.: Miliary aneurysms: relation of anomalies of the circle of Willis to formation of aneurysms, J. Neuropath. **1**:442, 1942.

403. Riggs, H. E., and Rupp, C.: Miliary aneurysms: relation of anomalies of the circle of Willis to formation of aneurysms, Arch. Neurol. Psychiat. **49**:615, 1943.

404. Riggs, H. E., and Rupp, C.: Variation in form of circle of Willis, Arch. Neurol. **8**:8, 1963.

405. Riser, M., Lazorthes, G., Géraud, J., and Anduze, H.: Deux cas de syndrome de Garcin par anévrysmes carotidien intra-caverneux, Rev. Neurol. **89**:373, 1953.

406. Ritchie, H.: Dissecting aneurysm of the left internal carotid and left middle cerebral arteries, Wisconsin Med. J. **60**:556, 1961.

407. Roach, M. R.: Changes in arterial distensibility as a cause of poststenotic dilatation, Amer. J. Cardiol. **12**:802, 1963.

408. Roach, M. R., and Drake, C. G.: Ruptured cerebral aneurysm caused by micro-organisms, New Eng. J. Med. **273**:240, 1965.

409. Robert, F., Maltais, R., and Giroux, J. C.: Dissecting aneurysm of middle cerebral artery, J. Neurosurg. **21**:413, 1964.

410. Robertson, E. G.: Cerebral lesions due to intracranial aneurysms, Brain **72**:150, 1949.

411. Roe, H.: Aneurism of the anterior cerebral artery, Trans. Path. Soc. London **3**:46, 1850-1851.

412. Rose, F. C., and Sarner, M.: Epilepsy after ruptured intracranial aneurysm, Brit. Med. J. **1**:18, 1965.

413. Rosen, S. R., and Kaufmann, W.: Aneurysm of the circle of Willis with symptom-free interval of 27 years between initial and final rupture, Arch. Neurol. Psychiat. **50**:350, 1943.

414. Ross, R. T.: Multiple and familial intracranial vascular lesions, Canad. Med. Ass. J. **81**:477, 1959.

415. Roy, V. C., Sundt, T. M., and Murphey, F.: Experimental subarachnoid hemorrhage: a study for spasm with the production of aneurysms, Stroke **1**:248, 1970.

416. Rubinstein, M. K., and Cohen, N. H.: Ehlers-Danlos syndrome associated with multiple intracranial aneurysms, Neurology **14**:125, 1964.

417. Rumbaugh, C. L., Bergeron, R. T., Talalla, A., and Kurze, T.: Traumatic aneurysms of the cortical cerebral arteries, Radiology **96**:49, 1970.

418. Runnels, R. A., Monlux, W. S., and Monlux, A. W.: Principles of veterinary pathology, Iowa, 1960, Iowa University Press.

419. Russell, D. S.: The pathology of spontaneous intracranial haemorrhage, Proc. Roy Soc. Med. **47**:689, 1954.

420. Sadik, A. R., Budzilovich, G. N., and Shulman, K.: Giant aneurysm of middle cerebral artery, J. Neurosurg. **22**:177, 1965.

421. Sahs, A. L.: Intracranial aneurysms and polycystic kidneys, Arch. Neurol. Psychiat. **63**:524, 1950.

422. Sahs, A. L.: Hypotension and hypothermia in the treatment of intracranial aneurysms, J. Neurosurg. **25**:593, 1966.

423. Sahs, A. L., Perrett, G., Locksley, H. B., Nishioka, H., and Skultety, F. M.: Preliminary remarks on subarachnoid hemorrhage, J. Neurosurg. **24**:782, 1966.

424. Salmon, J. H., and Blatt, E. S.: Aneurysm of the internal carotid artery due to closed trauma, J. Thorac. Cardiovasc. Surg. **56**:28, 1968.

425. Sargent, P.: Haemangeioma of the pia mater causing compression paraplegia, Brain **48**:259, 1925.

426. Sarner, M., and Crawford, M. D.: Ruptured intracranial aneurysm, Lancet **2**:1251, 1965.

427. Schact, F. W.: Hypertension in cases of congenital polycystic kidney, Arch. Intern. Med. **47**:500, 1931.

428. Scheie, H. G., and Hogan, T. F.: Angioid streaks and generalized arterial disease, Arch. Ophthal. **57**:855, 1957.

429. Schmidt, M.: Intracranial aneurysms, Brain **53**:489, 1930.

430. Schneck, S. A.: On the relationship between ruptured intracranial aneurysm and cerebral infarction, Neurology **14**:691, 1964.

431. Schneck, S. A., and Kricheff, I. I.: Intracranial aneurysm rupture, vasospasm, and infarction, Arch. Neurol. **11**:668, 1964.

432. Schnitker, M. A., and Bayer, C. A.: Dissecting aneurysm of the aorta in young individuals, particularly in association with pregnancy. With report of a case, Ann. Intern. Med. **20**:486, 1944.

433. Scholefield, B. G.: A case of aneurysm of the basilar artery, Guy's Hosp. Rep. **74**:485, 1924.

434. Schoolman, A., and Kepes, J. J.: Bilateral spontaneous carotid-cavernous fistulae in Ehlers-Danlos syndrome, J. Neurosurg. **26**:82, 1967.

435. Schorstein, J.: Carotid ligation in saccular intracranial aneurysms, Brit. J. Surg. **28**:50, 1940-1941.

436. Schürmann, K., Brock, M., and Samii, M.: Circumscribed hematoma of the lateral ventricle following rupture of an intraventricular saccular arterial aneurysm, J. Neurosurg. **29**:195, 1968.

437. Schwartz, M. J., and Baronofsky, I. D.: Ruptured intracranial aneurysm associated with coarctation of the aorta, Amer. J. Cardiol. **6**:982, 1960.

438. Scott, G. E., Neubuerger, K. T., and Denst, J.: Dissecting aneurysms of intracranial arteries, Neurology **10**:22, 1960.

439. Scott, R. W., and Sancetta, S. M.: Dissecting aneurysm of aorta with hemorrhagic infarction of the spinal cord and complete paraplegia, Amer. Heart J. **38**:747, 1949.

440. Seftel, D. M., Kolson, H., and Gordon, B. S.: Ruptured intracranial carotid artery aneurysm with fatal epistaxis, Arch. Otolaryng. **70**:52, 1959.

441. Seltzer, J., and Hurteau, E. F.: Bilateral symmetrical aneurysms of internal carotid artery within the cavernous sinus, J. Neurosurg. **14**:448, 1957.

442. Selverstone, B.: Aneurysms at middle cerebral "trifurcation": treatment with adherent plastics, J. Neurosurg. **19**:884, 1962.

443. Selverstone, B., Dehghan, R., Ronis, N., Deterling, R. A., and Callow, A. D.: Adherent synthetic resins in experimental arterial surgery, Arch. Surg. **84**:80, 1962.

444. Shaw, C., and Foltz, E. L.: Traumatic dissecting aneurysm of middle cerebral artery and carotid-cavernous fistula with massive intracerebral hemorrhage, J. Neurosurg. **28**:475, 1968.

445. Shenkin, H. A., Cabieses, F., van den Noordt, G., Sayers, P., and Copperman, R.: The hemodynamic effect of unilateral carotid ligation on the cerebral circulation of man, J. Neurosurg. **8**:38, 1951.

446. Shennan, T.: Dissecting aneurysms, Med. Res. Council Spec. Rep. Ser. No. 193, 1934.

447. Sherlock, S. P. V., and Learmonth, J. R.: Aneurysm of the splenic artery: with an account of an example complicating Gaucher's disease, Brit. J. Surg. **30**:151, 1942-1943.

448. Shnider, B. I., and Cotsonas, N. J.: Embolic

mycotic aneurysms, a complication of bacterial endocarditis, Amer. J. Med. **16:**246, 1954.

449. Shumacker, H. B., and Wayson, E. E.: Spontaneous cure of aneurysms and arteriovenous fistulas, with some notes on intrasaccular thrombosis, Amer. J. Surg. **79:**532, 1950.

450. Sigerist, H. E.: A history of medicine, New York, 1951, Oxford University Press, vol. 1.

451. Simon, H. B., and Thompson, G. J.: Congenital renal polycystic disease, J.A.M.A. **159:**657, 1955.

452. Sinclair, W.: Dissecting aneurysm of the middle cerebral artery associated with migraine syndrome, Amer. J. Path. **29:**1083, 1953.

453. Sirois, J., Lapointe, H., and Côté, P. E.: Unusual local complication of percutaneous cerebral angiography, J. Neurosurg. **11:**112, 1954.

454. Skultety, F. M., and Nishioka, H.: Report on the cooperative study of intracranial aneurysms and subarachnoid hemorrhage, Section VIII, Part 2. The results of intracranial surgery in the treatment of aneurysms, J. Neurosurg. **25:**683, 1966.

455. Slany, A.: Anomalien des Circulus arteriosus Willisi in ihrer Beziehung zur Aneurysmenbildung an der Hirnbasis, Virch. Arch. **301:**62, 1938.

456. Sloan, R. D., and Colley, R. N.: Coarctation of the aorta. The roentgenologic aspects of one hundred and twenty-five surgically confirmed cases, Radiology **61:**701, 1953.

457. Slosberg, P. S.: Medical treatment of intracranial aneurysm, Neurology **10:**1085, 1960.

458. Slosberg, P. S.: Subarachnoid hemorrhage with vertebro-basilar aneurysm, Acta Neurol. Scand. **42:**515, 1966.

459. Smith, D. E., and Windsor, R. B.: Embryologic and pathogenic aspects of the development of cerebral saccular aneurysms, In Fields, W. S.: Pathogenesis and treatment of cerebrovascular disease, Springfield, Ill., 1961, Charles C Thomas, Publisher, p. 367.

460. Snapper, I., and Forminje, P.: Aneurysm of the cerebral arteries and polycystic kidneys, Acta Med. Scand. **101:**105, 1939.

461. Sosman, M. C., and Vogt, E. C.: Aneurysm of the internal carotid artery and the circle of Willis, from a roentgenological viewpoint, Amer. J. Roentgen. **15:**122, 1926.

462. Souques, A.: Anévrysme, volumineux d'une branche de l'artère cérébrale moyenne ou Sylvienne, Nouv. Iconogr. Salpêtrière **21:**108, 1908.

463. Spudis, E. V., Scharyj, M., Alexander, E., and Martin, J. F.: Dissecting aneurysms in the neck and head, Neurology **12:**867, 1962.

464. Stark, D. C. C.: Effects of giving vasopressors to patients on monoamine-oxidase inhibitors, Lancet **1:**1405, 1962.

465. Steelman, H. F., Hayes, G. J., and Rizzoli, H. V.: Surgical treatment of saccular intracranial aneurysms, J. Neurosurg. **10:**564, 1953.

466. Steelman, H. F., Hayes, G. J., and Rizzoli, H. V.: Surgical treatment of saccular intracranial aneurysms, J. Neurosurg. **10:**564, 1953.

467. Stehbens, W. E.: Intracranial arterial aneurysms, Aust. Ann. Med. **3:**214, 1954.

468. Stehbens, W. E.: History of aneurysms, Med. Hist. **2:**274, 1958.

469. Stehbens, W. E.: Intracranial arterial aneurysms and atherosclerosis, Thesis, University of Sydney, 1958.

470. Stehbens, W. E.: Focal intimal proliferation in the cerebral arteries, Amer. J. Path. **36:**289, 1960.

471. Stehbens, W. E.: Hypertension and cerebral aneurysms, Med. J. Aust. **2:**4, 1962.

472. Stehbens, W. E.: Cerebral aneurysm and congenital abnormalities, Aust. Ann. Med. **11:**102, 1962.

473. Stehbens, W. E.: Aneurysms and anatomical variation of cerebral arteries, Arch. Path. **75:**45, 1963.

474. Stehbens, W. E.: Cerebral aneurysms of animals other than man, J. Path. Bact. **86:**161, 1963.

475. Stehbens, W. E.: Histopathology of cerebral aneurysms, Arch. Neurol. **8:**272, 1963.

476. Stehbens, W. E.: The renal artery in normal and cholesterol-fed rabbits, Amer. J. Path. **43:**969, 1963.

477. Stehbens, W. E.: Localization of spontaneous lipid deposition in the cerebral arteries of sheep, Nature **203:**1294, 1964.

478. Stehbens, W. E.: Intimal proliferation and spontaneous lipid deposition in the cerebral arteries of sheep and steers, J. Atheroscler. Res. **5:**556, 1965.

479. Stehbens, W. E.: Atypical cerebral aneurysms, Med. J. Aust. **1:**765, 1965.

480. Stehbens, W. E.: Blood vessel changes in chronic experimental arteriovenous fistulas, Surg. Gynec. Obstet. **127:**327, 1968.

481. Stehbens, W. E.: Discussion. In Toole, J. F., Moosy, J., and Janeway, R.: Cerebral vascular diseases, Seventh Princeton Conference, New York, 1971, Grune & Stratton, Inc., pp. 216, 246.

482. Stehbens, W. E.: Unpublished observations, 1971.

483. Stengel, A., and Wolferth, C. C.: Mycotic (bacterial) aneurysms of intravascular origin, Arch. Intern. Med. **31:**527, 1923.

484. Stern, K.: Über Kreislaufstörungen im Gehirn bei Wandeinrissen in extracerebralen Arterien, Z. Ges. Neurol. Psychiat. **148:**55, 1933.

485. Stern, W. E.: Mechanisms in the production of hemiparesis associated with intracranial aneurysm, Brain **78:**503, 1955.

486. Strully, K. J.: Successful removal of intraventricular aneurysm of the choroidal artery, J. Neurosurg. **12:**317, 1955.

487. Sugai, M., and Shoji, M.: Pathogenesis of so-called congenital aneurysms of the brain, Acta Path. Jap. **18:**139, 1968.

488. Summer, G. K.: The Ehlers-Danlos syndrome, Amer. J. Dis. Child. **91:**429, 1956.

489. Sweet, W. H., and Bennett, H. S.: Changes in internal carotid pressure during carotid and jugular occlusion and their clinical significance, J. Neurosurg. **5:**178, 1948.

490. Symonds, C.: Discussion, Proc. Roy. Soc. Med. **45:**20, 1952.

491. Symonds, C. P.: Contribution to the clinical

study of intracranial aneurysms, Guy's Hosp. Rep. **73**:139, 1923.

492. Szabó, J.: Jobboldali csigolyaveröér csöves hasadása (aneurysma dissecans), Budapest Orv. Ujs. **37**:201, 1939. Cited by Spudis et al.[463]

493. Tapp, E., and Hickling, R. S.: Renal artery rupture in a pregnant woman with neurofibromatosis, J. Path. **97**:398, 1969.

494. Taylor, A. B., and Whitfield, A. G. W.: Subarachnoid haemorrhage, Quart. J. Med. **5**:461, 1936.

495. Taylor, G. W.: Ehlers-Danlos syndrome with vertebral artery aneurysm, Proc. Roy. Soc. Med. **62**:734, 1969.

496. Taylor, P. E.: Delayed postoperative hemorrhage from intracranial aneurysm after craniotomy for tumor, Neurology **11**:225, 1961.

497. Thapedi, I. M., Ashenhurst, E. M., and Rozdilsky, B.: Spontaneous dissecting aneurysm of the internal carotid artery in the neck, Arch. Neurol. **23**:549, 1970.

498. Thompson, G. B.: Dissecting aortic aneurysm with infarction of the spinal cord, Brain **79**:111, 1956.

499. Tindall, G. T., Goree, J. A., Lee, J. F., and Odom, G. L.: Effect of common carotid ligation on size of internal carotid aneurysms and distal intracarotid and retinal artery pressures, J. Neurosurg. **25**:503, 1966.

500. Tindall, G. T., and Odom, G. L.: Treatment of intracranial aneurysms by proximal carotid ligation, Progr. Neurol. Surg. **3**:66, 1969.

501. Todd, E. M., and Crue, B. L.: The coating of aneurysms with plastic materials. In Fields, W. S., and Sahs, A. L.: Intracranial aneurysms and subarachnoid hemorrhage, Springfield, Ill., 1965, Charles C Thomas, Publisher, p. 357.

502. Todd, E. M., Shelden, C. H., Crue, B. L., Pudenz, R. H., and Agnew, W. F.: Plastic jackets for certain intracranial aneurysms, J.A.M.A. **179**:935, 1962.

503. Tomlinson, B. E.: Brain changes in ruptured intracranial aneurysm, J. Clin. Path. **12**:391, 1959.

504. Tridon, P., Renard, M., Picard, L., Weber, M., and André, J. M.: Malformation vasculaire cérébrale et syndrome d'Ehlers-Danlos, Rev. Neurol. **121**:615, 1969.

505. Troupp, H., and Rinne, T.: Methyl-2-cyanoacrylate (Eastman 910) in experimental vascular surgery with a note on experimental arterial aneurysms, J. Neurosurg. **21**:1067, 1964.

506. Tsuchiya, G., Sugar, O., Yashon, D., and Hubbard, J.: Reactions of rabbit brain and peripheral vessels to plastics used in coating arterial aneurysms, J. Neurosurg. **28**:409, 1968.

507. Turnbull, F., and Dolman, C. L.: Simultaneous hemorrhage from multiple intracerebral aneurysms: a case report. Canad. J. Surg. **5**:87, 1962.

508. Turnbull, H. M.: Alterations in arterial structure and their relation to syphilis, Quart. J. Med. **8**:201, 1915.

509. Turnbull, H. M.: Intracranial aneurysms, Brain **41**:50, 1918.

510. Tyler, H. R., and Clark, D. B.: Neurologic complications in patients with coarctation of aorta, Neurology **8**:712, 1958.

511. Ullrich, D. P., and Sugar, O.: Familial cerebral aneurysms including one extracranial internal carotid aneurysm, Neurology **10**:288, 1960.

512. Van 'T Hoff, W.: Hypopituitarism associated with intracranial aneurysms, Brit. Med. J. **2**:1190, 1961.

513. Ver Brugghen, A.: Pathogenesis of ophthalmoplegic migraine, Neurology **5**:311, 1955.

514. Voris, H. C.: Complications of ligation of the internal carotid artery, J. Neurosurg. **8**:119, 1951.

515. Voris, H. C., and Basile, J. X. R.: Recurrent epistaxis from aneurysm of the internal carotid artery, J. Neurosurg. **18**:841, 1961.

516. Wagenvoort, C. A., Harris, L. E., Brown, A. L.: and Veneklaas, G. M. H.: Giant-cell arteritis with aneurysm formation in children, Pediatrics **32**:861, 1963.

517. Walb, D., Redondo-Marco, J. A., and Beneke, G.: Aneurysma dissecans intrakranieller Arterien, Med. Welt **67**:1043, 1967.

518. Walker, A. E., and Allègre, G. W.: The pathology and pathogenesis of cerebral aneurysms, J. Neuropath. Exp. Neurol. **13**:248, 1954.

519. Walker, J. B., and Livingstone, F. D. M.: Coarctation of the aorta, Lancet **2**:660, 1938.

520. Walsh, F. B., and King, A. B.: Ocular signs of intracranial saccular aneurysms, Arch. Ophthal. **27**:1, 1942.

521. Walton, J. N.: The late prognosis of subarachnoid haemorrhage, Brit. Med. J. **2**:802, 1952.

522. Walton, J. N.: Subarachnoid haemorrhage in pregnancy, Brit. Med. J. **1**:869, 1953.

523. Walton, J. N.: Subarachnoid haemorrhage, Edinburgh, 1956, E. & S. Livingstone Ltd.

524. Wappenschmidt, J., and Holbach, K. H.: Zur Frage posttraumatischer Aneurysmen der Meningealarterien, Fortschr. Roentgenstr. **106**:555, 1967.

525. Wartman, W. B., and Laipply, T. C.: The fate of blood injected into the arterial wall, Amer. J. Path. **25**:383, 1949.

526. Watson, A. J.: Dissecting aneurysm of arteries other than the aorta, J. Path. Bact. **72**:439, 1956.

527. Wechsler, H. L., and Fisher, E. R.: Ehlers-Danlos syndrome, Arch. Path. **77**:613, 1964.

528. Weibel, J., Fields, W. S., and Campos, R. J.: Aneurysms of the posterior cervicocranial circulation: clinical and angiographic considerations, J. Neurosurg. **26**:223, 1967.

529. Weisman, A. D., and Adams, R. D.: The neurological complications of dissecting aortic aneurysm, Brain **67**:69, 1944.

530. Welch, K., and Eiseman, B.: Arterial graft and endarterectomy in reconstitution of the common carotid artery two years following ligation, J. Neurosurg. **14**:575, 1957.

531. Wells, A. L.: Cerebellar necrosis in a case of subarachnoid haemorrhage, Brit. Med. J. **2**:1356, 1953.

532. Wells, H. G.: Intracranial aneurysm of the

vertebral artery, Arch. Neurol. Psychiat. **7:** 311, 1922.

533. White, J. C., and Adams, R. D.: Combined supra- and infraclinoid aneurysms of internal carotid artery, J. Neurosurg. **12:**450, 1955.

534. White, J. C., and Ballantine, H. T.: Intrasellar aneurysms simulating hypophyseal tumours, J. Neurosurg. **18:**34, 1961.

535. White, J. C., Sayre, G. P., and Whisnant, J. P.: Experimental destruction of the media for the production of intracranial arterial aneurysms, J. Neurosurg. **18:**741, 1961.

536. Wichern, H.: Klinische Beiträge zur Kenntnis der Hirnaneurysmen, Deutsch. Z. Nervenheilk. **44:**220, 1912.

537. Williams, R. R., Bahn, R. C., and Sayre, G. P.: Congenital cerebral aneurysms, Proc. Staff Meet. Mayo Clin. **30:**161, 1955.

538. Wilson, G., Riggs, H. E., and Rupp, C.: The pathologic anatomy of ruptured cerebral aneurysms, J. Neurosurg. **11:**128, 1954.

539. Wilson, S. A. K.: In Bruce, A. B., editor: Neurology, London, 1940, Edward Arnold & Co., vol. 2, p. 1110.

540. Winkelman, N. W., and Eckel, J. L.: The brain in bacterial endocarditis, Arch. Neurol. Psychiat. **23:**1161, 1930.

541. Wise, B. L., and Palubinskas, A. J.: Per-sistent trigeminal artery (carotid-basilar anastomosis), J. Neurosurg. **21:**199, 1964.

542. Wisoff, H. S., and Rothballer, A. B.: Cerebral arterial thrombosis in children, Arch. Neurol. **4:**258, 1961.

543. Wolf, A. V.: Demonstration concerning pressure-tension relations in various organs, Science **115:**243, 1952.

544. Wolff, H. G.: Headache and other head pain, New York, 1948, Oxford University Press.

545. Wollschlaeger, G., and Wollschlaeger, P. B.: The primitive trigeminal artery as seen angiographically and at postmortem examination, Amer. J. Roentgen. **92:**761, 1964.

546. Wolman, L.: Cerebral dissecting aneurysms, Brain **82:**276, 1959.

547. Woodhall, B., Odom, G. L., Bloor, B. M., and Golden, J.: Direct measurement of intravascular pressure in components of the circle of Willis, Ann. Surg. **135:**911, 1952.

548. Wright, R. L.: Intraaneurysmal pressure reduction with carotid occlusion, J. Neurosurg. **29:**139, 1968.

549. Wyburn-Mason, R.: The vascular abnormalities and tumours of the spinal cord and its membranes, St. Louis, 1944, The C. V. Mosby Co.

10/Telangiectases, hemangiomas, arteriovenous aneurysms, and allied disorders

Vascular anomalies of the brain

Our knowledge of the so-called vascular malformations or anomalies is assuredly in a most confused state—more so than any other entity in the entire field of cerebrovascular pathology. Though sundry classifications have been proposed, no agreement has been reached. There is wide variation in both the morphology and structure of the lesions and a dearth of information relative to the pathogenesis. Nor is there consensus regarding the nomenclature for the lesions variously called angiomas, hemangiomas, hamartomas, arteriovenous aneurysms, arteriovenous malformations or anomalies, telangiectases, cavernous angiomas, arteriovenous angiomas, cirsoid angiomas, serpentine angiomas, racemose varix, venous and arterial racemose angiomas, arterial angiomas, venous angiomas, varices, and hemorrhoids of the meninges. Confusion surrounds the diagnosis and differentiation of the various types. Many and different lesions have been recorded under the same title, and similar lesions have been given a wide variety of titles.[238] Emphasis has been on descriptive terminology rather than on the fundamental pathology responsible for the lesions and quite conflicting hypotheses regarding their cause have been current. Knowledge of the etiology remains meagre.

For lack of a better term, the group as a whole will be classified under the heading of *vascular anomalies,* the term being used in the sense of an abnormality rather than a malformation. The term "malformation" presupposes that all the lesions are based on a developmental fault, a theory that is best avoided, as it is by no means proved or universally accepted. Not all should be classed as tumors or angiomas, for though some may be true hemangiomas, many are not neoplastic in any sense. The term "arteriovenous" should likewise be restricted to lesions primarily caused by an arteriovenous shunt.

The committee established by the Advisory Council for the National Institute of Neurological Diseases and Blindness[61] to study the classification of cerebrovascular diseases considered all these lesions to be essentially arteriovenous communications and felt the further differentiation of the lesions into capillary, venous, or arterial types was unwarranted. Conceding that etiologically all are arteriovenous communications, a point neither proved nor accepted, we find that the lesions do not all behave in a similar manner, which fact necessitates classification into subtypes. Thus, the results of the Cooperative Study[264] on vascular anomalies were limited because all vascular anomalies were treated as one group. Vascular anomalies will be dealt with in the present text under the following terms—telangiectases, cavernous hemangiomas, venous angiomas, and arteriovenous aneurysms, with a possible transitional form between telangiectasia and cavernous hemangioma.

Frequency of occurrence

Common practice in the past has been to indicate the prevalence of vascular anomalies as a numerical fraction of all intracranial tumors, thus Cushing and Bailey[70] found vascular anomalies constituted 1.1% of 1522 intracranial tumors. Olivecrona and Ladenheim[246] found 5000 verified brain tumors and 125 arteriovenous aneurysms at the Neurological Clinic, Serafimerlasarettet (Sweden), between 1923 and

1955, a frequency of approximately 2%. Perret and Nishioka[264] gave the frequency as 1.5% to 4% of intracranial tumors, and similarly Zimmerman[394] found 3.9% among 5199 cerebral tumors. Craig and associates,[65] on the other hand, reported that hemangiomas occurred too infrequently to list among 427 children with verified intracranial tumors. Their comparison is not quite fitting, particularly as arteriovenous aneurysms are far from being neoplastic and only in a broad sense are they occasionally highly malignant.

Russell[295] found vascular anomalies accounted for 21 (4.6%) of a total of 461 cases of intracerebral hemorrhage of significant size at the London Hospital (1912 to 1952). There were only eight among 126 similar cases at the National Hospital,[32] Queen Square (1909 to 1956), a frequency of 6.3%. Their figures account only for lesions complicated by hemorrhage. Mackenzie[191] estimated that they form approximately 1% of all neurological admissions. Table 7-2 provides the comparative causes of subarachnoid hemorrhage. Vascular anomalies account for anything from 0.2% to 9.6%.

In the Cooperative Study,[264] a total of 549 congenital or acquired arteriovenous aneurysms were reported in all. There were 453 "intracranial angiomatous malformations"* (421 supratentorial and 32 subtentorial), 37 coexistent intracranial arterial aneurysms and vascular anomalies, 39 carotid-cavernous sinus fistulas, and 20 miscellaneous vascular anomalies (including five aneurysms of the vein of Galen, four extracranial anomalies, seven combined intracranial-extracranial vascular anomalies, one iatrogenic vertebral arteriovenous fistula, two spinal angiomas, and one retinal angioma). These results give some indication of the relative frequency of the lesions, but they are of limited value because the main group of 453 anomalies, mostly arteriovenous in type, was nevertheless not homogeneous.

The prevalence of cerebral hemangiomas is unknown at present. Geschickter and Keasby[102] estimated that they constituted 7.6% of all hemangiomas, but this is an overestimate because the ubiquitous cutaneous hemangioma was mostly excluded from the series. A valuable and fairly reliable estimate could be obtained from a thorough (planned) autopsy search of brains and spinal cords from subjects in different age groups. In brains examined post mortem over a period of 21 years at the Jefferson Medical College (Philadelphia), the prevalence of telangiectases was 0.4%, of cavernous hemangiomas 0.02%, and of arteriovenous aneurysms 0.03%.[27]

Epidemiology

These vascular anomalies occur in the Negro, the Asian, and the Caucasian. Little information is present concerning their prevalence in the races of man and there has been no interest in their geographical distribution although quite possibly epidemiological studies could bring important but as yet unknown facts to light.

In a review of spontaneous neoplasm of the nervous system in animals, Lüginbühl and associates[190] found no instances of either hemangioma or arteriovenous aneurysm in the brains of other animals. However they referred to a case of venous angioma compressing the cervical spinal cord in a 9-year-old horse.

Pathology of vascular anomalies

Telangiectases. Telangiectases are characteristically small solitary lesions rarely larger than 3 cm. in their largest diameter. Usually found incidentally in adults at autopsy,[202,379] they are probably not as rare as the literature would suggest, for they are readily overlooked.[296]

They are found most frequently in the pons[70,354,379] where White and associates[379] found nine of 18 intracranial telangiectases. The remaining nine were in the cerebrum

---

*It was indicated by Perret and Nishioka[264] that in this group referred to as arteriovenous malformations neither cavernous hemangiomas, venous angiomas, nor telangiectases were excluded.

(frontal lobe, five; temporal lobe, two; parietal lobe, two), where they are known to involve the cerebral cortex or white matter[296] Those in the cerebral white matter may involve all white matter of a gyral fold. Teilmann[340] made a study of pontine hemangiomas and found that 22 of 45 cases in the literature probably had telangiectases. Six of nine telangiectases encountered by Russell and Rubinstein[296] were pontine in position. In a recent study of vascular anomalies of the posterior fossa, 38 lesions out of a total of 164 vascular anomalies were classified as telangiectases (Table 10-1), and of these, 27 were pontine, six were in the cerebellum, and five in the

medulla.[205] Pontine telangiectases constituted 56.3% of the pontine vascular anomalies.[205] Within the pons, they are usually near the median raphe.[296] Turner and Kernohan[354] assert they are also prevalent in the floor of the fourth ventricle.

The average age of patients with telangiectases has been estimated at 44 years, when the lesion is supratentorial, and 56, when it is subtentorial in position (Table 10-2). None of the lesions were found in the first decade and only 5% of the 45 before the age of 30 years. Thrash[345] recorded intracerebellar and subarachnoid hemorrhage from a hemangiomatous tumor of dilated budding capillaries in a premature infant on the eighth day after spontaneous delivery (5 months of gestation). This, of course, may not be a telangiectasis, but it appears to be the only mention of a possible occurrence in the newborn or an infant even though it is regarded as a congenital lesion.

Multiplicity of lesions is seen only on rare occasions and the few instances in the literature are thought to be cavernous angiomas rather than telangiectases.[296] Additional lesions occur in other parts of the brain including the cerebrum and also in the cord.[70] Hosoi[142] reported the case of a woman of 34 years with eight capillary hemangiomas (1 to 8 mm. in diameter) of the cerebrum. There were numerous large vessels with fibrous and hyaline thickening of the walls about each vascular anomaly.

Table 10-1. Distribution of 510 vascular anomalies according to type*

Type of vascular anomaly	Number above the tentorium	Number below the tentorium
Arteriovenous aneurysm	217	70
Telangiectases	22	38
Cavernous angiomas	59	21
Venous angiomas†	46	31
Varices†	2	4
Total	346	164

*Adapted from McCormick, W. F., Hardman, J. M., and Boulter, T. R.: Vascular malformations ("angiomas") of the brain, with special reference to those occurring in the posterior fossa, J. Neurosurg. **28**:241, 1968.
†In this text venous angiomas and varices are not differentiated but are classified as one group.

Table 10-2. Tabulation of average ages of vascular anomalies according to site at autopsy*

Type of vascular anomaly	Average age in years		
	Supratentorial	Subtentorial	Combined series
Arteriovenous aneurysm	32	33	
Venous angioma	48	50	
Cavernous hemangioma	50	45	
Telangiectasis	44	56	
Cerebellar anomalies (all types)			40
Brain stem (all types)			49
Posterior fossa (all types)			43.6

*Adapted from McCormick, W. F., Hardman, J. M., and Boulter, T. R.: Vascular malformations ("angiomas") of the brain, with special reference to those occurring in the posterior fossa, J. Neurosurg. **28**:241, 1968.

Other microscopic foci of similar hemangiomatous tissue were present in the frontal lobes, and small meningiomas were found attached to the dura. Evidence for hereditary factors is not very good.

Telangiectases are fairly small lesions, not well circumscribed, and in appearance pink or with pink-grey speckled areas. With somewhat larger and engorged vessels, they may appear as clusters of petechial hemorrhages (Figs. 10-1 and 10-2). Noran[238] asserted that they rarely reach the surface of the brain, although in Jaffé's[148] case and one other,[379] multiple telangiectases were found in the meninges and spinal nerve rootlets. Hemorrhage, either subarachnoid or intracerebral, is seldom a factor to be contended with,[238,296] although fatal bleeding has been reported.[213,340] Hemorrhage has not been attributed to telangiectases in reviews of the so-called cryptic angiomas.

Blackwood[30] described in the cerebral white matter, two capillary telangiectases that extended from the deep layers of the cortex tapering toward but not quite reaching the ventricle. They consisted of multiple capillary channels and dilatations with a trivial degree of gliosis. Hemorrhage was not a prominent feature. Pickworth preparations (benzidine test for hemoglobin on 200 μ thick frozen sections) revealed variations ranging from a mild fusiform to prominent vascular dilatation of the capillaries without apparent numerical increase in their incidence. Venous channels were enlarged but did not exhibit aneurysmal dilatations. A similar lesion (Fig. 10-3) was presented by Potter[272] and examples are illustrated in Figs. 10-4 to 10-6. The above could be specific entities, for all varieties illustrated in the literature or seen personally have involved the cerebrum. Other lesions referred to as telangiectases do not necessarily have the requisite microscopic structure described by Blackwood[30] for they have not been investigated thus.

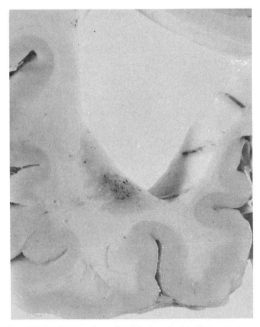

Fig. 10-1. An early telangiectasis in the caudate nucleus appearing as a cluster of dark pinpoint dots.

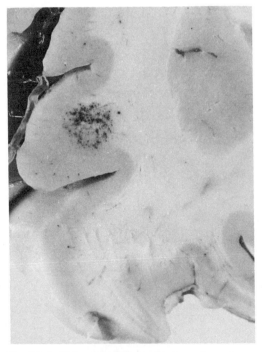

Fig. 10-2. Telangiectasis at the junction of cerebral cortex and white matter. The vessels are larger and more closely packed than that in Fig. 10-1.

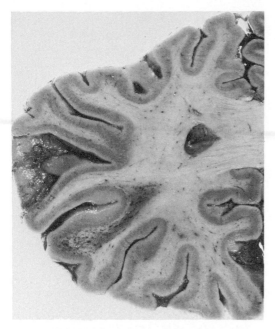

Fig. 10-3. Telangiectasis involving white matter of a gyrus and deep portion of the cortex. It is extending centrally toward ventricle in the line of venous drainage. (From Potter, J. M.: Angiomatous malformations of the brain: Their nature and prognosis, Ann. Roy. Coll. Surg. Eng. **16:**227, 1955.)

In general, telangiectatic vessels are thin walled, devoid of elastica and plain muscle, and are not closely packed together. They are separated by relatively normal brain parenchyma in which to a small extent gliosis may be found. The veins draining the lesion toward the ventricles are enlarged and may be tortuous. The very rare evidence of old hemorrhage or vascular occlusions substantiates the impression that they are benign lesions unlikely to cause serious hemorrhage or local neurological disturbances.

Farrell and Forno[95] reported a telangiectasis involving extensively the lower pons and upper third of the medulla oblongata of a man of 63 years who had symptoms of 8 years' duration. The lesions consisted of numerous thin-walled vessels of varying size with little tendency to packing and some notably large veins (Fig. 10-7). A few vessels exhibited some calification and there was gliosis of the intervening parenchyma at the center of the lesion. Though there was no evidence of hemorrhage, the subject suffered progressive disturbances of gait and bulbar signs.

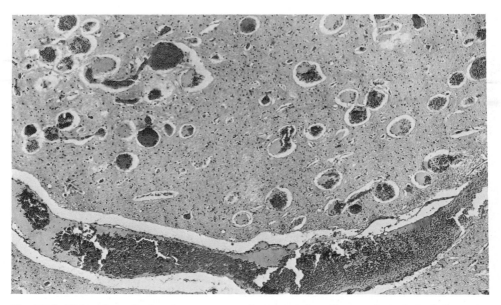

Fig. 10-4. Telangiectasis showing numerous large vessels and an enlarged draining vein. (Hematoxylin and eosin, ×45.)

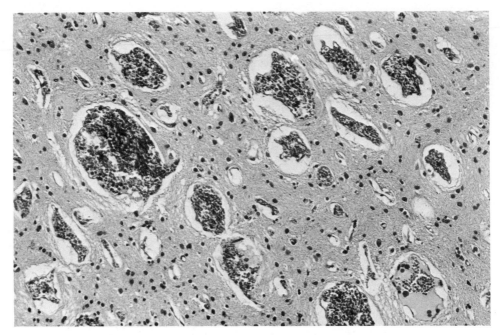

Fig. 10-5. Thin-walled vessels of a telangiectasis. (Hematoxylin and eosin, ×110.)

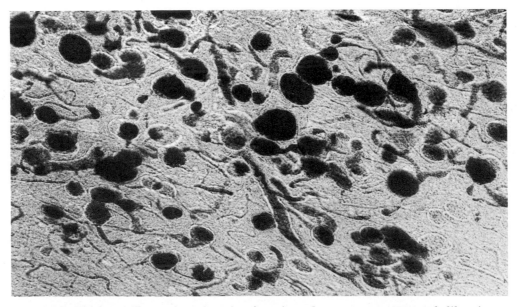

Fig. 10-6. Thick paraffin section of a telangiectasis to demonstrate aneurysmal dilatations of the small vessels. (Fuchsin, ×45.)

A male of 4 months, with congenital heart disease, had multiple cerebral hemangiomas of the type depicted in Fig. 10-8, *A*. The areas of brain involved were extensively infiltrated by numerous small vessels with evidence of previous hemorrhage and destruction of tissue (Fig. 10-8, *B*). Such diffuse lesions do not conform to any of the usual types of vascular anomaly and at present should be classified simply as hemangiomas.

Cavernous hemangioma (cavernoma). Cavernous hemangiomas have attracted considerable attention lately because like pontine lesions they are now recognized as a potential cause of massive intracerebral hemorrhage and can also cause cranial nerve lesions.[340] Clinically, they not infrequently produce Jacksonian epilepsy because of their frequent relationship to the

motor area of the cerebral cortex. Hypothalamic disturbances can result when sizable lesions are situated near the third ventricle.[238]

Like telangiectases, many workers consider them more prevalent than is generally believed because when small they can be overlooked, and if they have caused hemorrhage, they can be easily mistaken for part of the hematoma. They are most frequent in the cerebrum (Table 10-1), where they are often subcortical in position particularly in the region of the Rolandic fissure. Another preferred site is in the basal ganglia.[296] When in the wall of the third ventricle, they may partially or completely occlude the cavity. Noran[238] attributed the production of somnolence, obesity, and polyuria in a 10-year-old boy to a cavernous hemangioma involving the hypothalamus

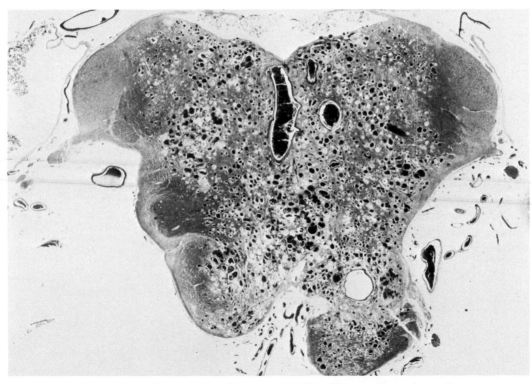

Fig. 10-7. Extensive telangiectasia of upper medulla. Abnormal vessels replace a considerable amount of parenchyma. Note large veins. (From Farrell, D. F., and Forno, L. S.: Symptomatic capillary telangiectasis of the brainstem without hemorrhage, Neurology 20:341, 1970.)

and third ventricle with obstructive hydrocephalus. Russell and Rubinstein[296] considered the pons to be the next most frequent site of involvement whereas the cerebellum is rarely involved. McCormick and colleagues,[205] however, found the cerebellum to be the site most often affected in the posterior fossa. Of 21 cavernous hemangiomas, 12 involved the cerebellum, seven the pons, one the midbrain, and one the medulla. White and associates[379] found that of the 50 intracranial vascular anomalies or tumors found incidentally at autopsy, 10 (20%) were cavernous hemangiomas. Of

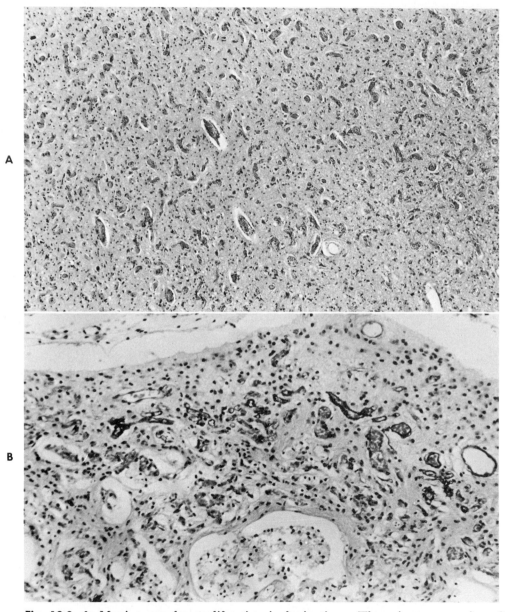

Fig. 10-8. A, Massive vascular proliferation in brain tissue. There is no suggestion of aneurysmal dilatation of vessels. Lesion has been classified as a hemangioma. **B,** Portion of hemangioma in **A** near a region of old hemorrhage. Iron incrustation of vessel walls. (Hematoxylin and eosion; **A,** ×45; **B,** ×110.)

these, five were in the cerebrum, two in the pons, one in the meninges, and two in the cerebellum. Of the 45 pontine hemangiomas reviewed by Teilmann,[340] 16 were cavernous in type (35.6%). On rare occasions, the dura[204] and cranial nerve roots may be involved.[296] Dandy[72] wrote of a young male infant with a large extracranial cavernous hemangioma in the suboccipital region. The mass, thought originally to be a meningocele, pulsated and was continuous through a porous and thinned occipital bone with a large mass of similar tissue displacing the cerebellum forward and obstructing the fourth ventricle. Hydrocephalus was the inevitable result with apparently no direct involvement of brain tissue by the hemangioma. Ohlmacher[244] described a case in which there were two cerebral cavernous hemangiomas, and a third in the cervical spinal cord had caused hematomyelia. Some cutaneous cavernous hemangiomas develop arteriovenous shunts and, according to Watson and McCarthy,[370] erode the cranial vault, causing fatal bleeding. Alternatively, they may involve the intracranial vessels in the arteriovenous shunt.

Multiple cavernous hemangiomas are found repeatedly,[142,244] as shown by Russell and Rubinstein[296] who estimated the frequency of multiplicity as about 16% or 17% of the patients. In one quite exceptional case, 42 hemangiomas were found in the brain.[296] Geschickter and Keasby[102] state that approximately one-third of the cavernous hemangiomas are associated with multiple angiomas in the central nervous system or elsewhere. Their estimate seems high, although definite statistics are not available. Burke and associates[46] encountered two newborn infants with innumerable cutaneous hemangiomas. Many of them involuted or showed signs of regression during the first 2 years of life. One child had multiple hemangiomas (2 mm. to 3 cm. in diameter) of the brain and some were believed to be undergoing involution by cyst formation, but an upper pontine lesion caused hydrocephalus by ob-

structing the aqueduct. In the other case, which was not fatal, the child was believed to have cerebral involvement after a calcified lesion in the cerebrum was detected on radiological examination of the skull.

The average age of supratentorial cavernous hemangiomas (Table 10-2) has been given as 50 years and of subtentorial lesions as 45 years,[205] but the range of the age distribution is wide. They are more prevalent in the male[296] and although there has been an occasional instance of an alleged familial factor,[213] no significant frequency has been established.

Macroscopically, cavernous hemangiomas are usually dark red or black in cross section, very well circumscribed, and at times lobulated. Most vary in size from a few millimeters to 3 or 4 cm. in diameter, with the majority less than 2 cm. Occasionally, the edges may be a little indefinite because of the presence of enlarged vascular channels at a distance from the main mass. Schneider and Liss[308] reported two massive cavernous hemangiomas, each being at least 8 cm. in diameter. They were well encapsulated and readily shelled out at operation. Most cavernous hemangiomas are not encapsulated, but perhaps the size of the mass and/or the rate of growth have bearing on capsule formation. Though readily mistaken for small hematomas, unlike them, cavernous hemangiomas cannot be evacuated and the cut surface is often depressed slightly below the surrounding brain substance. Pale areas, in reality fibrotic areas and organizing thrombi, may be seen in the substance of the hemangioma. On cutting, calcification[294] and bone[381] may be detectable, or additionally there may be evidence of old hemorrhage (yellow-brown pigmentation about the tumor, in the neighboring brain, or in the leptomeninges). On occasions, gliosis in the neighboring tissue imparts an undue firmness on palpation[296] with perhaps a degree of atrophy.[238]

At operation, these hemangiomas are known to pulsate with a cranial bruit audi-

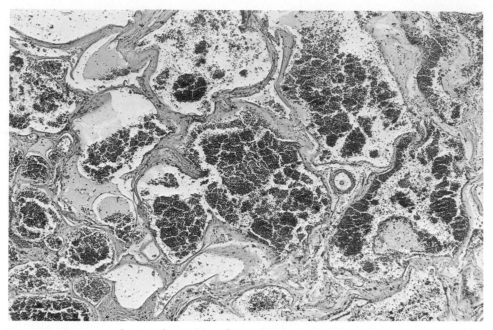

Fig. 10-9. Cavernous hemangioma. Note large closely packed irregular cavernous cavities separated by fibrous tissue, most of which is hyaline. (Hematoxylin and eosin, ×45.)

ble on auscultation[238] despite the fact that their blood supply is held to be not unduly large.[296,308] Noran[238] found enlarged tortuous vessels on the surface of the brain immediately overlying the hemangiomas in two of his cases. Cavernous hemangiomas in extracranial sites at times have a distinct arteriovenous shunt. There is apparently need for detailed examination of the blood supply both anatomically and functionally.

Histologically, the lesions have the characteristic appearance of cavernous hemangiomas, with many large vascular spaces packed closely together toward the center (Fig. 10-9). They are lined by a single layer of endothelium and arterioles and small arteries do not form a prominent feature of the lesion. Relatively normal brain tissue may extend inward between the cavernous spaces, especially at the periphery, but at other times only fibrous tissue or hyaline collagen exists in the intervening tissue. Such collagenous trabeculae vary in width and occasionally contain calcification or more rarely ossification.

The vascular spaces range in size between wide limits, and as the direct result of mutual pressure between contiguous spaces, their outlines often appear as if faceted rather than round or oval. In these cavernous hemangiomas in which the spaces are separated by hyaline trabeculae as in the liver, the margin of the hemangioma is usually far from being sharply defined. Gliosed brain parenchyma extends inward between the vascular spaces to partially or occasionally surround the peripheral blood spaces. Thrombosis within the vascular spaces is not an infrequent finding. Various stages of organization of thrombi may be seen, whereas some spaces are filled with loose hyaline fibrous tissue in which siderophages remain. Phleboliths as in Marfucci's syndrome[50] have not been recorded in the vascular spaces of these hemangiomas.

Evidence of hemorrhage is not infrequent, as the presence of siderophages in the interstitial tissue attests (Fig. 10-10) and even extravasated red cells may be observed histologically. The precise frequency

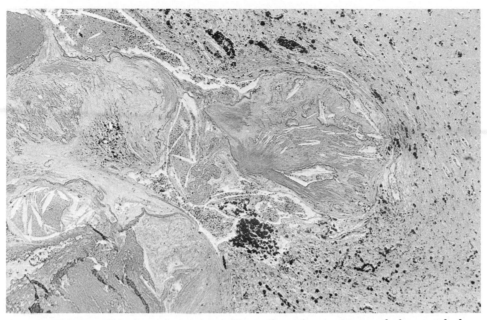

Fig. 10-10. Edge of a cavernous hemangioma of cerebrum. Many of the vessels have necrotic walls and are filled with unorganized thrombi containing many cholesterol clefts. There are large numbers of siderophages in the neighboring brain suggestive of hemorrhage though they can also result from organization of thrombi. (Hematoxylin and eosin, ×45.)

with which these cavernous hemangiomas actually bleed is not known and neither does the presence of calcification in the lesion preclude severe hemorrhage.[383]

The term "cavernous hemangioma" has been restricted by many authors to encompass only hemangiomas in which no brain tissue extends between the large dilated vascular spaces. This circumscribed use is unjustified for the term "cavernous" refers to the large cavernous spaces only, irrespective of the intervening tissue. In extracranial hemangiomas certainly the application is not restricted thus. There is the possibility that one variety may ultimately, as the spaces enlarge, transform to the other. Authors have referred to those hemangiomas in which brain parenchyma extends between the spaces as telangiectases, and for this reason the pathology of these vascular lesions may well be rewritten as uncertainties are resolved by further detailed study.

In telangiectases, it is not unusual to find adjacent aneurysmal dilatations in proximity and some thickening and hyalinization of the walls of the vascular spaces. Further enlargement of vascular spaces could result in lesions, such as those in Figs. 10-11 and 10-12, which could be regarded as transitional forms in which there has occurred further thickening and hyalinization of the cavernous walls, retrogressive changes in the intervening parenchyma, and even some hemorrhage as indicated by the presence of siderophages. Further progression (Fig. 10-13) can bring about typical cavernous hemangiomas. In the literature, these transitional forms have been variously classified, thus indicating the unreliable nature of some of the alleged clinical features of telangiectases and cavernous hemangiomas (such as age distribution and preferential locations).

Russell and Rubinstein[296] agree that distinction between telangiectases and cavernous hemangiomas is not always clear, but because of the age distribution, they con-

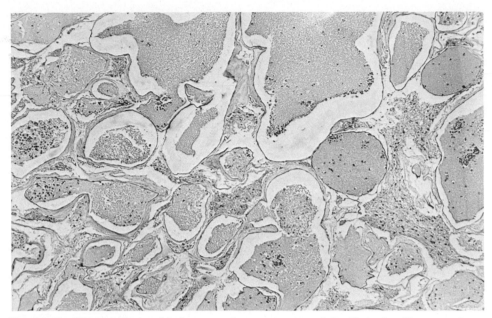

Fig. 10-11. Hemangioma with large cavernous spaces and hyalinized collagenous inter-vening trabeculae though there is also gliosed brain in the interstitial tissue in places. This is a transitional form between a telangiectasis and a cavernous hemangioma. (Hematoxylin and eosin, ×45.)

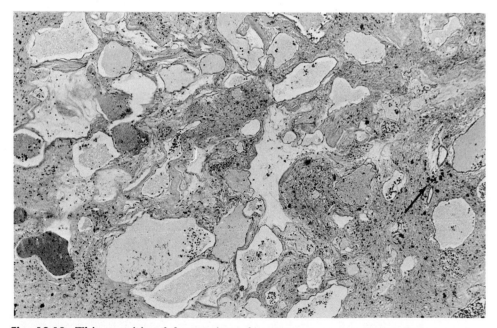

Fig. 10-12. This transitional hemangioma has many cavernous spaces that are not so tightly packed as those in Fig. 10-11. Arrow indicates siderophages suggestive of previous hemorrhage. (Hematoxylin and eosin, ×45.)

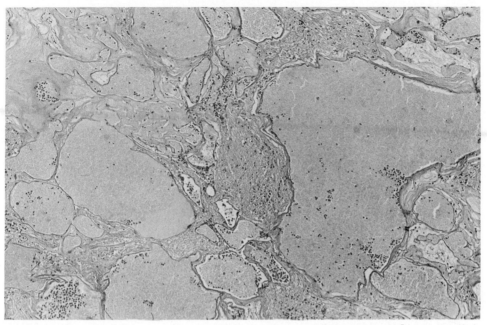

Fig. 10-13. Transitional hemangioma with extensive degenerative areas and gross hyalinization of interstitial tissue and trabeculae, but still some brain tissue is present between some cavernous spaces. (Hematoxylin and eosin, ×45.)

sider that the lesions should not be classified together and that cavernous hemangiomas are not a late stage in the development of telangiectases. However, reference to Table 10-2 indicates that age differences are hardly significant.

Russell and Rubinstein[296] discuss the relationship of these hemangiomas with similar lesions (cutaneous and visceral) elsewhere in the body, noting a tendency towards this association and that with other developmental faults. In three cases, two were in association with cutaneous hemangiomas, and the third with a renal hemangioma, renal cysts, and an adrenal gland within the renal capsule. White and associates[379] reported cavernous hemangiomas in the brain, lung, and liver of a man of 45 years of age who died from an astrocytoma and an instance of multiple hemangiomas of the pons, cerebellum, spinal cord, and thalamus. Schneider and Liss[308] wrote of a hemangioma of the tibia in association with a massive cavernous hemangioma of the cerebrum. In an 87-year-old woman,

Wood and associates[389] reported cavernous hemangiomas with lesions in the brain, spinal cord, kidney, heart, skin, and calvarium. This would indicate a compatibility with longevity. They further asserted that the liver was the site most often involved by associated extracranial hemangiomas. To assess the implications of such an association is difficult. Cavernous hemangiomas of the liver are very prevalent at routine autopsy and increase in frequency with age, and though the association of hemangiomas with extracranial lesions of a similar nature is regarded as being of some significance, only additional detailed study can verify the hypothesis.

Thrombocytopenia and an abnormal tendency to bleed sometimes accompany a cavernous hemangioma. The pathogenesis of the syndrome is obscure, but it is believed that sequestration of platelets occurs in thrombi within the hemangiomas. Multiple hemangiomas and telangiectases may be encountered in the skin and occasionally visceral lesions are found. As yet,

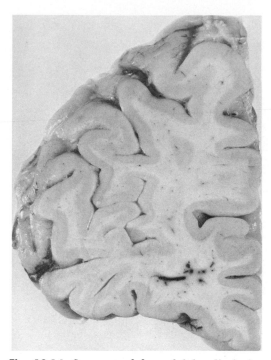

Fig. 10-14. Segment of frontal lobe displaying several enlarged veins constituting a venous angioma.

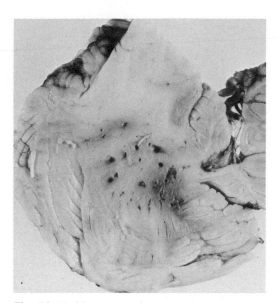

Fig. 10-15. Venous angioma of cerebellar hemisphere.

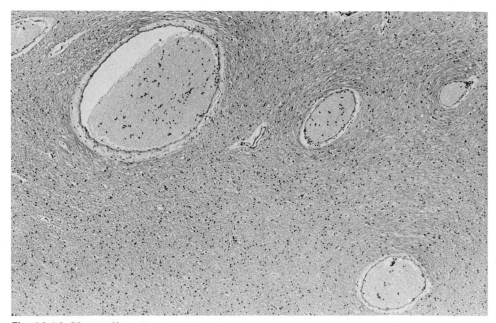

Fig. 10-16. Unusually enlarged veins of a venous angioma of the cerebellum. (Hematoxylin and eosin, ×45.)

no alterations in platelet count or function have been demonstrated in association with cerebral hemangiomas.

Venous angioma. Many authors do not recognize varix as a separate category,[296] but others[202,203,205] regard it as an entity distinct from venous angioma. Both could be included under venous angioma. The varix is said[202,203,205] to consist of a single dilated vein, or occasionally several such veins, within the neural parenchyma or in the leptomeninges. Microscopically, they are enlarged thin-walled veins, usually with little local disturbance and without cal-

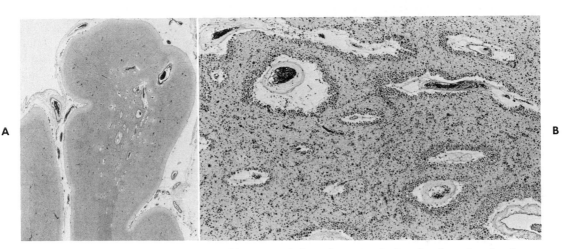

Fig. 10-17. A, Cerebral venous angioma consisting almost entirely of enlarged veins in the white matter and to a lesser extent the cortex. **B,** Numerous thick-walled veins of the cerebral venous angioma in **A.** Note multitudinous corpora amylacea about the vessels. (Hematoxylin and eosin; **A,** ×3.5; **B,** ×32.)

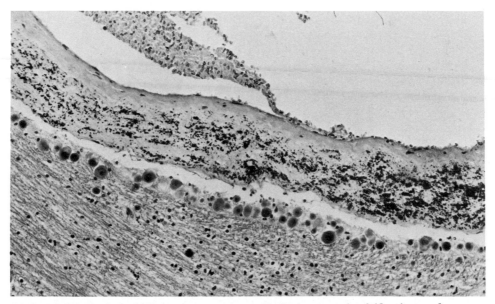

Fig. 10-18. Wall of cerebellar venous angioma displaying mural calcification and corpora amylacea in neighboring parenchyma. (Hematoxylin and eosin, ×110.)

cification. The infrequent complications consist of hemorrhage[202,238] and thrombosis with hemorrhagic infarction.[238] McCormick and associates[205] found two varices in the cerebrum, two in the cerebellum, and two in the pons (Table 10-1). Instances of aneurysmal dilatation of the vein of Galen[202] and of some dural sinuses with local bone erosion[238] have been regarded as varices but all are probably manifestations of arteriovenous aneurysms.

Small venous angiomas consist of single or several enlarged veins sometimes exhibiting tortuosity. They may arise within the parenchyma of the cerebrum or cerebellum (Figs. 10-14 and 10-15) and present a macroscopic appearance of multiple petechial hemorrhages. Histologically, the numerous veins may appear relatively normal (Fig. 10-16), though at times there is considerable thickening and even calcification of their walls (Figs. 10-17 to 10-18). Degenerative changes may be observed in the intervening parenchyma but are not common nor is hemorrhage. A thorough search reveals arteries in the neighborhood, but the enlarged vessels are predominantly venous in type.

Large venous angiomas, involving the large pial vessels, are considered akin to arteriovenous aneurysms but without the arterial element. They consist of single or several enlarged veins sometimes exhibiting pronounced tortuosity. Some lesions may form wedge- or cone-shaped vascular masses with the base at the meninges and the apex reaching to the ventricle.[238] The diagnosis of these lesions used to depend more on the macroscopic appearance than on histological analysis. Dandy[72] stated that the blood in these vessels is of low oxygen saturation (venous blood) with neither pulsation nor a thrill (or bruit) evident. Degenerative changes can also come about in the neural parenchyma, for thrombi and hemorrhage are not infrequent complications. These lesions are now generally regarded as variants of arteriovenous aneurysms.

Russell and Rubinstein[296] contend that the venous angiomas are much more frequent in the spinal cord and its meninges. McCormick and his colleagues[205] found that these angiomas comprised 19% of subtentorial and 13% of supratentorial vascular anomalies. Found in the main in the distribution of the middle cerebral artery in the cerebrum, they may be chanced upon in the distribution of the vein of Galen and the cerebellum. These lesions, it is believed, do not produce significant arteriovenous shunting, but their circulatory dynamics and precise anatomical relationships to the surrounding circulation are unresolved.

Arteriovenous aneurysms. There remains much to learn about arteriovenous aneurysms or "malformations." They are said to be vascular hamartomas in which there is an arteriovenous shunt of variable degree. Similar lesions consisting entirely of arteries have been described, but their existence is in doubt. Enlarged tortuous spinal arteries in coarctation of the aorta (Fig. 2-8) cannot be so classified for these arteries merely participate in a collateral circulation and as such are compensatorily enlarged and eventually become tortuous as do most collaterals. Noran[238] regards the existence of an authentic arterial vascular anomaly as a theoretical possibility only, and combined anatomical and hemodynamic studies may one day place venous angiomas in this same category.

Table 10-3. Sex distribution of arteriovenous aneurysms

Author	Males	Females	Total
Mackenzie (1953)[191]	25	25	50
Paterson & McKissock (1956)[259]	62	47	109
Olivecrona & Ladenheim (1957)[246]	83	42	125
af Björkesten & Troupp (1959)[2]	11	11	22
Sabra (1959)[298]	48	52	100
Sharkey (1965)[313]	14	6	20
Svien & McRae (1965)[334]	51	44	95
Cooperative Study (1966)[264]	236	217	453
Total	530	444	974

Prevalence. Arteriovenous aneurysms occur more particularly in the brain than elsewhere in the body[272] and in addition are the most common of all the vascular anomalies of the central nervous system (Table 10-1). Because many of the vascular anomalies remain clinically quiescent, being found only incidentally at autopsy, arteriovenous aneurysms constitute a much larger proportion of clinical material than postmortem material. In the Cooperative Study, arteriovenous malformations accounted for 6% of the subarachnoid hemorrhages studied (Table 7-2).

Sex distribution. There has been considerable emphasis on the preponderance of males among patients with vascular anomalies, and the ratio of males to females[276,296] is usually given as 2:1 to 3:1. The ratio, however, varies considerably (Table 10-3). Olivecrona and Ladenheim[246] found the ratio to be 2:1, whereas in Mackenzie's[191] series it was 1:1. In the Cooperative Study,[264] the ratio of males to females was 1.1:1, 1.05:1 among those who had presented with subarachnoid hemorrhage, and 1.17:1 in those without hemorrhage, the difference being of little practical or clinical significance. On academic grounds, however, it is interesting that factors responsible for the slight female preponderance seen in intracranial arterial aneurysms do not prevail with the vascular anomalies here under discussion.

Age distribution. Patients with cerebral arteriovenous aneurysms present clinically at an earlier age than do those with cerebral aneurysms. In the Cooperative Study, for instance, it was found that 64% of arteriovenous aneurysms were diagnosed before the age of 40 years, as against 26% of cerebral aneurysms diagnosed by that time. Paterson and McKissock[259] found that 70% of their patients had the lesions diagnosed before the age of 40. Approximately one-third (31%) of the vascular anomalies in the Cooperative Study[264] were found between 40 and 60 years of age. Table 10-4 gives the age distribution of patients at the time of diagnosis of their lesion and Table 10-5, the age distribution at the onset of symptoms.

Paterson and McKissock[259] in 50 patients found the average age at the onset of symptoms to be 24 years and at the time of diagnosis 32 years, indicating a time lapse of 8 years. Olivecrona and Riives[247] found a time lapse of 6 years. Some patients present clinically for the first time with intracranial hemorrhage only in the third or fourth decade. Often there is a long history of focal or general convulsions.

Location. The middle cerebral artery is the most frequent site for arteriovenous an-

Table 10-4. Age distribution of arteriovenous aneurysms of the brain at the time of diagnosis

Author	1-10 or 0-9	11-20 or 10-19	21-30 or 20-29	31-40 or 30-39	41-50 or 40-49	51-60 or 50-59	61-70 or 60-69	70 and over	Total
Bassett (1951)[20]	1	3	5	5	4				18
Mackenzie (1953)[191]		10	13	8	12	7			50
Paterson & McKissock (1956)[259]	2	20	29	25	23	9	1		109
Gurdjian et al. (1965)[118]		4	6	8	9	7	2	2	38
Sharkey (1965)[313]	2	1	3	7	6	1			20
McCormick et al. (1968)[205] (Posterior fossa anomalies only)	6	9	29	25	16	28	19	16	148
Meier-Violand (1969)[212]	2	3	12	13	14	10	4	1	59
Total	13	50	97	91	84	62	26	19	442
Cooperative Study* (1966)[264]	23	66	91	108	83	59	18	5	453

*These include an unstated number of hemangiomas.

Table 10-5. Age distribution of arteriovenous aneurysms of the brain at onset of symptoms

Author	1-10 or 0-9	11-20 or 10-19	21-30 or 20-29	31-40 or 30-39	41-50 or 40-49	51-60 or 50-59	61-70 or 60-69	70 and over	Total
Wyburn-Mason (1943)[390]	8	6	13	3			1		31
Mackenzie (1953)[191]	5	24	6	9	5	1			50
Paterson & McKissock (1956)[259]	11	38	26	23	7	4			109
Olivecrona & Ladenheim (1957)[246]	7	39	40	23	14	2			125
af Björkesten & Troupp (1959)[2]	2	4	9	3	2	1	1		22
Svien & McRae (1965)[334]	13	22	26	19	11	4*			95
Meier-Violand (1969)[212]	3	12	15	15	6	6	2		59
Total	49	145	135	95	45	18	4		491

*Four patients said to be over 50 years of age were placed in this decade for convenience, but their inclusion does not alter the results significantly.

Table 10-6. Location of encephalic arteriovenous aneurysms

Site	Cooperative Study[264]	Anderson & Korbin[8]	Sharkey[313]	Gurdjian et al.[118]	Krayenbühl & Yaşargil[161]	Total
Frontal	64 (14%)	7	4	6	8	89
Frontoparietal	28 (6%)		3	2	12	45
Frontotemporal	10 (2%)		1			11
Temporal	51 (11%)		4	1	14	70
Temporoparietal	26 (6%)	7	3	3	10*	49
Temporo-occipital	5 (1%)			1		6
Parietal	104 (23%)	12	2	9	17	144
Parieto-occipital	18 (4%)	6	1	4		29
Occipital	23 (5%)	3	1	3	11	41
Intraventricular or paraventricular	81 (18%)	2		1		84
Brain stem	11 (2%)			1	3	15
Cerebellum	21 (5%)		1		8	30
Whole hemisphere	3 (1%)				4	7
Multiple sites	3 (1%)					3
Site not mentioned	5 (1%)					5
Other sites				7	4	11
Total	453	37	20	38	91	639

*Ten lesions located in the Sylvian fissure were interpreted as temporoparietal.

eurysms and the location of the most extensive lesions. Supratentorial lesions are much more frequent than subtentorial and the majority of arteriovenous aneurysms are fed by branches of the internal carotid artery.[246] Contributions from one or more major cerebral arteries may augment the supply. The cerebellum and spinal cord are much less often affected.

In the Cooperative Study of 453 intracranial vascular anomalies,[264] it would appear that mostly vascular anomalies with a distinct arteriovenous shunt were considered. Of the lesions, 421 were supratentorial (93%) and 32 were subtentorial (7%). Little difference was noted between left- and right-sided involvement and only 8% were midline in location. In 2%, there was simultaneous involvement of both cerebral hemispheres. Table 10-6 sets out the distribution of the lesions reported in the literature, the parietal regions being the most commonly involved site. An unexpected left-sided predominance (60:41) was found in the Cooperative Study.[264] Angiographically, as far as could be determined the majority of anomalies was supplied by the middle cerebral artery. Most frontal and

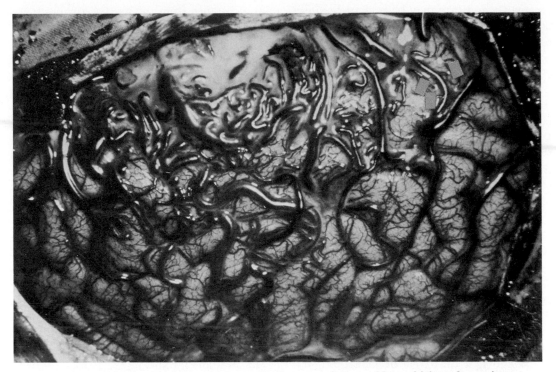

Fig. 10-19. Arteriovenous aneurysm exposed at craniotomy. Note thickened meninges and closely packed enlarged tortuous and turgid vessels. (Courtesy Dr. W. Feindel, Montreal, Quebec.)

parietal anomalies were fed by the branches of the anterior and middle cerebral arteries. The frontal region was involved on 105 occasions and the temporal in 95 cases. Multiple small anomalies were found bilaterally in only three patients.

Of a total of 183 arteriovenous aneurysms, Wappenschmidt and associates[368] found 170 situated above the tentorium and nine below. The remaining four cases were combined extracranial and intracranial arteriovenous aneurysms, located in the soft tissue of the temporal and occipital regions and involving the posterior fossa. Of 170 supratentorial lesions, vertebral angiography demonstrated that 19 were supplied by the vertebrobasilar system. Vertebral angiography was not performed in every case, and so the authors believe the latter sites are more often involved. Eight were in the region of the lateral ventricles and basal ganglia, four were related to the splenium of the corpus callosum and mid-

brain (with aneurysmal dilatation of the vein of Galen), and seven were cortical or subcortical in location presumably in the occipital lobe.

Macroscopic appearance. In patients suspected of harboring an intracranial arteriovenous aneurysm, a careful examination for vascular nevi is essential. Increased vascularity of the scalp can be accentuated in vivo by infrared photography.[276] The scalp vessels, diploic channels of the calvarium, and the dural vessels (both meningeal vessels and venous sinuses) should be carefully scanned for unusual enlargement and increased vascularity or seemingly aberrant vascular pathways. The changes may be bilateral. The subdural space may be bridged by small vessels, arteries, or veins (up to 2 mm. or more in diameter) that anastomose pial vessels with those of the dura when middle meningeal or extracranial vessels participate in the shunt. Enlarged foramina in the skull (such as the foramen spinosum) may be present because of the increased caliber of the vessels (such as the middle meningeal artery).

Arteriovenous aneurysms, after reflection of the dura mater, are more impressive when viewed at craniotomy (Fig. 10-19) than at autopsy when the vessels are collapsed and no longer turgid and pulsating. When seen post mortem, the overlying leptomeninges may be shriveled and exhibit considerable fibrotic thickening and siderotic pigmentation indicative of previous bleeding, or with recent bleeding, subdural or subarachnoid hemorrhage may be present. An area of the cerebral surface covered by a plexus of tortuous vessels is variable as is the caliber of the vessels. Arterial feeders extend into the plexus and are as a rule larger than usual. Vessels more proximally situated may likewise be enlarged and tortuous and such a shunt is a cause of the asymmetrical caliber of the components of the circle of Willis and its major branches. Dissection to demonstrate the arteriovenous relationships is difficult as is the macroscopic differentiation of arteries from veins. Injection preparations as illustrated by Russell and Rubinstein[296] and Rodda and Calvert[284] probably demonstrate best the in vivo appearance as well as the afferent and efferent vessels. The conglomerate of tortuous and intertwining vessels involves the sulci and many unusually large channels may penetrate the cortex. The carotid arteries in the neck may be so enlarged that prominent pulsations are visible.[70] Grossly enlarged and tortuous veins extending from the plexus may be recognizable channels such as the superficial Sylvian vein or veins and the greater and lesser anastomotic veins (of Trolard or Labbé respectively). The large size of some channels, otherwise small or insignificant, may give the impression of a gross anatomical departure from the usual vascular configuration, but the patterns are usually secondary manifestations of the vascular shunt. The same explanation applies to the vessels of the dura mater. The pathological enlargement of some veins occurs

at a distance from the matted, tortuous, and intertwining vessels, probably because of the absence of valves in the cerebral veins. Seljeskog and associates[311] attributed to an arteriovenous aneurysm in one frontal lobe, a massive aneurysmal dilatation of the inferior longitudinal sagittal sinus in an infant. The most frequent site for massive enlargements of an intracranial vein or dural sinus is the great cerebral vein of Galen. Occasionally, not only is the vein of Galen grossly dilated, but the straight sinus also or the superior longitudinal saggital sinus.[108,133]

Information on the occurrence of multiple intracranial arteriovenous aneurysms is sparse[20,289] and less than 1% of the cases reported in the Cooperative Study[264] proved to be multiple.

Perret and Nishioka[264] found that in 72% of the cases submitted to the Cooperative Study the anomaly was larger than 2 cm. in diameter and in 8% it was less, with no information available on the remaining 20%. Of 72 arteriovenous aneurysms surgically excised, 32 were less than 2 cm. in diameter, 16 measured 2 to 4 cm. in diameter, and 24 were larger than 4 cm.[251]

The cerebral hemisphere is frequently atrophied in part or in whole and in contrast with the contralateral hemisphere, the reduction in size is often extreme. In coronal section, the arteriovenous aneurysms tend to present as a triangular lesion extending from the base at the meninges to an apex at or close to the ventricles in the line of the transcerebral veins. The affected parenchyma may be honeycombed with large vessels, many of which collapse, and some are obviously aneurysmal. In association with the pathological vessels, old or recent hemorrhage, softening, and extensive gliosis are usual in fatal cases (Fig. 10-20). Calcification of the vessels and parenchyma may be apparent and changes associated with atherosclerosis superadded in older individuals.

Dandy[71] asserted that the mass of small vessels, the so-called angioma, connecting the arterial and venous channels supplying

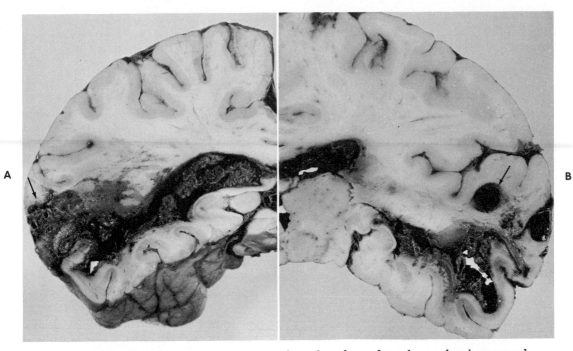

Fig. 10-20. A, Arteriovenous aneurysm on lateral surface of cerebrum showing several enlarged vessels (*arrow*). There is considerable softening of white matter, and intracerebral and ventricular hemorrhage occurred. **B,** In another plane of section an intracerebral aneurysm is present (*arrow*).

the lesion is usually deep within the brain parenchyma. No detailed study of large numbers of these lesions has put his allegation to the test. Postmortem microangiography with three-dimensional reconstruction would indicate whether he is correct.

Small arteriovenous aneurysms may fill from one major cerebral artery alone, usually the middle cerebral, whereas the arteriovenous shunt can be likened to an ever-enlarging drain. A collateral circulation develops, and by means of naturally occurring pial anastomoses, the anomaly may come to be supplied by two, three, or even more major arteries. Parietal lesions can readily be supplied from the anterior, middle, and posterior cerebral arteries. Less frequently the supply issues from the contralateral cerebral circulation as is the case when the anomaly is frontal, occipital, or midline in position. Involvement of the extracranial circulation, as evidenced by the enlargement of scalp, middle meningeal, and orbital vessels is known.

With progressive increase in the shunt and the enlargement of afferent vessels feeding the arteriovenous aneurysm, the corresponding efferent vessels (veins and sinuses) undergo compensatory and extensive enlargement. The enlargement of the vein is usually many times greater than that of the arteries. In some lesions, the tortuosity and aneurysmal enlargement of the veins overshadows the arterial changes. The additional venous drainage required may be reflected in the orbit (proptosis) and in the retina (venous tortuosity and engorgement with well-oxygenated blood).

Moersch and Kernohan[215] reported a series of events concerning a young girl of 18 years who, in a serious automobile accident, sustained a contusion to the right side of the head. There was progressive deterioration over the next 2 years and death occurred after an exploratory operation. After death it was discovered that the right middle cerebral artery coursed around the posterior surface of a large bilocular aneurysmal sac (approximately 7 cm. in its longest dimension) in the Sylvian fissure despite a direct communication between the artery and the sac. The much enlarged petrosquamous sinus* communicated freely with the aneurysm laterally. The sac had ruptured into the posterior part of the frontal lobe, the temporal lobe, the right lateral ventricle, and also into the subarachnoid space. The Sylvian vein was much enlarged and communicated with the aneurysmal sac. Other large tortuous cortical veins extended from the Sylvian fissure. The fistula was regarded as congenital but the history and the structure of the sac wall (without remnants of vessel wall), are suggestive of a traumatic origin.

An arteriovenous aneurysm occasionally involves the choroid plexus alone,[235,360] in which case it may be regarded as an intraventricular lesion causing variously a filling defect on ventriculography[352] or an intraventricular hemorrhage or occasionally hydrocephalus.[203] McGuire and associates[207] found bilateral hemangiomas of the lateral choroid plexuses with hydrocephalus, which was relieved after bilateral plexectomy. The type of vascular anomaly was uncertain. More frequently, the choroid plexuses of the lateral ventricles are involved as part of a more extensive arteriovenous aneurysm incorporating the neighboring midline structures including the thalamus, hypothalamus, and basal ganglia. Arteriovenous aneurysms in this location are comparatively uncommon.

Arteriovenous aneurysms of the midbrain. Wolf and Brock[387] reported a male of 21 years with an angiomatous nevus over the right cheek since birth and a loud temporal bruit extending down into the neck. On the right side, the ear and the temporal and carotid arteries pulsated energetically. Bilateral exophthalmos (more so on the right side) was noted. The patient was blind in the right eye because of angioma-

tous involvement of the retina, and this extended posteriorly to involve the right optic nerve, optic chiasm, the right side of the midbrain (with compression of the aqueduct and hydrocephalus), the right superior cerebellar peduncle, and the dentate nucleus of the right side of the cerebellum. The angioma was believed to be venous in type, but in view of the bruit, the arterial pulsation, the pulsating right ear,[42] and the exophthalmos, the lesion must have been associated with an arteriovenous shunt of considerable size.

Wyburn-Mason[390] reviewed arteriovenous aneurysms involving the midbrain as in the foregoing case. Some displayed in addition an anomaly of the retina and cutaneous nevi. These lesions in association occurred primarily in patients under 30 years of age. In the instances of the fully developed arteriovenous aneurysm, abnormal vessels extend as a tract of dilated and tortuous vessels on one side of the retina, covering and permeating the optic nerve, optic chiasm, and optic tract and lying above the cavernous sinus. They reach the dorsum of the midbrain posteriorly chiefly on one side and involve the quadrigeminal bodies, the brachia conjunctiva, and red nucleus (Fig. 10-21). There are extensions to the pulvinar and posterior part of the hypothalamus, backward to involve the cerebellum, laterally to the choroid plexus of the lateral ventricles, and caudally to the upper part of the pons. Enlarged afferent vessels were noted in a few cases, the increase in size being commensurate with both the size and duration of the shunt. In one of Wyburn-Mason's cases, a special branch from the basilar was involved, but in other instances the basilar and vertebral arteries were seldom enlarged. Enlarged efferent vessels were numerous, and even fairly remote veins and sinuses were so affected. Involvement of the cavernous sinus no doubt is responsible for proptosis and even bilateral exophthalmos can then result. The enlargement of the sinuses causes secondary deepening of the grooves in which they lie (especially the petrosal

---

*The petrosquamous sinus, when present, runs in a groove or a canal along the line of the petrosquamous suture to terminate in the transverse (lateral) sinus.

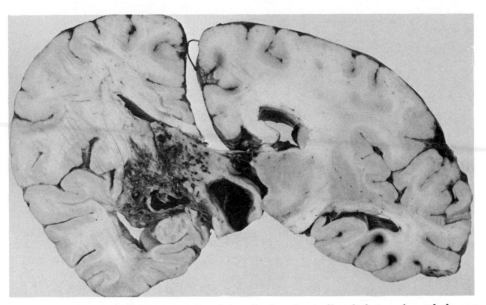

Fig. 10-21. Arteriovenous aneurysm involving the basal ganglia, thalamus, hypothalamus, and midbrain. Note abnormal vessels of variable size and a large aneurysmal vessel extending into the basis pedunculi.

and lateral sinuses) and radiologically the diploic vascular channels can be prominent. The eye, apart from being proptosed, also pulsates. In the fundus, there is usually (on the temporal aspect inferiorly) enlargement and tortuosity of both arteries and veins giving the impression of grossly increased retinal vascularity. The vessels protrude for some distance into the vitreous cavity. Histologically, degenerative changes in the retina have been observed. In 27 cases of retinal arteriovenous aneurysms or similar lesions, 81% were associated with evidence of an intracranial arteriovenous aneurysm, and where the neurological examination had been adequate, Wyburn-Mason believed it was probably in the midbrain. Conversely, in 20 cases of arteriovenous aneurysm of the midbrain, 70% had a retinal vascular anomaly.

In several cases, vascular nevi were associated with these lesions, usually in the homolateral trigeminal area, the fronto-parietal area in particular being mentioned. In one instance, a mother and grandmother were said to be similarly affected. A few of the patients had pigmented nevi also. Wyburn-Mason found other developmental defects (spina bifida, absence of one kidney, malformed phalanges) to support his contention that the association of lesions is caused by a maldevelopment. This syndrome has received little notice since Wyburn-Mason drew attention to it and to the related *formes frustes*.

Aneurysm of the vein of Galen. Aneurysmal dilatation of the great cerebral vein of Galen is relatively uncommon. Hirano and Terry,[133] in 1958, garnered in all only 17 cases from the literature. However, by 1964, Gold and associates[106] had collected 43 and stated that during the previous 3 years, 10 children, representing 1% of all neurological admissions, had been seen with verified cerebral vascular anomalies at the pediatric neurology division at the Columbia-Presbyterian Medical Center (New York). Half of these cases were aneurysmal dilatations of the vein of Galen (frequency 0.5% of pediatric neurology admissions). The majority of the afflicted patients were less than 2 years of age and showed a slight male preponderance.[106,133,297]

An aneurysm of the vein of Galen is an

aneurysmal dilatation of the great Galenic vein consequent upon the presence of an arteriovenous aneurysm. McCormick[202] considers that some may be instances of congenital varix but this is doubtful. In any case, varices themselves are probably the result of arteriovenous shunts. The arteriovenous shunt is due either to a direct anastomosis of neighboring arteries, such as the posterior cerebral, posterior communicating, superior cerebellar, basilar, anterior cerebral (callosal branches), and the anterior choroidal arteries, with the vein of Galen or alternatively, it can be due to the indirect drainage of a nearby arteriovenous aneurysm into the vein of Galen via dilated veins.[99] Gagnon and Boileau[100] reported that there were nine arteries opening directly into an enormously dilated venous sac, which extended anteriorly to the anterior extremity of the corpus callosum and posteriorly was continuous with a widely dilated straight sinus. The vein of Galen was almost half the width of the skull.[359] The dilatation may be irregular[6] as in the irregular dilatation of the veins in the case reported by Hirano and Terry,[133] in which the straight sinus exhibited a fusiform dilatation with a constriction between it and the vein of Galen at the junction of the free margins of the falx cerebri and tentorium cerebelli. In a case of Boldrey and Miller,[37] the straight sinus was enlarged but was considerably smaller than the vein of Galen, whereas the torcular Herophili formed a spherical aneurysmal dilatation. The thickened wall of the aneurysmal sac[6] may become sufficiently calcified to produce a radiographic shadow of its outline.[37] Tributaries and the more proximal sinuses (lateral sinuses) may also be pathologically enlarged and their walls thickened. Retrograde flow may be demonstrable angiographically in the superior longitudinal sagittal sinus, which can also be grossly dilated.[108] Involvement of extracranial veins of the scalp is a common feature, being prominent in one case when associated with secondary thrombo-

sis of the sigmoid sinus.[3] Proptosis is also frequent.

The feeding arteries, as in all arteriovenous aneurysms, are likely to be grossly enlarged and at least in one instance the afferent artery has been known to undergo spontaneous thrombosis.[133] Partial or complete thrombosis of draining veins may occur.[3,106,133] In one patient, the Galenic aneurysm underwent spontaneous thrombosis and the symptoms were related to the hydrocephalus.[376] In another patient, $4\frac{1}{2}$ years of age, the straight sinus was occluded presumably because of thrombosis and the venous drainage of the Galenic aneurysm had been assumed by circuitous superficial channels.[297]

The usual course is for the enormously dilated vein of Galen to compress the midbrain and aqueduct of Sylvius with, in many instances, a resultant hydrocephalus and hypoglycemia.[106] Another major complication is subarachnoid hemorrhage, and Cohen and associates[60] reported an arteriovenous aneurysm involving the great vein of Galen with intraventricular rupture of a large thin-walled efferent vessel extending anteriorly into the lateral ventricle.

Gold and associates[106] divide patients presenting with Galenic aneurysms into three major clinical groups according to the severity of the shunt. In the first category, the newborn infant at or shortly after birth is in cardiac and respiratory distress because of the large arteriovenous shunt from which the child will almost certainly die. Other features and complications are manifested to a lesser extent in this group than in the other categories. In the second type, the onset occurs at any age from birth to 9 months, frequently in association with hydrocephalus, convulsions, a cranial bruit, distended scalp veins, and subarachnoid hemorrhage. It is believed that the shunt is of intermediate severity, but the prognosis is poor because of naturally occurring complications, the high risk of surgery, and mental retardation. In the third type, the shunt is believed to be the least severe and occurs in older children and adults even up to the fifth decade. The average age of onset is about 13 years, with the diagnosis being made approximately 14 years later. The subjects suffer from headaches, fatigue, vertigo, hemiparesis, and subarachnoid hemorrhage. Calcification in the wall of the aneurysm is frequent and the prognosis is the least serious of the three groups.

Most authors have classified these lesions as congenital malformations and have described hemangiomas or telangiectases of the face, cervical hygroma, hemangioma of the lung, and even multiple small cerebral arteriovenous anomalies. Several patients had a history of a severe head injury[37] but this aspect has usually been disregarded.

In addition to that of the vein of Galen, Litvak and associates[178] drew attention to aneurysmal dilatation of other veins or sinuses in or near the midline. In each case it was caused by an arteriovenous aneurysm near to or remote from the midline but with drainage toward the deep midline venous system. Thus, a widely dilated torcular fed by cerebellar, posterior communicating, and internal carotid arteries, or an aneurysmal dilatation of the basal vein, eventuated and simulated an aneurysm of the vein of Galen. The division of the lesions into three categories may help clinically but is of little consequence for the basic pathology.

Arteriovenous aneurysms of the posterior fossa. Large arteriovenous aneurysms of the posterior fossa are infrequent.[296] In a recent review,[206] only 10% of large arteriovenous angiomas were subtentorial whereas smaller "cryptic" arteriovenous aneurysms were considerably more common in the posterior fossa than were the larger anomalies.[206] Of 164 vascular anomalies in the posterior fossa, 70 were found to be arteriovenous angiomas, 55 involved the cerebellum, and the remainder involved the mesencephalon, pons, and medulla, or all combined.[205] Reuter and associates[280] explained a low frequency of arteriovenous aneurysms

in the posterior fossa (2.5% of 247 angiographically demonstrable arteriovenous aneurysms) by the infrequent use of vertebral angiography previously. The frequency in surgical cases was said to be from 5.5% to 9%. There was no significant difference in the mean age of patients with supratentorial and subtentorial arteriovenous angiomas (Table 10-2).

Many arteriovenous angiomas are quite small and are referred to as "cryptic." They may lie deep in a sulcus and a few enlarged vessels nearby disclose their presence. Larger lesions can involve almost the whole of the cerebellum and enlarged veins may be seen above the tentorium. Some extend into the spinal canal and the dural sinuses related to the posterior fossa become enlarged. The blood supply is derived not only from branches of the vertebrobasilar system, but from the posterior communicating and posterior cerebral arteries.[280] Occasionally, an extracranial supply will be provided via defects in the cranium. Both the scalp and the overlying bone can exhibit grossly increased vascularity. Lesions like those above the tentorium bleed[205,280] with hydrocephalus the result of those involving the brain stem.

By angiography, Di Chiro[78] discovered in a blind man of 26 years two deeply situated vascular anomalies posterior to the third cervical vertebra, and two in the cerebellum. The anomalies, probably arteriovenous aneurysms, were associated with bilateral retinal angiomatosis with no obvious familial involvement.

Arteriovenous aneurysms of the brain stem can be small (cryptic) and lie wholly within the parenchyma, otherwise lying partly on the surface with part of the brain stem actually pulsating.[181] Aneurysmal dilatation of vessels can be confused with the berry type of aneurysm and enlarged tortuous veins may extend up to the hypothalamus and floor of the third ventricle.[181]

Bruits. In cerebral arteriovenous aneurysms, there may be a bruit (Table 2-6). Potter found bruits in 22% of his series of

arteriovenous aneurysms whereas Mackenzie[191] reported a frequency of 48%. Present perhaps for only a part of the natural
history of the lesions, their intensity can
vary and is accentuated by emotion, exercise, and the like. Paterson and McKissock[259] found a bruit in 67% of those whose
initial symptom was periodic migrainous
headache, in 50% of those with epilepsy,
and in only 12% of those with hemorrhage.
There was no correlation between the presence of a bruit and the position of the
lesion. Size was the most significant factor
in determining the audibility of the bruit.
They are less likely to occur in the small
arteriovenous aneurysms, which are more
prone to bleed, and this explains the infrequency of bruits associated with lesions
that have bled.[191,259]

Radiological findings. Radiological investigations are of the utmost importance
in arteriovenous aneurysms. The following
are radiological findings to be expected and
confirmed at autopsy:

1. Increased vascular markings of the skull
   vault caused by involvement of the meningeal vessels or dural sinuses
2. Enlarged foramina attributed to the enlargement of afferent arteries or efferent
   veins
3. Defects in the skull attributed to communicating channels between the extracranial
   and intracranial circulation
4. Enlarged foramina transversaria of the
   upper cervical vertebrae and of grooves in
   the arch of the atlas in posterior fossa
   lesions
5. Displacement of normal structures caused
   by space-occupying effects of dilated vessels
   or hematomas
6. Encroachment on or dilatation of the ventricular system
7. Calcification in the vessels of the vascular
   anomaly or the environs
8. Manifestations of raised intracranial pressure.
9. Angiographic demonstration of abnormally
   large vessels closely associated with or quite
   remote from the lesion, aneurysmal formation within the arteriovenous aneurysm or
   of the arteries supplying the lesions, and
   obstruction at times of afferent or efferent
   channels; angiography also reveals a short

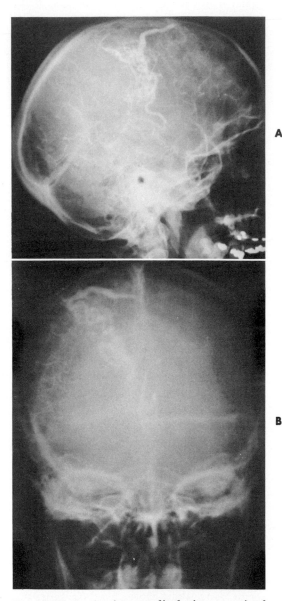

Fig. 10-22. A, Angiogram displaying a parietal
arteriovenous aneurysm with early filling of
veins and poor demonstration of arterial pattern. **B,** Anteroposterior view of an arteriovenous aneurysm (see **A**). Note that veins are
draining both to the superior longitudinal sagittal sinus and also centripetally via the deep
transcerebral veins toward the Galenic system.
(Courtesy Dr. J. E. Mincy, Albany, N. Y.)

arterial phase and rapid filling of the draining veins (Figs. 10-22 to 10-23)

10. Infrequently, a localized thinning or defect of the skull overlying enlarged vessels of the lesion[39],[387]; there is thickening of the cranial vault overlying the arteriovenous aneurysm, possibly with reduction in the size of the hemicranium[293] in a small number of cases
11. The enlargement of normally insignificant collateral vessels
12. Multiplicity of lesions
13. The location of hematomas
14. Cerebral atrophy and asymmetry of the skull
15. Enlarged diploic channels

Microscopic appearance. Histologically, arteriovenous aneurysms consist of many enlarged vessels of variable diameter. Many are in the confines of the subarachnoid space (Fig. 10-24). Others are in the parenchyma and are characteristically abnormal in size and number (Fig. 10-25). Some bulge into the ventricular system. Arteries with or without intimal thickening and elastic tissue degenerative changes can be recognized. The majority of vessels, however,

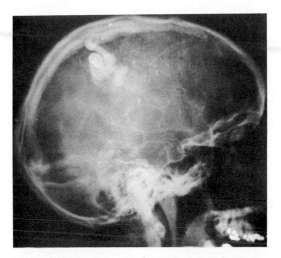

Fig. 10-23. Angiogram of another arteriovenous aneurysm displaying a large voluminous and tortuous vein draining into superior longitudinal sagittal sinus. (Courtesy Dr. J. E. Mincy, Albany, N. Y.)

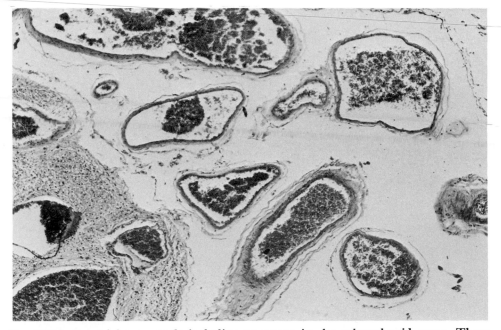

Fig. 10-24. Several large vessels including an artery in the subarachnoid space. These vessels were part of an arteriovenous aneurysm. Note large vessels in superficial portion of cortex. (Hematoxylin and eosin, ×45.)

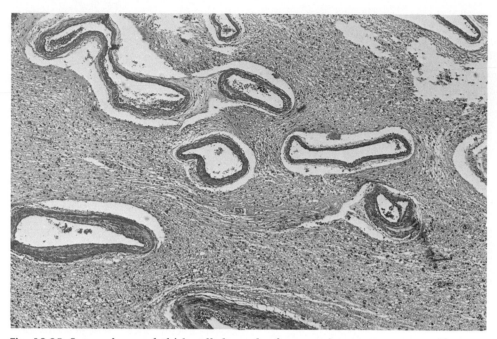

Fig. 10-25. Large abnormal thick-walled vessels of an arteriovenous aneurysm. Note vessels are wholly within white matter. (Hematoxylin and eosin, ×45.)

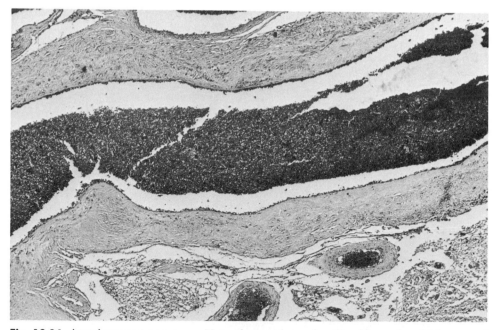

Fig. 10-26. Arteriovenous aneurysm. Note abnormal vessel walls of irregular thickness and consisting primarily of fibromuscular tissue with little elastica. (Hematoxylin and eosin, ×45.)

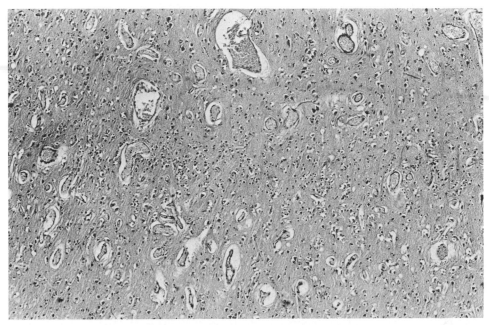

Fig. 10-27. Numerous thin-walled vessels from parenchyma neighboring an arteriovenous aneurysm. Note similarity to a telangiectasis (see Fig. 10-5). (Hematoxylin and eosin, ×45.)

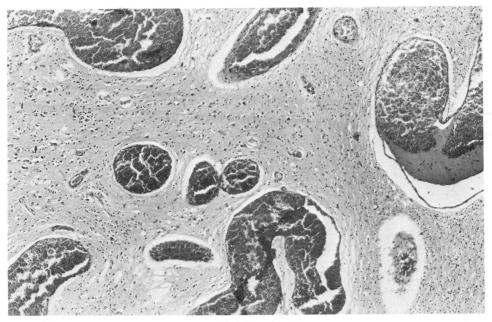

Fig. 10-28. Numerous large thin-walled vessels, mostly veins, from neighborhood of an arteriovenous aneurysm. Appearance resembles that of a venous angioma. (Hematoxylin and eosin, ×45.)

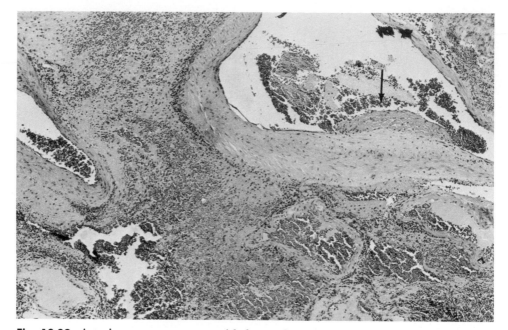

Fig. 10-29. Arteriovenous aneurysm with hemorrhage into the intervening brain tissue with small mural thrombus (*arrow*). (Hematoxylin and eosin, ×45.)

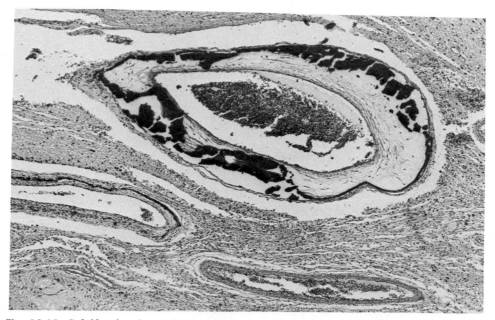

Fig. 10-30. Calcification in walls of vessels of an arteriovenous aneurysm. (Hematoxylin and eosin, ×45.)

possess walls of irregular thickness, mostly of fibromuscular tissue and a variable amount of elastica (Fig. 10-26). In places, the intimal proliferation is prominent and resembles intimal pads and plaques at forks and branchings. When collapsed, the contour of vessels in section is at times remarkably irregular. Many vascular channels are obviously dilated thin-walled veins, some with intimal thickening. Other large vessels possess walls histologically identical to aneurysmal walls, being mainly collagenous with some muscle demonstrable with phosphotungstic acid hematoxylin. Others consist merely of hyalinized collagen and can be regarded as aneurysmal dilatations. Recanalized vessels may be observed[284] and there may be siderosis of the surrounding tissues. Perivascular fibrosis is sometimes a feature. Smaller vessels often at the periphery are thin-walled channels in close apposition, resembling areas of telangiectasis (Figs. 10-27 and 10-28) or hemangioma of small vessels. In the adjoining parenchyma, there are often areas containing an excess of capillaries.

Thrombosis may occlude the vessel, or the thrombi may be mural (Fig. 10-29) with the reaction of the vessel wall similar to that of vessels elsewhere. Calcification is often present (Fig. 10-30), but frankly atherosclerotic changes, such as lipophages and cholesterol clefts, are seldom seen.

Paillas and associates[251] examined 72 surgical specimens of arteriovenous aneurysms and found sclerosis of the vessels to be universal. The presence of macroscopic atheroma could not be demonstrated. Histologically in five cases they found histiocytes with clear but nonfoamy cytoplasm deep to intimal pads. They believed the cells contained cholesterol, but no fat stains were mentioned nor was the feature adequately illustrated. No distinctly atherosclerotic areas (crystalline clefts and amorphous necrotic areas) were observed. Amyloid material may be demonstrable in vessels with thickened hyaline walls.[202,265] Ossification is infrequent.[331]

The intervening brain tissue exhibits varying degrees of edema, gliosis, demyelination, and calcification. The vascular enlargement replaces extensive amounts of parenchyma in larger lesions, and degenerative changes can be expected. Evidence of old or recent hemorrhage and softening is frequent. The brain, remote from the lesion, may exhibit some gliosis, loss of neurones, and possibly some siderotic staining of the meninges.

Hemorrhage. Hemorrhage can be considered the most important complication of the encephalic vascular anomalies. Perret and Nishioka[264] reported that of 453 patients in the Cooperative Study, 307 (or 68%) suffered hemorrhage some time prior to admission to hospital. In other words, 32% of those with vascular anomalies were admitted without a history or evidence of previous bleeding. This is in direct contrast to the patients with intracranial arterial aneurysms for of these only 9.7% were admitted without a history of hemorrhage. Thus aneurysms seem more prone to bleed than arteriovenous aneurysms. Perhaps a more important factor is the age distribution of patients with vascular anomalies at the time of their first hemorrhage (Fig. 10-31). The peak of the distribution falls between 10 and 30 years. Although 47% of all patients experienced this complication during these two decades, 72% had their first hemorrhage before the age of 40. The vascular anomalies in 40% of the entire series had bled at some time or other before the age of 40 years.[264]

Northfield[241] observed that in his series of "angiomas" (mostly arteriovenous aneurysms) the patients could be divided into those that presented with headache and epilepsy and those that suffered an intracranial hemorrhage. Headache, a frequent symptom, is extremely difficult to evaluate and is severe when the arteriovenous aneurysm bleeds. The relationship of convulsions to hemorrhage is of considerable practical importance because 272 of the 307 patients in the Cooperative Study[264] who

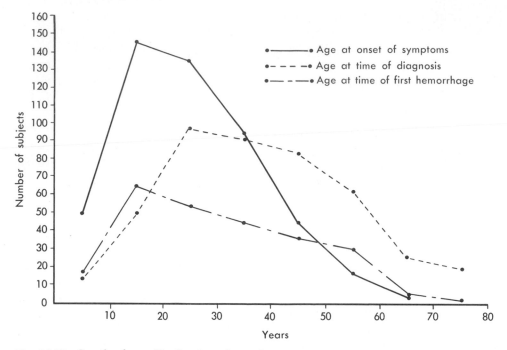

Fig. 10-31. Graph of age distribution of arteriovenous aneurysms at the time of onset of symptoms (491 cases from Table 10-5), at the time of diagnosis (442 cases from Table 10-4), and at the time of first hemorrhage (254 cases from the Cooperative Study[264]). (Plotted at middecade for each 10-year period.)

experienced hemorrhage from their anomaly (88%), had no history of convulsions either before or after the hemorrhage. On the other hand, only 18% of patients with convulsions subsequently suffered a hemorrhage. Tönnis and associates[348] reported a similar figure.

In Table 10-6, it can be seen that there were only 32 patients in the Cooperative Study with vascular anomalies below the tentorium, and of these, 26 were admitted to the Study because of a subarachnoid hemorrhage, a greater frequency of hemorrhage (81.3%) than in the group as a whole. In 337 or 61% of all the arteriovenous aneurysms in the Cooperative Study,[264] hemorrhage occurred at some time or other up to the end of the period of observation and the mortality therefrom was 10%. The rate of recurrence was 23%, and of this group, 12% died. The interval between hemorrhages, unlike aneurysmal bleeding, varied from a few days to 20

years. Svien and McRae[334] found that a second hemorrhage occurred in 34% of the survivors of the first hemorrhage and that of those who survived the second, 36% suffered a third episode. In the Cooperative Study,[264] bleeding was associated with 281 cases of supratentorial vascular anomaly.* Of these patients, 64 had a second episode (23%), 13 a third hemorrhage, and 4 a fourth hemorrhage.

Hemorrhage, be it subarachnoid, intracerebral, or intraventricular, can be the first manifestation of these arteriovenous aneurysms. Yet the frequency with which hemorrhage initiates the first symptom changes with different authors, such as Olivecrona and Riives[247] 40%, Mackenzie[191] 30%, Paterson and McKissock[259] 42%, and Henderson and Gomez[130] 76%.

Mackenzie[191] found that in patients with

*In the Cooperative Study,[264] this figure was incorrectly stated as 381 cases.

hemorrhage the arteriovenous aneurysm was usually deeply placed in the cerebral hemisphere and that no correlation between the size of the lesion and the onset of hemorrhage existed. However, in recent years the remarkable propensity to bleeding displayed by small arteriovenous aneurysms has been emphasized. Henderson and Gomez[130] noted that 100% of small arteriovenous aneurysms (2 cm. or less in size) presented clinically with hemorrhage as the cause of the first symptom, compared with 85.7% for medium-sized lesions (2 to 6 cm.) and 36.8% for large lesions (6 to 10 cm.). The severity of the hemorrhage and the prevalence of intracerebral hematoma is greater in individuals with small or medium-sized vascular anomalies.

Caram and associates[49] discovered a small aneurysm 3 mm. in diameter within the thalamus of a young man with intraventricular hemorrhage. The aneurysm was believed to be part of a small arteriovenous aneurysm supplied by the anterior choroidal artery. Association of intracerebral aneurysms of moderately large size and small arteriovenous aneurysms is discussed in Chapter 9.

Significant bleeding from an arteriovenous aneurysm usually results in blood reaching the subarachnoid space, permitting confirmation of the hemorrhage by lumbar puncture. In seven of the 60 cases studied by Paterson and McKissock[259] the hemorrhage did not extend to the subarachnoid space (11.7%), and in five of the 14 patients with intracerebral hemorrhage analyzed by Henderson and Gomez[130] the cerebrospinal fluid was normal. The presence of clear cerebrospinal fluid soon after the onset of any intracranial hemorrhage is well recognized, but often it will be blood stained or xanthochromic a day or two later and doubtless such is the case with arteriovenous aneurysms also.

As most arteriovenous aneurysms are related to the middle cerebral artery, subarachnoid hemorrhage from these lesions will be most severe over the lateral surface of the hemisphere. If the bleeding is extensive or if the blood tracks down along the lateral fissure, the subarachnoid hemorrhage is prominent at the base and the effect is similar to that of a ruptured arterial aneurysm. If the bleeding reaches the ventricular system, the escape of blood from the fourth ventricle into the posterior fossa can resemble a primary intracerebral or intraventricular hemorrhage. Arteriovenous aneurysms occur at other sites including the posterior fossa when the greatest concentration of blood is likely to be in the vicinity of the main mass of tortuous vessels rather than at some distance. Only a very few patients[130,259] have evidenced no extension to the cerebrospinal fluid, which adds to the difficulty of early diagnosis. However, at autopsy, the finding that a rapid demise has been caused by hemorrhage from an arteriovenous aneurysm is infrequent.

Tönnis and associates[348] asserted that patients presenting with convulsions were primarily those with lesions located chiefly in the central and precentral regions, areas where hemorrhage is less frequent than with lesions situated elsewhere in the cerebrum. Convulsions, they said, were only rarely associated with frontal and occipital lesions.

Arteriovenous aneurysms about the midline in the cerebrum can readily produce intraventricular hemorrhage. Blood ruptures through into the ventricle, or else the bleeding stems from varicose vessels bulging into the ventricles. It can also be derived from the involved choroid plexus.

In the Cooperative Study, 53% of the patients with subarachnoid hemorrhage from arteriovenous aneurysms suffered some neurological deficit as the result of their first hemorrhage, and it is likely that intracerebral hemorrhage occurred in a significant number.[264] A detailed analysis of the autopsy findings in large series of arteriovenous aneurysms is not available as it is in the case of saccular or berry aneurysms, and so the frequency of intracerebral and intraventricular hemorrhage can be gauged only by deduction or from small series. Those lesions situated deeply in the parenchyma will obviously produce intracerebral hematomas, but those abutting the pial or ventricular surface produce only insignificant intraparenchymatous hematomas or none at all. In large arteriovenous aneurysms extending from a wide base on the lateral cerebral surface almost to the ventricle, blood can track along the potential space between the parenchyma and the lesion to reach the cerebrospinal fluid, or it can form a localized intracerebral hematoma.[130] These anomalies do not often produce arterial spasm or cerebral infarction[130] and so the frequency of cerebral deficit is a rough gauge of the prevalence of the hematomas. Olivecrona and Riives[247] found that almost half of their patients had a hemiparesis or hemiplegia of sudden or gradual onset. In a series of 58 patients, Henderson and Gomez[130] found at operation 14 with intracerebral hematomas, a frequency of 24%, almost certainly an underestimate.

Subdural hemorrhage is an uncommon complication of a bleeding arteriovenous aneurysm.[57,239,339] Norlén[239] encountered one instance in 10 cases, Christensen[56] three in 80 cases, and Paterson and McKissock[259] three in 110 cases. In some large series no cases have been found.[191,247]

Subdural hemorrhage may occur with the first clinical episode of bleeding or during a recurrence.[57] It may be up to 2 cm. thick and extensive. Unless evacuated as in Norlén's case,[239] it can contribute substantially to the swift demise of the patient.[57] The three patients encountered by Paterson and McKissock[259] were operated on and in each case the hematoma was chronic. Two were situated over the arteriovenous aneurysm and one was located at a distance from the vascular anomaly. Some arteriovenous aneurysms bleed directly into the subdural space, whereas others do so presumably by inducing local tension with secondary tearing of the arach-

noid. The bleeding from an arteriovenous aneurysm is more likely to be derived from a dilated tortuous and sclerotic vein or an aneurysmal dilatation therefrom, and if the experimental animal is any criterion, bleeding occurs with a gush or deluge but not with a spurt or jet as in the case of arterial or aneurysmal bleeding (saccular or berry type). Arachnoidal adhesions may be a factor in the production of subdural hemorrhage.

Factors precipitating hemorrhage. In the Cooperative Study,[180] the onset of hemorrhage from arteriovenous aneurysms began during sleep in 36% of the patients with a complicating subarachnoid hemorrhage. In 30.5%, the hemorrhage commenced during lifting, bending, urination, defecation, coitus, or coughing, or when under emotional strain. These factors do not account for a corresponding proportion of the day. As in the case of saccular arterial aneurysms, such events may be of importance in that they precipitate hemorrhage because of their effect on the blood pressure and flow. In only 4.4% of the cases, trauma was related to the onset of hemorrhage, and in 0.5%, surgery apparently was the initiating factor. It is likely that trauma may precipitate the hemorrhage[7] of a lesion about to rupture. However, if the injury is more severe, it could cause tearing of the vessels in the arteriovenous aneurysm and Hamby[123] has observed that these vessels are particularly susceptible to injury at operation.

There have been reports of the onset of symptoms of hemorrhage from an arteriovenous aneurysm during pregnancy.[87,180,259] Of historical interest is that the spontaneous onset of the carotid-cavernous fistula reported by Travers[351] occurred during pregnancy. There were two cases in the Cooperative Study[180] and Dunn and Raskind[87] found only 10 in the literature. The initial symptoms of hemorrhage have occurred in similar lesions involving the spinal cord.[56] The relationship of pregnancy to vascular lesions such as cerebral arterial aneurysms was discussed in Chapter 9 but is pertinent to these lesions as well, though at present no statistical evidence proves that the inception of bleeding is initiated by either pregnancy or labor.[87] In the Cooperative Study, females presenting with bleeding from an arteriovenous aneurysm were younger than males.[264]

Progression of the lesion. It is believed that most intracranial arteriovenous aneurysms are present at birth and since the symptoms do not usually become obvious until the second decade, the assumption is that the lesions are slowly progressive. Traumatic fistulas in man and experimental arteriovenous fistulas are usually progressive, and though some small traumatic arteriovenous fistulas involving the meningeal vessels may undergo spontaneous thrombosis, in the case of cerebral arteriovenous aneurysms the series of symptoms portrayed suggests progression. Arteriovenous aneurysms appear to remain relatively quiescent after surgery or spontaneous partial regression for many years, but complications can be anticipated and the progressive enlargement of the vessels and the interference with the function of the neighboring cerebral parenchyma are the factors no doubt responsible for the symptoms the patients endure. They include epilepsy (26% to 32%), periodic migrainous headache (15% to 24%), progressive hemiparesis (7% to 12%), headaches (6%), and other sensory disturbances.[259]

In all probability, the arteriovenous shunt continues to increase. It is doubtful whether it ever reaches an equilibrium. Olivecrona and Riives[247] noted an increase in the caliber of afferent and efferent vessels of an arteriovenous aneurysm during a 10-year interval. Höök and Johanson[139] investigated 12 patients with 13 arteriovenous aneurysms. The patients were followed for 3½ to 21 years. Of the 13 lesions studied angiographically, in eight there was an increase in size and a ninth had undergone thrombosis; the remainder of the lesions had apparently reached a stage of equilibrium as far as size was concerned, but it does not follow that complications or further cerebral damage would not ensue.

However, the reliability of this angiographic evidence is uncertain. Significantly the results demonstrated that symptoms could progress in the absence of angiographic increase in the size of the lesion.

Regression or spontaneous cure. Conforti[62] reported spontaneous occlusion of an arteriovenous aneurysm and found two other instances in the literature and five with partial regression. Shumaker and Wayson[318] found that numbers of extracranial traumatic arteriovenous aneurysms have an associated saccular dilatation at the site of injury, very often between the artery and the vein as well. Mural thrombosis, not necessarily occlusive, was a common feature of these sacs. In 245 arteriovenous fistulas reviewed, they found that only five had demonstrated spontaneous, satisfactory cure by thrombosis. In three instances, the involved vein became thrombosed though a saccular aneurysm persisted. Thus, in only eight patients (3.3%), the arteriovenous shunt closed spontaneously and this should be compared with the ten peripheral saccular aneurysms mostly of traumatic origin that underwent spontaneous occlusion in a total of 122 cases (8.2%).[318]

Dandy[73] estimated that 10% of carotid-cavernous fistulas underwent spontaneous occlusion, and more recently in seven of the 50 cases of carotid-cavernous fistula analyzed by Whalley[378] spontaneous thrombosis supervened with clinical arrest of symptoms. Potter[271] recorded that in five of the 15 cases of carotid-cavernous fistula seen at the Radcliffe Infirmary, Oxford, between 1938 and 1953, spontaneous occlusion ensued. He conceded that carotid arteriography and hypotension may have contributed to the thrombosis in three instances.

In the case of a traumatic arteriovenous aneurysm, the surfaces of the injured vessels can initiate thrombosis until the endothelium extends over the thrombus and injured parts to provide intimal continuity from artery to vein. If an intervening false aneurysm or pulsating hematoma exists at the site of the shunt, the thrombus produced therein can initiate the formation of an occlusive thrombus. However, once these surfaces are endothelialized, further trauma or an intimal tear are probable prerequisites for the possible formation of an occlusive thrombus to seal the shunt. In chronic arteriovenous fistulas in experimental animals, intimal tears in the vein are not uncommon. They may be multiple, constituting the nidus of mural thrombi, which can occlude if the diameter of the vessel is small enough.[377] The intimal tears formed as the result of mechanical fatigue of the venous wall[326] may be sufficiently deep as to cause extramural extravasation of blood. Such a process is in all likelihood the mechanism of rupture of the cavernous sinus as it occurs in carotid-cavernous fistula. If the tear is incomplete, or presumably is against the bony surface, a mural thrombus only is likely to result. Ultimately, this could occlude the cavernous sinus. Little information is available to indicate how often the internal carotid artery is simultaneously occluded in these cases of spontaneous cure or thrombosis of the cavernous sinus. A like series of events can accompany blindness of the homolateral eye.[124] In experimental aortocaval fistulas in rabbits, it is not unusual for the fistula alone to close off and leave both the aorta and the inferior vena cava patent.

With intracranial arteriovenous aneurysms, spontaneous cure is rare. In the small traumatic lesions between the meningeal arteries and veins[146] or in the cortical arteries and veins, spontaneous thrombosis is likely to occur shortly after the traumatic communication has been established, in particular because of the small size of the vessels involved. However, the very existence of this entity is only now being appreciated as the result of the increasing use of angiography. Neither their frequency in head injury nor the rate of spontaneous cure is known. In the larger lesions believed to be congenital, spontaneous cure is extremely rare and no authentic cases are on record. Nevertheless, the spontaneous thrombosis of some veins may lead to

modification of the lesion and the shunt.

Surgical extirpation of the main lesion is followed by a progressive reversion of the vessels to their normal angiographic appearance.[239,348] Comparative study of preoperative and postoperative angiograms in 15 cases revealed a significant reduction in the caliber of the afferent arteries in 13 (86%) and a similar decrease or disappearance of dilated veins in 10 (67%).[51] Histological changes in these vessels have not been investigated.

Thrombosis. Hemorrhage from arteriovenous aneurysms appears to arise as the result of mural tears in the veins and from aneurysms of vessels participating in the arteriovenous shunt. If the patient survives, the site of the leakage will serve as the nidus for thrombus formation. Occlusive thrombosis may ensue, followed by a degree of propagation. The thrombus formation as it occurs in the carotid-cavernous fistula and in the aneurysmal dilatation of the vein of Galen[376] is the mechanism of self-cure. Thrombosis, however, is not necessarily curative. There is no information available on the subject of secondary infarction in arteriovenous aneurysms, but occlusion of veins is likely to produce hemorrhagic softening.

Thrombosis in afferent arteries has occasionally been reported[284] but it is uncertain whether there is any special tendency to arterial thrombosis. However, in instances of an aneurysm situated on the afferent artery, mural thrombus may be found in the sac.

Taveras and Poser[337] referred to a thrombosis of the middle cerebral artery in a child with the Sturge-Weber syndrome but gave no details of the relationship between the two vascular lesions. In this syndrome, the vascular anomaly is not currently believed to be arteriovenous in nature.

Associated intracranial saccular arterial aneurysms. Aneurysmal dilatation may occur in the vessels participating in an arteriovenous aneurysm and can be demonstrated by angiography. The dilatations can be multiple[347] and experimentally gross aneurysmal dilatation is to be found in the vein participating in the arteriovenous shunt.[326] In man also, it is the vein that is particularly prone to enlarge to aneurysmal proportions. The afferent artery undergoes dilatation and becomes tortuous. However, saccular arterial aneurysms of the berry type have frequently been found on the cerebral arteries in association with arteriovenous aneurysms[40,48,347] and less frequently the aneurysms are multiple.[259,264] Of 455 patients with subarachnoid hemorrhage, McKissock and associates[210] found only one case of a combined aneurysm and arteriovenous aneurysm. Of the nine patients with cerebral arteriovenous aneurysms seen at autopsy at the National Hospital (Queen Square, London) between 1950 and 1957, five were found[9] to have intracranial arterial saccular aneurysms in addition. This frequency seems to be too high but could well be applicable to very large arteriovenous aneurysms of long standing. Cronqvist and Troupp[67] found saccular aneurysms in 9% of 150 patients with arteriovenous aneurysms. Perrett and Nishioka[264] found 37 instances of the association in the Cooperative Study, a frequency of 14.8%. Details were available in only 34 with the following findings:

1. The patients were older than those presenting with an arteriovenous aneurysm alone. Of cases of arteriovenous aneurysms reported in the Cooperative Study, 63.6% were under 40 years of age, whereas only 32.3% of those with an associated saccular aneurysm were in this age group.
2. Of the 34 patients, 20 were male and 14 were female.
3. Six patients had two aneurysms, and two had three (23.5% with multiplicity).
4. Fifteen aneurysms (37%) were located on a major feeding artery of the arteriovenous aneurysm, 18 had aneurysms (43%) unrelated anatomically to the vascular anomaly, and the remainder (20%) were on the proximal portion of the feeding system.
5. Subarachnoid hemorrhage was a presenting symptom in 29 patients. In seven, the bleeding was attributed to rupture of the aneurysm whereas in the remainder the source was unknown or adjudged to be the arteriovenous aneurysm.

The discovery of a saccular aneurysm of the cerebral arteries in association with an intracranial arteriovenous aneurysm is of great practical importance to the neurosurgeon. Otherwise, the significance of the coexistence has been the topic for spirited debate. Since both lesions are developmental anomalies, it was said, the association supports the hypothesis that cerebral aneurysms are caused by developmental defects.[9]

In a woman, Ross[289] reported two cerebral arteriovenous aneurysms and an aneurysm on the middle cerebral artery feeding the larger, symptom-producing vascular anomaly. Her mother had died previously of a ruptured aneurysm. However, an isolated familial case adds little support to the congenital hypothesis, and concerning the etiology of arteriovenous aneurysms, the issue has not been settled, for at least some appear to be acquired lesions. Intracranial arterial aneurysms have been discussed in Chapter 9 and the evidence strongly supports an acquired etiology rather than hypothetical congenital factors. Boyd-Wilson[38] did not consider that patients with arteriovenous aneurysms had saccular aneurysms with any undue frequency although the prevalence in the Cooperative Study (14.8%) appears to be high.

Paterson and McKissock[259] suggested that hemodynamic stresses consequent upon the increased arterial blood flow to the aneurysm could be a factor in their etiology. Anderson and Blackwood[9] dismissed this possibility, yet more than two-thirds of the aneurysms in the cases they reviewed were on vessels feeding the arteriovenous aneurysm. In nine of the 13 patients discussed by Cronqvist and Troupp,[67] the arterial aneurysm was located on a vessel feeding the arteriovenous shunt. In the Cooperative Study, 57% of aneurysms were located on arteries proximal to the arteriovenous aneurysm. Moreover, selective angiography would be necessary to investigate the flow in vessels not clearly feeding the vascular anomaly. In view of the multiplicity of vessels feeding many of these arteriovenous aneurysms and the augmented flow in others acting as a collateral circulation to the deprived cerebral parenchyma, it is difficult to assess accurately the precise role of individual cerebral arteries in the presence of a sizable arteriovenous shunt. Blood flow estimations reveal that the flow is increased on both sides but particularly on the side of the arteriovenous aneurysm. Boyd-Wilson[38] contends that when the aneurysms are situated on the feeding vessels it is difficult to believe that hemodynamic factors are not influential in the production of the aneurysm. Sometimes a saccular aneurysm is on the feeding vessel immediately proximal to the arteriovenous aneurysm.[38,149] This relationship of aneurysm and arteriovenous aneurysm can be observed both above and below the tentorium.[103] Although such cases are most persuasive, they do not provide proof that the development of the aneurysms is dependent on hemodynamic factors. The older age distribution of patients with both an aneurysm and an anomaly would suggest that a time factor is important, that is, the arteriovenous aneurysms are of longer duration than those not associated with an aneurysm. Alternatively, the association might be fortuitous.

To date, no detailed histological study of the cerebral arterial tree has been undertaken in patients with long-standing cerebral arteriovenous aneurysms despite the need for the correlation of such findings with detailed arterial flow arrangements in relation to the vascular anomaly. However, in extracranial arterial aneurysms, be they spontaneous or traumatic in origin, it is known that dilatation of the proximal artery is a characteristic feature of a long-standing shunt and that aneurysmal dilatation of the artery can occur.[84, 177,361] In chronic experimental arteriovenous fistulas, the proximal artery exhibits gross medial thinning and elastic tissue degeneration sufficient to produce aneurysmal dilatation.[326] Thus, the formation of aneu-

rysms on the cerebral arteries proximal to the arteriovenous aneurysm is in all probability caused by the superadded hemodynamic stress associated with the shunt. The exact nature of the stress responsible is uncertain, but one can surmise that it is related to the grossly augmented flow rate and associated flow disturbance. Paterson[258] mentioned an arteriovenous aneurysm in the parieto-occipital region of a patient who subsequently developed a spontaneous carotid-cavernous fistula presumably because of rupture of an aneurysm of that segment of the internal carotid artery. Its development could well have been illustrative of the course outlined above. If the association were not caused by such a shunt, it might be expected that telangiectasis or a hemangioma would frequently be found with an aneurysm. Berry, Alpers, and White[27] found two instances of saccular arterial aneurysm of the cerebral arteries in association with a cerebral telangiectasis. Another patient had a fusiform aneurysm of the basilar artery and a cavernous hemangioma of the cerebellum, and two additional patients with telangiectasis had aortic aneurysms. The low frequency is not significant and in all probability the association is more prevalent than the dearth of information in the literature would lead one to believe, for telangiectases and small cavernous hemangiomas are frequently overlooked at autopsy.

Associated variations of the cerebral vasculature. Anatomical variations of the cerebral blood vessels (particularly veins) have not infrequently been attributed to the same basic developmental fault allegedly responsible for the vascular anomaly. Such variations are almost certainly secondary phenomena attributable to the arteriovenous shunt, for gross enlargement of vessels otherwise insignificant in size occurs in experimental arteriovenous fistulas.

Eight cases of an arteriovenous aneurysm in association with a persistent trigeminal artery (Table 1-4) have been found. Details were not always available and the association seems to be fortuitous.

Cardiovascular effects. In the traumatic or experimentally induced arteriovenous fistula, there is essentially a side-to-side shunt, blood being diverted from the afferent artery into the vein. The volume actually diverted depends on the dimensions of the fistula and the size of the afferent and efferent vessels (both arteries and veins). A small communication causes slight, barely detectable change.[135] In the distal artery, the blood flow may be either toward or away from the fistulous opening, and consequently it can be appreciated how a collateral circulation develops through peripheral anastomoses with arteries of adjoining territories. The vein dilates progressively until huge aneurysmal dilatations develop in conjunction with a collateral venous flow. Experimentally in carotid-jugular arteriovenous fistulas, not only does the homolateral vein enlarge but eventually even the contralateral vein exhibits increase in girth. Many of the small neighboring vessels enlarge and become tortuous. The general increase in vascularity is extremely troublesome in any attempt to reopen the neck to examine the fistula in vivo.

Several investigators have been interested in the hemodynamic effects of arteriovenous fistulas.[136,227] In the acute extracranial arteriovenous fistula, the systolic and diastolic pressures in the proximal artery (afferent) are slightly less than the contralateral normal artery, whereas the pressures in the artery distal to the fistula are lower still, though the lowest mean pressure is found in the vicinity of the fistula.[330] The quality of the pulse has been likened to that associated with aortic regurgitation (Corrigan's pulse).[42] The venous pulsations rarely exceed 5 mm. Hg, and the pressures vary between 0 and 15 mm. Hg. Negative pressure has been recorded in the vein proximal to the fistula[136,305,330] and as such is believed to be a function of high velocity flow in the proximal vein.[330] The pressure may rise to moderately high values in the vein while distally it remains below that of the proximal arterial pressure. At times, it

can exceed that of the artery distal to the fistula.[305,330]

Blood flow through the proximal artery increases considerably to as much as 12.6 times[305] and the diastolic flow might approach 80% to 90% of the maximum systolic flow.[145] The increase is progressive with time although local changes may account for a diminution.[305] Flow in the distal artery is complex and may be reversed, with the diameter not necessarily being proportionate to the flow, whereas with the passage of time, there can be a marked increase in flow in both distal limbs of the experimental fistula.[305] In the proximal vein, which is usually responsible for the bulk of the shunt, the flow is increased. In femoral arteriovenous fistulas, Schenk and associates[305] demonstrated a significant increase in the volume of the shunt with an increase in the lapse of time but this varied in cervical fistulas.

The circulation distal to the experimental fistula is dependent on the size of the fistula, the extent of the collateral circulation, and the volume of retrograde flow in the distal artery. It may be quite adequate with small fistulas, but with large fistulas the distal flow is diminished, the reduction being as great as 50% or more.[330] Congestion may be present but stasis is a prominent feature. In cerebral angiograms filling of the remainder of the cerebral arteries is usually poor, but extirpation of the arteriovenous aneurysm restores the filling to normal. The development of a collateral circulation related to the fistula is intriguing[136] and, in view of the reduced peripheral blood flow, not unexpected. The collateral circulation that develops participates in the shunt to a degree difficult to quantitate.

Peripheral arteriovenous aneurysms cause chronic increase in cardiac output and congestive cardiac failure occurs in man and in experimental animals. The hemodynamic effects of intracranial arteriovenous aneurysms are basically similar to those in extracranial sites[315,365] and include cardiac failure particularly in children. The size of the shunt and rate of progression are the principal determining factors.

Intracranial vascular anomalies associated with a sizable shunt in the newborn cause cardiac decompensation and the failure may be very severe. The event in the newborn is typified in aneurysmal dilatation of the vein of Galen.[136,173] The heart may be enormously enlarged (both hypertrophied and dilated), the veins to the head and neck may be grossly distended, the liver and lungs may exhibit signs of severe chronic venous congestion, and death may ensue. In a newborn baby, Silverman and associates[320] discovered a large arteriovenous aneurysm that almost replaced the right cerebral hemisphere and involved the right frontal bone and scalp, appearing on the surface as multiple cutaneous hemangiomas. The child died of cardiac insufficiency and at autopsy the heart weighed more than twice as much as normal. Failure to appreciate the presence of the shunt may lead to a misdiagnosis of cyanotic heart disease.[136]

Cardiac failure is less likely to eventuate during childhood and seldom occurs in the adult.[307] Some patients with intracranial arteriovenous aneurysms have enlarged hearts certainly, but one can rarely be positive that the cardiomegaly is of cerebral origin. However, in view of the greatly increased cardiac output associated with some shunts, it is likely that in some patients arteriovenous aneurysms will be contributory factors in the development of congestive cardiac failure. The failure is the effect of a progressively increasing shunt through the fistula or arteriovenous aneurysm culminating in a corresponding increase in the cardiac output and load. The increased output is achieved by means of an augmented stroke volume and also by a quickened pulse rate. Experimental arteriovenous fistula constitutes an experimental model for the study of cardiac insufficiency.

There has been little investigation of the hemodynamics in newborn infants with arteriovenous shunts, although in one 10-week-old male with an aneurysm of the vein of Galen the cardiac output was 2.2 liters per minute before surgery and only 1.9 liters per minute postoperatively. In the adult, vascular anomalies with small shunts may have no demonstrable effect on the heart but with large arteriovenous shunts the output is decidedly enhanced. In a recent study of three patients with carotid-cavernous fistulas,[117] it was demonstrated that the cardiac output was elevated in each patient. In two of the patients subjected to carotid ligation, the bruit disappeared though the cardiac output remained elevated. In another patient,[121] it has been found that the cardiac output was elevated to 9.2 liters per minute because of the presence of a carotid-cavernous fistula. Larson and Worman[170] found a flow rate of 800 cc. per minute in one patient with a carotid-cavernous fistula and 400 and 200 cc. in two others. In yet another subject, the flow rate was 845 cc. per minute on the ipsilateral side and 500 cc. on the healthy side.[164] Shenkin and colleagues[315] estimated that in one patient the cardiac output increased to 30% above normal in the horizontal position and to 61% when the patient was standing.[171] Nathanson and associates,[224] however, found a normal cardiac output in their patient, where presumably the shunt was small.

Wallace and associates[365] examined six patients with intracranial arteriovenous aneurysms and ascertained from the cardiac output that the blood flow through the shunt was at the level of 2904 ml. per minute at rest. Quite apart from the finding that there is reduced arteriovenous oxygen difference and increased oxygen saturation of jugular venous blood,[315] other investigations have demonstrated a considerable increase in cerebral blood flow.[171,222,315] Table 10-7 tabulates the estimated cerebral blood flow (sometimes several times greater than normal) and the size of the shunts in patients with arteriovenous aneurysms. Lassen and Munck[171] contend that the technique of estimating cerebral blood flow does not detect shunts less than 200 cc. per minute and that angiography is an unsatis-

Table 10-7. Measurements of cerebral flow and estimated size of shunts in patients with arteriovenous aneurysms

Author	Case	Sex	Age in years	Site of A-V aneurysm	Cerebral blood flow (cc./100 gm./min.)	Normal cerebral blood flow for technique (cc./100 gm./min.)	Estimated size of shunt (cc./min.)
Shenkin et al.[315]	1	Female	43	Frontoparietal	143	54	1250
	2	Male	28	Frontoparietal	185	54	1830
Lassen & Munck[171]	1	Male	42	Frontal	92	45	600
	2	Male	43	Occipital	155	50	1500
Nakamura et al.[222]	1		14	Occipitotemporal	151		
	2		48	Temporal	116		
	3		27	Frontotemporal	85		
	4		28	Frontal	68		
Bessman et al.[28]	1	Female	69	Parietal	156*	43	
	2	Male	28	Parietal	106†	54	
Tönnis, Schiefer & Walter†[348]	1			Parietal	239		
	2			Temporoparietal	180		
	3			Frontal	163		
	4			Central	145		
	5			Frontoparietal	105		
Bernsmeier & Siemons‡[26]	1				195	53	
	2				110	53	
	3				76.2	53	

*Estimated on side of lesion. Contralateral side 99 cc./100 gm./min.
†Estimated on side of lesion. Contralateral side 61 cc./100 gm./min.
‡Selected cases only.

factory method of determining the presence of a shunt because deductions from angiograms are at variance with cerebral blood flow measurements and volumetric estimates of the arteriovenous shunts.

Surgery on the arteriovenous aneurysms has resulted in the actual diminution of both cerebral blood flow and the estimated size of the shunt[28,171,222] although reduction is not always complete[171] and is associated with a postoperative increase in peripheral resistance as well as arteriovenous oxygen difference. Bessman and associates[28] found that postoperatively the blood flow on the side of the lesion fell from 106 to 50 cc./100 gm./min. and on the opposite side from 61 to 48 cc./100 gm./min. (normal value 54 cc./100 gm./min.). These results indicate that vessels on the contralateral side were contributing to the fistula or to the blood supply of the homolateral cerebral parenchyma, and it seems that in the presence of large arteriovenous shunts, the brain suffers some degree of vascular insufficiency. Furthermore, it was demonstrated that the cerebral metabolic rate was depressed preoperatively. McKissock[209] pointed out that in patients with arteriovenous aneurysms, preoperative angiography resulted in poor filling of the vessels in the remainder of the arterial tree, but that normal filling occurred after surgical excision of the lesion. The poor filling is restricted to the area about the arteriovenous aneurysm.[348]

Taveras and Poser[337] recorded in an infant of 7 months an arteriovenous fistula draining into an enormously dilated vein of Galen. The child's head had been enlarging, the neck veins were prominent, a bruit was audible over one eye and the heart was enlarged. Surgical attempts at ligating feeding vessels resulted in reduction in the size of the heart, of the aneurysmal venous dilatation (vein of Galen), and of the caliber of the internal carotid artery. In addition, it was estimated theoretically that flow through the fistula had been reduced by a factor of 8 to 10 times. In some large lesions, there is an *ipsilateral* reduction in retinal pressure.[334] Bloor and

associates[34] measured the intravascular pressures in arteries both proximal to and in one subject right in the vascular anomaly. They were able to demonstrate a drop in pressure in all vessels after occlusion of the arterial circulation at a site proximal to the anomaly.

The need is glaring for more extensive studies of cerebral blood flow both general and regional in patients with all varieties of vascular anomalies including the venous angiomas and the Sturge-Weber syndrome and the correlation of findings with postmortem microangiography should prove rewarding.

Possible tendency to bacterial endocarditis. Patients with coarctation of the aorta are peculiarly subject to the development of bacterial endocarditis. The infection may occur at the site of stenosis or in the poststenotic area. An arteriovenous fistula has a gross but essentially similar flow disturbance and the valves in animals with experimentally produced arteriovenous fistulas are susceptible to the development of bacterial endocarditis either spontaneously or after the intravenous injection of bacteria.[172,176,223] Furthermore, Lee and associates[172] demonstrated that in rats with arteriovenous fistulas, experimentally injected bacteria failed to clear from the bloodstream as rapidly as in the normal animal. The high frequency of bacterial endocarditis in patients with congenital fistulous heart disease (septal defects and patent ductus arteriosus) is well known. Systemic effects have been postulated in explanation, but there are also important local factors, and pathological changes in the cardiac valves themselves[223] may be pertinent. No cases have been found of bacterial endocarditis in association with intracranial arteriovenous aneurysm or fistula nor has any local susceptibility to infection been noted at the site of the vascular anomaly itself though these are all possibilities. However, there has been an instance of an arteriovenous aneurysm being infiltrated with an unusually large number of inflammatory cells.

Dementia. Olivecrona and Riives[247]

found mental changes in 50% of their patients with arteriovenous aneurysm. Of the changes, half were mild but the other 25% of patients had sustained severe mental impairment. Paterson and McKissock[259] reported definite intellectual impairment in 16 of their patients (14.5%) and two were attributed to hydrocephalus, although usually this is occasioned by cerebral atrophy attributable to cerebral ischemia and circulatory stagnation[119] distal to the vascular anomaly that has been caused by the hemodynamic shunt.[348] However, direct damage as well as replacement of cerebral parenchyma must also be contributory. The mental impairment can be coincidental and is not an essential component of the disease.

Pressure effects. Arteriovenous aneurysms can readily cause local pressure effects if situated advantageously and also when the affected vessels undergo aneurysmal dilatation. Paterson[258] encountered a case of bitemporal visual field defects attributable to compression of the optic chiasm by an aneurysmal vessel of the arteriovenous aneurysm. Some large arteriovenous aneurysms are associated with thinning and erosion of the overlying bone (a pressure effect), permitting the dilated tortuous vessels to protrude through the cranial defect and initiate a swelling on the forehead.[387]

Papilledema and raised intracranial pressure are most likely to be found in association with recent subarachnoid or intracerebral hemorrhage. Internal hydrocephalus in a small proportion of cases results from obstruction of the ventricular system by the vascular anomaly or from hemogenic meningitis due to recurrent subarachnoid hemorrhage. Rarely does the vascular anomaly cause raised intracranial pressure on account of its bulk alone although aneurysms of the vessels participating in the shunt can act as space-occupying lesions. Secondary pressure effects follow severe intracerebral hemorrhage and in some cases secondary pontine hemorrhage can be expected.

Tumors and aneurysms of the cerebellopontine angle can present clinically with symptoms of trigeminal neuralgia. There have been rare cases of arteriovenous aneurysms in this region causing the same symptoms.[152,357] Johnson and Salmon[152] pointed out that trigeminal neuralgia is normally rare before the age of 40 years and in such instances angiography is warranted. This is probably a local pressure manifestation of the lesion.

Miscellaneous associated lesions. Warren[369] encountered the unique coexistence of intracranial and pulmonary arteriovenous aneurysms with a glioblastoma multiforme, and Chandler[52] reported an intracranial arteriovenous aneurysm in a daughter and a pulmonary arteriovenous aneurysm and hereditary hemorrhagic telangiectasia in the mother. Instances of an arteriovenous aneurysm in association with polycystic disease of the kidneys or congenital heart disease have come to light.[27] In patients with cerebral vascular anomalies a cavernous hemangioma of the liver may be noted.[381] The statistical significance of such an association is unknown, and at present, the association of such lesions must be regarded as coincidental.

Lichtensteiger[174] reported the death of an 18-year-old youth from cerebellar hemorrhage attributable to an arteriovenous aneurysm of the left cerebellar hemisphere. The erythrocyte count was 6.6 million per cu. mm., the hematocrit 61 to 64.5 vol.%, and the hemoglobin value 20.5 to 21.4 gm. per 100 ml. No evidence of hemangioblastoma was discovered. This is an extremely rare association and in view of the prominent arteriovenous shunt associated with hemangioblastomas, the presence of such a tumor should be very carefully excluded before diagnosing polycythemia secondary to an arteriovenous aneurysm.

Prognosis. The prognosis of patients with arteriovenous aneurysms depends on several different factors, not only on size and location of the lesion but also on the size of the shunt. Undoubtedly, it is a major hazard to life, though not in comparison with intracranial arterial aneurysms of the berry type for then the prognosis is much less favorable. The major risk, discussed above, is hemorrhage. Neurological and mental deficits incapacitate the survivors to a variable degree. Patients who commence with a headache have basically a better prognosis, with approximately 50% living for more than 30 years. Improved neurosurgical techniques have changed the prognosis for these patients and remarkably little neurological impairment follows.

Etiology of the vascular anomalies

Although some arteriovenous fistulas of the scalp or cranial contents are accepted as being traumatic in origin, the remainder are generally attributed to a developmental fault. Not usually regarded as true neoplasms, they are assumed to be hamartomatous or developmental abnormalities in which the normal differentiation of the primitive capillary plexus into afferent and efferent channels fails to transpire.

Lesions classified as hemangiomas of the central nervous system whether capillary or cavernous in type are most often classified as hamartomas, in the belief that they are the result of perverse development of embryonic vessels that either undergo angiomatous proliferation in utero or remain quiescent for a variable period of time into postnatal life before proliferating. Hamartomas are tumorlike masses or a "mass of tissue that has gone wrong." Willis[382] defines them as minor malformations characterized by an improper admixture of tissues and tumorlike excess of one or more component tissues. As examples, simple angiomas, pigmented moles, neurofibroma, and some congenital lipomas are used. The assertion is contentious and the dividing line between hamartomatous and neoplastic lipomas is difficult to draw. No convincing evidence indicates that hemangiomas are hamartomatous any more than lipomas, papillomas, colonic polyps, etc., can be held to be. That the hemangioma is continuous with the general circulation is unimportant because the epithelium of papillomas is continuous with the adjacent normal epithelium. The etiology of neoplasia only begins to be elucidated, and it is im-

possible to state dogmatically with any degree of accuracy that these hemangiomatous lesions are not neoplastic. Again, it is a case of the credulous taking for granted the seeming infallibility of the written word.

The spontaneous resolution of some cutaneous hemangiomas in children lends nö more support to Willis's postulate than the spontaneous regression of some malignant melanomas. The spontaneous regression of either hemangiomas or arteriovenous aneurysms of the central nervous system has not been recorded, but it is pertinent that Rigdon[281] found hemangiomas in eight of 15 ducks at the site of local application of a carcinogen (methylcholanthrene) suggesting that at least some may be neoplastic. In view of the large size of some cavernous hemangiomas within the brain,[294,308] they are obviously capable of considerable growth as is consistent with the neoplastic concept.

Along with the other hemangiomas, Willis[383] has included Campbell de Morgan spots, or ruby spots, as angiomatoid malformations. The bright red color of these lesions strongly suggests an arteriovenous shunt[327] and quite recently in England[89,312] there have been outbreaks of Campbell de Morgan spots in epidemic form.

Willis[382,383] quite categorically groups all nonmalignant hemangiomatous lesions as hamartomas, reserving the term "tumor" for those that metastasize. Yet with pathologists accepting lipomas, fibromas, adenomas, and papillomas, etc., as tumors, there seems to be no convincing reason for denying that hemangiomas are true benign neoplasms. Unquestionably in many vascular lesions, particularly in arteriovenous aneurysms, it is difficult or impossible to differentiate between the initial primary lesion and the secondary manifestations of the hemodynamic disturbance. Such lesions now described as varices, or telangiectases, may be merely a stage in the natural history of an arteriovenous fistula, and one in which the shunt is not as vigorous as in arteriovenous formations with their loud bruit, palpable thrills, and red veins.

Landing and Farber[168] asserted that the distinction between malformations, hamartomas, and benign neoplasms of blood vessels is almost always impossible to define and that their etiology in various forms rests not so much on clinical or pathological grounds as on the opinion of the pathologist.

Willis,[382] believing them all to be hamartomatous in nature, stated that no sharp line of distinction could be drawn between angiomas and such lesions as cirsoid aneurysms or plexiform angiomatoses. Potter,[272] on the other hand, believes that an arteriovenous aneurysm, communication, or fistula is the basic pathological fault underlying these lesions and that the development of the congeries of tortuous vessels, whether predominantly arterial, venous, or of vessels of small caliber, is secondary. The possibility that telangiectases and cavernous hemangiomas are the result of an arteriovenous communication at a capillary or precapillary level cannot be excluded. In this respect, the observation that similar angiomatous tissue with telangiectasia and aneurysmal dilatation of small vessels accompanies the arteriovenous shunt in glioblastoma multiforme suggests that such vascular changes either with or without a tumor might be a secondary manifestation of a hemodynamic disturbance. Despite the attractiveness of this theory, there is no direct evidence to substantiate the concept.

In Fine's patient[97] with multiple hemangiomatous nevi in association with a spinal arteriovenous aneurysm, angiography revealed arteriovenous shunts in conjunction with the skin lesions. In some hemangiomas of the limb, the entire member may enlarge,[102] a development highly suggestive of an arteriovenous shunt. Arteriovenous shunts arise about experimentally produced implantation dermal cysts[217] and in association with chronic lung disease. The shunts with cerebral tumors are of no mean order. It is conceivable, therefore, that a hemangioma (transitional or cavernous) could be a tumor associated with an arteriovenous shunt as a secondary phenomenon. Dandy[71]

asserts that both Dupuytren and Virchow were aware of an arteriovenous shunt through cavernous hemangiomas and also that dilatation and tortuosity were features of the afferent artery as in the case of an arteriovenous aneurysm. A substantial arteriovenous shunt may be chanced upon in association with hemangiomas (such as Matas' case[100]).

Some assert that all vascular anomalies are in essence arteriovenous communications with secondary proliferation or overgrowth of some segment of the vascular tree. Padget[250] considered that on embryological grounds a fistula is the likeliest explanation of even capillary telangiectases. Evans and Courville[94] dismissed these anomalies as merely local perversions of development from the embryonic mesenchyme. A localized superficial plexiform angioma was attributed to the development of several smaller channels instead of one, and a varix was explained as an excessive development of a single vessel. The cavernous hemangioma was believed to be the perverse development of a group of vessels that became incompletely detached from the circulation. However, all is surmise for the relationship of many of these vascular anomalies to the general circulation is unknown as yet. The concept of the hamartomatous or developmental origin of many of the arteriovenous aneurysms of the brain has rested partly on an inability to understand the disturbed architecture of the pathologically dilated afferent and efferent vessels, changes, in all probability, secondary to the hemodynamic disturbance. In experimentally induced arteriovenous fistulas, gross changes are found in the walls of the afferent artery and the vein,[326] and an extensive collateral circulation develops. The fibrosis, elastic tissue damage, loss of tensile strength of the connective tissues, and aneurysmal dilatation are prominent features of the experimental lesion, and as such are analogous to the changes seen in the vessels of cerebral arteriovenous aneurysms. Focal intimal thickenings seen in dilated vessels are almost certainly the intimal pads or cushions seen at arterial forks of cerebral arteries (Chapter 3) rather than evidence of dysplasia of the vascular wall. Multiple large superficial veins and solitary superficial veins, rather than being instances of overdevelopment,[94] are merely the secondary manifestations of an arteriovenous shunt.

Reinhoff[278] believed that all such vascular anomalies are the result of the persistence of parts of the primitive vascular anlage, which, remaining latent for a time, subsequently open up. Kaplan and associates[154] concurred, believing that the maldevelopment stemmed from a very early stage of embryonic existence. But for arteriovenous aneurysms there seems to be no reason to postulate such an early inception, for the basic defect would be masked ultimately by all the secondary vascular changes associated with the shunt. Moreover, acquired disease during uterine life has not been excluded. Bailey[15] substantiated the developmental hypothesis of arteriovenous aneurysms by finding evidence of parenchymal dysgenesis in the neighborhood of the vascular anomaly. The dysgenesis could well be secondary to the arteriovenous shunt.

Currently no valid evidence suggests that these vascular anomalies are caused by inherited genetic factors although an occasional familial occurrence may be cited. Some vascular anomalies have a pronounced familial tendency, such as hereditary hemorrhagic telangiectasia, which is known to affect the brain. Much less certainty exists concerning other varieties of vascular derangement affecting the central nervous system. Michael and Levin[213] discovered multiple cavernous hemangiomas with calcification and ossification in the brain of a woman of 34 years and assumed a familial origin because of the presence in a few relatives of epilepsy or radiological intracranial calcification. Kidd and Cumings[158] recorded the death of a young Icelandic woman (33 years of age) from intracerebral hemorrhage caused by an arteriovenous aneurysm. Nine other members of the family died suddenly at an early age, with the suggestion being that all died from familial hemangiomas. The evidence from such reports as these is much too tenuous to accept seriously.

Most arteriovenous aneurysms outside the cranial cavity are said to be traumatic in origin, yet intracranially they are almost universally considered to be congenital. Of those arteriovenous aneurysms affecting the scalp, many are known to be acquired and the trauma need not be severe.[116,324] They are often multiple.[332] It is feasible that many more of the lesions could be traumatic with secondary involvement of the intracranial circulation. It is interesting that Dillard and associates[81] found that symptoms of traumatic arteriovenous fistulas commenced from 6 months to 12 years after injury, yet most patients with intracranial lesions of this type develop no symptoms until the second decade or later (Table 10-5).

Naturally occurring arteriovenous anastomoses varying in caliber from 20 to 160 μ can be demonstrated in the pial circulation.[290] Rowbotham and Little[290] have suggested that these shunts could be of importance in the etiology of cerebral arteriovenous aneurysms, which could be initiated by (1) the fortuitous occurrence of an unduly large arteriovenous cortical shunt, (2) the obstruction of the flow to the normal capillary bed with obligatory shunting of all blood through the naturally occurring arteriovenous anastomosis, or (3) the chance occurrence of two or more closely situated shunts sufficient to cause gross enlargement of the draining vein and the commencement of a vicious cycle.

In recent years, it has been recognized that traumatic arteriovenous aneurysms can develop between meningeal arteries and veins, meningeal arteries and diploic veins, meningeal arteries and pial veins, and pial arteries and pial veins.[292] It would seem that many undergo spontaneous thrombosis on account of the small size of the vessels concerned and probably also because the vessels are contused. Such arteriovenous aneurysms may be more common than has been previously recognized with a few persisting and progressing to the large, well-recognized lesions. Then again, Penfield[250] observed a man who had a fracture of the occipital lobe in childhood and a severe hemorrhage in later life from a vascular anomaly on the surface of the brain immediately beneath the old fracture site. This is not to say that all arteriovenous aneurysms are traumatic, for some of them are obviously initiated in utero, for example, an aneurysm of the vein of Galen for which the underlying pathogenesis continues to be obscure. It is likely, however, that trauma could well play a greater etiological role in the production of intracranial arteriovenous aneurysms than is generally believed.

The possible role of pregnancy and steroid hormones in the natural history of arteriovenous aneurysms as well as saccular aneurysms of the berry class has been mentioned. Watson and McCarthy[370] noted that hemangiomas not infrequently appear or increase rapidly in size with the onset of the menses or of a pregnancy. Furthermore, pregnancy is known to cause palmar erythema and spider nevi[22] in a substantial number of women. Keen students of ladies' legs can frequently observe linear hairlike or branched telangiectases often with a cyanotic hue or clusters of small unusually dilated veins in the legs of young parous women and also in older individuals of either sex. If these lesions can occur so readily without being attributed to developmental defects, the possibility that such vascular changes can occur postnatally within the cranium deserves serious consideration. Nothing is known of the pathogenesis of these extravascular lesions to date.

It must be concluded that these intracranial vascular anomalies require three-dimensional reconstruction of serial sections of the brain, together with postmortem microangiography and histological studies. Caution is urged in both etiological interpretation and dogmatic classification of these lesions until much more is known of their nature and pathogenesis.

Small or "cryptic" vascular anomalies. Although most primary intracerebral hemorrhages occur in subjects over the age of 40 years, clinicians and pathologists have observed that occasionally intracerebral bleeding occurs in young subjects without demonstrable cause[129] and in the absence of hypertension. Elkington[91] recorded cerebrovascular accidents in which the pathogenesis was in doubt because of the youthfulness of the patient and the absence of obvious cardiovascular disease. One patient died of a hemorrhage involving the pons and right brachium pontis, the bleeding being attributed to a telangiectasis of the pons and cerebellum. Elkington[91] suggested that other cases of this nature might be caused similarly by bleeding vascular anomalies. Other cases of intracerebral hemorrhage have been reported in which bleeding was attributed to a small vascular anomaly discovered by microscopy.[128,238] Hawkins and Rewell[128] advised a careful search for small hemangiomas or arteriovenous aneurysms in the walls of unexplained intracerebral hemorrhage in young people. Subsequently, Margolis and associates[195] published an account of six cases in which fatal hemorrhage was attributed to small arteriovenous or venous angiomas (the cryptic angiomas of Crawford and Russell[66]). Potter[272] considered that the small vascular anomalies exhibited a greater tendency to bleed than the larger lesions. Crawford and Russell[66] found 20 "cryptic" angiomas in a necropsy series of 461 samples of spontaneous intracerebral hemorrhage.[295] Of the series, all patients were under 40 years of age and 15 were under 20. Of the latter, the anomalies in 10 were related to the cerebral hemispheres and were found mostly in the territory of supply of the middle cerebral artery. One patient was pregnant. The lesions were often recognized from the cortical surface as clusters of small tortuous and dilated vessels related to the underlying hematoma, but sometimes they were buried in the depths of a sulcus, or were subcortical in location. They overlay the hematoma, which measured up to 10 cm. in diameter. Intraventricular hemorrhage was frequent and two cases exhibited subdural hematomas also. Another four were situated centrally in the cerebrum and macroscopically appeared entirely or predominantly venous although microscopically they consisted of both arteries and veins. Massive intraventricular hemorrhage was readily produced by these lesions. In one case, the anomaly involved the lesser vein of Galen with its tributaries and arteries supplying the thalamus. Plexiform dilated vessels were found in the meninges between the crus cerebri and the adjacent hippocampus. Many dilated vessels were seen on cut section through the pulvinar and the adjacent choroid plexus was similarly affected. A small thalamic hematoma and massive intraventricular hemorrhage accounted for the rapid demise of this 15-year-old girl.

The remaining six cases of Crawford and Russell[66] were cerebellar "cryptic angiomas" causing either rapid death or symptoms suggestive of "swiftly" growing cerebellar tumor. A few of these lesions microscopically appear to be entirely venous in type, not infrequently they are found as incidental findings at autopsy and may be less prone to rupture than cerebral lesions. Other cerebellar angiomas are distinctly arteriovenous in type. One of Crawford and Russell's angiomas was located in the superior medullary velum and caused extensive intraventricular hemorrhage. Others caused extensive intracerebellar and subarachnoid hemorrhage, and one was also associated with subdural hematoma. Although 12 of their cases proved to be rapidly fatal, some survived with the benefit of surgical intervention. The following lessons are to be learnt from their series of interesting cases:

1. The cryptic angioma can be and undoubtedly is readily and frequently overlooked because of cursory examination of the brain, the small size of the lesion, which may be buried in a *sulcus,* or the angioma being buried in the hematoma and therefore, difficult to recognize.
2. The intracerebral hemorrhage may be relatively small and the hemorrhage mainly intraventricular and subarachnoid, as in the small centrally located angiomas in the cerebrum, and the authors' case[66] in which the angioma was found in the superior medullary velum.
3. As Crawford and Russell[66] emphasized, these lesions are of considerable medicolegal importance because of possible misinterpretation of results unless the autopsy examination of the brain has been painstaking.

McConnell and Leonard[201] reported two cases of intraventricular hemorrhage due to small microangiomatous lesions; one 4 mm. lesion was subependymal in the medial surface of the caudate nucleus and the other, a 5 mm. lesion, was found in the choroid plexus of a lateral ventricle. There have been many other case reports illustrating hemorrhage from these small vascular anomalies,[16,160,388] which Gerlach and Jensen[101] have called microangiomas *(Mikroangiome).* Gerlach and Jensen found that the hematomas were most often in the posterior half of the cerebrum. Jensen and associates[151] demonstrated them by serial angiography in several cases.

McCormick and Nofzinger[206] briefly analyzed 48 "cryptic" lesions of their own. Most were arteriovenous aneurysms. The lesions varied in size from 1 mm. to 2.8 cm. An additional 260 cases were collected from the literature. The locations for the combined series are given in Table 10-8. The average age in their own series was 49 years and the frequency of hemorrhage was lower than that suggested by authors who stressed the importance of "cryptic angiomas" in intracerebral hemorrhage. It seems that the cavernous hemangioma and the small arteriovenous aneurysm are the two varieties mostly responsible for these hemorrhages. To attribute to them all cases of unexplained intracerebral hemorrhage unaccompanied by hypertension, however, is probably to overstate their importance. Failure to demonstrate cryptic angiomas in vivo after a bleeding episode can be attrib-

Table 10-8. Location of 308 "cryptic" hemangiomas and arteriovenous aneurysms*

Location	Number	
Supratentorial		161
Frontal lobe	45	
Temporal lobe	43	
Parietal lobe	23	
Occipital lobe	9	
Basal ganglia and insula	25	
Site uncertain	16	
Subtentorial		147
Mesencephalon, pons, medulla	85	
Cerebellum	44	
Spinal cord	18	
Total		308

*Adapted from McCormick, W. F., and Nofzinger, J. D.: "Cryptic" vascular malformations of the central nervous system, J. Neurosurg. **24**:865, 1966.

uted to thrombosis of vessels although it is doubtful that the entire blood supply would be interrupted. Even in patients with hypertension, an assiduous search for other causes of bleeding including hemangiomas and small arteriovenous aneurysms is desirable. Much emphasis has been placed on the destruction of the cryptic angioma when it bleeds but this is an unlikely occurrence. If it becomes incorporated in the hematoma, its demonstration may be more difficult. In the fresh state, the hematoma is most readily found by evacuating the blood clot and carefully examining the wall of the cavity. Without this, examination of a liberal number of blocks through the edge of the hematoma is the only recourse, short of postmortem microangiography. Additional detailed examination of large numbers of these small vascular anomalies is required to determine with certainty their natural history.

One additional case is worthy of note. Neumann[227] reported terminal intracerebral hemorrhage in the brain of a mentally retarded woman of 45 years with plaques and amyloid deposits in cerebral arterioles. The bleeding was attributed to small arteriovenous anomalies considered part of a syndrome of imbecility, a metabolic dis-

order accounting for the amyloid deposits and small vascular anomalies.

Sturge-Weber syndrome. The Sturge-Weber syndrome is so called after the English clinicians William Allen Sturge (1850 to 1919) and William Parkes Weber (1863 to 1962).[380] A historical account of the syndrome is offered by Wohlwill and Yakovlev,[385] Bean,[23] and Alexander and Norman.[5]

Synonyms for the entity include the Sturge-Weber-Dimitri syndrome, meningofacial angiomatosis, encephalofacial or encephalotrigeminal angiomatosis, the Sturge-Kalischer disease, the encephalotrigeminal variety of neurocutaneous angiomatosis, nevus flammeus with angiomatosis and encephalosis calcificans,[286] and many others.[175] Many eponyms have been used (Sturge, Kalischer, Weber, Krabbe, and Dimitri) leading to confusion, and avoiding them altogether would be better but the term Sturge-Weber syndrome is in very common use.

The syndrome[329,373,374] is generally considered to be unilateral and to consist of (1) an angiomatous nevus or port-wine stain at birth with a distribution corresponding to one or more of the areas supplied by branches of the fifth cranial nerve (Fig. 10-32) and (2) angiomatosis of the homolateral cerebral leptomeninges (Fig. 10-33) with progressive calcification in the underlying cerebral cortex. There are often divers features present that make it a much more complex syndrome. Some deem it necessary to restrict the syndrome to cases that exhibit a facial angioma in association with either intracranial angioma or angioma of the choroid of the eye.[185,240] Others espouse different criteria and argue whether there are *formes frustes* of the disease. Poser and Taveras[269] classified the Sturge-Weber syndrome into three types: *Type 1* constituted the typical Sturge-Weber encephalotrigeminal angiomatosis with a port-wine nevus and at least two other features of the syndrome such as convulsions (focal or general), hemiparesis, hemiatrophy or hemihypertrophy, mental retardation, or congenital glaucoma. *Type 2* was the incomplete form in which skin manifestations were absent, but other classical features were present including the typical radiological calcification as seen in a patient reported by Brock and Dyke.[42] *Type 3* included atypical cases with some type of vascular anomaly (not the port-wine stain) of the face in association with other features of the syndrome. In one instance, the facial lesion consisted of a raised hemangioma, in another a network of grossly enlarged cutaneous and subcutaneous veins in the trigeminal area, and in yet another there was

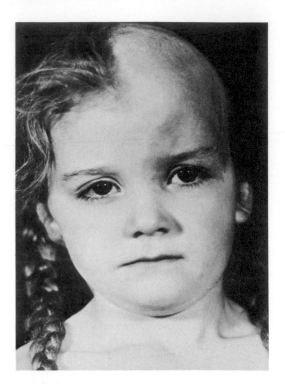

Fig. 10-32. Face of a young girl with the Sturge-Weber syndrome. There is a port-wine stain over scalp and forehead and about the left eye. (From Craig, J. M.: Encephalo-trigeminal angiomatosis [Sturge-Weber's disease], J. Neuropath. 8:305, 1949.)

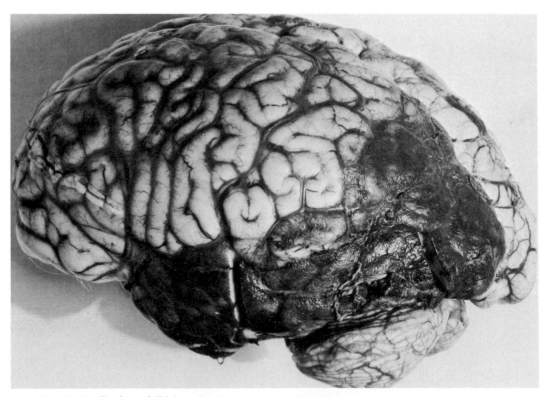

Fig. 10-33. Brain exhibiting the leptomeningeal angiomatosis of the temporal and occipital regions (Sturge-Weber syndrome). (From Craig, J. M.: Encephalo-trigeminal angiomatosis [Sturge-Weber's disease], J. Neuropath. 8:305, 1949.)

hyperpigmentation of the skin in the zone of the trigeminal nerve.

A differential sex ratio with a preponderance of males has been reported,[114,265] but in general it is of little significance.[5] Negroes do not escape[59,265] but most cases on record have been in Caucasians, there being no statistics available on racial trends for this comparatively rare disease.

The hemangiomatous nevi are present at birth and mostly the untoward clinical manifestations of the syndrome can be identified within the first decade and rarely after the third. The onset of clinical manifestations was precipitated by a head injury in Green's patient[112] at the early age of 6 months. Complications are predominantly cerebral encompassing mental retardation, hemiparesis, focal or general convulsions (in an estimated 89%),[265] visual field defects, and acute cerebral episodes suggestive of ischemia or hemorrhage. The affected cerebral cortex displays remarkable electrical inactivity.[5]

Pathology. The classic description of the angiomatous nevus in the Sturge-Weber syndrome is that of a port-wine stain of the skin. The skin, often bright red at birth, may fade a little and at times have a slight bluish tinge. To stimuli (heat, cold, pressure), it generally reacts differently from normal skin although its responses are consistent with the greater vascularity and augmented flow. The angiomatous area is not always flat and may be raised considerably above the normal surface as if the skin were rough and hypertrophied, despite a softness on palpation. These regions are attributed to a cavernous type of tissue and can be very disfiguring. A few small nodules or polyps are soft but more fibrous than elsewhere. Yakovlev and Guthrie[393] provided no histology but likened them to the sebaceous adenomas of tuberous sclerosis (epiloia) and the cutaneous nodules of von Recklinghausen's neurofibromatosis. The distribution involves the face and is said to correspond to the territory supplied by branches of the trigeminal nerve. Most authors believe the

topography is in accordance with the metameres, though Yakovlev and Guthrie[393] suggest it is determined by the sympathetic innervation, but metameric boundaries of the cutaneous angiomatous lesions are by no means anatomically accurate.[69] However, the lesion may affect the ophthalmic, maxillary, and mandibular divisions, or be bilateral. Involvement of the forehead and upper eyelid has recently been found to be of import, for in reviewing the literature, Alexander and Norman[5] did not disclose a single case in which either cerebral angiomatosis or gyriform calcification was present in association with an angiomatous nevus limited to other areas of the face.[5,240] They consider the relationship of the distribution of the cutaneous nevus to the trigeminal nerve to be merely fortuitous.

In a few patients, the characteristic cerebral features including the radiological appearance are exhibited with a total absence of skin manifestations.[42,265,269] Brock and Dyke[42] described a case closely resembling the Sturge-Weber syndrome except that the cutaneous lesion appeared to have a distinct arteriovenous shunt with a strong pulsation and bruit. It is likely that the cerebral and the cutaneous lesions possessed a direct vascular continuity. Some authors exclude such cases.[240]

Cutaneous lesions elsewhere on the body are fairly common.[265] In the historic case described by Sturge[329] in 1879, there was an extensive hemangioma of the right side of the head and neck, extending down to the fourth dorsal vertebra posteriorly and the second costal cartilage anteriorly with patches over the left side of the head. Weber[373,374] described gross involvement of half of the trunk in an afflicted patient. In 1906, Cushing[69] gave an account of three cases in which there were vascular birthmarks on the face associated with episodes suggestive of intracranial bleeding. He emphasized the trigeminal distribution of these angiomatous lesions of the skin, but of his three patients, two had involvement of the trunk or extremities also.

Not all patients with the syndrome are

mentally retarded and port-wine stains of the face are not conclusive evidence of the presence of leptomeningeal angiomatosis. The lips, gums, tongue, roof, and floor of the mouth, the pharynx, the uvula,[329] and even the nose may be affected and epistaxis can be troublesome. A thickening of the soft tissue of the face in the affected part coarsens the features. In the case of an ophthalmic distribution merely, thickening of the subcutaneous tissue in the region of the affected eyebrow and upper lid may be observed.[393] More extensive lesions are associated with a decided enlargement of half of the face, affecting even the bones.[69] The eyeballs are commonly exaggerated in size and proptosed on the affected side. The iris is of greater diameter (pupil too) and ophthalmoscopy reveals an increased vascularity and tortuosity of retinal vessels. The choroid is darker and redder than its counterpart and glaucoma (buphthalmos) is frequent.

Yakovlev and Guthrie[393] observed café-au-lait spots on the trunk as well as pigmented nevi although the association may not be statistically significant. Pigmentation of the skin in the territory of the trigeminal nerve has been noted in lieu of angiomatosis. Smith[222] states that the subcutaneous component of the syndrome can be a hygroma.

The calvarium on the affected side may be slightly smaller than on the contralateral side, appearing slightly depressed[69] and also imparting asymmetry to the head and face. The capacity of that half of the skull is also reduced.[5] The limbs on the side contralateral to the cerebral lesion are of reduced size, particularly when the patient is afflicted early in life because of the long-standing hemiplegia or hemiparesis. The dimensional asymmetry has been well illustrated by Bielawski and Tatelman.[29] A limb affected by the hemangiomatous state may be disproportionately large.

Features observed at the time of surgical exploration of the brain[69,393] are (1) an increased vascularity of the scalp of the affected part, (2) thickening, sponginess, and redness of the underlying calvarium and a tendency to hemorrhage and (3) augmented vascularity of the dura mater (angiomatosis) often with some adhesions to the arachnoid presumably the sequel of repeated vascular disturbances. At autopsy, it becomes much more difficult to appreciate the vascularity of the tissues because blood is drained off and usually vessels have collapsed. Affected areas in the bone may be accentuated by transillumination, the angiomatous areas being bright pink. Involvement of the dura and the bone is unusual[240] though diploic veins may be prominent[287] and the frontal sinuses enlarged.[286]

The affected hemisphere may be considerably smaller than the contralateral cerebral hemisphere as a result of gross atrophy. The cerebral hemiatrophy, cranial hemiatrophy with contralateral atrophy of the limbs, and hemiparesis occurring in concert constitute a striking pathological picture.[269]

The angiomatous area of the brain, most often in the parietal or occipital areas of a cerebral hemisphere,[269,287] sometimes extends further anteriorly to involve the temporal lobe and on occasions affects the entire hemisphere. In general, the lesion is fairly sharply demarcated and on the side of the most extensive facial nevus though it can occur on the contralateral side and, as in facial angiomatosis, both cerebral hemispheres can be involved. The cerebellum is rarely affected.[287] The leptomeninges may be thickened in places over the shrunken gyri and sometimes pial fibrosis is extensive.[265] The subarachnoid space in the affected zone contains a large number of small tortuous veins imparting a purplish color that completely coats the affected cortex. The angiomatous vessels are darker than normal veins. All vessels are of relatively similar caliber except perhaps for the larger drainage channels, and involvement of the arterial circulation is not usual. The vessels of the angiomatous area may be predominantly capillary in size[296] and the lesion is then held to be leptomeningeal telangiectasia. The grossly increased vascularity gives the meninges an injected appearance. The meningeal lesion is occasionally a distinct arteriovenous aneurysm. In Chao's patient,[53] bilateral vascular nevi over the face and trunk were accompanied by bilateral arteriovenous aneurysms of the brain.

The cortex, unless the subject is very young, will be gritty when cut because of the presence of calcification. If the mineralization is extensive, the specimen can be demonstrated radiologically to have the classical ("tram-line") parallel zones of density that conform to the gyral patterns.[265] Atrophy of the gyri is particularly noticeable on section and there is a corresponding loss of white matter. The cerebral atrophy may be localized to the parieto-occipital region or involve the entire hemisphere. In volume, the homolateral ventricle may exhibit moderate increase commensurate with the cerebral atrophy. Roizin and associates[286] described hemiatrophy of the cerebellum and medulla, with degeneration of the related corticospinal tracts.

The choroid plexus too may be affected and enlarged because of the presence of a conglomerate of enlarged distended veins or angiomatous tissue of cavernous type.[175, 385] A small angioma of the pituitary stalk has actually been found. The trigeminal ganglion may be smaller or larger than normal.

There may be hemangiomatous involvement of the viscera, and though it is usually asymptomatic, it can be associated with severe hemorrhage.[393] Hemangiomatous lesions have been observed in the lung,[286,393] gastrointestinal tract,[53,393] thymus, spleen, the testes,[286] and ovary.[385] Associated lesions of uncertain significance found with the Sturge-Weber syndrome include coarctation of the aorta,[53] pes cavus,[286] a high arched palate,[53,286] and obesity.[287]

Microscopic appearance. Histologically, the leptomeninges show a gross increase in the number of vessels, usually of the small venous type and of relatively uniform caliber (Fig. 10-34). Alexander and Norman[5] found the average diameter to be about 140 μ with several large veins present. The vessels lie several layers deep, sometimes completely filling the subarachnoid space including the sulci. The pial arteries frequently exhibit considerable intimal thickening and narrowing (consistent with arteriosclerosis) and mural calcification. The

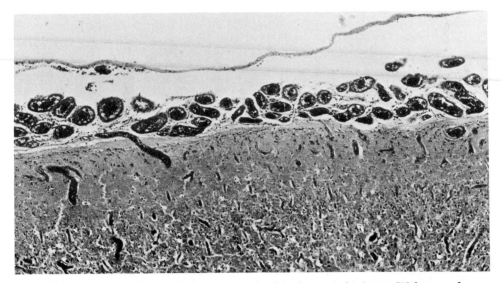

Fig. 10-34. Numerous enlarged pial vessels of affected cortex in Sturge-Weber syndrome. (Hematoxylin and eosin, ×45.)

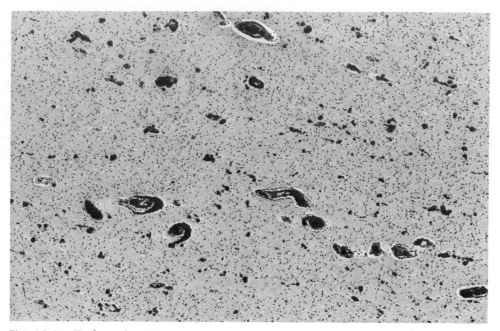

Fig. 10-35. Early and mild calcification of vessels in brain underlying leptomeningeal angiomatosis in Sturge-Weber syndrome. (Hematoxylin and eosin, ×45.)

latter, seen in a 3-month-old infant, has been considered an early manifestation of the syndrome.

Abnormal vessels rarely penetrate the cortex, although some increase in vascularity or the presence of a few unduly large and perhaps tortuous vessels is occasionally noted.[5,64,240] Beneath the meningeal hemangiomatosis, the second and third layers of the cerebral cortex[59] can be replaced by extensive calcium deposits. Initially, there is granular incrustation of small cortical blood vessels, and this ultimately extends to form vascular sheaths though some may appear in the parenchyma as well (Fig. 10-35). There is degeneration and disappearance of neurones and gliosis, and more extensive calcification ensues. Many small vessels appear to be obliterated. Spherical laminated calcific concretions (calcospherites) and calcified vessels become increasingly numerous with progressive coalescence of calcific deposits until numerous calcified plaques are formed. Calcified nerve cells and prominent perivascular fibrosis are also found in the cortex,[175] and there is calcifi-

cation of larger vessels with similar changes in the subcortical white matter. In a brain described by Krabbe[159] the cortical calcification was most prominent at the sides of the sulcus with relative sparing of the summits of the gyri. Tram-line calcification of the cerebral cortex is not pathognomonic of the Sturge-Weber syndrome. The calcification is less frequently observed in the very young but is almost a constant feature in the adult.[385] Poser and Taveras[269] found radiological evidence of cortical calcification as early as the eighteenth month of age, and though it may not be present when the patient is first examined, it is likely to develop within a relatively short period of time.

The calcium deposits give a variable result when stained for iron.[175] Chemical analysis reveals that the mineral deposits consist mainly of calcium phosphate and carbonate with no excess of iron.[240,346,363] Norman[240] suggests that the positive Prussian blue reaction is probably caused by absorption of available iron normally present in the tissues and that prolonged formalin fixation increases the amount of iron found chemically. The reason for the calcification is not apparent and Norman[240] suggests some underlying functional abnormality.

Though obliteration of small cortical vessels is frequent, larger vessels may undergo thrombosis. Poser and Taveras[269,337] found evidence of occlusion of a middle cerebral artery. Such lesions can lead to necrotic changes in the cortex with resolution and secondary cavitation.

Little attention has been paid to the spinal cord in the Sturge-Weber syndrome, apart from mere mention of small clusters of dilated pial vessels and hyalinization of vessel walls.[385] Examination of the cord seems worthwhile, particularly in those cases that present in association with angiomatosis of the trunk and extremities. Wohlwill and Yakovlev[385] discovered ectopic ganglion cells in the dorsal roots with some at a distance from the ganglia. Ectopic neurones were also observed in the subcortical white matter. These and other indications of dysplasia accounting for enlargement of the Gasserian ganglion are the basis for the authors' premise that the disease is probably a defect in the motor innervation of the malformed vessels of the affected metamere.

Radiological findings. The typical findings,[80] of asymmetry of the skull (most pronounced posteriorly), enlarged diploic channels in the skull, the characteristic sinuous double-contoured lines (occasionally bilateral), and cerebral atrophy with widening of the subarachnoid space and enlargement of the homolateral lateral ventricle are features demonstrable at autopsy.

Poser and Taveras[269] classified the angiographic changes into six groups: In the first group, a diffuse homogeneous increase in density is believed to represent an increase in the capillary bed. There is an increment in both size and number of veins and large capillaries but no alteration in the arteries supplying the affected area, the typical manifestations of classical Sturge-Weber syndrome. In the second group, the

arteries and veins are enlarged and abnormal and so constitute an arteriovenous malformation, a category rarely seen in the Sturge-Weber syndrome. The third group is associated with thrombosis of a major branch or smaller vessels supplying the area with a zone of avascularity as the result. The fourth group displays large veins coursing through the brain in unusual locations though not forming a conglomeration of abnormal vessels. Thrombosis of dural sinuses may also be seen. In the fifth group abnormalities composed of arteries and veins or actual angiomas are located in the territory normally supplied by the external carotid artery but now supplied by either the internal or external carotid artery. In the sixth group, miscellaneous radiological findings, such as subdural hematoma and cerebral atrophy, are present. Although it is believed that the venous angioma is the characteristic feature of the syndrome, Poser and Taveras[269] could demonstrate it in only 24% of cases. It was the most frequent angiographic abnormality found, for no pathological findings were detectable in 50% of the series.

One patient seen by Poser and Taveras[269] at 5½ months was found to have no calcification although angiographically bilateral capillary-venous angiomas were present. Fifteen months later massive calcification of the Sturge-Weber type was found bilaterally. Another infant in their series developed calcification after a 21-month interval.

Prognosis. The prognosis for these patients with the Sturge-Weber syndrome is quite poor because of the progressive destruction of the cerebral cortex, the consequent increase in the convulsions, and the progressive mental deterioration. Alexander and Norman[5] report a remarkable intellectual improvement in some patients after surgical resection of the pathological cortex. Institutional care is needed as the neurological deficit increases and most untreated patients die before middle age in status epilepticus.[5] Spontaneous bleeding from the lesion is unexpectedly uncommon although severe hemorrhage may occur when the lesion is damaged at craniotomy.

Etiology. The etiology is quite unknown and is not generally associated with a cranial bruit. Circulation through the lesion as demonstrated by angiography is not unduly fast although there is variation with the different phases of the disease. One cannot say for certain that there is a pronounced arteriovenous shunt, although Alexander and Norman[5] contend that the flow through the affected area of the cortex may be rapid early in life but considerably retarded in later years. Angiography might demonstrate this.

Lichtenstein[175] regarded the syndrome as a partial or regional manifestation of a generalized neurocutaneous hemangiomatosis. Bean[23] considered it to be related to Marfucci's syndrome in which hemangiomas and phlebectasia occur in association with dyschondroplasia.[50]

There has been the usual tumor-versus-hamartoma argument and most authors favor the concept of a vascular hamartoma or dysgenesis of the vessel development at the stage of differentiation of cerebral vessels from those of the extracranial circulation. The involvement of face, scalp, bone, dura, and the leptomeninges supports this hypothesis. The disease is sometimes associated with the Klippel-Trénaunay-Weber syndrome (large cutaneous hemangiomas with hypertrophy of related bones and soft tissues) though neither display Mendelian inheritance.[211]

The topographical similarity of the facial nevi to the territory supplied by the branches of the trigeminal nerve so impressed Cushing[69] that he suggested that an antenatal lesion (infectious or developmental) might account for the central (cerebral) and the peripheral lesions (face) of blood vessels in much the same manner as herpes zoster is associated with central and peripheral manifestations. Weber[375] believed that some accidental local injury to the embryo was responsible during early intrauterine life.

Yakovlev and Guthrie[393] considered the Sturge-Weber syndrome and the von Hippel-Lindau syndromes as probable variants of the same congenital malformation. They also supported a relationship between these syndromes and tuberous sclerosis and neurofibromatosis, although in recent times the Sturge-Weber syndrome is not thought to have any such relationship and it has no distinct hereditary tendency,[186] whereas tuberous sclerosis and neurofibromatosis are hereditary disorders.[211] The father of one of Chao's[53] patients with the syndrome had the peripheral nodular type of neurofibromatosis and the patient himself developed tuberous sclerosis while under observation. The patient's young brother possessed a small hemangioma of the shoulder and numerous café-au-lait spots on the trunk. Another of her patients had an unaffected identical twin.

There is some evidence that the syndrome is caused by partial chromosomal trisomy, although mostly the translocated segment is not demonstrable microscopically.[257]

Divry and van Bogaert[82] described two brothers with cutaneous telangiectases and a noncalcifying leptomeningeal angiomatosis not unlike that seen in the Sturge-Weber syndrome, only more diffuse and involving one cerebral hemisphere and the cerebellum (Fig. 10-35). It was regarded as heredofamilial and associated with dementia and epilepsy. Moreover, also there were present a leukodystrophy and areas of cortical necrosis. Pathological material was available in only one case but additional similar cases have been described.[44]

Hereditary hemorrhagic telangiectasia. Hereditary hemorrhagic telangiectasia has several synonyms: Osler's disease, Rendu-Osler's disease, Osler-Rendu-Weber disease, or Osler-Weber-Rendu disease. It is transmitted as a dominant Mendelian trait but apparently can appear as a chance mutation affecting, as far as is known, Caucasians, Negroes, and horses.[23] The extracranial manifestations of this malady with its frequent bleeding episodes[249,279,372] are well known. The cutaneous telangiectases often do not tend to appear until early adult life or even later, although epistaxes may become recurrent at a somewhat earlier age. Hemorrhages complicating this disease occur in adults, and other diagnostic manifestations are visible on the skin and on the mucous membranes of the lips, mouth, and nose.

Intracranial hemorrhage occurs only rarely and there have been vague records of stroke or a ruptured vessel in the brain[107] and few pathological studies. Walton[367] reported one instance in his review of subarachnoid hemorrhage. Quickel and Whaley[274] successfully resected from a young male (17 years) with hereditary hemorrhagic telangiectases a small vascular anomaly in the anterior horn of a lateral ventricle. The lesion was believed to be a small capillary hemangioma, demonstrated angiographically, and causing subarachnoid hemorrhage. Courville[63] reported the autopsy findings of a 61-year-old woman with the disease. No intracranial bleeding was discovered, but microscopically small clusters of enlarged tortuous veins of small caliber were present in the subarachnoid space and enlarged veins within the white matter. Russell and Rubinstein[296] found the brain of another afflicted patient to be perfectly normal, but in this disease involvement of the central nervous system need not occur in every instance. Rowley and associates[291] recently reported aggravation of the telangiectases by oral contraceptives, but no noticeable increase in reported cases of intracranial bleeding is apparent.

Telangiectases in the heart, lungs, alimentary tract, genitourinary system, and liver have been well recognized and arteriovenous aneurysms in the splanchnic area have been reported.[54,221] Arnould and associates[11] found a patient with this disease and vascular anomalies suggestive of arteriovenous aneurysms. The possibility is that the intracranial bleeding could be caused by an arteriovenous anomaly rather than a telangiectasis.

Ataxia telangiectasia (Louis-Bar syndrome). Ataxia telangiectasia, first described by Louis-Bar[187] in 1941 is a familial

syndrome of progressive cerebellar ataxia accompanied by oculocutaneous telangiectasia and featuring a propensity for pulmonary infections.[35] The telangiectasia consists of a faint hairlike network on the bulbar conjunctiva, the butterfly area of the face, the ear,[23] and other parts of the body[319]; apraxia of the eye movements simulating ophthalmoplegia; progeric hair and skin changes[4]; dull masklike face; equable disposition[23]; and normal intelligence but mental deterioration in late stages of the disease. More than 150 cases have been described but results of only a few pathological examinations are available. Aguilar and associates[4] have included in the pathological findings the following:

1. Cerebellar cortical atrophy
2. Chronic degeneration of neurones in the dentate and inferior olivary nuclei
3. Demyelination of the posterior spinal columns
4. Dystrophia and degeneration of anterior horn cells of the cord
5. Neuroaxonal dystrophy in the tegmentum of the medulla oblongata
6. Neuromelanosis and ballooning degeneration of neurones in the spinal ganglia
7. Acute and chronic inflammatory changes in the lung, including bronchiectasis
8. Absence or atrophy of the thymus
9. Generalized hypoplasia of lymphoid tissue
10. Reticuloendothelial malignancy
11. Left ventricular hypertrophy
12. Widespread bizarre nucleomegaly (aneuploidy) of several viscera, endocrine glands, and other tissues including the nervous tissue
13. Gonadal abnormalities

More recently, atypical diabetes mellitus and hepatic dysfunction[303] have been described. It is now apparent that endocrine disturbances (including those of pituitary and hypothalamic lesions) are not infrequent.[138,323] Terplan and Krauss[343] observed ectasia of the veins and capillaries in the white matter especially in frontal lobes, internal capsule, and some subependymal veins, together with evidence of small perivascular hemorrhages. The pial veins and some arteries were found to be uniformly dilated, particularly in the cerebral sulci.

Others have observed microscopic enlargement of pial veins between the cerebellar folia,[35] but such vascular changes are not universal.[4] Sourander and associates[325] described telangiectases in the spinal meninges. Solitare[323] found at the autopsy of a woman of 22 years with ataxia-telangiectasia and bilateral club feet, demyelination of the fasciculus gracilis, abnormal cell types in the pituitary and an absence of follicular activity in the ovaries.

Bean[23] classifies this syndrome as a possible variant of the congenital dysplastic angiectases (Sturge-Weber syndrome and von Hippel-Lindau disease) although evidence now suggests that the primary abnormality is an immunological deficiency.[138]

Miscellaneous cerebral vascular lesions

Potter's leptomeningeal hemangiectasia. Potter[270] reported meningeal hemangiectasis in two female infants. One died during labor and the other lived a day. In each case, innumerable tortuous and coiled venous channels with the histological structure of capillaries and venules covered the entire surface of the brain. The arteries were normal and the underlying brain was not involved. Both infants exhibited severe cardiac hypertrophy. Potter speculated that the cardiac hypertrophy could be secondary to the increased vascular bed in the leptomeninges as could well be the case if the unusual venous pial circulation were caused by the equally possible diffuse arteriovenous shunting. The unusual pattern of pial vessels cannot easily be attributed with any degree of accuracy to the cardiac hypertrophy and augmented cardiac output and blood pressure. A third case, included in the group, concerned an infant whose left innominate vein joined the left atrium of a slightly hypertrophied heart. The principal pial veins were considerably enlarged and the smaller vessels were tortuous to a lesser extent than in the two preceding cases. The liver exhibited prominent subcapsular veins, enlarged centrilobular veins, and periportal and interlobular fibrosis. The third case is not a clear instance of a primary meningeal vascular

abnormality, for the hemodynamic effects of such a cardiac abnormality complicate the issue. The pial vascular pattern exemplifies rather severe prolonged cerebral congestion although there may have been a concomitant arteriovenous shunt. A similar instance of diffusely tortuous and coiled pial vessels over the cerebral hemispheres was observed recently in a female neonate with an aneurysmal dilatation of the vein of Galen caused by a large arteriovenous shunt.

One girl (4 years of age) was reported by Jaffé[148] to have approximately 100 cutaneous hemangiomas and bilateral leptomeningeal hemangiomatosis (apparently not unlike the vascular changes of the Sturge-Weber syndrome). There were multiple small telangiectases in the viscera and death was attributed to unrelated causes. These cases and the familial noncalcifying leptomeningeal angiomatosis described by Divry and van Bogaert[82] and by Bruens and associates[44] cannot be conclusively classified but are probably related to the Sturge-Weber syndrome.

Hemangioma calcificans. Penfield and Ward[261,262] collected a small series of patients with temporal lobe epilepsy caused by vascular anomalies, mostly relatively small arteriovenous aneurysms, and hemangiomas displaying radiological calcification that occurred in both the vessels and the interstitial tissue. The lesions, appearing to be of long standing, exhibited evidence of clinical progression that contrasted with the prominent degenerative changes pathologically. They do not warrant any specific classification.

Klippel-Trénaunay-Weber syndrome. The Klippel-Trénaunay-Weber syndrome[43,371] (nevus varicosus osteohypertrophicus, hemangiectasia hypertrophicans, or angioosteohypertrophy) is characterized by a triad of symptoms: (1) nevi usually unilateral, (2) varicose veins, and (3) hypertrophy of the soft tissue and bone.[43] Although the cutaneous hemangioma, which can be extensive in distribution, is usually present at birth, the varicose veins and hypertrophy of bone and soft tissues need not appear till later in childhood. An arteriovenous shunt is associated with the nevi in many cases and is perhaps the prime cause of the tissue enlargement and the varicosities. In any individual with widespread cutaneous hemangiomatous nevi, involvement of the central nervous system should be suspected.

Collateral vascular network and subarachnoid hemorrhage. Nishimoto and colleagues[236,237] believe they have described a clinical syndrome occurring in young Japanese children or adults. It is associated with stenosis or occlusion of the internal carotid arteries (usually bilateral) and angiographic evidence of a "cerebral rete mirabile" or hemangiomatous collection of vessels at the base of the brain. Subarachnoid hemorrhage was prevalent among those over 21 years of age. The autopsy information is remarkably deficient and the authors consider the "vascular network" to be a congenital vascular anomaly but do not explain the association of carotid stenoses. However, on present evidence it is more likely that the rete mirabile is simply a collateral circulation secondary to bilateral occlusion of the internal carotid arteries. The preeminent problem then is the cause of arterial occlusions in the young subjects.

Carotid-cavernous fistula. The unusual anatomical relationship of the cavernous segment of the internal carotid artery to the cavernous sinus enhances the possibility of the development of an arteriovenous fistula after trauma or the rupture of an aneurysm of this arterial segment. Among other complications such frightful facial disfigurement can succeed the fistula that the lesions have attracted much more attention than their incidence warrants. Though not the sole cause of pulsating exophthalmos, the term is frequently used as a synonym of carotid-cavernous fistula or aneurysm. Travers[351] first recognized and treated the lesions by carotid ligation in the neck.

Prevalence. Carotid-cavernous aneurysm, a relatively uncommon entity, is simply diagnosed because of the distressing bruit,

exophthalmos, chemosis, and diplopia. In 1924, Locke[179] collected 588 cases from the literature. The Cooperative Study of Intracranial Aneurysms and Subarachnoid Hemorrhage[264] gives further indication of the frequency, for 39 carotid-cavernous aneurysms were recorded in 549 verified arteriovenous aneurysms (6.1%). Walker and Allègre[364] reported 24 instances, about one per year, an incidence of approximately one in 20,000 hospital admissions. These carotid-cavernous fistulas are occasionally bilateral.[198,309]

Age and sex distribution. The age and sex distribution depend on the etiology of the lesions. Two major causative factors are trauma and rupture of an arterial aneurysm of that segment of the internal carotid artery, hence the traumatic and so-called spontaneous groupings.

In the traumatic group of carotid-cavernous aneurysms or fistulas, males, being more exposed to trauma, outnumber the females. In Locke's study of 418 cases,[179] 76.8% were males and 23.2% were females, whereas in Hamby's series of 23 cases, there were 12 males and 11 females. In the group of 126 spontaneous fistulas, Locke found that 25.9% occurred in males and 74.1% in females, and Hamby[124] found three of the 19 cases were males and 16 were females. This is consistent with the preponderance of females among patients with saccular aneurysms of the internal carotid artery.[180] The peak of the age distribution falls in the third decade in the traumatic group, but in those that were spontaneous, the distribution is more even (Table 10-9).

Signs and symptoms. In carotid-cavernous aneurysms or fistulas, there are three cardinal findings:

1. EXOPHTHALMOS. The degree of exophthalmos may be quite extreme, even sufficient to prevent the closing of the eyelids. Dandy[73] said it varied from 4 to 20 mm. but usually averaged about 8 or 10 mm. The eyeball frequently protrudes eccentrically because of enlarged orbital veins (generally downward and outward). When bilateral (20% in the traumatic group and

Table 10-9. Age distribution of spontaneous and traumatic carotid-cavernous fistulas

Author	1-10	11-20	21-30	31-40	41-50	51-60	61-70	71-80	81-90	Total
Spontaneous										
Locke (1924)[179]	2	4	10	8	7	12	5	9	1	58
Perret & Nishioka (1966)[264]			2	3	6	5	4	3	1	23
Total	2	4	12	11	13	17	9	12	1	81
Traumatic										
Locke (1924)[179]	7	29	41	30	27	14	2			150
Perret & Nishioka (1966)[264]		3	5	2	1	3	2			16
Total	7	32	46	32	28	17	4			166

8% in the spontaneous group),[302] the degree of exophthalmos and the position differ on the two sides. Usually the exophthalmos occurs on the side of the lesion or is most severe on the ipsilateral side. Occasionally, the reverse is true, and although the explanation of such phenomena was discussed by Dandy,[73] the reason is yet uncertain. Sattler[302] suggested that the position of the fistula in the artery was responsible, but it could just as readily depend on anatomical variations of the cavernous sinuses and their structural reinforcement.[73]

The exophthalmos usually begins to manifest itself within 24 hours. In some patients, it is delayed for much longer intervals possibly because of the formation and rupture of a false sac some weeks later. It may be accentuated after thrombosis of the cavernous sinus or ophthalmic veins but will subsequently recede.

2. PULSATION. Pulsation of the eyeballs synchronous with the pulse is best detected when viewed from the side. Similar pulsations may be associated with prominent veins over the forehead or in the neck. Dandy[73] regards this as a cardinal sign, but Hamby[124] found it in only one-third of his cases.

3. BRUIT. With the onset of the fistula, the patient notices a murmur of varying intensity and quality, at times terribly distressing. The murmur is heard on auscultation; however, over the ipsilateral orbit and temporal region it is usually continuous with systolic intensification and frequently accompanied by a palpable thrill. Martin and Mabon[197] found murmurs in 85% of 224 cases reviewed. Dandy[73] regards this as the one absolutely constant sign of a carotid-cavernous fistula.

Other manifestations include headache, often intense chemosis, conjunctival congestion and possibly ulceration, extraocular palsies, papilledema, and optic atrophy.[1,73,124] Cardiac changes are unusual in carotid-cavernous aneurysm probably because it is not often seen in children and infants and because surgical therapy is instituted before the lesion becomes chronic.

Pathogenesis. The number of autopsies performed on these patients is considerably fewer than the number encountered clinically. In Locke's 544 cases in which the etiology was known, 126 (or 23.2%) were spontaneous and 418 (or 76.85%) were caused by trauma. Hamby[124] encountered 19 spontaneous and 23 traumatic fistulas.

Pool and Potts[268] believe that approximately 5% of carotid-cavernous fistulas are congenital and will be found occasionally in infants and young children without a history of head injury. However, there is no case of a newborn infant with a carotid-cavernous fistula in the literature and no infant or child learns to walk and climb without sustaining head injuries. The presence of an aneurysm on the internal carotid artery in young adults is hardly evidence that carotid-cavernous fistulas are at times congenital.

TRAUMATIC ONSET. The traumatic arteriovenous aneurysm usually results from a severe (anterior) head injury sufficient in most cases to cause a basal skull fracture.[137] Alternatively, the arterial injury can follow a perforating injury be it attributable to a knife, bullet, wire, piece of straw, or a spicule of bone. The injury may tear the artery completely or only enough to produce a false aneurysm, which accounts for the delayed onset of the fistula in some cases. Fistulas have complicated surgery on the trigeminal ganglion and paranasal air sinuses (ethmoid and sphenoid).[73]

In 17 autopsies on cases of traumatic carotid-cavernous fistula, 16 were attributed to a traumatic communication and one was aneurysmal; whether there was a traumatic aneurysmal sac or not was not clearly stated. The trauma may have had little or no bearing on a preexisting aneurysm.

A high proportion of fractures involving the base of the skull pass through the body of the sphenoid bone and to this is attributed the occasional involvement of the internal carotid artery. Furthermore, the artery is likely to tear at the junction of a fixed segment (petrous portion of the internal carotid) with the relatively less fixed cavernous segment. The position of the aperture, however, varies and pathological material is scanty. The aperture in the artery may be 2 to 9 mm. in diameter[73,74] and occasionally more than one aperture may be present or the artery avulsed. The margins of the fistula are smooth.

Carotid-cavernous aneurysm has occurred after carotid endarterectomy in two patients,[19] and in two cases a fracture through the base of the skull involving the clivus has resulted in a fistula between the internal carotid artery and the basilar venous plexus.[111]

SPONTANEOUS ONSET. The etiology of spontaneous arteriovenous fistula is well established as being caused in most instances by rupture of an infraclinoid aneurysm of the internal carotid artery. Bilateral arterial aneurysms can be found in this situation but their spontaneous, independent rupture at approximately the same time to produce bilateral exophthalmos is unlikely,

though it has been reported.[124] Sattler[302] found 8% of the spontaneous fistulas to have bilateral exophthalmos. Spontaneous fistulas are allegedly more frequent on the left side and those attributed to trauma favor the right side.[12]

Pregnancy has been regarded as an important factor in the onset of these fistulas or in the rupture of the causative aneurysm. Sattler[302] found that 17 of 41 cases occurred during pregnancy. Walker and Allègre[364] estimated that 25% to 30% of afflicted women develop their fistulas during the later half of pregnancy, and when one considers the age distribution of these cases, the effect of gestation is even more pronounced. Hamby[124] reported only two pregnancies among 16 women with spontaneous fistulas.

Dandy[73] suggested that trauma might precipitate the rupture of an infraclinoid aneurysm of the internal carotid artery. Others have suggested that a residual remnant of the primitive trigeminal artery could be a *locus minoris resistentiae*.[124] Such hypotheses are based on assumption only. Any tendency to rupture under increased static pressure could be acquired change, for fusiform dilatation at this site is not infrequent.

Hamby[124] believes that the majority of spontaneous fistulas are caused by rupture of preexisting arterial aneurysms. He found 31 intact infraclinoid aneurysms among a total of 508 intracranial arterial aneurysms and during the same interval encountered 19 spontaneous arteriovenous carotid-cavernous fistulas. This suggests that less than 40% of infraclinoid aneurysms rupture to cause carotid-cavernous fistulas. Cases in the literature allegedly of rupture of sclerotic internal carotid arteries[73] might have been of fusiform aneurysms. Apropos of this, Delens[77] found that the cavernous segment of the internal carotid artery was a common site of rupture after arterial injections were given under pressure. Locke[179] reported that in 50 autopsies, tumors of the orbit were the cause of pulsating exophthalmos in seven cases (14%). Presumably they were not attended by a carotid-cavernous fistula. Murphy[220] included tumor emboli as a cause of the fistulas and refers to an instance in a young woman with an ovarian carcinoma.

Spontaneous carotid-cavernous fistulas have been reported in patients suffering from Ehlers-Danlos syndrome,[98,110,309] in one case it was bilateral. The vessels in this connective tissue disorder are remarkably fragile and may rupture spontaneously without preceding aneurysmal dilation.

Mild arteriovenous shunts of spontaneous onset between the meningeal branches of the internal or external carotid artery and dural veins in the vicinity of the cavernous sinus can cause dilated conjunctival and ophthalmic veins, proptosis, and a bruit in middle-aged women.[233] It has been alleged that many of these lesions are misdiagnosed clinically as carotid-cavernous fistulas. Spontaneous resolution is frequent.

Vascular changes. If the fistula is of sufficiently long duration, the ipsilateral internal carotid artery may become enlarged. Tearing of an ectatic internal carotid artery has followed attempted intracranial clipping[74] but it is not known if the vessel is unduly fragile. Small saccular aneurysms of the cerebral arteries were found in two patients[74] but their presence could have been incidental.

The ophthalmic artery is likely to be enlarged and the collateral circulation may reach the fistula by means of the cerebral arteries, the circle of Willis, and many small carotid branches.[127,328] Parkinson[254,255] reviewed the anatomy of these branches of the cavernous segment of the internal carotid artery. The chief branches apart from an ophthalmic artery in some patients were (1) the meningohypophyseal trunk whose branches have anastomoses with the ophthalmic meningeal branches, hypophyseal and tentorial branches from the contralateral internal carotid and meningohypophyseal arteries, and meningeal branches of the vertebral end of cervical arteries, (2) the artery to the inferior cavernous sinus, which forms anastomoses with

the middle meningeal and accessory meningeal arteries near the foramen spinosum, and (3) capsular arteries anastomosing with corresponding branches of the opposite internal carotid. However, collateral circulation from the middle meningeal artery contributed to the shunt in one posttraumatic carotid-cavernous fistula.[273]

The cavernous sinus becomes grossly dilated, trabeculae disappear, and the wall is visibly thicker. There may be evidence of a mural tear and thrombus. There is dilatation of the venous channels communicating with the cavernous sinus and the passage of time is the prerequisite for the enlargement and tortuosity. Avenues of venous drainage include (1) the ophthalmic veins, (2) the intercavernous sinuses, (3) the petrosal sinuses, (4) the basal vein of Rosenthal, (5) the sphenoparietal sinus, (6) the Sylvian vein with its anastomotic channels, (7) the basilar plexus of sinuses, and (8) the emissary veins to the pharyngeal and pterygoid plexuses.

The ophthalmic veins are especially prone to enlarge, and with similar involvement of the intercavernous sinuses, the contralateral cavernous sinus may be affected, together with its corresponding drainage channels. Bilateral exophthalmos develops. Varicosities may be prominent about the orbit, the nose, and the forehead and bleeding therefrom can be profuse. At surgery, numerous enlarged tortuous veins may be visible over the frontal lobe. Thrombi may be found not only in the sinus but also in the drainage channels.[74]

In the carotid-cavernous fistula investigated by Parsons and associates,[256] angiography demonstrated the main venous drainage to the ophthalmic veins and thence to facial veins into the general circulation. The contrast medium disappears from the cerebral circulation in less than 4 seconds. Erosion of the sella turcica, the sphenoid, and the orbital walls may be demonstrated in plain X-rays of the skull[1] because of pressure effects of the enlarged pulsating veins.

Microscopically, the walls of the cavernous sinus exhibit considerable thickening, particularly in the intima, and calcification is a possibility.[74] No doubt the histological changes are similar to those produced in experimental animals.[326]

Untreated patients, if the fistulous shunt is not too severe and the subjective symptoms tolerable, can live for many years.[73,124] However, fistulas tend to progress, the symptoms are very distressing and complications such as disturbances of vision are frequent (30%).[73]

Complications. Hamby[124] considers that some cases of carotid-cavernous fistula escape detection probably because the patient dies of associated injuries. Alternatively, if the fistula is small, the patient may tolerate the unpleasant consequences.

Death may follow from hemorrhage. Some of the traumatic ruptures of the internal carotid artery are associated with extension into the sphenoid sinus and even fatal hemorrhage into the pharynx at an interval after the injury. In his review of 322 carotid-cavernous aneurysms, Sattler[302] discovered three cases in which fatal intracranial hemorrhage occurred and six bled from the nose. Thenceforth, the frequency of hemorrhage was usually accepted as 3%. However, this is probably an underestimate, for many if not most patients have in the past been treated surgically at least by carotid ligation. The true frequency of hemorrhage cannot be accurately assessed, but it is of interest that the only two untreated patients of a series of 14 with carotid-cavernous aneurysm[88] both died from rupture of the cavernous sinus. The bleeding may also arise from one of the enlarged communicating sinuses or veins within the cranium. Secondary infection of the eye and orbit can result in severe if not fatal hemorrhage from enlarged orbital veins.[124] Subdural hemorrhage can occur after rupture of the cavernous sinus.[127]

Spontaneous cure of these lesions occurs sporadically because of thrombosis of the pertinent vessels attended by a sudden pronounced increase in the proptosis and vascular engorgement of the orbit. The latter

should subside. Sattler[302] recorded 16 instances of spontaneous cure in 322 cases. Dandy[73] believed the figure was nearer to 10% but only the exceptional case is not subjected to some surgical procedure when the diagnosis is made. Holman[136] on the other hand has estimated that 16% will close spontaneously. Though carotid ligation in the neck may not be curative, it can nevertheless so modify the circulation that thrombosis presumably of the cavernous sinus can ensue. Echols and Jackson[88] found a cure rate of 27% after carotid ligation, and only three of the six patients submitted to the trapping operation were cured. Perhaps more often than not such a procedure is followed by further development of the collateral circulation.

Recently, a man who sustained a perforating injury to the left orbit at the age of 9 years[121] suffered headaches and complained of easy fatigue until at the age of 33 years he was found to have a carotid-cavernous fistula with unilateral exophthalmos and diplopia. The internal carotid artery was ligated intracranially proximal to the posterior communicating artery and the ophthalmic artery was ligated separately. Subsequently, the cervical segment of the internal carotid artery was likewise surgically occluded. One month later the patient noticed the return of an intracranial bruit. This was traced to enlargement of small hypophyseal and dural arteries that fed the fistula.

The complications of carotid ligation are essentially similar to those discussed in relation to the therapy of intracranial arterial aneurysms except that the fistula may have stimulated the development of an intracranial collateral circulation with backflow in the terminal segment of the internal carotid artery. In this case, carotid ligation may be less prone to result in cerebral ischemia.

Shaw and Foltz[314] reported the traumatic onset of a carotid-cavernous fistula and a dissecting aneurysm of the middle cerebral artery in a man of 20 years. Twelve years later the patient, subjected to a trapping operation, died 1 day postoperatively from a massive intracerebral hemorrhage attributed to altered hemodynamics after the clipping of the internal carotid artery. Jaeger[147] reported intracerebral hemorrhage in two patients in both instances several years after carotid ligation.

The insertion of muscle into the cavernous segment of the internal carotid artery is designed to induce vascular thrombosis within the artery. The muscle, acting as a foreign body, induces platelet aggregation and adhesion to its surface, and an occlusive thrombus is likely to ensue. Ultimately organization of the thrombus occurs later and the muscle is absorbed progressively. Propagation of the thrombus is less likely in the carotid artery than in the veins and a considerable reduction in the size of the enlarged venous channels follows occlusion of the fistula. The injection of sclerosing fluids is intended to initiate intravascular thrombosis and the process is instigated by damaging and perhaps even denuding the vessel wall of endothelium. However, there is little control over the localization of damage by such a procedure, and for the use of acrylics[90] and other plastics see Chapter 9.

Hemangioma of the dura mater. Angiomas and vascular anomalies of the dura mater are rare, although involvement of vessels in the dura with lesions primarily of the cerebrum are more frequent. McCormick and Boulter[204] recently recorded two localized cavernous hemangiomas of the dura mater. Both were symptomless and localized in the right half of the tentorium cerebelli of middle-aged men. Both were raised above the dural surface and one rested in an indentation within the occipital lobe to which there was no attachment. Only three instances of authentic hemangiomas of the dura mater were found in a review of the literature. Two were cavernous hemangiomas and the other was an arteriovenous aneurysm. Cases excluded were regarded as angioblastic meningiomas or lesions involving the brain or the Galenic venous system.

Vertebral arteriovenous aneurysms. Arteriovenous aneurysms, the fistulous communications between the vertebral artery and vein in the neck, are not common lesions. Tsuji and associates[353] collected 67 cases from the literature, four of which were believed to be congenital, 44 of traumatic origin, and in 19 no cause was advanced. Robles[283] reported an alleged congenital form in a woman of 59 years who at the age of 44 became aware of the sudden onset of a bruit after an abrupt change of head position. Trauma is the most frequent cause of these lesions and a penetrating wound is more often than not responsible; thus most arteriovenous aneurysms stem from war injuries.[55] A sliver from exploding glassware has been known to injure the vein and penetrate the artery and to lead to the formation of two false aneurysms of the artery in concert with an arteriovenous fistula to the vein. A minority of the traumatic cases of vertebral arteriovenous aneurysm accrue from vertebral angiography[150, 264] and are not necessarily severe, as Jamieson[150] had no difficulty in closing the fistula without impairing vertebral flow. Tsuji and associates[353] included four in their series of 67 cases and there was one case in the Cooperative Study.[264] Newton and Darroch[231] reported five cases in one of which bilateral lesions occurred after attempts at vertebral angiography. Markham[196] reported the spontaneous onset of such a fistula in a man of 50 years. He excluded a congenital etiology on account of the patient's age.

Mainly because of the disturbing bruits and attendant headaches, the lesions have not been permitted to progress to advanced stages of varicosity and grossly increased vascularity. Retrograde flow down the vertebral artery from the basilar has been seen angiographically, often in association with a relative degree of cerebral ischemia. Enlargement and tortuosity of the spinal vessels also feature.

Carotid-jugular fistula. Carotid-jugular arteriovenous fistula appears to be an extremely rare entity and usually occurs after trauma.[358] Of prime interest in this lesion is its experimental possibilities for it has become a common experimental model for the study of hemodynamics and for investigations of the chronic histological changes in the walls of vessels involved in the arteriovenous shunt. The experimental fistula between the common carotid artery and external jugular vein in the rabbit is rapidly followed by homolateral exophthalmos, which can become extreme. The proptosis, caused by gross enlargement of an intraorbital vein, is seen only occasionally in man and in sheep.

A carotid-jugular fistula has been produced on a number of occasions in the vain hope that the change wrought in the cerebral circulation would improve the intelligence of mentally retarded children[208,335] with the rationale based on the false premise that any increase in limb size caused by an arteriovenous aneurysm was caused by augmented flow in the limb distal to the fistula. Rather than instituting improvement in the cranial circulation, the procedure is more likely to diminish it despite vascular engorgement. The intelligence of the children so treated evidenced no amelioration and on the contrary a number developed subarachnoid, intracerebral, and intraventricular hemorrhage. Enlarged tortuous veins were found at the base of the brain, and histologically, small intracerebral vessels exhibited endothelial proliferation, medial thinning with luminal narrowing, and intravascular thrombi.[335]

Bleasel and Frew[33] created an arteriovenous fistula between the common carotid artery and the internal jugular vein in three patients with compression of the ipsilateral optic nerve caused by (1) an intracranial saccular aneurysm of the internal carotid artery immediately after its emergence from the cavernous sinus, (2) an aneurysm at the junction of the anterior cerebral artery and the anterior communicating artery and (3) by an ectatic and tortuous ophthalmic artery. Improvement of ocular symptoms followed although there was a subsequent fatal rupture of one carotid aneurysm. No mention was made of complications of the arteriovenous fistulas, which are essentially the same as those occurring in the experimental animal.[326]

Extracranial arteriovenous anomalies. Arteriovenous aneurysms may be confined solely to the vessels of the scalp and recently a case was reported of a male developing such a lesion after punch scalp–autograft transplantation for alopecia.[324] The lesions, though rare, may progress to enormous proportions with the enlarged tortuous veins being grossly disfiguring and the bruit very disconcerting.[71,72] Guida and Moore[116] finding only 23 instances of arteriovenous aneurysm involving the temporal artery in a survey of literature up to 1968 were puzzled since scalp wounds are so frequent.

In the Cooperative Study,[264] four cases ostensibly extracranial lesions with prominent tortuous pulsating vessels, possibly with a palpable thrill and audible bruit, were purported to be of this type. The blood supply appeared to come from both external carotid arteries, and there was the usual difficulty in occluding a sufficient number of afferent vessels to obliterate the shunt, short of complete excision of the main mass of vessels. In one of the cases, the patient suffered from transient episodes of blindness and had bilateral papilledema, which in the absence of other causes suggests simultaneous intracranial involvement, especially since numerous prominent perforating vessels between the scalp and the calvarium were found. As these perforating branches enlarge, the intracranial vessels may eventually come to participate in the efferent flow from an arteriovenous aneurysm. Intracranial arterial blood rarely supplies afferent blood to extracranial arteriovenous aneurysms from the middle meningeal artery.

Verbiest[358] reported 12 extracranial and cervical arteriovenous aneurysms of the carotid and vertebral arteries. Of these, four had vascular anastomoses with the dura or the cranium and two intraorbital lesions had communications with the external or internal carotid arteries. In the experience of Olivecrona and Riives[247] arteriovenous aneurysms involving the scalp, though often believed to be exclusively in the territory of the external carotid artery, involved equally the branches of the internal carotid artery. In all probability, if the lesion is allowed to proceed unchecked, intracranial involvement will eventually ensue.

Most of these lesions are attributed to congenital malformations[358] because they appear to develop spontaneously. However, most of the afflicted patients are adults and the history is of fairly short duration, suggesting that many of these so-called spontaneous lesions could be acquired and be the result of some forgotten trauma.

Cavernous hemangiomas of the scalp, forehead, or orbital region can exhibit an arteriovenous shunt of considerable proportions with drainage to the dural sinuses. However, these lesions are quite different in that the gross enlargement and tortuosity of afferent and efferent vessels displayed by the foregoing arteriovenous aneurysms are usually absent.

Associated intracranial and extracranial arteriovenous aneurysms. Not very often extracranial arteriovenous aneurysms occur in association with intracranial lesions of similar nature. The extracranial lesion may be situated in any area, inclusive of the head and neck. Only seven instances of separate and distinct arteriovenous aneurysms, one intracranial and one in the scalp, were found in the Cooperative Study.[264] However, whenever an arteriovenous aneurysm is encountered in the forehead and scalp, the association should be considered.

A 3-year-old boy in the Cooperative Study[264] had a lesion in the posterior fossa and another involving the forehead and orbits. In such cases where the arteriovenous aneurysms are well separated, it is likely that they are separate and distinct. However, another patient had a scalp lesion over the left occipital region and one in the cerebrum involving the left occipito-temporal region in which the intracranial and extracranial findings could be manifestations of a single vascular anomaly. In other words, such an arteriovenous aneu-

rysm could be supplied by branches of both the internal and external carotid arteries and angiography could demonstrate the vascular relationship.

The external carotid artery and intracranial arteriovenous aneurysms. The external carotid artery may involve the cerebral vasculature in three different ways.

1. There may be *venous drainage* from extracranial arteriovenous aneurysms of branches of the external carotid artery *into the dural sinuses* via emissary, diploic, or orbital veins. The dural sinuses are only secondarily involved in the organization, which has been discussed in the foregoing sections. A blood cyst or a hemangioma of the pericranium with vascular communications between it and the intracranial dural sinuses is a sinus pericranii[122] although other terminology has also been used to describe it. Hahn[122] supported the concept that the lesion was primarily an arteriovenous aneurysm, which seems feasible, but it is also likely that the term has been used loosely to include true hemangiomas.

2. Branches of the external carotid artery (whether extracranially or intracranially situated) may form *arteriovenous anastomoses with dural sinuses or meningeal veins.* Communication between the occipital artery and the transverse sinus is an unusual lesion that is associated with a pulsatile noise in the head and bruit on auscultation.[232,356] Enlarged tortuous and pulsating vessels may be visible behind the ear with a palpable bony defect in the skull through which the vessels pass. Angiography revealed that branches of the occipital artery anastomosed with the lateral sinus and in two instances the sigmoid sinus as well, whereas the middle meningeal arteries participated in the shunt in two cases. Meningeal branches of the occipital artery can contribute to the fistula. Branches of the external carotid artery form anastomoses with emissary veins. Reversal of flow and enlargement of vessels soon give the lesion the appearance of a direct communication between the artery and the sinus. The sinuses were not grossly aneurysmal. Second-

ary enlargement of veins over the cerebrum and cerebellum follows if the shunt is chronic and of any size. Kunc and Bret[166] estimated that these arteriosinusal fistulas as they called them constituted 6.25% of the arteriovenous aneurysms seen between 1951 and 1968. They included arteriovenous shunts between meningeal and tentorial branches from the internal carotid artery. Additional small arteriovenous aneurysms were demonstrated in each of their five patients.

The lateral sinus appears to be the sinus most frequently involved. A shunt between scalp vessels and the superior longitudinal sinus is likely to have afferent vessels from both external carotid arteries.[166]

Mingrino and Moro[214] reported the case of a woman of 67 years who suffered the spontaneous development of an arteriovenous communication between a branch of the internal maxillary artery and the cavernous sinus. The patient presented with proptosis, conjunctival congestion, papilledema, and unilateral loss of vision. The lesion was treated early, presumably before the shunt developed to large proportions, at which stage no doubt it would have closely resembled a carotid-cavernous fistula. Sachs and associates[300] recorded unilateral exophthalmos caused by an arteriovenous aneurysm in the middle cranial fossa fed by the middle meningeal artery.

Nicola and Nizzola[234] reported three dural arteriovenous malformations of the posterior fossa with no obvious involvement of scalp vessels but a preponderance of the blood supply coming from the external carotid artery (occipital artery). In two cases, there was also an enlarged meningeal branch of the internal carotid artery (artery of Bernasconi and Cassinari) participating in the shunt. Enlarged pial arteries were a prominent feature of one case, doubtless a secondary manifestation of the vascular anomaly. At times, however, these dural arteriovenous aneurysms are supplied by the meningeal arteries and may be of traumatic origin.[96,252] Suwanwela[332] emphasized that the middle meningeal

veins communicate with the sphenoparietal and the superior longitudinal sagittal sinuses, and so arteriovenous aneurysms that involve the dural vessels are likely to derange these sinuses. Arteriovenous shunts between the meningeal arteries and veins occur after trauma,[292,332] and in view of their close apposition and their anatomical enclosure between the calvarium and the dura are not very frequent. Jackson and Du Boulay[146] reported a case of arteriovenous fistula that underwent spontaneous closure within 5 months between the middle meningeal artery and a diploic vein after fracture of a parietal bone. At craniotomy in a boy of 10 years, Sachs[299] discovered what was apparently an arteriovenous aneurysm of the dura mater in the temporal area. There were numerous vascular connections traversing the subdural space to anastomose with pial vessels. The clinical symptoms were probably caused by vascular involvement of the cerebral cortex. There was also a pale telangiectatic nevus over the forehead but no mention of the scalp vessels.

3. Branches of the external carotid artery may constitute *an accessory afferent vessel or an important collateral to arteriovenous aneurysms* that involve primarily the internal carotid and vertebrobasilar systems. Olivecrona[245] found such an event in 10% of his cases.

The external carotid artery may be the major source of blood to the arteriovenous aneurysms. Cantu and associates[47] reported an unusual case—an elderly woman with an arteriovenous aneurysm involving the cerebrum. The afferent blood supply arose predominantly from the external carotid (middle meningeal, superficial temporal, and external occipital arteries), and after bilateral ligation of the external carotid arteries, it was demonstrated that the afferent supply arose from an anastomosis from the vertebral to the external carotid artery above the ligation. These anastomoses between muscular branches of the vertebral and those of the occipital artery can occasionally be demonstrated by angiography. They are probably present in most individuals and enlarge when near an arteriovenous shunt. Ramamurthi and Balasubramanian[275] briefly reviewed the literature and reported two cases in which the supply was predominantly from the external carotid artery. The most common contribution from the external carotid is via the middle meningeal artery, enlargement of the vascular markings of which can be demonstrated not infrequently by X-ray films of the skull.

Vascular anomalies of the spinal cord

Vascular anomalies of the spinal cord are less frequent than those within the cranium by virtue of the smaller size of the cord and the infrequency with which the spinal cord is examined at autopsy. However, in this age of angiography and aggressive neurosurgery, these vascular lesions are more readily demonstrated and the frequency of their clinical diagnosis is increasing. The task would be formidable for any one person to obtain pathological material in sufficient quantity for the detailed postmortem microangiography so essential for their adequate investigation. Precise estimation of the prevalence of these cord lesions is difficult, but some inkling of their infrequency can be gleaned from the Cooperative Study of subarachnoid hemorrhage.[264] There were but two instances of spinal "angioma" in a total of 510 verified vascular anomalies (excluding carotid-cavernous fistulas).

Palmer and Hickman[253] described a hemangioma (calling it a venous angioma) in the dorsal and dorsolateral areas of the spinal cord of a mare, but beyond this little is known of the vascular anomalies in lower animals.

Telangiectases and cavernous hemangiomas. Telangiectases are rarely seen in the spinal cord, and in a review of vascular anomalies and tumors of the cord, Turner and Kernohan[354] mentioned not a single case. Svien and Baker[333] reported two instances of spinal telangiectasis in 32 vascular anomalies of the cord. Morphologically

they consist of dilatations of capillary blood vessels and macroscopically they resemble those within the brain. Wyburn-Mason[391] believes that cavernous hemangiomas develop from telangiectases and asserts that there is no justification for differentiating between the two. The morphological overlap between these lesions in the brain can also be seen within the cord.

Odom and associates[243] reported three cases of telangiectases that had caused hematomyelia with expansion of the cord and the blood tracking for a distance up and down the cord. Subarachnoid hemorrhage had occurred in one case. Another was a cavernous hemangioma,[242] which is known to cause hemorrhage more frequently than telangiectases. Odom described yet another case[242] in which there was radicular pain, backache, paresthesia, and progressive paraparesis but no gross hemorrhage. The hemangioma contained areas of calcification and ossification, which suggested that the lesion was a cavernous hemangioma not a telangiectasis. In the absence of a clear distinction between the two and in view of the small number of cases so far found in the cord, it seems better at this stage to group the two types together under the simple heading "hemangioma."

These hemangiomas occur for the most part wholly within the cord, usually in the posterior columns,[242,391] and expand the part of the cord involved. Small hemorrhages may lead to siderosis of the neighboring tissues[242] but hemorrhage sufficient to cause severe cord disturbances is not uncommon.[132,242,243] Pial vessels may be unusually prominent.[109,391] Damage to the cord quite apart from hemorrhage and sufficient to cause paraplegia is not exceptional.[10,391]

As with vascular anomalies, elsewhere, the lesions are occasionally multiple. In Ohlmacher's case,[244] multiple hemangiomas were found in the brain, whereas another in the cervical cord had caused extensive hematomyelia in which the blood had dissected upward 4 to 4.5 cm. and downward 17 to 18 cm. from the hemangioma. In one instance[391] a spinal hemangioma had caused paraplegia and the girl died 15 months after laminectomy from pontine hemorrhage secondary to a cavernous hemangioma in that location. In Wyburn-Mason's review of 14 intramedullary hemangiomas, three patients had cutaneous hemangiomas. There were no cases of hereditary hemorrhagic telangiectasia with spinal cord involvement.

Extradural hemangiomas are very unusual. They may produce spontaneous spinal extradural hemorrhage and bleeding is often troublesome at operation. Involvement of the skin is a common feature, and less frequently there may be an associated spinal cord hemangioma.[391] In some, infiltration of the extradural fat may be prominent and angiolipoma is diagnosed. In some instances, the hemangioma appears to be an extension of a hemangioma within one or more vertebrae.[228] Karshner and associates[155] told of a boy of 14 years with hemangiomatous involvement of the sixth, seventh, and eighth thoracic vertebrae accompanied by extradural extension and compression of the cord. In addition, the youth had multiple cutaneous hemangiomas over the dorsal aspect of the trunk. These hemangiomas like the intramedullary hemangiomas, rarely cause subarachnoid hemorrhage but when large enough produce spinal block and compression. Pregnancy may accentuate the symptoms.[56,228]

Venous angiomas and arteriovenous aneurysms. The so-called intradural racemose angioma, said to be venous (that is, venous angioma) and arterial (that is, arteriovenous aneurysm) in type, is the most common variety of vascular anomaly affecting the spinal cord, and many authors have treated the two simultaneously[189,229,354] because of difficulty in distinguishing one type from the other. The venous angioma is the more prevalent. It may exhibit pulsations and well-oxygenated blood[120,229] so that any differentiation from the obvious arteriovenous aneurysm is probably artificial and unwarranted. Furthermore, compres-

sion of one vessel often alters the color of the blood circulating in the tortuous mass of vessels, suggesting that the color of the vessels is only an indication of the severity of the shunt. Macroscopic examination and angiography are both unsatisfactory methods of determining the presence and degree of the arteriovenous shunting, in all probability the underlying cause of both lesions. Luessenhop and Cruz[189] assert that only one type of lesion, the arteriovenous aneurysm, can be demonstrated by angiography. Once again detailed postmortem microangiographic investigations are necessary to confirm or negate the opposing contentions. In this text, the two allegedly distinct types will be dealt with together as arteriovenous aneurysms.

Prevalence. Constituting as they do the majority of the vascular anomalies of the spinal cord, Lombardi and Migliavacca[183] found intracranial arteriovenous aneurysms to be four times more frequent in their experience and spinal tumors 11 times more common. When considered with spinal cord tumors they are said to constitute anything from 3.3% to 11% of the total.[79] Wyburn-Mason[391] states that venous angioma is found in 2% to 5% of successive laminectomies.

There were two arteriovenous aneurysms and 107 primary tumors of the cord at the Manchester Royal Infirmary (England)[229] between 1936 and 1946 compared with 19 and 121 respectively between 1946 and 1956. This manifold increase in the ratio of arteriovenous aneurysm to primary spinal cord tumors mirrors no doubt the improved diagnostic methods rather than an actual increase in frequency in the patient population. Caucasians, Negroes, and Mongoloids are affected but to date there has been no mention of their occurrence in the Australoids, though there is no reason to believe they are unaffected by the disorder.

Age and sex distribution. The age distribution of the cord lesions is given in Table 10-10, which is a nonexhaustive compilation of 371 cases from the liter-

Table 10-10. Age distribution of arteriovenous aneurysms of the spinal cord

Author	1-10 or 0-9	11-20 or 10-19	21-30 or 20-29	31-40 or 30-39	41-50 or 40-49	51-60 or 50-59	61-70 or 60-69	70 and over	Total
Turner & Kernohan (1941)[354]			7	2	6	1	2		18*
Wyburn-Mason (1944)†[391]	1	7	19	24	16	20	7	1	95
Arseni & Samitca (1959)[13]			4	7	2	5			18
Gross & Ralston (1959)[115]		1			1	4	4		10
Lombardi & Migliavacca (1959)[183]		2	2	3	4	4	3		18
Newman (1959)[229]	2			1	6	6	4		19
Teng & Papatheodorou (1964)[341]			1	2	5	7			15
Shephard (1965)[317]	1	1	2	1	1	4		1	11
Hurth et al. (1968)[144]		1	1	2	5	2			11
Krayenbühl et al. (1969)[162]		1	3	2	4	2	5		17
Ommaya et al. (1969)[248]		2		4	6	1	4	1	18
Series from literature‡	7	20	24	22	26	13	7	2	121
Total	11	35	63	70	82	69	36	5	371
Wyburn-Mason[391] (at onset of symptoms)	5	12	22	17	19	13	4	1	93

*Two of this series were extradural.

†Personal cases from the literature; ages are those at admission to hospital.

‡Series collected from literature since Wyburn-Mason's review[391]; references: 10, 18, 21, 24, 25, 36, 41, 78, 83, 85, 86, 93, 97, 104, 120, 126, 131, 134, 140, 141, 143, 156, 167, 169, 184, 188, 189, 200, 219, 228, 230, 242, 243, 263, 267, 285, 310, 331, 338, 342, 344, 352, 355, 362, 366, 384.

ature. The ages at admission to a hospital when the diagnosis was established are given, but there is a distinct shift to the left for age at the onset of symptoms.

Many authors have commented on the extreme rarity of these lesions in infancy,[354] a feature that Table 10-10 confirms. Houdart and associates[143] collected 15 cases in which the spinal vascular anomaly had been studied by angiography. In 11, the symptoms commenced before the age of 12 years, and in two the history dated back prior to the third birthday. One of Newman's patient was paraplegic from birth although sciatic pain did not develop until 46 years of age and the author suggested that the paraplegia may have been caused by a separate congenital lesion. Another of Newman's patients developed leg weakness at 1 year of age and this child must be one of the youngest on record. In Wyburn-Mason's review, 82% of the cases occurred between 20 and 60 years, and in 67% of cases the onset was between 26 and 55 years. For the series, the youngest age of onset was 8 years and the oldest 71 years. Such a very late age of onset is significant

and, in view of the pernicious character of arteriovenous aneurysms, casts doubt indeed on the congenital theory of the etiology.

Table 10-11 gives the sex distribution, and in most reports in the literature, males predominate. In Table 10-11, the ratio of males to females is approximately 3:1.

Macroscopic appearance. These lesions manifest themselves in two ways. Firstly, the extramedullary component consists of either several or many tortuous vessels on the surface of the cord often causing deep impressions in its surface. At times gross dilatation and ectasia sufficient to obstruct the spinal canal ensue, and some of the vessels form saccular aneurysms from which serious pressure effects arise. Neurosurgeons have often classified these aneurysms according to color. Those containing dark or venous blood have been classified as venous and conversely those with a high oxygen saturation as arteriovenous aneurysms. As no satisfactory estimations of arteriovenous shunts are available in these lesions, the absence of a shunt cannot be denied, and most neurosurgeons treat these

Table 10-11. Sex distribution of arteriovenous aneurysms of the spinal cord

Author	Males	Females	Total
Turner & Kernohan (1941)[354]	15	3	18
Wyburn-Mason (1944)*[391]	69	27	96
Arseni & Samitca (1959)[13]	13	5	18
Gross & Ralston (1959)[115]	8	2	10
Lombardi & Migliavacca (1959)[183]	14	4	18
Newman (1959)[229]	17	2	19
Taveras & Dalton (1961)[336]	21	4	25
Bergstrand et al. (1964)[25]	8	4	12
Teng & Papatheodorou (1964)[341]	9	6	15
Shephard (1965)[317]	6	5	11
Hurth et al. (1968)[144]	8	3	11
Krayenbühl et al. (1969)[162]	15	2	17
Ommaya et al. (1969)[248]	14	4	18
Others from literature†	76	38	114
Total	293	109	402

*Personal cases and from the literature.
†Nonexhaustive series collected from literature subsequent to the review by Wyburn-Mason.[391]
(See Table 10-10.)

differences simply as variations of arteriovenous aneurysms. Ommaya and associates[248] classified them into the following three major morphological types:

1. SINGLE-COILED VESSEL. Usually only one or two afferent arteries feed the anomaly, which consists essentially of one long exceedingly tortuous vessel along the dorsal surface of the cord, and often over its entire length. This variety has a slow flow rate, is found in adults only, and is the type most frequently encountered and most often regarded as a venous angioma.

2. GLOMUS TYPE OF ARTERIOVENOUS ANEURYSM. This lesion, found only in adults, consists of a small localized plexus of small coiled vessels usually fed by a single afferent artery. Blood flow through the lesion is slow.

3. JUVENILE TYPE OF ARTERIOVENOUS ANEURYSM. This variety has been observed almost exclusively in children and young adults. Multiple feeders from both sides of the cord supply an extensive and voluminous lesion often filling the spinal canal and enveloping the cord. Blood flow through dilated tortuous veins extending up and down the cord is extremely rapid. This type, unlike the two preceding varieties, more closely resembles the arteriovenous aneurysms within the cranium.

The second major component of these lesions is an associated intramedullary proliferation of small vessels in number and size suggestive of telangiectasis that is at times extreme. The gray matter is often severely affected but the vessels are not limited to this portion of the cord. Whereas in the brain large vessels traverse the parenchyma, in the cord they are mostly on its surface or indent it, with the intramedullary vessels being usually quite small. The overlying leptomeninges may be considerably thickened with fibrosis exhibiting brown pigmentation.

Similar changes seldom occur in the extradural space, though in the case of Newquist and Mayfield[230] the extradural fat overlying the arteriovenous aneurysm was replaced by exceedingly vascular fibrous tissue.

A predominantly intramedullary arteriovenous aneurysm is extremely rare and fails to produce the characteristic appearance on myelography. With further progression of the lesion, pial vessels invariably become involved.

Radiological findings. The principal method of investigating these vascular anomalies is by radiology and the following findings derived therefrom are dependent on the obvious pathological changes:

1. Hemangioma of the vertebrae may be associated with enlarged extradural veins or extension into the extradural space with cord compression; an associated spinal lesion is uncommon.[336]

2. Calcification is rarely associated with spinal arteriovenous aneurysms.[310]
3. The spinal canal is enlarged and possibly the vertebrae eroded.[162]
4. On myelography, a complete spinal block, irregular wormlike filling defects particularly centrally situated,[97] or enlarged tortuous vessels are outlined; myelography does not necessarily indicate the limits of the lesion and pulsations in the oil column synchronous with the heart beat can be observed.[336]
5. Angiographically, the afferent and efferent vessels may be demonstrated together with the main mass of anomalous vessels, in more than half the cases, only a single arterial feeder has been demonstrated by selective arteriography[79]; this does not preclude the possibility of an alternative supply after ligation of the single afferent.

Distribution. Houdart and associates[143] found 10% of lesions in their material to be in the cervical region, 30% in the upper dorsal, and the remaining 60% of cases below the eighth thoracic vertebra. In Newman's series of 19 cases,[229] 12 were thoracic and about one-sixth occurred in the cervical cord.

In distribution, Wyburn-Mason[391] contended that venous angiomas affected the lower part of the cord below the fifth or sixth thoracic segment occurring mostly on the posterior surface of the cord. By contrast, the arteriovenous aneurysm was especially likely to affect the posterior aspect of the cord from the seventh thoracic to the upper lumbar segments in addition to the anterior part of the cervical enlargement. No explanation provides for these topographical differences.

Microscopic appearance. Histologically, the features that characterize the arteriovenous aneurysms within the cranium are observed in the cord. The arteries are considerably enlarged and tortuous with much loss of elastic tissue and medial thinning. Veins are grossly dilated with thickened walls. Some vessels have the structure of aneurysms and macroscopically are recognized as such. The intramedullary vessels have thick hyaline walls with narrowed lumens.[105,391] Rarely is calcification observed. The vessels are subject to thrombosis.

The spinal cord exhibits a considerable degree of gliosis, though at the level of the main portion of the lesion the architecture may be destroyed. Loss of nerve cells varies in degree and there is secondary degeneration of nerve tracts after extensive compression or softening of the cord and hematomyelia. The overlying leptomeninges exhibit fibrosis, siderosis, and possibly obliteration of the subarachnoid space.

Natural history. Newman[229] found that once disabling symptoms appeared, the progression to complete cord transection was more or less rapid. Eleven of his 19 patients were unable to walk 6 months to 4 years (average of about 2 years) after first noticing weakness of the lower limbs. Another five patients, though severely disabled, were still able to walk $1\frac{1}{2}$ to $4\frac{1}{2}$ years afterward. However, preceding such symptoms, characteristic of this phase of progressive paraplegia, pain in the back and radicular pain were often very distressing.

These arteriovenous aneurysms constitute the commonest individual cause of spinal subarachnoid hemorrhage, and some patients present with such an episode. Newman[229] found subarachnoid hemorrhage in 17 of 150 cases from the literature (11.3%). The episodes are often recurrent, being rarely fatal in themselves and most infrequently the cause of severe hematomyelia. The bleeding may be so profuse that it is mistaken for intracranial subarachnoid hemorrhage,[243] especially in the case of cervical lesions. The mechanism of rupture of vessels has been discussed in relation to the cerebral lesions and the pathogenesis of the bleeding is assuredly identical. Trauma in some cases appears to have been related to the onset of symptoms, but the vessels, if the lesion is present already, are probably unduly susceptible to injury. Lumbar puncture does not appear to provoke undue hemorrhage from these lesions involving the cauda equina.

One woman with a spinal subarachnoid hemorrhage from a spinal anomaly had a symptomatic attack of herpes zoster.[131]

Myelomalacia is the serious and irreversible complication[10] and is an ostensibly more common event than in the case of the corresponding lesions in the cranium. When hemorrhage occurs from vessels in the vascular anomaly (most probably veins), thrombosis will be initiated at the site of rupture, and in view of the relatively small caliber of these vessels, occlusion may well materialize. Lately neurosurgeons have been dissecting these vascular anomalies off the cord with relative impunity, and so occlusion of those surface vessels seems an unlikely explanation for the frequent myelomalacia. Spasm is rarely found in association with intracranial arteriovenous aneurysms and so should not be a factor in softening in the cord. Shephard[317] considers that the lesions frequently cause significant compression of the cord and nerve roots. However, other factors also come into play. Krayenbühl and associates[162] believe that most of the symptoms of these vascular anomalies are caused by depriving the cord of its blood supply, a type of "spinal steal syndrome." This is consistent with the known facts about arteriovenous shunts beyond which there may be congestion even though stasis predominates and ischemia ensues. Acute episodes can arise when there is an added strain on the circulation. In this respect it is of interest that a male of 62 years[10] with a vascular anomaly developed a flaccid paresis only after exertion until subsequently a complete paraplegia followed severe circulatory insufficiency. Krayenbühl and associates[162] have suggested that spinal decompression serves only to augment the spinal steal syndrome and so aggravate the spinal ischemia and the clinical deterioration.

Brion and associates[41] found nine cases presenting as transverse or diffuse myelitis that were in fact caused by myelomalacia secondary to vascular anomalies involving the cord. They also stated that the Foix-Alajouanine syndrome of "subacute necrotic myelopathy" can be attributed to a diffuse cord lesion associated with a vascular anomaly causing flaccid paraplegia.

The relapse and remission of symptoms in relation to pregnancy, not confined to vertebral angiomas,[228] has been found on several occasions in association with arteriovenous aneurysms (and venous angiomas) of the cord.[97,228-230] Newman[228] has suggested that the enlarged gravid uterus might obstruct venous drainage with delivery bringing relief. He conceded that this explanation is probably inadequate because at times the vascular anomaly is thoracic or gives rise to symptoms before the uterus is much enlarged. The factor responsible is liable to be hormonal.

The frequent occurrence of scoliosis with diseases of the spinal cord is well known, and three cases associated with spinal arteriovenous aneurysms were reported by Boldrey and associates.[36] In each instance, the spinal curvature was the first symptom of the spinal lesion, the onset being within the first decade.

The syndrome of Foix and Alajouanine. Subacute necrotic myelitis of Foix and Alajouanine, also called progressive necrosis of the spinal cord,[216] is characterized by amyotrophic paraplegia that progresses from an early spastic condition to flaccidity with loss of tendon reflexes and sphincter control. The sensory changes appear later and are at first disassociated then subsequently become complete, while the cerebrospinal fluid evinces a rise in protein without an increase in cells. The lower part of the cord (particularly the lumbosacral segments) exhibits necrotic degeneration affecting predominantly the gray matter, hypertrophy of vessels, and "mesoendovascularitis."[113] The course of the illness is generally subacute ending in death within 1 and 2 years of the onset.[113]

Greenfield and Turner[113] presented two subacute cases and a third regarded as acute. They emphasized the enlargement and gross intimal thickening of pial arteries and veins and also the prominence of the small intramedullary vessels that had thickened hyaline walls and narrowed lumens. Inflammatory changes in the vessels were not in evidence. These authors believed that the disease was primarily an obliterative sclerosis of small intramedullary and meningeal vessels of the lower segments of the spinal cord in conjunction with the pathological changes in the pial vessels mentioned above and that degenerative changes in the cord were consequent upon the vascular changes.

Wyburn-Mason[391] has it that necrotic myelitis is but a form of venous angioma of the cord "angioma racemosum venosum." Neuburger and associates[226] presented two additional cases emphasizing that the principal meningeal vascular changes were thickening and hyalinization of the walls of vessels, mainly veins and venules. The meninges were thickened and they believed that the intramedullary vessels had undergone proliferation in addition to exhibiting hyalinization and sclerosis. In one case, the disease terminated with hematomyelia and the vascular changes were regarded as all important. Mair and Folkerts[193] presented a case with thickened and tortuous veins about the affected segments of the cord. Some veins displayed changes of recanalization, which the authors attributed to thrombophlebitis. The vein accompanying the tenth thoracic nerve was exceptionally large and calcified and the thickened anterior spinal vein indented the thoracic segments. The architecture of the lower thoracic and lumbosacral segments was almost completely destroyed, and features usual to this syndrome in the cord appeared with calcification of many of the intramedullary vessels. Mair and Folkerts[193] said an idiopathic thrombophlebitis caused the disease and denied the presence of any vascular anomaly. Their illustrations do not uphold this statement but affirm the presence of an unusual degree of round cell infiltration. Blackwood[31] did not believe that a "varicose" condition of the meningeal veins, being absent in two of his four cases, was always present in subacute necrotic myelitis. He deplored the lack of information on the state of the paravertebral and lumbar veins and considered that insufficient

information was at hand for anyone to be certain of the pathogenesis. Subsequent authors consider the syndrome to be caused essentially by arteriovenous aneurysms with secondary ischemic manifestations in the cord itself.[10,229] The increase in inflammatory cells occasionally seen in the cerebrospinal fluid or in the cord could be associated with the necrotic changes in the cord and phlebothrombosis.[384] Then again inflammatory cell infiltration has been observed in one cerebral arteriovenous aneurysm where it could conceivably have been caused by a secondary infection associated with the hemodynamic disturbance as with poststenotic dilatations and patent ductus arteriosus. Such might explain the case of Mair and Folkerts,[193] whereas meningeal fibrosis or evidence of mild arachnoiditis has been attributed to the repeated leakage of blood[316] and underlying ischemic changes in the cord.

Associated findings

CEREBROSPINAL FLUID. Arseni and Samitca[13] found the cerebrospinal fluid protein increased in 50% of their cases, with levels ranging from 40 to 320 mg. though most were below 100 mg. per 100 ml. of fluid. When hemorrhage occurs naturally, the fluid is blood stained and xanthochromic staining persists for days.

CUTANEOUS HEMANGIOMAS. Cobb[58] described the case of an 8-year-old boy with a port-wine stain on the left side of the back and three on the right side of the trunk at the level of the umbilicus. Symptoms and signs were consistent with pressure on the cord, a consequence of a large arteriovenous aneurysm. Cobb[58] suggested that the cutaneous nevi may be of considerable diagnostic value though they are by no means always metameric in location. Most cord lesions associated with segmental cutaneous hemangiomas are found in the lower thoracic and lumbar segments. Several similar cases have since been reported.[68,104,321] Of 18 spinal or extradural lesions studied by Turner and Kernohan,[354] only one was associated with a hemangioma involving the skin and muscles of the corresponding metameres. Two were found in Wyburn-Mason's series of 32 cases, and Newman[229] collected only six instances of spinal arteriovenous aneurysm with a cutaneous angioma in the corresponding segment of skin in more than 150 cases.

Fine[97] reported the case of a young woman of 26 years with a history extending over 11 years including exacerbations during a pregnancy and after a fall. The right upper limb had extensive involvement by reddish blue vascular nevi particularly over the ulnar surface of the hand and forearm. They were of irregular size, and some were compressible, raised above the skin, and associated with a variable degree of hyperkeratinization. A few small lesions were present over the extensor surface of the arm and forearm corresponding to the fifth to eighth cervical (C) segments. An additional nevus (4½ by 6 inches) was present to the right of the midline of the back analogous to the thoracic (T) segments T2 to T4. The temperature of the right forearm was higher than that of the left. Neurological deficit was prominent in both lower limbs. In the spinal canal, a mass of enlarged pulsating arteries and veins lay over the cord, some vessels entering it at the level of C5. An audible bruit was present over the back. Several of the lesions in the right forearm were demonstrated by angiography to be arteriovenous fistulas complicated by ulceration and bleeding.

Doppman and his colleagues[86] found vascular nevi in six of a series of 28 patients with arteriovenous aneurysms of the spinal cord. They uncovered 10 similar instances in the literature up to 1969 and found that poorly discernible vascular nevi became very congested and prominent during the Valsalva maneuver. They went on to point out that the cutaneous hemangioma, when in the same metamere as the spinal lesion, was supplied by the same segmental artery. It seems that the anatomical connections of the venous drainage system with the vertebral would more likely result in the congestion during the Valsalva maneuver

than it would in an augmentation of arterial flow.

The association of these cutaneous hemangiomas with spinal aneurysms (and venous angiomas) has yet to be explained satisfactorily. The concurrence has been likened to the Sturge-Weber syndrome and so it would seem that examination of the spinal cord is essential in cases in which the cutaneous hemangioma extends over the trunk or a limb.

OTHER CARDIOVASCULAR LESIONS. No hemodynamic studies have been performed on these arteriovenous aneurysms of the spinal cord, and the vessels involved are probably too small to cause cardiac embarrassment. Before vessels progress to such a stage, spinal cord symptoms probably supervene. Though not common, bruits are known to occur with these spinal lesions.[200] Ommaya and associates[248] reported an incidence of only one in 26 cases.

Di Chiro[78] has recorded the case of a 19-year-old youth who lost the sight of both eyes because of retinal angiomatoses. At age 26, he was found to have at least two arteriovenous aneurysms in the posterior fossa and two in the cervical region.

Vascular lesions associated with spinal arteriovenous aneurysms include hemangioma of a vertebra,[229] cerebral arterial aneurysm,[41,85] arteriovenous aneurysm of the lung, arteriovenous aneurysm of the liver, and a probable renal arteriovenous aneurysm.[79] Wyburn-Mason[391] reported three cases associated with a patent ductus arteriosus.

Etiology. The etiology of arteriovenous aneurysms is believed to be similar to that of intracranial lesions. The maldevelopment is thought to originate at the stage of differentiation of the primitive capillary plexus of vessels destined to supply the cord and the more superficial structures supplied by the segmental vessels. This theory persists primarily for want of a better hypothesis.

Within the cranium, trauma is a likely cause of many lesions currently believed to be congenital, and so it is possible that trauma is also the cause of lesions of the cord. Elsberg[92] tells of a 13-year-old boy who after a fall suffered spinal concussion that confined him to bed for several days. One year later symptoms of spinal cord compression developed because of an arteriovenous aneurysm.

Reference to Table 10-10 indicates that a remarkable number of the afflicted are well past the age when most congenital developmental defects manifest themselves, and in view of the pernicious, progressive nature of these lesions the long lag period inherent in the age distribution cannot be accepted without question. The possibility that the development of an arteriovenous shunt is secondary to some other unrecognized lesion cannot be completely disregarded either, for the latter may ultimately become hidden or superceded by the progression of the former. Cutaneous hemangiomas are difficult to explain, but their existence lends support to the developmental theory.

Enlarged collaterals in the spinal cord. Elsberg[92] attributed some spinal varicosities to obstruction of drainage channels, removal of which relieves the venous congestion. MacLean[192] showed that enlargement of the anterior spinal veins with secondary compression and destruction of the spinal cord (cervical segment) followed thrombosis of the superior longitudinal sinus, the lateral sinuses, and the torcular Herophili in an infant. The accompanying illustration was of a large vein lying within a deep indentation in the cord, comparable in this instance, to a simple venous varix.[354] It is doubtful whether the entity exists, because the venous collateral circulation is rich in anastomoses and alternative pathways, except in the presence of gross obstructive vascular disease. More probably, MacLean's case had two distinct lesions, with that of the spine being a vascular anomaly. Wyburn-Mason[391] emphasized that the spinal arteries participate in the collateral circulation in coarctation of the aorta, and a greatly expanded and tortuous anterior spinal artery may be formed as in Fig. 2-9.

Such is a secondary phenomenon and not a vascular anomaly in itself. An aneurysm may be found along the course of the enlarged artery.

Pial varicosities can occur in association with hemangioblastomas of the cord.[163]

Extradural arteriovenous aneurysms. Extradural arteriovenous aneurysms are encountered less often than are those which implicate the cord, though secondary involvement of cord vessels could occur if the lesion were sufficiently chronic, but this aspect has not been investigated. Hemorrhage results in an extradural hemorrhage and spinal cord compression without subarachnoid hemorrhage.

Johnston[153] discovered an extradural vascular anomaly in a 5-year-old boy with a cutaneous hemangioma (8 cm. in diameter) just below the left scapula. The anomaly, described as a hemangioma, was in all probability an arteriovenous aneurysm, hemorrhage from which had caused a transverse pressure lesion of the cord at about the tenth thoracic segment of the cord. The child died 3 years later from renal failure secondary to pyelonephritis associated with the paraplegia.

Hemangiomas of the vertebral column. Hemangioma of the vertebral column was once thought to be a rare tumor, but since then postmortem studies of the vertebral column have yielded a frequency of 12% in 2154 necropsies.[349] Mostly, they do not cause serious clinical disturbances. Between 1935 and 1956, there were 15 (4.4%) vertebral hemangiomas in the 340 patients with vertebral tumors (admitted to a neurosurgical clinic in Bucharest).[14] Macroscopically, they are dark red in contrast with paler surrounding tissues. Characteristically they consist of a mass of thin-walled vascular channels in the form of a capillary hemangioma, or they are closely packed dilated channels constituting the more common type, the cavernous hemangioma. Microscopically, there is evidence both of bone absorption and new bone formation. The architecture of the bony trabeculae is grossly disturbed and thickened. Vertically oriented trabeculae are seen in the vertebral bodies.[45] Encroachment upon the vertebral canal occurs as the result of thickening and ballooning of the cortex of the vertebral bodies posteriorly and of spread into and thickening of the pedicles and laminae. The angioma may extend to the extradural space. Compression of the spinal cord or of the nerve roots is virtually unavoidable and is the major complication.[17,45] Actual spinal block occurs occasionally.[125] The most common vertebrae involved[165] are those from the third to the tenth thoracic, particularly the fourth thorracic although any part of the spine including the sacrum can be affected. Cervical vertebrae are rarely involved.[14,45] From one to four adjacent vertebrae may be involved, and although there is considerable osteolytic activity, there is little tendency to compression of the vertebral bodies, though this has been reported.[282]

Enlargement of paravertebral and extradural veins may be noted.[165] Hemorrhage into the extradural space can produce a spinal extradural hematoma and even the subarachnoid space may be involved.[14] Postoperative hemorrhage is frequent and can be difficult to control.

Arseni and Simionescu[14] found the average age to be 30 years. However, in Töpfer's study[349] of 257 hemangiomas at autopsy, less than 10% were under the age of 40 years, and 40% of all the lesions occurred in subjects over the age of 70. In the absence of information concerning the age distribution of the necropsy population studied, definite conclusions should not be drawn, but the results suggest that many of these hemangiomas could be acquired. Clinically they are more prevalent in females than males, and in one instance the clinical onset was precipitated by pregnancy.[14] Another patient of 35 years became paraplegic in her eighth month of pregnancy because of an intradural racemose angioma. She recovered, and 2 years later, after a relapse, a concomitant hemangioma of a lumbar vertebra was found. Occasionally other bones or viscera may

be incorporated by a form of hemangiomatosis,[165] and Nemours-Auguste[225] encountered the probable simultaneous involvement of skin and brain in one case.

Hemangiomas of the calvarium. Hemangiomas of the calvarium, though rare entities, are nevertheless the second most frequent site of intraosseous hemangiomas. Wyke[392] estimated that they constitute approximately 0.2% of all bone neoplasms and 10% of all primary benign neoplasms of the skull. Hemangiomas may arise in the skin and brain; trauma, followed immediately by pain, tenderness, and frequently swelling, is their usual mode of onset.[45,288] These hemangiomas, similar to those of the vertebrae, are for the most part cavernous and less often capillary in type. Small blood cysts may be visible macroscopically on the surface.[301]

The parietal and frontal bones are their most frequent sites[45,392] although other bones of the skull including the occipital and petrous portion of the temporal and mandible may be involved. Multiple cranial lesions are present in an estimated 15% of cases,[301] and they can be bilateral.[350] The hemangioma causes a biconvex swelling of the flat bone and pulsation of the center may be noted. The bony cortex may be eroded, but the periosteum usually remains intact, even though distended, and breaching of the pericranium or dura mater never comes to pass. The underlying brain is compressed. Hemangiomas may occur in the skin, brain, and liver.[194] Scheinberg and Elkin[304] reported a hemangioma of the occipital bone in association with an arteriovenous aneurysm of the left parietal zone without vascular communication between them.

Radiologically a characteristic "sunburst" appearance of the trabeculations is to be seen. There may be stippling of the translucent zone and a sclerotic rim may be a feature in a round to oval area of translucency.[45,288] Bucy and Capp[45] asserted that one hemangioma, believed to arise from the meninges, secondarily invaded the parietal bone with osseous changes similar to those seen in primary hemangiomas of the calvarium. In a case reported by Rosenbaum and associates,[288] the lesion of the parietal bone was supplied by the superficial temporal artery and to a lesser extent by the middle meningeal artery as demonstrated by external carotid angiography. Distribution of the contrast medium within the lesion was patchy and the circulation slow. The blood supply is only infrequently derived from the internal carotid artery as may be the case when the middle meningeal artery emerges from the ophthalmic artery. Enlargement and tortuosity of feeding vessels is seldom seen and is probably associated with large hemangiomas.[182] Davis and associates[75] considered the circulation of these hemangiomas to be relatively fast but this too seems to be variable.[288] The underlying intracranial vessels can be extensively displaced,[301] although the patient seen by Lombardi and Larini[182] exhibited considerable cortical atrophy with neurological signs. These signs occur only sporadically. Kessler and associates[157] recorded massive extradural hemorrhage from a cavernous hemangioma of the petrous portion of the temporal bone, together with bleeding from the external auditory canal.

Pool and Potts[268] described the case of a young girl with a corrected Fallot's tetralogy, progressive unilateral proptosis, and bulging of the adjacent temporal and frontal aspects of the skull. A bruit was audible over the lesion, and prominent pulsating arteries were clearly visible in the overlying scalp. A large almost spherical enlargement of the bone bulged into the orbit and displaced the eye. The lesion, which was supplied by the external carotid artery, was removed and considered to be an arteriovenous hemangioma or malformation. The rapid circulation of blood through some hemangiomas[288] and the palpable pulsation over some of these calvarial lesions suggest that the distinction between them and the arteriovenous aneurysms may be somewhat arbitrary.

References

1. Abrahamson, I. A., and Bell, L. B.: Carotid-cavernous fistula syndrome, Amer. J. Ophthal. **39:**521, 1955.
2. af Björkesten, G., and Troupp, H.: Arteriovenous malformations of the brain, Acta Psychiat. Neurol. Scand. 34:429, 1959.
3. Agee, O. F., Musella, R., and Tweed, C. G.: Aneurysm of the great vein of Galen, J. Neurosurg. 31:346, 1969.
4. Aguilar, M. J., Kamoshita, S., Landing, B. H., Boder, E., and Sedgwick, R. P.: Pathological observations in ataxia-telangiectasia, J. Neuropath. Exp. Neurol. 27:659, 1968.
5. Alexander, G. L., and Norman, R. M.: The Sturge-Weber syndrome, Bristol, 1960, John Wright and Sons Ltd.
6. Alpers, B. J., and Forster, F. M.: Arteriovenous aneurysm of great vein of Galen and arteries of circle of Willis, Arch. Neurol. Psychiat. **54:**181, 1945.
7. Ameli, N. O.: Brain angiomata and intracerebral haematoma. In Luyendijk, W.: Cerebral circulation, Progr. Brain Res. **30:**427, 1968.
8. Anderson, F. M., and Korbin, M. A.: Arteriovenous anomalies of the brain, Neurology **8:**89, 1958.
9. Anderson, R. McD., and Blackwood, W.: The association of arteriovenous angioma and saccular aneurysm of the arteries of the brain, J. Path. Bact. 77:101, 1959.
10. Antoni, N.: Spinal vascular malformations (angiomas) and myelomalacia, Neurology **12:**795, 1962.
11. Arnould, G., Dureux, J. B., Tridon, P., Picard, L., Weber, M., Thiriet, M., and Floquet, J.: Malformations vasculaires cérébrales et angiomatose de Rendu-Osler, Rev. Neurol. **119:**230, 1968.
12. Arseni, C., Ghitescu, M., Cristescu, A., Mihaila, G., and Dragotoiu, E.: Traumatic carotido-cavernous fistulas, Psychiat. Neurol. Neurochir. **73:**237, 1970.
13. Arseni, C., and Samitca, D. C.-T.: Vascular malformations of the spinal cord, Acta Psychiat. Neurol. Scand. 34:10, 1959.
14. Arseni, C., and Simionescu, M. D.: Vertebral hemangiomata, Acta Psychiat. Neurol. Scand. **34:**1, 1959.
15. Bailey, O. T.: The vascular component of congenital malformations in the central nervous system, J. Neuropath. Exp. Neurol. **20:**171, 1961.
16. Bailey, O. T., and Woodard, J. S.: Small vascular malformations of the brain: their relationship to unexpected death, hydrocephalus, and mental deficiency, J. Neuropath. Exp. Neurol. **18:**98, 1959.
17. Bailey, P., and Bucy, P. C.: Cavernous hemangioma of the vertebrae, J.A.M.A. **92:**1748, 1929.
18. Bailey, W. L., and Sperl, M. P.: Angiomas of the cervical spinal cord, J. Neurosurg. **30:**560, 1969.
19. Barker, W. F., Stern, W. E., Krayenbühl, H., and Senning, A.: Carotid endarterectomy com-

plicated by carotid cavernous sinus fistula, Ann. Surg. **167:**568, 1968.

20. Bassett, R. C.: Surgical experiences with arteriovenous anomalies of the brain, J. Neurosurg. **8:**59, 1951.

21. Bassett, R. C., Peet, M. M., and Holt, J. F.: Pial-medullary angiomas: clinicopathologic features and treatment, Arch. Neurol. Psychiat. **61:**558, 1949.

22. Bean, W. B.: Vascular changes of the skin in pregnancy: vascular spiders and palmar erythema, Surg. Gynec. Obstet. **88:**739, 1949.

23. Bean, W. B.: Vascular spiders and related lesions of the skin, Springfield, Ill., 1958, Charles C Thomas, Publisher.

24. Béraud, R., and Meloche, B. R.: À propos des malformation de deux cas et revue de littérature, Un. Med. Canada **94:**176, 1965.

25. Bergstrand, A., Höök, O., and Lidvall, H.: Vascular malformations of the spinal cord, Acta Neurol. Scand. **40:**169, 1964.

26. Bernsmeier, A., and Siemons, K.: Zur Messung der Hirndurchblutung bei intrakraniellen Gefässanomalien und deren Auswirkung auf den allgemeinen Kreislauf, Z. Kreislaufforsch. **41:**845, 1952.

27. Berry, R. G., Alpers, B J., and White, J. C.: The site, structure, and frequency of intracranial aneurysms, angiomas, and arteriovenous abnormalities. In: Cerebrovascular disease, Ass. Res. Nerv. Ment. Dis. **41:**40, 1966.

28. Bessman, A. N., Hayes, G. J., Alman, R. W., and Fazekas, J. F.: Cerebral hemodynamics in cerebral arteriovenous vascular anomalies, Med. Ann. District Columbia **21:**422, 1952.

29. Bielawski, J. G., and Tatelman, M.: Intracranial calcification in encephalotrigeminal angiomatosis, Amer. J. Roentgen. **62:**247, 1949.

30. Blackwood, W.: Two cases of benign cerebral telangiectasis, J. Path. Bact. **52:**209, 1941.

31. Blackwood, W.: Discussion on vascular disease of the spinal cord, Proc. Roy. Soc. Med. **51:**543, 1958.

32. Blackwood, W.: Vascular disease of the central nervous system. In Blackwood, W., McMenemey, W. H., Meyer, A., Norman, R. M., and Russell, D. S.: Greenfield's neuropathology, ed. 2, Baltimore, 1963, The Williams & Wilkins Co., p. 71.

33. Bleasel, K., and Frew, J.: Vascular compression of the optic nerves relieved by anastomosis of carotid artery to jugular vein, J. Neurol. Neurosurg. Psychiat. **32:**268, 1969.

34. Bloor, B. M., Odom, G. L., and Woodhall, B.: Direct measurement of intravascular pressure in components of the circle of Willis, Arch. Surg. **63:**821, 1951.

35. Boder, E., and Sedgwick, R. P.: Ataxia-telangiectasia: a familial syndrome of progressive cerebellar ataxia, oculocutaneous telangiectasia and frequent pulmonary infections, Pediatrics **21:**526, 1958.

36. Boldrey, E., Adams, J. E., and Brown, H. A.: Scoliosis as a manifestation of disease of the cervicothoracic portion of the spinal cord, Arch. Neurol. Psychiat. **61:**528, 1949.

37. Boldrey, E., and Miller, E. R.: Arteriovenous fistula (aneurysm) of the great cerebral vein (of Galen) and the circle of Willis, Arch. Neurol. Psychiat. **62:**778, 1949.

38. Boyd-Wilson, J. S.: The association of cerebral angiomas with intracranial aneurysms, J. Neurol. Neurosurg. Psychiat. **22:**218, 1959.

39. Bregman, L. E., and Mesz: Sur un cas d'angiome du crâne et du cerveau, Rev. Neurol. **2:**191, 1927.

40. Brihaye, J., and Blackwood, W.: Arteriovenous aneurysm of the cerebral hemispheres, J. Path. Bact. **73:**25, 1957.

41. Brion, S., Netsky, M. G., and Zimmerman, H. M.: Vascular malformations of the spinal cord, Arch. Neurol. Psychiat. **68:**339, 1952.

42. Brock, S., and Dyke, C. G.: Venous and arterio-venous angiomas of the brain: a clinical and roentgenographic study of eight cases, Bull. Neurol. Inst. N.Y. **2:**247, 1932.

43. Brooksaler, F.: The angioosteohypertrophy syndrome: Klippel-Trénaunay-Weber syndrome, Amer. J. Dis. Child. **112:**161, 1966.

44. Brucns, J. H., Guazzi, G. C., and Martin, J. J.: Infantile form of meningeal angiomatosis with sudanophilic leucodystrophy associated with complex abiotrophies. Study of a second family, J. Neurol. Sci. **7:**117, 1968.

45. Bucy, P. C., and Capp, C. S.: Primary hemangioma of bone with special reference to roentgenologic diagnosis, Amer. J. Roentgen. **23:**1, 1930.

46. Burke, E. C., Winkelman, R. K., and Strickland, M. K.: Disseminated hemangiomatosis: the newborn with central nervous system involvement, Amer. J. Dis. Child. **108:**418, 1964

47. Cantu, R. C., Ferris, E. J., and Baker, E. P.: Collateral circulation to a parietal arteriovenous malformation following bilateral external carotid artery ligation, J. Neurosurg. **28:**369, 1968.

48. Caram, P. C.: Simultaneous occurrence of intracranial aneurysm and angioma, J. Neurosurg. **16:**230, 1959.

49. Caram, P. C., Sharkey, P. C., and Alvord, E. C.: Thalamic angioma and aneurysm of the anterior choroidal artery with intraventricular hematoma, J. Neurosurg. **17:**347, 1960.

50. Carleton, A., Elkington, J. St. C., Greenfield, J. G., and Robb-Smith, A. H. T.: Maffucci's syndrome (dyschondroplasia with haemangeiomata), Quart. J. Med. **11:**203, 1942.

51. Carrasco-Zanini, J.: Arteriovenous malformations of the brain and their effect upon the cerebral vessels, J. Neurol. Neurosurg. Psychiat. **20:**241, 1957.

52. Chandler, D.: Pulmonary and cerebral arteriovenous fistula with Osler's disease, Arch. Intern. Med. **116:**277, 1965.

53. Chao, D. H.: Congenital neurocutaneous syndromes of childhood. III. Sturge-Weber disease, J. Pediat. **55:**635, 1959.

54. Childers, R. W., Ranniger, K., and Rabinowitz, M.: Intrahepatic arteriovenous fistula with pulmonary vascular obstruction in Osler-

Rendu-Weber disease, Amer. J. Med. **43**:304, 1967.

55. Chou, S. N., Story, J. L., Seljeskog, E., and French, L. A.: Further experience with arteriovenous fistulas of the vertebral artery in the neck, Surgery **62**:779, 1967.

56. Christensen, E., and Larsen, H.: Fatal subarachnoid haemorrhages in pregnant women with intracranial and intramedullary vascular malformations, Acta Psychiat. Neurol. Scand. **29**:441, 1954.

57. Clarke, E., and Walton, J. N.: Subdural haematoma complicating intracranial aneurysm and angioma, Brain **76**:378, 1953.

58. Cobb, S.: Haemangioma of the spinal cord, Ann. Surg. **62**:641, 1915.

59. Cohen, H. J., and Kay, M. N.: Associated facial hemangioma and intracranial lesion (Weber-Dimitri disease), Amer. J. Dis. Child. **62**:606, 1941.

60. Cohen, M. M., Kristiansen, K., and Hval, E.: Arteriovenous malformations of the great vein of Galen, Neurology **4**:124, 1954.

61. Committee of the Advisory Council for the National Institute of Neurological Diseases and Blindness, Public Health Service: A classification and outline of cerebrovascular diseases, Neurology **8**:395, 1958.

62. Conforti, P.: Spontaneous disappearance of cerebral arteriovenous angioma, J. Neurosurg. **34**:432, 1971.

63. Courville, C. B.: Encephalic lesions in hereditary hemorrhagic telangiectasis (Rendu-Osler-Weber disease), Bull. Los Angeles Neurol. Soc. **22**:28, 1957.

64. Craig, J. M.: Encephalo-trigeminal angiomatosis (Sturge-Weber's disease), J. Neuropath. **8**:305, 1949.

65. Craig, W. McK., Keith, H. M., and Kernohan, J. W.: Tumors of the brain occurring in childhood, Acta Psychiat. Neurol. **24**:375, 1949.

66. Crawford, J. V., and Russell, D. S.: Cryptic arteriovenous and venous hamartomas of the brain, J. Neurol. Neurosurg. Psychiat. **19**:1, 1956.

67. Cronqvist, S., and Troupp, H.: Intracranial arteriovenous malformation and arterial aneurysm in the same patient, Acta Neurol. Scand. **42**:307, 1966.

68. Cross, G. O.: Subarachnoid cervical angioma with cutaneous hemangioma of a corresponding metamere, Arch. Neurol. Psychiat. **58**:359, 1947.

69. Cushing, H.: Cases of spontaneous intracranial hemorrhage associated with trigeminal nevi, J.A.M.A. **47**:178, 1906.

70. Cushing, H., and Bailey, P.: Tumors arising from the blood-vessels of the brain, Springfield, Ill., 1928, Charles C Thomas, Publisher.

71. Dandy, W. E.: Arteriovenous aneurysm of the brain, Arch. Surg. **17**:190, 1928.

72. Dandy, W. E.: Venous abnormalities and angiomas of the brain, Arch. Surg. **17**:715, 1928.

73. Dandy, W. E.: Carotid-cavernous aneurysms. (Pulsating exophthalmos), Zbl. Neurochir. **2**:77, 165, 1937.

74. Dandy, W. E., and Follis, R. H.: On the pathology of carotid-cavernous aneurysms (pulsating exophthalmos), Amer. J. Ophthalmol. **24**:365, 1941.

75. Davis, D. O., Rumbaugh, C. L., and Petty, J.: Calvarial hemangioma: tumor stain and meningeal artery blood supply, J. Neurosurg. **25**:561, 1966.

76. Davis, R. A., Wetzel, N., and Davis, L.: An analysis of the results of treatment of intracranial vascular lesions by carotid artery ligation, Ann. Surg. **143**:641, 1956.

77. Delens, E.: De la communication de la carotide interne et du sinus caverneux, Thesis, Paris, 1870. Cited by Holman.[186]

78. Di Chiro, G.: Combined retino-cerebellar angiomatosis and deep cervical angiomas, J. Neurosurg. **14**:685, 1957.

79. Di Chiro, G., Doppman, J., and Ommaya, A. K.: Selective arteriography of arteriovenous aneurysms of spinal cord, Radiology **88**:1065, 1967.

80. Di Chiro, G., and Lindgren, E.: Radiographic findings in 14 cases of Sturge-Weber syndrome, Acta Radiol. **35**:387, 1951.

81. Dillard, B. M., Nelson, D. L., and Norman, H. G.: Review of 85 major traumatic arterial injuries, Surgery **63**:391, 1968.

82. Divry, P., and Van Bogaert, L.: Une maladie familiale caractérisée par une angiomatose diffuse cortico-méningée non calcifiante et une démyélinisation progressive de la substance blanche, J. Neurol. Neurosurg. **9**:41, 1946.

83. Djindjian, R., Dumesnil, M., Faure, C., and Tavernier, C.: Angiome médullaire dorsal (étude clinique et artériographique), Rev. Neurol. **108**:432, 1963.

84. Donald, J. M.: Aneurysm of the left common iliac artery secondary to a traumatic arteriovenous fistula of the left popliteal vessels, Ann. Surg. **127**:780, 1948.

85. Doppman, J., and Di Chiro, G.: Subtraction-angiography of spinal cord vascular malformations, J. Neurosurg. **23**:440, 1965.

86. Doppman, J. L., Wirth, F. P., Di Chiro, G., and Ommaya, A. K.: Value of cutaneous angiomas in the arteriographic localization of spinal-cord arteriovenous malformations, New Eng. J. Med. **281**:1440, 1969.

87. Dunn, J. M., and Raskind, R.: Rupture of a cerebral arteriovenous malformation during pregnancy, Obstet. Gynec. **30**:423, 1967.

88. Echols, D. H., and Jackson, J. D.: Carotid-cavernous fistula: a perplexing surgical problem, J. Neurosurg. **16**:619, 1959.

89. Editorial: A spot for Holmes? Lancet **1**:824, 1970.

90. El Gindi, S., and Andrew, J.: Successful closure of carotid cavernous fistula by the use of acrylic, J. Neurosurg. **27**:153, 1967.

91. Elkington, J. St. C.: Cerebral vascular accidents unassociated with cardiovascular disease, Lancet **1**:6, 1935.

92. Elsberg, C. A.: Surgical diseases of the spinal cord, membranes and nerve roots, New York, 1941, Paul B. Hoeber, Inc.

93. Epstein, J. A., Beller, A. J., and Cohen, I.:

Arterial anomalies of the spinal cord, J. Neurosurg. **6**:45, 1949.

94. Evans, N. G., and Courville, C. B.: Notes on the pathogenesis and morphology of new growths, malformations, and deformities of the intracranial blood-vessels, Bull. Los Angeles Neurol. Soc. **4**:145, 1939.

95. Farrell, D. F., and Forno, L. S.: Symptomatic capillary telangiectasis of the brainstem without hemorrhage, Neurology **20**:341, 1970.

96. Fincher, E. F.: Arteriovenous fistula between the middle meningeal artery and the greater petrosal sinus, Ann. Surg. **133**:886, 1951.

97. Fine, R. D.: Angioma racemosum venosum of spinal cord with segmentally related angiomatous lesions of skin and forearm, J. Neurosurg. **18**:546, 1961.

98. François, P., Woillez, M., Warrot, P., and Maillet, P.: Maladie d'Ehlers-Danlos avec anévrysme artério-veineux intra-crânien, Bull. Soc. Ophtal. France, no. 5, pp. 392, May 1955.

99. French, L. A., and Peyton, W. T.: Vascular malformations in the region of the great vein of Galen, J. Neurosurg. **11**:488, 1954.

100. Gagnon, J., and Boileau, G.: Anatomical study of an arteriovenous malformation drained by the system of Galen, J. Neurosurg. **17**:75, 1960.

101. Gerlach, J., and Jensen, H. P.: Die intracerebralen Haematome bei Mikroangiomen, Acta Neurochir. Suppl. **7**:367, 1961.

102. Geschickter, C. F., and Keasby, L. E.: Tumors of blood vessels, Amer. J. Cancer **23**:568, 1935.

103. Gibson, R. M., and da Rocha Melo, A. N.: Angiographic finding of an aneurysm and arteriovenous malformation in the posterior cranial fossa in a case of subarachnoid haemorrhage, J. Neurol. Neurosurg. Psychiat. **23**:237, 1960.

104. Gilbert, I.: Angioma venosum racemosum with angiomatous lesions of skin and omentum, Brit. Med. J. **1**:468, 1952.

105. Globus, J. H., and Doshay, L. J.: Venous dilatations and other intraspinal vessel alterations, including true angiomata, with signs and symptoms of cord compression, Surg. Gynec. Obstet. **48**:345, 1929.

106. Gold, A. P., Ransohoff, J., and Carter, S.: Vein of Galen malformation, Acta Neurol. Scand. **40** (suppl. 11):1, 1964.

107. Goldstein, H. I.: Hereditary epistaxis: with and without hereditary (familial) multiple hemorrhagic telangiectasia (Osler's disease), Int. Clin. **3**:148, 1930; **4**:253, 1930.

108. Gomez, M. R., Whitten, C. F., Nolke, A., Bernstein, J., and Meyer, J. S.: Aneurysmal malformation of the great vein of Galen causing heart failure in early infancy, Pediatrics **31**:400, 1963.

109. Goran, A., Carlson, D. J., and Fisher, R. G.: Successful treatment of intramedullary angioma of the cord, J. Neurosurg. **21**:311, 1964.

110. Graf, C. J.: Spontaneous carotid-cavernous fistula: Ehlers-Danlos syndrome and related conditions, Arch. Neurol. **13**:662, 1965.

111. Graf, C. J.: Carotid-basilar venous plexus fistula, J. Neurosurg. **33**:191, 1970.

112. Green, J. R.: Encephalo-trigeminal angiomatosis, J. Neuropath. Exp. Neurol. **4**:27, 1945.

113. Greenfield, J. G., and Turner, J. W. A.: Acute and subacute necrotic myelitis, Brain **62**:227, 1939.

114. Greenwald, H. M., and Koota, J.: Associated facial and intracranial hemangiomas, Amer. J. Dis. Child. **51**:868, 1936.

115. Gross, S. W., and Ralston, B. L.: Vascular malformations of the spinal cord, Surg. Gynec. Obstet. **108**:673, 1959.

116. Guida, P. M., and Moore, S. W.: Aneurysms and arteriovenous fistulas of the temporal artery, Amer. J. Surg. **115**:825, 1968.

117. Gupta, P. D., Fort, M. L., Barron, K. D., Baron, J. K., and Sharp, J. T.: Cardiac hemodynamics in intracranial arteriovenous fistula, Neurology **19**:198, 1969.

118. Gurdjian, E. S., Thomas, L. M., Herman, L. H., and Portnoy, H. D.: Angiographic findings in 300 cases of aneurysm, arteriovenous malformation, and subarachnoid hemorrhage. In Fields, W. S., and Sahs, A. L.: Intracranial aneurysms and subarachnoid hemorrhage, Springfield, Ill., 1965, Charles C Thomas, Publisher, p. 143.

119. Gurdjian, E. S., Webster, J. E., and Martin, F. A.: Carotid-internal jugular anastomosis in the rhesus monkey, J. Neurosurg. **7**:467, 1950.

120. Haberland, K.: Über ein spinales Angioma racemosum venosum, Arch. Psychiat. **184**:417, 1950.

121. Häggendal, E., Ingvar, D. H., Lassen, N. A., Nilsson, N. J., Norlén, G., Wickbom, I., and Zwetnow, N.: Pre- and postoperative measurements of regional cerebral blood flow in three cases of intracranial arteriovenous aneurysms, J. Neurosurg. **22**:1, 1965.

122. Hahn, E. V.: Sinus pericranii (reducible blood tumor of the cranium), Arch. Surg. **16**:31, 1928.

123. Hamby, W. B.: The pathology of supratentorial angiomas, J. Neurosurg. **15**:65, 1958.

124. Hamby, W. B.: Carotid-cavernous fistula, Springfield, Ill., 1966, Charles C Thomas, Publisher.

125. Hammes, E. M.: Cavernous hemangioma of the vertebrae, Arch. Neurol. Psychiat. **29**:1330, 1933.

126. Hauge, T.: Personal communication. Cited by Shephard.[316]

127. Hauser, K.: Das arterio-venöse Aneurysma der Arteria carotis interna im Sinus cavernosis. Ein therapeutisches Problem. Inaugural dissertation, University of Zürich, 1966.

128. Hawkins, C. F., and Rewell, R. E.: Unheralded fatal haemorrhages in haemangiomata of the brain, Guy's Hosp. Rep. **95**:88, 1946.

129. Hawthorne, C. O.: Cerebral and cerebellar haemorrhages in apparently healthy adolescents and children, Practitioner **109**:425, 1922.

130. Henderson, W. R., and Gomez, R. de R. L.: Natural history of cerebral angiomas, Brit. Med. J. **4**:571, 1967.

131. Henson, R. A., and Croft, P. B.: Spontaneous

spinal subarachnoid haemorrhage, Quart. J. Med. **25**:53, 1956.

132. Hieke, L.: Über Hämatomyelie bei intramedullären Teleangiektasien, Beitr. Path. Anat. **110**:433, 1949.

133. Hirano, A., and Terry, R. D.: Aneurysm of the vein of Galen, J. Neuropath. Exp. Neurol. **17**:424, 1958.

134. Hoffmann, G. R., and de Haene, A.: A propos de l'angiome médullaire; exérèse complète; guérison, Neurochirurgie **7**:138, 1961.

135. Holman, E.: Experimental studies in arteriovenous fistulas. III. Cardiac dilatation and blood vessel changes, Arch. Surg. **9**:856, 1924.

136. Holman, E.: Abnormal arteriovenous communications peripheral and intracardiac acquired and congenital, ed. 2, Springfield, Ill., 1968, Charles C Thomas, Publisher.

137. Holman, E., Gerbode, F., and Richards, V.: Communications between the carotid artery and cavernous sinus, Angiology **2**:311, 1951.

138. Hong, R., and Ammann, A. J.: Ataxia telangiectasia, New Eng. J. Med. **283**:660, 1970.

139. Höök, O., and Johanson, C.: Intracranial arteriovenous aneurysms: a follow-up study with particular attention to their growth, Arch. Neurol. Psychiat. **80**:39, 1958.

140. Höök, O., and Lindvall, H.: Arteriovenous aneurysms of the spinal cord. A report of two cases investigated by vertebral angiography, J. Neurosurg. **15**:84, 1958.

141. Hopkins, C. A., Wilkie, F. L., and Voris, D. C.: Extramedullary aneurysm of the spinal cord, J. Neurosurg. **24**:1021, 1966.

142. Hosoi, K.: Multiple intracranial angiomas, Amer. J. Path. **6**:235, 1930.

143. Houdart, R., Djindjian, R., and Hurth, M.: Vascular malformations of the spinal cord. The anatomic and therapeutic significance of arteriography, J. Neurosurg. **24**:583, 1966.

144. Hurth, M., Djindjian, R., and Houdart, R.: L'exérèse complète des anévrysmes artérioveineux de la moelle épinière. Intérêt de l'árteriographie médullaire sélective. A propos de 11 cas, Neurochirurgie **14**:499, 1968.

145. Ingebrigtsen, R., Krog, J., and Leraand, S.: Velocity and flow of blood in the femoral artery proximal to an experimental arteriovenous fistula, Acta Chir. Scand. **124**:45, 1962.

146. Jackson, D. C., and duBoulay, G. H.: Traumatic arterio-venous aneurysm of the middle meningeal artery, Brit. J. Radiol. **37**:788, 1964.

147. Jaeger, R.: Discussion, J. Neurosurg. **16**:626, 1959.

148. Jaffé, R. H.: Multiple hemangiomas of the skin and of the internal organs, Arch. Path. **7**:44, 1929.

149. Jamieson, K. G.: Aneurysms of the vertebrobasilar system, J. Neurosurg. **21**:781, 1964.

150. Jamieson, K. G.: Vertebral arteriovenous fistula caused by angiography needle, J. Neurosurg. **23**:620, 1965.

151. Jensen, H., Brumlik, J., and Boshes, B.: The application of serial angiography to diagnosis of the smallest cerebral angiomatous malformations, J. Nerv. Ment. Dis. **136**:1, 1963.

152. Johnson, M. C., and Salmon, J. H.: Arterio-

153. Johnston, L. M.: Epidural hemangioma with compression of spinal cord, J.A.M.A. **110**:119, 1938.

154. Kaplan, H. A., Aronson, S. M., and Browder, E. J.: Vascular malformations of the brain, J. Neurosurg. **18**:630, 1961.

155. Karshner, R. G., Rand, C. W., and Reeves, D. L.: Epidural hemangioma associated with hemangioma of the vertebrae, Arch. Surg. **39**:942, 1939.

156. Kaufman, H. H., Ommaya, A. K., Di Chiro, G., and Doppman, J. L.: Compression vs 'steal'. The pathogenesis of symptoms in arteriovenous malformations of the spinal cord, Arch. Neurol. **23**:173, 1970.

157. Kessler, L. A., Lubic, L. G., and Koskoff, Y. D.: Epidural hemorrhage secondary to cavernous hemangioma of the petrous portion of the temporal bone, J. Neurosurg. **14**:329, 1957.

158. Kidd, H. A., and Cumings, J. N.: Cerebral angiomata in an Icelandic family, Lancet **1**:747, 1947.

159. Krabbe, K. H.: Facial meningeal angiomatosis associated with calcifications of the brain cortex, Arch. Neurol. Psychiat. **32**:737, 1934.

160. Krayenbühl, H., and Siebermann, R.: Small vascular malformations as a cause of primary intracerebral hemorrhage, J. Neurosurg. **22**:7, 1965.

161. Krayenbühl, H., and Yaşargil, M. G.: Das Hirnaneurysma, Basel, 1958, J. R. Geigy S. A.

162. Krayenbühl, H., Yaşargil, M. G., and McClintock, H. G.: Treatment of spinal cord vascular malformations by surgical excision, J. Neurosurg. **30**:427, 1969.

163. Krishnan, K. R., and Smith, W. T.: Intramedullary haemangioblastoma of the spinal cord associated with pial varicosities simulating intradural angioma, J. Neurol. Neurosurg. Psychiat. **24**:350, 1961.

164. Kristiansen, K., and Krog, J.: Electromagnetic studies on the blood flow through the carotid system in man, Neurology **12**:20, 1962.

165. Krueger, E. G., Sobel, G. L., and Weinstein, C.: Vertebral hemangioma with compression of the spinal cord, J. Neurosurg. **18**:331, 1961.

166. Kunc, Z., and Bret, J.: Congenital arteriosinusal fistulae, Acta Neurochirurg. **20**:85, 1969.

167. Kunc, Z., and Bret, J.: Diagnosis and treatment of vascular malformations of the spinal cord, J. Neurosurg. **30**:436, 1969.

168. Landing, B. H., and Farber, S.: Tumors of the cardiovascular system. In: Atlas of tumor pathology, Section 3, Fascicle 7, Washington, 1956, Armed Forces Institute of Pathology.

169. Langmaid, C.: Personal communication. Cited by Shephard.[316]

170. Larson, S. J., and Worman, L. W.: Internal carotid artery flow rate during craniotomy and muscle embolization for carotid cavernous fistula, J. Neurosurg. **29**:1958, 1968.

171. Lassen, N. A., and Munck, O.: Cerebral blood flow in arteriovenous anomalies of the brain determined by the use of radioactive krypton

85, Acta Psychiat. Neurol. Scand. **31**:71, 1956.

172. Lee, S. H., Fisher, B., Fisher, E. R., and Little, A.: Arteriovenous fistula and bacterial endocarditis, Surgery **52**:463, 1962.

173. Levine, O. R., Jameson, A. G., Nellhaus, G., and Gold, A. P.: Cardiac complications of cerebral arteriovenous fistula in infancy, Pediatrics **30**:563, 1962.

174. Lichtensteiger, W. H.: Angioma arteriovenosum aneurysmaticum des Kleinhirns mit Polycythamie (Polyglobulie) und terminaler Massenblutung, Schweiz. Med. Wschr. **94**:720, 1964.

175. Lichtenstein, B. W.: Sturge-Weber-Dimitri syndrome: cephalic form of neurocutaneous hemangiomatosis, Arch. Neurol. Psychiat. **71**:291, 1954.

176. Lillehei, C. W., Shaffer, J. M., Spink, W. W., Bobb, J. R. R., Wargo, J. D., and Visscher, M. B.: Role of cardiovascular stress in the pathogenesis of endocarditis and glomerulonephritis, Arch. Surg. **63**:421, 1951.

177. Linder, F.: 30 Jahre bestehende arteriovenöse Fistel der A. femoralis mit sekundären Aneurysma der V. iliaca. Heilung durch Operation, Chirurg **22**:77, 1951.

178. Litvak, J., Yahr, M. D., and Ransohoff, J.: Aneurysms of the great vein of Galen and midline cerebral arteriovenous anomalies, J. Neurosurg. **17**:945, 1960.

179. Locke, C. E.: Intracranial arterio-venous aneurism or pulsating exophthalmos, Ann. Surg. **80**:1, 272, 1924.

180. Locksley, H. B.: Report on the cooperative study of intracranial aneurysms and subarachnoid hemorrhage. Section V, Part I. Natural history of subarachnoid hemorrhage, intracranial aneurysms and arteriovenous malformations, J. Neurosurg. **25**:219, 1966.

181. Logue, V., and Monckton, G.: Posterior fossa angiomas, Brain **77**:252, 1954.

182. Lombardi, G., and Larini, G. P.: Angioma of the skull, J. Canad. Ass. Radiol. **7**:33, 1956.

183. Lombardi, G., and Migliavacca, F.: Angiomas of the spinal cord, Brit. J. Radiol. **32**:810, 1959.

184. Losacco, G.: Zur Frage der Lokalisation der angiodysgenetischen Nekrotisierenden Myelopathic (Foix-Alajouaninesche Krankheit), Arch. Psychiat. Z. Neurol. **208**:360, 1966.

185. Louis-Bar, D.: Les limites nosographiques de l'angiomatose encéphalotrigéminée (Sturge-Weber-Krabbe), Confin. Neurol. **6**:1, 1944.

186. Louis-Bar, D.: Sur l'hérédité de la maladie de Sturge-Weber-Krabbe, Confin. Neurol. **7**:238, 1947.

187. Louis-Bar, Mme.: Sur un syndrome progressif comprenant des télangiectasies capillaires cutanées et conjunctivales symétriques, à disposition naevoïde et des troubles cérébelleux, Confin. Neurol. **4**:32, 1941.

188. Love, J. G., Svien, H. J., Baker, H. L., and Layton, D. D.: Intraspinal arteriovenous anomalies, Minn. Med. **49**:255, 1966.

189. Luessenhop, A. J., and Cruz, T. D.: The surgical excision of spinal intradural vascular malformations, J. Neurosurg. **30**:552, 1969.

190. Lüginbühl, H., Fankhauser, R., and McGrath, J. T.: Spontaneous neoplasms of the nervous system in animals, Prog. Neurol. Surg. **2**:85, 1968.

191. Mackenzie, I.: The clinical presentation of the cerebral angioma, Brain **76**:184, 1953.

192. MacLean, A. R.: Primary thrombosis of the superior longitudinal sinus with chronic obstruction, Thesis, 1937, Graduate School of the University of Minnesota.

193. Mair, W. G. P., and Folkerts, J. F.: Necrosis of the spinal cord due to thrombo-phlebitis (subacute necrotic myelitis), Brain **76**:563, 1953.

194. Major, R. H., and Black, D. R.: A huge hemangioma of the liver associated with hemangiomata of the skull and bilateral cystic adrenals, Amer. J. Med. Sci. **156**:469, 1918.

195. Margolis, G., Odom, G. L., Woodhall, B., and Bloor, B. M.: The role of small angiomatous malformations in the production of intracerebral hematomas, J. Neurosurg. **8**:564, 1951.

196. Markham, J. W.: Spontaneous arteriovenous fistula of the vertebral artery and vein, J. Neurosurg. **31**:220, 1969.

197. Martin, J. D., and Mabon, R. F.: Pulsating exophthalmos. Review of all reported cases, J.A.M.A. **121**:330, 1943.

198. Mason, T. H., Swain, G. M., and Osheroff, H. R.: Bilateral carotid-cavernous fistula, J. Neurosurg. **11**:323, 1954.

199. Matas, R.: Congenital arteriovenous angioma of the arm, Ann. Surg. **111**:1021, 1940.

200. Mathews, W. B.: The spinal bruit, Lancet **2**:1117, 1959.

201. McConnell, T. H., and Leonard, J. S.: Microangiomatous malformations with intraventricular hemorrhage, Neurology **17**:618, 1967.

202. McCormick, W. F.: The pathology of vascular ("arteriovenous") malformations, J. Neurosurg. **24**:807, 1966.

203. McCormick, W. F.: Vascular disorders of nervous tissue: anomalies, malformations, and aneurysms. In Bourne, G. H.: The structure and function of nervous tissue, New York, 1969, Academic Press Inc., vol. 3, p. 537.

204. McCormick, W. F., and Boulter, T. R.: Vascular malformations ("angiomas") of the dura mater, J. Neurosurg. **25**:309, 1966.

205. McCormick, W. F., Hardman, J. M., and Boulter, T. R.: Vascular malformations ("angiomas") of the brain, with special reference to those occurring in the posterior fossa, J. Neurosurg. **28**:241, 1968.

206. McCormick, W. F., and Nofzinger, J. D.: "Cryptic" vascular malformations of the central nervous system, J. Neurosurg. **24**:865, 1966.

207. McGuire, T. H., Greenwood, J., and Newton, B. L.: Bilateral angioma of choroid plexus, J. Neurosurg. **11**:428, 1954.

208. McKhann, C. F., Belnap, W. D., and Beck, C. S.: Cervical arteriovenous anastomosis in treatment of mental retardation, convulsive disorders, and cerebral spasticity, Ann. Surg. **132**:162, 1950.

209. McKissock, W.: Intracranial angiomata, Ann. Roy. Coll Surg. Eng. 7:472, 1950.

210. McKissock, W., Paine, K. W. E., and Walsh, L. S.: The treatment of ruptured intracranial aneurysms, Neurochirurgia 2:25, 1959.

211. McKusick, V. A.: Mendelian inheritance in man, ed. 2, Baltimore, 1968, Johns Hopkins Press.

212. Meier-Violand, K.: Das Schicksal nicht-operierter Patienten mit arteriovenösem Aneurysma des Gehirns, Inaugural dissertation, Zurich, 1969.

213. Michael, J. C., and Levin, P. M.: Multiple telangiectases of the brain, Arch. Neurol. Psychiat. 36:514, 1936.

214. Mingrino, S., and Moro, F.: Fistula between the external carotid artery and cavernous sinus, J. Neurosurg. 27:157, 1967.

215. Moersch, F. P., and Kernohan, J. W.: Cerebral arteriovenous aneurysms with report of a case, J. Nerv. Ment. Dis. 74:137, 1931.

216. Moersch, F. P., and Kernohan, J. W.: Progressive necrosis of the spinal cord, Arch. Neurol. Psychiat. 31:504, 1934.

217. Molyneux, G. S.: Personal communication, 1964.

218. Morris, L. Angioma of the cervical spinal cord, Radiology 75:785, 1960.

219. Moyes, P. D.: Intracranial and intraspinal vascular anomalies in children, J. Neurosurg. 31:271, 1969.

220. Murphy, J. P.: Cerebrovascular disease, Chicago, 1954, Year Book Publishers, Inc.

221. Nahum, H., Erlinger, S., Levesque, M., and Surcin, M.: Maladie de Rendu-Osler à localisation digestive. Diagnostic artériographique, Presse Med. 77:1663, 1969.

222. Nakamura, T., Kutsuzawa, T., Takahashi, S., Takahashi, S., Sato, T., and Iwabuchi, T.: Cerebral hemodynamics in arteriovenous aneurysm of the brain measured by the dye-dilution method, Tohoku J. Exp. Med. 95: 135, 1968.

223. Nakao, K., and Angrist, A. A.: Electron microscopy of nonbacterial valvular vegetations in rats with arteriovenous shunts, Brit. J. Exp. Path. 48:294, 1967.

224. Nathanson, M., Tobias, E., and Tinsley, M.: Carotid artery cavernous sinus fistula, Arch. Surg. 95:678, 1967.

225. Nemours-Auguste, M.: Un cas d'hémangiome vertébral. Trouvaille radiologique, Bull. Mem. Soc. Radiol. Med. France 22:565, 1934.

226. Neubuerger, K. T., Freed, C. G., and Denst, J.: Vasal component in syndrome of Foix and Alajouanine "subacute necrotizing myelitis," Arch. Path. 55:73, 1953.

227. Neumann, M. A.: Combined amyloid vascular changes and argyrophilic plaques in the central nervous system, J. Neuropath. Exp. Neurol. 19:370, 1960.

228. Newman, M. J. D.: Spinal angioma with symptoms in pregnancy, J. Neurol. Neurosurg. Psychiat. 21:38, 1958.

229. Newman, M. J. D.: Racemose angioma of the spinal cord, Quart. J. Med. 28:97, 1959.

230. Newquist, R. E., and Mayfield, F. H.: Spinal angioma presenting during pregnancy, J. Neurosurg. 17:541, 1960.

231. Newton, T. H., and Darroch, J.: Vertebral arteriovenous fistula complicating vertebral angiography, Acta Radiol. 5:428, 1966.

232. Newton, T. H., and Greitz, T.: Arteriovenous communication between the occipital artery and the transverse sinus, Radiology 87:824, 1966.

233. Newton, T. H., and Hoyt, W. F.: Dural arteriovenous shunts in the region of the cavernous sinus, Neuroradiology 1:71, 1970.

234. Nicola, G. C., and Nizzoli, V.: Dural arteriovenous malformations of the posterior fossa, J. Neurol. Neurosurg. Psychiat. 31:514, 1968.

235. Niemeyer, P.: Discussion des rapports sur « Les angiomes supratentoriels», Int. Congr. Neurol. Sci., Brussels, 1957, vol. 4.

236. Nishimoto, A., and Sugiu, R.: Hemangiomatous malformation of bilateral internal carotid artery at the base of the brain, Proc. Ann. Meet. Neuroradiol. Ass. Japan 5:2, 1964.

237. Nishimoto, A., and Takeuchi, S.: Abnormal cerebrovascular network related to the internal carotid arteries, J. Neurosurg. 29:255, 1968.

238. Noran, H. H.: Intracranial vascular tumors and malformations, Arch. Path. 39:393, 1945.

239. Norlén, G.: Arteriovenous aneurysms of the brain: report of ten cases of total removal of the lesion, J. Neurosurg. 6:475, 1949.

240. Norman, R. M.: Malformations of the nervous system, birth injury, and diseases of early life. In Blackwood, W., McMenemey, W. H., Meyer, A., Norman, R. M., and Russell, D. S.: Greenfield's neuropathy ed. 2, Baltimore, 1963, The Williams & Wilkins Co., p. 324.

241. Northfield, D. W. C.: Angiomatous malformations of the brain, Guy's Hosp. Rep. 90:149, 1940-1941.

242. Odom, G. L.: Vascular lesions of the spinal cord: malformations, spinal subarachnoid, and extradural hemorrhage, Clin. Neurol. 8:196, 1962.

243. Odom, G. L., Woodhall, B., and Margolis, G.: Spontaneous hematomyelia and angiomas of the spinal cord, J. Neurosurg. 14:192, 1957.

244. Ohlmacher, A. P.: Multiple cavernous angioma, fibrendothelioma, osteoma, and hematomyelia of the central nervous system in a case of secondary epilepsy, J. Nerv. Ment. Dis. 26:395, 1899.

245. Olivecrona, H.: Arteriovenous aneurysms in the brain, Nord. Med. 41:843, 1949. Cited by Ramamurthi and Balasubramanian.[275]

246. Olivecrona, H., and Ladenheim, J.: Congenital arteriovenous aneurysms of the carotid and vertebral arterial systems, Berlin, 1957, Springer-Verlag.

247. Olivecrona, H., and Riives, J.: Arteriovenous aneurysms of the brain, Arch. Neurol. Psychiat. 59:567, 1948.

248. Ommaya, A. K., Di Chiro, G., and Doppman, J.: Ligation of arterial supply in the treatment of spinal cord arteriovenous malformations, J. Neurosurg. 30:679, 1969.

249. Osler, W.: On multiple hereditary telangi-

ectases with recurring haemorrhages, Quart. J. Med. 1:53, 1907.

250. Padget, D. H.: The cranial venous system in man in reference to development, adult configuration, and relation to the arteries, Amer. J. Anat. 98:307, 1956.

251. Paillas, J. E., Berard, M., Sedan, R., Toga, M., and Alliez, B.: The relative importance of atheroma in the clinical course of arteriovenous angioma of the brain. In Luyendijk, W.: Cerebral circulation, Progr. Brain Res. 30:419, 1968.

252. Pakarinen, S.: Arteriovenous fistula between the middle meningeal artery and the spheno-parietal sinus, J. Neurosurg. 23:438, 1965.

253. Palmer, A. C., and Hickman, J.: Ataxia in a horse due to an angioma of the spinal cord, Vet. Rec. 72:611, 1960.

254. Parkinson, D.: Collateral circulation of cavernous carotid artery: anatomy, Canad. J. Surg. 7:251, 1964.

255. Parkinson, D.: A surgical approach to the cavernous portion of the carotid artery, J. Neurosurg. 23:474, 1965.

256. Parsons, T. C., Guller, E. J., Wolff, H. G., and Dunbar, H. S.: Cerebral angiography in carotid cavernous communications, Neurology 4:65, 1954.

257. Patau, K., Therman, E., Smith, D. W., Inhorn, S. L., and Picken, B. F.: Partial-trisomy syndromes. 1. Sturge-Weber's disease, Amer. J. Hum. Genet. 13:287, 1961.

258. Paterson, J. H.: Clinical aspects of intracranial angiomas. In William, D.: Modern trends in neurology, New York, 1957, Paul B. Hoeber, Inc., 2nd series, p. 105.

259. Paterson, J. H., and McKissock, W.: A clinical survey of intracranial angiomas with special reference to their mode of progression and surgical treatment: a report of 110 cases, Brain 79:233, 1956.

260. Penfield, W.: Discussion, Arch. Neurol. Psychiat. 35:716, 1936.

261. Penfield, W., and Ward, A.: Calcifying epileptogenic lesions (hemangioma calcificans); J. Neuropath. Exp. Neurol. 7:111, 1948.

262. Penfield, W., and Ward, A · Calcifying epileptogenic lesions. Hemangioma calcificans; report of a case, Arch. Neurol. Psychiat. 60:20, 1948.

263. Pennybacker, J.: Discussion on vascular disease of the spinal cord, Proc. Roy. Soc. Med. 51:547, 1958.

264. Perret, G., and Nishioka, H.: Arteriovenous malformations: an analysis of 545 cases of cranio-cerebral arteriovenous malformations and fistulae reported to the Cooperative Study, J. Neurosurg. 25:467, 1966.

265. Peterman, A. F., Hayles, A. B., Dockerty, M. B., and Love, J. G.: Encephalotrigeminal angiomatosis (Sturge-Weber disease), J.A.M.A. 167:2169, 1958.

266. Peterson, E. W., and Schulz, D. M.: Amyloid in vessels of a vascular malformation in brain, Arch. Path. 72:480, 1961.

267. Picard, L., Vert, P., Renard, M., Hepner, H., and Lepoire, J.: Aspects radio-anatomiques des angiomes médullaires. A propos de deux observations, Neurochirurgie 15:519, 1969.

268. Pool, J. L., and Potts, D. G.: Aneurysms and arteriovenous anomalies of the brain, New York, 1965, Harper & Row, Publishers.

269. Poser, C. M., and Taveras, J. M.: Cerebral angiography in encephalo-trigeminal angiomatosis, Radiology 68:327, 1957.

270. Potter, E. L.: Diffuse angiectasis of the cerebral meninges of the newborn infant, Arch. Path. 46:87, 1948.

271. Potter, J. M.: Carotid-cavernous fistula: five cases with "spontaneous" recovery, Brit. Med. J. 2:786, 1954.

272. Potter, J. M.: Angiomatous malformations of the brain: their nature and prognosis, Ann. Roy. Coll. Surg. Eng. 16:227, 1955.

273. Pradat, P., Piganiol, G., Navarro-Artiles, G., and David, M.: Revascularisation d'un anévrysme carotide-caverneux post-traumatique par l'intermédiare de l'artère méningée moyenne, Neurochirurgie 14:875, 1968.

274. Quickel, K. E., and Whaley, R. J.: Subarachnoid hemorrhage in a patient with hereditary hemorrhagic telangiectasia, Neurology 17:716, 1967.

275. Ramamurthi, B., and Balasubramanian, V.: Arteriovenous malformations with a purely external carotid contribution, J. Neurosurg. 25:643, 1966.

276. Ray, B. S.: Cerebral arteriovenous aneurysms, Surg. Gynec. Obstet. 73:615, 1941.

277. Reid, M. R.: The effect of arteriovenous fistula upon the heart and blood vessels: an experimental and clinical study, Johns Hopkins Hosp. Bull. 31:43, 1920.

278. Reinhoff, W. F.: Congenital arteriovenous fistula. An embryological study, with the report of a case, Johns Hopkins Hosp. Bull. 35:271, 1924.

279. Rendu, M.: Epistaxis répétées chez un sujet porteur de petits angiomes cutanés et muqueux, Bull. Mem. Soc. Hop. Paris 13:731, 1896.

280. Reuter, S. R., Newton, T. H., and Greitz, T.: Arteriovenous malformations of the posterior fossa, Radiology 87:1080, 1966.

281. Rigdon, R. H.: Tumors produced by methylcholanthrene in the duck, Arch. Path. 54:368, 1952.

282. Robbins, L. R., and Fountain, E. M.: Hemangioma of cervical vertebras with spinal-cord compression, New Eng. J. Med. 258:685, 1958.

283. Robles, J.: Congenital arteriovenous malformation of the vertebral vessels in the neck, J. Neurosurg. 29:206, 1968.

284. Rodda, R. A., and Calvert, G. D.: Post-mortem arteriography of cerebral arteriovenous malformations, J. Neurol. Neurosurg. Psychiat. 32:432, 1969.

285. Roger, H., Paillas, J.-E., Bonnal, J., and Vigouroux, R.: Angiomes de la moelle et des racines, Acta Neurol. Psychiat. Belg. 51:491, 1951.

286. Roizin, L., Gold, G., Berman, H. H., Bonafede, V. I.: Congenital vascular anomalies and their histopathology in Sturge-Weber-Dimitri

syndrome, J. Neuropath. Exp. Neurol. **18**:75, 1959.

287. Rønne, H.: A case of Sturge-Webers disease, Acta Dermatovener. **18**:591, 1937.

288. Rosenbaum, A. E., Rossi, P., Schechter, M. M., and Sheehan, J. P.: Angiography of haemangiomata of the calvarium, Brit. J. Radiol. **42**:682, 1969.

289. Ross, R. T.: Multiple and familial intracranial vascular lesions, Canad. Med. Ass. J. **81**:477, 1959.

290. Rowbotham, G. F., and Little, E.: A new concept of the circulation and the circulations of the brain, Brit. J. Surg. **52**:539, 1965.

291. Rowley, P. T., Kurnick, J., and Cheville, R.: Hereditary haemorrhagic telangiectasia: aggravation by oral contraceptives, Lancet **1**:474, 1970.

292. Rumbaugh, C. L.: Personal communication, 1970.

293. Rumbaugh, C. L., and Potts, D. G.: Skull changes associated with intracranial arteriovenous malformations, Amer. J. Roentgen. **98**:525, 1966.

294. Runnels, J. B., Gifford, D. B., Forsberg, P. L., and Hanbery, J. W.: Dense calcification in a large cavernous angioma, J. Neurosurg. **30**:293, 1969.

295. Russell, D. S.: The pathology of spontaneous intracranial haemorrhage, Proc. Roy. Soc. Med. **47**:689, 1954.

296. Russell, D. S., and Rubinstein, L. J.: Pathology of tumours of the nervous system, Baltimore, 1963, The Williams & Wilkins Co.

297. Russell, W., and Newton, T. H.: Aneurysm of the vein of Galen, Amer. J. Roentgen. **92**:756, 1964.

298. Sabra, F.: Observations on one hundred cases of cerebral angioma, J.A.M.A. **170**:1522, 1959.

299. Sachs, E.: Intracranial telangiectasis: symptomatology and treatment, with report of two cases, Amer. J. Med. Sci. **150**:565, 1915.

300. Sachs, M.: Posada, J. T., Doyon, D., Da Lage, C., and Andrainjatovo, J.: Exophthalmie unilatérale par anévrysme artério-veineux temporal de la méningée moyenne, Neurochirurgie, **15**:75, 1969.

301. Sargent, E. N., Reilly, E. B., and Posnikoff, J.: Primary hemangioma of the skull, Amer. J. Roentgen. **95**:874, 1965.

302. Sattler, C. H.: Pulsierender Exophthalmus, Handbuch der gesamten Augenheilkunde, Berlin, 1920, Julius Springer. Cited by Dandy.[73]

303. Schalch, D. S.: McFarlin, D. E., and Barlow, M. H.: An unusual form of diabetes mellitus in ataxia telangiectasia, New Eng. J. Med. **282**:1396, 1970.

304. Scheinberg, L., and Elkin, M.: Hemangioma of the skull associated with intracranial angioma, Neurology **8**:650, 1958.

305. Schenk, W. G., Bahn, R. A., Cordell, A. R., and Stephens, J. G.: The regional hemodynamics of experimental acute arteriovenous fistulas, Surg. Gynec. Obstet. **105**:733, 1957.

306. Schenk, W. G., Martin, J. W., Leslie, M. B., Portin, B. A.: The regional hemodynamics of chronic experimental arteriovenous fistulas, Surg. Gynec. Obstet. **110**:44, 1960.

307. Schlesinger, E. B., and Hazen, R.: The cardiovascular effects of arteriovenous fistulae above and below the heart, Trans. Amer. Neurol. Ass. **79**:214, 1954.

308. Schneider, R. C., and Liss, L.: Cavernous hemangiomas of the cerebral hemispheres, J. Neurosurg. **15**:392, 1958.

309. Schoolman, A., and Kepes, J. J.: Bilateral spontaneous carotid-cavernous fistulae in Ehlers-Danlos syndrome, J. Neurosurg. **26**:82, 1967.

310. Scoville, W. B.: Intramedullary arteriovenous aneurysm of the spinal cord, J. Neurosurg. **5**:307, 1948.

311. Seljeskog, E. L., Rogers, H. M., and French, L. A.: Arteriovenous malformation involving the inferior sagittal sinus in an infant, J. Neurosurg. **29**:623, 1968.

312. Seville, R. H., Rao, P. S., Hutchinson, D. N., and Birchall, G.: Outbreak of Campbell de Morgan spots, Brit. Med. J. **1**:408, 1970.

313. Sharkey, P. C.: Intracranial arteriovenous malformations, Arch. Neurol. **12**:546, 1965.

314. Shaw, C., and Foltz, E. L.: Traumatic dissecting aneurysm of middle cerebral artery and carotid-cavernous fistula with massive intracerebral hemorrhage, J. Neurosurg. **28**:475, 1968.

315. Shenkin, H. A., Spitz, E. B., Grant, F. C., and Kety, S. S.: Physiologic studies of arteriovenous anomalies of the brain, J. Neurosurg. **5**:165, 1948.

316. Shephard, R. H.: Observations on intradural spinal angioma: treatment by excision, Neurochirurgia **6**:58, 1963.

317. Shephard, R. H.: Some new concepts in intradural spinal angioma, Riv. Patol. Nerv. Ment. **86**:276, 1965.

318. Shumacker, H. B., and Wayson, E. E.: Spontaneous cure of aneurysms and arteriovenous fistulas, with some notes on intrasaccular thrombosis, Amer. J. Surg. **79**:532, 1950.

319. Siekert, R. G., Keith, H. M., and Dion, F. R.: Ataxia-telangiectasia in children, Proc. Staff Meet. Mayo Clin. **34**:581, 1959.

320. Silverman, B. K., Breckx, T., Craig, J., and Nadas, A. S.: Congestive failure in the newborn caused by cerebral A-V fistula, Amer. J. Dis. Child. **89**:539, 1955.

321. Silverman, S.: Vascular tumours of the spinal cord associated with skin haemangiomata, Brit. J. Surg. **33**:307, 1945-1946.

322. Smith, D. E.: Central nervous system. In Ackerman, L. V., and Butcher, H. R., Jr.: Surgical pathology, ed. 2, St. Louis, 1959, The C. V. Mosby Co., p. 922.

323. Solitare, G. B.: Louis-Bar's syndrome (ataxia-telangiectasia), Neurology **18**:1180, 1968.

324. Souder, D. E., and Bercaw, B. L.: Arteriovenous fistula secondary to hair transplantation, New Eng. J. Med. **283**:473, 1970.

325. Sourander, P., Bonnevier, J. O., and Olsson, Y.: A case of ataxia-telangiectasia with lesions in the spinal cord, Acta Neurol. Scand. **42**:354, 1966.

326. Stehbens, W. E.: Blood vessel changes in chronic experimental arteriovenous fistulas, Surg. Gynec. Obstet. **127**:327, 1968.

327. Stehbens, W. E., and Ludatscher, R. M.: Fine structure of senile angiomas of human skin, Angiology **19**:581, 1968.

328. Stern, W. E., Brown, W. J., and Alksne, J. F.: The surgical challenge of carotid-cavernous fistula: the chief role of intracranial circulating dynamics, J. Neurosurg. **27**:298, 1967.

329. Sturge, W. A.: A case of partial epilepsy apparently due to a lesion of one of the vasomotor centres of the brain, Trans. Clin. Soc. London **12**:162, 1879. Reprinted in Arch. Neurol. **21**:555, 1969.

330. Sumner, D. S.: Physiology and pathological anatomy. In Strandness, D. E.: Collateral circulation in clinical surgery, Philadelphia, 1969, W. B. Saunders Co., p. 40.

331. Suter-Lochmatter, H.: Die spinaler Varikose, Acta Neurochir. **1**:154, 1950-1951.

332. Suwanwela, C.: Traumatic epidural arteriovenous aneurysm, J. Neurosurg. **24**:576, 1966.

333. Svien, H. J.: and Baker, H. L.: Roentgenographic and surgical aspects of vascular anomalies of the spinal cord, Surg. Gynec. Obstet. **112**:729, 1961.

334. Svien, H. J., and McRae, J. A.: Arteriovenous anomalies of the brain, J. Neurosurg. **23**:23, 1965.

335. Tarlov, I. M., and Grayzel, D.: Brain hemorrhage after carotid-jugular anastomosis, Ann. Surg. **136**:250, 1952.

336. Taveras, J. M., and Dalton, C. J.: Myelographic aspects of vascular malformations of the spinal cord. In Rajewsky, B.: Ninth international congress of radiology, Stuttgart, 1961, Georg Thieme Verlag, vol. 1, p. 453.

337. Taveras, J. M., and Poser, C. M.: Roentgenologic aspects of cerebral angiography in children, Amer. J. Roentgen. **82**:371, 1959.

338. Taylor, J. R., and Van Allen, M. W.: Vascular malformation of the cord with transient ischemic attacks, J. Neurosurg. **31**:576, 1969.

339. Teabeaut, J. R.: Subdural hematoma of nontraumatic origin, New Eng. J. Med. **245**:272, 1951.

340. Teilmann, K.: Hemangiomas of the pons, Arch. Neurol. Psychiat. **69**:208, 1953.

341. Teng, P., and Papatheodorou, C.: Myelographic appearance of vascular anomalies of the spinal cord, Brit. J. Radiol. **37**:358, 1964.

342. Teng, P., and Shapiro, M. J.: Arterial anomalies of the spinal cord, Arch. Neurol. Psychiat. **80**:577, 1958.

343. Terplan, K. L., and Krauss, R. F.: Histopathologic brain changes in association with ataxia-telangiectasia, Neurology **19**:446, 1969.

344. Therkelsen, J.: Angioma racemosum venosum medullare spinalis, Acta Psychiat. Neurol. Scand. **33**:219, 1958.

345. Thrash, A. M.: Vascular malformations of the cerebellum, Arch. Path. **75**:65, 1963.

346. Tingey, A. H.: Iron and calcium in Sturge-Weber disease, J. Ment. Sci. **102**:178, 1956.

347. Tomlinson, B. E.: Brain changes in ruptured intracranial aneurysm, J. Clin. Path. **12**:391, 1959.

348. Tönnis, W., Schiefer, W., and Walter, W.: Signs and symptoms of supratentorial arteriovenous aneurysms, J. Neurosurg. **15**:471, 1958.

349. Töpfer, D.: Über ein infiltrierend wachsendes Hämangiom der Haut und multiple Kapillarektasien der Haut und inneren Organe. II. Zur Kenntnis der Wirbelangioma, Frankfurt. Z. Path. **36**:337, 1928.

350. Toynbee, J.: An account of two vascular tumours developed in the substance of bone, Lancet **2**:676, 1845.

351. Travers, B.: A case of aneurism by anastomosis in the orbit, cured by the ligature of the common carotid artery, Med.-Chir. Trans. **2**:1, 1809-1811.

352. Trupp, M., and Sachs, E.: Vascular tumors of the brain and spinal cord and their treatment, J. Neurosurg. **5**:354, 1948.

353. Tsuji, H. K., Redington, J. V., and Kay, J. H.: Vertebral arteriovenous fistula, J. Thorac. Cardiovasc. Surg. **55**:746, 1968.

354. Turner, O. A., and Kernohan, J. W.: Vascular malformations and vascular tumors involving the spinal cord, Arch. Neurol. Psychiat. **46**:444, 1941.

355. Tym, R.: Personal communication. Cited by Shephard.[316]

356. Van Wijngaarden, G. K., and Vinken, P. J.: A case of intradural arteriovenous aneurysm of the posterior fossa, Neurology **16**:754, 1966.

357. Verbiest, H.: Arterio-venous aneurysms of the posterior fossa, analysis of six cases, Acta Neurochir. **9**:171, 1961.

358. Verbiest, H.: Extracranial and cervical arteriovenous aneurysms of the carotid and vertebral arteries, Johns Hopkins Med. J. **122**:350, 1968.

359. Verdura, J., and Shafron, M.: Aneurysm of vein of Galen in infancy, Surgery **65**:494, 1969.

360. Vianello, A.: Angiome artério-veineux (A. A. V.) du glomus choroïdien gauche, Neurochirurgie **15**:327, 1969.

361. Vollmar, J.: Zentrale Gefässektasien bei lange bestehenden arteriovenösen Fisteln, Arch. Klin. Chir. **294**:627, 1960.

362. Vraa-Jensen, G.: Angioma of the spinal cord, Acta Psychiat. Neurol. **24**:709, 1949.

363. Wachsmuth, N., and Löwenthal, A.: Détermination chimique d'éléments minéraux dans les calcifications intracérébrales de la malade de Sturge-Weber, Acta Neurol. Psychiat. Belg. **50**:305, 1950.

364. Walker, A. E., and Allègre, G. E.: Carotid-cavernous fistulas, Surgery **39**:411, 1956.

365. Wallace, J. M., Nashold, B. S., and Slewka, A. P.: Hemodynamic effects of cerebral arteriovenous aneurysms, Circulation **31**:696, 1965.

366. Walton, J. N.: Subarachnoid haemorrhage of unusual aetiology, Neurology **3**:517, 1953.

367. Walton, J. N.: Subarachnoid haemorrhage, Edinburgh, 1956, E. & S. Livingstone Ltd.

368. Wappenschmidt, J., Grote, W., and Holbach, K. H.: Diagnosis and therapy of arteriovenous malformations shown by vertebral angiogra-

phy. In Luyendijk, W.: Cerebral circulation, Progr. Brain Res. **30:**411, 1968.

369. Warren, G. C.: Intracranial arteriovenous malformation, pulmonary arteriovenous fistula, and malignant glioma in the same patient, J. Neurosurg. **30:**618, 1969.

370. Watson, W. L., and McCarthy, W. D.: Blood and lymph vessel tumors, Surg. Gynec. Obstet. **71:**569, 1940.

371. Weber, F. P.: Angioma-formation in connection with hypertrophy of limbs and hemihypertrophy, Brit. J. Derm. **19:**231, 1907.

372. Weber, F. P.: Multiple hereditary developmental angiomata (telangiectases) of the skin and mucous membranes associated with recurring hemorrhages, Lancet **2:**160, 1907.

373. Weber, F. P.: Right-sided hemi-hypertrophy resulting from right-sided congenital spastic hemiplegia, with a morbid condition of the left side of the brain, revealed by radiograms, J. Neurol. Psychopath. **3:**134, 1922-1923.

374. Weber, F. P.: A note on the association of extensive haemangiomatous naevus of the skin with cerebral (meningeal) haemangioma, especially cases of facial vascular naevus with contralateral hemiplegia, Proc. Roy. Soc. Med. **22:**431, 1929.

375. Weber, F. P.: Rare diseases and some debatable subjects, ed. 2, London, 1947, Staples Press Ltd.

376. Weir, B. K. A., Allen, P. B. R., and Miller, J. D. R.: Excision of thrombosed vein of Galen aneurysm in an infant, J. Neurosurg. **29:**619, 1968.

377. Wessler, S., and Stehbens, W. E.: Thrombosis. In Bang, N. U., Beller, F. K., Deutsch, E., and Mammen, E. F.: Thrombosis and bleeding disorders, Stuttgart, 1971, Georg Thieme Verlag, p. 488.

378. Whalley, N.: Arteriovenous fistulous aneurysms, J. Neurol. Neurosurg. Psychiat. **24:**92, 1961.

379. White, R. J., Wood, M. W., and Kernohan, J. W.: A study of fifty intracranial vascular tumors found incidentally at autopsy, J. Neuropath. Exp. Neurol. **17:**392, 1958.

380. Wilkins, R. H., and Brody, I. A.: Sturge-Weber syndrome, J. Neurosurg. **21:**554, 1969.

381. Williams, A. W.: Ossifying haemangioma of the cerebrum, Brit. J. Surg. **38:**245, 1950-1951.

382. Willis, R. A.: The borderland of embryology and pathology, London, 1958, Butterworth and Co. Ltd.

383. Willis, R. A.: Pathology of tumours, ed. 4, New York, 1967, Appleton-Century-Crofts.

384. Wirth, F. P., Post, K. D., Di Chiro, G., Doppman, J. L., and Ommaya, A. K.: Foix-Alajouanine disease, Neurology **20:**1114, 1970.

385. Wohlwill, F. J., and Yakovlev, P. I.: Histopathology of meningo-facial angiomatosis (Sturge-Weber's disease), J. Neuropath. Exp. Neurol. **16:**341, 1957.

386. Wolf, A., and Brock, S.: Histopathologic study of two angiomas of the brain, Arch. Neurol. Psychiat. **29:**1362, 1933.

387. Wolf, A., and Brock, S.: The pathology of cerebral angiomas, Bull. Neurol. Inst. N.Y. **4:**144, 1935-36.

388. Wolf, P. A., Rosman, N. P., and New, P. F. J.: Multiple small cryptic venous angiomas of the brain mimicking cerebral metastases, Neurology **17:**491, 1967.

389. Wood, M. W., White, R. J., and Kernohan, J. W.: Cavernous hemangiomatosis involving the brain, spinal cord, heart, skin, and kidney, Proc. Staff Meet. Mayo Clin. **32:**249, 1957.

390. Wyburn-Mason, R.: Arteriovenous aneurysm of the mid-brain and retina, facial naevi, and mental changes, Brain **66:**163, 1943.

391. Wyburn-Mason, R.: The vascular abnormalities and tumours of the spinal cord and its membranes, St. Louis, 1944, The C. V. Mosby Co.

392. Wyke, B. D.: Primary hemangioma of the skull: a rare cranial tumor, Amer. J. Roentgen. **61:**302, 1949.

393. Yakovlev, P. I., and Guthrie, R. H.: Congenital ectodermoses (neurocutaneous syndromes) in epileptic patients, Arch. Neurol. Psychiat. **26:**1145, 1931.

394. Zimmerman, H. M.: Brain tumors: their incidence and classification in man and their experimental production, Ann. N.Y. Acad. Sci. **159:**337, 1969.

11 / Tumors

Hemangioblastomas of the brain and spinal cord

Hemangioblastomas, unlike telangiectases, hemangiomas, venous angiomas, and arteriovenous aneurysms, are almost universally regarded as true neoplasms. They were subdivided by Cushing and Bailey[33] into cystic and solid varieties, each of which has three subtypes (capillary, cellular, and cavernous) but the classification has not been generally accepted mainly because of the uncertain nature of these entities. Complex classifications at this stage seem unwarranted, and though electron microscopy may help to elucidate satisfactorily the identity of the stromal cell, the classification of Russell and Rubinstein[130] is preferable at this time.

Hemangioblastoma has been variously called angioreticuloma, cerebellar angioma, cerebellar or gliosing hemangioendothelioma, and Lindau tumor. The term "hemangioblastoma" has been regarded as a misnomer because the lesion does not display the implied degree of malignancy and anaplasia.[2] Moreover, though at present hemangioblastoma is generally accepted as a benign tumor,[130] there is debate on whether it is a tumor or a malformation. The clinical picture differs little from that of other cerebellar tumors, being dependent on local subtentorial symptoms and signs together with a raised intracranial pressure accentuated when the fourth ventricle is occluded.

Incidence. Hemangioblastomas are not common tumors of the central nervous system. In large series of tumors their prevalence has been estimated as 1.5% by Zülch[176] in 4000 cases, 1.9% by Zimmerman[175] in 5199 cases, and approximately 2% by Olivecrona[111] in 4188 verified intracranial tumors. In 446 intracranial tumors

of military personnel (aged 18 to 38 years) during World War II, Bennett[11] found 17 cases of hemangioblastoma (3.8%). These tumors occur predominantly in the posterior fossa of adults and constituted 7.3% of Olivecrona's tumors of the posterior fossa.[111] Mondkar and associates[99] assembled the largest series of cerebellar hemangioblastomas (112 cases), which comprised 1.8% of all their intracerebral tumors encountered between 1947 and 1965 and 12% of the neoplasms of the posterior fossa. Zülch[176] found in his series that they constituted 11.6% of 482 tumors of the cerebellum and fourth ventricle, 0.3% of 345 parietal lobe tumors, 0.4% of 282 pontocerebellar angle tumors, and 4.2% of 96 tumors of the spinal cord. Kernohan and associates[76] found four hemangioblastomas (7.8%) among 51 cases of intramedullary tumor. It is believed that in other animals hemangioblastomas with cyst formation and von Hippel-Lindau's disease do not occur,[72] but Lüginbühl and associates[88] have observed hemangioblastomas in a few isolated cases (dog and pig).

Age and sex distribution. The age distribution of these tumors is indicated in Table 11-1, the peak frequency being in the fourth decade. Hemangioblastoma is rare in the first decade, only 1.9% of those in Table 11-1 being in this age group. The mean age is usually given as between 35 and 40 years, and Olivecrona[111] drew attention to an earlier involvement in females than in males. In the female he found the maximum peak between 20 and 40 years whereas the peak for males fell between 40 and 60 years. Other investigations have not confirmed this assertion, but reports in the literature attest to the preponderance of males affected; the ratio of males to females in Table 11-2 is 3:2 for

Table 11-1. Age distribution of hemangioblastoma

Author	0-10 or 0-9	11-20 or 10-19	21-30 or 20-29	31-40 or 30-39	41-50 or 40-49	51-60 or 50-59	61-70 or 60-69	Total
Intracranial								
Cushing & Bailey (1928)[33]		1	3	4	2	1		11
Sargent & Greenfield (1929-1930)[134]			2	3	1	2		8
Noran (1945)[108]		1	3	2	2			8
Cramer & Kimsey (1952)[31]	2	3	14	14	11	4		48
Olivecrona (1952)[111]		6	13	14	14	20	3	70
Silver & Hennigar (1952)[140]	2	2	11	8	6	10	1	40
Meredith & Hennigar (1954)[95]		2	2	2	4	2	2	14
Pennybacker (1954)[115]			1	1	4			6
Stein et al. (1960)[144]	1	3	8	4	3	2		21
Mondkar et al. (1967)[99]	1	13	14	28	26	23	7	112
Wolpert (1970)[168]				3	2	2	1	8
Subtotal	6	31	71	83	75	66	14	346
Spinal								
Wyburn-Mason (1944)[172]	1	2	7	10	12	2		34
Total	7	33	78	93	87	68	14	380

Table 11-2. Sex distribution of patients with hemangioblastoma

Author	Male	Female	Total
Intracranial			
Cushing & Bailey (1928)[33]	8	3	11
Sargent & Greenfield (1929)[134]	5	3	8
Noran (1945)[108]	5	3	8
Perlmutter et al. (1950)[116]	10	15	25
Cramer & Wimsey (1952)[31]	23	19	42
Olivecrona (1952)[111]	41	29	70
Silver & Hennigar (1952)[140]	24	16	40
Meredith & Hennigar (1954)[95]	7	7	14
Pennybacker (1954)[115]	4	2	6
Zülch (1957)[176]	41	19	60
Stein et al. (1960)[144]	13	8	21
Mondkar et al. (1967)[99]	63	49	112
Subtotal	244	173	417
Spinal			
Wyburn-Mason (1944)[172]	22	12	34
Total	266	185	451

both intracranial and spinal lesions. Morello and Bianchi[100] reviewed supratentorial hemangioblastomas and found only six cases of fairly certain diagnosis and adequate detail. All were males with the age distribution similar to that cited above.

Location. By far the most common site of hemangioblastoma is the posterior fossa, though as yet no adequate explanation for this concentration has been proffered. In the cerebellum, they tend to appear in a paramedian position, but the lateral lobes and vermis are also frequently affected.[130] However, Stein and associates[144] found 16 of their 21 cases in the cerebellar hemispheres, the left of which is involved about twice as commonly as the right. The cerebellar tonsils are rarely affected.[130] Tumors of the vermis readily deform and infiltrate the cavity of the fourth ventricle,[130] but rarely does a lesion arise directly from the floor of the fourth ventricle and rarely is it located in the cisterna magna.[144] Olivecrona[111] found 56 tumors in the cerebellar hemispheres and nine in the vermis. Hemangioblastomas occur less frequently in the medulla oblongata, where they have been known to originate from the area postrema.[130]

Supratentorial hemangioblastomas[100,114] are extremely uncommon. Morello and Bianchi,[100] after reviewing the literature in 1963, concluded that there were only nine cases histologically proved to be supratentorial hemangioblastomas and that the diagnosis of these tumors is quite contentious. Russell and Rubinstein[130] pointed out that assessment of the frequency of supratentorial hemangioblastomas depends on whether angioblastic meningiomas are placed in a separate category (pp. 568 and 569). From 1947 to 1965 Mondkar and associates[99] encountered three supratentorial hemangioblastomas and found 112 cases in the cerebellum. Bailey and Ford[5] reported a smaller series with 15 in the cerebellum and only one in the cord. The spinal cord is nevertheless a more common site than the cerebrum. The spinal tumor is usually posteriorly situated either intramedullary or pial, whereas the nerve roots and cauda equina are less often affected. The regions of the cord most commonly involved are from the third cervical to the first thoracic and from the seventh thoracic to the first lumbar segments.[172]

Multiplicity. Hemangioblastomas are usually solitary tumors, though more than one may be found in the posterior fossa.[34,130] With supratentorial tumors there may also be a similar tumor in the posterior fossa, and associated tumors of the spinal cord are not infrequent. As Russell and Rubinstein[130] pointed out, multiplicity is one of the features of von Hippel-Lindau's disease. They cited the case of a hemangioblastoma of the area postrema accompanied by four small symptomless tumors of similar structures in the spinal pia mater (seventh cervical to fifth thoracic segments).

Hoff and Ray[69] reported von Hippel-Lindau's disease in a man with both cerebral and cerebellar hemangioblastomas. Approximately half of the familial cases have multiple hemangioblastomas.[2]

Pathology. Subtentorial hemangioblastomas are either solid or cystic tumors. In one series of 40 cerebellar hemangiomas,[140] only six were solid. Thirty consisted of a nodule with a single large cyst and four had a grossly multiloculated appearance. Stein and associates[144] found 16 cystic tumors in their 21 cases. Olivecrona[111] believed that the presence of a cyst had been overemphasized. He found 55 cystic and 15 solid tumors in a series of 70 cases. Cystic hemangioblastomas occur for the most part in the cerebellum and less frequently elsewhere such as in the pons[103] and above the tentorium.

The cystic lesions can be recognized by the fullness, flattening, or discoloration of the cerebellar surface or several large prominent vessels on the pial surface. Seldom are the pia mater and dura mater thickened or firmly adherent to the cyst.[140] The cyst may increase to 6 cm. in diameter and contain clear, colorless, but more usually xanthochromic fluid, which may coagulate spontaneously[108] and have a relatively high protein content (as high as 6 gm. per 100 ml.)[140,157] In the event of hemorrhage very seldom does blood extend into the cystic space. The volume of the fluid may be as much as 60 or even 100 ml.[144] The cyst quickly refills after aspiration of the fluid and in one instance a recurrent cyst contained 200 ml. of fluid.[144] Chemical analysis of fluid from cystic tumors within the central nervous system intimates that degenerative changes within the neoplasm initiate the accumulation of transudate from the blood vessels.[32] The fluid from cysts of hemangioblastomas is strikingly similar to that of pleural and peritoneal effusions, and hemorrhage is not considered to play a role in cyst formation. Greenfield[61] suggests that trauma might have precipitated cyst formation in some of his cases.

It has been noted that the cysts (large

and small) in the cerebellar hemangioblastomas are lined by a flattened type of epithelium, which rightly or wrongly, has been called endothelium. The presence of the lining cells is difficult to explain. It would suggest that either the tumor forms cyst-like spaces that fill with fluid or that the formation of lining cells is secondary to the formation of a space filled with transudate. If the lining cells are an integral part of the tumor, one would then expect that after removal of the mural nodule alone there would be a recurrence but, as such is not the case, their appearance is probably secondary.

The wall of the cyst is smooth, resembling the ependymal surface. A small tumor nodule, sessile or flattened, may project into the lumen most often from the posterior aspect of the cyst and is related to the pia and cortex.[6] Sometimes only careful or perhaps microscopic examination of the wall will reveal the hemangioblastic tissue.[111] The mural nodule consists of firm gray to red tissue occasionally with more than one nodule in a single cyst.[144] Acute large cysts can occur within the substance of the hemangioblastoma rather than at their periphery.[75] The involved cerebellar hemisphere is enlarged and compresses the brain stem and the remainder of the cerebellum. The cerebellar tonsils are then forced downward into the foramen magnum, except when the tumor is midline, for then the tonsils will be spread apart. Compression of the fourth ventricle is the rule, and hence internal hydrocephalus is likely to be prominent. Invasion of the floor of the fourth ventricle is rare.

The less common solid variety of hemangioblastoma is a well circumscribed, reddish or yellowish tumor often with a spongy texture attributed to the presence of small cysts. These cysts, varying in size, lie in the substance of the tumor and not necessarily at the periphery[75] although blood spaces can also give the neoplasm a spongy appearance and texture. Those in the superior part of the cerebellum and in the cerebrum are mostly solid.[111] A rare cystic tumor with multiple mural nodules in the left temporal lobe has been observed.[144] Rivera and Chason[122] reported a case of cerebral hemangioblastoma associated with splenic and adrenal amyloidosis. Raynor and Kingman[121] emphasized the enlarged tortuous vessels related to the fossa and considered that there was a vascular malformation associated with the tumor in this instance. Such vascular changes occur with both cystic and solid hemangioblastomas. In the cystic variety the enlarged vessels may be seen radiating from the mural nodule on the inner surface of the cyst. The increased vascularity, often extreme, simulates an arteriovenous aneurysm of considerable magnitude. Histologically the neighboring vessels are often consistent with such a view (Figs. 11-1 and 11-2). Meredith and Hennigar[95] referred to these vessels as angiomatous and indeed they bleed profusely when injured[6] and are a characteristic feature in angiograms.[168] A bruit has been detected with both hemangioblastoma[33] and angioblastic meningioma,[7] but there is no information concerning the frequency of such murmurs. Even retinal hemangioblastomas have been mistaken for arteriovenous aneurysms.[94] In cases of spinal hemangioblastomas myelography can reveal a picture similar to that of an arteriovenous aneurysm and arterial blood has been noted in tortuous spinal veins in a case of spinal hemangioblastoma.[12] The cardiac output in patients with these tumors has not been measured, but it probably increases particularly when several intracranial and spinal tumors occur concurrently. In view of the similarity of hemangiopericytoma to hemangioblastoma, the case of a woman[55] with a large highly vascular hemangiopericytoma of the thigh is of interest. A bruit and a large arteriovenous shunt were present and the cardiac output was 9.5 liters per minute preoperatively and 5.9 postoperatively.

The spinal cord tumors are morphologically similar to the intracranial lesion although some are extremely small.[130] Multiple tumors are not uncommon, and with

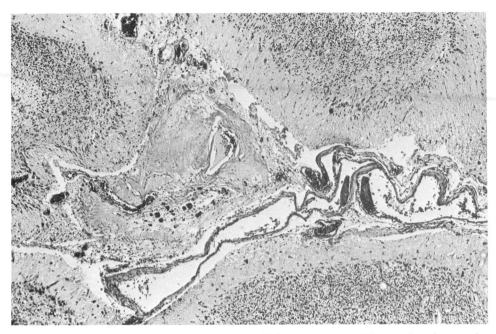

Fig. 11-1. Vessels of irregular contour and thickness near periphery of a hemangioblastoma. One vessel has been recanalized and surrounding cerebellum exhibits ischemic changes. (Hematoxylin and eosin, ×45.)

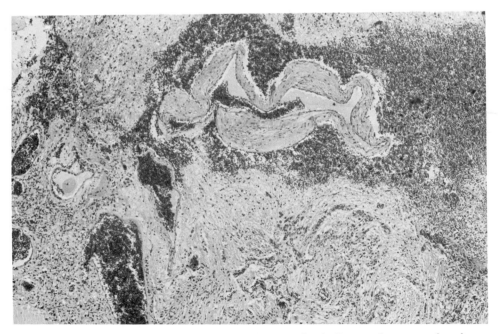

Fig. 11-2. Vessel from edge of a hemangioblastoma is similar to that occurring in an arteriovenous angioma. Extensive hemorrhage is present. (Hematoxylin and eosin, ×45.)

all spinal hemangioblastomas the brain should be carefully examined for additional lesions. These rounded, well-circumscribed but not encapsulated tumors have remnants of compressed cord about their periphery, whereas those irregular in shape may extend into the cord and sequester islands of cord parenchyma.[172] Spinal lesions may exhibit calcification[172] and there are a few small cysts. The variable degree of vascularity predetermines partly the color of the tumor. On the surface of the cord[80,131] and frequently detected by myelography are enlarged arteries and veins simulating an arteriovenous aneurysm. The vessels may be extensive and large covering the cord and producing a spinal block. Wyburn-Mason[172] reported pial varicosities in 15 of 40 adequately described cases, a conservative estimate. Hemangioblastoma of the cord may be overlooked if attention is focused solely on the tortuous and enlarged pial vessels.[80]

Syringomyelia, which occurs with other spinal cord tumors,[75] is inexplicably a frequent accompaniment of spinal hemangioblastomas,[75,172] with the cavity extending far above and below the level of the tumor or arising some distance away and even in the medulla (syringobulbia). It occurs only with the spinal hemangioblastomas, not with those of the pia, nerve roots, or brain. The syringomyelic cavity may be irregular and branching and lined by a zone of glial tissue or else it resembles a softening.[172] Wyburn-Mason[172] found syringomyelia in 11 of 25 cases of intramedullary tumor, that is, 44% of cases, and in 77% of cases of intramedullary hemangioblastoma. Theories, none of them satisfactory, abound concerning the pathogenesis of the associated syringomyelia.[172] The syringomyelic cavity has been likened to the cyst associated with cerebellar hemangioblastoma with transudate from the tumor supposedly tracking up and down the columns till it collects and forms an elongated cavity about which reactive gliosis occurs secondarily. This thesis would not explain syringomyelia associated with other intramedullary tumors.

The second suggestion is that the cavity is caused by myelomalacia secondary to circulatory disturbances engendered by the tumor, and the third is that the cavity results from hematomyelia caused by the tumor. However, even microscopically breakdown products of blood are absent in the cavity. Finally both syringomyelia and the hemangioblastoma are thought to result from congenital factors with neither causally related to the other. The maldevelopment concept neglects to account for both the occurrence of syringomyelia with other forms of spinal cord tumor and its absence with hemangioblastomas at other sites (pia mater, nerve roots, and cerebellum).

Radiologically with hemangioblastomas come signs of increased intracranial pressure and hydrocephalus with a dilated or blocked fourth ventricle. Angiography demonstrates the unusual vascularity[111,168] although cysts are avascular areas. In recent years spinal angiography has facilitated the diagnosis of hemangioblastomas of the cord in the absence of a laminectomy. Still, as both can produce fragmentation of the radiopaque dye and spinal block, they can be readily mistaken for an arteriovenous aneurysm.

Hemorrhage and softening. With their extreme vascularity and an apparently coexistent arteriovenous shunt of some magnitude, hemorrhage, usually mild but occasionally severe, is a complication. Globus[56] mentioned hemorrhage into a cerebellar cyst, and Meredith and Hennigar[95] mentioned a fatal subarachnoid hemorrhage in a 24-year-old woman who was 8½ months pregnant. Hemorrhage of lesser degree is considerably more common as evidenced by the presence of siderophages in or about the tumor microscopically. The xanthochromia of the cystic fluid has not been investigated chemically. Ischemic softening about cerebellar hemangioblastomas may be severe and may account for the syringomyelia associated with spinal lesions.

Microscopic appearance. Histologically the solid portion of the tumor consists of

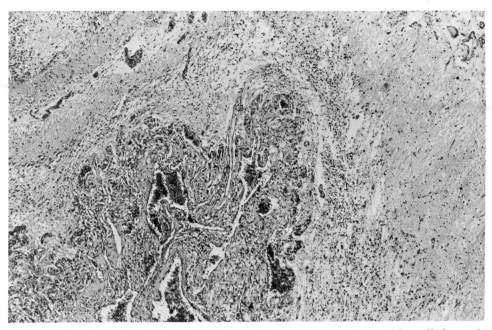

Fig. 11-3. Growing edge of hemangioblastoma. Note numerous, large, thin-walled vessels and gliotic and ischemic cerebellum nearby. (Hematoxylin and eosin, ×45.)

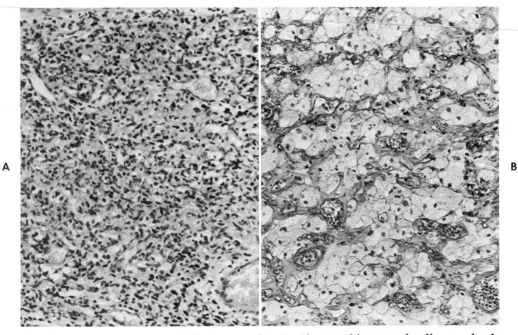

Fig. 11-4. Pattern of hemangioblastoma varies. **A,** Pleomorphic stromal cells are closely packed with few vessels and, **B,** the tumor consists of aggregates of xanthoma cells in a vascular stroma. (Hematoxylin and eosin, ×110.)

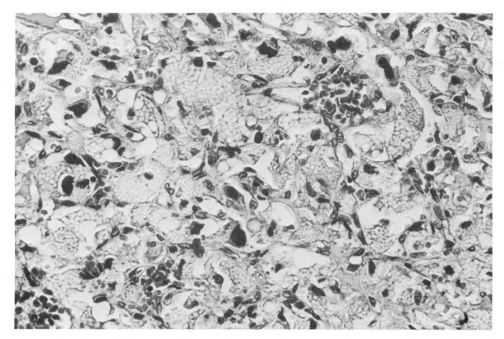

Fig. 11-5. Hemangioblastoma showing detail of foamy cytoplasm and pleomorphic and hyperchromatic nuclei. (Hematoxylin and eosin, ×275.)

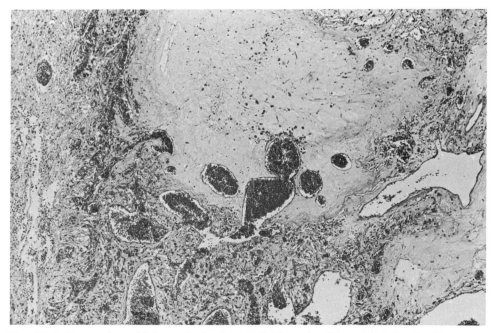

Fig. 11-6. Large sinusoidal vessels in hemangioblastoma. Note extensive hyaline areas containing some siderophages. (Hematoxylin and eosin, ×45.)

capillary and cavernous vascular channels throughout the neoplasm. Vessels at the periphery are often particularly large and prominent, with most vascular channels being thin-walled (Fig. 11-3). When cavernous blood spaces are particularly prominent, the tumor may superficially resemble a cavernous hemangioma. The intervening tissue is cellular and consists of small embryonic vessels that are usually empty, and pseudoxanthomatous stromal cells with oval stippled nuclei and often a nucleolus with a variable quantity of foamy cytoplasm from which the lipid has been extracted during the preparation of the histological slides (Fig. 11-4). The lipid, believed to be closely related to cholesterol ester,[174] is absent at times, and then the cytoplasm is pale and homogeneous. Multinucleated giant cells are occasionally seen and also hyperchromatic and atypical nuclei (Fig. 11-5). Mitotic figures are extremely rare. The ratio of vessels to cellular elements varies from area to area and tumor to tumor and with them no erythropoietic tissue has been seen.

Dense reticulin fibers, from which the term "angioreticuloma" is derived,[111] surround the vessels and permeate the intervening tissue to a variable extent between xanthoma cells and small groups of stromal cells[167] interrupted by zones of hyaline connective tissue. When the stromal or xanthomatous cells form large compact masses with a relatively small vascular component, reticulin fibers are scanty or even absent.[120] Hemorrhage and a consequent infiltration of the tissue with siderophages are not infrequent as well as areas of necrosis and hyalinization (Fig. 11-6) and more rarely calcification,[75] microscopic in quantity.

Blood vessels are usually prominent at the periphery, and small vessels appear to sprout into the surrounding neural tissue, which exhibits gliosis. The wall of the associated cyst consists of glial fibers with tumor only at the mural nodule.[108] The cyst is said to be imperfectly lined by a layer of flattened cells resembling endothelium.[144] Blood vessels, related to the mural nodule,

may extend into the wall of the cyst for a short distance. Occasionally a vessel is thrombosed and the pattern of the tumor is interrupted by lakes of protein-rich fluid irregular in size. Larger cystic spaces may be numerous.

Silver and Hennigar[140] classified hemangioblastomas into three histological types, juvenile, transitional, and clear cell varieties. The juvenile type, occurring in the first three decades of life, is characterized by the presence of thin-walled often distinctly cavernous capillaries. Pink-staining protein-containing fluid, believed to be transuded plasma, occurs in variable amounts in the interstitial spaces. This type is regarded as a capillary-cavernous hemangioma[95] and is histologically similar to extracranial hemangiomas. Silver and Hennigar[140] did not believe it underwent sclerosing and obliterative changes. The transitional type, found only in the third to sixth decades, is said to depict the response of the tumor to hemorrhage, the red cells and plasma being engulfed by endothelial cells that consequently develop a foamy cytoplasm. Such was thought to be a transition stage between the juvenile and the clear cell types, with multinucleated giant cells being more numerous. However the formation of xanthoma cells in abundance in the absence of siderophages would constitute a most unusual reaction to extravasated blood. The clear cell type (fourth decade onward) is comprised almost entirely of xanthoma cells in the vascular stroma. Silver and Hennigar[140] found transitional stages in postoperative recurrences. On histological grounds they differentiated the clear cell type from metastatic hypernephroma by the prevalence of mitotic figures and the prominence of the nuclei in the renal tumors.

Kernohan and Sayre[75] in a classification not generally accepted subdivided hemangioblastomas into capillary hemangioma, hemangioendothelioma, capillary hemangioendoblastoma, and hemangiosarcoma, according to increasing grades of malignancy. They have also been likened to sclerosing hemangiomas of extracranial sites[5,7] and have actually been called sclerosing hemangiomas because of the increase in lipid, hemosiderin, and giant cells, the associated manifestations of the sclerosis. The absence of cystic change in the extracranial variety was not explained.

In some angioblastic meningiomas, numbers of stromal cells may be arranged about the vessels producing a peritheliomatous appearance. Some authors assign these tumors to a separate category, the hemangiopericytoma, but Russell and Rubinstein[130] find no reason for such classification.

The source of the stromal cells in hemangioblastomas is unknown. They have been thought to be endothelial cells.[140] Russell and Rubinstein[130] consider that they originate from the pia mater or blood vessels and explain that the vascular element in some tumors is not prominent but stromal cells form large compact masses suggestive of a meningioma. It is also possible that the vascular changes are secondary manifestations of the tumor's potential to initiate an arteriovenous shunt.

Ultrastructure. Cancilla and Zimmerman,[16] examining the ultrastructure of a hemangioblastoma, found large cells with irregular hyperchromatic nuclei scattered throughout the cytoplasm, which contained membranous whorls, spirals, or concentric laminae with a radial periodicity of 60 Å between the laminae. Electron-dense amorphous material, thought to be lipid, lay in the cytoplasm adjoining the aggregates. In a late stage the aggregates of dense bodies were membrane bound and eventually released into the intercellular spaces. The stromal cells also contained cytoplasmic fibrils and were believed to be derived from endothelium that did not exhibit unusual features.

In a spinal hemangioendothelioma Ramsey[120] reported very numerous endothelial cells possessing numerous fingerlike processes that projected into the lumen and anastomosed to enclose vascular spaces and inclusions of an extracellular material. No fenestrae were present as in the cerebral

hemangiopericytoma also studied. The stromal cells contained cytoplasmic fibrils but were without the aggregates of dense bodies seen by Cancilla and Zimmerman.[16] The conclusion was that the hemangioendothelioma and hemangiopericytoma are quite distinct.

Castaigne and associates[19] after examining four hemangioblastomas were unable to determine the nature of the tumor cell. Stromal cells contained numerous nonstriated microfibrils (70 Å in diameter) often filling all profiles, abundant tubular agranular endoplasmic reticulum, lipid vacuoles (in three tumors), glycogen granules, lamellated membranous bodies or zebra bodies (membranes arranged in parallel fashion), and evidence of red cell phagocytosis. Fenestrated endothelium was observed in one instance. Endothelial cells could not be regarded as abnormal, and mast cells were encountered with inclusions similar to those observed by Cancilla and Zimmerman[16] These limited studies have not identified the stromal cell and much further work remains to be done.

Relationship to angioblastic meningiomas. Bailey and associates[7] touched off a dispute over the relationship of hemangioblastomas and angioblastic meningiomas when describing a group of tumors of blood vessel origin that they termed "angioblastic meningiomas." In defining angioblastic meningiomas they indicated that they did not mean a meningioma with a high degree of vascularity but rather a tumor macroscopically and in location similar to a meningioma with the same architectural features and reticular network as the cerebellar hemangioblastoma. Such tumors occur almost universally above the tentorium. Bailey and Ford[5] believed that except for site the two tumors were one and the same. Morello and Bianchi[100] considered that only nine definite supratentorial hemangioblastomas had been reported in the literature and much disagreement concerns the nature of individual case reports. Barnard and Walshe[8] reported a dark purple to plum-colored tumor 8 cm. in diameter attached to the dura mater in the temporal region of a woman of 47 years. It was spongy and contained an irregular multiloculated smooth-walled cyst. The patient had two small renal fibromas. Histologically the tumor was classified as a "capillary hemangioma" or a Lindau tumor. Russell and Rubinstein[130] called it a hemangioblastoma but considered that angioblastic meningioma was a reasonable interpretation. Morello and Bianchi[100] also were uncertain of its identity. Kernohan and Sayre[75] believe that angioblastic meningiomas are not true meningiomas but blood vessel tumors under the generic term "angioblastoma."

Topographical and macroscopic differences exist between hemangioblastomas and angioblastic meningiomas, but no single criterion provides absolute distinction.[129,130] Supratentorial tumors are generally angioblastic meningiomas, yet one temporal lobe tumor[8] was partly cystic and another[69] in a man with von Hippel-Lindau's disease was associated with a cyst 4 cm. in diameter. Subtentorial tumors are mostly hemangioblastomas and cystic although the solid variety is also represented. A subtentorial meningioma has caused a cerebellar cyst as Russell and Rubinstein[130] demonstrated. In a few cases of angioblastic meningioma Wolf and Cowen[164] found typically meningiomatous areas.

Corrandini and Browder,[25] discussing at length the difference between the tumors, pointed out that the angioblastic meningioma invariably had a distinct capsule and was attached to the dura mater. On the other hand, the usually intracerebral hemangioblastoma was neither encapsulated nor attached to the dura, though continuity with the pia mater can be demonstrated regularly upon careful examination,[129,130] which no doubt accounts for the rarity of involvement of the dentate nucleus. A similar continuity was found between spinal hemangioblastomas and the pia, and Russell illustrated a hemangioblastoma arising from the spinal pia mater in a case of the von Hippel-Lindau syndrome.[129] Russell and Rubinstein[130] contend that the hemangioblastoma is a true neoplasm of pial and vascular origin closely related to the angioblastic meningioma. Courville's case[27] of a man with a parasagittal angioblastic meningioma in the parietal region and a cystic cerebellar hemangioblastoma substantiates this relationship. The subject also had multiple renal angiomas, his blind father had a cerebellar hemangioblastoma, and his brother became blind 18 years after operation on a cerebellar cyst. Although in this instance von Hippel-Lindau's disease may have been present, the syndrome is virtually restricted to the subtentorial hemangioblastoma.[129] Moreover polycythemia has not been found in association with angioblastic meningiomas.

Malignancy and prognosis. Hemangioblastomas are generally slow-growing neoplasms, but their position and the frequent association of a cerebellar cyst induce compression and displacement of the cerebellum and brain stem with hydrocephalus readily occurring. Symptoms may be out of all proportion to the actual size and duration of the tumor. With spinal hemangioblastomas there is a long lag period between the onset of symptoms and diagnosis.[169] Hemangioblastomas are representative of the less severe varieties of brain tumor, particularly when cystic[71] despite their potential for both growth and invasion. Recurrence is generally regarded as being the result of inadequate removal or destruction of the tumor, in which event invasion of even extracranial tissues may follow postoperatively.[115] In Pennybacker's case[115] there were multiple recurrences over a period of 20 years from the onset of symptoms. Extension to the overlying muscle and skin as far down as the fifth cervical vertebra was established, yet hemangioblastomas are so frequently multiple that it may be difficult to distinguish between a recurrence and the prospect of a second tumor.

Horrax[71] recorded seven operative deaths in a series of 48 cystic cerebellar hemangioblastomas, a mortality of 14.5%, whereas of the patients 35 were alive and well 20 years postoperatively (73% of the total number or 85.3% of the 41 survivors). Forster[51] found the average survival to be 7 years, with the longest 24 years and 19% dying within 3 months postoperatively. Vinas and Horrax[155] reported a recurrent cerebellar hemangioblastoma after 22 years. The long interval indicates either slow or delayed growth of residual neoplastic tissue or alternatively a second tumor.

Mondkar and associates[99] found that, of 112 patients, three died preoperatively. The operative mortality was 15% and a few died of meningitis. Three months postoperatively 93 were alive. The 5-year survival was 90%, the 10-year survival 80%, and the 20-year survival 40%, whereas only two deaths were attributable to the tumor.

Spinal hemangioblastomas and associated syringomyelia are not so readily lethal, but paraplegia is the frequent serious accompaniment and in these patients intracranial lesions should be sought.

Kernohan and Sayre[75] believe that some vascular tumors are malignant but do not differentiate between hemangioblastomas, and angioblastic meningiomas. Russell and Rubinstein[130] consider the hemangioblastoma to be benign and expect angioblastic meningiomas to be malignant and metastasize.[1]

Associated phenomena. Hemangioblastomas in the posterior cranial fossa may produce hydrocephalus, which can appear early in the illness according to the size and position of the tumor. David and associates[34] emphasized the importance of medullary compression by these tumors and the accompanying cysts.

Trophic changes in the lower limb complicate spinal cord tumors, and bed sores and urinary tract infections remain serious problems in chronic paraplegias. With hemangioblastomas of the spinal cord and medulla oblongata, the cerebrospinal fluid protein is raised, sometimes to extremely high values. Those lesions within the cerebellum cause only an occasional elevation of the protein content.[94] Two very impor-

tant syndromes involving hemangioblastomas consist of those patients with von Hippel-Lindau's disease and those exhibiting an erythrocytosis in their peripheral blood.

Secondary polycythemia. Secondary polycythemia (erythrocytosis) occurs with various tumors, most frequently renal carcinoma, with cerebellar hemangioblastoma being second.[87] Polycythemia has been reported[31,95,157,159] in some 230 cases, occurring with cerebellar hemangioblastoma in 9% to 20%, a frequency considerably higher than that with other varieties of intracranial tumor. In some series of hemangioblastomas a high concentration of erythrocytosis has often been encountered,[95,140] but these cases might have been caused by hemoconcentration. The polycythemia is of the secondary type unaccompanied by splenomegaly, leukocytosis, and thrombocytosis; so the association is probably not a fortuitous concurrence of tumor with polycythemia rubra vera. There may be up to 9 million erythrocytes per cu. mm.[158] or more[13] with hematocrit values from 60 to 70 vol.%[155,160] and hemoglobin values from 20 to 25 gm. per 100 ml. of blood.[17,155,160] As only the hematocrit and the value of the red cell count are increased, the condition has also been termed "erythrocytosis."[149]

Many cases have come to light, and by 1964, 50 cases, not all in detail, had been reported.[87] In 21 patients the elevated red cell indices returned to normal values within a few weeks after extirpation of the tumor.[17] With recurrence of the tumor, the polycythemia tends to reappear.[157]

In a nonexhaustive review* of 38 cases (readily available and with adequate information) of polycythemia with hemangioblastoma, the mean average age was 37.1 years (with a range of 14 to 61 years). Quite unexpectedly there was found an unexplained and inordinately large prepon-

---

*The series consists of patients reported in the following references: 13, 14, 17, 31, 67, 93, 95, 135, 136, 143, 148, 149, 154-157, 159, 160, 170.

derance of this syndrome in males, with only 3 patients being female.

It is generally accepted that the oxygen content of arterial blood by means unknown has a direct influence over erythropoietic activity and that a humoral factor, hemopoietin, is involved. There is evidence that the kidney is a major site of production of erythropoietin[104,123,124] and indeed polycythemia has been associated with renal diseases (polycystic disease, hypernephroma, hydronephrosis, hemangioma, renal adenoma, and nephrocalcinosis attributed to hyperparathyroidism).[24,124] In 1961 Waldmann and associates[157] found a total of 40 instances of polycythemia in association with renal tumors. The presence of erythropoietin has been demonstrated in renal cystic fluid, hydronephrotic fluid, and tissue extracts of hypernephroma.[124] The red cell count generally returns to normal upon excision of the lesion.[24,53] The underlying mechanism has not been explained and erythropoietin may be demonstrated in renal cysts in polycythemic patients yet present in cystic fluid in the absence of polycythemia.[124] Moreover polycythemia has occurred with uterine fibroids[43,114,151] with reversion to normal blood counts after hysterectomy. It has been found in hepatic carcinoma,[92] glioblastoma multiforme, and cerebral metastases.[116] Jepson[74] compiled a lengthy list of miscellaneous diseases associated with secondary polycythemia, which can hardly be regarded as specific for hemangioblastoma. Furthermore, it can be seen in association with other neurological diseases (infections, degenerative lesions, and tumors other than hemangioblastoma).[39,70,83] Drew and Grant[39] reported a case of chronic subdural hematoma with polycythemia. The blood picture reverted to normal after drainage of the hematoma. In man, the diencephalon seems to be involved in the neurogenic production of polycythemia,[17,39] which has been produced experimentally by Schulhof and Matthies[137] by injecting siliceous earth into the diencephalic region of rabbits' brains.

Waldmann and associates[157] found in their patients a normal plasma volume but a very elevated total red cell volume (44 ml. per kg.). The life-span of the erythrocytes was within normal limits and no evidence of increased red cell destruction was detected, yet the rate of red cell synthesis was increased and the red cell iron turnover was considered to be proportional to the increase in red cell mass. There was no evidence of extramedullary erythropoiesis. In fasting rats cyst contents were found to stimulate erythropoiesis, whereas concentrated urine, plasma, and ventricular or spinal fluid from the patient failed to do so. It was found that the erythropoietin in the tumor fluid was stable on freezing and thawing, nondializable, and partially but not completely inactivated after being boiled for 5 minutes.

Race and associates[119] found that fluid from a hemangioblastic cyst produced a reticulocytosis and increase in circulating platelets. Fluid from each of three hemangioblastic cysts of the cerebellum has been shown to have distinct erythropoietic stimulating activity when assayed in rats by the iron (^{59}Fe)-uptake technique.[67] As only two of the three patients exhibited evidence of a secondary polycythemia, the tentative conclusion was that all hemangioblastomas might possess a similar propensity to stimulate erythrocytosis. Polycythemia is associated with both the cystic and the solid variety[67,94] but has not been found in association with angioblastic meningiomas. Apparently the cerebellar tumor is responsible for local production and accumulation of erythropoietin although tissue culture has not been utilized to test the neoplasm for the production of this humoral factor. In Cramer and Kimsey's[31] patient there was also a solitary renal cyst and in Sweeney's case[149] there was polycystic disease of the kidneys. Conceivably the renal lesions could have been responsible for the polycythemia.

It is unlikely that the arteriovenous shunt so frequently associated with cerebellar hemangioblastomas is responsible for the polycythemia. Polycythemia is not a feature of arteriovenous aneurysm of the central nervous system though Lichtensteiger[83] recorded the association. The vascular anomaly was situated in the cerebellum, and so a small hemangioblastoma may have been overlooked. On the basis of present evidence it seems very likely that the tumor produces a humoral factor, hemopoietin, which in some cases of hemangioblastoma causes secondary polycythemia.

Von Hippel-Lindau's disease. In 1926, Lindau,[6] when studying cerebellar cysts, observed that some had hemangiomatous nodules rather than gliomatous tissue in their walls. He also noted the frequency of an associated retinal angioma (von Hippel's disease). The afflicted patients often had raised intracranial pressure and a cerebellar cyst was revealed at autopsy in some instances.[6] Lindau[85] stated that 25% of patients with von Hippel's disease (retinal angioma) have symptoms of brain disorder. He concluded that the two lesions were etiologically related and called the condition "angiomatosis of the central nervous system," since referred to as Lindau's disease or von Hippel-Lindau's disease (or syndrome). Lichtenstein[84] contended that the classical triad of the disease consists of (1) a solid or cystic hemangioblastoma of the hindbrain or spinal cord, (2) retinal angioma (von Hippel's disease), and (3) cystic adenomas of the kidneys. In many cases the full triad is not present[30] and these are regarded as *formes frustes*. The term "von Hippel-Lindau's disease" denotes different things to different authors. Further confounding the problem is variation in the chronological order of appearance of the lesions. One can probably consider the syndrome to consist of hemangioblastomas of the brain and/or spinal cord in association with either retinal and/or visceral involvement. However any patient with a hemangioblastoma of the central nervous system or retina should be examined for the additional constituents of the syndrome and the relatives interrogated and checked for a similar involvement.

The pathological findings are as follows.

Central nervous system. The cerebellar hemangioblastoma (or Lindau's tumor), either solid or cystic, single or multiple, is the most important lesion. It is typically cystic with multiple tumors occurring in 10% of cases. Hemangioblastoma of the brain stem may be present, but a cerebral hemangioblastoma is very unusual.[69]

A number of the patients also have spinal cord hemangioblastomas,[78] perhaps multiple.[166] Russell and Rubinstein[130] found four spinal cord hemangioblastomas in one case. One of the tumors was only 2.5 mm. in its largest diameter and so could easily have been overlooked. Levin[82] asserted that the spinal cord was involved in every proved case of von Hippel-Lindau's disease in which the spinal cord was examined post mortem. Kinney and Fitzgerald[78] estimated that in the literature about 50% (11 cases) of 22 spinal cord hemangioblastomas were associated with von Hippel-Lindau's disease with syringomyelia in 10 of these 11 cases, a higher frequency than in those without. Wolf and Wilens[166] found both syringobulbia and syringomyelia in a male with von Hippel-Lindau's disease (33 years of age) and two hemangioblastomas of the spinal cord. Otenasek and Silver[112] reported a probable spinal hemangioblastoma in association with other manifestations of von Hippel-Lindau's disease in six members of one family. The grandfather was affected as were four of his seven children, and one of the affected daughters had five children, three of whom were afflicted. The fact may not be of significance but von Recklinghausen's disease (neurofibromatosis) and tuberose sclerosis have been described in relatives of patients with von Hippel-Lindau's disease.[94]

Eyes. Retinal hemangioblastoma (von Hippel's disease), histologically similar to those occurring in the posterior fossa, consists of a plexus of numerous thin-walled vessels and cystic spaces with intervening stromal and xanthoma cells.[23] In the lesion frequently referred to as a hemangioblastoma, the retinal artery and vein are dilated and the retinal angioma has been mistaken for an arteriovenous aneurysm.[94] The artery may be beaded and both eyes may be affected in the course of a few years leading to total blindness unless treated early.

Unlike hemangioblastomas of brain and cord, those involving the retina may exhibit considerable calcification and even ossification[35] sufficient to throw a radiological shadow. Retinal hemorrhages may also occur in the absence of papilledema.[4] Retinal detachment attributed to cyst formation[108] frequently follows.[165]

Kidneys. The renal lesions of von Hippel-Lindau's disease, simple cysts and renal cell carcinoma[94] appear in more than two-thirds of autopsy examinations.[121] Weber,[161] believing that the renal cysts differed from those usually seen as polycystic disease of the kidneys, referred to the renal and hepatic cysts as cystic dysplasia of the kidneys and liver.

The renal tumors or adenomas were once believed to be benign, but metastases have revealed that they are true hypernephromas. In a case reported by Melmon and Rosen[94] the hypernephromas were bilateral and metastases were present in the para-aortic lymph nodes.

Pancreas. The pancreas is frequently involved in Lindau's disease usually with multiple cysts that have been described as endothelial or lymphangiomatous cysts[84] although cystadenomas have been observed.[35]

Liver. Cysts of the liver[161] and occasionally an adenoma or cavernous hemangioma have been recorded, but the significance of the latter is open to question.

Epididymis. Simple cysts and cystadenomas of the epididymis are sometimes seen. Tumors resembling hypernephromas have been observed in the epididymis but they may be metastatic. In females there is no counterpart of the epididymal lesions of the male.

Miscellaneous. Melmon and Rosen,[94] listing innumerable other lesions found in association with von Hippel-Lindau's disease, include the following: splenic angioma,

pulmonary cysts lined by columnar or cubical epithelium, adenoma or hyperplasia of the adrenal cortex, cyst or pheochromocytoma of the adrenal medulla, paraganglioma, meningiomas, cyst or hemangioma of bones, pigmented or vascular nevi of the skin[64] (including port-wine stains of face),[161, 172] and hemangioblastoma of the bladder. Several of the lesions are not uncommon at routine autopsy and their incidence in von Hippel-Lindau's disease would have to be shown to be of significance, for the coexistence of an isolated rare lesion such as splenic angioma in a single case of von Hippel-Lindau's disease probably has few implications.

Pheochromocytoma has been reported in association with neurofibromatosis and retinal angiomatosis[20] and associated with von Hippel-Lindau's disease.[94] The association of pheochromocytoma with cerebellar hemangioblastoma has been encountered in a woman and her son[20] and also in a patient with familial pheochromocytoma.[101] In all the association of these two lesions has been recorded now in eight cases[101,107] so that in hypertensive patients with von Hippel-Lindau's disease pheochromocytoma should be excluded.

Other features of the syndrome. In no case to date has the onset appeared prior to puberty.[94] The first symptoms are related to either the cerebellar lesion or the retinal tumor usually in the fourth decade although in the kindred studied by Melmon and Rosen[94] the age range was 19 years to 53 (average 33 years). The sex distribution is said to be equal,[94] despite the male predominance in hemangioblastomas of the posterior fossa and of the spinal cord.[172]

Familial occurrences of hemangioblastoma have been noted.[111] Mondkar and associates[99] found six cases with a family history of hemangioblastoma in a series of 112 cases. With retinal and visceral lesions present, such cases are labeled von Hippel-Lindau's disease. In two sisters with hypernephromas Collier[22] found hemangioblastomas of the posterior fossa. The other manifestations of von Hippel-Lindau's disease being absent is suggestive of *formes frustes* and similarly with other instances of familial hemangioblastoma. Indeed if patients survive sufficiently long, the other manifestations (visceral and retinal) might well materialize.

Melmon and Rosen[94] found 12 subjects with von Hippel-Lindau's disease in three generations of a family tree. Tonning and associates[152] found three of four siblings with von Hippel-Lindau's disease and their mother, blind in one eye, had died of a brain tumor. Silver[139] traced the family tree from a union occurring in Virginia in 1788, and of 96 descendants, adequate information was obtainable on 61. Actual clinical verification of the vascular tumor was available in 19 cases and presumptive evidence in another eight, yielding 27 of 61 members. Though this approximates the anticipated 50% involvement, until 1948 the family had been unaware of the genetic trait, indicating that isolated or sporadic cases may only seem to be so. Christoferson and colleagues[21] found 11 cases of von Hippel-Lindau's disease in a family tree of 90 members. The lesions included five hemangioblastomas in the cerebellum, three in the brain stem, and three in the retina; six subjects had hypernephroma, and polycystic disease of the kidneys was found in four and of the pancreas in five. Goodman and associates[58] traced a family with von Hippel-Lindau's disease, and over three generations 13 members of the family exhibited evidence of the disease. In a parallel group stemming from the sister of the progenitor of the von Hippel-Lindau's disease, all eight people in the three generations suffered from bilateral cataracts of the senile type. In another family Wright[171] found six verified cases and four presumptive cases in four generations. Despite the difficulties inherent in tracing diseases such as this in family trees,[139] remarkable success has been achieved, and investigators consider that von Hippel-Lindau's disease is transmitted as an autosomal dominant gene.

Pathogenesis of hemangioblastoma. The familial incidence and occurrence of multiple lesions has led to the concept that hemangioblastomas arise from congenital rests and malformations. Bailey[6] emphasizes the rich blood supply found in the area postrema at the posterior end of the fourth ventricle. Finding a hemangioblastoma in that situation, he surmised that this variety of tumor arose from maldevelopments of the primitive vascular primordium in the third month of fetal life. The late age of onset (fourth decade) of the majority of cases conflicts with this hypothesis, but most authors have accepted the premise that though difficult to refute, it is equally difficult to substantiate.

The obscure pathogenesis of the various lesions in von Hippel-Lindau's disease obviously encompasses an unspecified inherited etiological factor. It may not necessarily be a tendency to the maldevelopment of the vascular primordium. Our meager knowledge of the pathogenesis limits the efficacy of further discussion of the etiology.

Extradural hemangioblastoma. Wyburn-Mason[172] collected a few cases of extradural hemangioblastoma that exhibited an equal sex ratio and similar age distribution to the preceding tumors and were generally related to the upper thoracic vertebrae. They were not attached to the dura mater or the periosteum or spinal ligaments, and local invasive properties were manifest when the tumors recurred.

Blood vessels and tumors of nonvascular origin

Tumors can be regarded as the excessive autonomous and uncoordinated proliferation of cells or tissue with an active metabolism differing from that of the parent tissue. The frequent progressive nature and high metabolic activity of the new growth demand adequate blood supply and drainage; so there is a simultaneous proliferation primarily of tumor cells and secondarily of blood vessels. The relationship of blood vessels to tumors is relatively unex-

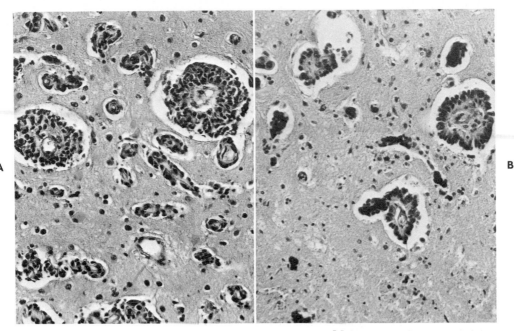

Fig. 11-7. Perivascular extension of metastatic tumors. **A,** Malignant melanoma. **B,** Metastatic carcinoma of the pancreas with palisading of the perivascular tumor cells. (Hematoxylin and eosin, ×110.)

plored territory though of fundamental importance in the proliferation of the tumor and the associated complications. Humoral factors are believed to be involved in angiogenesis in the tumor.[50,60]

The vascularity of intracranial and intraspinal tumors, varying considerably in degree, may even suggest neoplasia of the blood vessels themselves. Meningiomas in particular are often extremely vascular, and angioblastic meningiomas closely resemble the hemangioblastomas. Other tumors often have close architectural relationships to the blood vessels, for example, the pseudopalisading in glioblastomas, the perivascular pseudorosettes of ependymomas,[130] and the perivascular growth of metastatic carcinoma (Fig. 11-7).

The vascularity and stroma are frequently similar to those prevailing in the tissue of origin and particularly in papillomas of the choroid plexus, the vessels of which maintain a similar relationship to the proliferating tumor cells as in the original choroid plexus. The extent of this reproduction of the characteristics of the tissue of origin is as yet unknown. Hypernephromas and carcinomas of the thyroid gland and alimentary tract metastasize to the brain, but whether fenestrated endothelium occurs in the metastases (as is usually found in the kidney, endocrine glands, and alimentary tract) or the nonfenestrated continuous type of endothelium that usually prevails in the brain has not been ascertained.

Apart from implementing the sporadic perivascular round cell infiltration in both primary and secondary tumors of the central nervous system, blood vessels are involved in proliferation of the tumor and the frequent complications of neoplastic tissues.

Edema. Rapidly growing intracranial tumors are often associated with edema, which can be a local reaction in the environs of the tumor. The edema may affect one lobe or extend to the entire hemisphere, but extension to the cerebellum or opposite hemisphere is rare.[75] Edema significantly alters the course of the symptoms and aggravates the space-occupying effects of the tumor. Of uncertain cause, the edema is probably concerned with local pressure effects interfering with the circulation of blood and venous return through the deep transcerebral veins. Anoxia is no doubt contributory and increased capillary permeability ensues. The edema may be pronounced about rapidly growing tumors and is accentuated by trauma. It is more pronounced in the white matter than in the cortex and is characterized by enlargement of perivascular and pericellular spaces and loosening of the ground substance. Perret and Kernohan[117] also included swelling and proliferation of astrocytes and oligodendroglia and degeneration of nerve cells. There is evidence of some demyelination.[173] No doubt the degenerative changes are the consequence of anoxia from the circulatory disturbance caused by the tumor.

Vascular patterns. Hardman[65] investigated the angioarchitecture of the gliomas and found considerable disturbance to the normal vascular pattern. About the malignant tumors the brain has a normal pattern, though in injected specimens the vessels contained little of the infusate. In the margin of the tumor and in the adjoining white matter[42] the vessels were larger and more numerous than the surrounding brain, and those somewhat more deeply situated were large sinusoidal vessels exhibiting tortuosity and variation in caliber. The center was necrotic and contained extravasated blood and thrombosed vessels. Aneurysmal dilatation of capillary loops at the periphery of the tumor was noted with glomerulus-like formations (glomeruloids). In benign gliomas the vascular pattern was abnormal; the vessels were unusually numerous with some reduplication. Arieti[3] emphasized that the large tortuous peripheral vessels in the glioblastoma multiforme were sinusoidal and exhibited aneurysmal dilatations and irregular branching but had no capillary network or anastomoses. Their occlusion jeo-

pardizes a considerable quantity of tissue. Sahs and Alexander[132] likened their vascular configurations to a "wind-swept tree" and a "shrub" formation.

Meningiomas may be exceedingly vascular, with large blood vessels entering the capsule and present about the tumor and little else between the whorls and tumor cells. Many are irregular, thin-walled vessels up to 175 μ in diameter (average of about 80 μ).[132] Small blood vessels or sinusoids up to 100 μ diameter may be visible in the center of the whorls (Fig. 11-8). Their lumens may be obliterated, but they have hyaline and thickened walls as if arteriosclerotic and arteriolosclerotic (Fig. 11-9).

Monckton[98] examined the angioarchitecture of 25 supratentorial meningiomas by the Pickworth[118] method and divided the vascular patterns into five groups of ascending degrees of vascularity. There was no correlation between the vascular type and the age of the patient, the length of history, or the location of the tumor.

Sahs and Alexander[132] thought the vascular architecture of intracranial tumors fell into two main types. One type consists of an interstitial arrangement of vessels mainly restricted to zones about and in between the whorls or lobular subdivisions of the tumor. This arrangement was found in meningiomas and medulloblastomas although in the latter variety of tumor, bulbous dilatations, and loop formations also occurred. In the second group there was a fairly diffuse permeation of the tumor by a vascular stroma, the vessels being infrequently of capillary size and most often sinusoidal or cavernous. In this group were the astrocytomas and oligodendrogliomas. They considered the vascular configuration was characterized by a disorderliness as if the tumor interfered with the normal organization of blood vessels.

Endothelial proliferation. In glioblastoma multiforme (astrocytomas, grades 3 and 4),[75] vascular changes (endothelial proliferation) are particularly common. They occur in localized areas in approximately

95% of these tumors.[52,130] and are not distributed uniformly throughout the tumor. They can be seen in the neighboring brain tissue a short distance from the tumor, and Russell and Rubinstein[130] observed similar lesions in the brain on the side of a sulcus opposite to the infiltrated gyrus. Deery[37] considered the changes to be most prominent and extensive in the areas of most active tumor growth. They are less frequent in astrocytomas than in glioblastoma multiforme[130] and have also been ob-

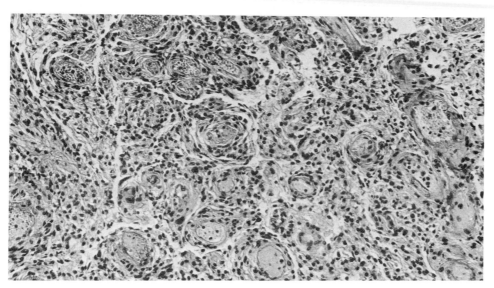

Fig. 11-8. Meningioma with sinusoidal vessels in center of whorls. (Hematoxylin and eosin, ×110.)

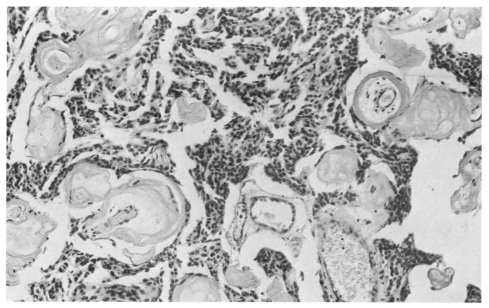

Fig. 11-9. Blood vessels in this meningioma exhibit hyalinized walls and narrowed lumens. Such vessels at times exhibit tortuosity. (Hematoxylin and eosin, ×110.)

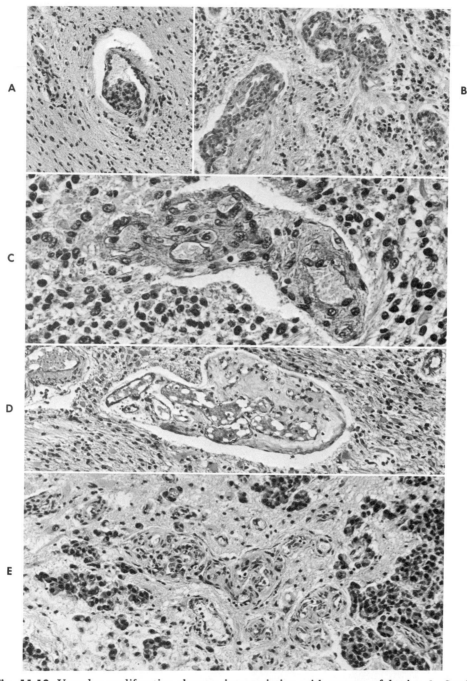

Fig. 11-10. Vascular proliferative changes in association with tumors of brain. **A,** Small clump of proliferated cells projects into lumen. **B,** Proliferation is more diffuse. **C** and **D,** Thickening appears to be outside endothelium. Note mitotic figure in **C** and the fibrosis about vessels in **D. E,** Proliferative changes are related to a metastatic tumor. (Hematoxylin and eosin; **A, B, D,** and **E,** ×110; **C,** ×275.)

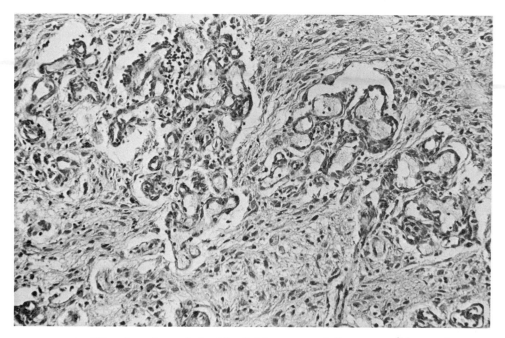

Fig. 11-11. Proliferation of vessels in this glioblastoma multiforme resembles angiomatous tissue. (Hematoxylin and eosin, ×110.)

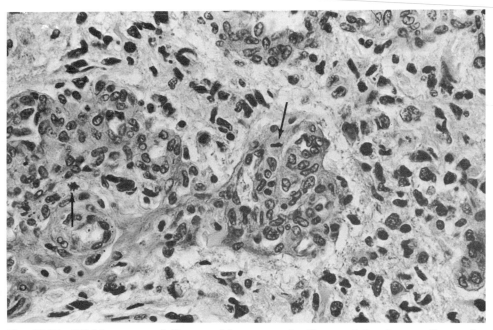

Fig. 11-12. Glioblastoma multiforme with a mass of cells containing few small vascular lumens. There are two mitotic figures (*arrows*). (Hematoxylin and eosin, ×275.)

served in the medulloblastoma,[37] ependymoma, oligodendroglioma, pinealoma, and
craniopharyngioma.[44] The changes are not
limited to glioblastoma multiforme but
occur in and about some metastatic tumors
of the brain. They are also seen in intracranial granulation tissue (especially in organizing hematomas) and in extracranial
tissues (breast and skin).[37] Similar though
only mild or early lesions of this type may
be observed in areas of repair about hematomas, in softenings, and also in the vicinity
of parenchymal damage caused by an arteriovenous aneurysm.

The vascular changes consist of considerable proliferation of the small parenchymal blood vessels so that in a given
area the vessels are exceptionally numerous. Pial vessels are usually not involved.
Some vessels are histologically normal and
others have mildly thickened walls, caused
by either cellular or connective tissue constituents. Still other vessels are a focus of
cellular proliferation or an irregularly
shaped mass, column, or sheet of cells with
plump vesicular nuclei, a moderate amount
of cytoplasm, and perhaps an occasional
giant cell.[37] Within the cellular structures
a few small lumens containing red cells
may be seen, giving the appearance of periendothelial proliferation. In some such
structures no lumen at all may be discernible, whereas in others the proliferation is
less cellular and contains more lumens suggestive of angiomatous tissue (Fig. 11-11).
In some large vessels the proliferation of
cells resembles an intimal pad often projecting into the lumen (Fig. 11-10, *A*). Endothelial cells actually lining the lumen may
have plump nuclei, but generally they are
somewhat more hyperchromatic than most
proliferated cells, which are unlike cells of
the tumor proper. Associated with the vascular proliferative lesions are occasional
mitotic figures (Fig. 11-12), and Deery[37] has
found amitotic forms. Some lesions contain variable numbers of round cells resembling lymphocytes, often with a scanty
stroma or hyaline fibrous tissue. Other vessels exhibit periadventitial proliferation of

connective tissue containing cells and capillaries with few thrombi.

Storring and Duguid[146] on quite inadequate evidence[59,130] attributed the vascular
proliferative lesions with multiple lumens
to thrombosis and recanalization. Deery[37]
regarded them as the subdivision of the
original lumen. Such interpretations mislead, for the original lumen was doubtless
the size of a capillary or venule and no-
where approached the dimensions of most
lesions, which are essentially proliferative
though a few or several lumens may develop and a moderate amount of reticulin
may be demonstrable.[37]

Deery[37] classified these vascular proliferative lesions into four types: those attributed
to overgrowth of endothelium, those attributed to proliferation of adventitia,
those exhibiting a combination of the previous two, and finally those with medial
fibrosis. Despite Deery's emphasis on endothelial proliferation,[37] the pathogenesis is
as yet unproved. Endothelial proliferation
is often used loosely and incorrectly to
mean thickening of vascular walls particularly of the intima, and in these tumors
the cellular proliferations frequently appear to be periendothelial, perhaps of periadventitial cells rather than overgrowth
of endothelium. Electron microscopic studies may identify the cell type. Nyström[109]
made an ultrastructural investigation of
the blood vessels of glioblastoma multiforme. The endothelium was somewhat hypertrophied, and he described an increase
in perivascular connective tissue, multiple
layers of basement membrane, penetration
of endothelial cells by extensions of connective tissue, and variation in the periodicity of collagen. There was no identification of the cells responsible for the vascular proliferative lesions. Conclusions
from electron microscopy and light microscopy were the same, that is, the vascular
changes represented endothelial hyperplasia. Luse[89] considered that proliferation
and thickening of the endothelial cells and
adventitial hyperplasia in varying proportions, with the incorporation in the wall

of neoplastic glial cells resulting from proliferation of the basement membrane, caused the vascular changes. Torack[153] believed that glial cells were not incorporated into the vessel wall but that the cell processes were adventitial cells interrupting and extending outward beyond the basement membranes. These vascular proliferative lesions occur widely, and beyond and independently of tumors; so it is unlikely that Luse's interpretation is correct.

The walls of large sinusoidal or cavernous channels nearer or between areas of necrosis may be thickened irregularly and exhibit some mild infiltration with round cells. The lumens contain thrombi and the wall of an occasional vessel is infiltrated with fibrin suggestive of fibrinoid necrosis.

The vascular proliferative lesions of glioblastoma multiforme are said to undergo sarcomatous change, with the tumors being called perivascular fibrosarcoma or gliosarcoma.[66,130] Russell and Rubinstein[130] asserted that in the examination of a large series of glioblastomas, transitional stages occur between the vascular proliferative lesions described above and sarcomatous proliferation.[45,126] In such tumors the malignant vascular component resembles a fibrosarcoma without evidence of vasoformative characteristics.

Associated vascularity and arteriovenous shunts. The vascularity of tumors whether primary or secondary is naturally abnormal (Fig. 11-13), but the topography of the large vessels angiographically is sometimes sufficiently distinctive to be of diagnostic value, particularly with glioblastomas and meningiomas.[162] There is now ample evidence to indicate that a considerable arteriovenous shunt occurs with many intracranial tumors particularly glioblastoma multiforme, vascular meningiomas, hemangioblastomas, papillomas of the choroid plexus, and even metastatic carcinoma.[46] In general one may say that the more vascular the tumor, the greater is the likelihood of an associated, if temporary, arteriovenous shunt. Possibly it is a feature of all intracranial tumors varying only in degree. Cer-

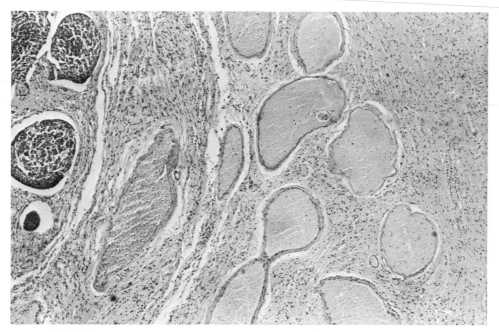

Fig. 11-13. Grossly enlarged thin-walled vessels surrounding metastatic tumor. (Hematoxylin and eosin, ×45.)

tainly it seems that arteriovenous shunts develop readily even with cortical scars.[46,125] Evidence of the shunts is dependent on the following:

1. Early filling of veins on angiography[138]
2. The presence of red arterial blood in veins corresponding to those exhibiting early filling in angiography
3. Actual blood analyses in at least one case confirmed the high oxygen saturation of the blood in these "red" veins
4. Demonstration of direct arteriovenous communications in glioblastoma multiforme by injection of the vessels.

Sanders[133] observed in tumor transplants in observation chambers that the differentiation of capillaries, arterioles, and venules was poorer than in normal tissues. The rapid growth of the tumor and vessels and the poor vascular differentiation permit the ready formation of arteriovenous shunts. Feindel and Perot[46] attributed the presence of blood with a high oxygen saturation in veins to poor oxygen utilization because of the low metabolic activity of the tissue. Both factors may play a role. Yet the arteriovenous shunt, by depriving the tumor of an adequate blood supply (a steal mechanism) may be responsible for the degenerative changes and necrosis within the neoplasm. Consistent with this concept is the observed circulatory stasis in the tumor, for dye in the tumor may persist long after the injection.[98] It has also been observed that these arteriovenous shunts are variable because veins may change from red to blue and back again under different conditions. The state of the transcerebral venous system is thought to influence cortical shunts,[46] and indicator dyes (Coomassie Blue or fluorescein) injected intravascularly have been used to provide comparative transit times for the dyes in different areas of cerebral tumors.[47,48]

The blood supply of meningiomas may come from the vessels normally supplying the scalp, skull, meninges, and brain, with those nearer the base supplied more particularly by vessels of the dura mater and bone. Those of the falx are supplied mostly from the brain. With tumors arising nearer the peripheral extent of the meningeal arterial tree, the dependence on the cerebral circulation is greater and on the extracranial blood supply is less.[98]

Meningiomas demonstrated angiographically produce a "blush" or "stain" caused by enlarged, often tortuous arteries in and about the tumor. This tumor "blush" fades into the capillary phase. The vessels may look frankly angiomatous[98] and because of their vascularity there may be increased vascular[86] markings in the overlying skull: enlarged venous grooves extending to the nearest dural sinus, enlarged emissary foramina, and an augmented vascularity of the bone perhaps with hyperostosis. The vascular changes are probably secondary to the sometimes large arteriovenous shunts and not to the circulatory needs of the neoplasm. For instance, a highly vascular meningioma involving the middle cranial fossa and the orbit, was originally thought to be a carotid-cavernous fistula because of the unilateral exophthalmos, an intracranial bruit, and a high cardiac output, which returned to normal after surgical removal of the tumor.[62]

With intracranial arterial aneurysms being so prevalent, some inevitably will coexist with cerebral tumors[81] and pose a difficult therapeutic problem. The association may be fortuitous, but the development of the aneurysm could occur proximally to an arteriovenous shunt associated with the tumor.

Hemorrhage and necrosis. Large brain tumors generally bleed (Fig. 11-14) into their substance.[57] Infrequently the hemorrhage is sudden and massive, and it was into the tumor or neighboring brain in 3.7% of 832 cases in Oldberg's series.[110] Lesser degrees of hemorrhage (Fig. 11-15) can jeopardize an already precarious cerebral circulation and abrupt clinical deterioration can eventuate. In some cases the sudden onset of profound unconsciousness is associated with hemorrhage into the

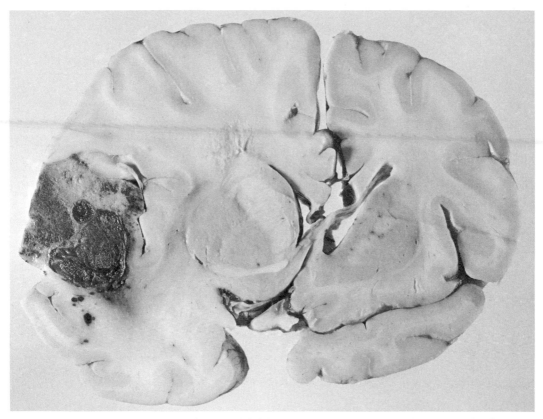

Fig. 11-14. Glioblastoma multiforme exhibiting hemorrhages into its substance and a few satellite parenchymal hemorrhages. Note enlargement of ipsilateral hemisphere because of edema, compression of ventricles, and shift of midline structure.

brain stem.[28] The exacerbation of symptoms may also occur with the development of ischemic necrosis of significant portions of the tumor.[110] Seepage of blood is more common than moderate or severe hemorrhage and can be precipitated by trauma.[29] The hemorrhage may be the first indication of the tumor. It may be subdural, subarachnoid, intracerebral, or intraventricular depending on the tumor location. Reaction of the brain and meninges to the extravasated blood does not differ from that in other pathological states, and superficial hemosiderosis of the central nervous systems has also been attributed to recurrent leakage.[79]

Tumor necrosis is frequently attributed to (1) tumor proliferation outstripping the blood supply, (2) thrombosis of supply vessels caused by toxic factors[37] or infiltra-

tion of the vessel wall by neoplastic cells, and (3) ischemia engendered by a significant arteriovenous shunt effecting a type of steal mechanism. Also such a shunt may possibly be a factor in the hemorrhage from veins

Hematogenous metastases. Most secondary neoplasms are the result of hematogenous spread. Willis[163] estimated that metastatic tumors of the brain occur in approximately 5% of fatal cases of malignant disease, whereas Russell and Rubinstein[130] found metastatic tumors in the brain in 1% of routine autopsies. Hematogenous metastases to the spinal cord are exceedingly rare, but spinal cords are seldom examined at autopsy. Hematogenous metastases constitute from 3% to almost 40% of all intracranial tumors,[75] with the prevalence being dependent on the source of

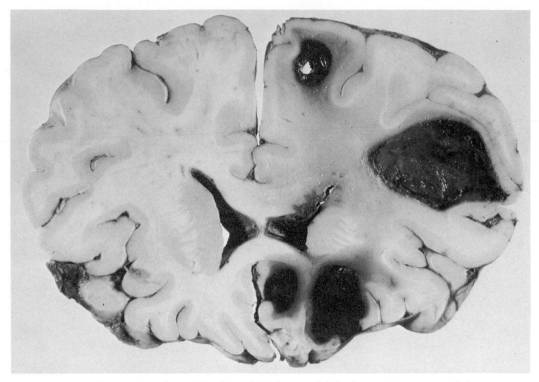

Fig. 11-15. Coronal section of brain exhibiting multiple hemorrhages caused by metastatic melanoma.

the material and the nature of the institution.[40]

Secondary involvement of the brain and its meninges may also occur by vascular permeation or by neoplasms affecting the bones, the nasopharynx, paranasal air sinuses, and even the ear (that is, direct spread).

Autopsy material is a misleading criterion for estimation of the frequency of metastases to the central nervous system. Bronchogenic carcinoma is the commonest cause of cerebral metastases (8% to 41% of cases).[37,163] In a male population Earle[40] reported that 57.5% were from the lung, with the squamous variety producing cerebral metastases less often than other cellular types.[54,130] Previously carcinoma of the breast predominated,[163] but recently, apparently because the afflicted patients do not come to autopsy, it has constituted a lesser proportion of autopsy material.[77] Willis[163] found that mammary cancer was

responsible for fewer cases than bronchogenic cancer, but it had produced secondary brain tumors in 20% of fatal cases. Hypernephromas produce cerebral metastases in 25% of fatal cases, and those of the thyroid are also frequent. Gastric carcinomas do not metastasize to the brain so often but, being so frequent, are relatively common causes of the metastases. Chorionepithelioma, though rare, generally involves the brain,[130] although it is estimated that at least half of all malignant melanomas metastasize to the central nervous system.[75] Rare, interesting metastases to the brain have been reported from primary tumors of the heart, both cardiac myxomas[106] and fibrosarcomas.[26] Metastases to the brain are multiple in 70% of cases[77] but from sarcomas are quite infrequent. Hematogenous metastases to the spinal cord, mostly with cerebral metastases, are usually from the lung and breast.[130,163]

Entry of tumor cells into the blood-

stream. The spread of malignant tumors by the bloodstream presupposes the entrance of neoplastic cells into the bloodstream through some deficiency in the vessel wall. Invasion of vessel walls is frequent, and Willis[163] considers it to be a property of most malignant neoplasms to a greater or lesser extent. Small blood vessels including venules often contain tumor cells, but Willis[163] believes that tumor invasion of large pulmonary veins is a more important source of metastases. The mechanism behind the neoplastic cell invasion of the bloodstream is generally presumed to be an active migration. Some fault in the vascular wall in the face of expanding pressures is no doubt a contributory factor. Trauma to neoplastic tissue and various diagnostic procedures[49] are believed to facilitate the entry of tumor cells into the bloodstream.

Passage of tumor emboli in the bloodstream. Provided that the vessel is not occluded by pressure, the tumor cells, gaining entrance, will act as a foreign surface to which platelets readily adhere. With the nidus of a thrombus thus established, emboli will ensue, with cells washing away or proliferating within the lumen. In the brain, tumor emboli originate variously from the lung, mediastinum, or left atrium, except for sporadic cases of paradoxical embolism from the peripheral circulation.[150] Retrograde venous embolism via the vertebral venous system[10,68] is discussed in Chapter 1. Circulation and uninterrupted passage of individual tumor cells through the pulmonary circulation is feasible[49] and would be facilitated by arteriovenous shunts.

Tumor emboli consist of single cells or more often clumps of cells or thrombi containing tumor cells. Willis[163] estimated that the caliber of pulmonary vessels obstructed by tumor emboli was 206 μ (range of 15 to 650 μ, as measured in paraffin sections) and concluded that most emboli had a diameter of 100 to 200 μ. Tumor emboli to the central nervous system are believed to be smaller than those reaching the lung from the peripheral circulation.[163]

Sites and fate of tumor emboli. Blood-borne tumor emboli will lodge in the cerebral arterial tree, and massive cerebral infarction or multiple small softenings can occur without invasion of the cerebral parenchyma.[90] However the embolism is generally silent or subclinical. Tumor emboli from the vertebral venous system will doubtless be in draining veins.

Tumor embolism of major arteries is rare, and pulmonary surgery is considered to be a major factor in precipitating the embolism. Such cases have been associated with chorionic carcinoma, testicular teratoma,[150] cardiac myxoma,[106] and pulmonary neoplasms.[38,97] Yet like most nonneoplastic emboli, these large tumor emboli occlude the middle cerebral artery[41,150] rather than the posterior or vertebrobasilar circulation.

Hematogenous metastases to the brain are most frequent in the cerebrum and the small ones occur particularly near the junction of the cortex and white matter. Willis,[163] in 168 cases recorded, found the cerebrum affected in 129, the cerebellum in 66, and the brain stem in only 2. Metastases are not often found in the pineal and pituitary glands[96] although Strang and Marsan[147] reported pituitary involvement in 15 cases of a total of 193. Meyer and Reah[96] found only two metastases in the spinal cord in 216 autopsies in which the central nervous system and meninges were secondarily involved by tumors. Barron and associates[9] analyzed 127 necropsies performed for symptomatic involvement of the spinal cord and cauda equina by extradural metastatic tumors and in only two cases were intramedullary metastases found.

A further but rare sequel of hematogenous spread of tumors to the brain is the formation of arterial aneurysms.

Neoplastic aneurysms. Aneurysmal dilatation of small vessels in the vicinity of cerebral tumors may be demonstrated by angiography[162] but irregularity in the caliber of these vessels may be the result of arteriovenous shunts. Murphy[102] asserted that arterial aneurysms could develop as the result of neoplastic invasion of the wall after tumor embolism at forks.

In recent years true neoplastic aneurysms associated with cardiac myxomas have been recognized as distinct entities. Cardiac myxomas have been reported in over 350 patients.[106] They are found mostly (75%) in the left atrium and in almost 50% of cases with systemic embolic manifestations emboli are found in the brain.[141] Stoane and associates[145] assert that other emboli derange the renal, splenic, and coronary arterial beds, but if an adequate search is made, it will be found that the mesenteric and iliac arterial trees are also involved. Cerebral angiography has recently revealed that the emboli do not merely obstruct branches of the arterial tree and cause infarction but that irregular dilatation of the lumen is also possible.[15,18,105,106] These aneurysms, which have been mostly multiple and bilateral, are on the terminal branches of the middle cerebral artery and are often associated with multiple stenoses and occlusions of the vessels. The vertebrobasilar circulation can be affected.[106] In an autopsy reported by New and associates, there were multiple aneurysms of the cerebral circulation (Fig. 11-16) and systemic arteries. The cerebral complications may arise with silent cardiac myxomas[91] or be-

come manifest after removal of the cardiac tumor. Macroscopically, these aneurysms secondary to emboli from a cardiac myxoma are irregularly fusiform and lobulated gray-white swellings along the course of the terminal branches of cerebral and cerebellar arteries. They are frequently located at or near bifurcations. The largest measured up to 25 mm. in its largest dimension.[106] Most are considerably smaller (up to 5 mm. in diameter). In association with the lesions the small peripheral vessels and even large arteries such as the basilar are partially or completely occluded.[106] Recent and old infarcts of varying age may be scattered throughout the brain. There may be some hemorrhage but it is not a prominent feature. The gamma globulin in the cerebrospinal fluid is increased.[106]

Microscopically arteries of all sizes may contain myxomatous deposits in the wall or occluding the lumen and, though destruction of the arterial wall results in dilatation, the walls are nevertheless thick because of the proliferation of the neoplastic tissue.[15,106] Connective tissue proliferation of the vessel wall and a mild inflammatory reaction may accompany the vascular lesions. False aneurysms have also been reported[106] and thrombi may be associated with some metastases. Myxomatous tissue may be found in the leptomeninges. These myxomatous metastases appear to exhibit low-grade invasive properties and indicate the necessity for early diagnosis and treatment of cardiac myxomas.

Hematogenous spread of tumors from the brain. Metastatic tumors to the central nervous system may in turn involve veins or even the dural sinuses, producing tertiary spread from these metastases. In such instances metastases from the primary site may be so numerous that tertiary spread is masked by the widespread tumor dissemination.

Despite still existing skepticism,[163] spread of primary tumors of the central nervous system to extracranial sites is now well recognized but the extreme rarity of such an event is enigmatic. Many intracranial tu-

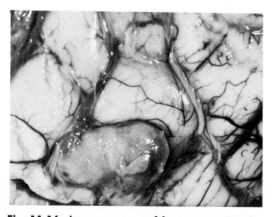

Fig. 11-16. Aneurysm caused by myxomatous infiltration of the wall by embolus from cardiac myxoma. (From New, P. F. J., Price, D. L., and Carter, B.: Cerebral angiography in cardiac myxoma, Radiology **96:**335, 1970.)

mors are highly anaplastic and locally invasive, yet distal metastases are exceedingly rare, whether because of the tumors or the cerebral blood vessels is unknown. The reasons frequently given for this characteristic of malignant tumors of the brain are (1) the absence of lymphatics, (2) the thin walls of cerebral veins, which are thought to collapse before invasion occurs, (3) the thick fibrous (dural) investment of the venous sinuses, and (4) the relatively short survival time of patients with malignant cerebral tumors.

Glioblastomas occasionally invade a blood vessel or a dural sinus, and Russell and Rubinstein[130] illustrated glioblastomatous permeation of veins in the wall of the superior longitudinal sagittal sinus. Similarly tumors of the pituitary can invade the cavernous sinus.[73] During surgical removal of the intracranial tumors, venous channels are opened and the negative intraluminal pressure is allegedly sufficient to draw viable tumor cells into the lumen[1] in a manner similar to the inspiration of air. Rubinstein[128] found some 50 cases of extracranial extension and metastasis in the literature up to 1967, but failed to find a well-documented case in which some surgical procedure had not preceded the complication. Rubinstein[127] reported a cerebellar medulloblastoma with both blood and lymphatic spread. The extracranial extension and metastases were ascribed to the invasion of the orbit and permeation of dural veins by a secondary in the frontal fossa 4 years after a diagnostic biopsy. He also encountered a malignant astrocytoma that had invaded the superior longitudinal sagittal sinus with consequent widespread metastases.

Patterson and colleagues[113] stated in 1961 that about 60 instances of metastasis from primary tumors of the central nervous system were known. All except two ependymomas of the cauda equina were exclusively intracranial. They added a case of ependymoma of the cauda equina with invasion of the dura mater, vertebral bodies, and retroperitoneal space, together with widespread metastases in viscera and lymph nodes. Of 11 ependymomas in the literature with spread to extracranial or extraspinal tissues, three had invaded soft tissues locally, and eight had distal metastases. Of 15 gliomas that had metastasized, one was oligodendroglioma, five were medulloblastomas, eight were glioblastomas, and two were unclassified. Considerable controversy has raged concerning their validity, yet metastases distant from meningiomas and sarcomas have been accepted with less skepticism. Other intracranial tumors that have metastasized are neoplasms of the pineal gland, pituitary tumor, hemangioblastoma, melanoma, and choroid plexus papillomas.

Smith and associates[142] found among some 8000 neuroectodermal tumors of the central nervous system only 35 cases with extracranial or extraspinal metastases. Of these 23 were glioblastomas, eight were medulloblastomas, and four were miscellaneous glial tumors. A craniotomy had been performed previously in every case and thus there is accord with Rubinstein's view[128] of how critical is the factor of surgical intervention.

The most frequent sites of extracranial metastases are the cervical lymph nodes and the axial skeleton,[63] although the lung, liver, and lymph nodes elsewhere (mediastinum and retroperitoneum) have been involved.

Perivascular spread of tumors. In their absence, spread along lymphatic spaces is not available to malignant tumors of the central nervous system. However the Virchow-Robin spaces may act in this capacity to a degree. Malignant tumors of extracranial sources that have reached the brain by direct or hematogenous spread not infrequently extend along the perivascular spaces (Fig. 11-7), and in leptomeningeal carcinomatosis or melanomatosis, the spread along them penetrates for a considerable distance into the cortex. Metastases to the cerebrum itself exhibit the same infiltration at the periphery, but peculiarly enough, this form of spread is not an element of primary tumors of the central nervous system.

References

1. Abbott, K. H., and Love, J. G.: Metastasizing intracranial tumors, Ann. Surg. 118:343, 1943.
2. Annotation: Cerebellar haemangioblastoma: a misnomer, Lancet 1:1095, 1967.
3. Arieti, S.: The vascularization of cerebral neoplasms studied with the fuchsin staining method of Eros, J. Neuropath. Exp. Neurol. 1:375, 1942.
4. Armstrong, M. V.: Angiomatosis retinae (von Hippel's disease, Lindau's disease) complicated by pregnancy, Amer. J. Obstet. Gynec. 34:494, 1937.
5. Bailey, O. T., and Ford, R.: Sclerosing hemangiomas of the central nervous system. Progressive tissue change in hemangioblastomas of the brain and in so-called angioblastic meningiomas, Amer. J. Path. 18:1, 1942.
6. Bailey, P.: Intracranial tumors, ed. 2, Springfield, Ill., 1948, Charles C Thomas, Publisher.
7. Bailey, P., Cushing, H., and Eisenhardt, L.: Angioblastic meningiomas, Arch. Path. 6:953, 1928.
8. Barnard, W. G., and Walshe, F. M. R.: Capillary haemangeioma of cerebrum, J. Path. Bact. 34:385, 1931.
9. Barron, K. D., Hirano, A., Araki, S., and Terry, R. D.: Experiences with metastatic neoplasms involving the spinal cord, Neurology 9:91, 1959.
10. Batson, O. V.: The function of the vertebral veins and their role in the spread of metastases, Ann. Surg. 112:138, 1940.
11. Bennett, W. A.: Primary intracranial neoplasms in military age groups—World War II, Milit. Surg. 99:594, 1946.
12. Bergstrand, A., Höök, O., and Lidvall, H.: Vascular malformations of the spinal cord, Acta Neurol. Scand. 40:169, 1964.
13. Blumberg, B., and Myerson, R. M.: Erythrocytosis associated with cerebellar hemangioblastoma, Neurology 7:367, 1957.
14. Brody, J. I., and Rodriguez, F.: Cerebellar hemangioblastoma and polycythemia (erythrocythemia), Amer. J. Med. Sci. 242:579, 1961.
15. Burton, C., and Johnston, J.: Multiple cerebral aneurysms and cardiac myxoma, New Eng. J. Med. 282:35, 1970.
16. Cancilla, P. A., and Zimmerman, H. M.: The fine structure of a cerebellar hemangioblastoma, J. Neuropath. Exp. Neurol. 24:621, 1965.
17. Carpenter, G., Schwartz, H., and Walker, A. E.: Neurogenic polycythemia, Ann. Intern. Med. 19:470, 1943.
18. Case Record of Massachusetts General Hospital: Case 481970, New Eng. J. Med. 283:1157, 1970.
19. Castaigne, P., David, M., Pertuiset, B., Escourolle, R., and Poirier, J.: L'ultrastructure des hémangioblastomes du système nerveux central, Rev. Neurol. 118:5, 1968.
20. Chapman, R. C., and Diaz-Perez, R.: Pheochromocytoma associated with cerebellar hemangioblastoma, J.A.M.A. 182:1014, 1962.
21. Christoferson, L. A., Gustafson, M. B., and Petersen, A. G.: Von Hippel-Lindau's disease, J.A.M.A. 178:280, 1961.
22. Collier, W. T.: Two cases of Lindau's disease, Brit. Med. J. 2:144, 1931.
23. Collins, E. T.: Ocular haemangiomatous formations associated with vascular tumours of the brain and spinal cord, Proc. Roy. Soc. Med. 24:372, 1931.
24. Cooper, W. M., and Tuttle, W. B.: Polycythemia associated with a benign kidney lesion: report of a case of erythrocytosis with hydronephrosis, with remission of polycythemia following nephrectomy, Ann. Intern. Med. 47:1008, 1957.
25. Corradini, E. W., and Browder, J.: Angioblastic neoplasms of the brain, J. Neuropath. Exp. Neurol. 7:299, 1948.
26. Coulter, J. A., and Gildenhorn, V. B.: Cerebral metastasis from a silent cardiac sarcoma, J. Neurosurg. 18:384, 1961.
27. Courville, C. B.: Histogenetic interrelationships between supratentorial angioblastic meningiomas and hemangioblastomas of the cerebellum, Bull. Los Angeles Neurol. Soc. 22:159, 1957.
28. Cox, L. B.: Haemorrhage of the brain stem as a significant complication of intracranial tumors, Med. J. Aust. 1:259, 1939.
29. Cox, L. B.: Trauma and intracranial tumours, Med. J. Aust. 1:256, 1939.
30. Craig, W. McK., Wagener, H. P., and Kernohan, J. W.: Lindau-von Hippel disease, Arch. Neurol. Psychiat. 46:36, 1941.
31. Cramer, F., and Kimsey, W.: The cerebellar hemangioblastomas. Review of fifty-three cases, with special reference to cerebellar cysts and the association of polycythemia, Arch. Neurol. Psychiat. 67:237, 1952.
32. Cumings, J. N.: The chemistry of cerebral cysts, Brain 73:244, 1950.
33. Cushing, H., and Bailey, P.: Tumors arising from the blood-vessels of the brain, Springfield, Ill., 1928, Charles C Thomas, Publisher.
34. David, M., Messimy, R., Sachs, M., and Chedru, F.: Hémangioblastomes cérébelleux et compression médullaire, Presse Med. 76:2413, 1968.
35. Davison, C., Brock, S., and Dyke, C. G.: Retinal and central nervous hemangioblastomatosis with visceral changes (von Hippel-Lindau's disease), Bull. Neurol. Inst. N.Y. 5:72, 1936.
36. Deeley, T. J., and Edwards, J. M. R.: Radiotherapy in the management of cerebral secondaries from bronchial carcinoma, Lancet 1:1209, 1968.
37. Deery, E. M.: Some features of glioblastoma multiforme, Bull. Neurol. Inst. N.Y. 2:157, 1932.
38. Dickens, W. N., Sayre, G. P., Clagett, O. T., and Goldstein, N. P.: Tumor embolism of the basilar artery: case report, Arch. Neurol 5:655, 1961.
39. Drew, J. H., and Grant, F. C.: Polycythemia as a neurosurgical problem, Arch. Neurol. Psychiat. 54:25, 1945.
40. Earle, K. M.: Metastatic and primary intracranial tumors of the adult male, J. Neuropath. Exp. Neurol. 13:448, 1954.

41. Eason, E. H.: A case of cerebral infarction due to neoplastic embolism, J. Path. Bact. **62:** 454, 1950.

42. Elsberg, C. A., and Hare, C. C.: The blood supply of the gliomas, Bull. Neurol. Inst. N.Y. **2:**210, 1912.

43. Engel, H. W., and Singer, K.: Polycythemia with fibroids, J.A.M.A. **159:**190, 1955.

44. Feigin, I., Allen, L. B., Lipkin, L., and Gross, S. W.: The endothelial hyperplasia of the cerebral blood vessels with brain tumors, and its sarcomatous transformation, Cancer **11:**264, 1958.

45. Feigin, I. H., and Gross, S. W.: Sarcoma arising in glioblastoma of the brain, J. Path. Bact. **31:**633, 1955.

46. Feindel, W., and Perot, P.: Red cerebral veins. A report on arteriovenous shunts in tumors and cerebral scars, J. Neurosurg. **22:**315, 1965.

47. Feindel, W., Yamamoto, Y. L., and Hodge, C. P.: Intracarotid fluorescein angiography: a new method for examination of the epicerebral circulation in man, Canad. Med. Ass. J. **96:**1, 1967.

48. Feindel, W., Yamamoto, Y. L., and Hodge, P.: The human cerebral microcirculation studied by intra-arterial radio-active tracers, Coomassie blue and fluorescein dyes, Proceedings of the Fourth European Conference on Microcirculation, Bibl. Anat. **9:**220, 1967.

49. Fisher, E. R., and Fisher, B.: Recent observations on concepts of metastasis, Arch. Path. **83:**321, 1967.

50. Folkman, J., Merler, E., Abernathy, C., and Williams, G.: Isolation of a tumor factor responsible for angiogenesis, J. Exp. Med. **133:** 275, 1971.

51. Forster, D. M. C.: Cystic cerebellar tumours: a clinico-pathological reappraisal, J. Neurol. Neurosurg. Psychiat. **28:**462, 1965.

52. Frankel, S. A., and German, W. J.: Glioblastoma multiforme. Review of 219 cases with regard to natural history, pathology, diagnostic methods and treatment, J. Neurosurg. **15:**489, 1958.

53. Frey, W. G.: Polycythemia and hypernephroma. Review and report of a case with apparent surgical cure, New Eng. J. Med. **258:** 842, 1958.

54. Galluzzi, S., and Payne, P. M.: Brain metastases from primary bronchial carcinoma: a statistical study of 741 necropsies, Brit. J. Cancer **10:**408, 1956.

55. Gensler, S., Caplan, L. H., and Laufman, H.: Giant benign hemangiopericytoma functioning as an arteriovenous shunt, J.A.M.A. **198:** 203, 1966.

56. Globus, J. H.: Hemorrhage into hemangiomatous cerebellar cyst, Arch. Neurol. Psychiat. **64:**741, 1950.

57. Globus, J. H., and Sapirstein, M.: Massive hemorrhage into brain tumor: its significance and probable relationship to rapidly fatal termination and antecedent trauma, J.A.M.A. **120:**348, 1942.

58. Goodman, J., Kleinholz, E., and Peck, F. C.: Lindau's disease—in the Hudson valley, J. Neurosurg. **21:**97, 1964.

59. Gough, J.: The structure of the blood vessels in cerebral tumours, J. Path. Bact. **51:**23, 1940.

60. Greenblatt, M., and Shubik, P.: Tumor angiogenesis: transfilter diffusion studies in the hamster by the transparent chamber technique, J. Nat. Cancer Inst. **41:**111, 1968.

61. Greenfield, J. G.: Discussion, Proc. Roy. Soc. Med. **24:**382, 1931.

62. Gupta, P. D., Fort, M. L., Barron, K. D., Baron, J. K., and Sharp, J. T.: Cardiac hemodynamics in intracranial arteriovenous fistula, Neurology **19:**198, 1969.

63. Gyepes, M. T., and D'Angio, G. J.: Extracranial metastases from central nervous system tumors in children and adolescents, Radiology **87:**55, 1966.

64. Hall, G. S.: Blood vessel tumours of the brain with particular reference to the Lindau syndrome, J. Neurol. Psychopath. **15:**305, 1935.

65. Hardman, J.: The angioarchitecture of the gliomata, Brain **63:**91, 1940.

66. Hawn, C. van Z., and Ingraham, F. D.: Blood vessel hyperplasia masking glioblastoma multiforme, J. Neuropath. Exp. Neurol. **4:**364, 1945.

67. Hennessy, T. G., Stern, W. E., and Herrick, S. E.: Cerebellar hemangioblastoma: erythropoietic activity by radioiron assay, J. Nucl. Med. **8:**601,1967.

68. Herlihy, W. F.: Revision of the venous system: the role of the vertebral veins, Med. J. Aust. **1:**661, 1947.

69. Hoff, J. T., and Ray, B. S.: Cerebral hemangioblastoma occurring in a patient with von Hippel-Lindau disease, J. Neurosurg. **28:**365, 1968.

70. Holmes, C. R., Kredel, F. E., and Hanna, C. B.: Polycythemia secondary to brain tumor, Southern Med. J. **45:**967, 1952.

71. Horrax, G.: Benign (favorable) types of brain tumor. The end results (up to twenty years), with statistics and useful survival, New Eng. J. Med. **250:** 981, 1954.

72. Innes, J. R. M., and Saunders, L. Z.: Comparative neuropathology, New York, 1962, Academic Press Inc.

73. Jefferson, G.: Extrasellar extensions of pituitary adenomas, Proc. Roy. Soc. Med. **33:**433, 1940.

74. Jepson, J. H.: Polycythemia: diagnosis, pathophysiology, and therapy, Canad. Med. Ass. J. **100:**271, 327, 1969.

75. Kernohan, J. W., and Sayre, G. P.: Tumors of the central nervous system. In: Atlas of tumor pathology, Section 10, Fascicles 35 and 37, Washington, 1952, Armed Forces Institute of Pathology.

76. Kernohan, J. W., Woltman, H. W., and Adson, A. W.: Intramedullary tumors of the spinal cord. A review of fifty-one cases, with an attempt at histologic classification, Arch. Neurol. Psychiat. **25:**679, 1931.

77. Kiefer, E. J.: Metastatic brain tumors. Thesis, University of Minnesota Graduate School, 1947.

78. Kinney, T. D., and Fitzgerald, P. J.: Lindau-

von Hippel disease with hemangioblastoma of the spinal cord and syringomyelia, Arch. Path. 43:439, 1947.

79. Kott, E., Bechar, M., Bornstein, B., Askenasy, H. M., and Sandbank, U.: Superficial hemosiderosis of the central nervous system, Acta Neurochir. 14:287, 1966.

80. Krishnan, K. R., and Smith, W. T.: Intramedullary haemangioblastoma of the spinal cord associated with pial varicosities simulating intradural angioma, J. Neurol. Neurosurg. Psychiat. 24:350, 1961.

81. Levin, P., and Gross, S. W.: Meningioma and aneurysm in the same patient, Arch. Neurol. 15:629, 1966.

82. Levin, P. M.: Multiple hereditary hemangioblastomas of the nervous system, Arch. Neurol. Psychiat. 36:384, 1936.

83. Lichtensteiger, W. H.: Angioma arteriovenosum aneurysmaticum des Kleinhirns mit Polycythämie (Polyglobulie) und terminaler Massenblutung, Schweiz. Med. Wschr. 94:720, 1964.

84. Lichtenstein, B. W.: Lindau's disease—pathological observations, J. Neuropath. Exp. Neurol. 10:103, 1951.

85. Lindau, A.: Discussion on vascular tumours of the brain and spinal cord, Proc. Roy. Soc. Med. 24:363, 1931.

86. Lindblom, K.: A roentgenographic study of the vascular channels of the skull, Acta Radiol. Scand., Suppl. 30, p. 1, 1936.

87. Lipsett, M. B., Odell, W. D., Rosenberg, L. E., and Waldmann, T. A.: Humoral syndromes associated with nonendocrine tumors, Ann. Intern. Med. 61:733, 1964.

88. Lüginbühl, H., Frankhauser, R., and McGrath, J. T.: Spontaneous neoplasms of the nervous system in animals, Progr. Neurol. Surg. 2:85, 1968.

89. Luse, S. A.: Electron microscopic studies of brain tumors, Neurology 10:881, 1960.

90. Madow, L., and Alpers, B. J.: Cerebral vascular complications of metastatic carcinoma, J. Neuropath. Exp. Neurol. 11:137, 1952.

91. Maroon, J. C., and Campbell, R. L.: Atrial myxoma: a treatable cause of stroke, J. Neurol. Neurosurg. Psychiat. 32:129, 1969.

92. McFadzean, A. J. S., Todd, D., and Tsang, K. C.: Polycythemia in primary carcinoma of the liver, Blood 13:427, 1958.

93. McGovern, V. J.: Personal communication, 1970.

94. Melmon, K. L., and Rosen, S. W.: Lindau's disease: review of the literature and study of a large kindred, Amer. J. Med. 36:595, 1964.

95. Meredith, J. M., and Hennigar, G. R.: Cerebellar hemangiomas; a clinicopathologic study of fourteen cases, Amer. Surg. 20:410, 1954.

96. Meyer, P. C., and Reah, T. G.: Secondary neoplasms of the central nervous system and meninges, Brit. J. Cancer 7:438, 1953.

97. Miller, A. A., and Jackson, F. B.: Gross arterial embolism by a myxosarcoma of pulmonary origin, J. Path. Bact. 68:221, 1954.

98. Monckton, G.: An investigation into the causes of failure of certain supratentorial meningiomata to show tumour vessels on angiography, Brain 76:149, 1953.

99. Mondkar, V. P., McKissock, W., and Russell, R. W. R.: Cerebellar haemangioblastomas, Brit. J. Surg. 54:45, 1967.

100. Morello, G., and Bianchi, M.: Cerebral hemangioblastomas. Review of literature and report of two personal cases, J. Neurosurg. 20: 254, 1963.

101. Mulholland, S. G., Nuzhet, O. A., and Walzak, M. P.: Familial pheochromocytoma associated with cerebellar hemangioblastoma, J.A.M.A. 207:1709, 1969.

102. Murphy, J. P.: Cerebrovascular disease, Chicago, 1954, Year Book Publishers, Inc.

103. Myers, J., Scott, M., and Silverstein, A.: Cystic hemangioblastoma of pons, J. Neurosurg. 18: 694, 1961.

104. Naets, J.-P.: The role of the kidney in the production of the erythropoietic factor, Blood 16:1770, 1960.

105. New, P. F. J.: Myxomatous emboli in brain, New Eng. J. Med. 282:396, 1970.

106. New, P. F. J., Price, D. L., and Carter, B.: Cerebral angiography in cardiac myxoma, Radiology 96:335, 1970.

107. Nibbelink, D. W., Peters, B. H., and McCormick, W. F.: On the association of pheochromocytoma and cerebellar hemangioblastoma, Neurology 19:455, 1969.

108. Noran, H. H.: Intracranial vascular tumors and malformations, Arch. Path. 39:393, 1945.

109. Nyström, S.: Pathological changes in blood vessels of human glioblastoma multiforme, Acta Path. Microbiol. Scand. 49: (suppl. 137):1, 1960.

110. Oldberg, E.: Hemorrhage into gliomas. A review of eight hundred and thirty-two consecutive verified cases of glioma, Arch. Neurol. Psychiat. 30:1061, 1933.

111. Olivecrona, H.: The cerebellar angioreticulomas, J. Neurosurg. 9:317, 1952.

112. Otenasek, F. J., and Silver, M. L.: Spinal hemangioma (hemangioblastoma) in Lindau's disease, J. Neurosurg. 18:295, 1961.

113. Patterson, R. H., Campbell, W. G., and Parsons, H.: Ependymoma of the cauda equina with multiple visceral metastases, J. Neurosurg. 18:145, 1961.

114. Payne, P., Woods, H. F., and Wrigley, P. F. M.: Uterine fibromyomata and secondary polycythaemia, J. Obstet. Gynaec. Brit. Comm. 76:845, 1969.

115. Pennybacker, J.: Recurrence in cerebellar haemangiomas. Zbl. Neurochir. 14:63, 1954.

116. Perlmutter, I., and Strain, R. E.: Polycythemia complicated by brain tumor, Neurology 4: 398, 1954.

117. Perret, G. E., and Kernohan, J. W.: Histopathologic changes of the brain caused by intracranial tumors (so-called edema or swelling of the brain), J. Neuropath. Exp. Neurol. 2:341, 1943.

118. Pickworth, F. A.: A new method of study of the brain capillaries and its application to

the regional localization of mental disorder, J. Anat. **69**:62, 1934.

119. Race, G. J., Finney, J. W., Mallams, J. T., and Balla, G. A.: Hematopoietic stimulating effect of a cerebellar hemangioblastoma, J.A.M.A. **187**:150, 1964.

120. Ramsay, H. J.: Fine structure of hemangiopericytoma and hemangioendothelioma, Cancer **19**:2005, 1966.

121. Raynor, R. B., and Kingman, A. F.: Hemangioblastoma and vascular malformations as one lesion, Arch. Neurol. **12**:39, 1965.

122. Rivera, E., and Chason, J. L.: Cerebral hemangioblastoma. Case report and review of the literature, J. Neurosurg. **25**:452, 1966.

123. Rosse, W. F., and Waldmann, T. A.: The role of the kidney in the erythropoietic response to hypoxia in parabiotic rats, Blood **19**:75, 1962.

124. Rosse, W. F., Waldmann, T. A., and Cohen, P.: Renal cysts, erythropoietin and polycythemia, Amer. J. Med. **34**:76, 1963.

125. Rowbotham, G. F., and Little, E.: A new concept of the circulation and the circulations of the brain. The discovery of surface arteriovenous shunts, Brit. J. Surg. **52**:539, 1965.

126. Rubinstein, L. J.: The development of contiguous sarcomatous and gliomatous tissue in intracranial tumours, J. Path. Bact. **71**:441, 1956.

127. Rubinstein, L. J.: Extracranial metastases in cerebellar medulloblastoma, J. Path. Bact. **78**:187, 1959.

128. Rubinstein, L. J.: Development of extracranial metastases from a malignant astrocytoma in the absence of previous craniotomy, J. Neurosurg. **26**:542, 1967.

129. Russell, D. S.: Meningeal tumours: a review, J. Clin. Path. **3**:191, 1950.

130. Russell, D. S., and Rubinstein, L. J.: Pathology of tumours of the nervous system, ed. 2, Baltimore, 1963, The Williams & Wilkins Co.

131. Sachs, M., Rancurel, G., Escourolle, R., and Poirier, J.: Maladie de von Hippel-Lindau. Hémangioblastomes médullaires simulant une malformation artério-veineuse, Neurochirurgie. **15**:575, 1968.

132. Sahs, A. L., and Alexander, L.: Vascular pattern of certain intracranial neoplasms, Arch. Neurol. Psychiat. **42**:44, 1939.

133. Sanders, A. G.: Microcirculation in grafts of normal and malignant tissue, J. Anat. **97**:631, 1963.

134. Sargent, P., and Greenfield, J. G.: Haemangiomatous cysts of the cerebellum, Brit. J. Surg. **17**:84, 1929-1930.

135. Schmid, R., and French, L. A.: Cerebellares Hämangioblastom mit Polycythämie, Schweiz. Med. Wschr. **85**:1274, 1955.

136. Schmidt, E. B.: Nevropat. i Psikhiat. **17**:53, 1948. Cited by Schmid and French.[135]

137. Schulhof, K., and Matthies, M. M.: Polyglobulia induced by cerebral lesions, J.A.M.A. **89**:2093, 1927.

138. Schurr, P. H., and Wickbom, I.: Rapid serial angiography: further experience, J. Neurol. Neurosurg. Psychiat. **15**:110, 1952.

139. Silver, M. L.: Hereditary vascular tumors of the nervous system, J.A.M.A. **156**:1053, 1954.

140. Silver, M. L., and Hennigar, G.: Cerebellar hemangioma (hemangioblastoma): a clinicopathological review of 40 cases, J. Neurosurg. **9**:484, 1952.

141. Silverman, J., Olwin, J. S., and Graettinger, J. S.: Cardiac myxomas with systemic embolization, Circulation **26**:99, 1962.

142. Smith, D. R., Hardman, J. M., and Earle, K. M.: Metastasizing neuroectodermal tumors of the central nervous system, J. Neurosurg. **31**:50, 1969.

143. Starr, G. F., Stroebel, C. F., and Kearns, T. P.: Polycythemia with papilledema and infratentorial vascular tumors, Ann. Intern. Med. **48**:978, 1958.

144. Stein, A. A., Schilp, A. O., and Whitfield, R. D.: The histogenesis of hemangioblastoma of the brain, J. Neurosurg. **17**:751, 1960.

145. Stoane, L., Allen, J. H., and Collins, H. A.: Radiologic observations in cerebral embolization from left heart myxomas, Radiology **87**:262, 1966.

146. Storring, F. K., and Duguid, J. B.: The vascular formations in glioblastoma, J. Path. Bact. **68**:231, 1954.

147. Strang, R., and Marsan, C. A.: Brain metastases, Arch. Neurol. **4**:8, 1961.

148. Stroebel, C. F., and Fowler, W. S.: Secondary polycythemia, Med. Clin. N. Amer. **40**:1061, 1956.

149. Sweeney, L.: Case reported of Lindau's disease with polycythemia and the relationship of erythropoietin, Amer. J. Roentgen. **95**:880, 1965.

150. Thompson, T., and Evans, W.: Paradoxical embolism, Quart. J. Med. **23**:135, 1929-1930.

151. Thomson, A. P., and Marson, F. G. W.: Polycythemia with fibroids, Lancet **2**:759, 1953.

152. Tonning, H. O., Warren, R. F., and Barrie, H. J.: Familial haemangiomata of the cerebellum, J. Neurosurg. **9**:124, 1952.

153. Torack, R. M.: Ultrastructure of capillary reaction to brain tumors, Arch. Neurol. **5**:416, 1961.

154. Trupp, M., and Sachs, E.: Vascular tumors of the brain and spinal cord and their treatment, J. Neurosurg. **5**:354, 1948.

155. Vinas, F. J., and Horrax, G.: Recurrence of cerebellar hemangioblastoma after 22 years—operation and recovery, J. Neurosurg. **13**:641, 1956.

156. Waldmann, T. A., and Levin, E. H.: The production of an erythropoiesis stimulating factor by a cerebellar hemangioblastoma, Clin. Res. **8**:19, 1960.

157. Waldmann, T. A., Levin, E. H., and Baldwin, M.: The association of polycythemia with a cerebellar hemangioblastoma, Amer. J. Med. **31**:318, 1961.

158. Walker, A. E.: Neurogenic polycythemia: re-

port of a case, Arch. Neurol. Psychiat. **53**:25, 1945.

159. Walker, A. E.: Discussion, J. Neuropath. Exp. Neurol. **10**:104, 1951.

160. Ward, A. A., Foltz, E. L., and Knopp, L. M.: "Polycythemia" associated with cerebellar hemangioblastoma, J. Neurosurg. **13**:248, 1956.

161. Weber, F. P.: Discussion, Proc. Roy. Soc. Med. **24**:386, 1931.

162. Wickbom, I.: Angiographic determination of tumour pathology, Acta Radiol. **40**:529, 1953.

163. Willis, R. A.: The spread of tumours in the human body, ed. 2, London, 1952, Butterworth and Co. (Publishers), Ltd.

164. Wolf, A., and Cowen, D.: Angioblastic meningiomas. Supratentorial hemangioblastomas, Bull. Neurol. Inst. N. Y. **5**:485, 1936.

165. Wolf, A., and Wilens, S. L.: Multiple hemangioblastomas of the spinal cord with syringomyelia and cysts of the pancreas and kidney (Lindau's disease), Arch. Path. **15**:604, 1933.

166. Wolf, A., and Wilens, S. L.: Multiple hemangioblastomas of the spinal cord with syringomelia, Amer. J. Path. **10**:545, 1934.

167. Wolman, L.: Cystic cerebellar tumours: a clinico-pathological reappraisal, J. Neurol. Neurosurg. Psychiat. **28**:461, 1965.

168. Wolpert, S. M.: The neuroradiology of hemangioblastomas of the cerebellum, Amer. J. Roentgen. **110**:56, 1970.

169. Woltman, H. W., Kernohan, J. W., Adson, A. W., and Craig, W. McK.: Intramedullary tumors of spinal cord and gliomas of intradural portion of filum terminale, Arch. Neurol. Psychiat. **65**:378, 1951.

170. Woolsey, R. D.: Hemangioblastoma of cerebellum with polycythemia, J. Neurosurg. **8**: 447, 1951.

171. Wright, R. L.: Familial von Hippel-Lindau's disease, J. Neurosurg. **30**:281, 1969.

172. Wyburn-Mason, R.: The vascular abnormalities and tumours of the spinal cord and its membranes, St. Louis, 1944, The C. V. Mosby Co.

173. Yanagihara, T., and Cumings, T. N.: Lipid metabolism in cerebral edema associated with human brain tumor, Arch. Neurol. **19**:241, 1968.

174. Zeitlin, H.: Hemangioblastomas of the meninges and their relation to Lindau's disease, J. Neuropath. Exp. Neurol. **1**:14, 1942.

175. Zimmerman, H. M.: Brain tumors: their incidence and classification in man and their experimental production, N. Y. Acad. Sci. **159**:337, 1969.

176. Zülch, K. J.: Brain tumors. Their biology and pathology (transl. by Rothballer, A. B., and Olszewski, J.), ed. 2, New York, 1957, Springer Publishing Co., Inc.

12/Miscellaneous diseases of the cerebral blood vessels

One has difficulty comprehending a disease of the central nervous system in which blood vessels do not participate. Their active role in inflammatory and destructive lesions as well as in repair processes is not necessarily different from the reaction of extracranial vessels although detailed investigations of their involvement under such pathological conditions are wanting. Perivascular cellular infiltrates are often found whether inflammatory cells as in the encephalitides, macrophages laden with lipid or otherwise hemosiderin in the repair of destructive or hemorrhagic lesions, or even epithelioid cells and multinucleated globoid bodies in Krabbe's disease. Then again the blood vessels are involved in parasitic diseases of the central nervous system primarily after hematogenous spread or secondarily in the destructive or space-occupying lesion so formed. Proliferation of small vessels is frequent in repair processes and could be associated with some degree of condensation of vessels because of a loss of intervening parenchyma. Such lesions will not be dealt with here. There are, however, several diseases (degenerative, inflammatory, etc.) in which there is significant involvement of the cerebral vessels. Degenerative disorders of the cerebral blood vessels is considered first.

Degenerations
Hypertensive vascular disease

It has long been considered that hypertension can be induced by a relative ischemia of vital centers in the lower pons and medulla oblongata ("the neurogenic theory of hypertension"). A cerebral occlusion is frequently associated with a temporary increase in blood pressure,[123] but evidence that a persistent hypertension can

be induced by ischemia[53] is far from convincing.[106,123]

Hypertension, by its effect on the heart, the coronary circulation, the aorta, and large vessels of the arch, together with the cerebral arteries, contributes very substantially to the pathogenesis of many lesions of the central nervous system. In the pathogenesis of cerebral hemorrhage, infarcts, and probably aneurysms, its role is significant and, apart from atherosclerosis and age, it is the single most important etiological factor in cerebrovascular disease. Just as the small arteries and arterioles elsewhere in the body undergo degenerative changes (arteriosclerosis and arteriolosclerosis) in the presence of hypertension, so do those of the central nervous system though to a less severe degree.

Arteriosclerosis. Arteriosclerosis is not used generically here but rather to indicate a disease of small arteries that is often overlooked in the classification of arterial disease and on other occasions is termed "diffuse hyperplastic sclerosis." In this sense, arteriosclerosis encompasses the changes in small peripheral arteries. They occur generally but are most severe in intracerebral vessels, the deep perforating arteries of the cerebrum. The arteries may exhibit thickening of the intima with degeneration of the elastic lamina and often of accessory and poorly formed elastic laminae within the newly proliferated fibromuscular intimal tissue. Consequently, the lumen may be severely narrowed. The media is correspondingly narrowed and fibrotic and eventually lost (Fig. 12-1). Such vessels usually have little adventitia. Elastic tissue degeneration becomes pronounced, more so by the end of the fifth decade but even then vessels of similar size are not

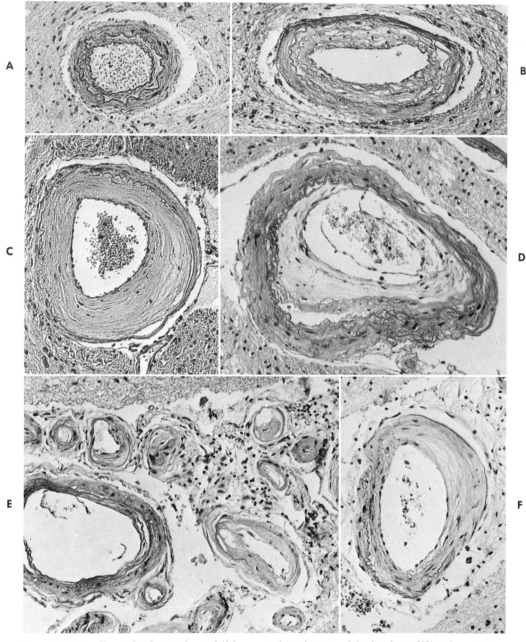

Fig. 12-1. Small cerebral arteries exhibit a varying degree of intimal proliferation. Note the wavy elastic laminae in **A** and **B** and the thinning and almost complete loss of media on one side of **B. C,** Intima is dense and collagenous, and media nonexistent in parts of circumference. **D,** Intimal connective tissue is rather loose and internal elastic lamina is deficient. **E,** Several small arteries and arterioles exhibit arteriosclerotic and arteriolosclerotic changes. **F,** Note fibrous part of the vessel wall, deficient internal elastic lamina, thinned media, and eccentric changes. (Hematoxylin and eosin, ×110.)

affected uniformly. Some vessels exhibit relatively little intimal proliferation and consequently their walls become fibrosed and are often hyaline and relatively acellular (Fig. 12-2). Amorphous material may be found in the intima of some vessels and tortuosity is often apparent. Lipid stains as with the corresponding intrarenal arteries occasionally reveal lipid deposits in the intima or outlining the elastic laminae and less frequently occur intracellularly in lipophages (Fig. 12-2). Accentuation of the perivascular spaces can be seen with increasing age. The significance is not known though it can be accentuated by fixation. Occasionally, the spaces are not visible.

Aggregates of lipophages may be found in severely sclerotic vessels even in paraffin sections and on rare occasions they have been said to narrow or obstruct the lumen.[66] Calcific stippling may be observed in the intima but more extensive calcification is uncommon. These vascular changes, that is, arteriosclerosis, are not peculiar to hypertension, occurring as they do in the kidney in normotensive individuals though in milder form. They are accentuated by hypertension and age, but the severity is

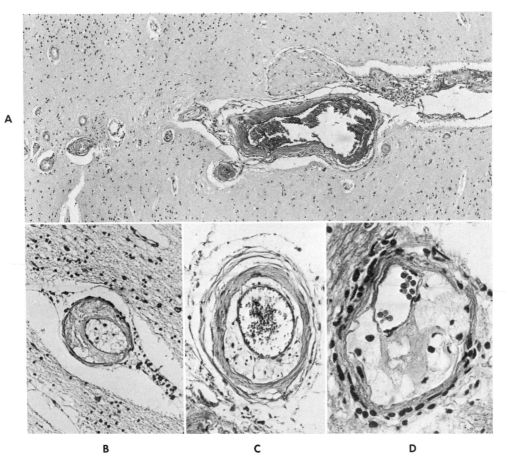

Fig. 12-2. A, Small pial artery in the depth of a sulcus has a hyaline wall of variable thickness (probably a miliary aneurysm). Immediately above is an irregularly oval fibrous nodule, probably an old healed miliary aneurysm. Several small vessels also exhibit arteriolosclerosis in **A. B** to **D,** Three small arteriosclerotic arteries: **B** exhibits amorphous material in its wall and **C** and **D** contain foam cells. (Hematoxylin and eosin; **A,** ×45; **B** to **D,** ×110.)

not as great as that seen in the kidney. Baker,[18] attributing such changes to age, asserted that they occurred in the vessels of the basal ganglia earlier than elsewhere.

The lipid deposits probably constitute an intergral part of arteriosclerosis, though as indicated elsewhere, there is overlap with atherosclerosis, and the differentiation between these diseases, when disparities in the caliber of the vessels are considered, is

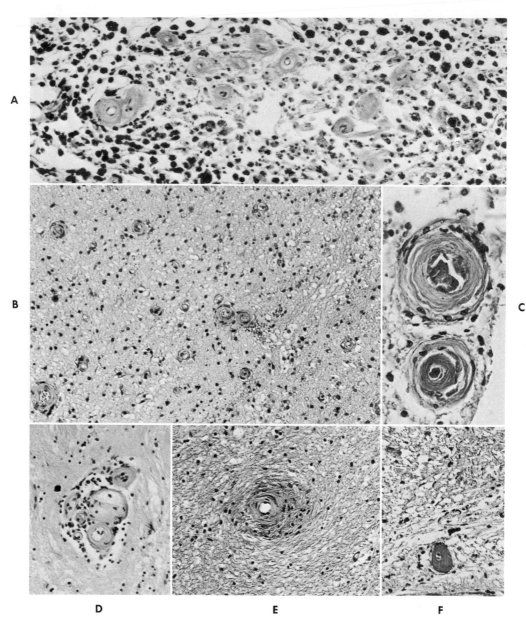

Fig. 12-3. Examples of arteriolosclerosis. Concentration of affected arterioles in **A** and **B.** Those in **A** are hyaline and in an old area of hemorrhage. **C,** Two severely affected arterioles. **D,** Hyaline arterioles and possibly a foam cell with surrounding siderophages. **E,** Concentric arrangement of fibrous tissue that merges with surrounding parenchyma. **F,** Fibrinoid degeneration of arteriolar wall. (Hematoxylin and eosin; **A, B, D** to **F,** ×110; **C,** ×275.)

far from distinct. It is likely that with age there is some degree of arteriectasis in these vessels especially within the parenchyma, though this aspect has not been investigated.

Progression of such lesions to form small aneurysmal dilatations is readily understood. The predilection displayed by miliary aneurysms for the brain can no doubt be attributed to the thinness of the arterial walls, the virtual absence of adventitia and the perivascular supporting connective tissues, and the unique hemodynamics of the cerebral circulation. Such arteriosclerotic changes are usually severe in those brains in which there are either miliary aneurysms, the walls of which are often lined or infiltrated by fibrin and red cells, or hyalinized structures believed to be thrombosed and organized microaneurysms (Fig. 12-2, A). Siderophages are frequently prevalent in and about such lesions, and this fact indicates that previous hemorrhage has occurred. Occluded lesions may be associated with lacunae.

Cerebral hemorrhage is believed to be more likely in subjects with very high blood pressures,[140] which would suggest that these advanced lesions, progressing to microaneurysm formation, are correspondingly more prevalent in those people with very severe hypertension though the duration of the hyperpiesis is doubtless a factor. Spinal arteries do not exhibit a similar degree of arteriosclerosis. In severely affected vessels, some proliferation of connective tissue may occur about the vessel as in extracranial arteriosclerosis, but such adventitial proliferation is not considered to be the prime degenerative change as Baker and Iannone[19] alleged.

Baker and Iannone[19] found little correlation in the frequency of the degenerative changes in small intracerebral arteries with that of atherosclerosis of the large basal arteries. Such a finding is surprising in view of the recognized fact that the degenerative changes in both sets of vessels are age dependent and also augmented by hypertension. Individual variations of course are

likely. Moreover, in some subjects, thickening of the arterial walls with arteriectasis and a tendency for the cut vessels to pout may be associated with degenerative changes but not necessarily with severe overt atheromatous plaques. The macroscopic grading of such vessels can be misleading.

Arteriolosclerosis. A variable degree of fibrosis, often acellular, thickening of the arteriolar walls is more frequent than hyaline arteriolosclerosis, and the reduction in the lumen is often considerable (Fig. 12-3). Concentric arrangement of the connective tissue, at times appearing to be periarteriolar as well, may present a mild onion-layer appearance. Affected vessels may have a patchy distribution and occur with variable frequency in the vicinity of old areas of infarction. Such lesions are considerably more frequent than hyaline arteriolosclerosis, which tends to affect slightly smaller arterioles.

Hyaline arteriolosclerosis occurs in normotensive subjects and its incidence increases with age. The hyaline, resembling basement-membrane material,[180] occurs primarily in the media replacing the muscle but may also be found in the intima. Some authors maintain that hyaline is precipitated plasma protein.[3] The arterioles also regularly contain lipid, but the relationship of lipid to the other constituents of hyalinized arteriolar walls is obscure. The frequency with which it is found in such viscera as the kidney, spleen, pancreas, adrenal glands, and liver is greatly augmented in the presence of hypertension, particularly in long-standing hyperpiesis, and in the severity of the lesions a similar trend is evident. The brain, in common with other vascular beds such as the heart, gastrointestinal tract, thyroid, and pituitary, rarely exhibits arteriolosclerosis, but its frequency and severity are increased with age and long-standing hypertension.[160] In practice, cerebral arteriolosclerosis is likely to be found primarily in the aged hypertensive person. It is also essential to remember that arteriolosclerosis is neither pathognomonic, nor an essential feature, of long-standing hypertension even in the kidney. Wartman[173] found that arteriosclerosis microscopically in the brain has a frequency and severity secondary only to the spleen and that cerebral arteriolosclerosis is correspondingly severe. Such results are difficult to explain and few authors concur. The spinal cord, as in the case of arteriosclerosis, is affected less frequently.

The remarkable frequency of hyaline arteriolosclerosis in the spleen even in normotensives suggests that some peculiarity of the splenic vascular bed predisposes to the development of these arteriolar degenerative changes. On the other hand, its infrequency and lesser severity in the brain and heart even in the presence of severe atherosclerosis of the major arteries of supply suggest that the hemodynamic conditions prevailing in these organs demonstrate little predisposition for these vascular lesions. In the kidney, hyaline arteriolosclerosis is found earliest at the corticomedullary junction near the arcuate arteries, but in the brain no preferential site has become apparent.

Fibrinoid arteriolonecrosis. Fibrinoid necrosis of arterioles (Fig. 12-3) with or without evidence of extravasation of blood is a frequent finding in malignant hypertension although it is nevertheless not as common within the brain and spinal cord as in the kidney. Fibrinoid changes in arterioles were present in only four of 59 cases of malignant hypertension compared to changes in the pancreas and adrenal glands in 27 and 24 subjects respectively.[95] Fibrinoid arteriolar necrosis is found at times at the margin of primary intracerebral hematomas[61] though not necessarily in association with malignant hypertension. The resolution of such vascular lesions with modern hypotensive therapy for malignant hypertension[139] makes it likely that these manifestations will be seen seldom if at all by pathologists in the future.

Byrom[31] provided no indication as to etiology but observed a small aneurysm on the middle cerebral arteries of two severely hypertensive rats.

In the experimental animal, arteriolar fibrinoid changes have consisted of the accumulation of fibrin beneath the endothelium in the absence of necrosis. Large interendothelial cell gaps were believed to be responsible for the apparently enhanced endothelial permeability leading to the deposition of fibrin.[180] Lipid is already demonstrable in these vessels and, like fibrin, is believed to be derived from the plasma. Initially, the lipid is medial and is contained within necrotic muscle cells though some is extracellular.[169]

Asscher and Anson,[17] having demonstrated necrotizing vascular lesions after doses of X-rays that were innocuous in normotensive animals, say that X-irradiation sensitizes the blood vessels of the cord to the effects of hypertension. A similar phenomenon is to be seen in the brain.[32]

In malignant hypertension, neurological disturbances are not at all singular and occur in from 40% to 70% of the patients. Types of vascular lesion demonstrable at autopsy[151] are (1) ischemia, (2) cerebral hemorrhage either massive, small, or perivascular, (3) subarachnoid hemorrhage,[38] and (4) hypertensive encephalopathy. Ischemic lesions are usually focal in type rather than being massive infarcts, and hemorrhages are quite variable. Massive hemorrhage accounts for death in 43% of the patients with neurological manifestations of malignant hypertension[38] and occurs in up to 20% of all patients with this disease.[95] The prevalence of small foci of ischemia or hemorrhage, either old or recent, depends to some extent on the thoroughness of the search.

The cerebrospinal fluid, either bloody or xanthochromic, is frequently elevated in malignant hypertension, particularly in the case of hypertensive encephalopathy when there is considerable cerebral edema. The cellular content of the fluid is generally normal, apart from the hemorrhage, and the protein is elevated in about 21% of cases.[38]

Hypertensive encephalopathy. Hypertensive encephalopathy has been described as an acute or subacute episode[4] occurring within the terminal weeks or months of severely hypertensive patients—usually in malignant hypertension and less frequently in benign or renal hypertension. The manifestations are severe headache, convulsions, amaurosis, mental confusion, stupor or coma, and, in some instances, transient neurological disturbances such as hemiplegia, monoplegia, hemianesthesia, and aphasia. This syndrome is consistent with Byrom's observations on hypertensive encephalopathy in rats with experimentally induced severe ("malignant") hypertension.[31] In man, it appears that in the past, transient ischemic attacks or possibly small hemorrhagic episodes have at times been mistaken for the rare hypertensive encephalopathy, for in these conditions the clinical symptomatology can be remarkably similar.

In severe hypertension in rats, focal, widespread vasospasm of cerebral pial arteries has been demonstrated[30] and the brain appeared pale. Byrom[30,31] considered the vasospasm to be the direct local response to the excessive intra-arterial pressure, the effects of the spasm in increasing order of severity being (1) a transient disturbance of function, (2) increased capillary permeability with attendant focal edema attributed to ischemia, and (3) local necrosis of the arterial wall and/or necrosis of the tissue supplied. The fibrinoid vascular lesions he attributed to a purely mechanical tear or disruption of the media.[32] Reduction of the arterial pressure abolished the vasospasm and it is likely that a similar sequence of events causes hypertensive encephalopathy in man. Pial arterial vasoconstriction has been confirmed in hypertensive cats and monkeys with resultant cerebral edema and perivascular hemorrhages.[121] More recently, Robertson and associates[148] found cortical microinfarcts, occasionally hemorrhagic, in 42% of hypertensive rats. Mostly the lesions were confined to the border zones of supply of the three major cerebral arteries and attributed to vasospasm because of the infrequency of fibrinoid change in the related vessels.

Capillary fibrosis. An increase in reticulin in the walls of cerebral capillaries is said to be a feature of hypertensive cardiovascular disease, but this aspect is generally neglected though reappraisal of its nature is warranted and ultrastructural studies could be enlightening.

One can conclude that cerebrovascular lesions are more prevalent in the hypertensive than in the normotensive[39] and that no vascular lesion can be categorically regarded as pathognomonic of hypertension. Hypertension merely aggravates to a varying degree the various vascular lesions discussed above and a reduction in arterial pressure probably influences the course of the vascular disease. The full effects of the widespread use of hypotensive drug therapy in hypertension are yet to be determined, and the application of this therapy to the normotensive may also prove instructive and beneficial.

Diabetic vascular disease

Generally atherosclerosis is greatly aggravated by diabetes mellitus, but because the frequency of hypertension and hypercholesterolemia in diabetics is unduly high, one has difficulty in being certain whether the metabolic disturbance associated with the diabetes or the associated phenomena are responsible for the augmented frequency.

The frequency of both cerebral hemorrhage and cerebral infarction is greater with diabetes mellitus than in the nondiabetic.[5] This could well be attributed to the prevalence of hypertension and the augmented severity of atherosclerosis in the diabetic. Alex and associates[5] assert that the arteriosclerosis (as well as arteriolosclerosis of parenchymal vessels) is accentuated to some degree by diabetes mellitus, which could well account for the increased frequency of focal softenings in diabetics. No ultrastructural study of the basement-membrane changes seen in diabetes has included investigation of the cerebral blood vessels. At present, no cerebrovascular lesion specific to diabetes mellitus is recognized.

Idiopathic symmetrical calcification of cerebral vessels

Calcification is common in the large arteries of man, and in general the mineral content progressively increases with age though in the cerebral arteries mineralization is less severe and less frequent than in the aorta or coronary arteries. The calcification, readily detected macroscopically, is most often found in atherosclerotic internal carotid and basilar and vertebral arteries, with lesser amounts observed histologically and mostly related to the internal elastic lamina or an atherosclerotic intima as early as the second decade. Gross calcification can be observed in aneurysms of long standing (Chapter 9) and in vascular anomalies (Chapter 10).

Calcification of small cerebral arteries, veins, and capillaries appears to be a response to varied pathological influences, which include various forms of encephalitis and endocrine disorders (particularly hypoparathyroidism) that account for the majority of instances.[129] Calcification has been found in 28% of cases of idiopathic hypoparathyroidism, in 48% of cases of pseudohypoparathyroidism,[24] and also in hypervitaminosis D and destructive bone lesions.[2]

In a number of instances, a distinct familial trend is apparent, with such cases often being associated with oligophrenia or microcephaly.[129] Melchior and associates[116] reported the disease in three siblings of one family and in two siblings of another. Subjects are mostly between the ages of 30 and 50 years and exhibit a progressive onset of organic dementia and extrapyramidal motor dysfunction.[70] The clinical picture can vary considerably. Often, however, there is no history of familial involvement and the cause is not apparent. Such cases are idiopathic. Involvement of small cortical vessels is also found in the rare Sturge-Weber syndrome (Chapter 10).

The localization of the calcification is remarkably uniform. It is most severe in the putamen and the central regions of the cerebellar hemispheres about the dentate nucleus. The globus pallidus, thalamus, parts of the cerebral cortex, and centrum ovale can also be implicated to a varying degree and a bilateral distribution is characteristic. It is sometimes known as symmetrical cerebral calcification or idiopathic nonarteriosclerotic cerebral calcification. Fahr's disease, another synonym, is not in current favor, for descriptions of the disease antedate Fahr by several decades.

The brain is generally small with atrophic gyri and massive calcification or brainstones in the basal ganglia, in the cerebral white matter, or about the dentate nucleus. Histologically, calcium is deposited near or in the walls of small blood vessels, often with severe narrowing or complete occlusion of the lumens. There is also massive mineralization of the parenchyma in the form of globular masses that coalesce. Diffuse demyelination and axonal degeneration occur in the affected zones. After decalcification, the matrix stains with the periodic acid–Schiff reagent, which staining is therefore believed to indicate the presence of an acid mucopolysaccharide (pseudocalcification or neurogel[129]). It has been suggested that the acid mucopolysaccharide is first deposited in the nuclei and perinuclear cytoplasm of glial cells (mostly the oligodendroglia). Spread occurs beyond the cell, and further accumulation of the matrix substance is observed in the parenchyma (to form noncalcified round bodies) and about blood vessels.[2] Calcification then occurs first in the blood vessels and subsequently in the parenchyma. Tiny granules surround the capillary walls and impart to them a beaded appearance on longitudinal section. Subsequently larger granules and globules coalesce to form solid pericapillary sheaths, and finally obliteration of the lumen by irregular, elongated, or mulberry-shaped concretions. In arterioles, arteries, and to a lesser extent veins, the granules first appear in the outer layer of the media and then the adventitia and perivascular spaces. The entire wall can be calcified finally.[56] Massive calcification is ultimately seen in the parenchyma with coalescence of the concretions to form a solid, irregular, calcified mass readily demonstrable radiologically.

The calcium content of the concretions has been found to be 11 mg.% of dry weight with a small quantity of iron (32 μg.% of dry weight).[2] The latter accounts for the weakly positive Prussian blue reaction to be found at the periphery and in recent deposits. In an analysis by Norman and Urich,[129] there was 16,800 mg.% of calcium and 25.5 mg.% of iron (wet basis). The calcium occurs mainly as the phosphate. Traces of magnesium and cystine have also been found.[93]

The etiology of this disease remains obscure, and obviously there is need for further information concerning the nature of the matrix or neurogel that precedes the calcification. Norman and Urich[129] assert that there is likely to be a vascular factor, possibly related to the capillary permeability, that is responsible for the peculiar localization of the lesions.

Geyelin and Penfield[73] described epilepsy in a father and all four of his children in association with nonsymmetrical areas of cortical calcification, which they referred to as "cerebral endarteritis calcificans," including the extensive involvement of blood vessels. Not only calcification but also considerable narrowing of the lumens of those vessels was observed, accounting no doubt for the patchy perivascular gliosis. Alexander and Woodhall[6] encountered a male epileptic with extensive calcification in the white matter of one temporal lobe and this too displayed extensive vascular calcification. It is likely that these cases are basically variants of idiopathic symmetrical cerebral calcification.

Vascular siderosis

Vascular siderosis, also known as pallidal siderosis, or calcinosiderosis, is an autogenous iron deposition in and about small blood vessels of the globus pallidus, hence the term "pallidal siderosis" (Fig. 12-4). Thus, Hurst[88] found siderosis in 50% of 100 brains and found that it was the anterior half of the globus pallidus particularly that was most severely affected. Neumann[128]

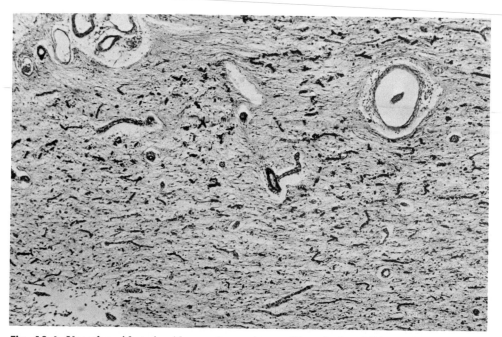

Fig. 12-4. Vascular siderosis. Almost the entire capillary bed exhibits pericapillary siderotic stippling. (Hematoxylin and eosin, ×45.)

recorded a frequency of 40% in the brains examined, whereas Slager and Wagner[159] found it in 68.5% of 200 consecutive brains. It occurs as early as the second and third decade, but it is more frequent in the aged, and 80% of subjects were affected by the age of 70 years.[159] Strassmann[164] asserted that vascular siderosis occurred regularly in those over 60 years of age and observed it in a 7-year-old idiot. Despite this remarkable frequency, the disease has been sadly neglected and its significance is far from clear.

As well as the globus pallidus, vessels of the putamen and caudate nucleus may also be affected, and in like manner, the striatum, dentate nucleus, and substantia nigra though less frequently and to a lesser degree than the globus pallidus.[164] It can, however, be seen beyond these areas as in Fig. 12-5 in which it is present in the cerebellar cortex. It may occur in oligodendrogliomas[164] and has been observed in metastatic tumors. The deposits are densely basophilic, invariably stain for iron, and in

a small percentage of cases (2.5%)[159] also contain demonstrable calcium. Hurst[88] asserted that the presence of calcium deposits in these vessels was unproved, indicating at least its infrequency. In those subjects in which calcium is demonstrable, it is not present in all deposits. The mineralization is thought to depend on a mucopolysaccharide ground substance, which stains with the periodic acid—Schiff reagent.[128]

Small stipples about capillaries are observed histologically, sometimes reaching pronounced proportions (Fig. 12-4). Larger granules develop primarily about the capillary. The iron deposits may also arise about the adventitia of arterioles and small arteries (Fig. 12-6), and possibly veins. In many instances, the deposits coalesce to form thick basophilic deposits around the full circumference of the arteriolar or arterial walls, which almost invariably exhibit degenerative changes, either a narrowed lumen or a grossly thickened arteriolosclerotic or arteriosclerotic wall. It is not unusual for the elastic laminae to be outlined

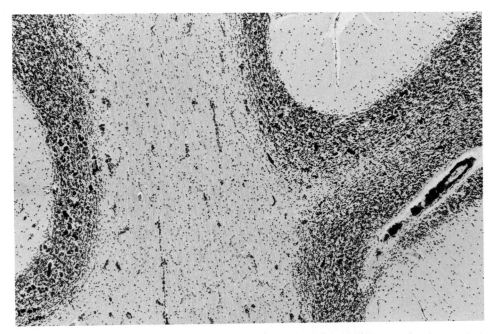

Fig. 12-5. Vascular siderosis involving small vessels and also a small artery in the cerebellar cortex and white matter of the folia. (Hematoxylin and eosin, ×45.)

and the vessels are not infrequently occluded. Spherules and mulberry-shaped deposits, not obviously related to blood vessels, may be free in the parenchyma.[159] In severe cases, ferrugination of glial and nerve cells has been noted.[164] A frequent association with arteriosclerosis[128] and cerebral softenings[159] has been affirmed and certainly small softenings in the neighboring tissue of the lenticular nucleus are not uncommon. However, in view of the age distribution of this disease, the significance of softenings and arteriosclerosis is yet to be determined and the etiology of vascular siderosis is quite unknown.

Amyloidosis

The central nervous system is rarely involved in generalized amyloidosis, but when the central nervous system is involved, the amyloid tends to be restricted to the pial vessels. Amyloid deposits are known to be demonstrable in advanced atherosclerosis but this is regarded only as a casual secondary manifestation of the disease. Amyloid may also be observed about capillaries and in the thickened walls of vessels in X-irradiation necrosis of the brain[104] and in the vessels of arteriovenous aneurysms.[138]

Schwartz[155] has recently drawn attention to massive mural deposits of amyloid in small pial and cortical arteries, sufficient to narrow or even occlude the lumen. Such changes were observed in seven brains. In senile dementia, amyloid degeneration of meningeal and cortical capillaries, arteries, and veins is not uncommon in association with senile plaques, etc. It may also involve

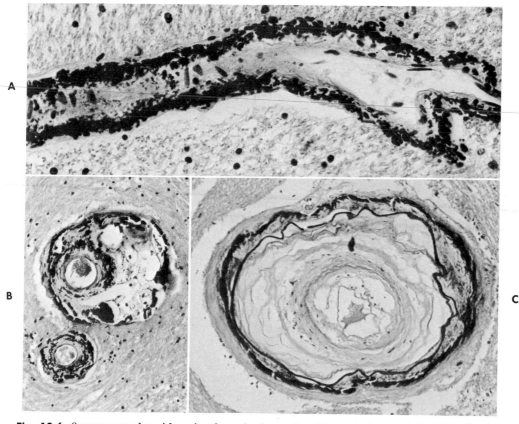

Fig. 12-6. Severe vascular siderosis of cerebral arteries. Note tendency to involve elastic lamina in **B** and **C** and the gross narrowing of the lumens. (Hematoxylin and eosin; **A**, ×275; **B, C**, ×110.)

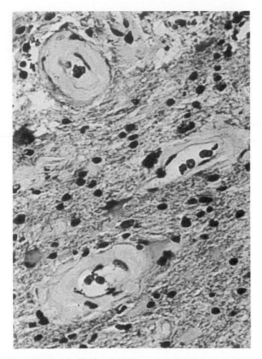

Fig. 12-7. Acellular hyaline amyloid in walls of three vessels near edge of a large primary tumorlike amyloid mass in the cerebrum. (Hematoxylin and eosin, ×275.)

the perivascular parenchymal tissue. Amyloid may at times occur in the brain as tumorlike masses, originating within either the brain or the choroid plexus.[97] In such rare conditions, amyloidosis of the vessels at the periphery may be observed (Fig. 12-7).

Inflammatory diseases of the cerebral blood vessels

Blood vessels play an integral part in any inflammatory reaction but the larger cerebral blood vessels manifest lesions in bacterial infections, fungal diseases, parasitic and viral diseases, specific hypersensitivity arteritides, and some miscellaneous inflammatory disorders.

Ishikawa[90] has suggested that a nonspecific arteritis may be responsible for the high incidence of nontraumatic and nonatherosclerotic thromboses of the internal carotid arteries in young adult Japanese males. Migratory phlebitis sometimes accompanies these occlusions. In general, little attention has been paid to cerebral

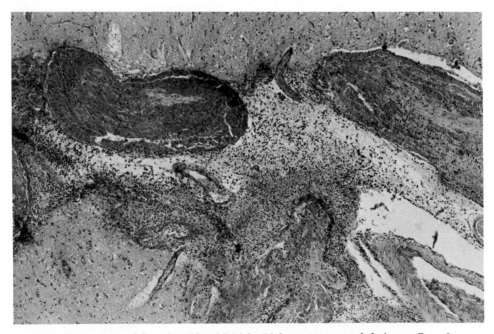

Fig. 12-8. Acute necrotizing thrombophlebitis. Pial artery at top left is unaffected except for a few inflammatory cells in the adventitia. There was no evidence of a primary leptomeningitis. (Hematoxylin and eosin, ×45. Courtesy Dr. V. J. McGovern, Sydney, Australia.)

phlebitis. Fig. 12-8 shows an acute widespread necrotizing thrombophlebitis. The venous walls were infiltrated with fibrin and leukocytes and a superadded thrombosis was usually present. The actual pathogenesis of such lesions and the reason for the peculiar sparing of the arteries are uncertain.

In recent years, a new disease entity has appeared—the necrotizing angiitis associated with drug abuse.[36,77] No specific drug has yet been incriminated and most of the users have had access to several varieties. The clinical picture is similar to that of polyarteritis nodosa and multiple small cerebral aneurysms have been demonstrated in arteriograms. Cerebral and pontine softenings have been observed and severe parenchymal hemorrhage or subarachnoid bleeding may ensue.[36]

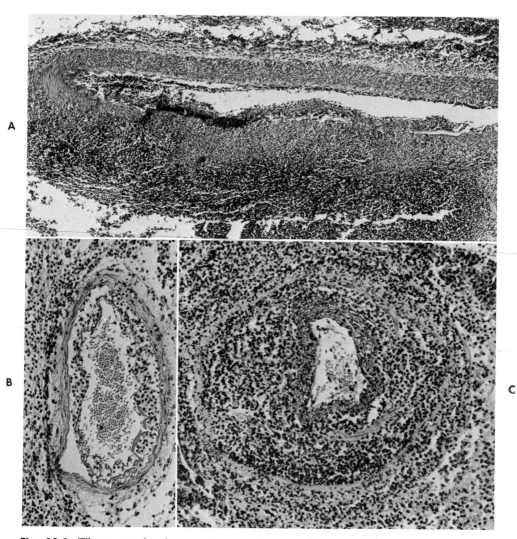

Fig. 12-9. Three arteries from patients with acute leptomeningitis. An acute arteritis affects entire lower wall of artery in **A,** and a bacterial aneurysm could form here. **B,** Endothelium is elevated by a subendothelial accumulation of leukocytes. **C,** Entire wall is infiltrated with polymorphs and is disorganized. (Hematoxylin and eosin; **A,** ×45; **B, C,** ×110.)

Bacterial infections

The central nervous system exhibits relatively less resistance to bacterial infections than other tissues, and the small blood vessels, during both the acute and chronic phases, naturally play a crucial role in any inflammatory process as well as in the stage of repair. The larger vessels, both arteries and veins, may be secondarily involved in leptomeningitis often with serious consequences.

Acute leptomeningitis. In acute leptomeningitis, it is not unusual to see the wall of cortical vessels (arteries and veins) focally or diffusely infiltrated with inflammatory cells (Fig. 12-9). The infiltration may be adventitial only but in some instances is more extensive and reaches the intima. The endothelium may be elevated by a crescentic mass of neutrophils. The media may be necrotic. Occasionally, red cells are observed in the media and frank subarachnoid hemorrhage follows. In rare instances, acute arteritis so damages the wall that an aneurysmal dilatation is the outcome (Chapter 9). A much more common complication of acute meningitis is the formation of a mural or occlusive thrombus in inflamed and damaged vessels. Stasis, difficult to recognize histologically, can cause cortical necrosis but more extensive infarcts follow thrombosis of larger vessels and account for some postmeningitic neurological sequelae. Disseminated intravascular thrombosis probably associated with septicemia can be a terminal event.

When arteritis and phlebitis are present and inadequate chemotherapy has been administered, the vascular lesions may progress to suppuration, and death, being merely delayed by the antibiotics, is inevitable. In chronic stages, proliferative changes with considerable narrowing of the lumen appear.

Tuberculous meningitis. Tuberculous meningitis is usually attributed to hematogenous spread to the subarachnoid space possibly by way of a small cortical or para-

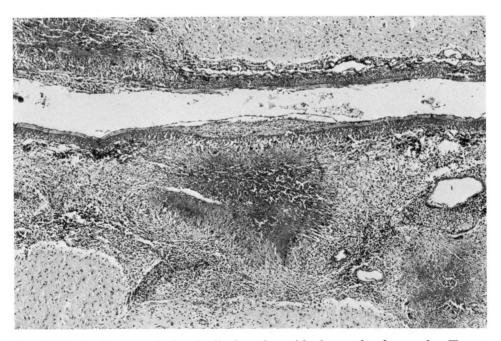

Fig. 12-10. A pial artery in longitudinal section with three tubercles nearby. Two tubercles actually involve the arterial wall, and in each instance the overlying intima is thickened and infiltrated with leukocytes. (Hematoxylin and eosin, ×45.)

ventricular tuberculoma. It is also possible that an arteritis or phlebitis may develop, with subsequent secondary spread to the cerebrospinal fluid, though a primary lesion in the choroid plexus can be responsible. In the well-developed tuberculous meningitis, tubercles are characteristically distributed along pial vessels. This constant finding suggests a predilection for the infection to localize in and about blood vessel walls[145] and in fact the experimental injection of tubercle bacilli into the cerebrospinal fluid is followed by localization of the infection about small meningeal vessels as in man.[145] It is not surprising, therefore, that arteritis and phlebitis may be prominent in tuberculous meningitis (Figs. 12-10 and 12-11). Intense perivascular infiltration of the meningeal vessels is frequent, with the adventitia being infiltrated by lymphocytes, plasma cells, and phagocytes. The media may exhibit coagulation necrosis, separation of fibers, and infiltration with inflammatory cells including polymorphonuclear leukocytes. The elastic lamina may be intact or disrupted. The endothelium may be elevated with inflammatory cells between it and the elastic lamina, and a superadded thrombus may partially or completely occlude the lumen. Incipient or actual aneurysms may form where the wall is destroyed though thrombosis and endarteritis protect against this. More often there is loose intimal thickening that considerably narrows the lumen. The wall may be directly involved by a tubercle and caseation may rapidly extend to the vessels. Giant cells are scattered in the inflammatory exudate

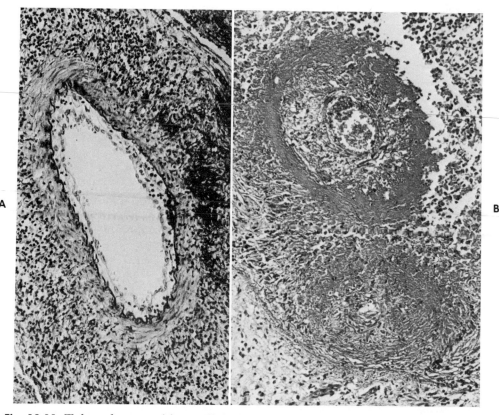

Fig. 12-11. Tuberculous arteritis. **A,** Fibrin infiltration of wall extending even to intima: the endothelium is elevated. **B,** Two necrotic vessels are disorganized and extensively infiltrated with fibrin. (**A,** Luxol blue fast and periodic acid–Schiff; **B,** hematoxylin and eosin, ×110.)

and here and there a distinct tubercle may be found. Goldzieher and Lisa[74] observed a tubercle with a giant cell in the subintima but this is unusual. Although the greatest degree of endarteritis is found in small- and medium-sized arteries, veins are often affected.

Secondary hemorrhage, although not well recognized, is a fairly frequent event in tuberculous meningitis. The hemorrhage, primarily subarachnoid, may be due to rupture of a bacterial aneurysm (Chapter 9) but can also be due to tuberculous arteritis. In Sheldon's[157] series of 50 autopsies of intracranial hemorrhage in children under 12 years of age, three deaths were caused by hemorrhage complicating tuberculous meningitis. Corresponding infarction also follows the occlusion of the many involved arteries.

Syphilitic arteritis. Cardiovascular syphilis and neurosyphilis have come to be almost of historical interest only to most pathologists because of an improvement in therapy of early syphilis. The cases likely to arise are from untreated or inadequately treated patients and the patients are usually between 30 and 60 years of age.[118] Most of the clinical symptoms of cerebral syphilis accrue directly or indirectly from disease of the cerebral blood vessels.[118] Syphilitic (Heubner's) arteritis is generally accompanied by syphilitic leptomeningitis or meningoencephalitis. In general, there is little more than a round cell infiltration of the adventitia of large- and medium sized cerebral arteries and possibly some thickening of the adventitia (Fig. 12-12). Lymphocytes and plasma cells tend to aggregate about vasa vasorum and may extend into the media but polymorphonuclear and giant cells are quite infrequent. Intimal thickening may be very prominent and the inflammatory reaction may progress to necrosis with a frank gummatous involvement of the media and adventitia. At this stage, polymorphs may be abundant, the elastic lamina disrupted, and the intima considerably narrowed (endarteritis obliterans) and infiltrated with inflammatory cells. Spiro-

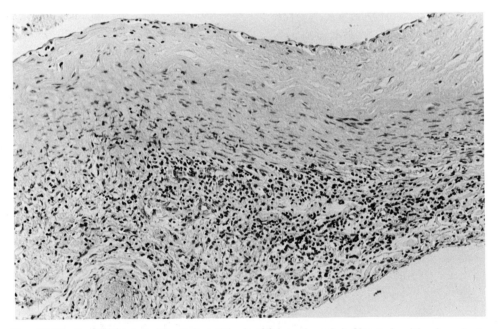

Fig. 12-12. Syphilitic arteritis. Adventitia is thickened and infiltrated with chronic inflammatory cells, which are extending into media. Intima is also thickened. (Hematoxylin and eosin, ×110.)

chetes may be demonstrable in the tissues. Macroscopically, the vessel is white, opaque, and thickened with a narrowed lumen.[167] Superadded thrombosis and organization may follow but the round cell infiltration persists long after healing has occurred. Hemorrhage is most infrequent and aneurysm formation even more rare.

The middle cerebral artery is the most frequent site. In 42 cases of thrombosis in cerebrovascular syphilis, it was involved 26 times. The basilar was thrombosed five times, the anterior cerebral, posterior cerebral, and posterior inferior cerebellar arteries each three times, and the internal carotid and anterior choroidal each once.[118] The spinal cord is less frequently involved.

Small arteries may exhibit endarteritis and periarteritis with some perivascular lymphocytic infiltration, all of which are more usual with other types of neurosyphilis. Syphilitic phlebitis of the brain and cord is rare and consists of endophlebitis and adventitial round cell infiltration, which can proceed to necrosis and gummatous change.

The cerebrospinal fluid is usually clear and under normal pressure. The cellular content is slightly raised but is seldom over 100 cells per cu. mm. The protein is elevated in two-thirds of the cases, and the colloidal gold curve is of the paretic or tabetic form. The specific tests for syphilis are essential and nearly always positive.

Mycoses

In fungal diseases, spread to the brain is often hematogenous. When the vessels are implicated in meningeal reactions, an angiitis or a loose intimal proliferation (endarteritis obliterans) as in coccidioidomycosis can arise. Spread in cryptococcosis appears to be via the Virchow-Robin space with early parenchymal lesions usually distinctly perivascular,[63] although in this disease some endarteritis also may be manifested.[174] A few mycoses tend to spread inside the cerebral vessels and may occasionally cause true mycotic aneurysms.

Mucormycosis (phycomycosis). Mucormy-cosis, also termed phycomycosis,[57] constitutes a group of rare mycoses in which broad, irregularly branching, nonpigmented, mostly nonseptate hyphae can be found in the tissues. The fungi implicated are members of the order Mucorales, that is, *Rhizopus oryzae, R. arrhizus,* and *Absidia corymbifera.* Species of the genus *Mucor* are infrequently responsible.[82] The fungi are widely distributed in nature (soil, dung, and vegetable matter) and are only potentially pathogenic to man and other mammals. However, in susceptible individuals, particularly those with poorly controlled diabetes mellitus, leukemia, debilitating diseases, or uremia, or those receiving radiation therapy, steroids, and modern chemotherapeutic agents,[20,89] the fungi can cause serious infections. An increase in the prevalence of the infection is anticipated with the growing implementation of modern drugs. There has been an instance in a heroin addict.[78]

Although mucormycosis may complicate amebiasis and malnutrition or skin lesions (burns, fractures, and wounds), the most usual manifestation is a rhinocerebral involvement commencing in the paranasal air sinuses or pharynx and spreading directly to neighboring structures including the orbit, meninges, and brain. Though the fungi can be found in the parenchyma usually superficially, the spread is mostly via the meninges and especially the arteries (**Fig.** 12-13.)

Histological demonstration of the characteristic hyphae (3 to 12 μ wide) in pathological material is essential for diagnosis (Fig. 12-14). It is advisable to attempt culture but identification of the species should be reserved for the expert.[82] Sporangia may be observed in necrotic tissue from the nose or sinuses.

Histologically, the characteristic vessel involvement (arteries and veins) results in necrosis of the vessel wall, elevation and desquamation of the endothelium, and the accumulation of acute inflammatory cells often with sufficient polymorphs to constitute pus and plentiful macrophages. Giant cells are not infrequent. The lumen is readily occluded by thrombus, debris, or purulent exudate. The hyphae, though present in the lumen and surrounding tissues, appear mostly in the walls. Signs of chronicity with round cell involvement and organization of clot and fibrosis are not usual. The characteristic microscopic appearance explains the widespread necrosis or infarction attributed to obstructed vessels, but hemorrhage is a frequent concomitant. Parenchymal hemorrhage, whether mild or fairly se-

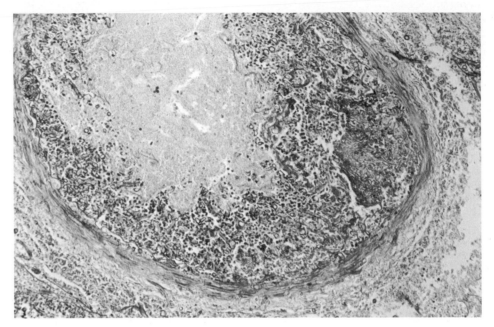

Fig. 12-13. Mucormycosis of a cerebral artery. There is extensive fungal infiltration of necrotic vessel wall and of lumen. The fungus is also present in surrounding tissue. Note inflammatory cells about fungus in lumen. (Hematoxylin and eosin, ×110.)

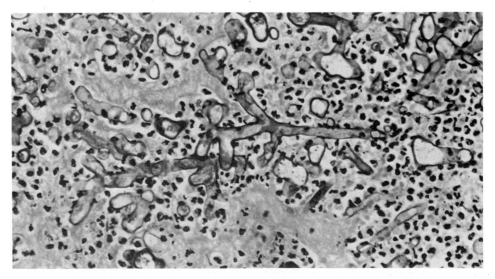

Fig. 12-14. Higher magnification of fungus showing branched hyphae, which are mostly nonseptate. (Hematoxylin and eosin, ×275.)

vere, can be mistaken for subarachnoid hemorrhage of aneurysmal origin. Though subdural hemorrhage has been observed,[162] it may be a complication of leukemia. The vessels involved are usually pale or hemorrhagic, friable, and necrotic, and if they are embedded in blood clot, dissection is difficult. On occasions, the segments of the vessels may be dilated, usually in an irregular or fusiform fashion.[162] They do not simulate saccular or berry aneurysms.

Cavernous sinus thrombosis and thrombosis of the internal carotid artery are often terminal events. The neighboring cranial nerves, especially those entering the orbit, may be widely infiltrated and necrotic. The brain is most severely affected anteriorly at the base, although involvement of the posterior fossa[34] or deep cerebral structures can develop.

The lung, the second most common site of mucormycosis, may be affected simultaneously though embolic spread to the brain can follow a primary lesion in the lung. On rare occasions, spread to the brain is by embolic dissemination from extrapulmonary foci.[107]

The disease is usually rapidly fatal, and though recovery under treatment has been reported, residual cerebral damage has been considerable.[108] The disease may not be suspected clinically or even at autopsy.

Aspergillosis. Few of the 350 recognized species of *Aspergillus* are pathogenic to man. The most common pathogen is *A. fumigatus.*[63] Aspergillosis mostly complicates the following:

1. Chronic debilitating diseases such as leukemia, lymphosarcoma, Hodgkin's disease, and carcinoma
2. Chemotherapy particularly with corticosteroids, antimetabolites, and cytotoxic drugs
3. Occupational exposure to abundant dust
4. In a few instances, drug addiction or even blood transfusions[63]

Aspergillosis only infrequently affects the central nervous system. The fungus reaches the brain usually by direct spread from paranasal air sinuses, bone, or the orbit or otherwise by hematogenous spread from the lung. Although blood vessels are affected most often, the remarkably strong affinity for the vessels exhibited by mucormycosis is nevertheless lacking. Vascular thromboses, small hemorrhages, and infarction make their appearance. The invaded vessels are for the most part small channels only and large vessels are affected much less often. In a recent survey of 33 cases deemed to be well documented,[124] there were three instances in which an internal carotid or middle cerebral artery was directly involved with secondary thrombosis. Rupture with hemorrhage[113] occurred in two. Involvement of venous sinuses is rare.

In histological sections, numerous small branching septate hyphae of fairly uniform size (3 to 6 μ in diameter) are surrounded by necrotic tissue and numerous polymorphonuclear leukocytes and less frequently a granulomatous reaction if the infection is prolonged. Spread in the central nervous system in experimental aspergillosis is believed to be due to spread along venous channels[58] which is consistent with the frequency of mycotic angiitis as noted in autopsy specimens of brain. Cerebral or spinal infection is usually part of a terminal infection and survival is exceptional.

Candidiasis. Candidiasis, a complication of diabetes mellitus or leukemia, usually affects mucosal surfaces and the skin. But it is an infrequent finding in the central nervous system, where it is caused most often by the species *Candida albicans,* which reaches the brain by hematogenous spread from the lungs or gastrointestinal tract.[63] Basal meningitis, abscesses, and granulomas of the brain are found. Invasion of the walls of cortical blood vessels is not unusual, and secondary thrombosis, infarction, and multiple petechiae are the result. Histologically, *Candida* is recognizable as yeast-like bodies with pseudohyphae. Small abscesses contain collections of neutrophils though granulomatous reactions have occurred.

Candida is a common cause of true mycotic endocarditis, which, though likely to be a terminal event, can complicate cardiac surgery. The vegetations are extremely soft and friable and hence multiple emboli are usually present in the cerebral arteries. At least one case of a candida mycotic aneurysm has been observed in such an instance.[12] It ruptured causing subarachnoid hemorrhage. Histologically the organisms are found in the embolus. The vessel wall is necrotic and infiltrated by polymorphs. Round cells, fibroblasts, an occasional foreign body giant cell, and siderophages appear later.

Viral and rickettsial diseases

Congenital rubella is an active contagious disease from which various abnormalities eventuate. Extracranial vascular lesions are frequent (75%) and consist predominately of fibromuscular proliferation of the intima,[59,60] which results in pulmonary and renal artery stenosis, the latter being possibly the cause of hypertension. The central nervous system is affected though not always severely in up to 81% of cases. Encephalitis and leptomeningitis can be expected, and often an acute vasculitis consisting of a diffuse round cell infiltration of the vessel wall[51] can also be expected. At autopsy, six of 13 infants had widespread perivascular calcification in the brain. One had a subarachnoid hemorrhage. The cerebral blood vessels have also been involved in experimental congenital rubella in ferrets.[150]

Lesions in the central nervous system are usual in both European and scrub typhus fevers. The brain exhibits edema and congestion and possibly petechial hemorrhages. Histologically, there is a disseminated acute vasculitis of small vessels with perivascular typhus nodules. Thrombi are frequent in the affected vessels. Larger vessels are involved in Rocky Mountain spotted fever, the medial muscle is invaded, and microinfarcts result.

Eosinophilic meningoencephalitis and parasitic aneurysms

Eosinophilic meningoencephalitis is characterized by (1) meningitis in which eosinophils and plasma cells are prominent, (2) tortuous tracks of varying size in the brain and spinal cord parenchyma surrounded by a variable reaction and degenerating neurons, (3) a granulomatous response to dead *Angiostrongylus cantonensis,* and (4) vascular lesions including perivascular infiltrates of lymphocytes and eosinophils, edema of vessel wall, rupture, and thrombosis of vessels with hemorrhage and aneurysm formation.[131] *Gnathostoma* is also a common cause of this disease and in some localities in Thailand is responsible for 14% to 30% of the deaths attributed to cerebral hemorrhage. The vascular lesions, it is thought, are possibly caused by meandering nematodes and their tracks are usually present near small vascular lesions. The parenchymal hemorrhages are multiple and the aneurysms on small peripheral arteries are often multiple and small and appear to be false sacs similar to the traumatic variety. In one instance the aneurysm had a fibrotic wall and was of longer duration.

Miscellaneous inflammatory disorders of cerebral blood vessels

Those arteritides that are not due to infectious causes are not common. They constitute a very diverse group of diseases and many are believed to be manifestations of an immune disorder.

Serum sickness manifests itself in the brain as focal areas of edema and also as a disseminated focal infiltrative vasculitis resulting in vascular thrombosis or rupture with hemorrhage.[122] Such lesions are said to be similar to those of polyarteritis nodosa.

Polyarteritis (periarteritis) nodosa. Focal and diffuse inflammation of medium and small arteries characterize polyarteritis nodosa. The clinical picture is most variable and the course is subacute or chronic. Two to three times more frequent in the male than in the female, the disease most commonly occurs between the ages of 20 and 50 years. Hypertension, believed to result from the renal involvement, is present in more than 50% of the victims.

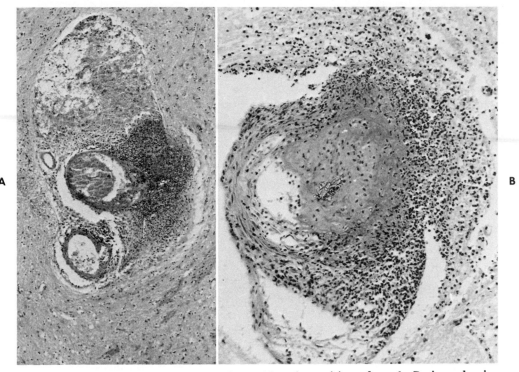

Fig. 12-15. Cerebral vessels from a patient with polyarteritis nodosa. **A,** Perivascular inflammation. **B,** Part of wall is destroyed and replaced by fibrin, which partially occludes vessel (an artifact is present in the center of **B**). (Hematoxylin and eosin; **A,** ×45; **B,** ×110.)

Arkin[15] divided the vascular lesions into four stages: The *first* is characterized by edema and fibrinous exudate in the media and about the internal elastic lamina. Necrosis follows, much elastica is destroyed, and leukocytic infiltration commences. The endothelium may be elevated and the adventitia unimpaired. In the *second* or acute inflammatory stage, there is pronounced infiltration by neutrophils, eosinophils, lymphocytes, and plasma cells not only of the wall but also of the perivascular tissues (Fig. 12-15). There may be a reactive proliferation of the intima or secondary thrombosis. Aneurysmal dilatation of part of the wall may be apparent and extravasation of blood is a frequent event. The lesions are segmental and the vessels exhibit nodularity. The *third* stage is a reparative one in which fibroblasts proliferate throughout the inflammatory zone with an increase in fibrous tissue, lymphocytes, and plasma cells in and about the vessel. The fibrin exudate and necrotic debris are replaced by granulation tissue and even new vessels. Thrombi become organized, and in patent vessels, the intima is usually considerably thickened. In the *final* stage, the inflammatory reaction progressively disappears as scar tissue replaces the destroyed vessel wall. Small aneurysms may heal by means of thrombosis and organization. The vessels are still nodular and periarterial fibrosis is prominent. In the second and third stages, siderophages give evidence of previous hemorrhage primarily from necrotic vessels or aneurysms.

The vascular lesions may be widespread, affecting particularly the splanchnic vessels, voluntary muscle, vasa nervorum, and less frequently the skin. The central nervous system is involved less often than peripheral nerves (8% to 20% of cases)[15,102,122] although transient neurological symptoms are more prevalent.[122] Of 114 patients from the Mayo Clinic, 53 (46%) had symptoms and signs referable to the central nervous system.[134] In 47%, they were late manifestations. Parker and Kernohan[134] found cerebral involvement in 11 of 16 cases (69%). The cerebral arteries, such as the internal carotid, vertebral, and basilar[52] may be affected, but usually more peripheral vessels such as the pial or even the parenchymal arteries are involved. Vascular occlusion can be expected and so ischemic infarcts of varying size may be present not only in the cerebrum but in the cerebellum and brain stem. Hemorrhage may be minor and petechial, though it is a cause of subarachnoid hemorrhage, both intracranial[177] and spinal.[83] Massive intracerebral hemorrhages are on record.[69,84] Small aneurysmal nodules may be found on the pial arteries, or alternatively, the lesions may be microscopically demonstrable only.

The vasa nervorum of cranial nerves may also be affected, most frequently the facial nerve and less often the retina and optic nerves.[177]

Involvement of the spinal vessels is encountered in sporadic cases. Complicating hemorrhage has occasioned interest but extensive infarction of the cord is also a possibility.[166]

The etiology of the disease is still uncertain. It is believed to be an immune reaction to foreign antigens, which may be of microbiological origin.[181] A very high incidence of similar diseases in a variety of animal species has raised the possibility of a viral etiology.

Wegener's granulomatosis. Wegener's granulomatosis or necrotizing respiratory granulomatosis, a rare disease of unknown etiology, is characterized by (1) necrotizing, giant cell granulomatous lesions involving the trachea, bronchi, and upper respiratory tract including the nose and paranasal air sinuses, (2) necrotizing vasculitis of lungs and other tissues with hemorrhage and infarction, and (3) a focal or widespread necrotizing glomerulitis. The patient usually dies in uremia. The vascular changes can be very acute, or, proceeding to a healing stage, can resemble in many ways polyarteritis nodosa of which Wegener's granulomatosis, though of unknown etiology, is considered a variant.

Involvement of the nervous system is frequent. Walton[172] in 1958 studied 54 cases from the literature and found that 7.4% had lesions of the brain and meninges. Drachman[54] more recently found that 56 of 104 reported cases in the literature had nervous or neuromuscular symptoms. The neurological manifestations were of three main types: (1) Invasion of the orbit and base of the skull from granulomatous lesions in the nose and paranasal air sinuses may involve the cranial nerves and vestibular apparatus, or with invasion of the skull, the pituitary, and the optic nerves and chiasm will be affected or a severe meningitis can develop. (2) In this very small group, granulomatous lesions affect the cranial nerves (two cases) or the parietal bone (one case). Multiple granulomatous lesions may be found in the brain. (3) Vasculitis of vasa nervorum accounts for many cases of peripheral neuritis and also at times for subarachnoid and intracerebral hemorrhage both of which are considered to be late manifestations of the disease. MacFadyen[101] encountered bilateral massive thalamic hemorrhage that was attributed to the fibrinoid necrosis of the perforating arteries. The vasculitis may be associated with multiple small infarcts[26] or sinus thrombosis. Even large branches of the major cerebral arteries can be necrotic and thrombosed with consequent softening of more extensive areas of the brain. An instance of an aneurysm on a branch of the vertebral artery has been reported.[112]

Systemic lupus erythematosus. Systemic lupus erythematosus is a systemic disease of connective tissues and blood vessels, affecting young adults and females more often than males (ratio 8:1). It is characterized by dermal photosensitivity, a typical erythematous facial rash, polyarteritis, pyrexia, anemia, lymphadenopathy, and frequently leukopenia and hyperglobulinema. The lupus erythematosus cell test is positive in more than 82% of afflicted patients and antinuclear antibodies are demonstrable in the serum in almost 90% of patients.[152] Renal involvement is common, and clinically in more than 50% the cardiovascular system is affected and the central nervous system in 25%.[37,152] Debilitation is progressive and within 5 years death usually eventuates from renal failure.

Although cerebral hemorrhage is said to occur because of thrombocytopenia,[156] the more common pathological manifestations in the brain and cord are vascular in origin. Fibrinoid necrosis of small arteries and arterioles (Fig. 12-16) is likely to lead to thrombosis with infarction, though some hemorrhage is not infrequent. Lupus tends to affect smaller vessels than those in polyarteritis nodosa and in general vascular nodosity and the intense inflammatory reaction of polyarteritis are not present. On occasions, small vessels may be thrombosed, and others exhibit atypical organization

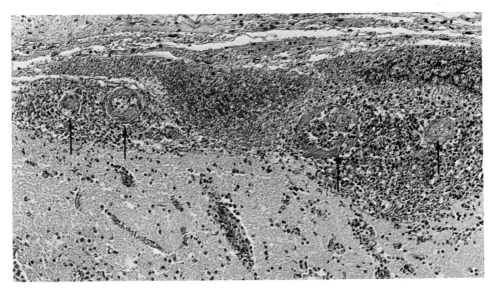

Fig. 12-16. Fibrinoid necrosis of four small pial vessels (*arrows*) in lupus erythematosus. Note surrounding hemorrhage and early red softening of cortex. (Hematoxylin and eosin, ×110.)

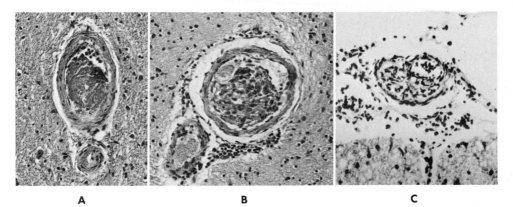

| A | B | C |

Fig. 12-17. Small cerebral vessels in lupus erythematosus exhibiting thrombosis in **A** and atypical organization of vessels in **B** and **C**. (Hematoxylin and eosin, ×110.)

(Fig. 12-17). As the result of the occlusion of multiple small vessels, often pial or cortical, microinfarcts, sometimes hemorrhagic, may be numerous and impart a granularity to the cortical surface. The basal ganglia may also be affected. Medium-sized vessels are infrequently affected but when they are larger, softenings are manifest. Petechial hemorrhages are also not an uncommon manifestation of the disease and subdural as well as subarachnoid hemorrhage is known to occur on occasions.[103] Piper[141] recorded the occurrence of vasculitis in the spinal cord with widespread thrombosis of the vessels related to the lumbar segments of the cord with some myelomalacia. The manifestations of a secondary infection may complicate the pathological picture.

Although systemic lupus erythematosus has been regarded as a typical autoimmune disease, the recent finding of possible viral inclusions in the endothelium of involved vessels and tissues[76,130] is of considerable interest even though the relationship of the inclusions to the disease has not been clarified.

Rheumatic fever. Patients dying from acute rheumatic fever have been found to have cerebral edema with widened perivascular spaces, capillary sclerosis, old and recent petechial hemorrhages, and multiple necrotic foci.[41] Although it is believed that there is a primary vascular lesion of small vessels in acute rheumatic fever, some of Costero's lesions may have been embolic, but to what extent embolism (from the rheumatic endocarditis) occurs at this stage of the disease is not known. Denst and Neubuerger[50] also attributed lesions of the cortical arteries in chronic rheumatic heart disease to a specific rheumatic factor. These lesions could have been embolic and appeared to be nonspecific. Winkelman and Eckel[184] observed a nonspecific productive endarteritis of small cortical vessels. Breutsch,[25] however, has emphasized the occurrence of obliterative arteritis of cerebral vessels in the pathogenesis of various neurological and psychiatric disturbances

in patients with recurrent attacks of rheumatic fever. Gardner[71] asserts that a widespread arteritis similar to polyarteritis nodosa can also affect the cerebral vessels in acute rheumatic fever. Autopsy material of this nature is so infrequent that a reappraisal of these lesions is desirable. Rheumatic meningoencephalitis may be associated with perivascular round cell cuffing, and in chronic rheumatic heart disease, cerebral embolism (major and minor) is a frequent complication, with or without a superadded bacterial endocarditis. Subarachnoid hemorrhage has been attributed to acute rheumatic fever,[55] but a superadded bacterial endocarditis should be excluded in such cases. Lindsay[99] attributed a peculiar fusiform aneurysm of a cerebellar artery to rheumatic arteritis in a subject with rheumatic heart disease, but insufficient detail was available for classification.

Rheumatoid arthritis. Specific cardiovascular lesions are rare in rheumatoid arthritis. Granulomatous lesions may arise in the heart, mitral and aortic cusps, and the root of the aorta. Acute myocarditis or cardiac amyloidosis can also occur, but clinically cardiovascular manifestations are much less in evidence than the pathological manifestations.[81] Gardner[71] indicated that intracranial hemorrhage or cerebral infarction may complicate an incidental hypertension. Bilateral vertebral artery thrombosis has occurred after severe rheumatoid arthritis of the cervical spine[175] but this was due to mechanical factors, probably stretch lesions and secondary infarction of the midbrain, medulla, and cerebellum.

There may be a diffuse vasculitis that affects small arteries, veins and arterioles, venules and capillaries and that primarily is associated with corticosteroid overdosage.[81] A ruptured aneurysm on the middle colic artery has been attributed to a necrotizing arteritis in rheumatoid arthritis[176] though as yet no specific involvement of the central nervous system has been reported.

Takayasu's arteritis. Takayasu's disease is a chronic progressive diffuse arteritis of the aorta and its main branches and usually proceeds to vascular occlusion.[154] Occurring in young women characteristically (female to male ratio 10-20:1), it is not peculiar to the Japanese. The aortic arch and the major vessels from the arch, the sites of predilection, are not necessarily those most severely involved.[154]

The clinical syndrome includes (1) vascular insufficiency of the head, neck, and upper extremities[16,147] including mental deterioration and emotional instability, (2) development of the collateral circulation sometimes simulating, but frequently dissimilar to, that of coarctation of the aorta, (3) carotid sinus syncope,[16] (4) cardiac involvement, including cardiomegaly, hypertension, coronary insufficiency, and valvular incompetence,[154] and (5) general symptoms, including an elevated erythrocyte sedimentation rate, and often a history of an acute fever. It is the commonest cause of the aortic arch syndrome, which has erroneously often been regarded as synonymous with Takayasu's arteritis.

Pathologically,[126] the arteritis involves the intima, the media, and the adventitia with focal or diffuse destruction of elastic tissue and muscle, resulting in extensive fibrosis of the media, considerable intimal thickening, and much periarterial fibrosis with round cell infiltration. Granulomatous tissue and new blood vessels may be prominent. Giant cells are generally few, but scarring and stenosis are prominent. Outside Japan, a superimposed atherosclerosis may aggravate the luminal narrowing. Calcification and aneurysm formation occur occasionally,[154] with thrombosis complicating the lesion and causing complete obstruction of the major aortic branches. This disease could be confused with syphilitic arteritis.

With each of the large vessels arising from the arch progressively becoming occluded, the fully developed aortic arch syndrome is manifest. The severity is dependent on the number of vessels occluded and of course the collateral circulation. In earlier stages of the disease, when one or two major cervical arteries to the brain may be affected, the steal phenomenon is demonstrable in some cases. As more vessels are obstructed, the severity of the cerebral vascular insufficiency increases. In 40 cases selected from the literature, it was found that 17 had a paralysis, 15 had sensory changes, 8 had aphasia, 5 had bulbar signs, and 29 had syncope and loss of consciousness. Convulsions are common and atypical, and coarctation of the aorta is not unusual,[147,154] but as yet the secondary development of a cerebral aneurysm has not been observed. Occasionally, small extracranial arteries are involved but arteritis has not been observed in the intracranial arteries. In 50% of cases there are changes in the retinal vessels[147] that are believed to be primarily ischemic. Vascular stasis in retinal vessels is a prominent feature[48] and could reflect a similar state in the cerebral circulation. Cerebral hemorrhage, reported in one patient, was attributed to the associated renal hypertension.[170] In this disease, the pathology of the cerebral vessels has not received attention. The disease, it is suspected, belongs to the autoimmune group. It is associated with a raised erythrocyte-sedimentation rate, a false positive serological test for syphilis often, a negative treponemal-immobilizing test (TPI), perhaps an altered electrophoretic pattern of serum proteins, and an altered albumin-globulin ratio. Occasionally, positive lupus erythematosus cell preparations and rarely pyrexia and leukocytosis lend some indirect support for the contention.[92,125] The possibility of an infective agent cannot be excluded.[126]

Giant cell or temporal arteritis. Giant cell arteritis is a subacute or chronic illness characterized by (1) a prodromal stage of general malaise and general symptoms extending from a few days to 18 months (usually 1 to 2 months)[80] followed by (2) headache, with the temporal arteries becoming acutely tender, tortuous, nodular, swollen, inflamed, and indurated soon after. Pulsation in the temporal artery is ultimately lost, tenderness and signs of inflammation

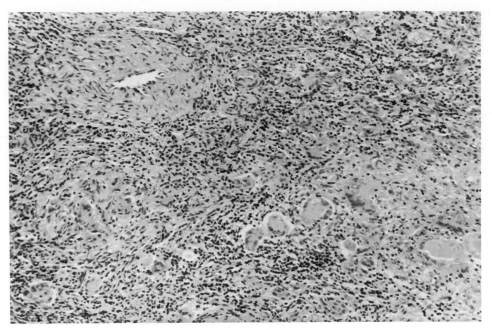

Fig. 12-18. Chronic inflammatory tissue of temporal arteritis. Note numerous giant cells. (Hematoxylin and eosin, ×110.)

subside, and the artery becomes hard and reduced in caliber. The course of the illness varies from 8 weeks to 30 months (mean 7.2 months).[80] Most patients are over 60 years and there is no sex predominance. The frequent though not invariable involvement of the temporal arteries has imparted the term "temporal" or "cranial arteritis." Yet the disease can affect any of the large or medium-sized arteries. Because of the widespread nature of the arterial involvement, the clinical picture may vary widely.[136] The erythrocyte-sedimentation rate and serum globulin[47] are generally raised, a mild hypochromic anemia is frequent, and a leukocytosis is occasional.

Biopsy of the temporal artery, sometimes leading to symptomatic relief, reveals that the artery is thickened, with little or no lumen and much perivascular fibrosis. The proliferation of the intima narrows the lumen grossly to a slit or irregular cavity.

In the innermost portions, the intima consists of a loose cellular fibrous tissue with relatively few inflammatory cells. In the outermost part of the intima, the in-

flammatory reaction may be florid with macrophages, round cells, polymorphonuclear leukocytes, giant cells, fibroblasts, and newly formed vessels in evidence (Fig. 12-18). Eosinophils are rare[80] and the foreign-body giant cells are at times related to the elastic tissue, which is markedly fragmented and deficient (Fig. 12-19). Frank necrosis may occur. The inflammatory reaction extends into the media where actual tubercle-like structures have been observed.[80] The adventitia exhibits a considerable fibrous tissue overgrowth and an infiltration of often perivascular inflammatory cells. Giant cells are absent and thrombosis is infrequent.

Electron microscopic examination of an involved temporal artery confirmed light microscopic findings and the relationship of the fragmented internal elastic lamina to macrophages and giant cells, which appeared to be phagocytosing masses of fibrillar material. This was thought to be either fibrin or altered elastica.[161]

Large arteries such as the aorta and carotid arteries exhibit changes primarily in

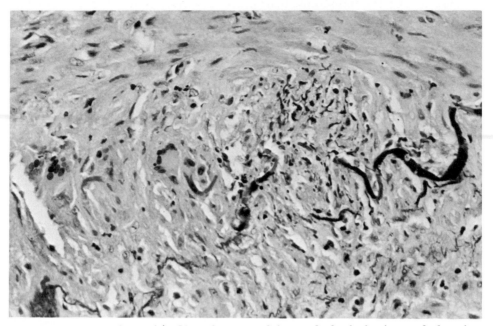

Fig. 12-19. Temporal arteritis. Note fragmented internal elastic lamina and the giant cells. (Verhoeff's elastic stain, ×275.)

the media. There is much destruction of elastica, an inflammatory reaction of lymphocytes, plasma cells, giant cells, and a few polymorphs. Intimal proliferation is generally mild as are adventitial changes. In arteries of intermediate size, intimal proliferation is more noticeable and thrombosis is usual.

The arteritis is a generalized one involving the aorta and other large arteries[40] and can be a cause of the aortic arch syndrome and dissecting aneurysm of the aorta. The brunt of the disease, however, falls upon the carotid system. Thus in 41 of 72 patients (57%) the first symptom was pain and tenderness of the scalp associated with temporal or occipital arteritis, which ultimately affects almost all patients.[179] About 68% of patients in the same series[179] developed visual symptoms though it has been estimated that about 50% develop permanent complete or partial blindness in one or both eyes because of involvement of the retinal arteries or the arteries supplying the optic nerves. The loss of vision is usually due to ischemic optic neuritis,[86] but in

other patients different manifestations of retinal ischemia have been found. Of 175 patients from the Mayo Clinic, 88 had symptoms suggestive of an intracranial lesion but only 19 had neurological findings. The relationship to giant cell arteritis was indefinite.[86]

Giant cell arteritis can involve the large branches of the aortic arch, and the carotid arteries also in their course in the neck may exhibit varying degrees of involvement with irregular narrowings and sometimes superadded thrombosis. The internal carotid and vertebral arteries[46,114] intracranially may likewise be involved with serious and even fatal cerebral infarction being the outcome, but since the disease is subacute, there may be time, unless thrombosis intervenes, for collaterals to compensate. The major cerebral arteries can be affected and so too the small meningeal vessels. Pial vessels have exhibited segmental grayish white thickening of the wall with narrowing of the lumen, in association with multiple, small widespread cerebral softenings and arteries histologically typical of giant-cell arteritis. Spinal medullary and pituitary arteries can be involved.[46]

In a child of 34 months who died of multiple aneurysms on systemic arteries complicating widespread giant cell arteritis, there were aneurysms of the internal carotid arteries immediately proximal to the circle of Willis.[171] These were also attributed to giant cell arteritis. The authors believed that the disease was distinct from that occurring in elderly adults and termed the entity "giant cell arteritis of children." Hinck and associates[85] observed angiographic beading of cerebral arteries occasioned by segmental stenoses alternating with areas of ectasia. The patient died with softenings, and histologically the vessels exhibited granulomatous inflammation of the media and intima with occasional giant cells. Vascular changes were restricted to the pial arteries primarily.

The mortality[47] has been estimated at 10%. In fatal cases of giant cell arteritis, cerebrovascular involvement is a major cause of death,[179] with either massive or multiple small infarcts in evidence, though cerebral hemorrhage has been alleged to be a complication.[11] Myocardial ischemia attributed to coronary arteritis is also a frequent cause of death.

The disease has been compared and contrasted with other arteritides, and although much speculation has surrounded the etiology, the cause remains quite unknown.

Granulomatous angiitis of the central nervous system. Granulomatous angiitis, a rare form or arteritis, exhibits a predilection for the central nervous system[87] though visceral vessels can be involved.[42,65] Synonyms include allergic angiitis, allergic granulomatosis, and giant cell arteritis of small vessels. Résumés of some 16 cases had been published by 1968 with an age range of 18 to 96 years (mean 50 years).[96] Headache, severe mental deterioration, and motor loss are usually in evidence. Some cases run a relatively short course (3 days to 6 weeks) but others survive for 9 months or almost 4 years.[96] The pressure of the cerebrospinal fluid is increased as are the protein levels (70 to 560 mg. per 100 ml.), and lymphocyte content (40 to 150 cells per cu. mm.).

Widespread granulomatous inflammation of small cerebral arteries and veins, mostly less than 200 μ in diameter, is characteristic of the disease. The lesions can occur in both the retinal and spinal vessels, with large arteries and even the capillary bed being involved occasionally. In a few instances, the veins are the more severely affected. Vessels occasionally exhibit necrosis with fibrinoid infiltration of the wall together with lymphocytes, histiocytes sometimes resembling epithelioid cells, fibroblasts, and giant cells of the foreign body and Langhans' type. Various vessels are affected asymmetrically. Others are occluded or replaced by a granulomatous inflammatory reaction, and the changes may be evident in only part of the vessel wall or otherwise in its entire thickness. There is widespread round cell infiltration of the leptomeninges, the adventitia of pial vessels, and Virchow-Robin spaces in the absence of other evidence of meningitis. The vascular changes on occasions involve the cranial nerves and furthermore can be associated with ischemic or hemorrhagic infarcts.

A similarity to Takayasu's arteritis and giant cell arteritis[111,127] has been stressed, but such diseases tend to affect larger vessels especially the extracranial arteries. More difficulty has been experienced in differentiation from sarcoidosis. The emphasis has been on the presence of necrosis and fibrinoid necrosis in granulomatous angiitis and the absence of necrotic lesions in sarcoidosis. However, Meyer and associates[120] reported a case in which noncaseating sarcoidlike granulomas were found in the lungs, liver, kidneys, and lymph nodes in association with perivascular granulomas in the leptomeninges. The presence of vascular necrosis and superadded thrombosis in pial vessels was more suggestive of granulomatous angiitis than acute sarcoidosis. Fisher[65] indicated that such arteritic lesions are exceedingly rare in sarcoidosis and that the case reported by Meyer and associates[120] is in all probability granulomatous angiitis. Involvement of visceral vessels, he asserts, is probably not as unusual as has been alleged.[96] Fisher[65] considers granulomatous angiitis a generalized arteritis evincing a predilection for the cerebrospinal vessels. He included allergic granulomatosis, described by Churg and Strauss,[35] as disseminated granulomatous vasculitis associated with asthma and a pronounced eosinophilia in which the vessels of the central nervous system were at times affected. It is uncertain, however, whether this is related to granulomatous angiitis, which according to most authors is virtually confined to the brain and cord.[96] In view of the difficulty in separating these diseases, it seems desirable for the establishment of some mechanism for pooling data and material from such cases so that subsequently larger numbers can be expertly analyzed and reappraised.

Though granulomatous angiitis has occurred in association with Hodgkin's disease[144] and a similarity to sarcoidosis has been mentioned, the etiology is unknown. It has been generally regarded as an autoimmune disease and a beneficial effect from corticosteroids has been observed.

Thromboangiitis obliterans. Thromboangiitis obliterans (Buerger's disease or von Winiwarter-Buerger's disease) has long been considered a localized panarteritis and panphlebitis of medium and small arteries and veins of the lower limb affecting, in particular, young adult Jews of Polish and Russian extraction. Several reports have purported to demonstrate a similar involvement of the internal carotid arteries in the neck,[10,91] the cerebral arteries,[13,185] and even the veins and dural sinuses.[13] Vessels of the lower limbs in such cases are not affected significantly[13] until several years after the cerebral involvement. Zülch[187] considers that the cerebral form of the disease is rare, affecting vessels predominantly 250 to 750 μ in diameter and causing granular atrophy and the proliferation of small collateral vessels mainly in the border zones of the cerebral cortex.

Recently there has been doubt that thromboangiitis obliterans is a specific disease entity.[64,75] Buerger[27] thought originally that the disease was primarily thrombotic in nature with little inflammatory reaction. Later he alleged it was an inflammatory disease with both acute and chronic stages including microabscesses, endothelioid cell proliferation, and giant cells histologically.[28,29] Fisher[64] in a critical review argued that the evidence for an inflammatory basis for this disease was remarkably ill founded and that the facts as they existed favored atherosclerosis as the primary cause of the arterial thrombosis in extracranial sites. No definite cases of Buerger's disease were encountered at a Jewish Hospital over a 10-year period,[178] but since some authors[142,182] still maintain that the disease is a separate entity, the controversy continues.

Fisher[64] pointed out that the major and typical features of cerebral thromboangiitis obliterans consisted of (1) shrunken, yellowish (siderotic) areas of patchy infarction in the territories of the anterior and middle cerebral arteries with maintenance of the gross pattern and without cavitation or complete dissolution of the brain tissue, (2) numerous white obliterated vessels on the surface of the infarcted region in contrast to the patent blood-containing vessels related to infarcts of the usual variety, (3) infarcts and white vessels usually coextensive, (4) generally an occluded artery proximal to the infarcted zone in which the peripheral branches of the middle and anterior cerebral arteries are of a fairly uniform age, with normal vessels intervening, (5) white vessels occluded by fine, sometimes loose, connective tissue containing siderophages or lipophages and sinusoidal vessels of recanalization without evidence of inflammation, (6) noninvolvement of cerebral veins, and (7) conventional infarcts at times coexistent. Granular atrophy of the cerebral cortex has also been described in cerebral thromboangiitis obliterans,[100,187] but the atrophy is far from specific.

Fisher[64] contended that an explanation

other than arteritis should be sought and that the cerebral infarcts were the result of a proximal occlusion of a vessel with failure of the collateral flow, which had been adequate for a time. The stagnation of vessels over the ischemic zone resulted in thrombosis and recanalization, with the infarct, under these circumstances, of a patchy nature. In some cases, the internal carotid artery in the neck is obstructed, and another possible explanation is that the patchy infarct might be due to a shower of small emboli possibly associated with a complete occlusion of the artery proximally. This would also provide an explanation for (1) the siderotic pigmentation of the patchy infarct, which no doubt was hemorrhagic initially, and (2) the presence of transient cerebral ischemic attacks in some cases. The absence of a plausible explanation for the vascular occlusion is an inadequate reason for labeling such cases as Buerger's disease. Romanul and Abramowicz[149] have described similar white pial arteries associated with infarcts in the border zones and have attributed them to thrombi formed during periods of relative stasis, but microembolism seems a more likely explanation. At present, the evidence is insufficient to support a concept of Buerger's disease as a specific entity within the cranium, for the vascular changes are nonspecific.

Miscellaneous disorders of cerebral blood vessels

Scleroderma (progressive systemic sclerosis). Scleroderma, a chronic generalized disease of connective tissue more common in women, is characterized by an insidious but progressive sclerosis of the skin and subcutaneous tissues and impaired mobility of the affected parts. A similar involvement occurs in the submucosa of the alimentary tract with ulceration, inflammation, and stricture. The renal lesions can be identical with those of malignant nephrosclerosis. There may be congestive cardiac failure or pulmonary fibrosis and cystic change (honeycomb lung). Cachexia with intercur-

rent infection is the usual mode of death. Vascular lesions may be widespread in scleroderma, since there are sclerotic changes in all coats of arterioles and small arteries and narrowing of the lumen, possibly preceded by acute fibrinoid necrosis. The vascular changes, which are remarkably similar to those of malignant hypertension, are most prominent in the viscera, especially the kidney. Involvement of large arteries such as the aorta and carotids is rare. Hypertension is usual.

The peripheral nerves and much less often the central nervous system may be affected. Richter[146] reported scleroderma in a man who had generalized convulsions and a severe confusional psychosis. At autopsy, extracranial vessels exhibited perivascular fibrosis, and in the brain there was grossly increased reticulin in and about cortical capillaries. In one series of seven cases, four hypertensive patients exhibited cerebral involvement. One had vascular changes in the cord[14] consisting of thickening and hyalinization of cerebral arteries, fibrinoid arteriolar necrosis, and capillary thickening. Associated with the vascular changes were small ischemic softenings, focal demyelination, and the loss of neurones. Lee and Haynes[98] encountered a 33-year-old woman whose left internal carotid artery was thickened and narrowed. The media was fibrotic and indistinct and the intima very thick: vasa vasorum were surrounded by inflammatory cells and there was fibrinoid arteriolar necrosis in the dense connective tissue surrounding the carotid. Much of the left cerebral hemisphere was infarcted and multiple small softenings were found in the right. There was evidence of arteriolar and capillary fibrosis and old occlusion of small cerebral arteries. The left anterior cerebral artery was thrombosed, the left middle cerebral artery had been recanalized, and in the perivascular connective tissue, small arteries exhibited degenerative and inflammatory changes.

Currently, the pathogenesis of scleroderma is uncertain and involvement of the brain and cord too infrequent for analysis.

There is no pathological evidence to suggest cerebral involvement in circumscribed scleroderma.

Focal nonseptic necrosis of cerebral arteries. Focal nonseptic necrosis of the vertebral and cerebellar arteries was found[94] in four middle-aged or elderly patients who died a few days after uncomplicated abdominal operations. Three were slightly hypertensive and the fourth was normotensive. Each patient died of massive subarachnoid hemorrhage, and the source of the bleeding was attributed to a small perforation in either a vertebral or a posterior inferior cerebellar artery. Histologically, there was little in the way of inflammatory reaction and this was mainly restricted to zones of necrosis in the adventitia. The arteries had apparently perforated relatively abruptly through zones of necrosis to cause adventitial dissection. Evidence of sepsis was absent and none of the systemic changes of polyarteritis nodosa were observed in the splanchnic areas. The illustrations did not adequately demonstrate necrosis, and the possible relationship of these lesions to dissecting aneurysms must be kept in mind although structurally they are atypical. Cases similar to those of Kernohan and Woltman[94] have not been reported, and so classification of their observations is not at present possible.

Thrombotic thrombocytopenic purpura. Thrombotic thrombocytopenic purpura, Moschcowitz's disease, and thrombotic microangiopathy are synonyms for a rare disease. Only 99 acceptable cases had been reported up to 1956.[165] It is thought to be primarily a vascular disease manifested by an acute febrile illness, hemolytic anemia, thrombocytopenic purpura, hyperglobulinemia,[33] and bizarre neurological disturbances.[165]

Every organ in the body may be affected. The vascular lesions are usually widespread and most numerous in the myocardium, subcapsular zone of the adrenal cortex, hepatic portal tracts, bone marrow, kidneys, and the cerebral gray matter[165] to the relative exclusion of the lungs.[23] The lesions in the central nervous system are often responsible for the patient's death. Characteristically, the lesions affect the arterioles and capillaries and occasionally the venules, which are partially or completely obstructed by granular or hyaline masses in various stages of organization (Fig. 12-20). The thrombi may be endothelialized and similar material appears to infiltrate the wall. Endothelial hyperplasia has been described, but there has been no identification of these cells at an ultrastructural level. Small aneurysmal dilatations (often thrombosed) of small arteries and of the arteriolar-capillary junction[115,132] and glomeruloid structures are held to be salient features. The thrombotic material is said to be fibrinoid[23] with a small admixture of platelets and fibrin. Perivascular infiltration of periodic acid Schiff–positive material has been noted in the brain of one patient.[23] There is no evidence of an angiitis but a few round cells may be related to the lesions. Small hemorrhages and infarcts, either microscopic or visible to the naked eye,[165] are common and are succeeded by glial proliferation and demyelination.

The cause is unknown and though thought to be related to the collagen diseases, the disease could be a nonspecific syndrome of multiple etiologies.[168] Associations with rheumatoid arthritis and drug therapy have been reported,[165] but concomitant lupus erythematosus or glomerulonephritis is more frequent. In most adults, the condition is rapidly fatal, few surviving 1 year. Chronicity and recovery are more frequent in children.[7]

Fibromuscular hyperplasia. Fibromuscular hyperplasia of the renal arteries producing renal artery stenosis and secondary hypertension is now a well-recognized entity occurring mostly in young females. Nonatherosclerotic renal arterial disease has generally been termed "fibromuscular hyperplasia" although various morphological subclassifications exist.[45,110] These subtypes, however, may be merely variants in which there is (1) profound elastic tissue destruction, (2) gross thinning of the media, as

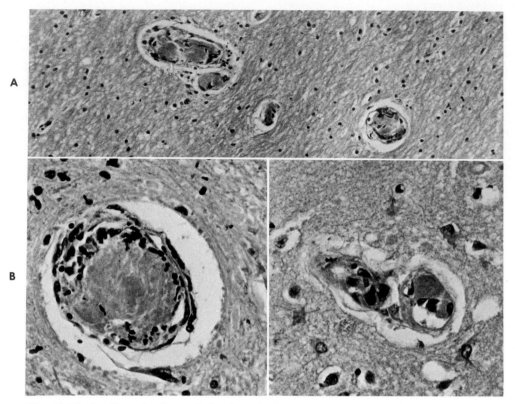

Fig. 12-20. Small cerebral vessels in thrombotic thrombocytopenic purpura. Lumens are occluded by eosinophilic somewhat granular thrombi and some atypical cellular proliferation. Hyaline eosinophilic material appears to lie within the wall in **C**. (Hematoxylin and eosin; **A**, ×110; **B, C**, ×275.)

when atrophic or simulating transverse tears occurring after the administration of methyl cellulose,[163] (3) medial muscular hyperplasia, often with much fibrosis, and (4) adventitial fibrosis sometimes resulting in stenosis. Other splanchnic arteries are frequently affected and the extracranial segments of the internal carotid and vertebral arteries may likewise be involved.[21,133] The classic appearance in arteriograms is like a "string of beads" or standing waves. Bruits and poststenotic aneurysmal dilatations occur in association with narrowing and irregularity of the arterial lumen, and there have been seven instances of saccular aneurysms of the cerebral arteries in association with this vascular disease.[21,133] Two sisters with fibromuscular hyperplasia of renal and other visceral arteries died from subarachnoid hemorrhage, but neither cere-

bral aneurysms nor fibromuscular hyperplasia of cerebral arteries were divulged at autopsy.[79] When cerebral angiography was performed, cerebral aneurysms were found in five of 10 patients with fibromuscular hyperplasia,[133] and so possibly a significant relationship exists between these two diseases. A 14-year-old boy with malignant hypertension, abdominal coarctation, and a cerebral aneurysm[67] also had bilateral renal arterial stenosis, and the illustration was suggestive of fibromuscular hyperplasia. Secondary severe hypertension may be responsible for the interrelationship, but detailed histological examination of the intracranial arteries including the petrous and cavernous segments of the internal carotid is wanting in this unusual disease. Neither has there been a pathological study of the cerebral aneurysms. Secondary hemodynamic disturbances are responsible for some of the aneurysmal dilatations of the extracranial arteries. Sandok and associates[153] reviewed 11 instances of cerebral aneurysms associated with fibromuscular hyperplasia with or without subarachnoid hemorrhage. Transient ischemic attacks may be associated with involvement of the cervical carotid and vertebral arteries,[22,143] whereas occlusive thrombosis is only an occasional finding. Fibromuscular hyperplasia of intracranial arteries (not commonly manifested angiographically) has been reported in association with electroencephalographic evidence of widespread cortical atrophy in the insular regions.[9]

Since the etiology and the natural history of fibromuscular hyperplasia are yet unknown, it is unwise to place too much significance on the coexistence of these two diseases. However, fibromuscular hyperplasia appears to be a widespread vascular abnormality possibly related to diseases of connective tissue. Functional studies of the vessel walls for elasticity and tensile strength would seem desirable. In summation, most patients are female, hypertension is the rule, elastic tissue loss in the arteries is severe,[186] and grossly disturbed hemodynamics (hypertension and bruits) accompany the vascular changes.

Effect of X-irradiation on cerebral blood vessels. Radiation therapy for intracranial tumors can cause necrosis of the neighboring brain. The neurological deficit is usually delayed several months to several years. Associated with these changes are severe vascular lesions consisting of fibrinoid necrosis of perforating vessels with superadded thrombosis, and possibly perivascular fibrinous exudate or even hemorrhage.[137] Some vessels on the other hand exhibit considerable fibrous thickening of their walls with disruption of their normal architecture, and possibly organization and recanalization of intravascular thrombi. Amyloid can be demonstrated in the walls of thickened vessels and about capillary walls.[104] Increased permeability is mani-

fested by the arterioles and capillaries, and fibrinoid necrosis follows. The pial vessels may display adventitial thickening. If the dose is sufficiently large, death may occur within hours or days after being irradiated and the cerebral vessels may exhibit an acute vasculitis.[183]

Recent evidence indicates that X-irradiation sensitizes or potentiates the effect of hypertension on blood vessels.[17,31]

Pathological effects of cerebral angiography. Cerebral angiography is perhaps the most important neurosurgical diagnostic technique in cerebrovascular disease. That it is not without risk has long been known, but in view of the ubiquitous use of cerebral angiography, the risks with modern radioopaque injection media are remarkably small. Hypersensitivity occasionally occurs, and this is usually but a mild reaction, though from time to time severe anaphylactic reactions occur and can be fatal. Sickling can be induced in individuals who are homozygous for sickle cell disease. The microcirculatory effects on the cellular constituents of the blood caused by the various agents used for angiograms have not been investigated in those without the sickle cell trait. The procedure is not without other effects, both local and general.

Local effects. A simple arterial puncture at arteriography results in perivascular hemorrhage, which may be quite extensive not only in the carotid sheath but also in the tissues of the neck and at times reaches as far down as the mediastinum. The hemorrhage is said to be minimal in the young and maximal in elderly hypertensives.[44] Laceration of the internal jugular or a vertebral vein can be responsible for severe bleeding, and a hematoma in the neck or thoracic inlet can result in compression of the trachea[8] or even of the oropharynx.[62] Traumatic arteriovenous aneurysms also result from local injury to the artery and vein in vertebral angiography (Chapter 10).

After injection of the artery, the needle track is filled by a thrombus and endothelial cells proliferate, covering the luminal surface by about the seventh day. Thereafter the plug becomes organized from both the luminal and adventitial ends of the needle track leaving a fibrous scar, with organization being complete by about 28 days.[43] Muscle and fine fibrillary elastica proliferate but there is no architectural reconstitution of the media and elastic lamellae.[43]

Crawford[43,44] found no instances of pyogenic infection but described acute inflammatory changes in the vicinity of the needle track, together with a few sterile abscesses. These were attributed to leakage of the contrast medium into the tissues because of the numerous foamy macrophages among the polymorphonuclear cells.

Mural thrombosis is to be expected at the site of puncture and also in relation to any other scratches or lacerations of the intimal surface. This is a source of small emboli, and the thrombus will become endothelialized and organized with a resulting intimal plaque containing fibrillary elastica, collagen, and smooth muscle. Crawford[44] reported five cases with multiple nonlethal cerebral infarcts, with the site of carotid puncture being the only likely site of origin of the emboli. Occlusive thrombosis rarely complicates angiography. Advanced atherosclerosis locally with severe local trauma is more likely to contribute to such a complication. Foreign bodies such as cotton fibers and particulate matter (starch powder) may have been introduced with a needle or a catheter to cause embolism, but such an event must be quite infrequent. The risks of cerebral air embolism are grave but well recognized. It is nevertheless possible that an occasional small quantity of air could be injected inadvertently. It is much more likely that intimal injury of the artery is the source of emboli, though of course some minor thrombosis may occur in the catheter or needle and thus lead to embolism. Such emboli can thus cause transient or, less frequently, permanent neurological deficits.

In one series of 604 carotid angiograms,[135] 4.6% of the subjects had neurological complications varying from tran-

sient neurological defects, from which recovery occurred within minutes, days, or weeks, to severe permanent (0.8%) defects, including death, hemiplegia, etc. Peculiarly enough the complications were most frequent (19%) in migrainous patients, next most frequent in those with occlusive vascular disease (11%), and least frequent in those with tumors (0.9%). In general, the neurological status of the patient before angiography was of paramount importance, with complications being more likely to occur in those already having a serious neurological deficit. In yet another series,[8] there were 21 complications in 538 angiograms (a frequency of 3.9%), including one death, one permanent hemiplegia, and 12 with transient neurological disturbances. The fatal case was due to the subintimal injection of the contrast medium. The complication rate varies considerably (up to 20%), but it seems that the risks of percutaneous vertebral angiography are greater than those of most other techniques.[62,158]

Crawford[44] found two traumatic false aneurysms among 75 subjects who came to angiography. These were small false aneurysms about 1 cm. in diameter. However, traumatic dissecting aneurysms are much more frequent, and nine were found among 75 autopsies. These dissecting aneurysms (see Chapter 9) varied from 0.5 to 4 cm. in length, and part of the false lumen became endothelialized in the few patients who died about 3 weeks after angiography. Allen and associates[8] consider that local arterial trauma is probably the commonest cause of complications. A rare but fatal instance of bilateral pneumothorax has complicated subclavian arteriography and thoracentesis.[62]

When the brachial, axillary, or subclavian artery is punctured, local bleeding may also occur and evidence of ischemia may be observed in the upper limb. Other injuries include brachial neuritis and recurrent laryngeal nerve palsy.[8]

Distal effects. Complete occlusion of the carotid in the neck attributed to intramural injection and dissection can result in an extensive cerebral infarct, which can be fatal. Emboli lodging in the brain can cause ischemic lesions, which on occasions can be severe. Other effects such as bleeding from a saccular or an arteriovenous aneurysm can occur during angiography, with the rupture being either coincidental or possibly precipitated by the injection of the material under pressure.

Toxicity. Some contrast media used in the past were fairly toxic. Sodium iodide (25%) had a high mortality[1] and iodopyracet (Diodrast) had a direct toxic effect on neurones as well as causing vasospasm.[68] Thorium dioxide (Thorotrast) has been used to a limited extent because of its radioactivity and potential dangers.[49] Modern contrast media are regarded as virtually nontoxic and fairly safe. However, Mersereau and Robertson[119] found that endothelial damage including desquamation of endothelial cells of the rat inferior vena cava and iliac vein could be produced by various radiographic contrast media. The severity of the damage varied with the medium and the duration of exposure. Similar endothelial damage and desquamation was produced in the cerebral blood vessels of rats after carotid perfusion with various contrast media,[109] and such endothelial damage is likely to initiate thrombus formation, but whether other changes are produced in the behavior of the cellular constituents of the blood is uncertain though tests could be carried out in rabbit ear chambers. Such changes could be associated with stasis and alterations in the bloodbrain barrier, but toxicity cannot be completely ignored. That neurotoxic activity is manifested by some contrast media is strongly suggested by the activation of epileptogenic foci for several hours and electroencephalographic abnormalities after angiography with Diodrast.[1,68] The toxic effect of a contrast medium has been shown to cause edema, sludging, and delay in the passage of the dye through the spinal circulation of experimental animals, although not all doses manifest such toxicity.[105]

There is need for further investigation of the action of all the contrast media, but the need for and diagnostic value of angiography must be considered in the evaluation of the ill effects of this important procedure.

References

1. Abbott, K. H., Gay, J. R., and Goodall, R. J.: Clinical complications of cerebral angiography, J. Neurosurg. 9:258, 1952.
2. Adachi, M., Wellmann, K. F., and Volk, B. W.: Histochemical studies on the pathogenesis of idiopathic non-arteriosclerotic cerebral calcification, J. Neuropath. Exp. Neurol. 27:483, 1968.
3. Adams, C. W. M.: Vascular histochemistry, Chicago, 1967, Year Book Medical Publishers, Inc.
4. Adams, R. D., and Vander Eecken, H. M.: Vascular diseases of the brain, Ann. Rev. Med. 4:213, 1953.
5. Alex, M., Baron, E. K., Goldenberg, S., and Blumenthal, H. T.: An autopsy study of cerebrovascular accident in diabetes mellitus, Circulation 25.663, 1962.
6. Alexander, L., and Woodhall, B.: Calcified epileptogenic lesions as caused by incomplete interference with the blood supply of the diseased areas, J. Neuropath. Exp. Neurol. 2:1, 1943.
7. Allanby, K. D., Huntsman, R. G., and Sacker, L. S.: Thrombotic microangiography, Lancet 1:237, 1966.
8. Allen, J. H., Parera, C., and Potts, D. G.: The relation of arterial trauma to complications of cerebral angiography, Amer. J. Roentgen. 95:845, 1965.
9. Andersen, P. E.: Fibromuscular hyperplasia of the carotid arteries, Acta Radiol. 10:90, 1970.
10. Andrell, P. O.: Thrombosis of the internal carotid artery, Acta Med. Scand. 114:336, 1943.
11. Andrews, J. M.: Giant-cell ("temporal") arteritis, Neurology 16:963, 1966.
12. Andriole, V. T., Kravetz, H. M., Roberts, W. C., and Utz, J. P.: Candida endocarditis, Amer. J. Med. 32:251, 1962.
13. Antoni, N.: Buerger's disease, thrombo-angiitis obliterans in the brain, Acta Med. Scand. 108:502, 1941.
14. Antonovych, T. J., and Steingaszner, L. C.: Pathologic changes in progressive systemic sclerosis, Georgetown Med. Bull. 16:27, 1962.
15. Arkin, A.: A clinical and pathological study of periarteritis nodosa, Amer. J. Path. 6:401, 1930.
16. Ask-Upmark, E.: On the pulseless disease outside of Japan, Acta Med. Scand. 149:161, 1954.
17. Asscher, A. W., and Anson, S. G.: Arterial hypertension and irradiation damage to the nervous system, Lancet 2:1343, 1962.
18. Baker, A. B.: Structure of the small cerebral arteries and their changes with age, Amer. J. Path. 13:453, 1937.

19. Baker, A. B., and Iannone, A.: Cerebrovascular disease: II. The smaller intra-cerebral arteries, Neurology **9**:391, 1959.

20. Baker, R. D.: Mucormycosis—a new disease? J.A.M.A. **163**:805, 1957.

21. Belber, C. J., and Hoffman, R. B.: The syndrome of intracranial aneurysm associated with fibromuscular hyperplasia of the renal arteries, J. Neurosurg. **28**:556, 1968.

22. Bergan, J. J., and MacDonald, J. R.: Recognition of cerebrovascular fibro-muscular hyperplasia, Arch. Surg. **98**:332, 1969.

23. Bornstein, B., Boss, J. H., Casper, J., and Behar, M.: Thrombotic thrombocytopenic purpura, J. Clin. Path. **13**:124, 1960.

24. Bronsky, D., Kushner, D. S., Dubin, A., and Snapper, I.: Idiopathic hypoparathyroidism and pseudohypoparathyroidism: case reports and review of the literature, Medicine **37**:317, 1958.

25. Bruetsch, W. L.: Rheumatic brain disease: late sequel of rheumatic fever, II. Int. Congr. Psychiat., Zürich, Sept. 1957.

26. Budzilovich, G. N., and Wilens, S. L.: Fulminating Wegener's granulomatosis, Arch. Path. **70**:653, 1960.

27. Buerger, L.: Thrombo-angiitis obliterans: a study of the vascular lesions leading to presenile spontaneous gangrene, Amer. J. Med. Sci. **136**:567, 1908.

28. Buerger, L.: Recent studies in the pathology of thrombo-angiitis obliterans, J. Med. Res. **31**:181, 1914-1915.

29. Buerger, L.: Thromboangiitis obliterans concepts of pathogenesis and pathology, J. Int. Chir. **4**:399, 1939.

30. Byrom, F. B.: The pathogenesis of hypertensive encephalopathy and its relation to the malignant phase of hypertension, Lancet **2**:201, 1954.

31. Byrom, F. B.: The hypertensive vascular crisis. An experimental study, London, 1969, W. Heinemann Medical Books Ltd.

32. Byrom, F. B.: Vascular lesions in malignant hypertension, Lancet **2**:495, 1969.

33. Cahalane, S. F., and Horn, R. C.: Thrombotic thrombocytopenic purpura of long duration, Amer. J. Med. **27**:333, 1959.

34. Carpenter, D. F., Brubaker, L. H., Powell, R. D., and Valsamis, M. P.: Phycomycotic thrombosis of the basilar artery, Neurology **18**:807, 1968.

35. Churg, J., and Strauss, L.: Allergic granulomatosis, allergic angiitis, and periarteritis nodosa, Amer. J. Path. **27**:277, 1951.

36. Citron, B. P., Halpern, M., McCarron, M., Lundberg, G. D., et al.: Necrotizing angiitis associated with drug abuse, New Eng. J. Med. **283**:1003, 1970.

37. Clark, E. C., and Bailey, A. A.: Neurological and psychiatric signs associated with systemic lupus erythematosus, J.A.M.A. **160**:455, 1956.

38. Clarke, E., and Murphy, E. A.: Neurological manifestations of malignant hypertension, Brit. Med. J. **2**:1319, 1956.

39. Cole, F. M., and Yates, P. O.: Comparative incidence of cerebrovascular lesions in normotensive and hypertensive patients, Neurology **18**:255, 1968.

40. Cooke, W. T., Cloake, P. C. P., Govan, A. D. T., and Colbeck, J. C.: Temporal arteritis: a generalized vascular disease, Quart. J. Med. **15**:47, 1946.

41. Costero, I.: Cerebral lesions responsible for death of patients with active rheumatic fever, Arch. Neurol. Psychiat. **62**:48, 1949.

42. Cravioto, H., and Feigin, I.: Noninfectious granulomatous angiitis with a predilection for the nervous system, Neurology **9**:599, 1959.

43. Crawford, T.: The healing of puncture wounds in arteries, J. Path. Bact. **72**:547, 1956.

44. Crawford, T.: The pathological effects of cerebral arteriography, J. Neurol. Neurosurg. Psychiat. **19**:217, 1956.

45. Crocker, D. W.: Fibromuscular dysplasias of renal artery, Arch. Path. **85**:602, 1968.

46. Crompton, M. R.: The visual changes in temporal (giant-cell) arteritis, Brain **82**:377, 1959.

47. Crompton, M. R.: Giant-cell arteritis, World Neurol. **2**:237, 1961.

48. Currier, R. D., DeJong, R. N., and Boles, G. G.: Pulseless disease: central nervous system manifestations, Neurology **4**:818, 1954.

49. da Silva Horta, J., Abbatt, J. D., da Motta, L. C., and Roriz, M. L.: Malignancy and other late effects following administration of Thorotrast, Lancet **2**:201, 1965.

50. Denst, J., and Neuberger, K. T.: Intracranial vascular lesions in late rheumatic heart disease, Arch. Path. **46**:191, 1948.

51. Desmond, M. M., Wilson, G. S., Melnick, J. L., Singer, D. B., Zion, T. E., Rudolph, A., J., Pineda, R. G., Ziai, M., and Blattner, R. J.: Congenital rubella encephalitis, J. Pediat. **71**: 311, 1967.

52. Diaz-Rivera, R. S., and Miller, A. J.: Periarteritis nodosa: a clinicopathological analysis of seven cases, Ann. Intern. Med. **24**:420, 1946.

53. Dickinson, C. J., and Thomson, A. D.: A post mortem study of the main cerebral arteries with special reference to their possible role in blood pressure regulation, Clin. Sci. **19**:513, 1960.

54. Drachmann, D. A.: Neurological complications of Wegener's granulomatosis, Arch. Neurol. **8**: 145, 1963.

55. Easby, M. H.: A case of rheumatic heart disease with subarachnoid hemorrhage, Med. Clin. N. Amer. **18**:307, 1934.

56. Eaton, L. M., Camp, J. D., and Love, J. G.: Symmetric cerebral calcification, particularly of the basal ganglia, demonstrable roentgenographically, Arch. Neurol. Psychiat. **41**:921, 1939.

57. Emmons, C. W., Binford, C. H., and Utz, J. P.: Medical mycology, Philadelphia, 1963, Lea & Febiger.

58. Epstein, S. M., Miale, T. D., Moosy, J., Verney, E., and Sidransky, H.: Experimental intracranial aspergillosis, J. Neuropath. Exp. Neurol. **27**:137, 1968.

59. Esterly, J. R., and Oppenheimer, E. H.: Vas-

cular lesions in infants with congenital rubella, Circulation **36**:544, 1967.

60. Esterly, J. R., and Oppenheimer, E. H.: Pathological lesions due to congenital rubella, Arch. Path. **87**:380, 1969.

61. Feigin, I., and Prose, P.: Hypertensive fibrinoid arteritis of the brain and gross cerebral hemorrhage, Arch. Neurol. **11**:98, 1959.

62. Feild, J. R., Robertson, J. T., and DeSaussure, R. L.: Complications of cerebral angiography in 2,000 consecutive cases, J. Neurosurg. **19**: 775, 1962.

63. Fetter, B. F., Klintworth, G. K., and Hendry, W. S.: Mycoses of the central nervous system, Baltimore, 1967, The Williams & Wilkins Co.

64. Fisher, C. M.: Cerebral thromboangiitis obliterans, Medicine **36**:169, 1957.

65. Fisher, C. M.: Ocular palsy in temporal arteritis, Minn. Med. **42**:1258, 1430, 1617; 1959.

66. Fisher, C. M.: The arterial lesions underlying lacunes, Acta Neuropath. **12**:1, 1969.

67. Fisher, E. R., and Corcoran, A. C.: Congenital coarctation of the abdominal aorta with resultant renal hypertension, Arch. Intern. Med. **89**:943, 1952.

68. Foltz, E. L., Thomas, L. B., and Ward, A. A.: The effects of intracarotid Diodrast, J. Neurosurg. **9**:68, 1952.

69. Ford, R. G., and Siekert, R. G.: Central nervous system manifestations of periarteritis nodosa, Neurology **15**:114, 1965.

70. Friede, R. L., Magee, K. R., and Mack, E. W.: Idiopathic nonarteriosclerotic calcification of cerebral vessels, Arch. Neurol. **5**:279, 1961.

71. Gardner, D. L.: Pathology of the connective tissue diseases, Baltimore, 1966, The Williams & Wilkins Co.

72. Gery, L., Fontaine, R., and Branzeu, P.: Les lésions chroniques oblitérantes des artères des membres (étude anatomo-clinique), J. Int. Chir. **4**:427, 1939.

73. Geyelin, H. R., and Penfield, W.: Cerebral calcification epilepsy, Arch. Neurol. Psychiat. **21**:1020, 1929.

74. Goldzieher, J. W., and Lisa, J. R.: Gross cerebral hemorrhage and vascular lesions in acute tuberculous meningitis and meningo-encephalitis, Amer. J. Path. **23**:133, 1947.

75. Gore, I., and Burrows, S.: A reconstruction of the pathogenesis of Buerger's disease, Amer. J. Clin. Path. **29**:319, 1958.

76. Györkey, F., Min, K.-W., Sincovics, J. G., and Györkey, P.: Systemic lupus erythematosus and myxovirus, New Eng. J. Med. **280**:333, 1969.

77. Halpern, M., and Citron, B. P.: Necrotizing angiitis associated with drug abuse, Amer. J. Roentgen. **111**:663, 1971.

78. Hameroff, S. B., Eckholdt, J. W., and Lindenberg, R.: Cerebral phycomycosis in a heroin addict, Neurology **20**:261, 1970.

79. Hansen, J., Holten, C., and Thorborg, J. V.: Hypertension in two sisters caused by so-called fibromuscular hyperplasia of the renal arteries, Acta Med. Scand. **178**:461, 1965.

80. Harrison, C. V.: Giant-cell or temporal arteritis: a review, J. Clin. Path. **1**:197, 1948.

81. Hart, F. D.: Rheumatoid arthritis: extra-articular manifestations, Brit. Med. J. **3**:131, 1969.

82. Hazen, E. L., Gordon, M. A., and Reed, F. C.: Laboratory identification of pathogenic fungi simplified, ed. 3, Springfield, Ill., 1970, Charles C Thomas, Publisher.

83. Henson, R. A., and Croft, P. B.: Spontaneous spinal subarachnoid haemorrhage, Quart. J. Med. **25**:53, 1956.

84. Hiller, F.: Cerebral hemorrhage in hyperergic angiitis, J. Neuropath. Exp. Neurol. **12**:24, 1953.

85. Hinck, V. C., Carter, C. C., and Rippey, J. G.: Giant cell (cranial) arteritis, Amer. J. Roentgen. **92**:769, 1964.

86. Hollenhorst, R. W., Brown, J. R., Wagener, H. P., and Shick, R. M.: Neurologic aspects of temporal arteritis, Neurology **10**:490, 1960.

87. Hughes, J. T., and Brownell, B.: Granulomatous giant-cell angiitis of the central nervous system, Neurology **16**:293, 1966.

88. Hurst, E. W.: On the so-called calcification in the basal ganglia of the brain, J. Path. **29**:65, 1926.

89. Hutter, R. V. P.: Phycomycetous infection (mucormycosis) in cancer patients: a complication of therapy, Cancer **2**:330, 1959.

90. Ishikawa, K.: Arterial disease in Japan, Jap. Heart J. **5**:199, 1964.

91. James, T. G. I.: Thrombosis of the internal carotid artery, Brit. Med. J. **2**:1264, 1949.

92. Judge, R. D., Currier, R. D., Gracie, W. A., and Figley, M. M.: Takayasu's arteritis and the aortic arch syndrome, Amer. J. Med. **32**: 379, 1962.

93. Kalamboukis, Z., and Molling, P.: Symmetrical calcification of the brain in the predominance in the basal ganglia and cerebellum, J. Neuropath. Exp. Neurol. **21**:364, 1962.

94. Kernohan, J. W., and Woltman, H. W.: Postoperative, focal, nonseptic necrosis of vertebral and cerebellar arteries, J.A.M.A. **122**:1173, 1943.

95. Kincaid-Smith, P., McMichael, J., and Murphy, E. A.: The clinical course and pathology of hypertension with papilloedema (malignant hypertension), Quart. J. Med. **27**:117, 1958.

96. Kolodny, E. H., Rebeiz, J. J., Caviness, V. S., and Richardson, E. P.: Granulomatous angiitis of the central nervous system, Arch. Neurol. **19**:510, 1968.

97. Lampert, P.: Tumorforming atypical amyloidosis of the choroid plexus with invasion of the cerebral white matter, J. Neuropath. Exp. Neurol. **17**:604, 1958.

98. Lee, J. E., and Haynes, J. M.: Carotid arteritis and cerebral infarction due to scleroderma, Neurology **17**:18, 1967.

99. Lindsay, S.: Subarachnoid hemorrhage due to intracranial rheumatic aneurysm, J. Nerv. Ment. Dis. **99**:717, 1944.

100. Lippmann, H. I.: Cerebrovascular thrombosis in patients with Buerger's disease, Circulation **5**:680, 1952.

101. MacFadyen, D. J.: Wegener's granulomatosis

with discrete lung lesions and peripheral neuritis, Canad. Med. Ass. J. **83**:760, 1960.

102. Malamud, N., and Foster, D. B.: Periarteritis nodosa, Arch. Neurol. Psychiat. **47**:828, 1942.

103. Malamud, N., and Saver, G.: Neuropathologic findings in disseminated lupus erythematosus, Arch. Neurol. Psychiat. **71**:723, 1954.

104. Mandybur, T. I., and Gore, I.: Amyloid in late postirradiation necrosis of brain, Neurology **19**:983, 1969.

105. Margolis, G., Griffin, A. T., Kenan, P. D., Tindall, G. T., Riggins, R., and Fort, L: Contrast-medium injury to the spinal cord. The role of altered circulatory dynamics, J. Neurosurg. **16**:390, 1959.

106. Marshall, J.: Evidence upon the neurogenic theory of hypertension, Lancet **2**:410, 1966.

107. McBride, R. A., Corson, J. M., and Dammin, G. J.: Mucormycosis. Two cases of disseminated disease with cultural identification rhizopus; review of literature, Amer. J. Med. **28**:832, 1960.

108. McCall, W., and Strobos, R. R. J.: Survival of a patient with central nervous system mucormycosis, Neurology **7**:290, 1957.

109. McConnell, F., and Mersereau, W. A.: The effect of angiographic contrast media on arterial endothelium: an experimental study, J. Canad. Assoc. Radiol. **15**:14, 1964.

110. McCormack, L. J., Poutasse, E. F.: Meaney, T. F., Noto, T. J., and Dustan, H. P.: A pathologic-arteriographic correlation of renal arterial disease, Amer. Heart. J. **72**:188, 1966.

111. McCormick, H. M., and Neubuerger, K. T.: Giant-cell arteritis involving small meningeal and intracerebral vessels, J. Neuropath. Exp. Neurol. **17**:471, 1958.

112. McCormick, W. F.: Problems and pathogenesis of intracranial arterial aneurysms. In Toole, J. F., Moosy, J., and Janeway, R.: Cerebral vascular diseases, New York, 1971, Grune & Stratton, Inc., p. 219.

113. McKee, E. E.: Mycotic infection of brain with arteritis and subarachnoid hemorrhage, Amer. J. Clin. Path. **20**:381, 1950.

114. McMillan, G. C.: Diffuse granulomatous aortitis with giant cells. Arch. Path. **49**:63, 1950.

115. Meacham, G. C., Orbison, J. L., Heinle, R. W., Steele, H. J., and Schaefer, J. A.: Thrombotic thrombocytopenic purpura: a disseminated disease of arterioles, Blood **6**:706, 1951.

116. Melchior, J. C., Benda, C. E., and Yakovlev, P. I.: Familial idiopathic cerebral calcifications in childhood, Amer. J. Dis. Child. **99**:787, 1960.

117. Menser, M. A., Dorman, D. C., Reye, R. D., and Reid, R. R.: Renal-artery stenosis in the rubella syndrome, Lancet **1**:790, 1966.

118. Merritt, H. H., Adams, R. D., and Solomon, H. C.: Neurosyphilis, New York, 1946, Oxford University Press.

119. Mersereau, W. A., and Robertson, H. R.: Observations on venous endothelial injury following the injection of various radiographic conrast media in the rat, J. Neurosurg. **18**:289, 1961.

120. Meyer, J. S., Foley, J. M., and Campagna-Pinto D.: Granulomatous angiitis of the meninges in sarcoidosis, Arch. Neurol. Psychiat. **69**:587, 1953.

121. Meyer, J. S., Waltz, A. G., and Gotoh, F.: Pathogenesis of cerebral vasospasm in hypertensive encephalopathy. II. The nature of increased irritability of smooth muscle of pial arterioles in renal hypertension, Neurology **10**:859, 1960.

122. Miller, H.: Clinical consideration of cerebrovascular disorders occurring during the course of general diseases of an inflammatory or allergic nature, Proc. Roy. Soc. Med. **44**:852, 1951.

123. Moore, W. S., and Hall, A. D.: Pathogenesis of arterial hypertension after occlusion of cerebral arteries, Surg. Gynec. Obstet. **131**:885, 1970.

124. Mukoyama, M., Gimple, K. and Poser, C. M.: Aspergillosis of the central nervous system, Neurology **19**:967, 1969.

125. Nakao, K., Ikeda, M., Kimata, S., Niitani, H., Miyahara, M., Ishimi, Z., Hashiba, K., Takeda, Y., Ozawa, T., Matsushita, S., and Kuramochi, M.: Takayasu's arteritis, Circulation **35**:1141, 1967.

126. Nasu, T.: Pathology of pulseless disease, Angiology **14**:225, 1963.

127. Neubuerger, K. T.: Giant cell arteritis with involvement of small intracranial arteries and arterioles, J. Neuropath. Exp. Neurol. **17**:515, 1958.

128. Neumann, M. A.: Iron and calcium dysmetabolism in the brain, J. Neuropath. Exp. Neurol. **21**:148, 1962.

129. Norman, R. M., and Urich, H.: The influence of a vascular factor on the distribution of symmetrical cerebral calcification, J. Neurol. Neurosurg. Psychiat. **23**:142, 1960.

130. Norton, W. L.: Endothelial inclusions in active lesions of systemic lupus erythematosus, J. Lab. Clin. Med. **74**:369, 1969.

131. Nye, S. W., Tangchai, P., Sundarakiti, S., and Punyagupta, S.: Lesions of the brain in eosinophilic meningitis, Arch. Path. **89**:9, 1970.

132. Orbison, J. L.: Morphology of thrombotic thrombocytopenic purpura with demonstration of aneurysms, Amer. J. Path. **28**:129, 1952.

133. Palubinskas, A. J., Perloff, D., and Newton, T. H.: Fibromuscular hyperplasia, an arterial dysplasia of increasing clinical importance, Amer. J. Roentgen. **98**:907, 1966.

134. Parker, H. L., and Kernohan, J. W.: The central nervous system in periarteritis nodosa, Proc. Staff Meet. Mayo Clin. **24**:43, 1949.

135. Patterson, R. H., Goodell, H., and Dunning, H. S.: Complications of carotid arteriography, Arch. Neurol. **10**:513, 1964.

136. Paulley, J. W., and Hughes, J. P.: Giant-cell arteritis, or arteritis of the aged, Brit. Med. J. **2**:1562, 1960.

137. Pennybacker, J., and Russell, D. S.: Necrosis of the brain due to radiation therapy, J. Neurol. Neurosurg. Psychiat. **11**:183, 1948.

138. Peterson, E. W., and Schulz, D. M.: Amyloid

in vessels of a vascular malformation in brain, Arch. Path. **72**:480, 1961.

139. Pickering, G.: Reversibility of malignant hypertension, Lancet **1**:413, 1971.

140. Pickering, G. W.: High blood pressure, London, 1955, J. & A. Churchill Ltd.

141. Piper, P. G.: Disseminated lupus erythematosus with involvement of the spinal cord, J.A.M.A. **153**:215, 1953.

142. Prusik, B., and Reiniš, Z.: Does Buerger's disease exist? Angiologica **1**:94, 1964.

143. Rainer, W. G., Cramer, G. G., Nemby, J. P., and Clarke, J. P.: Fibromuscular hyperplasia of the carotid artery causing positional cerebral ischemia, Ann. Surg. **167**:444, 1968.

144. Rewcastle, N. B., and Tom, M. I.: Non-infectious granulomatous angiitis of the nervous system associated with Hodgkin's disease, J. Neurol. Neurosurg. Psychiat. **25**:51, 1962.

145. Rich, A. R., and McCordock, H. A.: The pathogenesis of tuberculous meningitis, Johns Hopkins Hosp. Bull. **52**:5, 1933.

146. Richter, R. B.: Peripheral neuropathy and connective tissue disease, J. Neuropath. Exp. Neurol. **13**:168, 1954.

147. Riehl, J.: The idiopathic arteritis of Takayasu, Neurology **13**:873, 1963.

148. Robertson, D. M., Dinsdale, H. B., and Hayashi, T., and Tu, J.: Cerebral lesions in adrenal regeneration hypertension, Amer. J. Path. **59**:115, 1970.

149. Romanul, F. C. A., and Abramowicz, A.: Changes in brain and pial vessels in arterial border zones, Arch. Neurol. **11**:40, 1964.

150. Rorke, L. B., Fabiyi, A., Elizan, T. S., and Sever, J. L.: Experimental cerebrovascular lesions in congenital and neonatal rubella-virus infections of ferrets, Lancet **2**:153, 1968.

151. Rosenberg, E. F.: The brain in malignant hypertension, Arch. Intern. Med. **65**:545, 1940.

152. Rowell, N. R.: Systemic lupus erythematosus, Brit. Med. J. **2**:427, 1969.

153. Sandok, B. A., Houser, O. W., Baker, H. L., and Holley, K. E.: Fibromuscular dysplasia, Arch. Neurol. **24**:462, 1971.

154. Schrire, V.: Arteritis of the aorta and its major branches, Aust. Ann. Med. **16**:33, 1967.

155. Schwartz, P.: New aspects of cardiovascular disease: senile cardiovascular amyloidosis (fluorescence microscopic investigations), Trans. N. Y. Acad. Sci. **30**:22, 1967.

156. Sedgwick, R. P., and Von Hagen, K. O.: The neurological manifestations of lupus erythematosus and periarteritis nodosa, Bull. Los Angeles Neurol. Soc. **13**:129, 1948.

157. Sheldon, W. P. H.: Intracranial haemorrhage in infancy and childhood, Quart. J. Med. **20**:353, 1927.

158. Silverstein, A.: Arteriography of stroke. III. Complications, Arch. Neurol. **15**:206, 1966.

159. Slager, U. T., and Wagner, J. A.: The incidence, composition, and pathological significance of intracerebral vascular deposits in basal ganglia, J. Neuropath. Exp. Neurol. **15**:417, 1956.

160. Smith, J. P.: Hyaline arteriolosclerosis in

spleen, pancreas, and other viscera, J. Path. Bact. **72**:643, 1956.

161. Smith, K. R.: Electron microscopy of giant-cell (temporal) arteritis, J. Neurol. Neurosurg. Psychiat. **32**:348, 1969.

162. Stehbens, W. E.: Atypical cerebral aneurysms, Med. J. Aust. **1**:765, 1965.

163. Stehbens, W. E., and Silver, M. D.: Arterial lesions induced by methyl cellulose, Amer. J. Path. **48**:483, 1966.

164. Strassman, G.: Iron and calcium deposits in the brain; their pathologic significance, J. Neuropath. Exp. Neurol. **8**:428, 1949.

165. Symmers, W. St. C.: Thrombotic microangiopathy (thrombotic thrombocytopenic purpura) associated with acute haemorrhagic leucoencephalitis and sensitivity to oxophenarsine, Brain **79**:511, 1956.

166. Thenabadu, P. N., Wickremasinghe, H. R., and Rajasuriya, K.: Acute ascending ischaemic myelopathy in polyarteritis nodosa, Brit. Med. J. **1**:734, 1970.

167. Turnbull, H. M.: Alterations in arterial structure and their relation to syphilis, Quart. J. Med. **8**:201, 1914-1916.

168. Umlas, J., and Kaiser, J.: Thrombohemolytic thrombocytopenic purpura (TTP), Amer. J. Med. **49**:723, 1970.

169. Veress, B., Jellinek, Kóczé, A., and Venesz, I.: The distribution of lipids in malignant hypertensive fibrinoid necrosis, J. Atheroscler. Res. **10**:55, 1969.

170. Vinijchaikul, K.: Primary arteritis of the aorta and its main branches (Takayasu's arteriopathy), Amer. J. Med. **43**:15, 1967.

171. Wagenvoort, C. A., Harris, L. E., Brown, A. L., and Veeneklaas, G. M. H.: Giant-cell arteritis with aneurysm formation in children, Pediatrics **32**:861, 1963.

172. Walton, E. W.: Giant-cell granuloma of the respiratory tract (Wegener's granulomatosis), Brit. Med. J. **2**:265, 1958.

173. Wartman, W. B.: The incidence and severity of arteriosclerosis in the organs from five hundred autopsies, Amer. J. Med. Sci. **186**:27, 1933.

174. Watts, J. W.: Torula infection, Amer. J. Path. **8**:167, 1932.

175. Webb, F. W. S., Hickman, J. A., and Brew, D. St. J.: Death from vertebral artery thrombosis in rheumatoid arthritis, Brit. Med. J. **2**:537, 1968.

176. Webb, J., and Payne, W. H.: Abdominal apoplexy in rheumatoid arthritis, Aust. Ann. Med. **19**:168, 1970.

177. Wechsler, I. S., and Bender, M. B.: The neurological manifestations of periarteritis nodusa, J. Mount Sinai Hosp. **8**:1071, 1941.

178. Wessler, S., Ming, S., Gurewich, V., and Freiman, D. G.: A critical evaluation of thromboangiitis obliterans, New Eng. J. Med. **262**:1149, 1960.

179. Whitefield, A. G. W., Bateman, M., and Cooke, W. T.: Temporal arteritis, Brit. J. Ophthal. **47**:555, 1963.

180. Wiener, J. Spiro, D., and Lattes, R. G.: The cellular pathology of experimental hyperten-

Table 13-1. Death rates per 100,000 population for vascular disease of the central nervous system (both sexes)*

Country	1955	1956	1957	1958	1959	1960	1961
Australia	119.9	122.6	119.0	115.4	118.4	115.2	113.9
Austria	151.9	153.4	167.7	171.0	173.6	179.8	175.7
Belgium	65.3	70.7	73.7	74.1	76.8	77.3	77.2
Canada	90.8	90.0	91.3	88.7	89.7	86.6	83.9
Czechoslovakia		93.7	100.8	99.4	105.1	95.1	93.3
Denmark	122.2	114.5	118.2	119.1	116.0	116.2	118.5
England and Wales	166.6	166.8	176.4	168.9	165.6	166.5	166.7
Finland	120.3	142.0	136.4	132.8	117.5	119.5	120.7
France	144.0	147.9	138.1	136.7	136.4	136.8	134.5
Germany (West)	167.6	176.4	175.7	169.6	171.1	174.0	173.5
Hungary	121.3	135.8	138.4	136.4	142.4	144.1	140.1
Israel†	61.1	70.3	68.9	65.1	63.9	60.0	59.7
Italy	122.8	138.5	137.7	129.8	128.3	132.0	128.3
Japan	136.1	148.4	151.7	148.6	153.7	160.7	165.4
Netherlands	101.3	105.1	101.6	99.8	95.4	92.8	98.4
New Zealand	108.7	106.1	112.8	114.0	110.1	106.7	113.4
Northern Ireland	151.6	152.2	147.6	153.2	148.2	154.2	159.5
Norway	132.7	132.8	136.9	150.7	146.8	150.3	151.0
Poland							
Portugal							
Scotland	187.2	188.2	185.7	193.1	190.0	189.1	189.8
Sweden	139.7	138.8	144.3	140.3	137.9	134.7	132.0
Switzerland	134.6	138.3	121.8	122.9	122.1	110.1	119.8
United States of America	106.0	106.3	110.2	110.1	108.5	108.0	105.4
Venezuela	21.4	22.3	23.8	24.4	24.6	25.1	22.6

*Information obtained from the World Health Organization (Epidem. Vital Statistics Rep., vol. 20, 1967, and
†Jewish population.

decrease in the frequency of cerebral hemorrhage and a simultaneous increase in that of cerebral infarction in England and Wales during this century. Hospital autopsy figures in Manchester confirmed the finding. Yates suggested that there might be a tendency to a general increase in thrombosis of veins, diseased arteries, and damaged heart valves. He further suggested that there could have been a real increase in the frequency of occlusion of the cervical segment of the internal carotid, on the one hand increasing the prevalence of cerebral infarct and on the other hand allegedly protecting against cerebral hemorrhage and thereby decreasing the frequency of this disease. Kurtzke[12] considers the difference attributable to a change in diagnosis, nomenclature, and constitution of the hospital population studied by Yates rather than a change in disease per se. Anderson and MacKay[1] observed changes in the prev-

1962	1963	1964	1965	1966	1967	1968	1969
113.7	115.2	117.8	120.4	120.6	114.5	127.7	
184.8	179.1	169.7	187.1	178.4	188.8	189.9	198.4
90.4	94.7	89.5	101.4	158.2	152.2		
82.4	81.6	78.1	80.1	78.2	75.7	74.8	
85.6	103.7	101.0	114.1	115.0	116.9	141.9	
120.0	125.4	125.6	120.1	120.5	105.1	104.8	
167.8	170.8	156.0	163.6	164.0	159.7	165.4	163.3
127.1	127.1	128.6	134.5	133.3	131.6	137.0	
139.7	139.2	128.9	132.3	128.3	129.6	144.0	150.9
183.1	178.3	173.9	182.5	182.2	175.2		
150.3	136.5	141.5	165.6	156.7	158.9	164.4	169.1
65.0	75.5	77.4	84.0	80.1	91.9	90.0	97.1
135.5	134.1	129.1	136.3	136.3	131.4		
169.4	171.4	171.7	175.8	173.8	172.0		
99.2	97.3	93.3	98.7	98.9	94.6	101.5	94.1
109.5	109.2	106.1	108.6	114.6	103.5	112.8	
153.5	153.2	151.7	154.9	144.0	139.3	154.7	153.9
153.3	156.3	148.9	153.8	153.6	153.5	154.8	
45.4	35.9	29.9	31.7	31.3	32.9	33.7	35.0
139.2	151.7	153.8	155.0	109.2	172.3	174.5	193.2
188.8	190.9	194.4	201.6	198.8	189.1	197.8	
131.4	128.1	120.9	120.9	117.9	116.9	116.3	
123.0	121.9	116.8	120.4	114.4	115.0	113.0	
106.3	106.7	103.6	103.7	104.6	102.2		
22.6	24.2	25.0	26.6	28.3	27.2	30.1	28.7

World Health Statistics Rep., vol. 22, 1969, and vol. 24, 1971.)[23-25]

alence of cerebral hemorrhage and thrombosis in Ontario from 1901 to 1962 similar to that observed for England and Wales[29] but because there was no alteration in the time interval between onset of the "stroke" and death, they concluded that no significant change in death rates had occurred. The widespread use of antihypertensive drug therapy should bring in its wake a reduction in mortality, at least for cerebral hemorrhage.

The major problem of atherosclerosis, which is responsible for more deaths (cardiac, cerebral, and others) than any other single factor, remains. It has been suggested that cerebral atherosclerosis and hence cerebral thrombosis and infarction are less dependent on environmental factors (stress, strain, and diet) than coronary artery disease because the cerebral arteries are more consistent in size, being less subject to vasomotor variation in caliber.[28]

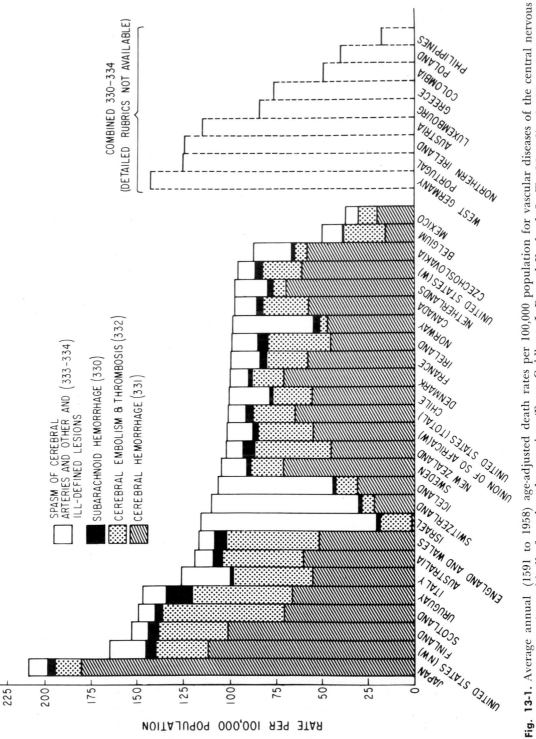

Fig. 13-1. Average annual (1591 to 1958) age-adjusted death rates per 100,000 population for vascular diseases of the central nervous system are represented graphically for selected countries. (From Goldberg, I. D., and Kurland, L. T.: Mortality in 33 countries from diseases of the nervous system, World Neurol. 3:444, 1962.)

Table 13-2. Death rates per 100,000 population according to age for selected countries in 1966*

Country	0-34	35-44	Age groups in years 45-54	55-64	65-74	75+
Australia	1.5	18.9	55.7	164.5	566.6	2159.5
Austria	0.8	7.7	31.2	131.2	570.4	2361.5
Belgium	1.7	6.9	31.1	133.8	520.1	2109.5
Bulgaria	0.9	11.0	52.9	238.9	893.8	2685.6
Canada	1.1	8.3	29.5	104.3	362.8	1665.7
China (Taiwan)	1.7	26.5	114.4	382.4	1027.9	2152.2
Czechoslovakia	1.1	6.7	27.4	125.8	522.8	1938.7
Denmark	1.0	7.7	18.9	91.5	401.4	1903.5
England and Wales	1.6	11.7	42.0	145.6	546.4	2158.0
Finland	2.7	24.6	69.5	188.9	703.3	2575.4
France	1.4	8.7	34.8	119.3	406.5	1619.7
Germany (West)	0.8	6.8	30.2	146.7	649.2	2682.4
Greece	1.9	5.8	30.6	121.8	460.0	1681.7
Hong Kong	2.0	14.2	65.9	220.2	578.1	1761.4
Hungary	1.2	9.2	43.6	174.1	671.9	2485.4
Ireland	2.1	16.4	50.4	174.6	580.0	2044.7
Israel†	0.6	7.6	32.7	138.0	573.6	1988.3
Italy (1965)	1.1	9.3	42.1	161.9	628.9	2077.3
Japan	2.2	26.0	113.2	413.5	1325.6	3414.5
Malta	2.0	19.7	91.8	233.3	890.1	2342.1
Netherlands	1.4	7.2	22.1	86.2	392.2	1821.0
New Zealand	2.1	19.0	46.8	147.3	486.6	2192.9
Norway	1.5	7.7	26.8	103.2	500.5	2265.1
Poland	1.6	7.5	21.0	65.9	205.0	527.6
Portugal	0.9	12.4	56.7	275.5	970.0	2807.7
Romania	1.8	13.7	55.3	203.6	688.4	2215.1
Scotland	2.1	15.4	59.1	204.0	733.3	2874.7
Spain	3.9	10.5	39.4	154.1	591.6	2124.0
Sweden	1.1	7.7	27.0	87.3	359.0	1570.8
Switzerland	1.1	6.0	21.5	86.2	421.6	1967.6
Thailand	1.6	6.4	15.4	25.6	51.0	62.5
Trinidad and Tobago	3.7	35.4	153.7	400.0	1095.2	2381.0
United States	1.8	15.6	43.4	124.1	432.0	1711.8
Venezuela‡	1.6	15.7	45.3	136.8	360.6	1074.4
Yugoslavia	1.6	8.2	39.7	142.7	472.1	1261.8

*Adapted from World Health Statistics Rep., vol. 22, 1969.
†Jewish population.
‡Excluding tribal Indians.

Geographic distribution

The quite obvious geographic variation in death rates for cerebrovascular disease has long intrigued epidemiologists. Tables 13-1 and 13-2 reveal astonishing differences even in adjoining countries where populations are relatively homogeneous. The remarkable difference between the rate for England and Wales and of that for Scotland has not been explained. Kurtzke[12] stressed the similarity in age-specific annual death rates within Denmark, Eire, England and Wales, Norway, Sweden, and the United States in which medical and reporting standards appear reliable. It is most unlikely that such standards differ significantly from those prevailing in Scotland, so that other explanations, not forthcoming as yet, should be sought. Although interest has been concentrated mainly on the high death rates, some countries such as Poland (Table 13-2) have such low death rates that the reasons for the low incidence require complete investigation.

The death rates within some countries display regional differences though their significance is difficult to appraise. In the United States, geographic variation in

Table 13-3. Death rates per 100,000 population for vascular lesions affecting the central nervous system for geographic divisions in the U.S.A. (1967)*

Geographic division	Death rate per 100,000 population
New England	105.7
Middle Atlantic	93.2
East North Central	103.8
West North Central	126.5
South Atlantic	104.2
East South Central	124.4
West South Central	101.1
Mountain	74.0
Pacific	91.6

*Extracted from Vital Statistics of the United States, 1967, Vol. 2, Mortality, Washington, 1969, U. S. Public Health Service.[22]

death rates has attracted considerable interest, the death rate being highest in the southeast central and northwest central divisions (Table 13-3) and lowest in the southwestern and mountain regions.[21] However, individual states in other divisions also have high rates. The rate in some states is more than four times that prevailing in Alaska. Kurtzke[12] considered that there was a focus of high prevalence of cerebrovascular disease for males in the deep South but that the distribution for females was more random. The frequency of cerebrovascular disease appeared to be inversely proportional to the regional physician population[12] suggesting that some variation in death rates could be spurious. Similar findings, though less striking, were apparent in the Scandinavian studies. However, an extensive morbidity study in the United States[10] refutes that the American geographic variation is attributable to artifacts of certification practices or diagnostic inaccuracies.

In Japan, the mortality for cerebrovascular disease (in particular cerebral hemorrhage) has been consistently reported as being higher than any other country (Fig. 13-1 and Table 13-2).[4,12] It has been estimated that cerebrovascular disease constitutes 59% of all cardiovascular deaths.[18]

The death rate has been reported as being particularly high in the prefectures of the northeastern part of the main island,[19,20] particularly the Akita prefecture. This has generally been attributed to the prevalence of hypertension allegedly caused by a high salt intake attributed to consumption of miso (soybean) soup and pickled vegetables, both of which have a high salt content. In 1952, 92% of all cerebrovascular deaths in Japan were classified as cerebral hemorrhage, and in 1962 they comprised 71% whereas deaths caused by cerebral thromboembolism rose from four to 28 per 100,000 in the same interval.[12] Expressed in another way, the ratio of the frequency of cerebral hemorrhage to that of cerebral infarction decreased from 29:1 in 1951 to 4:1 in 1962.[8] Katsuki and Hirota[8] reported an investigation of deaths in a small Japanese town in which the autopsy rate was very high and cerebral thrombosis was more than twice as frequent as cerebral hemorrhage (1961 to 1965). These differences in mortalities within such a short span of time are rather suggestive of a change in diagnostic fashion. It is perhaps significant too that cerebral hemorrhage as a cause of death in Japan has been regarded as socially desirable and supposedly indicative of the superior intellect of the deceased.[11,13]

Among the survivors of Hiroshima and Nagasaki, Johnson and associates[7] reported that cerebrovascular disease was twice as prevalent as coronary heart disease and that their findings were in accord with the known high incidence of cerebrovascular disorders. In another study of these survivors,[6] it was concluded that deaths from cerebrovascular disease probably outnumber those from heart disease by a factor of 2 or 3:1. Yet, in a recent Japanese series of consecutive autopsies, cerebral thrombosis was more frequent than cerebral hemorrhage,[16] and Kurtzke[12] believes that the high mortality for cerebral hemorrhage and cerebrovascular disease in general is fictitious and due to diagnostic fashion.

Kurtzke[12] concluded from the study of

the geographic distribution of cerebrovascular disease that no deductions could be made regarding the relationship of environmental factors to the pathogenesis. However, treating all cerebrovascular diseases together is likely to mask otherwise prominent differences in national, geographic, or racial mortalities for the basic subdivisions or rubrics.

The relative frequency of types of cerebrovascular disease has been dealt with in previous chapters, and Kurtzke[12] considers that hospital series and population surveys are too variable to give reliable estimates of the death rates for the various types. Community studies also exhibit considerable discrepancies, and an estimate of the relative frequencies of the subtypes of cerebrovascular disease has been made (Table 7-1). It must be emphasized that they are but estimates. Kurtzke[12] concluded that the death rates for the subdivisions of cerebrovascular disease are incorrectly differentiated in 30% to 80% of cases, and inaccuracies in the mortality data were such that he considered differentiation between hemorrhage and thrombosis as hazardous.

Racial death rates

The American Negro has a higher mortality for cerebrovascular disease per 100,000 population for each sex than do American whites,[11,12] particularly is this so in the southeastern part of the United States. Kurtzke[12] believes that the inverse relationship between cerebrovascular disease and physician population is more pronounced for the black than for the white population. Furthermore, the discrepancy in death rates between black and white people is less pronounced in those states best supplied with physicians. Several hospital series suggest that there is little real racial difference in the death rates.[12] It would seem, therefore, that any racial differences in mortalities are as yet unproved. The unusually high rate of hypertension and cerebral hemorrhage in the American Negro has been discussed in Chapter 8.

Climatic influence

Deaths from several diseases including those of the cardiovascular system vary with the seasons. It has long since been recognized that deaths from cardiovascular disease are more frequent during the winter months. McDowell and associates[14] reported that hospital admissions for nonembolic cerebral infarction were most numerous during winter months despite considerable variation in their figures. In the United States, the 1967 mortality for cerebrovascular disease exhibited a peak during the December-January period.[22] For each of the rubrics (subarachnoid hemorrhage, cerebral hemorrhage, cerebral embolism and infarction, and other vascular lesions), the peak incidence occurred consistently during these months. Such factors as atmospheric pressure, humidity, and air temperature have been incriminated.[2] It is natural that pneumonia and upper respiratory tract infections display similar seasonal variation. The mortality in the United States[22] for neoplasms, syphilis, diseases of blood and blood-forming organs, and allergic endocrine system, metabolic, and nutritional diseases exhibited a peak in December. The reasons for the seasonal variation are obscure. There is no proof that climatic factors are directly involved though the cold climates of Japan and Scotland have been incriminated in the high mortality figures for these countries. The higher blood pressure during winter months may be a factor for consideration.

Validity of mortality statistics

Epidemiology is concerned with the distribution, mortality, and morbidity of a disease with respect to frequency, time, geography, race, age, sex, environment, the economy, weather, and the social and other habits of the population as well as individual and genetic peculiarities of the victims. Analysis and interpretation of mortality statistics in respect of the above factors are difficult enough, but when the given data are inaccurate, as certainly appears to be the case, the conclusions reached must be guarded to say the least.

Low death rates from some countries appear to be due to overdiagnosis. Some low rates are caused by underreporting and misclassification. In the United States, it has been estimated that the official mortality figures for cerebrovascular disease in 1965 represented only about 73% of the actual rate[3] with further correction necessary to compensate for errors in diagnosis. Even in the densely populated centers of the United States, only a small percentage of deaths is followed by autopsy. Thus the death rates for cerebrovascular disease are based primarily on clinical diagnoses that currently have an error of 30% to 80%.[12] The difficulties in the clinical differentiation of the major cerebrovascular diseases, the widespread use of nonspecific terms (such as stroke, apoplexy, cerebrovascular diseases), together with the already known sources of error inherent in mortality data,[15] introduce errors of uncertain magnitude into epidemiological studies.

In a survey conducted in 75 hospitals of the British National Health Service in 1959 to obtain information on the accuracy of the certification of deaths, the conclusion was that the clinician tended to overdiagnose cerebrovascular disease.[5] In 539 cases diagnosed as primary intracerebral hemorrhage, the diagnosis was confirmed at autopsy in only 43%. In only 59% of 351 cases in which the cause of death had been attributed to cerebral thrombosis or embolism, was confirmation made at autopsy. Two-thirds of the clinical diagnoses of subarachnoid hemorrhage were verified at autopsy. During the same period, there were 276 cases certified as dead because of cerebrovascular disease. The autopsies revealed a variety of causes, such as neoplasms (35 cases), cardiac disease (78 cases), pneumonia (25 cases), trauma (24 cases), and 114 miscellaneous noncerebral causes. Ninety-two cases proved at autopsy to be due to cerebrovascular disease had been diagnosed clinically as neoplasms (13 cases), cardiac diseases (18 cases), pneumonia (8 cases), and trauma (12 cases), whereas miscellane-

ous noncerebral causes made up the remainder. These revealing figures indicate not only how unreliable the mortality figures for cerebrovascular disease derived from hospitals can be, but also how the tendency to overdiagnose cerebrovascular disease can affect the mortality figures for cardiac disease and even carcinoma of the lung. Such figures hardly engender confidence in the validity of current national death rates, and there is no reason to believe that the results from other countries would be substantially better, and in fact it is likely that in many instances they may be considerably worse. Pathologists with considerable autopsy experience in major teaching hospitals are accustomed to the lack of correlation between the clinical diagnosis and the autopsy report. However, the inaccuracy of diagnosis on death certificates from country areas and underdeveloped countries must undoubtedly be far worse than the above figures from hospitals in which the services of at least one pathologist are available. Furthermore, death certificates are not always amended in accordance with additional information made available by autopsy in all countries. Significant epidemiological findings are more likely to result from the following:

1. A vast improvement in the reliability of the clinical diagnosis of the cerebrovascular diseases
2. Improvement in the international classification of diseases
3. An improved autopsy rate
4. Avoidance of international semantic difficulties

Treating all cerebrovascular diseases as one is hardly likely to provide significant epidemiological findings. With the unreliability of the input, interpretations of the data are peculiarly fraught with error of such a magnitude as to raise doubt about the validity of epidemiological conclusions concerning cerebrovascular disease.

References

1. Anderson, T. W., and MacKay, J. S.: A critical reappraisal of the epidemiology of cerebrovascular disease, Lancet 1:1137, 1968.

2. Bokonjić, R., and Zec, N.: Strokes and the weather, J. Neurol. Sci. **6**:483, 1968.

3. Florey, C. du V., Senter, M. G., and Acheson, R. M.: A study of the validity of the diagnosis of stroke in mortality data. 1. Certificate analysis, Yale J. Biol. Med. **40**:148, 1967.

4. Goldberg, I. D., and Kurland, L. T.: Mortality in 33 countries from diseases of the nervous system, World Neurol. **3**:444, 1962.

5. Heasman, M. A., and Lipworth, L.: Accuracy of certification of cause of death. In the series: Studies on medical and population subjects. No. 20, London, 1966, Her Maj. Stat. Off.

6. Jablon, S., Angevine, D. M., Matsumoto, Y. S., and Ishida, M.: On the significance of causes of death as recorded on death certificates in Hiroshima and Nagasaki, Japan, Nat. Cancer Inst. Monograph. **19**:445, 1966.

7. Johnson, K. G., Yano, K., and Kato, H.: Cerebral vascular disease in Hiroshima, Japan, J. Chronic Dis. **20**:545, 1967.

8. Katsuki, S., and Hirota, Y.: Current concept of the frequency of cerebral hemorrhage and cerebral infarction in Japan. In Millikan, C. H., Siekert, R. G., and Whisnant, J. P.: Cerebral vascular diseases, New York, 1966, Grune & Stratton, Inc., p. 99.

9. Kay, D. W. K., Beamish, P., and Roth, M.: Old age mental disorders in Newcastle upon Tyne, Part I: A study of prevalence, Brit. J. Psychiat. **110**:146, 1964.

10. Kuller, L., Anderson, H., Peterson, D., Cassel, J., et al.: Nationwide cerebrovascular disease morbidity study, Stroke **1**:86, 1970.

11. Kurland, L. T., Choi, N. W., and Sayre, G. P.: Current studies of the epidemiology of cerebrovascular diseases. In Fields, W. S., and Spencer, W. A.: Stroke rehabilitation: Basic concepts and research trends, St. Louis, 1967, Warren H. Green, Inc., p. 3.

12. Kurtzke, J. F.: Epidemiology of cerebrovascular disease, Berlin, 1969, Springer Verlag.

13. Kurtzke, J. F., and Kurland, L. T.: Epidemiology of cerebrovascular disease. In Siekert, R. G., editor: Cerebrovascular survey report for Joint Council Subcommittee on Cerebrovascular disease, National Institute of Neurological Diseases and Stroke, and National Heart and Lung Institute, 1970, p. 163.

14. McDowell, F. M., Louis, S., and Monahan, K.: Seasonal variation of nonembolic cerebral infarction, J. Chronic Dis. **23**:29, 1970.

15. Newell, G. R., and Waggoner, D. E.: Cancer mortality and environmental temperature in the United States, Lancet **1**:766, 1970.

16. Otsu, S.: The incidence of cardio- and cerebrovascular diseases in autopsy cases, Jap. Circulation J. **33**:1459, 1969.

17. Riishede, J.: Cerebral apoplexy, Acta Psychiat. Neurol. Scand. (suppl. 108) p. 347, 1956.

18. Stallones, R. A.: Epidemiology of cerebrovascular disease, J. Chronic Dis. **18**:859, 1965.

19. Takahashi, E., Kato, K., Kawakami, Y., et al.: Epidemiological studies on hypertension and cerebral haemorrhage in north-east Japan, Tohoku J. Exp. Med. **74**:188, 1961.

20. Takahashi, E., Sasaki, N., Takeda, J., and Itō, H.: The geographic distribution of cerebral hemorrhage and hypertension in Japan, Hum. Biol. **29**:139, 1957.

21. The U. S. President's commission on heart disease, cancer, and stroke. Report to the President. A national program to conquer heart disease, cancer, and stroke, Vol. 1, Washington, 1964, U. S. Government Printing Office.

22. United States Department of Health, Education, and Welfare: Vital statistics of the United States, 1967, Vol. II. Mortality, Washington, 1969, Public Health Service, Surgeon General.

23. World Health Organization: Epidem. Vital Stat. Rep. 20, 1967.

24. World Health Organization: World Health Stat. Rep. 22, 1969.

25. World Health Organization: World Health Stat. Rep. 24, 1971.

26. Wylie, C. M.: Recent trends in mortality from cerebrovascular accidents in the United States, J. Chronic Dis. **14**:213, 1961.

27. Wylie, C. M.: Cerebrovascular accident deaths in the United States and in England and Wales, J. Chronic Dis. **15**:85, 1962.

28. Yablonski, M., Behar, A., Ungar, H., Resch, J., and Alter, M.: Cerebral atherosclerosis among Israeli Jews of European and Afro-Asian origin, Neurology **18**:550, 1968.

29. Yates, P. O.: A change in the pattern of cerebrovascular disease, Lancet **1**:65, 1964.

30. Yates, P. O.: The changing pattern of cerebrovascular disease in the United Kingdom. In Millikan, C. H., Siekert, R. G., and Whisnant, J. P.: Cerebral vascular diseases, New York, 1966, Grune & Stratton, Inc., p. 67.

Index